Emergency Medical Services

Clinical Practice and Systems Oversight

Emergency Medical Services

Clinical Practice and Systems Oversight

Volume 1: Clinical Aspects of EMS

Second Edition

Editor-in-Chief

David C. Cone, MD

Professor of Emergency Medicine
Yale University School of Medicine
New Haven, Connecticut, USA

Editors

Jane H. Brice, MD, MPH

Orange County EMS Director
Professor of Emergency Medicine
University of North Carolina at Chapel Hill
Chapel Hill, North Carolina, USA

Theodore R. Delbridge, MD, MPH

Professor of Emergency Medicine
Brody School of Medicine
East Carolina University
Greenville, North Carolina, USA

J. Brent Myers, MD, MPH

Director and Medical Director
Wake County EMS System
Raleigh, North Carolina, USA

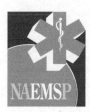

WILEY

Materials appearing in this book prepared by individuals as part of their official duties as United States government employees are not covered by the above mentioned copyright, and any views expressed therein do not necessarily represent the views of the United States government. Such individuals' participation in the Work is not meant to serve as an official endorsement of any statement to the extent that such statement may conflict with any official position of the United States Government. This applies to Chapters 4, 32, 33, 35, 39 in Volume 1 and Chapters 1, 17, 29, 39, 42 in Volume 2.

Registered Office
John Wiley & Sons, Ltd, The Atrium, Southern Gate, Chichester, West Sussex, PO19 8SQ, United Kingdom

For details of our global editorial offices, for customer services and for information about how to apply for permission to reuse the copyright material in this book please see our website at www.wiley.com.

The right of the author to be identified as the author of this work has been asserted in accordance with the Copyright, Designs and Patents Act 1988.

Library of Congress Cataloging-in-Publication Data

Emergency medical services (Cone)
    Emergency medical services : clinical practice and systems oversight / edited by David C. Cone, Jane H. Brice, Theodore R. Delbridge, J. Brent Myers. – Second edition.
        p. ; cm.
    Includes bibliographical references and index.
    ISBN 978-1-118-86530-9 (pbk.)
I. Cone, David C., editor. II. Brice, Jane H., editor. III. Delbridge, Theodore R., editor. IV. Myers, J. Brent, editor. V. Title.
    [DNLM: 1. Emergency Medical Services. 2. Emergency Medicine. WX 215]
    RA645.5
    362.18–dc23
                                                                                                2014039737

A catalogue record for this book is available from the British Library.

Set in 9.5/12pt Minion pro by SPi Publisher Services, Pondicherry, India

Printed in Singapore by C.O.S. Printers Pte Ltd

1   2015

Contents

Contributors

Maria B. Abrahamsen
Dykema Gossett PLLC
Bloomfield Hills, Michigan

James G. Adams, MD
Professor of Emergency Medicine
Northwestern University Feinberg School of Medicine
Chicago, Illinois

Brendan Anzalone, DO
Special Operations Surgical/Critical Care Evacuation Team
Air Force Special Operations Command
Clinical Assistant Professor of Emergency Medicine
University of Alabama School of Medicine
Birmingham, Alabama

James Atkins, MD
Professor of Medicine and Surgery
University of Texas Southwestern Medical Center
Dallas, Texas

Robert R. Bass, MD
Executive Director
Maryland Institute for EMS Systems
Clinical Associate Professor of Emergency Medicine
University of Maryland School of Medicine
Baltimore, Maryland

Gerald (Wook) Beltran, DO, MPH
Associate Medical Director
Kalamazoo County Medical Control Authority
Assistant Professor of Emergency Medicine
Western Michigan University School of Medicine
Kalamazoo, Michigan

Molly Berkoff, MD, MPH
Associate Professor of Pediatrics
University of North Carolina at Chapel Hill
Chapel Hill, North Carolina

Michael C. Beuhler, MD
Medical Director
Carolinas Poison Center
Associate Professor of Emergency Medicine
University of North Carolina
Chapel Hill, North Carolina

Blair L. Bigham, MSc ACPf
Advanced Care Flight Paramedic,
Ornge Transport Medicine
Missisauga, Canada
Collaborating Investigator, Rescu, St Michael's Hospital
Toronto, Canada

Scott S. Bourn, PhD, RN, EMT-P
Vice President of Clinical Practices and Research
American Medical Response
Greenwood Village, Colorado
Arizona Emergency Medicine Research Center
University of Arizona
Tucson, Arizona

Sabina A. Braithwaite, MD, MPH, EMT-P
Medical Director
Wichita-Sedgwick County EMS System
Clinical Associate Professor of Emergency Medicine
University of Kansas
Wichita, Kansas

Jane H. Brice, MD, MPH
Professor of Emergency Medicine
University of North Carolina at Chapel Hill
Chapel Hill, North Carolina

Jonnathan Busko, MD, MPH
EMS Director
Eastern Maine Medical Center
Assistant Professor
Maine Maritime Academy
Bangor, Maine

José G. Cabañas, MD, MPH
Deputy Medical Director
Austin-Travis County EMS System
Austin, Texas

Micha Campbell, MD, EMT-P
Clinical Instructor of Emergency Medicine
University of Pittsburgh
Pittsburgh, Pennsylvania

Thomas V. Caprio, MD
Associate Professor of Medicine
University of Rochester School of Medicine
and Dentistry
Rochester, New York

Jestin N. Carlson, MD, MSc
Director of Resident Research
Saint Vincent Hospital System
Erie, PA
Adjunct Assistant Professor of Emergency Medicine
University of Pittsburgh School of Medicine
Pittsburgh, Pennsylvania

Alix J.E. Carter, MD, MPH
Research Medical Director
EHS Nova Scotia
Director, Division of EMS
Dalhousie University
Halifax, Nova Scotia
Canada

Aaron Case, MD
Oregon Health and Science University
Portland, Oregon

Jennifer Cook, GCPH
Senior Research Assistant
Oregon Health and Science University
Portland, Oregon

Derek R. Cooney, MD, EMT-P
Associate Professor of Emergency Medicine
State University of New York Upstate Medical University
Syracuse, New York

Stephanie A. Crapo, MD
Assistant Professor of Emergency Medicine
University of North Carolina
Chapel Hill, North Carolina

Todd J. Crocco, MD
Professor of Emergency Medicine
West Virginia University School of Medicine
Morgantown, West Virginia

Jeremy T. Cushman, MD, MS, EMT-P
EMS Medical Director
Monroe County and City of Rochester
Associate Professor of Emergency Medicine
University of Rochester School of Medicine and Dentistry
Rochester, New York

Neil B. Davids, MD
Major, US Army
San Antonio Military Medical Center
Fort Sam Houston, Texas

Stephen M. Davis, MPA, MSW
Adjunct Associate Professor of Emergency Medicine
West Virginia University School of Medicine
Morgantown, West Virginia

Mohamud Daya, MD, MS
EMS Medical Director
Tualatin Valley Fire and Rescue
Associate Professor of Emergency Medicine
Oregon Health & Science University
Portland, Oregon

Lynne Dees, PhD, EMT-P
Associate Professor of Emergency Medicine Education
University of Texas Southwestern Medical Center at Dallas
Dallas, Texas

Jocelyn M. De Guzman, MD
Associate Medical Director
Pitt County EMS
Clinical Assistant Professor of Emergency Medicine
Brody School of Medicine
East Carolina University
Greenville, North Carolina

Theodore R. Delbridge, MD, MPH
Professor of Emergency Medicine
Brody School of Medicine
East Carolina University
Greenville, North Carolina

T.J. Doyle, MD, MPH
Associate Medical Director
STAT MedEvac
Clinical Assistant Professor of Emergency Medicine
University of Pittsburgh School of Medicine
Pittsburgh, Pennsylvania

Ian R. Drennan, PhDc, ACP
Institute for Medical Science
University of Toronto
Toronto, Ontario, Canada

Jorge L. Falcon-Chevere, MD
Assistant Professor of Emergency Medicine
University of Puerto Rico
Carolina, Puerto Rico

Jeffrey D. Ferguson, MD
Medical Director
Pitt County EMS
Assistant Professor of Emergency Medicine
East Carolina University
Greenville, North Carolina

Deborah Flowers, MSN
Program Coordinator
Child Medical Evaluation Program
University of North Carolina at Chapel Hill
Chapel Hill, North Carolina

Raymond L. Fowler, MD
Professor of Emergency Medicine, Surgery, Health Professions,
and Emergency Medicine Education
University of Texas Southwestern Medical Center
Dallas, Texas

Anthony J. Frank Jr, MD
Clinical Assistant Professor of Emergency and Hyperbaric Medicine
East Carolina University
Greenville, North Carolina

Benjamin T. Friedman, EMT-P (deceased)
University of California San Francisco
San Francisco, California

Adam Frisch, MD, MS
Albany Medical Center Hospital
Albany, New York

Susan Fuchs, MD
Associate Head,
Pediatric Emergency Medicine
Ann & Robert H. Lurie Children's Hospital of Chicago
Chicago, Illinois

Dia Gainor, MPA
Executive Director
National Association of State EMS Officials
Falls Church, Virginia

Douglas R. Gallo, MD
Medical Director
Stamford EMS
Stamford, Connecticut

Gregory H. Gilbert, MD
San Mateo EMS Medical Director
Clinical Assistant Professor
Stanford University Hospital
Stanford, California

W. Scott Gilmore, MD, EMT-P
Medical Director
St Louis Fire Department
Assistant Professor of Emergency Medicine
Washington University School of Medicine
St Louis, Missouri

Jeffrey M. Goodloe, MD, EMT-P
Medical Director
EMS System for Metropolitan Oklahoma City
and Tulsa
Professor of Emergency Medicine
University of Oklahoma School of Community Medicine
Tulsa, Oklahoma

Toni Gross, MD, MPH
Medical Director of Emergency Preparedness and
Prehospital Coordination
Phoenix Children's Hospital Emergency Department
Clinical Associate Professor of Child Health
University of Arizona College of Medicine-Phoenix
Phoenix, Arizona

Francis X. Guyette, MD, MPH
Medical Director
STAT MedEvac
Associate Professor of Emergency Medicine
University of Pittsburgh School of Medicine
Pittsburgh, Pennsylvania

Eric Hawkins, MD, MPH
Assistant Professor of Emergency Medicine
Carolinas Medical Center
Charlotte, North Carolina

Michael T. Hilton, MD, MPH
Clinical Assistant Professor of Emergency Medicine
University of Pittsburgh
Pittsburgh, Pennsylvania

David J. Hirsch, MD, MPH
EMS Medical Director
Concord Hospital
Concord Emergency Medical Associates
Concord, New Hampshire

J. Stephen Huff, MD
Professor of Emergency Medicine
University of Virginia Health Sciences Center
Charlottesville, Virginia

Angus M. Jameson, MD, MPH
Medical Director
Pinellas County EMS
Largo, Florida

Brent D. Kaziny, MD, MA
Assistant Professor of Pediatrics
Baylor College of Medicine
Houston, Texas

Andrew King, MD
Assistant Professor of Clinical Medicine
Wayne State University
Detroit, Michigan

Bryan B. Kitch, MD
Brody School of Medicine
East Carolina University
Greenville, North Carolina

Sean Kivlehan, MD, MPH
University of California San Francisco
San Francisco, California

Christian C. Knutsen, MD
Medical Director
Upstate EMS Educational Programs
Assistant Professor of Emergency Medicine
SUNY Upstate Medical University
Syracuse, New York

Carla Kohoyda-Inglis, MPA
Program Director
International Center for Automotive Medicine
University of Michigan
Ann Arbor, Michigan

Rachel Liu, MD
Instructor in Emergency Medicine
Yale University School of Medicine
New Haven, Connecticut

Robert Lowe, MD
EMS Medical Director
Doctors Hospital
Columbus, Ohio
Clinical Professor of Emergency Medicine
Ohio University Heritage College of Osteopathic Medicine
Athens, Ohio

Dave W. Lu, MD, MBE
Assistant Professor of Emergency Medicine
Northwestern University Feinberg School of Medicine
Chicago, Illinois

Jeffrey Lubin, MD, MPH
Associate Professor of Emergency Medicine
Penn State Milton S. Hershey Medical Center
Hershey, Pennsylvania

Robert L. Mabry, MD
Lieutenant Colonel, US Army
San Antonio Military Medical Center
Fort Sam Houston, Texas

Russell D. MacDonald, MD, MPH
Medical Director,
Ornge Transport Medicine
Associate Professor of Emergency Medicine
University of Toronto
Toronto, Canada

Kevin E. Mackey, MD
Medical Director
Mountain Valley EMS Agency
Modesto, CA
Kaiser Permanente
South Sacramento, CA

Christian Martin-Gill, MD, MPH
Associate Medical Director
STAT MedEvac & UPMC Prehospital Care
Assistant Professor of Emergency Medicine
University of Pittsburgh
Pittsburgh, Pennsylvania

John McManus, MD, MBA, MCR
Professor of Emergency Medicine
Georgia Regents University
Augusta, Georgia

Bryan McNally, MD, MPH
Associate Medical Director
Emory Flight
Associate Professor of Emergency Medicine
Emory University School of Medicine
Atlanta, Georgia

Greg Mears, MD
Medical Director
ZOLL
Broomfield, Colorado
Adjunct Professor of Emergency Medicine
University of North Carolina at Chapel Hill
Chapel Hill, North Carolina

Mary P. Mercer, MD, MPH
Medical Director
San Francisco Base Hospital
Assistant Professor of Emergency Medicine
University of California San Francisco
San Francisco, California

Paul M. Middleton, MBBS, MD
Discipline of Emergency Medicine
University of Sydney
Sydney, New South Wales, Australia

Ken Miller, MD, PhD
Medical Director
Emergency Medical Services Section
Orange County Fire Authority
Irvine, California

Michael D. Mills, MD
Lakeridge Health, Oshawa and Credit Valley Eye Care
Mississauga, Ontario, Canada

Jennifer Monroe, DO
East Carolina University
Greenville, North Carolina

Laurie J. Morrison, MSc, MD, FRCPC
Professor of Emergency Medicine
University of Toronto
Toronto, Ontario, Canada

Vincent N. Mosesso Jr, MD, EMT-P
Medical Director
UPMC Prehospital Care
Professor of Emergency Medicine
University of Pittsburgh
Pittsburgh, Pennsylvania

Hawnwan Philip Moy, MD
Assistant Medical Director
St Louis City EMS
Clinical Instructor of Emergency Medicine
Washington University School of Medicine
St Louis, Missouri

Christine M. Murphy, MD
Assistant Professor of Emergency Medicine
Carolinas Medical Center
Charlotte, North Carolina

J. Brent Myers, MD, MPH
Director | Medical Director
Wake County EMS System
Raleigh, North Carolina

Petra Norris, RN
Sexual Assault/Domestic Violence Nurse Examiner
Women's College Hospital
Toronto, Ontario, Canada

Kraigher O'Keefe, MD
Clinical Assistant Professor of Emergency Medicine
Brody School of Medicine
East Carolina University
Greenville, North Carolina

Marcus Ong, MBBS, MPH
Associate Professor
Duke-National University of Singapore Graduate Medical School
Singapore

Jason Oost, MD
Department of Emergency Medicine
Oregon Health & Science University
Portland, Oregon

Joseph P. Ornato, MD
Professor of Emergency Medicine
Virginia Commonwealth University
Richmond, Virginia

Stephanie Outterson, RN
Albany Medical Center Hospital
Albany, New York

Alim Pardhan, MD, MBA
Assistant Clinical Professor of Emergency Medicine
McMaster University
Hamilton, Ontario, Canada

Paul M. Paris, MD
Professor of Emergency Medicine
University of Pittsburgh
Pittsburgh, Pennsylvania

Hiren Patel, MD
Emory University School of Medicine
Atlanta, Georgia

P. Daniel Patterson, PhD, EMT-P
Assistant Professor of Emergency Medicine
University of Pittsburgh School of Medicine
Pittsburgh, Pennsylvania

Debra G. Perina, MD
Division Director, Prehospital Care
Professor of Emergency Medicine
University of Virginia Health Sciences Center
Charlottesville, Virginia

Mark R. Quale, MD
Medical Director
Alamance County Emergency Medical Services
Wake Forest Baptist Health
Winston-Salem, North Carolina

Jay H. Reich, MD
EMS Medical Director
City of Kansas City, Missouri
Assistant Professor of Emergency Medicine
University of Missouri-Kansas City School of Medicine
Kansas City, Missouri

Jon C. Rittenberger, MD, MS
Associate Professor of Emergency Medicine
University of Pittsburgh School of Medicine
Pittsburgh, Pennsylvania

Ronald N. Roth, MD
Medical Director, City of Pittsburgh Department of Public Safety
Professor of Emergency Medicine
University of Pittsburgh
Pittsburgh, Pennsylvania

Jeffrey P. Salomone, MD
Trauma Medical Director
Maricopa Medical Center
Phoenix, Arizona

Joseph A. Salomone, MD
Medical Director, Kansas City Fire Department (retired)
St Croix, US Virgin Islands

Scott M. Sasser, MD
Associate Professor of Emergency Medicine
National Center for Injury Prevention and Control
Centers for Disease Control
Atlanta, Georgia

Michael R. Sayre, MD
Associate Medical Director
Seattle Fire Department
Professor Emergency Medicine
University of Washington
Seattle, Washington

Terri A. Schmidt, MD, MS
Professor of Emergency Medicine
Oregon Health and Sciences University
Portland, Oregon

David J. Schoenwetter, DO
Medical Director
Geisinger EMS and Geisinger Life Flight
Geisinger Health System
Danville, Pennsylvania

Richard B. Schwartz, MD
Professor of Emergency Medicine and Hospitalist Services
Georgia Regents University
Augusta, Georgia

Manish I. Shah, MD
Assistant Professor of Pediatrics
Baylor College of Medicine
Houston, Texas

Manish N. Shah, MD, MPH
Associate Professor of Emergency Medicine
University of Rochester School of Medicine and Dentistry
Rochester, New York

Ronald D. Stewart, MD
Professor of Anesthesia and Emergency Medicine
Dalhousie University
Halifax, Nova Scotia, Canada

Aaron Stinton, MD
University of Missouri-Kansas City School of Medicine
Kansas City, Missouri

Robert Swor, DO
Professor of Emergency Medicine
Oakland University William Beaumont School of Medicine
Royal Oak, Michigan

James I. Syrett, MD, MBA
Director of Prehospital Care
Rochester General Health System
Rochester, New York

Allison Tadros, MD
Associate Professor of Emergency Medicine
West Virginia University School of Medicine
Morgantown, West Virginia

David P. Thomson, MS, MD, MPA
Medical Director
Vidant Medical Transport
Clinical Professor of Emergency Medicine
East Carolina University Brody School of Medicine
Greenville, North Carolina

Andrew Travers, MD, MSc
Provincial Medical Director
Emergency Health Services, Nova Scotia
Associate Professor of Emergency Medicine
Dalhousie University
Dartmouth, Nova Scotia, Canada

P. Richard Verbeek, MD
Centre for Prehospital Medicine
Sunnybrook Health Sciences Centre
University of Toronto
Toronto, Ontario, Canada

Henry E. Wang, MD, MS
Professor of Emergency Medicine
University of Alabama School of Medicine
Birmingham, Alabama

Stewart C. Wang, MD, PhD
Director
International Center for Automotive Medicine
Professor of Surgery
University of Michigan
Ann Arbor, Michigan

Michelle Welsford, MD
Medical Director
HHS Centre for Paramedic Education and Research
Associate Professor of Emergency Medicine
McMaster University
Hamilton, Ontario, Canada

Jefferson G. Williams, MD, MPH
Deputy Medical Director
Wake County EMS System
Clinical Assistant Professor of Emergency Medicine
University of North Carolina
Chapel Hill, North Carolina

Joseph L. Wright, MD, MPH
Professor of Pediatrics and Child Health
Howard University College of Medicine
Washington, DC

Donald M. Yealy, MD
Professor of Emergency Medicine
University of Pittsburgh School of Medicine
Pittsburgh, Pennsylvania

Dana Zive, MPH
Research, Senior Instructor
Center for Health Policy and Research in Emergency Medicine
Oregon Health & Sciences University
Portland, Oregon

Foreword

As this book is published, the National Association of EMS Physicians® has finished celebrating its 30th anniversary. This is a great sign that the association is maturing. This is our fifth edition of the textbook, and the previous editions have served as a key resource for EMS medical directors, fellowship directors, and managers. The association has grown in size, has an established and well-attended annual meeting, and serves as a key resource for the EMS community as a whole. As always, we remain focused on patient outcomes and providing the best possible patient care.

In other ways, this is just the beginning. This is the first edition of the textbook published since EMS has become a recognized medical subspecialty. This fact alone makes this book a landmark edition. Within its pages, the reader will find the definitive reference for the core content in EMS. This book will serve as the foundation for our young specialty. The editors and authors who contributed to this work understand the key role this book plays in preparing our new subspecialists.

I want to thank Drs Cone, Brice, Delbridge, and Myers for their hard work as editors of this text. It is their passion for and incredible contributions to our specialty that made them the perfect choice for leading this endeavor.

Ritu Sahni, MD, MPH
President, National Association
of EMS Physicians®

Preface

Since the earliest versions of this textbook in 1989, the subspecialty of EMS has evolved dramatically. In addition to increasing sophistication and application of expertise, EMS has developed to encompass a unique body of knowledge. Recognizing these features and an ongoing need to nurture the professionalism of those who are and might become committed to EMS, the American Board of Medical Specialties recognized EMS as a subspecialty in 2010. The American Board of Emergency Medicine administered the first certification examination in 2013, leading to the very first board-certified EMS subspecialists. The Accreditation Council for Graduate Medical Education has accredited 41 EMS fellowship programs as of this writing.

This second edition of *Emergency Medical Services: Clinical Practice and Systems Oversight* builds on the foundations of its predecessors, *EMS Medical Directors Handbook* (1989), *Prehospital Systems and Medical Oversight* (1994, 2002), and the first edition of this book in 2009. At the same time, planning this to be the primary textbook for those EMS fellowship programs, it is intended to be more concise and focused, reducing redundancy and making it an ideal source for reliable information. Within its pages is the core content thought to be relevant to EMS fellows and that which forms the basis for the certification examination. The Appendix shows this core content, previously published by the American Board of Emergency Medicine [1].

We are, of course, proud of this textbook's authors. They were careful to ensure that the right information is included in their topic areas, meaning reliable and appropriately comprehensive. However, we are also indebted and most grateful to the authors and editors of the prior books noted above. They have served our subspecialty well by creating a foundation upon which we have been able to build a solid structure of unique knowledge, academic integrity, and clinical expertise. We share with the authors of this edition a sense of deep gratitude and sincere appreciation for the contributions made by authors of previous editions of this text. In many cases, their knowledge has been retained in this edition while in others their frameworks and underpinnings were used by the current authors as they updated content to reflect current best practices. To all who have contributed to this textbook, to all who contributed to prior versions, to all who commit parts of their professional lives to improving the delivery of EMS, and to all who will glean for themselves new knowledge through this textbook, we thank you!

D. Cone
J. Brice
T. Delbridge
B. Myers

Reference

1 EMS Examination Task Force, American Board of Emergency Medicine. The core content of emergency medical services medicine. *Prehosp Emerg Care* 2012;16(3):309–22.

Abbreviations

AAOS	American Academy of Orthopedic Surgeons
AAP	American Academy of Pediatrics
ABEM	American Board of Emergency Medicine
AC	assist control/acromioclavicular
ACEP	American College of Emergency Physicians
ACF	alternative care facility
ACLS	Advanced Cardiac Life Support
ACPE	acute cardiogenic pulmonary edema
ACS	American College of Surgeons/acute coronary syndrome
ADHF	acute decompensated heart failure
AED	automated external defibrillator
AEMS	Advocates for EMS
AEMT	advanced emergency medical technician
AGE	arterial gas embolism
AHA	American Heart Association
AICD	automatic implantable cardioverter defibrillator
AIS	abbreviated injury scale
AKI	acute kidney injury
ALOC	altered level of consciousness
ALS	Advanced Life Support
ALTE	apparent life-threatening event
AMI	acute myocardial infarction
AMS	altered mental status/acute mountain sickness/air medical services
ANOVA	analysis of variance
ARC	American Red Cross
ASA	American Society of Anesthesiologists/American Stroke Association
ASPR	Assistant Secretary of Preparedness and Response
ASTM	American Society for Testing and Materials
ATA	atmosphere absolute
atm	atmosphere
AWLS	Advanced Wilderness Life Support
BAC	blood alcohol concentration
BBP	blood-borne pathogen
BiPAP	bilevel positive airway pressure
BIVAD	biventricular assist device
BLS	Basic Life Support
BMI	body mass index
BNP	B-type natriuretic peptide
BSA	body surface area
BVM	bag-valve-mask
CAD	coronary artery disease/computer-aided dispatch
CAMTS	Commission on Accreditation of Medical Transport Systems
CDC	Centers for Disease Control and Prevention
CDE	continuing dispatch education
CERT	community emergency response team
CHF	congestive heart failure
CI	confidence interval
CISD	critical incident stress debriefing
CISM	critical incident stress management
CKD	chronic kidney disease
CLIA	Clinical Laboratory Improvement Amendments
CNS	central nervous system
CO	carbon monoxide
COPD	chronic obstructive pulmonary disease
CPAP	continuous positive airway pressure
CPP	coronary/cerebral perfusion pressure
CPR	cardiopulmonary resuscitation
CSF	cerebrospinal fluid
CSM	confined space medicine
CT	computed tomography
DCS	decompression sickness
DFI	drug-facilitated intubation
DFSA	drug-facilitated sexual assault
DHEW	Department of Health, Education, and Welfare
DHHS	Department of Health and Human Services
DHS	Department of Homeland Security
DKA	diabetic ketoacidosis
DLS	dispatch life support
DMAT	disaster medical assistance team
DMORT	disaster mortuary response team
DNR	do not resuscitate
DOT	Department of Transportation
DSMB	data and safety monitoring board
DVT	deep vein thrombosis
EAP	employee assistance program
ECG	electrocardiogram
ECLS	extracorporeal life support
ECMO	extracorporeal membrane oxygenation
ED	emergency department
EEG	electroencephalogram
eGFR	estimated glomerular filtration rate
EMA	emergency management agency
EMAC	Emergency Management Assistance Compact
EMD	emergency medical dispatch
EMR	emergency medical responder
EMSC	Emergency Medical Services for Children
EMT	emergency medical technician
EMT-A	emergency medical technician- ambulance
EMTALA	Emergency Medical Treatment and Active Labor Act
EMT-I	emergency medical technician-intermediate
EOC	emergency operations center
EPA	Environmental Protection Agency
ESAR-VHP	Emergency System for Advanced Registration of Volunteer Health Professionals
ESC	European Society of Cardiology
ESF	emergency support function

ESRD	end-stage renal disease	**KPI**	key performance indicator
ETC	esophageal tracheal Combitube	**LEOC**	local emergency operations center
EtCO$_2$	end-tidal carbon dioxide	**LLD**	left lateral decubitus
ETI	endotracheal intubation	**LMA**	laryngeal mask airway
FAST	focused assessment with sonography in trauma	**LVAD**	left ventricular assist device
FCC	Federal Communications Commission	**LZ**	landing zone
FCS	Fireground Command System	**MAP**	mean arterial pressure
FDA	Food and Drug Administration	**MCHB**	Maternal and Child Health Bureau
FEMA	Federal Emergency Management Agency	**MCI**	mass casualty incident
FFP	fresh frozen plasma	**MDI**	metered dose inhaler
ffw	feet of freshwater	**MI**	myocardial infarction
FICEMS	Federal Interagency Committee on EMS	**MOI**	mechanism of injury
fsw	feet of seawater	**MRC**	Medical Reserve Corps
GABA	gamma-aminobutyric acid	**MRSA**	methicillin-resistant *Staphylococcus aureus*
GCS	Glasgow Coma Scale	**MSDS**	Material Safety Data Sheet
GI	gastrointestinal	**MTA**	medical threat assessment
HACE	high altitude cerebral edema	**MUCC**	Model Uniform Core Criteria
HAPE	high altitude pulmonary edema	**MVC**	motor vehicle collision
HBIG	hepatitis B immune globulin	**NAEMSP**	National Association of EMS Physicians
HBO	hyperbaric oxygen	**NAEMT**	National Association of EMTs
HBV	hepatitis B virus	**NASEMSD**	National Association of State EMS Directors
HCFA	Health Care Financing Administration	**NASEMSO**	National Association of State EMS Officials
HCP	health care provider	**NAS-NRC**	National Academy of Sciences National Research Council
HCV	hepatitis C virus		
HEMS	helicopter EMS	**NCT**	narrow-complex tachydysrhythmia
HF	hydrofluoric acid	**NDMS**	National Disaster Medical System
HIPAA	Health Insurance Portability and Accountability Act	**NEDARC**	National EMSC Data Analysis Resource Center
HIV	human immunodeficiency virus	**NEMSIS**	National EMS Information System
HRSA	Health Resources and Services Administration	**NFDD**	noise/flash diversionary device
HSP	Henoch–Schönlein purpura	**NFPA**	National Fire Protection Association
IABP	intraaortic balloon pump	**NGO**	non-governmental organization
IAP	incident action plan	**NHTSA**	National Highway Traffic Safety Administration
IBW	ideal body weight	**NICU**	neonatal intensive care unit
IC	incident commander	**NIH**	National Institutes of Health
ICD	implanted cardioverter-defibrillator	**NIMS**	National Incident Management System
ICH	intracranial hemorrhage	**NIOSH**	National Institute for Occupational Safety and Health
ICP	intracranial pressure	**NIPPV**	non-invasive positive pressure ventilation
ICS	incident command system	**NKHS**	non-ketotic hyperosmolar state
ICU	intensive care unit	**NMDA**	n-methyl-D-asparate
IDLH	immediately dangerous to life and health	**NMRT**	national medical response team
I/E	inspiratory-to-expiratory	**NNT**	number needed to treat
IED	improvised explosive device	**NREMT**	National Registry of Emergency Medical Technicians
IJ	internal jugular	**NSAID**	non-steroidal antiinflammatory drug
IL	interleukin	**NSTEMI**	non-ST-elevation MI
IM	intramuscular	**NVG**	night vision goggles
IMS	incident management system	**NVRT**	National Veterinary Response Team
IMSURT	international medical/surgical response team	**OHCA**	out-of-hospital cardiac arrest
IN	intranasal	**OR**	operating room/odds ratio
IO	intraosseous	**OSHA**	Occupational Safety and Health Administration
IOM	Institute of Medicine	**PAD**	public access defibrillation
IPE	immersion pulmonary edema	**PAI**	prearrival instructions
IPV	intimate partner violence	**PALS**	Pediatric Advanced Life Support
IRB	institutional review board	**PASG**	pneumatic antishock garment
ISS	injury severity score	**PAT**	Pediatric Assessment Triangle
ITD	impedance threshold device	**PCI**	percutaneous coronary intervention
IV	intravenous	**PCR**	patient care report
JTTR	Joint Theater Trauma Registry	**PD**	peritoneal dialysis
JVD	jugular venous distension	**PDI**	postdispatch instruction
KED	Kendrick Extrication Device	**PDSA**	Plan-Do-Study-Act

PE	pulmonary embolus		**SSC**	secondary stroke center
PEA	pulseless electrical activity		**SSM**	system status management
PEEP	positive end-expiratory pressure		**STEMI**	ST-segment elevation myocardial infarction
PEL	permissible exposure limit		**SVR**	systemic vascular resistance
PEP	postexposure prophylaxis		**SVT**	supraventricular tachycardia
PFAST	prehospital FAST		**SWAT**	special weapons and tactics
PI	performance improvement		**TAC**	Technical Assistance Center
PID	pelvic inflammatory disease		**TB**	tuberculosis
PIO	public information officer		**TBI**	traumatic brain injury
PIP	peak inspiratory pressure		**TBSA**	total body surface area
PMCS	perimortem cesarean section		**TBW**	total body weight
POC	point of care		**TCCC**	tactical combat casualty care
POLST	Physician Orders for Life-Sustaining Treatment		**TdP**	torsades de pointes
PPE	personal protective equipment		**TECC**	Tactical Emergency Casualty Care
PRA	patient reception area		**TEMS**	tactical emergency medical support
PS	pressure support		**TIA**	transient ischemic attack
PSC	primary stroke center		**TM**	tympanic membrane
PSO	patient safety organization		**TOA**	tuboovarian abscess
PTSD	posttraumatic stress disorder		**TOR**	termination of resuscitation
PVC	premature ventricular contraction		**t-PA**	tissue plasminogen activator
QA	quality assurance		**TQM**	total quality management
QALY	quality-adjusted life-year		**TTJV**	transtracheal jet ventilation
QI	quality improvement		**TV**	tidal volume
QM	quality management		**TXA**	tranexamic acid
RCT	randomized controlled trial		**US&R**	urban search and rescue
REBOA	reverse endovascular balloon occlusion of the aorta		**UTI**	urinary tract infection
ROSC	return of spontaneous circulation		**UXO**	unexploded ordnance
RR	respiratory rate		**VAD**	ventricular assist device
RSA	rapid sequence airway		**VF**	ventricular fibrillation
RSI	rapid sequence intubation		**VL**	video laryngoscope
RSV	respiratory syncytial virus		**VNS**	vagus nerve stimulator
RTS	Revised Trauma Score		**VOAD**	Voluntary Organizations Active in Disaster
RVAD	right ventricular assist device		**VoIP**	voice over internet protocol
SABA	short-acting inhaled beta$_2$-agonist		**VP**	ventriculoperitoneal
SAEM	Society for Academic Emergency Medicine		**VT**	ventricular tachycardia
SAR	search and rescue		**VTE**	venous thromboembolism
SARS	severe acute respiratory syndrome		**VZV**	varicella zoster virus
SBP	systolic blood pressure		**WCT**	wide-complex tachydysrhythmia
SC	sternoclavicular		**WEMS**	wilderness EMS
SCA	sudden cardiac arrest		**WEMT**	wilderness EMT
SCBA	self-contained breathing apparatus		**WFA**	wilderness first aid
SGA	supraglottic airway		**WFR**	wilderness first responder
SIMV	synchronized intermittent mandatory ventilation		**WHO**	World Health Organization
SMS	Simplified Motor Scale/safety management system		**WMD**	weapon of mass destruction
SOG	standard operating guideline		**WMS**	Wilderness Medical Society
SRR	survival risk ratio		**WPHEC**	wilderness prehospital emergency care

About the companion website

This series is accompanied by a companion website:

www.wiley.com\go\cone\naemsp

The website includes:

- video clips
- interactive MCQs
- link to the EMS Examination Task Force, American Board of Emergency Medicine.

CHAPTER 1

History of EMS

Robert R. Bass

Before 1966: historical perspectives

Early hunters and warriors provided care for the injured. Although the methods used to staunch bleeding, stabilize fractures, and provide nourishment were primitive, the need for treatment was undoubtedly recognized. The basic elements of prehistoric response to injury still guide contemporary EMS programs. Recognition of the need for action led to the development of medical and surgical emergency treatment techniques. These techniques in turn made way for systems of communication, treatment, and transport, all geared toward reducing morbidity and mortality.

The Edwin Smith Papyrus, written in 1500 BC, vividly describes triage and treatment protocols [1]. Reference to emergency care is also found in the Babylonian Code of Hammurabi, where a detailed protocol for treatment of the injured is described [2]. In the Old Testament, Elisha breathed into the mouth of a dead child and brought the child back to life [3]. The Good Samaritan not only treated the injured traveler but also instructed others to do likewise [4]. Greeks and Romans had surgeons present during battle to treat the wounded.

The most direct root of modern prehospital systems is found in the efforts of Jean Dominique Larrey, Napoleon's chief military physician. Larrey developed a prehospital system in which the injured were treated on the battlefield and horse-drawn wagons were used to carry them away [5]. In 1797 Larrey built "ambulance volantes" of two or four wheels to rescue the wounded. Larrey had introduced a new concept in military surgery: early transport from the battlefield to the aid stations and then to the frontline hospital. This method is comparable to the way that modern physicians modified the military use of helicopters in Korea and Vietnam. Larrey also initiated detailed treatment protocols, such as the early amputation of shattered limbs to prevent gangrene.

The Civil War is the starting point for EMS systems in the United States [6]. Learning from the lessons of the Napoleonic and Crimean Wars, military physicians led by Joseph Barnes and Jonathan Letterman established an extensive system of prehospital care. The Union Army trained medical corpsmen to provide treatment in the field; a transportation system, which included railroads, was developed to bring the wounded to medical facilities. However, the wounded received suboptimal treatment in these facilities, stirring Clara Barton's crusade for better care [7].

The medical experiences of the Civil War stimulated the beginning of civilian urban ambulance services. The first were established in cities such as Cincinnati, New York, London, and Paris. Edward Dalton, Sanitary Superintendent of the Board of Health in New York City, established a city ambulance program in 1869. Dalton, a former surgeon in the Union Army, spearheaded the development of urban civilian ambulances to permit greater speed, enhance comfort, and increase maneuverability on city streets [8]. His ambulances carried medical equipment such as splints, bandages, straitjackets, and a stomach pump, as well as a medicine chest of antidotes, anesthetics, brandy, and morphine. By the turn of the century, interns accompanied the ambulances. Care was rendered and the patient left at home. Ambulance drivers had virtually no medical training. Our knowledge of turn-of-the-century urban ambulance service comes from the writings of Emily Barringer, the first woman ambulance surgeon in New York City [9].

Further development of urban ambulance services continued in the years before World War I. Electric, steam, and gasoline-powered carriages were used as ambulances. Calls for service were generally processed and dispatched by individual hospitals, although improved telegraph and telephone systems with signal boxes throughout New York City were developed to connect the police department and the hospitals.

During World War I, the introduction of the Thomas traction splint for the stabilization of patients with leg fractures led to a decrease in morbidity and mortality. Between the two world wars, ambulances began to be dispatched by mobile radios. In the 1920s, in Roanoke, Virginia, the first volunteer rescue squad was started. In many areas, volunteer rescue or ambulance squads gradually developed and provided an alternative to the local fire department or undertaker. After the entry of America

Emergency Medical Services: Clinical Practice and Systems Oversight, Second Edition. Volume 1: Clinical Aspects of EMS.
Edited by David C. Cone, Jane H. Brice, Theodore R. Delbridge, and J. Brent Myers.
© 2015 NAEMSP. Published 2015 by John Wiley & Sons, Inc. Companion Website: www.wiley.com\go\cone\naemsp

into World War II, the military demand for physicians pulled the interns from ambulances, never to return, resulting in poorly staffed units and non-standardized prehospital care. Postwar ambulances were underequipped hearses and similar vehicles staffed by untrained personnel. Half of the ambulances were operated by mortuary attendants, most of whom had never taken even a first aid course [10].

Throughout the 1950s and 1960s, two geographic patterns of ambulance service evolved. In cities, hospital-based ambulances gradually coalesced into more centrally coordinated city wide programs, usually administered and staffed by the municipal hospital or fire department. In rural areas, funeral home hearses were sporadically replaced by a variety of units operated by the local fire department or a newly formed rescue squad. Additionally, in both urban and rural areas, a few profit-making providers delivered transport services and occasionally contracted with local government to provide emergency prehospital services and transport. Before 1966, very little legislation and regulation applicable to ambulance services existed. Providers had relatively little formal training, and physician involvement at all levels was minimal.

A number of factors combined in the mid-1960s to stimulate a revolution in prehospital care. Advances in medical treatments led to a perception that decreases in mortality and morbidity were possible. Closed-chest cardiopulmonary resuscitation (CPR), reported as successful in 1960 by W.B. Kouwenhoven [11] and Peter Safar [12], was eventually adopted as the medical standard for cardiac arrest in the prehospital setting. New evidence that CPR, pharmaceuticals, and defibrillation could save lives immediately created a demand for physician providers of those interventions in both the hospital and prehospital environments. Throughout the 1960s, fundamental understanding of the pathophysiology of potentially fatal dysrhythmias expanded significantly. The use of rescue breathing and defibrillation was refined by Peter Safar, Leonard Cobb, Herbert Loon, and Eugene Nagel [13]. Safar persuaded many others that defibrillation and resuscitation were viable areas of medical research and clinical intervention.

In 1966 Pantridge and Geddes pioneered and documented the use of a mobile coronary care unit ambulance for prehospital resuscitation of patients in Belfast, Ireland. Their treatment protocols, originally developed for the treatment of myocardial infarction in intensive care units, were moved into the field [14]. Because the medical team was often with the patient at the time of cardiac arrest, the resuscitation rate was a remarkable 20%. Their "flying squads" added a dimension of heroic excitement to the job of being an ambulance attendant, and their performance data helped convince American city health officials and physicians that a more medically sophisticated prehospital advanced life support (ALS) system was possible.

1966: the NAS-NRC report

The modern era of prehospital care in the United States began in 1966. In that year, the recognition of an urgent need, the crucial element necessary for development of prehospital systems

nationwide, was heralded by a report generated by the National Academy of Sciences National Research Council (NAS-NRC), a non-profit organization chartered by Congress to provide scientific advice to the nation. *Accidental Death and Disability: The Neglected Disease of Modern Society* documented the enormous failure of the United States health care system to provide even minimal care for the emergency patient. The NAS-NRC report identified key issues and problems facing the United States in providing emergency care (Figure 1.1). Its summary report listed recommendations that would serve as a blueprint for EMS development, including such things as first aid training for the lay public, state-level regulation of ambulance services, emergency department improvements, development of trauma registries, single nationwide phone number access for emergencies, and disaster planning [15]. This document established a benchmark against which to measure subsequent progress and change.

The 1966 NAS-NRC document described both prehospital services and hospital emergency departments as being woefully inadequate. In the prehospital arena, treatment protocols, trained medical personnel, rapid transportation, and modern communications concepts, such as two-way radios and emergency call numbers, were all identified as necessities that were simply not available to civilians. Although there were more than 7,000 accredited hospitals in the country at the time, very few were prepared to meet the increased demand that developed between 1945 and 1965. From 1958 to 1970, the annual number of emergency department visits increased from 18 million to more than 49 million [15]. In addition, emergency departments were staffed by the least experienced personnel, who had little education in the treatment of multiple injuries or critical medical emergencies. Early efforts of the American College of Surgeons (ACS) and the American Academy of Orthopedic Surgeons (AAOS) to improve emergency care were largely unsuccessful because medical interest was essentially non-existent [16–19].

The 1966 NAS-NRC document was the first to recommend that emergency facilities be categorized. It also emphasized aggressive clinical management of trauma, suggesting that local trauma systems develop databases, and that studies be instituted to designate select injuries to be incorporated in the epidemiological reports of the US Public Health Service. Changes were also recommended concerning legal problems, autopsies, and disaster response reviews. Trauma research was especially emphasized, with the ultimate goal of establishing a National Institute of Trauma [15]. Another problem identified in the report was the broad gap between existing knowledge and operational activity.

The NAS-NRC was not the first report in which many of these issues were raised. The President's Commission on Highway Safety had previously published a report entitled *Health, Medical Care, and Transportation of Injured* [20], which recommended a national program to reduce deaths and injuries caused by highway accidents. Its findings were complemented by and consistent with the NAS-NRC report. The recommendations

Inadequacies of Prehospital Care in 1966

1. The general public is insensitive to the magnitude of the problem of accidental death and injury.

2. Millions lack instruction in basic first aid.

3. Few are adequately trained in the advanced techniques of cardiopulmonary resuscitation, childbirth, or other life-saving measures, yet every ambulance and rescue squad attendant, policeman, fire fighter, paramedical worker, and worker in high-risk industry should be trained.

4. Local political authorities have neglected their responsibility to provide optimum emergency medical services.

5. Research on trauma has not been supported or identified at the National Institutes of Health on a level consistent with its importance as the fourth leading cause of death and a primary cause of disability.

6. The potentials of the U.S. Public Health Service Program in accident prevention and emergency medical services have not been fully exploited.

7. Data are lacking on how to determine the number of individuals whose lives are lost through injuries compounded by misguided attempts at rescue and first aid, absence of physicians at the scene of the injury, unsuitable ambulances with inadequate equipment and untrained attendants, lack of traffic control, or the lack of voice communication facilities.

8. Helicopter ambulances have not been adapted to civilian peacetime needs.

9. Emergency departments of hospitals are overcrowded, some are archaic, and there are no systematic surveys on which to base requirements for space, equipment, or staffing for present, let alone future, needs.

10. Fundamental research on shock and trauma is inadequately supported; medical and health-related organizations have failed to join forces to apply knowledge already available to advanced treatment of trauma, or educate the public and inform Congress.

Figure 1.1 Key findings of the 1966 NAS-NRC report. Adapted from *Accidental Death and Disability: The Neglected Disease of Modern Society*. Washington, DC: National Academy of Sciences, 1966, National Academy Press.

in both documents were used when the Highway Safety Act of 1966 was drafted. This law established the cabinet-level Department of Transportation (DOT) and gave it legislative and financial authority to improve EMS. Specific emphasis was placed on developing a highway safety program, including standards and activities for improving both ambulance service and provider training [21].

The Highway Safety Act of 1966 also authorized funds to develop EMS standards and implement programs that would improve ambulance services. Matching funds were provided for EMS demonstration projects and studies. All states were required to have highway safety programs in accordance with the regulatory standards promulgated by DOT. The standard on EMS required each state to develop regional EMS systems that could handle prehospital emergency medical needs. Ambulances, equipment, personnel, and administration costs were funded by the highway safety program. Regional financing, as opposed to county or state funding, was a new concept that would be echoed in federal health legislation throughout the remainder of the decade [21].

With the Highway Safety Act as a catalyst, DOT contributed more than $142 million to regional EMS systems between 1968 and 1979. A total of roughly $10 million was spent on research alone, including $4.9 million for EMS demonstration projects. A number of other federal EMS initiatives in the late 1960s and early 1970s poured additional funds into EMS, including $16 million in funding from the Health Services and Mental Health Administration, which had been designated as the lead EMS

agency of the Department of Health, Education, and Welfare (DHEW), to areas of Arkansas, California, Florida, Illinois, and Ohio for the development of model regional EMS systems [22].

In 1969 the Airlie House Conference proposed a hospital categorization scheme [23]. The AMA Commission on EMS urged facility categorization and published its own scheme, which identified staffing, equipment, services, and personnel types [24]. This became known as "horizontal categorization." Although it was supported by professional and hospital associations, many hospitals and physicians feared hospitals in lower categories would suffer a loss of prestige, patients, or reimbursement. DHEW EMS program developed a categorization scheme based on hospital-wide care of specific disease processes. Known as "vertical categorization," this concept was ultimately embraced by many regional programs as a major theme in the development of EMS systems.

By the late 1960s, drugs, defibrillation, and personnel were available to improve prehospital care. As early as 1967, the first physician responder mobile programs morphed into "paramedic" programs using physician-monitored telemetry as a modification of the approach by Pantridge in Belfast.

The "Heartmobile" program, begun in 1969 in Columbus, Ohio, initially involved a physician and three EMTs. Within 2 years, 22 highly trained (2,000 hours) paramedics provided the field care, and the physician role became supervisory. Similarly, in Seattle, physicians supervised highly trained paramedics, increasing the survival rate from 10% to 30% for prehospital cardiac arrest patients whose presenting rhythm was ventricular fibrillation. The Seattle story was also one in which fire department first responders played a crucial role in building what is now called a chain of survival. In Dade County, Florida, rapid response of mobile paramedic units was combined with hospital physician direction via radio and telemetry for the first time [25]. In Brighton, England, non-physician personnel provided field care without direct medical oversight. Electrocardiographic data were recorded continuously to permit retrospective review by a physician [26].

National professional organizations such as the ACS, the AAOS, the American Heart Association (AHA), and the American Society of Anesthesiologists (ASA), in concert with other groups, provided extensive medical input into the early development of EMS. New organizations were formed to focus on EMS, including the AMA's Commission on EMS, the AHA's Committee on Community Emergency Health Services, the American Trauma Society, the Emergency Nurses Association, the Society of Critical Care Medicine, the National Registry of Emergency Medical Technicians (NREMT), and the American College of Emergency Physicians (ACEP). In the years prior to 1973, such groups made significant but uncoordinated efforts toward the reorganization, restructure, improvement, expansion, and politicization of EMS [23,24,27,28].

In 1972, the NAS-NRC published *Roles and Resources of Federal Agencies in Support of Comprehensive Emergency Medical Services*, which asserted that the federal government had not kept pace with efforts by professional and lay health organizations to upgrade EMS. The document endorsed a vigorous federal government role in the provision and upgrading of EMS. It recommended that President Nixon acknowledge the magnitude of the accidental death and disability problem by proposing action by the legislative and executive branches to ensure optimum universal emergency care. It urged the integration of all federal resources for delivery of emergency services under the direction of a single division of DHEW, which would have primary responsibility for the entire emergency medical program. It also recommended that the focal point for local emergency medical care be at the state level, and that all federal efforts be coordinated through regional EMS programs [29].

1973: the Emergency Medical Services Systems Act

By 1973 several major lessons had emerged from the demonstration projects and the various studies undertaken during the preceding 7 years. Although the federal initiative had been limited to the 1968 DHEW regional demonstration projects mentioned earlier, significant progress had been made toward clearly defining a potential program goal. The projects proved that a regional EMS system approach could work. However, because systems research was not a component of DHEW program, the demonstration projects did not prove that a regional approach, or for that matter any particular approach, was more effective than another.

By early 1973 many national organizations supported further federal involvement, both in establishing EMS program goals and in providing direct financial support. The first efforts at passing federal EMS legislation were defeated, but a later modified EMS bill passed with support from numerous public and professional groups. President Nixon vetoed this bill in August 1973. The standard conservative philosophy was that EMS was a service that should be provided by local government, and the federal government should neither underwrite operations nor purchase equipment. Additional congressional hearings led to the reintroduction of a bill proposing an extensive federal EMS program, based on the rationale that individual communities would not be able to develop regional systems without federal encouragement, guidelines, and funding. Finally, in November 1973, the Emergency Medical Services Systems Act was passed and signed. It was added as Title XII to the Public Health Service Act, wherein it addressed EMS systems, research grants, and contracts. It also added a new section to the existing Title VII concerning EMS training grants [30].

Although the law was amended to reauthorize expenditures in 1976, 1978, and again in 1979, its goal remained to encourage development of comprehensive regional EMS systems throughout the country. The available grant funds were divided among the four major portions of the EMS Systems Act: Section 1202 – Feasibility studies and planning; Section 1203 – Initial operations; Section 1204 – Expansion and improvement; and Section 1205 – Research. Applicants were encouraged to use existing health resources, facilities, and personnel. The EMS regions were ultimately expected to become financially self-sufficient. Therefore, a phase-out of all federal funding was targeted for 1979 but later extended to 1982. The program was administered in DHEW through the Division of Emergency Medical Services (DEMS), with David Boyd, the medical director of the Illinois demonstration project, named as director. The law and subsequent regulations emphasized a regional systems approach, a trauma orientation, and a requirement that each funded system address the 15 "essential components" (Figure 1.2). It should be noted that medical

```
 1. Manpower
 2. Training
 3. Communications
 4. Transportation
 5. Facilities
 6. Critical care units
 7. Public safety agencies
 8. Consumer participation
 9. Access to care
10. Patient transfer
11. Coordinated patient record-keeping
12. Public information and education
13. Review and evaluation
14. Disaster plan
15. Mutual aid
```

Figure 1.2 *The Fifteen Essential EMS Components.* Washington, DC: Department of Health, Education, and Welfare, Division of EMS, 1973.

oversight was not one of the 15 components, although subsequent regulations encouraged medical oversight.

1973–1978: rapid growth of EMS systems

In 1974 the Robert Wood Johnson Foundation allocated $15 million for EMS-related activities, the largest single contribution for the development of health systems ever made in the United States by a non-profit foundation. Forty-four areas received grants of up to $400,000 to develop EMS systems [31]. This money was intended to encourage communities to build regional EMS systems, emphasizing the overall goal of improving access to general medical care. The money was provided over a 2-year period to establish new demonstration projects and develop regional emergency medical communications systems [32].

In early 1974 a newly reorganized DHEW-DEMS began implementing the legislative mandate. Adopted from earlier experiences, the basic principles were that an effective and comprehensive system must have resources sufficient in quality and quantity to meet a wide variety of demands, and the discrete geographic regions established must have sufficient populations and resources to enable them to eventually become self-sufficient.

Each state was to designate a coordinating agency for state-wide EMS efforts. Ultimately, 304 EMS regions were established nationwide. By 1979, 17 regions were fully functional and independent of federal money. However, of the 304 geographic areas, there were 22 that had no activity and 96 that were still in the planning phase [33]. Testimony was given before the congressional committee considering extension of funding, and an additional year of funding was authorized as the 1202b program for planning.

In the regulations, David Boyd strictly interpreted the congressional legislative intent of the EMS Systems Act to mandate that all communities adopt the 15 essential components. Regions were limited to five grants, and with each year of funding, progress toward more sophisticated operational levels was expected. By the end of the third year of funding, regions were expected to have basic life support (BLS) capabilities, which required no physician involvement. ALS capability, which was expected to perform traditional physician activities, was expected at the end of the fifth year. The use of BLS and ALS terminology in the regulations spread widely. However, the original definitions that corresponded directly to the funded emergency medical technician- ambulance (EMT-A) and paramedic levels of training quickly became elusive as variations in the EMT-A and paramedic levels emerged. The EMT-A level required no medical input, but some states such as Kentucky did extend medical oversight to BLS because of insurance laws – laws making medical care and transportation across a county line virtually impossible without a physician's approval over the radio.

Developing the geographic regions required to secure federal funding through the EMS Systems Act usually necessitated new EMS legislation at the state level. The state laws that developed throughout the 1970s varied markedly in regard to the issues of medical oversight, overall operational authority, and financing. In some states, physician involvement was required. In others, medical oversight was not even mentioned. Often, the responsibility for coordinating activities was assigned to a regional EMS council of physicians, prehospital providers, insurance companies, and consumers who often had interests to protect. Commonly, physician input was somewhat removed from the medical mainstream.

Personnel

A lack of appropriately trained emergency personnel at every level of care had been identified in the NAS-NRC document [15]. After 1973, extensive effort and money were directed at correcting this educational deficiency, and serendipity played a role. A large number of medical corpsmen, physicians, and nurses, who understood that trained non-physicians could perform life-saving tasks in the field, were returning from Vietnam. Many argued that rapid transport and early surgery could improve civilian trauma practice.

Physicians

In 1966 the NAS-NRC document stated, "No longer can responsibility be assigned to the least experienced member of the medical staff, or solely to specialists, who, by the nature of their training and experience, cannot render adequate care without the support of other staff members." [15] Thus the importance of physician leadership and training in EMS was identified early. During the 25 years following World War II, increasing demands for care were placed on hospital emergency departments. Not surprisingly, a branch of medicine evolved with its focus on the critically ill. The academic discipline and scientific rigor necessary to define a separate medical specialty began to develop.

In 1968 ACEP was founded by physicians interested in the organization and delivery of emergency medical care. In 1970 the first emergency medicine residency was established at the University of Cincinnati, and the first academic department of emergency medicine in a medical school was formed at the University of Southern California. Soon the directors of medical school hospital emergency departments founded the University Association for Emergency Medical Services. Between 1972 and 1980 more than 740 residents completed training at 51 emergency medicine residencies throughout the country [34–36]. The first major step toward certification as a specialty occurred in 1973 when the AMA authorized a provisional Section of Emergency Medicine. In 1974 a Committee on Board Establishment was appointed, and a liaison Residency Endorsement Committee was formed [36]. Further impetus toward expansion of residency programs in emergency medicine occurred with the formation of the American Board of

Emergency Medicine (ABEM) in 1976 [37]. Before that time there was some hesitancy to create residency programs that might not lead to board certification.

In September 1979, emergency medicine was formally recognized as a specialty by the AMA Committee on Medical Education and the American Board of Medical Specialties. One of the strongest arguments in favor of the new specialty was that emergency physicians had a unique role in the oversight of prehospital medicine. The ABEM gave its first certifying examination in 1980, which incidentally did not touch on any areas of prehospital care.

Although emergency medicine, emergency nursing, and prehospital care were all nourished by the funds distributed between 1973 and 1982, the interest of ACEP in EMS activities lagged, perhaps because individual physician interest lagged. The first full-time EMS medical director was not appointed until April 1981. Previously, all had been part-time, and some had simply been functionaries. Shortly thereafter, cities like Salt Lake City and Houston followed New York's lead, and appointed full-time EMS medical directors. Even then, EMS as a physician career choice was perceived by many as too limited and perhaps a risky career undertaking.

Prehospital providers

The Highway Safety Act of 1966 funded EMT-A training and curriculum development. By 1982, there were approximately 100,000 providers trained at the EMT-A level. They were trained to provide basic, non-invasive emergency care at the scene and during transport, including such skills as CPR, control of bleeding, ventilation, oxygen administration, fracture management, extrication, obstetrical delivery, and patient transport. The educational requirements, which began as a 70-hour curriculum published by the AAOS in 1969, soon grew to 81 hours of lectures, skills training, and hospital observation, with most of the increase in hours being due to the addition of training in the use of pneumatic anti-shock garments. After working for 6 months, graduates were allowed to take a national certifying examination administered by the NREMT. Founded in 1970, the NREMT developed a standardized examination for EMT-A personnel as one requirement for maintaining registration. Many states began to recognize NREMT registration for the purposes of reciprocity or state certification or licensure [28].

While the EMT-A quickly became a nationally recognized standard, the development of national consensus at the paramedic level lagged behind, with marked differences in training from locality to locality. Paramedic practices became somewhat formalized with the adoption of DOT emergency medical technician – paramedic (EMT-P) curriculum. By 1982, EMT-P training ranged from a few hundred to 2,000 hours of educational and clinical experience. Typical clinical skills included cardiac defibrillation, endotracheal intubation, venepuncture, and the administration of a variety of drugs. The use of these skills was based on interpretation of history, clinical signs, and rhythm strips. Telemetric and voice communications with physicians

were usually required. In the early days of paramedics, extensive "online" medical oversight was mandatory for all calls in most systems. With time, this requirement was modified by the introduction of protocols allowing for greater use of standing orders [38]. However, a great deal of variation in the use of direct medical oversight remained. As early as 1980, paramedics in decentralized systems such as New York's used many clinical protocols, most of which had few indications for mandatory direct medical oversight. On the other hand, as late as 1992, many centralized systems, such as the Houston Fire Department, had only a few standing orders (mainly for cardiac arrest) that did not require contemporaneous instruction from direct medical oversight.

The concept of the EMT-Intermediate (EMT-I) evolved as a provider level located somewhere between EMT-A and EMT-P. Airway management, IV therapy, fluid replacement, rhythm recognition, and defibrillation were the most common "advanced" skills included in the EMT-I curriculum, though significant variation existed (and still does) from state to state. Many states developed several levels of EMT-I, often in a modular progression with formal bridge courses. By 1979, formally recognized prehospital providers existed at dozens of levels, with highly variable requirements for medical oversight.

Public education

Cardiopulmonary resuscitation training gradually became more widely accepted, as evidenced by participation in training programs throughout the country. As early as 1977, a Gallup Poll reported that 12 million Americans had taken CPR courses and another 80 million were familiar with the technique and wanted formal training [6]. The success of public training was documented by many studies [39,40]. The issues of whom to train and how to improve skill retention continue to be explored, as reflected in the AHA/International Liaison Committee on Resuscitation's *Guidelines 2010* document, which contains significant changes in how the techniques of CPR and emergency cardiac care are taught to laypersons [41].

Communications

Before 1973, there were few communication systems available for emergency medical care. Only one in 20 ambulances had voice communications with a hospital, a universal emergency telephone number was not operational, and telephones were not available on highways and rural roads. Centralized dispatch was uncommon and there were problems in communications because of community resistance, cost, and insufficient technology. With DOT funding, major steps were taken toward overcoming these communication problems. National conferences, seminars, and public awareness programs advocated diverse methodologies for EMS communication systems. A communications manual published in 1972 provided technical systems information [42]. In 1973, the 9-1-1 universal emergency number was advocated as a national standard by DOT and the White House Office of Telecommunications. The Federal Communications Commission (FCC) established rules and regulations for EMS communication and dedicated a limited number of radio frequencies for emergency systems. In 1977 DHEW issued guidelines for a model EMS communications plan [43].

Emergency medical services medical directors gradually began to appreciate the importance of more structured call receiving, patient prioritizing, and vehicle dispatching. Physicians were forced to look seriously at EMS operational issues that had previously been seen as neither critical nor medical [44]. On the other hand, telemetry as it had been pioneered by Gene Nagel in Florida was generally seen to be impractical, expensive, and unnecessary, and essentially disappeared over time.

Transportation

Transportation of the critically ill or injured patient rapidly improved after 1973. Although national standards for ambulance equipment were developed in the early 1960s, a 1965 survey of 900 cities reported that fewer than 23% had ordinances regulating ambulance services. An even smaller percentage required an attendant other than the driver, and only 72 cities reported training at the level of an American Red Cross advanced first aid course, the nearest thing to a standard ambulance attendant course before the advent of EMT-A in 1969 [45]. The hearses and station wagons used in the 1960s did not allow personnel room to provide CPR or other treatments to critically ill patients. The vehicles were designed to carry coffins and horizontal loads, not a medical team and a sick patient. In the 1960s, two reports focused national attention on the hazardous conditions of the nation's ambulances [15,46]. In addition to inadequate policies, staff training, and communications, ambulance design was faulty and equipment absent or inadequate. Morticians ran 50% of the ambulance services because they owned the only vehicles capable of carrying patients horizontally. No US manufacturer built a vehicle that could be termed an ambulance.

As early as 1970, DOT and the ACS had developed ambulance design and equipment recommendations [47,48]. In 1973, DHEW released the comprehensive guide, *Medical Requirements for Ambulance Design and Equipment*, and a year later the General Services Administration issued federal specifications KKK-A 1822 for ambulances [49]. Although the KKK specifications were originally developed for government procurement contracts, local EMS agencies were often politically obligated to meet or exceed the specifications when ordering new ambulances. A 1978 study of 183 EMS regions described the status of ambulance services within 151 of the regions. Only 65% of the 13,790 ambulances in those regions met the federal KKK standards. Eighty-one regions used paramedics and 72

had some type of air ambulance capability. Response time was often longer than 10 minutes in urban areas and as much as 30 minutes in rural areas [50].

Hospitals

When awarding grants for EMS under the EMS Systems Act, DHEW required regions to develop standards and guidelines for categorization of emergency departments in the following eight critical clinical groups: trauma, burns, spinal cord injuries, poisoning, cardiac, high-risk infants, alcohol and drug abuse, and behavioral emergencies. Regions were required to identify the most appropriate hospitals for each of these clinical problems.

In reality, only a small portion of emergency facilities was functionally categorized and in many cases the system did not work as described on paper. Hospital administrators resisted losing control, physicians feared surrendering clinical judgment, and both feared losing patient revenues. Despite this resistance, DHEW used EMS hospital categorization fairly effectively to restructure acute patient distribution along the lines of clinical capability rather than market share.

1978–1981: EMS at midpassage

By 1978 many of the original problems and questions concerning EMS had come into focus. Most of the deficiencies identified in the 1966 NAS-NRC report had been addressed, and progress was being made in many areas. Economic resources and political support were being contributed by local and state governments, private foundations, non-profit organizations, and professional groups. However, there was still tremendous geographic variability regarding distribution of services, access, accessibility, quality, and quantity of EMS resources. Basic questions concerning the effectiveness of the various components, system designs, and relationships still existed, and future funding was uncertain.

In 1978, the NAS-NRC released *Emergency Medical Services at Midpassage*, which stated, "EMS in the United States in midpassage [is] urgently in need of midcourse corrections but uncertain as to the best direction and degree." The report was sharply critical of how the EMS Systems Act had been implemented by DHEW, and recommended "research and evaluation directed both to questions of immediate importance to EMS system development and to long-range questions. Without adequate investment in both types of research, EMS in the United States will be in the same position of uncertainty a generation hence as it is today" [51]. The report documented coordination problems among various governmental agencies, focusing particular concern on the multiple standards promulgated as a condition of funding. Some of the standards were conflicting; often they had never been evaluated [51].

Between 1974 and 1981, there were various sources of federal and private funds, and each grant often came with a new set of requirements. DOT established standards for ambulance design, provider training, and other transportation elements, and DHEW announced seven critical care areas as the basis for a systems approach and 15 components as modular elements for EMS design. A variety of private organizations also produced standards. With regard to the technique of CPR, the American Red Cross and the AHA established slightly different standards, criteria, and training requirements. By 1978 some states still had not enacted EMS legislation, whereas others had legislated exactly what prehospital providers could do, potentially hampering the flexibility needed for successful local development. Lack of national conformity or agreement precluded the development of universally accepted national standards in most areas of EMS.

On 26 October 1978, a memorandum of understanding was signed by DOT and DHEW describing each organization's responsibilities relating to development of EMS systems [48]. The agreement was an attempt to coordinate government activities and assign national level responsibility for EMS development and direction. DOT, in coordination with DHEW, was to "develop uniform standards and procedures for the transportation phases of emergency care and response." DHEW was responsible, in coordination with DOT, for developing "medical standards and procedures for initial, supportive, and definitive care phases of EMS systems." Research and technical assistance were to be performed cooperatively, and both agencies agreed to exchange information and "establish joint working arrangements from time to time" [52].

Because the roots, constituencies, and operating philosophies of the agencies were markedly different, the 1978 agreement quickly failed. Over the four subsequent years the lack of coordination continued [53].

In 1980 the EMS directors from each state banded together to form the National Association of State EMS Directors (NASEMSD). With membership from all 50 states and the territories, it attempted to take a leadership role with regard to national EMS policy, and to collaborate on the development of effective, integrated, community-based, and consistent EMS systems. Its strategy was to "achieve our mission by the participation of all the states and territories, by being a strong national voice for EMS, an acknowledged key resource for EMS information and policy, and a leader in developing and disseminating evidence-based decisions and policy" [54].

Financing

By 1978, termination of federal funding in most regions was imminent, and the potential effect on operations and future development began to raise concerns. The 1976 and 1979 amendments to the EMS Systems Act reflected concerns about future funding and had consequently demanded evidence of financial self-sufficiency as one basis for further support. Significant disagreement in describing financial self-sufficiency was apparent in the testimony and documents provided by the various agencies. DOT estimates of non-federal monies spent annually between 1968 and 1980 ranged up to $800 million.

In 1979, DHEW officials estimated in testimony that 90% of regions with paramedic service had achieved financial self-sufficiency by 1978 [43]. However, the Comptroller General, in a 1976 report entitled *Progress in Developing Emergency Medical Services Systems*, cited considerable inconsistency in the degree and duration of support provided by community resources [55]. A few years later, in 1979, the Comptroller General testified on the financial status of the EMS regions after analyzing grant applications under the 1976 amendments. Regions were required to document commitment by local governments to continue financial support after federal funds were terminated under Title XII. By the 1980s, the discrepancy between DHEW's and the Comptroller General's estimates of financial self-sufficiency of EMS systems suggested serious unrecognized difficulties in the continued underwriting of EMS systems.

The financial demands on an EMS system were considerable, related to four major elements: prehospital care, hospital care, communications, and management. The specific costs varied by community. The original 1966 NAS-NRC report estimated that ambulance services accounted for about one-fourth of total EMS system costs, with 75% of that amount for personnel. Communications costs varied from 7% of total cost when there was integration with existing public services, to 35% when completely new systems needed to be established. Although management costs were high during the development phases, they were originally expected to account for less than 2% of the total cost during the operational phase [51].

Health insurance reimbursement did not keep pace with EMS costs, which presented a real problem for EMS providers. Health care benefits were often limited to hospital care and had maximum fixed reimbursements. For example, 20% of Blue Cross patients were not covered for emergency transport, and, of those covered, one-third were only covered after an accident. By 1982, the NAS-NRC wrote, "Availability of advanced emergency care throughout the nation is a worthy objective, but the cost of such services may prohibit communities from obtaining them" [51].

Research

A total of $22 million was appropriated between 1974 and 1979 for EMS research. The National Center for Health Services Research, in coordination with DHEW, funded various clinical and systems research projects. During the 1979 legislative hearings, testimony from DHEW and the leadership of academic research centers stressed the need for continued EMS research. Annual reports from DHEW detailed the type of research under way, questions being studied, and the scope of long-term and short-term research projects funded under Section 1205 of Title XII [50]. These projects included "methods to measure the performance of EMS personnel, evaluate the benefits and the costs of advanced life support systems, examine the impact of categorization efforts, determine the clinical significance of response time, and explore the consequences of alternative system configurations and procedures" [56]. Other projects focused on "developing systems of quality assurance, designing and testing clinical algorithms, and examining the relationships between Emergency Departments and their parent hospitals (including rural-urban differences)" [56].

In early 1979, the Center for the Study of Emergency Health Services at the University of Pennsylvania urged continued support of EMS research, claiming "Dollars spent in EMS research have great potential to help control rising health care costs, [and can] have a significant and visible effect in preventing death and enhancing the quality of patient life following emergency events" [57]. The center suggested research identifying EMS cost control potentials because the phasing out of federal funds, coupled with the effects of local tax revolts, would certainly reduce financing. As the 1980s progressed, the demand for more efficient, effective systems would become universal. Managers of EMS systems, just like their counterparts elsewhere, needed to know which components of the system were crucial and which could be deleted if funding was limited. The answers to those questions were anything but clear.

1981: the Omnibus Budget Reconciliation Act

Late in the summer of 1981, President Reagan signed comprehensive cost containment legislation that converted 25 Department of Health and Human Services (DHHS) funding programs into seven consolidated block grants [58]. EMS was included in the Preventive Health Block Grant, along with seven other programs such as rodent control and water fluoridation. In effect, individual states were left to determine how much money from the block grants would be distributed locally. Although existing EMS programs were temporarily guaranteed minimal support, a state could later decide to withdraw all block grant money from one or more regional EMS programs. This concept, simply a fundamental premise of conservative federal government, evolved quite differently in each of the states. As with decisions regarding how to implement provider levels and assure competence, the funding process was generally quite political, with little direct input from the public or the medical community.

The 1976 *Forward Plan for the Health Services Administration* made it clear that by 1982, all federal EMS system financial support would end, and regional EMS programs would be the responsibility of the regional agencies. The federal role was to be "one of technical assistance and coordination" [59].

1982–1996: changing federal roles

The public health initiative for developing a national EMS system came to a gradual, quiet, and unceremonious demise after 1981. In most regions the remnants of the old DHEW program were left to die off slowly under the cloud of confusion occasioned by the Preventive Health Block Grants formula. In most, but not all, states EMS regional programs were lost in the shuffle of competing health programs while the Reagan administration was systematically eliminating federal support for all such programs. In fact, in most jurisdictions the regional EMS momentum present throughout the 1970s simply evaporated. Paradoxically, some individuals involved in EMS saw the end of DHEW era as an opportunity to develop and implement alternative approaches that would not previously have been permitted [60].

Organizations such as the NREMT, National Association of EMTs (NAEMT), and NASEMSD stepped into the vacuum and endeavored to provide some degree of national infrastructure and EMS identity. At the state level, state EMS agencies managed to keep the momentum by sponsoring well-attended state-wide provider conferences.

In 1984 the Emergency Services Bureau of the National Highway Traffic Safety Administration (NHTSA) was instrumental in creating the American Society for Testing and Materials (ASTM) Committee F-30. Through the ASTM, NHTSA sought to legitimize the promulgation of standards in many areas of EMS. Through a complex consensus process, thousands of ASTM technical standards were arrived at in many different industries, including construction and building. Although these standards have no federal mandate, they were often enforced at the local level, for example, in building codes. Since a confusing but enthusiastic beginning in 1984, more than 30 EMS-related standards have been developed, including those for the EMT-A curriculum, rotary and fixed-wing medical aircraft, and EMS system organization. This last document outlines the roles and responsibilities of state, regional, and local EMS agencies. The resultant standards, although mandated by no authority, were considered by several state legislatures when state EMS laws or guidelines, written to obtain federal funding in the mid-1970s, required updating.

The F-30 Committee prospered as long as physician involvement was evident and decisive, but it was clearly NHTSA's decision what standard to expedite and when. the NREMT, NAEMT, and other interest groups joined the physicians, each to protect themselves. Although many physicians and physician groups eventually tired of the F-30 exercise, NHTSA preserved some semblance of a central authority.

As early as 1983, NHTSA began assuming some roles previously associated with the old DHEW program. Many of the original evaluation staff were hired on a part-time basis to promote use of EMS management information systems. Management conferences were arranged for regional EMS system grantees. Saddled with growing financial problems under block grants, few could attend. In 1988, NHTSA attempted to organize the electronic exchange of information among surviving EMS clearing houses, but those efforts eventually failed after 3 years. Because NHTSA had no specific legislative mandate to assume many of the roles previously performed by DHEW, some states tried to assume those roles but were often unsuccessful. One area that received less attention at the federal level was trauma research and systems development. That would remain so until the passage of the Trauma Care Systems Planning and Development Act in 1990 (Public Law 101-590).

It would be incorrect to view the period since 1982–1996 as simply stagnant. It might be better characterized as a time when centrifugal forces played havoc with attempts by the federal government and national organizations to define and standardize EMS. During this time, neither an operational consensus nor a discrete EMS development philosophy emerged. Across the country, local activists battled others in pursuit of diminishing funds. By 1992, patients had clearly emerged as customers, and, by the beginning of the Clinton administration, EMS was just as conceptually unified, standardized, efficient, expensive, and confused as the rest of American health care. The Clinton health care plan of 1993 barely mentioned ambulance services, and it did not address EMS systems at all.

The Emergency Medical Services for Children (EMSC) program was first authorized and funded by the US Congress in 1984 as a demonstration program under Public Law 98-555. Administration of the EMSC program is jointly shared by the Health Resources and Services Administration's Maternal and Child Health Bureau (MCHB) and NHTSA. This program is a national initiative designed to reduce child and youth disability and death caused by severe illness or injury [61], and serves as an example of a successful collaboration between government and academic forces.

In the late 1970s, the Hawaii Medical Association laid the groundwork for the EMSC program. It urged members of the American Academy of Pediatrics (AAP) to develop multifaceted EMS programs that would decrease morbidity and mortality in children. It worked with Senator Daniel Inouye (D-HI) and his staff to write legislation for a pediatric EMS initiative.

In 1983, a particular incident demonstrated the need for these services. One of Senator Inouye's senior staff members had an infant daughter who became critically ill. Her treatment showed the serious shortcomings of an average emergency department when caring for a child in crisis. A year later, Senators Orrin Hatch (R-UT) and Lowell Weicker (R-CT),

backed by staff members with disturbing experiences of their own, joined Senator Inouye in sponsoring the first EMSC legislation.

Initial funding from the EMSC program supported four state demonstration projects. These state projects developed some of the first strategies for addressing important pediatric emergency care issues, such as disseminating educational programs for prehospital and hospital-based providers, establishing data collection processes to identify significant pediatric issues in the EMS system, and developing tools for assessing critically ill and injured children. In later years, additional states were funded to develop other strategies and to implement programs developed by their predecessors. This work progressed through the 1990s when all 50 states and the territories received funding to improve EMSC and integrate it into their existing EMS systems. In response to the available money, in many areas prehospital care of children became the focus of all EMS innovation.

After several years, with projects developing many useful and innovative approaches to taking care of children in the prehospital setting, a mechanism was needed to make these ideas and products more easily accessible to interested states. In 1991, two national resource centers were funded to provide technical assistance to states and to manage the dissemination of information and EMSC products. In 1995, the EMSC National Resource Center in Washington, DC was designated the single such center for the nation. Additionally, with the recognition of the dire need for research and the lack of qualified individuals in each state to perform it, a new center was funded, the National EMSC Data Analysis Resource Center (NEDARC) located at the University of Utah School of Medicine. Created through a cooperative agreement with the Maternal and Child Health Bureau, the NEDARC was established to "help states accelerate adoption of common EMS data definitions, and to enhance data collection and analysis throughout the country" [62].

As the 1980s ended, members of Congress requested information that justified continued funding of the EMSC program. The Institute of Medicine (IOM) of the National Academy of Sciences was commissioned in 1991 to conduct a study of the status of pediatric emergency medicine in the nation. A panel of experts was convened to review existing data and model systems of care, and to make recommendations as appropriate. The findings from this national study revealed continuing deficiencies in pediatric emergency care for many areas of the country and listed 22 recommendations for the improvement of pediatric emergency care nationwide [63]. These recommendations fell into the following categories: education and training, equipment and supplies, categorization and regionalization of hospital resources, communication and 9-1-1 systems, data collection, research, federal and state agencies and advisory groups, and federal funding. These findings convinced Congress to raise funding for the EMSC program.

In response to the IOM report, the EMSC program developed a strategic plan. With the assistance of multiple professionals, including physicians, nurses, and prehospital providers, major goals and objectives were identified. The EMSC 5-year plan for 1995–2000 served as a guideline for further development of the program [64]. The plan had 13 goals and 48 objectives. Each objective had a specific plan that identified national needs, suggested activities and mechanisms to achieve the objective, and listed potential partners. In 1998, the plan was updated with baseline data, refined objectives, and progress in completing activities [65].

EMS physicians 1982–1996

Throughout the 1970s, emergency physicians and the fledgling ACEP supported regional EMS programs. Unfortunately, by 1983, emergency physicians and the embryonic state chapters of ACEP were primarily focused on developing their new specialty. During this period, medical directors for EMS systems around the country increasingly began to publish articles in scientific journals on prehospital research and on their respective experiences with prehospital care. Gradually, they began to meet and in the process found many areas of common interest. After a series of organizational meetings that began in Hilton Head, South Carolina, in 1984, the National Association of EMS Physicians (NAEMSP) was created in 1985, with Dr Ron Stewart as its first president. By the late 1980s, emergency physician groups such as ACEP and the Society for Academic Emergency Medicine (SAEM) placed more emphasis on EMS and began to encourage EMS-related activities among their members.

Training 1982–1996

In the early 1980s, NHTSA developed an EMT-I curriculum and by 1992 developed the EMT-B curriculum, which was a qualified success and adopted by most states. The EMT-B curriculum included the use of automated external defibrillators as recommended by the AHA [41] and assisting patients with their medications. The National EMS Training Blueprint Project Task Force sponsored by the NREMT began a process to more clearly define the scope of practice of EMS providers in 1993 [66].

Transportation 1982–1996

Encouraging the use of voluntary ambulance standards was common from 1983 to 1990. By 1990, issues of ambulance operations, safety, and optimal mode of response were starting to be a risk management concern and more services began to use medical priority dispatch systems. The number and availability of medical helicopters increased, but with as many as 44 such crashes in one year, safety concerns began to increase as well.

1996–2008: the role of the federal government matures, the United States faces terrorism, and EMS is at breaking point

EMS Agenda for the Future

In 1996, NHTSA and the Health Resources and Services Administration (HRSA) published the *EMS Agenda for the Future* [67]. This document was the culmination of a year-long process to develop a common vision for the future of EMS. The federally funded project was coordinated by NAEMSP and NASEMSD, but involved hundreds of other organizations and EMS-interested individuals who provided input to the spirit and content of the agenda. In addition to describing a vision for the future of EMS, the document discusses 14 attributes of the EMS system and outlines steps that will enable progress toward realizing that vision. Shortly after its initial publication, thousands of copies of the *EMS Agenda for the Future* had been distributed to guide EMS system-related planning, policy creation, and decision making.

EMS Education for the Future: A Systems Approach

In December 1996, NHTSA held a conference to address EMS education recommendations of the *EMS Agenda for the Future* report published earlier in the year. Over the next 2 years an EMS Education Task Force was established and the goals were expanded to include defining the essential elements of a national EMS education system as well as the interrelationships necessary to achieve the recommendations in the agenda.

The outcome of the Task Force was the document entitled the *EMS Education for the Future: A Systems Approach* [68], which called for the development of five components of an overall EMS education system: a national EMS core content, a national EMS scope of practice blueprint, national EMS education standards, national EMS education program accreditation, and national EMS certification.

National ambulance fee schedule

Complaints about Medicare reimbursement for ambulance services increasingly became an issue during the 1990s. Specifically, there were concerns about the lack of uniformity in reimbursement from region to region. The Balanced Budget Act of 1997 required the Health Care Financing Administration (HCFA) to commence a negotiated rule-making process with industry groups and develop a national fee schedule for ambulance services. That process began in 1999 when the HCFA established a rules committee that included the HCFA, the American

Ambulance Association, the International Association of Fire Chiefs, the International Association of Firefighters, the National Volunteer Fire Council, the AHA, the National Association of Counties, the NASEMSD, the Association of Air Medical Services, and a single physician representing both ACEP and NAEMSP.

The regulations and national fee schedule that resulted from the negotiated rule-making process became effective on 1 April 2002 [69]. The fee schedule established seven national categories of reimbursement for ground ambulances: BLS (emergency and non-emergency), ALS (emergency and non-emergency), a second level of ALS for complex cases, paramedic ALS intercept, and specialty care transport. In addition, there were two categories for air medical transport: fixed winged and rotary winged. The final rule also included adjustments for regional wage differences as well as for services provided in rural areas where the cost per transport is generally higher due to the lower overall numbers of transports.

A medical committee was established during the negotiated rule-making process to develop a coding system for ambulance billing that would better convey to the HCFA the medical necessity for transport and the need for ALS. This document was not an official component of the rule-making process. However, the coding system was eventually adopted in 2005 by the Centers for Medicare and Medicaid Services as an "educational tool." It was never made a requirement for reimbursement as was originally proposed [70].

National EMS Information System

In 2001 the NASEMSD, in conjunction with its federal partners at NHTSA and the Trauma/EMS Systems program at the HRSA, began developing a national EMS database, the National EMS Information System (NEMSIS). By 2003, a detailed data dictionary was completed. Information about each of the data elements, the variables, and the definitions associated with the data elements as well as how to deploy the elements in a database were described [71].

With funding from NHTSA, EMSC, and CDC, the NEMSIS Technical Assistance Center (TAC) was established at the University of Utah School of Medicine in 2005. The mission of the TAC is to partner with the University of North Carolina at Chapel Hill to provide support to the NEMSIS project [72].

11 September 2001

The attacks on the World Trade Center and the Pentagon on 11 September 2001 changed the way that Americans think about the world as well as the way they live. Efforts to enhance the capability to prevent and respond to terrorist attacks have become routine. Shortly after 9/11, the Department of Homeland Security (DHS) was established, which represented the largest and most expensive reorganization of the federal government in history. Congress began funding preparedness efforts with billions of dollars going to federal agencies, state and local

governments, and private entities such as hospitals. Despite the massive funding for public safety and medical preparedness, reports have indicated that only a small percentage (less than 4%) of this funding has gone to EMS [73]. Advocacy efforts to increase federal funding for EMS, for both day-to-day services and preparedness, were largely unsuccessful.

Advocates for EMS

Recognizing the need for greater national advocacy for EMS, the NASEMSD and NAEMSP formed a non-profit organization, Advocates for EMS (AEMS), on 22 October 2002, for promoting, educating, and increasing awareness among decision makers in Washington on issues affecting EMS [74]. Although there had been previous efforts to establish national EMS advocacy coalitions, none were able to sustain their efforts for more than a few years.

Federal Interagency Committee on EMS

The Federal Interagency Committee on EMS (FICEMS) has coordinated efforts between federal agencies on related EMS issues for several decades. Although this forum provided an opportunity for collaboration between federal agencies on EMS issues, the FICEMS lacked statutory authority and its representatives were not senior officials, which often led to policy and implementation challenges. In 2005, Congress created a new FICEMS with senior representatives from DOT, DHS, DHHS, the Department of Defense, the Federal Communications Commission, and a single state EMS director. The role of the FICEMS is to identify state and local EMS needs, to recommend new or expanded programs for improving EMS at all levels, and to streamline the process through which federal agencies support EMS. The first meeting of the new FICEMS was held in December 2006. In 2007, the National EMS Advisory Council was established to provide advice and consult with the FICEMS and the Secretary of Transportation relating to EMS issues affecting DOT.

Trends in air medical services

Air medical services in the United States struggled financially for a number of decades and the industry as a whole experienced only modest growth until 2000. However, by 2005, an estimated 700 air ambulances were in operation, more than double the number from a decade before. Unfortunately, that same growth was associated with a more than 200% increase in helicopter crashes. From 2000 to 2005, 60 people died in 84 crashes, and an estimated 10% of air ambulances in the United States had experienced crashes [75]. At the same time, the number of flights paid for by Medicare was up 58% from 2001, and during the same period Medicare payments for air ambulance transports doubled to $103 million [76]. This has led to a belief that the improved reimbursement for air medical services that came with the implementation of the national fee schedule in 2002 was a factor that contributed to this increase in helicopter utilization.

Efforts by states to regulate air ambulance services have been hampered by legal challenges from the industry related to the Airline Deregulation Act of 1978. The act preempts states from regulating FAA-licensed air transport services in ways that affect their rates, routes, or services. Although the FAA recognizes the role of states in regulating the medical aspects of air ambulance services, questions frequently arise as to what is medical and what is related to rates, routes, or services [77].

Institute of Medicine report on the future of emergency care

In the decade from 1993 to 2002, the number of emergency departments and hospital inpatient beds in the United States declined at the same time that the number of patients coming to emergency departments (EDs) increased by 26%. As emergency medicine has matured as a specialty, patients have increasingly come to EDs as a place to get what is perceived as good care at a convenient time. Additionally, they are frequently referred to EDs by private physicians for unscheduled care. There is also evidence that patients without insurance use EDs as a safety net for obtaining care that they cannot get elsewhere. The result of these intersecting issues, combined with an aging population, is hospital and ED overcrowding. When hospitals are full, admitted patients are frequently "boarded" in the ED until an inpatient bed becomes available. ED boarding, as well as elective admissions, are felt to be the major factors contributing to ambulance diversion. In 2003 there were more than 500,000 ambulance diversions in the United States.

The IOM began a study of hospital-based emergency care in 2003 that rapidly expanded to address long-standing and significant issues related to EMS and emergency care for children. In particular, EMS systems were viewed as increasingly overburdened and underfunded. The result was a three-volume IOM report titled *The Future of Emergency Care*, which was released in 2006 [78]. Key findings of the report included the following: many EDs and trauma centers are overcrowded; emergency care is highly fragmented; critical specialists are often unavailable to provide emergency and trauma care; EMS and EDs are not well equipped to handle pediatric care. Key recommendations of the report included the following: create coordinated, regionalized, and accountable emergency care systems; create a lead (federal) agency for emergency care; end ED boarding and diversion; increase funding for emergency care; enhance emergency care research; promote EMS workforce standards; enhance pediatric presence throughout emergency care.

The IOM report was the first major report on emergency care since the 1966 NAS-NRC report and included a number of recommendations for EMS that, if adopted, would have a major impact. One recommendation of particular relevance to EMS physicians is the recommendation to create a subspecialty for EMS physicians. Other recommendations of specific interest to EMS include developing national standards for the categorization of emergency care facilities; developing evidence-based national model EMS protocols; increased funding for EMS preparedness; states should require national accreditation of paramedic education programs and national certification for state licensure; EMS agencies should have pediatric coordinators to ensure appropriate equipment, training, and services for children.

2009–2013: a period of incremental progress

Subspecialty in EMS medicine

Following decades of efforts and bolstered by a recommendation in the 2006 IOM report *The Future of Emergency Care*, them ABEM successfully petitioned and the American Board of Medical Specialties approved a physician subspecialty in EMS on 23 September 2010. The ABEM website has the following description of the subspecialty.

> Emergency Medical Services (EMS) is a medical subspecialty that involves prehospital emergency patient care, including initial patient stabilization, treatment, and transport in specially equipped ambulances or helicopters to hospitals. The purpose of EMS subspecialty certification is to standardize physician training and qualifications for EMS practice, improve patient safety and enhance the quality of emergency medical care provided to patients in the prehospital environment, and facilitate further integration of prehospital patient treatment into the continuum of patient care [79].

A task force developed and published an article entitled "The core content of EMS medicine" on 10 January 2012 [80]. The first certification examination was administered in October 2013.

EMS provider education

In 2009, NHTSA published the National EMS Education Standards. These are consistent with the principles of the 1996 *EMS Education Agenda for the Future: A Systems Approach* [68] and establish the entry-level educational competencies for the levels of EMS providers outlined in the National EMS Scope of Practice Model [81]. The current model has four levels of providers: emergency medical responder, emergency medical technician, advanced emergency medical technician, and paramedic. The emergency medical technician-intermediate that was established in 1999 was eliminated. The National EMS Education Standards are replacing the National Standard Curricula and will enable more diverse implementation methods and more frequent updates.

Community paramedicine

There has been growing interest in the United States in expanding the role of paramedics to include the management of urgent low-acuity illnesses, monitoring patients with chronic illnesses at home, and performing other functions that do not involve the traditional EMS role of treating and transporting patients to emergency departments. While scientific evidence of the safety and effectiveness of such expanded roles is limited, the success of programs in Canada, England, and Australia has drawn the attention of governments and others interested in innovative models of health care delivery and incorporating non-physician providers, who are sometimes viewed as under-utilized, into these models [82]. Legislation passed in Minnesota in 2011 (2011 Minn. Laws, Chap. #12) defines community paramedics and establishes a process for educating and certifying them. In 2012 a law was passed to enable reimbursement for community paramedic services under the medical assistance program and to study the cost and quality of the program (2012 Minn. Laws, Chap. #169). Also in 2012, the Maine legislature passed a law to establish pilot community paramedic projects (Chapter 562, Sec. 1 §84). Community paramedic programs also function in Western Eagle County, Colorado, and Fort Worth, Texas [83].

National EMS Culture of Safety Project

Emergency medical services is known to be a high-risk profession; EMS providers are 2.5 times more likely than the average worker to be killed on the job [84], and their transportation-related injury rate is five times higher than average [85]. Additionally, there are patient safety concerns as outlined in the 1999 IOM report *To Err is Human* as well as concerns about risks to EMS personnel, patients, and the community from ambulance crashes. In 2009 the National EMS Advisory Council recommended that NHTSA create a strategy for building a culture of safety in EMS. With support from the EMS for Children Program at the HRSA, NHTSA contracted with ACEP to develop a National EMS Culture of Safety Strategy that was published in October 2013 [86].

EMS research

In response to the recommendations to improve research in emergency care that were included in the 2006 IOM report *The Future of Emergency Care*, the National Institutes of Health (NIH) established an Emergency Care Research Working Group in 2007. The purpose of the working group is to coordinate research in emergency care across the NIH in an effort to improve efficiency, realize scientific opportunities, and enable the rigorous training of new investigators. In November 2010, the NIH published four papers in the *Annals of Emergency Medicine* summarizing the progress, promise, and process of emergency care research and reporting on the outcomes of three roundtables. An Office of Emergency Care Research has been established and Jeremy Brown MD was appointed the first permanent director in July 2013.

Acknowledgments

We wish to offer special recognition to Carl Post PhD and Marsha Treiber MPS for their extensive contributions to the original writing of this chapter.

References

1 Breasted JH. Historical medicine. *Bull Hist Med* 1923;3:58–78.
2 Major RH. *A History of Medicine*, vol. 1. Springfield, IL: Charles C. Thomas, 1954.
3 *1 Kings* 17:17–24.
4 *Luke* 10:25–37.
5 Garrison FH. *An Introduction to the History of Medicine*, 4th edn. Philadelphia: W.B. Saunders, 1929.
6 The Gallup Poll, Field Newspaper Syndicate, June 30, 1977.
7 Post CJ. Red Crossader. *EMS* 1997;64.
8 Haller JS Jr. The beginnings of urban ambulance service in the United States and England. *J Emerg Med* 1990;8(6):743–55.
9 Barringer ED. *Bowery to Bellevue*. New York: W.W. Norton & Co., 1950.
10 Barkley KT. The history of the ambulance. *Proc Int Cong Hist Med* 1974;23:456–66.
11 Kouwenhoven WB, Jude JR, Knickerbocker GB. Closed chest cardiac massage. *JAMA* 1960;173: 1064–7.
12 Safar P, Brown TC, Holtey WJ, Wilder RJ. Ventilation and circulation with closed-chest cardiac massage in man. *JAMA* 1961;176:574–6.
13 Eisenberg MS. *Life in the Balance: Emergency Medicine and the Quest to Reverse Sudden Death*. New York: Oxford University Press, 1997.
14 Pantridge JF, Geddes JS. A mobile intensive care unit in the management of myocardial infarction. *Lancet* 1967;2(7510):271–3.
15 Committee on Trauma and Committee on Shock. *Accidental Death and Disability: The Neglected Disease of Modern Society*, September 1966, Washington, DC. Fifth printing by the Commission on Emergency Medical Services, January 1970, American Medical Association.
16 Committee on Trauma. Minimal equipment for ambulances. *Bull Am Coll Surgeons* 1961;46:136–7.
17 Committee on Trauma. Minimal equipment for ambulances. *Bull Am Coll Surgeons* 1967;52:92–6.
18 Hampton OP. The systematic approach to emergency medical services. *Arch Environ Health* 1970;21(2):214–17.
19 Hampton OP. Transportation of the injured: a report. *Bull Am Coll Surgeons* 1960;45:55–9.
20 President's Commission on Highway Safety. *Health, Medical Care, and Transportation of Injured*. Washington, DC: US Government Printing Office, 1965, pp.10–19.
21 National Highway Safety Act of 1966 (US), PL No. 89–564.
22 Jelenko C, Frey CF. *Emergency Medical Services: An Over View*. Bowie, MD: Brady Company, 1976.
23 Committee on Trauma. *Recommendations for an Approach to an Urgent National Problem. Proceedings of the Airlie Conference on Emergency Medical Services*. Chicago: American College of Surgeons, American Academy of Orthopedic Surgeons, 1969.
24 Commission of Emergency Medical Services. *Recommendations of the Conference on the Guidelines for the Categorization of Hospital Emergency Capabilities*. Chicago: American Medical Association, 1971.
25 Nagel EL, Hirschman JC, Nussenfeld SR, Rankin D, Lundblad E. Telemetry medical command in coronary and other mobile emergency care systems. *JAMA* 1970;214(2):332–8.
26 Lewis RP, Stang JM, Fulkerson PK, Sampson KL, Scoles A, Warren JV. Effectiveness of advanced paramedics in a mobile coronary care system. *JAMA* 1979;241(18):1902–4.
27 American Heart Association, National Academy of Sciences, National Research Council. Cardiopulmonary resuscitation. *JAMA* 1966;198(4):372–9.

28 Boyd DR, Edlich RF, Micik S. *Systems Approach to Emergency Care.* Norwalk, CT: Appleton-Century-Crofts, 1983.

29 Committee on Emergency Medical Services. *Roles and Resources of Federal Agencies in Support of Comprehensive Emergency Medical Services.* Washington, DC: National Research Council, 1972.

30 Emergency Medical Services Systems Act of 1973 (US), PL No. 93–154, Title XII of the Public Health Service Act.

31 Diehl D. The Emergency Medical Services Program. *Robert Wood Johnson Foundation Special Report*, Number 2, 1977.

32 Robert Wood Johnson Foundation. *National Competitive Program Grants for Regional Emergency Medical Communications Systems Administered in Cooperation with National Academy of Sciences.* Program guidelines, 1973.

33 Lythcott GI. Statement before the Subcommittee on Health and Scientific Research Committee on Labor and Human Resources. In: *United States Senate Hearing Report 24*, Feb 1979.

34 Anwar AH, Hogan MH. Residency-trained physicians: where have all the flowers gone? *JACEP* 1979;8(2):84–7.

35 Emergency Medicine Residents Association. A survey by EMRA, May 1980.

36 Liaison Residency Endorsement Committee. American College of Emergency Physicians. Information supplied June 1980.

37 American Board of Emergency Medicine. *Eligibility Requirements.* East Lansing, MI: ABEM, 1976.

38 Joint Review Committee on Educational Programs for EMT-Paramedics. *Essentials and Guidelines of an Accredited Educational Program for the Emergency Medical Technician-Paramedic.* Essentials adopted 1978, guidelines approved 1979.

39 Eisenberg MS, Berger L, Hallstrom A. Epidemiology of cardiac arrest and resuscitation in a suburban community. *JACEP* 1979;8(1):2–5.

40 McElroy CR. Citizen CPR: the role of the layperson in prehospital care. *Top Emerg Med* 1980;1(4):37–46.

41 American Heart Association in collaboration with International Liaison Committee on Resuscitation. Guidelines 2000 for Cardiopulmonary Resuscitation and Emergency Cardiovascular Care. *Circulation* 2000;102(suppl):I1–I384.

42 National Highway Traffic Safety Administration. *Communication: Guidelines for Emergency Medical Services.* Washington, DC: US Department of Transportation, 1972.

43 Emergency Medical Services Division, Department of Health, Education, and Welfare. HSA 77–2036, March 1977.

44 Kuehl AE, Kerr JT, Thompson JM. Urban emergency medical system: a consensus. *Am J Emerg Med* 1984;2(6):559–63.

45 Hampton OP. Present status of ambulance services in the United States. *Bull Am Coll Surgeons* 1965;50:177–9.

46 *Summary Report of the Task Force on Ambulance Services.* Washington, DC: National Academy of Sciences, National Research Council, 1967.

47 American College of Surgeons Committee on Trauma. Essential equipment for ambulances. *Bull Am Coll Surgeons* 1970;55(5):7–13.

48 National Highway Traffic Safety Administration. *Ambulance Design Criteria.* Washington, DC: US Government Printing Office, 1971.

49 Roemer R, Kramer C, Frink JE. *Planning Urban Health Services: Jungle to System.* New York: Springer Publishing, 1975.

50 Answers to questions submitted by members of Subcommittee on Health and Scientific Research of the Committee on Labor and Human Resources. In: *United States Senate Hearing Report 98–100*, Feb 1979.

51 Committee on Emergency Medical Services. *Emergency Medical Services at Midpassage.* Washington, DC: National Research Council, 1978.

52 Memorandum of understanding between the US Department of Transportation and the US Department of Health, Education, and Welfare. *Procedures Relating to Emergency Medical Services Systems.* Washington, DC: US Government Printing Office, 1978.

53 Post CJ. *Omaha Orange: A Popular History of EMS in America.* Boston, MA: Jones and Bartlett, 1992.

54 National Association of State EMS Directors. Available at: www.nasemso.org

55 Comptroller General of the United States. *Progress in Developing Emergency Medical Services Systems.* Washington, DC: US Government Accountability Office, 1976: HRD 76–150;13.

56 Boyd DR. Emergency medical services systems evaluation. Statement submitted to the Subcommittee on Health and Scientific Research, Committee on Labor and Human Resources. In: *United States Senate Hearing Report 47–57*, Feb 1979.

57 Cayten GC. Testimony to the Subcommittee on Health and Scientific Research of the Committee on Labor and Human Resources. In: *United States Senate Hearing Report 156–166*, Feb 1979.

58 The Omnibus Budget Reconciliation Act of 1981 (US), PL No. 97–35.

59 US Department of Health, Education and Welfare. *The Forward Plan for the Health Services Administration.* Washington, DC: US Government Printing Office, 1976.

60 Page J. History and Legislation Panel. Phoenix, AZ: EMS Medical Directors' Course, 1993.

61 Ball J. Emergency medical services for children. In: Foltin G, Tunik M, Cooper A, Markenson D, Treiber M, Karpeles T (eds) *Teaching Resource for Instructors in Prehospital Pediatrics.* New York: Center for Pediatric Emergency Medicine, 2000.

62 Who is NEDARC? The National EMSC Data Analysis Resource Center. Available at: www.nedarc.org/nedarcCanHelp/whoIsNEDARC.html

63 Durch JS, Lohr KN (eds). *Emergency Medical Services for Children.* Washington, DC: National Academy Press, 1993.

64 US Department of Health and Human Services, Health Resources and Services Administration, Maternal and Child Health Bureau. *5-Year Plan: Emergency Medical Services for Children, 1995-2000.* Washington, DC: Emergency Medical Services for Children National Resource Center, 1995.

65 US Department of Health and Human Services, Health Resources and Services Administration, Maternal and Child Health Bureau. *5-Year Plan: Midcourse Review, Emergency Medical Services for Children, 1995-2000.* Washington, DC: Emergency Medical Services for Children National Resource Center, 1998.

66 National EMS Training Blueprint (working draft). Columbus, OH: National Registry of EMTs, 1993.

67 Emergency Medical Services. *Education Agenda for the Future: A Systems Approach.* Washington, DC: Department of Transportation, National Highway Traffic and Safety Administration (US), 1996.

68 Emergency Medical Services. *Education Agenda for the Future: A Systems Approach.* Washington, DC: Department of Transportation, National Highway Traffic and Safety Administration (US), 2000.

69 Centers for Medicare and Medicaid Services. *Medicare Program: Payment of Ambulance Services, Fee Schedule; and Revision to Physician Certification Requirements for Coverage of Nonemergency Ambulance Services.* 42 CFR Parts 410 and 414. Final Rule, 2002.

70 Department of Health and Human Services, Centers for Medicare and Medicaid Services. *CMS Manual System, Pub 100-4 Medicare Claims.* Transmittal 395, Dec 2004.

71 Dawson DE. National Emergency Medical Services Information System (NEMSIS). *Prehosp Emerg Care* 2006;10(3):314–16.

72 NEMSIS Technical Assistance Center. Available at: www.nemsis.org

73 US Department of Justice, Office of Domestic Preparedness. ODP Information Bulletin No. 110, May 2004.

74 Advocates for EMS. *2008 Annual Report.* Falls Church, VA. Available at: www.advocatesforems.org.

75 Surge in crashes scars air ambulance industry. *USA Today,* Jul 17, 2005.

76 Air ambulances are multiplying, and costs rise. *New York Times,* May 3, 2005.

77 McGinnis KK, Judge T, Nemitz B, et al. Air medical services: future development as an integrated component of the emergency medical services (EMS) system: a guidance document by the Air Medical Task Force of the National Association of State EMS Officials, National Association of EMS Physicians, Association of Air Medical Services. *Prehosp Emerg Care* 2007;11(4):353–68.

78 Committee on the Future of Emergency Care in the United States Health System. Future of Emergency Care series, including: *Emergency Medical Services: At the Crossroads; Emergency Care for Children: Growing Pains; Hospital-Based Emergency Care: At the Breaking Point.* Washington, DC: National Academies Press, 2006. Available at: www.nap.edu

79 American Board of Emergency Medicine. Available at: www.abem.org

80 EMS Examination Task Force, American Board of Emergency Medicine, Perina DG, et al. The core content of emergency medical services medicine. *Prehosp Emerg Care* 2012;16(3):309–22.

81 National Highway Traffic Safety Administration. *National EMS Scope of Practice Model.* Washington, DC: Department of Transportation, National Highway Traffic Safety Administration (US), DOT HS 810 657; February 2007. Available at: www.ems.gov/educationstandards.htm

82 Bigham BL, Kennedy SM, Drennan I, Morrison LJ. Expanding paramedic scope of practice in the community: a systematic review of the literature. *Prehosp Emerg Care* 2013;17(3):361–72.

83 Responding before a call is needed. *New York Times,* September 18, 2011.

84 Maguire BJ, Hunting KL, Smith GS, Levick NR. Occupational fatalities in emergency medical services: a hidden crisis. *Ann Emerg Med* 2002;40(6):625–32.

85 Maguire BJ. Transportation-related injuries and fatalities among emergency medical technicians and paramedics. *Prehosp Disaster Med* 2011;26(5):346–52.

86 American College of Emergency Physicians. *Strategy for a National EMS Culture of Safety.* 2013. Available at: www.emscultureofsafety.org

SECTION I

Airway

CHAPTER 2

EMS airway management

Francis X. Guyette and Henry E. Wang

The skills of airway management

RJ is a 34-year-old, 6ft, 100 kg, unhelmeted male operator of an ATV who was thrown from the vehicle. The flight crew arrived, completed their survey, placed the patient on the monitor, established a 20G peripheral IV, and hung normal saline. The patient's GCS was 7, BP 104/50, pulse 128, respiratory rate 24, and oxygen saturation 94% on 15L NRB.

The patient's airway was assessed using the LEMON method. **Look** externally – noting a possible fractured jaw. **Evaluate** using the 3-3-2 rule, noting that three fingers could not be placed in the mouth, three fingers could be placed from the angle of the jaw to the mentum, and two fingers could be placed from the thyroid cartilage to the bottom of the jaw. The **Mandible** was not receding. **Obstruction** was assessed using a modified Mallampati, which provided a clear view of the posterior oropharynx and uvula when the blood was suctioned. Lastly, the patient's **Neck mobility** was limited by the cervical collar, which was removed and inline stabilization was held while providing a jaw thrust. Etomidate and succinylcholine were drawn up. Drug choices and dosing were verbalized aloud and confirmed using a challenge–response method and visual inspection by both crew members. A checklist was read aloud while the flight crew prepared for intubation. The BVM and O_2 were checked, the suction device was functional, the IV patency confirmed, and the patient's pulse oximetry, pulse, and BP were checked. Oxygen via nasal cannula at 6 LPM was placed on the patient to provide passive oxygenation. An 8.0 and 7.5 ETT were placed next to the patient. The 8.0 balloon was inspected and a stylet was lubricated and inserted. The video laryngoscope (VL) was turned on and was recording. A waveform capnograph was connected as was a commercial tube holder. A #5 King LTD-S was placed on the patient's chest as a contingency.

The RSI medications were administered and the patient was oxygenated with a BVM. After fasciculation, the VL was placed while suctioning and the ETT was visualized to pass through the cords. The balloon was inflated and placement confirmed by $EtCO_2$ and five-point auscultation. The tube was secured with a commercial tube holder and the patient was reassessed to ensure stable vitals. The patient was sedated and placed in restraints to preclude self-extubation.

Introduction

Airway management is one of the most essential interventions in the prehospital care of the critically ill or injured [1,2]. Many scientific efforts have highlighted the difficulty of endotracheal intubation (ETI) in the prehospital setting, the adverse events associated with the procedure, and the challenges in attaining and maintaining clinical proficiency. Other studies highlight the uncertain connections with improved patient outcomes [3]. These observations underscore that airway management is not simply a discrete procedure but a comprehensive strategy of care that requires close, system-level medical oversight. The most successful prehospital airway management programs incorporate multiple elements including training, skills verification, equipment selection, decision support, continuing education, and total quaility management.

The goal of this chapter is to describe the medical direction paradigms and considerations necessary for a high-quality airway management program. The practicing EMS physician must also be aware of these issues, and must be an expert in out-of-hospital airway management.

The challenges of airway management in the prehospital setting

Airway management in the prehospital setting comes with unique challenges. Prehospital airway management occurs in an uncontrolled environment where patients are severely ill, undifferentiated in presentation and medical history, and may be situated in awkward positions (e.g. on the floor, in a bed, or in the wreckage of a car). Prehospital providers, including EMS physicians, have fewer monitoring and pharmacological options

---

Emergency Medical Services: Clinical Practice and Systems Oversight, Second Edition. Volume 1: Clinical Aspects of EMS.
Edited by David C. Cone, Jane H. Brice, Theodore R. Delbridge, and J. Brent Myers.

than exist in the hospital. Unlike the hospital setting, there are very limited resources with respect to personnel and equipment. These factors significantly increase the complexity and difficulty of airway management and underscore the need for simple and efficient field approaches.

While the individual components may resemble techniques performed in the hospital, prehospital airway management often requires approaches different from the hospital setting. The medical director must be keenly aware of these distinctions and provide appropriate guidance. When it is the EMS physician who is managing the airway in the field, he or she must be aware of the differing resources and conditions from those in a hospital where the bulk of his or her experience might have been garnered.

Which airway, when, and how?

Successful prehospital airway management relies on the optimized combination of basic, advanced, and rescue airway interventions. Medical directors must choose strategies appropriate for the needs of their services based on available personnel, resources, and environment. An exclusive focus on any one management technique will limit the providers' abilities to adapt to difficult situations and failed procedures.

Basic airway interventions

Basic airway interventions include measures to provide supplemental oxygen and/or ventilation without the use of an advanced invasive airway device. Basic airway interventions are used by providers of all skill levels. While they lack protection from aspiration (and in fact may increase aspiration risk through inadvertent gastric insufflation), they are the essential foundation of any successful airway management program. Providers of all levels – even practitioners who perform more advanced airway interventions – must master basic airway techniques. Practitioners will rely on basic airway intervention skills when advanced airway interventions fail.

The medical director may define conditions for which basic airway management is the preferred technique. These situations may include scenarios with short transport times where the time and risk necessary to perform advanced airway maneuvers outweigh the benefits of a secure airway. Another example is pediatric respiratory arrest, where most providers are more experienced with bag-valve-mask ventilation than endotracheal intubation.

Endotracheal intubation

Endotracheal intubation is the most widely recognized method of invasive airway management and has been performed by paramedics in the United States for over 25 years [4–7]. ETI has many theoretical advantages, including isolation of the airway from secretions or gastric contents and the provision of a direct conduit to the trachea without separate airway opening maneuvers. However, equipoise exists with respect to the clinical benefit of ETI in the prehospital environment.

Endotracheal intubation is associated with several risks, including failed intubation, unrecognized esophageal intubation, hypoxia, hypotension, bradycardia, aspiration, and airway trauma. Many of the risks of ETI can be mitigated through proper training and equipment. However, prehospital systems are often unable to make the substantial investments necessary to ensure a high degree of safety in the procedure. Medical directors who choose ETI as a method of airway management must be prepared to properly educate and train their providers, ensuring that they have the decision-making and psychomotor skills necessary to perform the procedure. This must include a minimum of didactic training on the indications, contraindications, and techniques for endotracheal intubation, and simulated and live intubations in supervised environments.

The medical director must determine how best to provide suitable training to providers performing ETI. Strategies may include mandatory minimums for yearly ETI experience supplemented by simulation and supervised experience in the operating room (OR) or emergency department (ED). In order to concentrate limited field experiences, it may be necessary to restrict the skill to a few selected providers. A commitment to continuous quality improvement is also necessary, requiring rigorous review of all airway cases. Direct observation in the field or through video review is often desirable. Quantitative assessment of ETI should include not only procedural success rates but also physiological measurements. ETI attempts should be confirmed by end-tidal carbon dioxide ($EtCO_2$) and monitored for vital sign abnormalities including hypoxia, hypotension, and bradycardia. When available, quality assurance should also include time to intubation and review of video images [8].

Several adjunctive techniques are available to facilitate ETI, each with distinct advantages and disadvantages. For example, the tracheal introducer or gum elastic bougie has been widely described as a device either for blind intubation or as an adjunct for difficult intubation. While use of such devices may improve intubation success, the medical director must consider their added complexity as well as the need for additional training and skills maintenance. The latter point deserves emphasis. Each newly acquired tool intended to improve the likelihood of successful or optimal airway management also increases the burden or obligation to maintain skills regarding its use. This reality is too easily overlooked in the enthusiasm to deploy something new which is perceived to make circumstances easier.

Does prehospital ETI improve survival?

Few studies link prehospital ETI to improved patient survival. Gausche et al. performed the only randomized, controlled trial of prehospital ETI, finding no differences in survival or neurological outcome between children receiving ETI and those receiving bag-valve-mask (BVM) ventilation [9]. Davis et al.

evaluated patient survival after paramedic rapid sequence intubation (RSI) for traumatic brain injury, associating prehospital RSI with an increased risk of death compared with matched historical controls [10]. A variety of other studies encompassing a range of different patient subsets observed equivocal or worsened outcomes associated with prehospital ETI [3,11]. While most cases of prehospital ETI occur for patients in cardiac arrest, there have been only observational analyses of this subset. This is primarily due to the large sample sizes (>10,000 patients) that would be required to detect survival differences or equivalence in this population. Thus, while ETI is common prehospital practice, its survival benefit remains unproven.

Do adverse events occur during prehospital ETI?

Recent studies have drawn attention to previously unrecognized adverse events associated with prehospital ETI. Successful prehospital airway management programs have placed strong emphasis on minimizing these and other adverse events. Many of these adverse events have been detected only through the advent of monitoring technology and rigorous airway management review.

Katz and Falk described 108 paramedic-placed endotracheal tubes brought to an Orlando trauma center, finding that the tube was misplaced in 25% of the cases [12]. Other studies have identified lower but not insignificant incidences of endotracheal tube misplacement [13,14]. Other efforts describe the frequency of endotracheal tube dislodgment during prehospital care [15]. Use of continuous $EtCO_2$ has reduced the incidence of the unrecognized misplaced endotracheal tube.

Dunford et al. examined a subset of patients receiving prehospital RSI and found that a considerable portion experienced iatrogenic oxygen desaturation or bradycardia during intubation attempts [16]. Hypoxia and bradycardia may be prevented by continuous monitoring of pulse oximetry with the provision of oxygen and supplemental ventilation during any period of hypoxia. Episodes of hypoxia can be mitigated using apneic oxygenation through a high-flow nasal cannula applied during the endotracheal intubation attempt.

Prehospital ETI can also interact or interfere with other important resuscitation tasks. For example, Davis et al. linked post-RSI hyperventilation with worsened TBI outcomes [17]. Aufderhiede et al. showed that hyperventilation after successful ETI of cardiac arrest patients can compromise coronary perfusion during cardiopulmonary resuscitation (CPR) chest compressions [18,19]. Studies on human simulators suggest that conventional ETI efforts may increase CPR "hands-off" or no-flow time (pauses in CPR to facilitate endotracheal intubation) compared with other airway devices [20]. Models of high-performance CPR now teach providers to defer airway management in favor of providing uninterrupted compressions.

Should emergency medical technicians perform ETI?

The prior national EMT curriculum included ETI as an optional module [21]. However, the ability of EMTs to acquire and maintain clinical ETI skills remains unclear. Two independent studies of EMT ETI found suboptimal success rates (<50%) [22,23]. Most medical directors are not comfortable with EMTs performing ETI. However, several series describe the ability of basic EMTs to use supraglottic airways (SGA) (e.g. Combitube) [24–26]. The current National EMS Education Standards do not list either ETI or SGA as EMT skills; SGAs are listed for advanced EMTs.

Should EMS providers limit the number of ETI attempts?

While many prehospital EMS personnel define an ETI "attempt" as an effort to insert the endotracheal tube, national consensus guidelines suggest that an ETI "attempt" should be defined as an insertion of the laryngoscope blade, to maintain consistency with other airway management definitions used in other medical disciplines. Selected studies indicate that a substantial portion of prehospital ETI require multiple attempts [27]. Evaluations of inhospital ETI efforts suggest that more than one ETI attempt is associated with an increased risk of developing cardiac arrest [28]. Some EMS agencies use a "three attempts and out" rule, limiting intubation efforts to no more than three attempts. Given the low probability of success following the second attempt, medical directors may choose to limit providers to two attempts, followed by immediate use of a supraglottic rescue airway.

Drug-facilitated intubation

Drug-facilitated intubation (DFI) is the use of intravenous sedative and/or neuromuscular blocking agents to facilitate ETI of patients with intact protective airway reflexes [29]. The most common forms of DFI include RSI, also termed "neuromuscular blockade-assisted intubation," and sedation-assisted intubation. Most medical directors regard DFI as an advanced technique that should be reserved for only the most qualified practitioners. The National Association of EMS Physicians has published national consensus standards for drug-facilitated intubation [29].

Rapid sequence intubation denotes the use of a neuromuscular blocking (paralytic) agent combined with a sedative or induction agent to facilitate ETI. The key challenge of RSI is that administered paralytic agents will result in rapid and complete loss of airway reflexes. EMS personnel (including EMS physicians) performing prehospital RSI must possess exceptional ETI skills. The consequence of failed RSI may be a patient who cannot be intubated nor ventilated, with ensuing cardiac arrest from hypoxia.

Agencies performing RSI must use monitors capable of continuous physiological monitoring, including cardiac rhythm, heart rate, blood pressure, pulse oximetry, and waveform capnography. These measures are important to warn of physiological decompensation such as oxygen desaturation and bradycardia. Finally, there must be a plan and appropriate preparation for those times when RSI fails, including a rescue airway.

Many medical directors believe that intensive continuing training is essential for maintaining a prehospital RSI program. Some medical directors require that paramedics perform at least 12 ETIs annually, either on prehospital or in-hospital (ED or OR) patients [30]. Others have integrated human simulator-based training to provide exposure to difficult airway scenarios [31]. The requirement for live ETI training remains controversial, with some proponents citing the value of live airway experience and opponents citing the absence of supporting data [29].

Experts recommend restricting RSI to EMS agencies with the highest standards of clinical airway management practice, including a comprehensive commitment to airway management quality. Colloquially speaking, "RSI is not just about the drugs." As with ETI, medical directors and providers considering RSI must place an emphasis on clinical decision making, not just procedural technique [29].

A modification of RSI is rapid sequence airway (RSA), which replaces ETI with placement of a SGA [32]. RSI is difficult because of the need to rapidly accomplish tracheal intubation after the administration of paralytics. The appeal of RSA is that SGA insertion is simpler and contains fewer pitfalls than ETI. This approach is theoretically safer than traditional RSI. RSA case reports using the Combitube and King LT have demonstrated the feasibility of this approach. In a simulation study, when compared to RSI, Southard demonstrated that RSA reduced time to airway placement and reduced hypoxia episodes [33]. When examined in an air medical system, however, no difference was detected between the two techniques [34]. While other anecdotal reports exist, RSA has not been described in larger scientific series. However, in systems using traditional RSI, RSA may provide an important alternative option in the face of an anticipated or encountered airway management difficulty.

Sedation-assisted intubation is a common approach that uses a sedative agent only, without concurrent neuromuscular blocking agents [29,35–39]. Most medical directors discourage this technique. The anesthesia community has promoted sedation-assisted intubation as being safer than RSI, citing that patients receiving only sedatives may retain adequate native reflexes to preserve airway patency in the event of unsuccessful ETI efforts. However, it is not clear if this principle can be generalized to the prehospital setting. Prehospital EMS personnel often do not possess the laryngoscopy skills of anesthesiologists, and the environments are at opposite ends of the spectrum in terms of optimal control.

Adverse events associated with RSI (e.g. iatrogenic oxygen desaturation and bradycardia) may be at least as likely with sedation-assisted ETI [16,17]. Sedation-assisted intubation with etomidate has been demonstrated to have lower success rates when compared to RSI [40]. While etomidate results in more profound sedation than benzodiazepines, a formal comparison of etomidate with midazolam for prehospital sedation-assisted intubation identified similar ETI success rates [37].

Many EMS systems use other combinations of slow-onset benzodiazepines and opiates to facilitate endotracheal intubation, such as combinations of diazepam, morphine, or other agents. This practice is particularly unsafe since the single or combination use of these agents has a rather slow onset and unpredictable sedative effects, as well as strong potential for causing hypotension. From a medical oversight point of view, the system-level measures necessary to ensure airway management quality with sedation-assisted intubation are essentially equal to those required for RSI programs.

Video laryngoscopy

Video laryngoscopy is increasingly being adopted for use in training and difficult airway scenarios in both the OR and ED [41–44]. Prehospital application of this tool has resulted in improved laryngscopic view, increased intubation success, and decreased time to tracheal intubation [45,46]. However, these devices, while useful, are not a replacement for basic intubation training and skills. In addition, practitioners must be familiar with the skills particular to the device. Complications associated with video laryngoscopy are similar to those for traditional intubation, including multiple intubation attempts and airway perforation [47].

Key considerations for the medical director are the need for specialized training with the video larygoscope and skill maintenance requirements similar to ETI. If video laryngoscopy is employed, the medical director must also decide whether it is used as the primary intubation method, which may erode skills associated with direct laryngoscopy, or if it is used as a rescue technique, which will require greater efforts at skill maintenance given the relative infrequency of use. Cost is also a factor as many of these devices cost several thousands of dollars to acquire and maintain. If the number of airway interventions in the service is low, the medical director may consider applying those resources to training or more frequently used equipment.

Supraglottic airways

Supraglottic airways facilitate ventilation without the use of a conventional endotracheal tube [30]. The medical director's choice to utilize supraglottic devices will vary with service type, provider level, and nature of the jurisdiction.

Supraglottic airways are typically used as rescue devices for failed ETI [48,49]. They are generally easier to insert and have greater success rates than surgical airway techniques, especially in situations potentially involving difficult airway anatomy. National consensus guidelines recommend that all EMS personnel carry at least one type of SGA (e.g. Combitube, King LT, or LMA) for airway management in the event of failed ETI efforts [50]. Medical directors should develop airway management paradigms that include clear indications for failed intubation and an alternative management strategy which may include SGAs.

The 2010 Advanced Cardiac Life Support guidelines emphasize the delivery of uninterrupted chest compressions during CPR [51]. Espousing this principle, a growing number of EMS agencies have elected to substitute ETI with the rapid insertion of an SGA in patients suffering cardiopulmonary arrest [52,53]. Some experts point to the additional benefits of using SGAs as the primary invasive airway device, including the simplicity of operation, the reduced risk of significant adverse events (such as inadvertent airway dislodgment), and the reduced baseline and skills maintenance burdens. Additionally, SGA insertion skills may be more easily translated from mannequin training to clinical application on live patients.

Limited data verify the ability of EMS personnel to place SGAs during cardiac arrest without interrupting compressions and in less time than an endotracheal tube [54]. However, the outcomes related to SGA use in cardiac arrest remain unclear [55,56].

Some EMS agencies have allowed BLS providers to insert SGAs. Previous studies have demonstrated the use of SGAs with a high degree of success [25,57]. One study compared the first-pass success rates during cardiac arrest of BLS providers using SGAs and ALS providers using ETI. First-pass success was five times more likely with the SGA [54]. BLS use of SGAs outside of cardiac arrest has not been studied.

Surgical airways

When developing alternatives for failed laryngoscopy, the medical director should consider the option of surgical airway management. In rare circumstances, when the patient cannot be intubated or ventilated, surgical airway management may be the only viable option. Prehospital surgical airway procedural success is highly variable, ranging from 77% to 93% [58–60]. However, survival after prehospital surgical airway placement is poor, ranging from 15% to 37%. Limited data describe the complications associated with prehospital cricothyrotomy [61–64]. Some medical directors question the role of crico-thyrotomy in the prehospital setting, citing the difficulty of the procedure and the rarity of the intervention with associated need to maintain appropriate clinical skills.

Non-invasive positive pressure ventilation

Non-invasive positive pressure ventilation (NIPPV), including both continuous positive airway pressure (CPAP) and bilevel positive airway pressure (BiPAP), is used to reduce the work of breathing and to improve oxygenation. The clinical indications for prehospital CPAP or BiPAP include patients with acute respiratory distress who possess intact ventilatory drive, protective airway reflexes, and mental status. NIPPV is safe and can be used to treat a variety of respiratory problems even in the face of diagnostic uncertainty. NAEMSP recommends the use of NIPPV for the treatment of acute dyspnea [65]. Although not a replacement for ETI, NIPPV reduces the need for ETI in many patients with acute congestive heart failure, chronic obstructive pulmonary disease, or respiratory failure from other causes [66]. CPAP is feasible for use in BLS systems and may provide an important tool to services where ALS is unavailable or too remote [67]. The medical director should incorporate NIPPV into an airway management scheme with specific indications for use.

Pediatric airway management

Gausche et al.'s study demonstrated no survival or neurological benefit from prehospital pediatric ETI [9]. Given the strength of these data and the relatively low number of pediatric procedures performed by individual prehospital providers, some physicians recommend using BVM ventilation instead of ETI for critically ill children. However, many medical directors have dismissed the generalizability of the Gausche study, citing that the paramedics in that trial did not have adequate experience with pediatric ETI. Consequently, there appears to be variation in prehospital ETI practices nationally.

Pediatric airways have unique features that may pose difficulties for those not accustomed to caring for critically ill children. Since pediatric patients comprise a small proportion of all prehospital ETI, medical directors must weigh the benefits of pediatric ETI against the challenges of providing adequate pediatric airway training and clinical experience.

Some SGAs come in pediatric sizes. Pilot and simulator series describe the viability of SGA use in children [68,69]. There are no large-scale studies of prehospital pediatric SGA use.

Preventing common pitfalls of airway management

Avoidable errors in airway management may include failures of training, preparation, technique, confirmation, or device management. Insufficient training is an inherent problem in EMS given the cost of training, relative infrequency of the procedure, and limited access to live patient training and high-fidelity educational tools [70].

Who should manage the airway?

The degree to which EMS providers participate in airway management is determined by their scope of practice and the discretion of their medical directors. EMS protocols for airway management may vary based on the level of available provider and the system architecture. While all providers should be adept at basic airway management, invasive airway management may be limited to ALS providers. The medical director must choose which providers receive advanced airway training, taking into account the ability to acquire and maintain airway skills, as well as distance to the hospital and the availability of back-up personnel. For instance, some jurisdictions may allow for SGA placement by BLS providers when transport times are long or back-up is remote.

Some systems may employ a tiered response, providing additional providers for airway calls. The additional provider may be a supervisor or a more experienced provider capable of a wider range of airway management techniques. In systems where this type of back-up is readily available, protocols may specify that the providers responding for back-up have additional tools or skills which would be impractical for training or cost-prohibitive if deployed among the entire service. In systems where ETI is a low-frequency event, it may be beneficial to focus education on BLS interventions or supraglottic techniques. Limiting ETI to supervisors or a specific cohort of providers has the benefit of concentrating field experience for the procedure and decreasing the resources necessary for training and competency verification. In some regions it may be possible to train the second-tier providers in advanced adjunctive techniques such as RSI, video laryngoscopy, or use of the bougie. The ideal airway management paradigm for a given service may vary based on the level of provider, available resources, coverage area, and volume of calls requiring airway management.

Provider training and competency

Endotracheal intubation is a complex and difficult procedure that requires substantial training to attain and maintain proficiency. Recent studies highlight the difficulties of providing prehospital providers with adequate ETI training. These observations underscore the importance of medical director involvement in developing and maintaining airway management skills. Provider training requires three components: baseline acquisition of skill, maintenance of skill, and an iterative process of quality assurance used to identify deficits and guide skills maintenance.

Provider competency requires a program of initial training followed by periodic skill verification and continuing education. Training should begin with didactics to review basic airway management. Advanced airway procedures should be introduced by discussing indications and contraindications for airway management, an algorithm for airway management, procedural complications, relevant pharmacology, local protocols, and special considerations.

Psychomotor skills should also be taught and verified using a model or low-fidelity simulator. Skills reviewed should include all those necessary for the airway management algorithm, including BLS airway skills, invasive airways, and surgical airways when applicable. High-fidelity simulators may provide added realism for teaching psychomotor skills and also provide the ability to run scenarios to test decision making and practice the procedures needed to move through the airway management algorithm. High-fidelity simulators can also be used to assess protocol knowledge, teamwork dynamics, and adherence to policies.

Obtaining live intubation training in the OR or other controlled environment is the gold standard of airway training. However, access to ORs is often limited by availability, liability, and cost. The prevalence of non-invasive forms of airway management in the OR combined with an increase in the number of trainees and professionals seeking intubation experience (residents, nurse anesthetists, respiratory therapists, etc.) has reduced the opportunity for prehospital providers to obtain ETI experience in controlled environments. Furthermore, selection bias introduced by the supervising professional may limit the trainee to only less challenging airways [71]. Liability concerns about allowing minimally trained

providers into the OR have further curtailed intubation experiences for EMS providers [72]. The current national standards recommend that paramedic students perform at least five ETIs before graduation [73]. However, one study suggests that paramedic students need at least 20–25 ETIs to attain baseline ETI proficiency [70]. Most successful prehospital airway management programs require EMS personnel to perform at least 12 ETIs annually; these programs have access to ORs to provide supplemental training [62]. Although live training supervised by an expert operator is ideal, experience may also be gained through field intubations during actual calls. Unfortunately, or fortunately depending on one's perspective, field intubation is a relatively rare event, with paramedics in one state indicating that they perform on average only one intubation per year.

Whenever possible, the medical director should seek opportunities for EMS practitioners to obtain live patient intubation experience. Ideally, this would be done in ORs and EDs under close supervision. The medical director should develop relationships with local hospitals to allow for live intubation training. Contracts and memoranda of understanding may help limit medicolegal exposure, define expectations, and improve access to procedures.

Many training programs and EMS agencies use mannequins and human simulators for ETI training [74]. Simulators do not accurately recreate the "feel," range, or variability of live human airway anatomy [18]. However, they are convenient, widely available, flexible, and can be relatively less expensive than other methods of airway training. Low-fidelity human simulators, which often consist of just a mannequin head, are useful for limited psychomotor training. Some medical directors advocate integrating high-fidelity human simulator-based training to recreate complex "difficult airway" situations [31]. The rationale for this additional training is to develop airway management decision making skills, which cannot be fostered in the controlled OR setting. These experts believe that it is essential that paramedics develop good airway management decision-making skills, not just good laryngoscopy skills.

Protocol development and equipment selection

Airway management protocols may include several components including inclusion and exclusion criteria, an airway management algorithm, descriptions of mandatory procedures, benchmarks for quality assurance, and parameters for difficult or failed management. Protocols should clearly delineate inclusion and exclusion criteria based on physiological parameters, which indicate failures of ventilation or oxygenation. These may include vital signs (including respiratory rate, oxygen saturation, end-tidal carbon dioxide), respiratory mechanics (fatigue, accessory muscle use), and mental status (Glasgow Coma Scale). An airway management algorithm

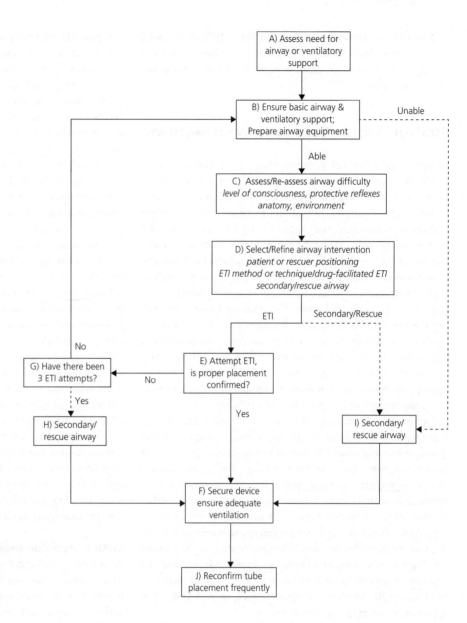

Figure 2.1 Airway management algorithm.

needs to be specific to the equipment and skills available within the system.

One example of an airway management algorithm is shown in Figure 2.1 [75]. Airway management algorithms should begin with providers performing an initial assessment including the ABCs and initiation of BLS airway management. If the personnel are not able to provide ventilation or oxygenation, then they proceed directly to a rescue airway. If they are able to ventilate and oxygenate using BLS skills, then they reassess the patient to determine if invasive airway management will be necessary. If ETI fails, then the provider determines if he can ventilate the patient. Adequately ventilated patients would warrant a second attempt with actions designed to improve intubating conditions (better positioning, different laryngoscope blade, different operator). Those who cannot be ventilated

prompt the need for additional resources and for the airway to be managed with a supraglottic device or surgical airway. Airway attempts should be limited to two per operator or three total, as the probability of success drops dramatically after the second attempt [76]. In some jurisdictions and patient populations (e.g. pediatrics), medical directors advocate for no attempts at ETI given a lack of field experience or low probability of success.

How to proceed through the airway algorithm is often a matter of judgment. Furthermore, providers may have to alter the response to the algorithm based on patient (lack of reserve) or scene (unsafe environment) conditions. Provider judgment can be developed through case review of errors and best practices, as well as practice with high-fidelity simulation [77,78]. Key among these skills is the ability to recognize a difficult airway and preplanning contingencies for a difficult or failed airway. Given the challenges inherent in prehospital airway management, it may be prudent to anticipate all prehospital airways as difficult.

Strategic approaches to airway management

In addition to the airway management algorithm described above, the medical director may employ a variety of tools to reduce risk in airway management. Some systems choose to automatically dispatch a second unit to airway calls, providing additional equipment and operators to facilitate successful airway management. Medical directors may also choose to focus the use of ETI on patients with a high probability of success. Those who fail a single attempt might be transitioned to BLS or SGA management to reduce the risk of secondary injury due to hypoxia or direct airway trauma. Given the equipoise surrounding the use of ETI, the choice to forego ETI entirely may be predicated on the available resources and skill of the provider. A pilot study in rural EMS demonstrated SGA use as the primary means for invasive management [79]. Such an approach may be appropriate based on an analysis of risk and benefit of invasive airway management in a particular EMS system.

Equipment choices are also critical to successful airway management. The medical director should consider devices based on efficacy, reliability, ease of use, and cost. To the extent possible, devices that have been demonstrated to be effective in out-of-hospital studies are preferable. The prehospital environment is austere, and equipment that functions only within limited ranges of environmental conditions may not be desirable. As advanced airway management is a relatively infrequent need in the field, devices should be chosen that are easy to use and for which it is easier to retain proficiency. In general, the equipment chosen for the airway algorithm should include a full range of BLS devices, a method for ETI, an SGA and, when appropriate, a surgical airway technique.

Total quality management

In order to maintain a highly functioning system of airway management, the medical director must develop a system of total quality management (TQM). TQM is an iterative process of training, continuing education, data collection, assessment, and reeducation. This process begins with initial training and skills verification, ensuring that each provider can perform airway management skills for his or her level of training. Providers should then be educated on the application of those skills in simulation and scenario-based education. Skill maintenance should occur at regular intervals for all providers with special attention to providers who have been unsuccessful in field airway management or who have not had the opportunity to manage airways in the field.

If possible, all airway management cases should be reviewed with an emphasis on failed airway, misplaced or dislodged invasive airway devices, number of attempts, and death [80,81]. Continuous physiological data should also be reviewed as abnormalities may draw attention to unrecognized adverse events. Case review requires the reliable abstraction of pertinent data elements as described in NAEMSP position statement on recommended guidelines for uniform reporting of data for out-of-hospital intubation [82]. Review of airway cases should be used to inform directed feedback to the provider, assessment of system processes that may have contributed to the error, and future continuing education so that all providers can learn from the error. Directed provider feedback may include case review, skill reassessment, or additional scenario-based training. In order to encourage self-report of errors and a culture of safety, discipline should be reserved only for careless or reckless behavior that has been refractory to reeducation. System-based assessment should allow the medical director to examine the protocols and procedures asking the question, "Would other providers make the same error in the same situation?" In rare cases, it may be necessary to send an immediate system-wide message out to prevent such an error from recurring. Lastly, in order to prevent a recurrence of the same type of error, incorporation into simulation or scenario-based training will allow others to learn from the event in a safe environment.

Ensuring quality airway management requires the medical director to develop a strategy that is tailored to the skills and resources of the system. The airway program necessitates strategies that are simple to follow, built on a foundation of good initial training, use reliable equipment, and benefit from close scrutiny informing iterative continuing education and training.

Critical decision making

Paramedics are dispatched to a patient with respiratory distress who is noted to have swelling and pain involving the submental tissues, which began within the last 24 hours. He has been suffering from a tooth infection and was recently placed on penicillin and advised to see a dentist for an extraction. The crew arrives to find the man with trismus, drooling, and limited mouth opening. His vital signs are BP 136/84, pulse 110, RR 26, SpO_2 97% on room air. The crew assesses the patient's airway and elects to perform RSI, as they are concerned that he will not be able to protect his airway for the 20-minute transport to the emergency department. The crew prepares medications and paralyze the patient. They are unable to advance a 4 Macintosh blade into the patient's mouth and switch to a 3 Miller. Over three more attempts, they note significant swelling in the airway and have difficulty identifying structures and cannot clearly visualize the vocal cords. They place an endotracheal tube but quickly remove it when it does not return $EtCO_2$. They are forced to abandon the attempts when the patient's oxygen saturation falls to 60% and he becomes bradycardic. They place a SGA and are able to ventilate and to recover the patient's oxygen saturation.

The medical director reviews the case and the crew is reeducated on the following points.

1 Given the patient's ability to protect his own airway, it may have been better to manage the patient conservatively, keeping him upright with humidified oxygen and suction (know when not to intubate).

2 When it is clear that there will be a difficult airway, ask for additional resources including, perhaps, a second unit, supervisor, EMS physician, or critical care team (call for help).

3 Intubation attempts should be discontinued if they are not likely to be successful. The conditions of the intubation (positioning, equipment, or provider) should be changed after a failed attempt.

4 The back-up plan should be discussed prior to the attempt and prepared for implementation.

The crew was sent to rerun this scenario in a high-fidelity simulation to review alternative actions, which could have resulted in a better outcome. The simulation included multiple iterations of the scenario and debriefing to discuss the points noted above. The scenario was then used to build a simulation demonstrating and evaluating decision making for all the paramedics in the service during the following year's education sessions.

References

1 Thomas JB, Abo BN, Wang HE. Paramedic perceptions of challenges in out-of-hospital endotracheal intubation. *Prehosp Emerg Care* 2007;11(2):219–23.

2 Pollock MJ, Brown LH, Dunn KA. The perceived importance of paramedic skills and the emphasis they receive during EMS education programs. *Prehosp Emerg Care* 1997;1(4):263–8.

3 Wang HE, Yealy DM. Out-of-hospital endotracheal intubation: where are we? *Ann Emerg Med* 2006;47(6):532–41.

4 Stewart RD, Paris PM, Winter PM, Pelton GH, Cannon GM. Field endotracheal intubation by paramedical personnel. Success rates and complications. *Chest* 1984;85(3):341–5.

5 Jacobs LM, Berrizbeitia LD, Bennett B, Madigan C. Endotracheal intubation in the prehospital phase of emergency medical care. *JAMA* 1983;250(16):2175–7.

6 Guss DA, Posluszny M. Paramedic orotracheal intubation: a feasibility study. *Am J Emerg Med* 1984;2(5):399–401.

7 DeLeo BC. Endotracheal intubation by rescue squad personnel. *Heart Lung* 1977;6(5):851–4.

8 Carlson JN, Quintero J, Guyette FX, Callaway CW, Menegazzi JJ. Variables associated with successful intubation attempts using video laryngoscopy: a preliminary report in a helicopter emergency medical service. *Prehosp Emerg Care* 2012;16(2):293–8.

9 Gausche M, Lewis RJ, Stratton SJ, et al. Effect of out-of-hospital pediatric endotracheal intubation on survival and neurological outcome: a controlled clinical trial. *JAMA* 2000;283(6):783–90.

10 Davis DP, Hoyt DB, Ochs M, et al. The effect of paramedic rapid sequence intubation on outcome in patients with severe traumatic brain injury. *J Trauma* 2003;54(3):444–53.

11 Wang HE, Peitzman AB, Cassidy LD, Adelson PD, Yealy DM. Out-of-hospital endotracheal intubation and outcome after traumatic brain injury. *Ann Emerg Med* 2004;44(5):439–50.

12 Katz SH, Falk JL. Misplaced endotracheal tubes by paramedics in an urban emergency medical services system. *Ann Emerg Med* 2001;37(1):32–7.

13 Jemmett ME, Kendal KM, Fourre MW, Burton JH. Unrecognized misplacement of endotracheal tubes in a mixed urban to rural emergency medical services setting. *Acad Emerg Med* 2003;10(9):961–5.

14 Jones JH, Murphy MP, Dickson RL, Somerville GG, Brizendine EJ. Emergency physician-verified out-of-hospital intubation: miss rates by paramedics. *Acad Emerg Med* 2004;11(6):707–9.

15 Wang HE, Kupas DF, Paris PM, Bates RR, Yealy DM. Preliminary experience with a prospective, multi-centered evaluation of out-of-hospital endotracheal intubation. *Resuscitation* 2003;58(1):49–58.

16 Dunford JV, Davis DP, Ochs M, Doney M, Hoyt DB. Incidence of transient hypoxia and pulse rate reactivity during paramedic rapid sequence intubation. *Ann Emerg Med* 2003;42(6):721–8.

17 Davis DP, Dunford JV, Poste JC, et al. The impact of hypoxia and hyperventilation on outcome after paramedic rapid sequence intubation of severely head-injured patients. *J Trauma* 2004;57(1):1–8; discussion 8–10.

18 Aufderheide TP, Lurie KG. Death by hyperventilation: a common and life-threatening problem during cardiopulmonary resuscitation. *Crit Care Med* 2004;32(9 Suppl):S345–51.

19 Aufderheide TP, Sigurdsson G, Pirrallo RG, et al. Hyperventilation-induced hypotension during cardiopulmonary resuscitation. *Circulation* 2004;109(16):1960–5.

20 Abo BN, Hostler D, Wang HE. Does the type of out-of-hospital airway interfere with other cardiopulmonary resuscitation tasks? *Resuscitation* 2007;72(2):234–9.

21 United States Department of Transportation National Standard Curricula. 2007. Available at: www.nhtsa.gov/people/injury/ems/pub/emtbnsc.pdf

22 Bradley JS, Billows GL, Olinger ML, Boha SP, Cordell WH, Nelson DR. Prehospital oral endotracheal intubation by rural basic emergency medical technicians. *Ann Emerg Med* 1998;32(1):26–32.

23 Sayre MR, Sakles JC, Mistler AF, Evans JL, Kramer AT, Pancioli AM. Field trial of endotracheal intubation by basic EMTs. *Ann Emerg Med* 1998;31(2):228–33.

24 Ochs M, Vilke GM, Chan TC, Moats T, Buchanan J. Successful prehospital airway management by EMT-Ds using the combitube. *Prehosp Emerg Care* 2000;4(4):333–7.

25 Lefrancois DP, Dufour DG. Use of the esophageal tracheal combitube by basic emergency medical technicians. *Resuscitation* 2002; 52(1):77–83.

26 Cady CE, Pirrallo RG. The effect of Combitube use on paramedic experience in endotracheal intubation. *Am J Emerg Med* 2005;23(7):868–71.

27 Wang HE, Yealy DM. How many attempts are required to accomplish out-of-hospital endotracheal intubation? *Acad Emerg Med* 2006;13(4):372–7.

28 Mort TC. The incidence and risk factors for cardiac arrest during emergency tracheal intubation: a justification for incorporating the ASA Guidelines in the remote location. *J Clin Anesth* 2004;16(7):508–16.

29 Wang HE, Davis DP, O'Connor RE, Domeier RM. Drug-assisted intubation in the prehospital setting (resource document to NAEMSP position statement). *Prehosp Emerg Care* 2006;10(2):261–71.

30 Wayne MA, Friedland E. Prehospital use of succinylcholine: a 20-year review. *Prehosp Emerg Care* 1999;3(2):107–9.

31 Davis DP, Buono C, Ford J, Paulson L, Koenig W, Carrison D. The effectiveness of a novel, algorithm-based difficult airway curriculum for air medical crews using human patient simulators. *Prehosp Emerg Care* 2007;11(1):72–9.

32 Braude D, Richards M. Rapid Sequence Airway (RSA) – a novel approach to prehospital airway management. *Prehosp Emerg Care* 2007;11(2):250–2.

33 Southard A, Braude D, Crandall C. Rapid sequence airway vs rapid sequence intubation in a simulated trauma airway by flight crew. *Resuscitation* 2010;81(5):576–8.

34 Frascone RJ, Russi C, Lick C, et al. Comparison of prehospital insertion success rates and time to insertion between standard endotracheal intubation and a supraglottic airway. *Resuscitation* 2011;82(12):1529–36.

35 Wang HE, O'Connor RE, Megargel RE, et al. The utilization of midazolam as a pharmacologic adjunct to endotracheal intubation by paramedics. *Prehosp Emerg Care* 2000;4(1):14–18.

36 Dickinson ET, Cohen JE, Mechem CC. The effectiveness of midazolam as a single pharmacologic agent to facilitate endotracheal intubation by paramedics. *Prehosp Emerg Care* 1999;3(3):191–3.

37 Jacoby J, Heller M, Nicholas J, et al. Etomidate versus midazolam for out-of-hospital intubation: a prospective, randomized trial. *Ann Emerg Med* 2006;47(6):525–30.

38 Bozeman WP, Kleiner DM, Huggett V. A comparison of rapid-sequence intubation and etomidate-only intubation in the prehospital air medical setting. *Prehosp Emerg Care* 2006;10(1):8–13.

39 Bozeman WP, Young S. Etomidate as a sole agent for endotracheal intubation in the prehospital air medical setting. *Air Med J* 2002;21(4):32–5.

40 Kociszewski C, Thomas SH, Harrison T, Wedel SK. Etomidate versus succinylcholine for intubation in an air medical setting. *Am J Emerg Med* 2000;18(7):757–63.

41 Cooper RM. Use of a new videolaryngoscope (GlideScope) in the management of a difficult airway. *Can J Anaesth* 2003;50(6):611–13.

42 Greenland KB, Brown AF. Evolving role of video laryngoscopy for airway management in the emergency department. *Emerg Med Australas* 2011;23(5):521–4.

43 Raja AS, Sullivan AF, Pallin DJ, Bohan JS, Camargo CA Jr. Adoption of Video Laryngoscopy in Massachusetts Emergency Departments. *J Emerg Med* 2012;42(2):233–7.

44 Sakles JC, Mosier JM, Chiu S, Keim SM. Tracheal Intubation in the Emergency Department: A Comparison of GlideScope((R)) Video Laryngoscopy to Direct Laryngoscopy in 822 Intubations. *J Emerg Med* 2012;42(4):400–5.

45 Wayne MA, McDonnell M. Comparison of traditional versus video laryngoscopy in out-of-hospital tracheal intubation. *Prehosp Emerg Care* 2010;14(2):278–82.

46 Guyette FX, Farrell K, Carlson JN, Callaway CW, Phrampus P. Comparison of video laryngoscopy and direct laryngoscopy in a critical care transport service. *Prehosp Emerg Care* 2013;17(2):149–54.

47 Cooper RM. Complications associated with the use of the GlideScope videolaryngoscope. *Can J Anaesth* 2007;54(1):54–7.

48 Guyette FX, Wang H, Cole JS. King airway use by air medical providers. *Prehosp Emerg Care* 2007;11(4):473–6.

49 Schalk R, Byhahn C, Fausel F, et al. Out-of-hospital airway management by paramedics and emergency physicians using laryngeal tubes. *Resuscitation* 2010;81(3):323–6.

50 Guyette FX, Greenwood MJ, Neubecker D, Roth R, Wang HE. Alternate airways in the prehospital setting (resource document to NAEMSP position statement). *Prehosp Emerg Care* 2007;11(1):56–61.

51 Committees on Emergency Cardiac Care. 2005 American Heart Association Guidelines for Cardiopulmonary Resuscitation and Emergency Cardiovascular Care. Part 1: Introduction. *Circulation* 2005;112(24_suppl):IV-1–5.

52 Fales W, Farrell R. Impact of New Resuscitation Guidelines on Out-of-hospital Cardiac Arrest Survival. *Acad Emerg Med* 2007; 14(5):S157–8.

53 Wang HE, Mann NC, Mears G, Jacobson K, Yealy DM. Out-of-hospital airway management in the United States. *Resuscitation* 2011;82(4):378–85.

54 Gahan K, Studnek JR, Vandeventer S. King LT-D use by urban basic life support first responders as the primary airway device for out-of-hospital cardiac arrest. *Resuscitation* 2011;82(12):1525–8.

55 Wang HE, Szydlo D, Stouffer JA, et al. Endotracheal intubation versus supraglottic airway insertion in out-of-hospital cardiac arrest. *Resuscitation* 2012;83(9):1061–6.

56 Kajino K, Iwami T, Kitamura T, et al. Comparison of supraglottic airway versus endotracheal intubation for the pre-hospital treatment of out-of-hospital cardiac arrest. *Crit Care* 2011;15(5):R236.

57 Shin SD, Ahn KO, Song KJ, Park CB, Lee EJ. Out-of-hospital airway management and cardiac arrest outcomes: a propensity score matched analysis. *Resuscitation* 2012;83(3):313–19.

58 Hubble MW, Wilfong DA, Brown LH, Hertelendy A, Benner RW. A meta-analysis of prehospital airway control techniques part II: alternative airway devices and cricothyrotomy success rates. *Prehosp Emerg Care* 2010;14(4):515–30.

59 Spaite DW, Joseph M. Prehospital cricothyrotomy: an investigation of indications, technique, complications, and patient outcome. *Ann Emerg Med* 1990;19(3):279–85.

60 Robinson KJ, Katz R, Jacobs LM. A 12-year experience with prehospital cricothyrotomies. *Air Med J* 2001;20(6):27–30.

61 Leibovici D, Fredman B, Gofrit ON, Shemer J, Blumenfeld A, Shapira SC. Prehospital cricothyroidotomy by physicians. *Am J Emerg Med* 1997;15(1):91–3.

62 Boyle MF, Hatton D, Sheets C. Surgical cricothyrotomy performed by air ambulance flight nurses: a 5–year experience. *J Emerg Med* 1993;11(1):41–5.

63 Gerich TG, Schmidt U, Hubrich V, Lobenhoffer HP, Tscherne H. Prehospital airway management in the acutely injured patient: the role of surgical cricothyrotomy revisited. *J Trauma* 1998;45(2):312–14.

64 Xeropotamos NS, Coats TJ, Wilson AW. Prehospital surgical airway management: 1 year's experience from the Helicopter Emergency Medical Service. *Injury* 1993;24(4):222–4.

65 Daily JC, Wang HE. Noninvasive positive pressure ventilation: resource document for the National Association of EMS Physicians position statement. *Prehosp Emerg Care* 2011;15(3):432–8.

66 Thompson J, Petrie DA, Ackroyd-Stolarz S, Bardua DJ. Out-of-hospital continuous positive airway pressure ventilation versus usual care in acute respiratory failure: a randomized controlled trial. *Ann Emerg Med* 2008;52(3):232–41.

67 Cheskes S, Thomson S, Turner L. Feasibility of continuous positive airway pressure by primary care paramedics. *Prehosp Emerg Care* 2012;16(4):535–40.

68 Ritter SC, Guyette FX. Prehospital pediatric King LT-D use: a pilot study. *Prehosp Emerg Care* 2011;15(3):401–4.

69 Mitchell MS, Lee White M, King WD, Wang HE. Paramedic King Laryngeal Tube airway insertion versus endotracheal intubation in simulated pediatric respiratory arrest. *Prehosp Emerg Care* 2012;16(2):284–8.

70 Wang HE, Kupas DF, Hostler D, Cooney R, Yealy DM, Lave JR. Procedural experience with out-of-hospital endotracheal intubation. *Crit Care Med* 2005;33(8):1718–21.

71 Warner KJ, Sharar SR, Copass MK, Bulger EM. Prehospital management of the difficult airway: a prospective cohort study. *J Emerg Med* 2009;36(3):257–65.

72 Johnston BD, Seitz SR, Wang HE. Limited opportunities for paramedic student endotracheal intubation training in the operating room. *Acad Emerg Med* 2006;13(10):1051–5.

73 National Highway Traffic Safety Administration. Emergency Medical Technician Paramedic: National Standard Curriculum (EMT-P). 1998. Available at: www.nhtsa.dot.gov/people/injury/ems/EMT-P.

74 Hall RE, Plant JR, Bands CJ, Wall AR, Kang J, Hall CA. Human patient simulation is effective for teaching paramedic students endotracheal intubation. *Acad Emerg Med* 2005;12(9):850–5.

75 Wang HE, Kupas DF, Greenwood MJ, et al. An algorithmic approach to prehospital airway management. *Prehosp Emerg Care* 2005;9(2):145–55.

76 Wang HE, O'Connor RE, Schnyder ME, Barnes TA, Megargel RE. Patient status and time to intubation in the assessment of prehospital intubation performance. *Prehosp Emerg Care* 2001;5(1):10–18.

77 Steadman RH, Coates WC, Huang YM, et al. Simulation-based training is superior to problem-based learning for the acquisition of critical assessment and management skills. *Crit Care Med* 2006;34(1):151–7.

78 Barsuk D, Ziv A, Lin G, et al. Using advanced simulation for recognition and correction of gaps in airway and breathing management skills in prehospital trauma care. *Anesth Analg* 2005;100(3):803–9.

79 Russi CS, Hartley MJ, Buresh CT. A pilot study of the King LT supralaryngeal airway use in a rural Iowa EMS system. *Int J Emerg Med* 2008;1(2):135–8.

80 Wang HE, Abella BS, Callaway CW. Risk of cardiopulmonary arrest after acute respiratory compromise in hospitalized patients. *Resuscitation* 2008;79(2):234–40.

81 Wang HE, Simeone SJ, Weaver MD, Callaway CW. Interruptions in cardiopulmonary resuscitation from paramedic endotracheal intubation. *Ann Emerg Med* 2009;54(5):645–52.

82 Wang HE, Domeier RM, Kupas DF, Greenwood MJ, O'Connor RE. Recommended guidelines for uniform reporting of data from out-of-hospital airway management: position statement of the National Association of EMS Physicians. *Prehosp Emerg Care* 2004;8(1):58–72.

CHAPTER 3
Airway procedures

Jestin N. Carlson and Henry E. Wang

Introduction

Airway management is one of the most essential interventions in the prehospital care of the critically ill or injured. This chapter provides an overview of the techniques and current controversies surrounding prehospital airway management.

Basic airway interventions

Basic airway interventions include measures to provide supplemental oxygen and/or ventilation without the use of an advanced airway device. These techniques are practiced by all prehospital providers, including first responders, EMTs, paramedics, and EMS physicians.

Oxygen cannulas and face masks

In spontaneously breathing patients, prehospital EMS personnel may deliver supplemental oxygen using nasal cannulas or oxygen masks. The nasal cannula provides low-flow (2–5 L/min) oxygen in inhaled fractions (FiO_2) from 21% to 40%. Oxygen masks used in the prehospital setting include simple face masks (6–10 L/min oxygen delivery, 40–60% FiO_2) and non-rebreather masks (10–15 L/min oxygen delivery, close to 100% FiO_2).

Oxygen cannulas and masks are designed for patients with spontaneous respiratory drive and intact protective airway reflexes. Patients with frank respiratory compromise or apnea should receive bag-valve-mask ventilation support or advanced airway management. The standard teaching for EMS personnel is to provide oxygen to all patients with actual or potential for hypoxia. In practice, it is best to base supplemental oxygen protocols and practices on clinical findings. While some EMS agencies use pulse oximetry to titrate oxygen therapy for specific oxygen saturation deficits, this approach may shift EMS personnel focus to oxygen saturation readings, rather than the patient's physical findings. Many patients with acute respiratory compromise present with increased respiratory rates (over 40–50 breaths/minute), not necessarily hypoventilation, hypoxia, or apnea.

Bag-valve-mask ventilation

Bag-valve-mask (BVM) ventilation is the primary method for providing active ventilatory support without the use of an advanced airway device (Figure 3.1). The key BVM device components include a self-inflating bag, oxygen reservoir, and conforming face mask. The primary indications for BVM ventilation include hypoventilation (inadequate respiratory drive or effort) or frank apnea.

The technique of BVM ventilation is difficult, requiring rescuers to open the airway and maintain a mask seal with one hand while squeezing the ventilation bag with the other hand. Seasoned providers often recommend performing BVM using a two-person technique, with one rescuer opening the airway and holding the mask with both hands, and the other squeezing the bag [1]. Two-handed BVM techniques provide greater tidal volumes than one-handed techniques [2]. Several studies have demonstrated the difficulty of performing effective BVM ventilation, particularly in a moving ambulance or during prolonged resuscitation efforts; this is one of the motivations for the use of advanced airway in many prehospital patients [3].

An important potential adverse effect associated with BVM ventilation is gastric insufflation, which may result in regurgitation and aspiration of gastric contents into the airway. Many anesthesiologists use Sellick's maneuver (cricoid pressure) to minimize gastric insufflation during operating room BVM ventilation [4–7]. While probably not harmful, this technique has not been proven to be helpful in the prehospital setting.

Demand valve ventilation

The demand valve is an oxygen-powered resuscitator that delivers high-flow oxygen through a mask via a trigger valve. The valve is actuated by a single finger, allowing the rescuer to use both hands to seal the mask and open the airway. The

Emergency Medical Services: Clinical Practice and Systems Oversight, Second Edition. Volume 1: Clinical Aspects of EMS.
Edited by David C. Cone, Jane H. Brice, Theodore R. Delbridge, and J. Brent Myers.
© 2015 NAEMSP. Published 2015 by John Wiley & Sons, Inc. Companion Website: www.wiley.com\go\cone\naemsp

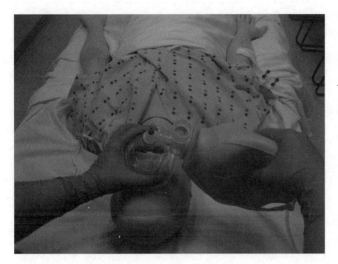

Figure 3.1 Bag-valve-mask (BVM) ventilation.

major limitation of this device is the inability to sense lung compliance, which may be important in the presence of barotrauma or pneumothorax. Formal comparisons to BVM ventilation or other ventilatory devices remain limited [8,9]. Although once popular, fewer agencies appear to be using these devices.

Oropharyngeal and nasopharyngeal airways

Oropharyngeal and nasopharyngeal airways are important adjuncts for basic airway support. The oropharyngeal airway is a curved plastic device that is inserted into the oropharynx, maintaining airway patency by lifting the tongue forward from the posterior wall of the pharynx. The nasopharyngeal airway is a soft plastic tube that is inserted through the nose, similarly facilitating airway patency. EMS personnel should use one of the adjuncts during BVM ventilation. Many clinicians report the simultaneous use of both devices in selected patients. While either adjunct may be suitable with a non-rebreather mask for a spontaneously breathing patient, insertion of the oropharyngeal airway should be reserved for patients without a gag reflex.

Advanced airway management

Advanced airway management involves the insertion of an airway tube into the oropharynx and hypopharynx to facilitate oxygen delivery and ventilatory support. Advanced airway management is indicated in hypoventilating or apneic patients or individuals with actual or potential airway compromise. Current options for prehospital airway management include endotracheal intubation (ETI), supraglottic airways (SGA), and surgical airways. While advanced providers typically perform these techniques, ETI was an optional module in the prior national emergency medical technician curriculum; it is not listed as an emergency medical technician (EMT) or AEMT skill in the current National EMS Education Standards. In some areas EMTs may use SGAs [10,11]. SGAs are not included at the EMT level, but are included at the AEMT level, in the National EMS Education Standards.

Endotracheal or tracheal intubation

Endotracheal intubation is the most widely recognized method of advanced airway management. Paramedics have performed ETI in the United States for over 30 years [12–15]. ETI has many theoretical advantages, including the isolation of the airway from secretions or gastric contents and the provision of a direct conduit to the trachea without separate airway opening maneuvers.

Orotracheal intubation

Direct orotracheal intubation is the most common method of ETI (Figure 3.2). In this approach the rescuer uses a lighted laryngoscope to displace the patient's tongue and expose the epiglottis and vocal cords, permitting direct insertion of the endotracheal tube into the trachea.

The most common laryngoscope blades used for orotracheal intubation include Macintosh (curved) and Miller (straight) blades, which require slight variations in laryngoscopic technique [16]. The rescuer places the curved Macintosh blade into the vallecula (the space immediately anterior to the epiglottis), facilitating indirect lifting of the epiglottis and exposure of the vocal cord structures. In contrast, the rescuer uses the broad side of the straight Miller blade to displace the oropharyngeal structures, using the tip of the blade to directly lift the epiglottis. Blade selection is a matter of personal preference; there are no data indicating the superiority of either blade in prehospital ETI.

Orotracheal intubation optimally requires the absence or near-absence of protective airway reflexes. It is extremely difficult in patients who are awake or have intact airway reflexes. In these situations, drug-facilitated intubation techniques are often necessary to facilitate access to the oropharynx.

In scenarios with potential cervical spine fracture or injury, EMS personnel must perform orotracheal intubation with "manual in-line stabilization" of the cervical spine, without hyperextension of the head or neck during laryngoscopy (Figure 3.3). This approach requires a second rescuer to manually hold the cervical spine "in line" during laryngoscopy attempts. Laryngoscopy and exposure of the vocal cord structures are relatively difficult while maintaining cervical spine stabilization. A critical review questions the value of manual in-line stabilization, suggesting that it significantly impairs laryngoscopy while not affording adequate spinal cord protection [17]. However, video laryngoscopy may provide adequate visualization of the glottis while minimizing cervical spine movement during ETI [18].

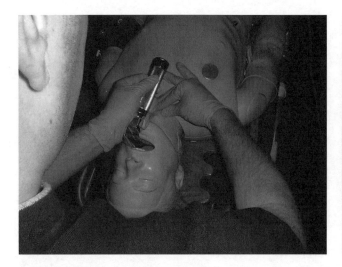

Figure 3.2 Orotracheal intubation.

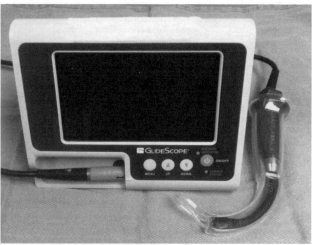

Figure 3.4 GlideScope video laryngoscope.

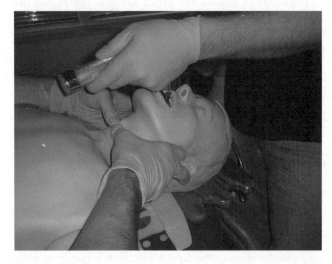

Figure 3.3 Manual in-line stabilization for intubation of the patient with suspected cervical spine injury.

Video laryngoscopy

Video laryngoscopy uses a camera attached to the distal end of the blade of the laryngscope to obtain images of the anatomy that are then displayed on a video screen. Newer generation video laryngoscopes include portable and disposable configurations that may be used in the prehospital setting. While video laryngoscopy has demonstrated equal or improved ETI success rates when compared to traditional laryngoscopy in nearly all clinical settings, its cost is higher than conventional laryngoscopy [19–21]. Some studies suggest that proficiency with video laryngoscopy may be obtained in as few as five ETIs [22]. Some video laryngoscopes also allow providers to record their ETI

efforts for offline review for quality improvement or educational initiatives [23].

Endotracheal intubation technique using video laryngoscopy depends upon the brand and model used. Although several different video laryngoscopes are available, the GlideScope® (Verathon, Bothell, WA) and C-MAC® (Karl Storz Corp., Tuttlingen, Germany) currently appear to be the most widely used. While some manufacturers provide standard Macintosh curved blades that allow for conventional direct laryngoscopy, such as the C-MAC, other manufacturers provide a hyper-curved blade, including the GlideScope (Figure 3.4). With the latter device, visualization of the vocal cords can only occur through the video screen; direct visualization of the vocal cords is not possible. In addition, because the pathway from the mouth to the vocal cords is no longer a straight line, the endotracheal tube and stylet must be bent with a slightly deeper curve. The GlideScope requires a specialized stylet for this application.

Nasotracheal intubation

Nasotracheal intubation involves insertion of an endotracheal tube through the nose and into the trachea. It is possible only in patients with intact respiratory efforts, for example, individuals with congestive heart failure or acute pulmonary edema. The approach may be possible for patients who cannot lay supine, for example, patients entrapped after a motor vehicle collision. In contrast with orotracheal methods, nasotracheal intubation is often possible in awake patients, and those with intact gag reflexes or trismus.

Successful nasotracheal intubation requires a skilled and experienced operator. The rescuer chooses an endotracheal tube one-half size smaller than customary for orotracheal intubation, inserting the tube into the nares without a stylet and directing the endotracheal tube inferiorly and anteriorly towards the vocal cords. Experts recommend first entering the right nostril, which is often larger than the left. The rescuer coordinates insertion of the tube through the vocal cords with patient inhalation.

The Endotrol® (Mallinckrodt, Inc., Hazelwood, MO) endotracheal tube has a special trigger device that flexes the tip of the tube, facilitating its direction toward the larynx as the tube is advanced [24]. A sometimes helpful adjunct is the Beck Airway Airflow Monitor (BAAM®, Great Plains Ballistics, Lubbock, TX). When placed on the connector end of the endotracheal tube, the device "whistles" as the tube approaches the vocal cords.

Important complications associated with nasotracheal intubation include nasal trauma and epistaxis, sinusitis (which may cause sepsis), and perforation of the cribiform plate with subsequent intracranial placement [25–29].

Other intubation techniques

Digital intubation is one of the original methods of endotracheal intubation [30]. In this technique, the rescuer places his/her second and third fingers into the patient's pharynx, forming a cradle extending to the epiglottis and the vocal cords. The rescuer then uses the other hand to guide an endotracheal tube along the cradle and through the vocal cords. Some clinicians recommend twisting the endotracheal tube into a corkscrew shape to facilitate the technique (Figure 3.5). Digital intubation may be viable in unresponsive patients where EMS personnel have limited access to the airway. The technique could result in rescuer injury should the patient bite down during the procedure [31]. Some clinicians advocate the concurrent use of a dental prod or mouth gag during digital intubation efforts.

The *lighted stylet* is a semi-rigid stylet equipped with a battery-powered lighted tip [31]. The rescuer inserts the stylet through the endotracheal tube and bends the combination into a "hockey stick" shape. The rescuer then inserts the stylet/endotracheal tube combination blindly into the oropharynx and uses the light to facilitate movement of the tube through the vocal cords. When properly placed, the bulb of the lighted stylet is visible through the patient's cricoid membrane. Few EMS agencies use lighted stylet intubation due to the cost of the device and difficulty of the technique. Further, the procedure is limited by the need for low ambient lighting.

In *retrograde intubation*, the rescuer places a large-bore needle through the cricothyroid membrane, pointing it cephalad, and then inserts a guidewire through the needle, advancing it superiorly until the wire tip comes out through the mouth. A conventional endotracheal tube can then be threaded over the guidewire and through the vocal cords. It is important that the wire be threaded through the "Murphy's eye" of the tube. Commercial kits exist for retrograde intubation. Only limited data support this technique in the prehospital environment [32].

The *gum elastic bougie,* an adjunct for orotracheal intubation, is essentially a semi-rigid stylet (Figure 3.6). The rescuer performs

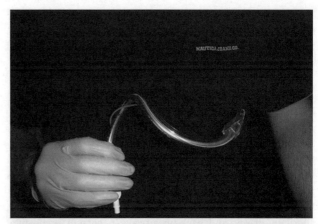

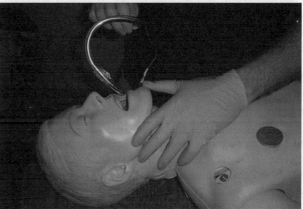

Figure 3.5 Corkscrew of endotracheal tube for digital intubation.

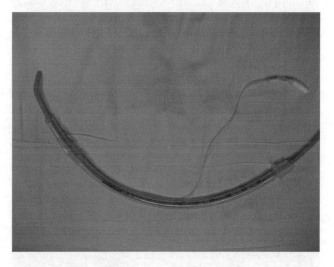

Figure 3.6 Gum elastic bougie.

conventional orotracheal laryngoscopy, placing the bougie through the vocal cords and into the trachea. Because the bougie is smaller and stiffer than an endotracheal tube, it is usually easier to place through the vocal cords. The angled, "hockey stick" tip also provides tactile feedback from the tracheal rings, assuring that the device is in the correct endotracheal position.

The rescuer can slide a conventional endotracheal tube over the bougie and through the vocal cords before removing the bougie. Limited data describe the use of the bougie in the prehospital setting but generally describe improved ETI success [33,34].

Supraglottic airways

Supraglottic airways are advanced airway devices used to facilitate ventilation without the use of conventional endotracheal tubes [35]. Other terms commonly used to describe SGAs include extraglottic airway, rescue airway, secondary airway, failed airway device, difficult airway device, salvage airway, alternate airway, and back-up airway. In current prehospital practice, EMS personnel typically reserve SGAs use for situations with failed ETI efforts, but recent reports suggest a potential primary role for SGAs [36].

The most common SGAs in current North American prehospital use are the esophageal tracheal Combitube™ (ETC), the King laryngotracheal (King LT™) airway, and the laryngeal mask airway (LMA™). When EMS personnel have inserted a SGA, instead of ETI, they should provide advance notification to the receiving ED. The SGA may require exchange to an endotracheal tube or surgical airway, and the receiving ED may need additional time to prepare or to assemble an appropriate team.

Esophageal tracheal Combitube

The ETC is a double-lumen tube with a distal and a proximal balloon [37] (Figure 3.7). The rescuer inserts the ETC blindly into the patient's mouth, typically positioning the smaller distal balloon in the esophagus and the larger proximal balloon in the oropharynx. If the distal part of the ETC is correctly positioned in the esophagus (the most common position), insufflation through the longer, blue-colored lumen will deliver oxygen indirectly to the trachea through holes in the blue-colored tube at the level of the vocal cords. If the distal part of the ETC is positioned in the trachea, insufflation through the shorter, white-colored tube will deliver oxygen directly to the trachea. Auscultation or visualization of chest rise may not correctly discriminate between esophageal and endotracheal placement of the airway. End-tidal carbon dioxide detection is recommended to help identify the correct port for insufflation.

Multiple studies have verified the adequacy of ventilation and feasibility of ETC insertion in the prehospital setting [37,38]. The ETC currently comes in two sizes, including a standard size (for patients >5'6") as well as a smaller (Combitube SA™) size for shorter individuals (<5'6"). The smaller SA size often works satisfactorily in taller patients. Pediatric ETC sizes do not exist. Complications attributed to ETC include oropharyngeal bleeding, esophageal perforation, and aspiration pneumonitis, among others [39]. Some agencies have trained EMTs to insert ETCs [10,11,40].

King laryngotracheal airway

The King LT is a SGA that resembles an ETC but consists of a single-lumen tube (Figure 3.8). A single insufflation port simultaneously inflates two balloon cuffs. Shorter and smaller than an ETC, the King LT design is supposed to facilitate more consistent placement in the esophagus. Insertion of the King LT airway is very similar to the Combitube. After balloon cuff inflation, the rescuer may need to withdraw the tube slightly to seal the balloon against the oropharyngeal structures.

Disposable versions of the device exist for prehospital application. There is also a version with an esophageal port permitting concurrent placement of an orogastric tube. In addition to three different adult sizes, pediatric sizes of the King LT are also available. Given the simplicity of its design, the King LT can be rapidly placed by providers with a range of skills in a variety of clinical settings [41].

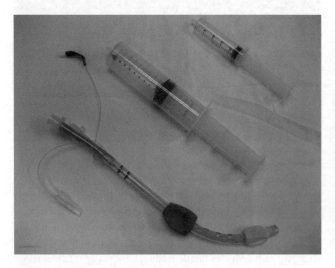

Figure 3.7 Esophageal tracheal Combitube.

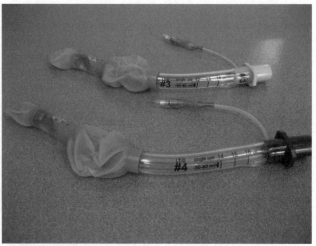

Figure 3.8 King LT airway.

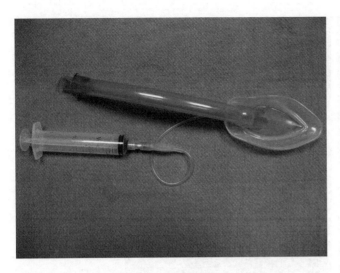

Figure 3.9 Laryngeal mask airway.

Laryngeal mask airway

The LMA is a SGA originally designed for use in the operating room [42] (Figure 3.9). The distal tip of the airway contains a spade-shaped balloon designed to seal around the vocal cord structures. The rescuer inserts the device blindly through the oropharynx, positioning the cuff around the laryngeal structures. Inflation of the cuff facilitates proper sealing of the device.

Limited studies describe LMA use by prehospital EMS personnel [43]. Prehospital use in the United States remains relatively limited, possibly due to concerns about the device's inability to prevent aspiration as well as its potential for inadvertent dislodgment. A variation is the LMA Fastrach, or Intubating LMA, which is designed to allow passage of an endotracheal tube. Disposable versions of both the LMA as well as the LMA Fastrach currently exist. Some EMS agencies favor the LMA due to the availability of pediatric sizes.

Other supraglottic airways

Supraglottic airways no longer used in contemporary prehospital EMS practice include the esophageal obturator airway, esophageal gastric tube airway, and pharyngotracheal lumen airway. Other SGAs currently available include the cuffed oropharyngeal airway (COPA), and the Cobra perilaryngeal airway™ (Engineered Medical Systems, Indianapolis, IN), among others. Some prehospital systems have reported success with the I-gel™, which resembles a solid LMA without an inflatable perilaryngeal cuff. Only limited data describe these techniques in the prehospital setting.

Surgical airways

Surgical airways involve the placement of the airway directly into the trachea through an incision in the neck. The primary prehospital surgical airway methods include cricothyroidotomy

and transtracheal jet ventilation (TTJV). EMS personnel typically use surgical airways in the event of failed endotracheal intubation efforts or where significant facial trauma precludes conventional intubation techniques.

Cricothyroidotomy

Cricothyroidotomy involves exposure and incision of the cricothyroid membrane (directly inferior to the thyroid cartilage) and direct insertion of a tracheostomy or endotracheal tube into the trachea (Figure 3.10). In the classic "open technique," the rescuer identifies the thyroid cartilage, uses a scalpel to place a longitudinal midline incision, then transversely incises the cricothyroid membrane, placing a tracheostomy tube or 6.0 endotracheal tube through the opening and into the trachea. Some providers prefer a transverse incision, although this approach may heighten the risk of inadvertent thyroid vessel laceration.

An alternative approach uses commercially packaged Seldinger-type devices. For example, the Pertrach™ kit consists of a needle, wire, dilator, and cannula. The rescuer makes a small skin incision and inserts a needle/dilator combination through the cricothyroid membrane, subsequently using the dilator to spread the tissues. The rescuer can then feed the tracheal tube over the guidewire and into the trachea.

Limited data describe the complications associated with prehospital cricothyroidotomy [44–47]. Medical directors question the role of cricothyroidotomy in the prehospital setting, citing the difficulty of the procedure and the rarity of the intervention with associated need to maintain appropriate clinical skills.

Transtracheal jet ventilation

Transtracheal jet ventilation, occasionally referred to as "needle cricothyroidotomy," involves the insufflation of high-pressure oxygen via a large-bore intravenous type catheter (16-gauge or larger) inserted through the cricothyroid membrane. This technique requires 50 psi oxygen equipment capable of delivering oxygen at >50 L/min through a catheter. This is equivalent to "wall" oxygen pressure. TTJV cannot successfully be performed using conventional BVM equipment or a standard 25 L/min flow meter.

While TTJV has many theoretical limitations, the clinical implications remain unclear. For example, because TTJV primarily facilitates oxygenation, most clinicians assume that the technique can only be used for short periods of time. However, extensive data underscore the utility of the technique for prolonged periods [48,49]. A 16 gauge catheter with a flow rate >50 L/min and a ventilatory rate of 20 breaths/min can deliver a tidal volume of 950 mL [50,51]. Aspiration is also a concern, but only limited data clinically quantify this phenomenon [52]. EMS personnel may also use a properly placed jet ventilation catheter to help convert to an open cricothyroidotomy.

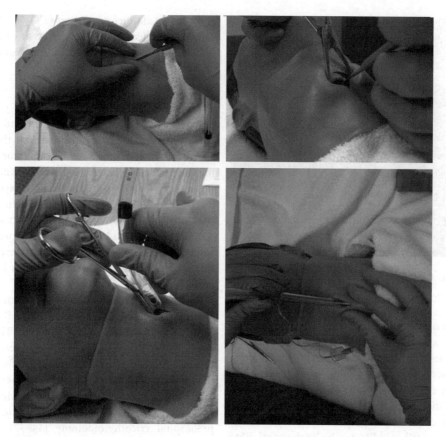

Figure 3.10 Cricothyroidotomy.

Confirmation of airway placement

After ETI, verification of endotracheal tube placement is essential [53]. Tube placement verification is particularly important given the uncontrolled nature of the prehospital environment and the risks of unrecognized tube dislodgment or misplacement [54–57]. Because of the amount of patient movement in prehospital care, EMS personnel must frequently (and preferably continuously) verify correct tube positioning. In addition to visualizing the endotracheal tube passing through the vocal cords into the trachea, endotracheal tube placement should be confirmed using multiple techniques.

Auscultation is the most common method for verifying endotracheal tube placement. In this technique the rescuer auscultates both lung fields to verify the presence of breath sounds, and also auscultates the epigastrium to verify the absence of gastric sounds.

Several adjunct devices are available for verifying correct endotracheal placement of the endotracheal tube. The *esophageal intubation detector (EID)* consists of a Toomey syringe with a special adaptor for the endotracheal tube. The rescuer attaches the EID to the end of the endotracheal tube and quickly withdraws the plunger. Easy plunger withdrawal suggests correct endotracheal tube placement. Conversely, plunger resistance suggests esophageal tube placement. The *esophageal detector device (EDD)* is a large, bulb-type device (Figure 3.11). The rescuer squeezes the bulb before attaching it to the endotracheal tube. Complete bulb inflation suggests correct endotracheal tube placement. Incomplete bulb reinflation suggests esophageal placement. Both of these devices are based on the concept that the esophagus will collapse, producing resistance to the vacuum, while the trachea will not collapse and will therefore not produce any resistance as the bulb or plunger produces suction.

The most important technique for verifying endotracheal tube placement is the detection of exhaled (or end-tidal) carbon dioxide. Patients exhale carbon dioxide through the bronchotracheal tree; the presence of carbon dioxide in the endotracheal tube indicates correct endotracheal tube placement. There are currently three types of devices used for detecting exhaled (or end-tidal) carbon dioxide: colorimetric end-tidal carbon dioxide detector, digital capnometer, and waveform end-tidal capnographer.

The *colorimetric end-tidal carbon dioxide detector* uses a chemically treated paper detector that changes color from purple to yellow when exposed to carbon dioxide (Figure 3.12).

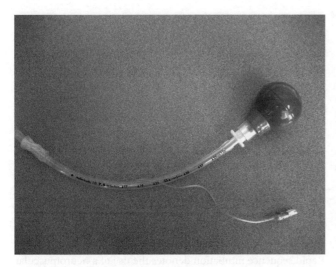

Figure 3.11 Esophageal detector device.

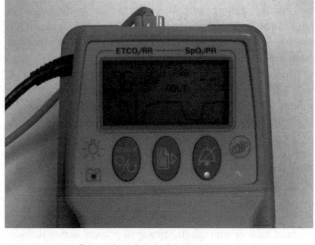

Figure 3.13 Waveform carbon dioxide detector.

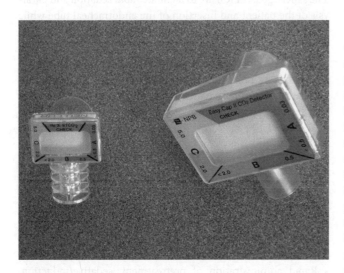

Figure 3.12 Colorimetric carbon dioxide detector.

If the paper color remains purple, this suggests esophageal tube placement. Designed for single use, these devices can be used for only a limited duration (<2 hours). Exposure to liquid (for example, vomitus or blood) renders these devices non-functional.

Digital end-tidal carbon dioxide capnometry samples exhaled gases, measuring and displaying carbon dioxide level. A positive carbon dioxide level connotes correct endotracheal tube placement.

Waveform end-tidal capnography is similar to digital capnometry, except that the exhaled carbon dioxide level is depicted continuously in graphical form (Figure 3.13). The "waveform" on the display makes it easier to observe changes in the exhaled carbon dioxide level. This also enables measurement of ventilation rate.

There are two primary designs for capnometers and capnographers: sidestream and mainstream [58]. Sidestream capnographers draw a sample of the exhaled gases from a port attached to the endotracheal tube. In mainstream capnography, the sensor is placed in the gas delivery line near the endotracheal tube. In general, with sidestream devices there is a short (<1 second) delay between gas sampling and delivery of a carbon dioxide level reading. In contrast, in-line devices provide instant carbon dioxide readings. The sensor for an in-line device is placed near the endotracheal tube. Some practitioners find this positioning awkward with the potential for tube dislodgment. However, the sensors for newer in-line devices are light and compact. Sidestream devices may be more prone to condensation. EMS personnel may use sidestream devices with a nasal cannula in spontaneously breathing patients, broadening their potential application.

Medical directors and EMS agencies should select a particular design based upon individual considerations. Waveform end-tidal capnography is the most accurate tube placement verification technique. However, waveform capnographers are expensive (over $3,000 per unit). However, most newer multiparameter monitors can be purchased with built-in capnography. In addition, in situations with low perfusion (e.g. cardiopulmonary arrest), there may be inadequate circulation of carbon dioxide to the lungs. In these situations, carbon dioxide detectors may incorrectly indicate a misplaced endotracheal tube. Some systems have made waveform capnography mandatory for all intubated patients.

An essential consideration is that prehospital patients undergo considerable movement during field care, which may heighten the risk for tube dislodgment. Many medical directors have emphasized the need for frequent reverification or continuous monitoring of endotracheal tube placement, especially after each patient movement sequence; for example, after moving the patient onto the stretcher or loading into an ambulance. Only capnometers and capnographers are currently capable of providing continuous tube placement information. EMS personnel using other confirmation techniques will need to pause and reconfirm tube placement frequently during care.

While some clinicians rely upon fogging of the endotracheal tube to indicate its correct placement, a well-executed animal study demonstrated the inaccuracy of this technique [59].

Methods for securing the endotracheal tube and supraglottic airways

Emergency medical services personnel must secure the endotracheal tube or supraglottic airway to prevent device dislodgment. The most common method for securing the tube is the use of adhesive tape wrapped around the neck and the tube (Lillehei method) [60]. Another method uses umbilical twill tape, which is a flat, woven cloth tape designed for tying off umbilical cords after childbirth. Some EMS personnel use intravenous or oxygen tubing to tie the endotracheal tube in place. A variety of commercial tube holders also exists, typically consisting of a plastic bite-block strapped to the patient's face using Velcro tape, and a plastic strap or screw clamp to hold the endotracheal tube in place.

Because of the theoretical risk of tube dislodgment with flexion-extension or lateral rotation of the head, some EMS providers also place the intubated patient on a spinal immobilization board and apply a cervical immobilization device to the patient's head.

Current advanced cardiovascular life support (ACLS) guidelines recommend the use of commercial tube holders. However, one cadaver study found that conventional adhesive taping of the endotracheal tube surpassed most commercial tube holders [60]. The one exception was the Thomas Tube Holder™ (Laerdal Medical, Inc., Stavanger, Norway) which performed better than taping. Only limited prehospital clinical data describe the effectiveness of endotracheal tube securing methods at preventing tube dislodgment [61]. There are also no data describing the effectiveness of spinal or cervical immobilization devices at preventing tube dislodgment.

Some EMS personnel manually hold the endotracheal tube in place without using tape or other tube securement methods. We do not recommend this method as anecdotal reports have associated this technique with inadvertent tube dislodgment.

EMS personnel should also secure alternative airway devices such as the Combitube, King LT airway, and LMA. The manufacturers recommend conventional taping methods for securing these airways. We have anecdotally observed that some commercial tube holders are not designed for supraglottic airways (which have wider outer diameters than endotracheal tubes) and do not adequately hold these devices in place.

Drug-facilitated intubation

Drug-facilitated intubation (DFI) is the use of intravenous sedative and/or neuromuscular blocking agents to facilitate ETI of patients with intact protective airway reflexes [62]. The most common forms of DFI include rapid sequence intubation (RSI, also termed neuromuscular blockade-assisted intubation) and sedation-assisted intubation. Most medical directors regard drug-facilitated intubation as an advanced technique that should be reserved for only the most qualified practitioners. The National Association of EMS Physicians has published national consensus standards for drug-facilitated intubation [62].

Rapid sequence intubation
Rapid sequence intubation denotes the use of a neuromuscular blocking (paralytic) agent combined with a sedative or induction agent to facilitate ETI of a patient with intact protective reflexes. The salient goals of RSI are to facilitate rapid sedation and paralysis of the patient and insertion of the endotracheal tube while effecting minimum physiological disturbances (heart rate, blood pressure, intracerebral pressure, etc.). Current prehospital RSI practices closely parallel ED practices. The general clinical indications for prehospital RSI include the need for airway and ventilatory control in patients with intact protective airway reflexes; for example, victims of traumatic brain injury.

RSI technique
The main elements of prehospital rapid sequence intubation include the following.
- Insertion of an intravenous line
- Attachment of continuous monitors (electrocardiogram, blood pressure, and pulse oximetry)
- Preoxygenation of the patient (non-rebreather mask or BVM ventilation)
- Rapid administration of pretreatment, sedative/induction, and neuromuscular blocking agents
- Performance of laryngoscopy and tube placement
- Verification of tube placement and securing of the endotracheal tube

Agents used for RSI
Pretreatment agents may be administered prior to attempting RSI; for example, intravenous lidocaine to attenuate the intracerebral pressure response to laryngoscopy. Because there are only limited data supporting the effectiveness of pretreatment regimens, protocols often exclude the use of these agents during prehospital RSI.

A wide range of sedative/induction and neuromuscular blocking agents exists. The most popular sedative/induction agent for RSI is etomidate. Most clinicians favor this agent because of its minimal effect upon blood pressure, heart rate, and intracerebral pressure. The typical induction dose for etomidate is 0.3 mg/kg intravenously (20 mg in a typical 70 kg patient). Recent studies raise concern regarding the clinical consequences of adrenosuppression resulting from etomidate administration [63,64]. Limited data describe the link between etomidate's adrenocortical suppression and patient outcomes [64].

Another commonly used agent for sedation/induction is midazolam administered at a dose of 0.1 mg/kg. However, because midazolam and other benzodiazepines may cause clinically significant hypotension, and because many prehospital patients requiring RSI have significant hemodynamic compromise, many EMS physicians prefer not to use these agents for prehospital RSI.

The neuromuscular blocking agent most commonly used for RSI is succinylcholine, typically administered at a dose of 1.0–2.0 mg/kg intravenously (70–140 mg in a typical 70 kg patient). Succinylcholine's rapid onset and short duration are ideal for RSI. The rationale for using a rapid-acting paralytic is to achieve intubating conditions as quickly as possible. The rationale for using a short-acting paralytic is to facilitate rapid recovery of the patient's spontaneous airway reflexes in the event of unsuccessful laryngoscopy and intubation efforts. Relative contraindications to succinylcholine include conditions with known hyperkalemia, such as acute renal failure or rhabdomyolysis. Succinylcholine-induced hyperkalemia in these settings may cause cardiopulmonary arrest. While burn injuries can cause hyperkalemia, this complication usually does not occur until 2–3 days after the acute injury. Succinylcholine can be safely used for the acute management of burn victims. Other relative contraindications to succinylcholine include muscular wasting diseases (which can cause hyperkalemia) and pseudocholinesterase deficiency (where succinylcholine may cause prolonged neuromuscular blockade).

While other neuromuscular blocking agents such as vecuronium and rocuronium are available, these agents have longer durations of action, making them less favorable for the prehospital setting.

After completion of the RSI procedure, it is essential to administer additional pharmacological agents to maintain sedation and paralysis. Therefore, EMS practitioners performing RSI should also carry longer-acting paralytics (for example, vecuronium or pancuronium), as well as longer-acting sedative agents (for example, lorazepam, midazolam, or diazepam).

Pediatric RSI

Pediatric practices for RSI often vary slightly from adult protocols. The pediatric literature raises concern regarding the possibility of unrecognized muscular myopathies, which would result in hyperkalemia with administration of succinylcholine [65]. Therefore, many specialty pediatric transport teams use non-depolarizing agents instead to facilitate paralysis. The use of etomidate for children remains unresolved. Prehospital RSI protocols appear to vary between the use of etomidate and midazolam for sedation. Because of paradoxical bradycardia with RSI agents in children, many practitioners pretreat these patients with intravenous atropine.

Additional RSI considerations

The administered paralytic agents will result in rapid and complete ablation of intact airway reflexes. Therefore, EMS personnel performing prehospital RSI must possess exceptional ETI skills. State-of-the-art practice requires utilization of waveform end-tidal capnography to immediately verify and continuously monitor correct endotracheal tube placement. Finally, SGAs should be readily available in the event of failed RSI efforts.

Sedation-assisted endotracheal intubation

Sedation-assisted intubation is a common approach using a sedative agent only without concurrent neuromuscular blocking agents [62,66–70]. Practitioners typically use benzodiazepines such as midazolam or diazepam for this technique. Recently, some agencies have used etomidate to facilitate intubation [68,69]. Sedation-assisted intubation is common due to the wide availability of benzodiazepines for other prehospital applications; for example, treatment of seizures or agitation. Furthermore, anesthesiologists in inhospital settings commonly use sedation-only regimens when facilitating airway management.

Sedation-assisted ETI technique

Except for the omission of a neuromuscular blocking agent, the clinical procedures for sedation-assisted intubation are similar to RSI. A typical regimen involves uses intravenous midazolam 0.1 mg/kg (7 mg in a 70 kg patient). While clinicians commonly use midazolam doses on the order of 2 mg for a 70 kg patient, anecdotal experience indicates the inadequacy of this low dose. While midazolam has rapid onset and short duration, it may cause clinically significant hypotension, potentially harming critically ill prehospital patients.

Etomidate 0.3 mg/kg IV (approximately 20 mg for a typical 70 kg patient) is another alternative for sedation-assisted intubation. Etomidate has extremely rapid onset (5–10 seconds) and short duration (5–10 minutes). Some clinicians believe that etomidate is a safer option compared with benzodiazepines given its more profound sedative effect as well as its lower propensity for causing hypotension. However, adverse events associated with single-dose etomidate include myoclonus (muscle spasms, specifically in the jaw) and adrenocortical suppression. The former development may theoretically impede airway management efforts should the patient develop trismus.

Other drug-facilitated techniques

Some practitioners parallel anesthesia practice by using *topical anesthetic sprays* (benzocaine, etc.) to facilitate ETI. Limited data support this technique in the prehospital setting [71].

Non-invasive positive pressure ventilation

Prehospital providers are more commonly using non-invasive ventilatory support, or non-invasive positive pressure ventilation (NIPPV), as an alternative to ETI or SGAs. This includes continuous positive airway pressure (CPAP) and bilevel positive airway pressure (BiPAP) [72–77]. These systems deliver high-pressure oxygen through a specially designed, tight-sealing face mask. CPAP provides continuous positive pressure throughout inspiration and exhalation phases. BiPAP separately controls inspiratory pressure support and positive end-expiratory pressure. Both modalities reduce work of breathing and improve physiological response through a variety of mechanisms, including increase of intrathoracic pressure, reduction of left ventricular afterload, and increase of functional residual capacity. Contrary to popular belief, NIPPV does not "blow fluids out of the lungs." Both CPAP and BiPAP have been used extensively in hospital settings to treat patients with respiratory failure, including congestive heart failure and pulmonary edema, among others.

Portable systems permit prehospital application of NIPPV. These systems typically use a separate oxygen delivery control unit coupled with a standard oxygen cylinder. The control unit requires a significant capital investment (of the order of $1,000, not including mask and tubing). A notable prehospital innovation is the Boussignac CPAP device, which uses turbulent oxygen flow to create a virtual CPAP valve [75]. The Boussignac system is simple, single use, and costs less than $75 per use, and does not require a separate control unit. Some prehospital ventilators used by air medical and critical care transport units can be configured to provide CPAP. The range of applicable CPAP pressure varies with each device.

The clinical indications for prehospital NIPPV include patients with acute respiratory distress who possess intact ventilatory drives, protective airway reflexes, and adequate mental status. In other situations, endotracheal intubation may prove more appropriate. While more common applications of NIPPV are for congestive heart failure or pulmonary edema, some clinicians have reported success with other conditions such as pneumonia or asthma.

Emergency medical services personnel may initially set CPAP to 7 cmH$_2$O pressure support, titrating to clinical effect. BiPAP systems permit independently set inspiratory and expiratory airway pressures. Common initial settings include inspiratory pressure at 10 cmH$_2$O and expiratory pressure at 5 cmH$_2$O, with titration to clinical effect. EMS personnel should provide concurrent pharmacological therapies with NIPPV; for example, nitrates, furosemide, morphine, beta-agonists, etc. EMS personnel may gauge the response to NIPPV through subjective assessment of work of breathing, respiratory rate, heart rate, and oxygen saturation. End-tidal capnography may provide another measure to gauge clinical response.

Communication with the receiving ED is essential when NIPPV is used. Hospital systems are often not interchangeable with prehospital systems so receiving EDs may require time to mobilize the appropriate equipment for an incoming patient. A prehospital NIPPV patient may deteriorate en route to the hospital; the receiving ED may require time to assemble the needed airway resources.

Considerable scientific data support the utility and effectiveness of NIPPV in the hospital. Multiple studies have documented the ability of NIPPV to decrease intubation rates, shorten hospital length of stays, and improve survival when used in the prehospital setting [73–76,78].

Conclusion

Airway management is one of the most important elements of prehospital emergency care. Prehospital airway management involves numerous clinical, educational and system-level complexities. EMS physicians and medical directors must be familiar with the many issues related to prehospital airway care.

References

1 Davidovic L, LaCovey D, Pitetti RD. Comparison of 1- versus 2-person bag-valve-mask techniques for manikin ventilation of infants and children. *Ann Emerg Med* 2005;46(1):37–42.

2 Otten D, Liao MM, Wolken R, et al. Comparison of bag-valve-mask hand-sealing techniques in a simulated model. *Ann Emerg Med* 2013.

3 Kurola J, Harve H, Kettunen T, et al. Airway management in cardiac arrest – comparison of the laryngeal tube, tracheal intubation and bag-valve mask ventilation in emergency medical training. *Resuscitation* 2004;61(2):149–53.

4 Salem MR, Wong AY, Mani M, Sellick BA. Efficacy of cricoid pressure in preventing gastric inflation during bag-mask ventilation in pediatric patients. *Anesthesiology* 1974;40(1):96–8.

5 Moynihan RJ, Brock-Utne JG, Archer JH, Feld LH, Kreitzman TR. The effect of cricoid pressure on preventing gastric insufflation in infants and children. *Anesthesiology* 1993;78(4):652–6.

6 Petito SP, Russell WJ. The prevention of gastric inflation – a neglected benefit of cricoid pressure. *Anaesth Intensive Care* 1988; 16(2):139–43.

7 Fanning GL. The efficacy of cricoid pressure in preventing regurgitation of gastric contents. *Anesthesiology* 1970;32(6):553–5.

8 Updike G, Mosesso VN Jr, Auble TE, Delgado E. Comparison of bag-valve-mask, manually triggered ventilator, and automated ventilator devices used while ventilating a nonintubated mannikin model. *Prehosp Emerg Care* 1998;2(1):52–5.

9 Menegazzi JJ, Winslow HJ. In-vitro comparison of bag-valve-mask and the manually triggered oxygen-powered breathing device. *Acad Emerg Med* 1994;1(1):29–33.

10 Ochs M, Vilke GM, Chan TC, Moats T, Buchanan J. Successful prehospital airway management by EMT-Ds using the combitube. *Prehosp Emerg Care* 2000;4(4):333–7.

11 Lefrancois DP, Dufour DG. Use of the esophageal tracheal combitube by basic emergency medical technicians. *Resuscitation* 2002; 52(1):77–83.

12 Stewart RD, Paris PM, Winter PM, Pelton GH, Cannon GM. Field endotracheal intubation by paramedical personnel. Success rates and complications. *Chest* 1984;85(3):341–5.

13 Jacobs LM, Berrizbeitia LD, Bennett B, Madigan C. Endotracheal intubation in the prehospital phase of emergency medical care. *JAMA* 1983;250(16):2175–7.

14 Guss DA, Posluszny M. Paramedic orotracheal intubation: a feasibility study. *Am J Emerg Med* 1984;2(5):399–401.

15 DeLeo BC. Endotracheal intubation by rescue squad personnel. *Heart Lung* 1977;6(5):851–4.

16 Levitan RM. *The Airway Cam Guide to Intubation and Practical Emergency Airway Management.* Salt Lake City, UT: Airway Cam Technologies, 2004.

17 Manoach S, Paladino L. Manual in-line stabilization for acute airway management of suspected cervical spine injury: historical review and current questions. *Ann Emerg Med* 2007;50(3):236–45.

18 Turkstra TP, Craen RA, Pelz DM, Gelb AW. Cervical spine motion: a fluoroscopic comparison during intubation with lighted stylet, GlideScope, and Macintosh laryngoscope. *Anesth Analg* 2005; 101(3):910–15.

19 Wayne MA, McDonnell M. Comparison of traditional versus video laryngoscopy in out-of-hospital tracheal intubation. *Prehosp Emerg Care* 2010;14(2):278–82.

20 Kim YM, Kim JH, Kang HG, Chung HS, Yim HW, Jeong SH. Tracheal intubation using Macintosh and 2 video laryngoscopes with and without chest compressions. *Am J Emerg Med* 2011; 29(6):682–6.

21 Guyette FX, Farrell K, Carlson JN, Callaway CW, Phrampus P. Comparison of video laryngoscopy and direct laryngoscopy in a critical care transport service. *Prehosp Emerg Care* 2012;17(2): 149–54.

22 Bradbury CL, Hillermann C, Mendonca C, Danha R. Analysis of the learning curve with the C-MAC video laryngoscope: a manikin study. *J Anesthe Clin Res* 2011;2(10):167.

23 Carlson JN, Quintero J, Guyette FX, Callaway CW, Menegazzi JJ. Variables associated with successful intubation attempts using video laryngoscopy: a preliminary report in a helicopter emergency medical service. *Prehosp Emerg Care* 2012;16(2):293–8.

24 O'Connor RE, Megargel RE, Schnyder ME, Madden JF, Bitner M, Ross R. Paramedic success rate for blind nasotracheal intubation is improved with the use of an endotracheal tube with directional tip control. *Ann Emerg Med* 2000;36(4):328–32.

25 Holdgaard HO, Pedersen J, Schurizek BA, Melsen NC, Juhl B. Complications and late sequelae following nasotracheal intubation. *Acta Anaesthesiol Scand* 1993;37(5):475–80.

26 Rhee KJ, Muntz CB, Donald PJ, Yamada JM. Does nasotracheal intubation increase complications in patients with skull base fractures? *Ann Emerg Med* 1993;22(7):1145–7.

27 Tintinalli JE, Claffey J. Complications of nasotracheal intubation. *Ann Emerg Med* 1981;10(3):142–4.

28 Aebert H, Hunefeld G, Regel G. Paranasal sinusitis and sepsis in ICU patients with nasotracheal intubation. *Intensive Care Med* 1988;15(1):27–30.

29 Dinner M, Tjeuw M, Artusio JF Jr. Bacteremia as a complication of nasotracheal intubation. *Anesth Analg* 1987;66(5):460–2.

30 Mahajan R, Kumar S, Kumar Batra Y. Digital assistance of nasotracheal intubation – another way to prevent trauma during nasotracheal intubation. *Paediatr Anaesth* 2007;17(7):703.

31 Davis L, Cook-Sather SD, Schreiner MS. Lighted stylet tracheal intubation: a review. *Anesth Analg* 2000;90(3):745–56.

32 Van Stralen DW, Rogers M, Perkin RM, Fea S. Retrograde intubation training using a mannequin. *Am J Emerg Med* 1995;13(1): 50–2.

33 Jabre P, Combes X, Leroux B, et al. Use of gum elastic bougie for prehospital difficult intubation. *Am J Emerg Med* 2005;23(4):552–5.

34 Combes X, Jabre P, Margenet A, et al. Unanticipated difficult airway management in the prehospital emergency setting: prospective validation of an algorithm. *Anesthesiology* 2011;114(1): 105–10.

35 Guyette FX, Greenwood MJ, Neubecker D, Roth R, Wang HE. Alternate airways in the prehospital setting (resource document to NAEMSP position statement). *Prehosp Emerg Care* 2007;11(1): 56–61.

36 Fales W, Farrell R. Impact of new resuscitation guidelines on out-of-hospital cardiac arrest survival. *Acad Emerg Med* 2007;14 (5Supplement 1):S157–8.

37 Agro F, Frass M, Benumof JL, Krafft P. Current status of the Combitube: a review of the literature. *J Clin Anesth* 2002;14(4): 307–14.

38 Davis DP, Valentine C, Ochs M, Vilke GM, Hoyt DB. The Combitube as a salvage airway device for paramedic rapid sequence intubation. *Ann Emerg Med* 2003;42(5):697–704.

39 Vezina MC, Trepanier CA, Nicole PC, Lessard MR. Complications associated with the Esophageal-Tracheal Combitube in the prehospital setting. *Can J Anaesth* 2007;54(2):124–8.

40 Cady CE, Pirrallo RG. The effect of Combitube use on paramedic experience in endotracheal intubation. *Am J Emerg Med* 2005; 23(7):868–71.

41 Guyette FX, Wang H, Cole JS. King airway use by air medical providers. *Prehosp Emerg Care* 2007;11(4):473–6.

42 Pollack CV Jr. The laryngeal mask airway: a comprehensive review for the Emergency Physician. *J Emerg Med* 2001;20(1):53–66.

43 Murray MJ, Vermeulen MJ, Morrison LJ, Waite T. Evaluation of prehospital insertion of the laryngeal mask airway by primary care paramedics with only classroom mannequin training. *CJEM* 2002; 4(5):338–43.

44 Leibovici D, Fredman B, Gofrit ON, Shemer J, Blumenfeld A, Shapira SC. Prehospital cricothyroidotomy by physicians. *Am J Emerg Med* 1997;15(1):91–3.

45 Boyle MF, Hatton D, Sheets C. Surgical cricothyrotomy performed by air ambulance flight nurses: a 5-year experience. *J Emerg Med* 1993;11(1):41–5.

46 Gerich TG, Schmidt U, Hubrich V, Lobenhoffer HP, Tscherne H. Prehospital airway management in the acutely injured patient: the role of surgical cricothyrotomy revisited. *J Trauma* 1998;45(2):312–14.

47 Xeropotamos NS, Coats TJ, Wilson AW. Prehospital surgical airway management: 1 year's experience from the Helicopter Emergency Medical Service. *Injury* 1993;24(4):222–4.

48 Spoerel WE, Narayanan PS, Singh NP. Transtracheal ventilation. *Br J Anaesth* 1971;43(10):932–9.

49 Jacobs HB, Smyth NP, Witorsch P. Transtracheal catheter ventilation: clinical experience in 36 patients. *Chest* 1974;65(1):36–40.

50 Yealy DM, Stewart RD, Kaplan RM. Myths and pitfalls in emergency translaryngeal ventilation: correcting misimpressions. *Ann Emerg Med* 1988;17(7):690–2.

51 Yealy DM, Stewart RD, Kaplan RM. Clarifications on translaryngeal ventilation. *Ann Emerg Med* 1988;17(10):1130.

52 Yealy DM, Plewa MC, Reed JJ, Kaplan RM, Ilkhanipour K, Stewart RD. Manual translaryngeal jet ventilation and the risk of aspiration in a canine model. *Ann Emerg Med* 1990;19(11):1238–41.

53 O'Connor RE, Swor RA. Verification of endotracheal tube placement following intubation. National Association of EMS Physicians Standards and Clinical Practice Committee. *Prehosp Emerg Care* 1999;3(3):248–50.

54 Katz SH, Falk JL. Misplaced endotracheal tubes by paramedics in an urban emergency medical services system. *Ann Emerg Med* 2001;37(1):32–7.

55 Jemmett ME, Kendal KM, Fourre MW, Burton JH. Unrecognized misplacement of endotracheal tubes in a mixed urban to rural emergency medical services setting. *Acad Emerg Med* 2003;10(9): 961–5.

56 Wang HE, Kupas DF, Paris PM, Bates RR, Yealy DM. Preliminary experience with a prospective, multi-centered evaluation of out-of-hospital endotracheal intubation. *Resuscitation* 2003;58(1):49–58.

57 Jones JH, Murphy MP, Dickson RL, Somerville GG, Brizendine EJ. Emergency physician-verified out-of-hospital intubation: miss rates by paramedics. *Acad Emerg Med* 2004;11(6):707–9.

58 Jaffe MB. Mainstream or Sidestream Capnography? 2002. Available at: http://oem.respironics.com/Downloads/Main%20vs%20Side.pdf

59 Kelly JJ, Eynon CA, Kaplan JL, de Garavilla L, Dalsey WC. Use of tube condensation as an indicator of endotracheal tube placement. *Ann Emerg Med* 1998;31(5):575–8.

60 Carlson J, Mayrose J, Krause R, Jehle D. Extubation force: tape versus endotracheal tube holders. *Ann Emerg Med* 2007;50(6): 686–91.

61 Kaufmann KF, Kupas DF, Wang HE. Do different tube securing methods affect endotracheal tube dislodgement in a prehospital setting? (abstract). *Prehosp Emerg Care* 2007;11:104.

62 Wang HE, Davis DP, O'Connor RE, Domeier RM. Drug-assisted intubation in the prehospital setting (resource document to NAEMSP position statement). *Prehosp Emerg Care* 2006;10(2):261–71.

63 Zed PJ, Mabasa VH, Slavik RS, Abu-Laban RB. Etomidate for rapid sequence intubation in the emergency department: is adrenal suppression a concern? *CJEM* 2006;8(5):347–50.

64 Jackson WL Jr. Should we use etomidate as an induction agent for endotracheal intubation in patients with septic shock?: a critical appraisal. *Chest* 2005;127(3):1031–8.

65 Sullivan M, Thompson WK, Hill GD. Succinylcholine-induced cardiac arrest in children with undiagnosed myopathy. *Can J Anaesth* 1994;41(6):497–501.

66 Wang HE, O'Connor RE, Megargel RE, et al. The utilization of midazolam as a pharmacologic adjunct to endotracheal intubation by paramedics. *Prehosp Emerg Care* 2000;4(1):14–18.

67 Dickinson ET, Cohen JE, Mechem CC. The effectiveness of midazolam as a single pharmacologic agent to facilitate endotracheal intubation by paramedics. *Prehosp Emerg Care* 1999;3(3):191–3.

68 Jacoby J, Heller M, Nicholas J, et al. Etomidate versus midazolam for out-of-hospital intubation: a prospective, randomized trial. *Ann Emerg Med* 2006;47(6):525–30.

69 Bozeman WP, Kleiner DM, Huggett V. A comparison of rapid-sequence intubation and etomidate-only intubation in the prehospital air medical setting. *Prehosp Emerg Care* 2006;10(1):8–13.

70 Bozeman WP, Young S. Etomidate as a sole agent for endotracheal intubation in the prehospital air medical setting. *Air Med J* 2002;21(4):32–5.

71 Kenny JF, Molloy K, Pollack M, Ortiz MT. Nebulized lidocaine as an adjunct to endotracheal intubation in the prehospital setting. *Prehosp Disaster Med* 1996;11(4):312–13.

72 Caples SM, Gay PC. Noninvasive positive pressure ventilation in the intensive care unit: a concise review. *Crit Care Med* 2005; 33(11):2651–8.

73 Hubble MW, Richards ME, Jarvis R, Millikan T, Young D. Effectiveness of prehospital continuous positive airway pressure in the management of acute pulmonary edema. *Prehosp Emerg Care* 2006;10(4):430–9.

74 Kosowsky JM, Stephanides SL, Branson RD, Sayre MR. Prehospital use of continuous positive airway pressure (CPAP) for presumed pulmonary edema: a preliminary case series. *Prehosp Emerg Care* 2001;5(2):190–6.

75 Templier F, Dolveck F, Baer M, Chauvin M, Fletcher D. 'Boussignac' continuous positive airway pressure system: practical use in a prehospital medical care unit. *Eur J Emerg Med* 2003;10(2):87–93.

76 Kallio T, Kuisma M, Alaspaa A, Rosenberg PH. The use of prehospital continuous positive airway pressure treatment in presumed acute severe pulmonary edema. *Prehosp Emerg Care* 2003;7(2):209–13.

77 Collins SP, Mielniczuk LM, Whittingham HA, Boseley ME, Schramm DR, Storrow AB. The use of noninvasive ventilation in emergency department patients with acute cardiogenic pulmonary edema: a systematic review. *Ann Emerg Med* 2006;48(3):260–9.

78 Wong DT, Tam AD, van Zundert TC. The usage of the Boussignac continuous positive airway pressure system in acute respiratory failure. *Minerva Anestesiol* 2013;79(5):564–70.

CHAPTER 4

Airway management: special situations

Brendan Anzalone and Henry E. Wang

Introduction

The prehospital environment presents unique challenges or barriers to patient care. Airway management in these situations may be difficult or impossible. For example, airway management may need to be carried out with the patient on the floor or upright while entrapped in a vehicle. This chapter describes considerations and strategies for airway management in special prehospital situations.

Ground-level airway management

The classic position for intubation has the patient supine at the level of the rescuer's xiphoid. However, prehospital patients requiring airway management are often found in unusual positions, such as on the ground. Conventional approaches to laryngoscopy and intubation must be modified in these scenarios.

There are several approaches to rescuer positioning for ground-level endotracheal intubation (ETI).

- **Prone**. The rescuer lies prone on the ground in line with the patient's head (Figure 4.1). The rescuer places both elbows on the ground. With this approach, laryngoscopy requires lifting at the wrist rather than with the forearm. Placement of the tracheal tube must be accomplished using movements of the wrist.
- **Left lateral decubitus position.** With this approach, the rescuer lays on his or her left side, perpendicular to the head of the patient (Figure 4.2). As with the prone position, the rescuer stabilizes the left elbow on the ground, relying upon wrist movement to perform laryngoscopy. However, the right arm is free to facilitate tube placement in a conventional fashion.

- **Kneeling**. The rescuer kneels at the patient's head. The left elbow and forearm may be supported by the rescuer's knee. In this position, the rescuer assumes a slightly more vertical position over the patient's head, and thus the angle for glottis visualization may be steeper than usual (Figure 4.3).
- **Sitting**. The rescuer sits at the patient's head with legs either crossed or extended to each side of the patient's head. The left arm may be braced against the rescuer's leg (if sitting with crossed legs) (Figure 4.4).
- **Straddling the patient**. The rescuer straddles the patient in a face-to-face position. The rescuer holds and inserts the laryngoscope with the right hand, and passes the tube with the left hand (Figure 4.5).

Because prehospital patients are frequently found and treated at ground level, rescuers should learn each of these techniques. Note that compared with traditional positioning, the rescuer's face is closer to the patient's oropharynx with ground-level intubation, and thus visualization of glottic structures may differ from conventional approaches. Pinchalk et al. describe a technique involving tilting the patient upwards (using the stretcher back or a backboard) to afford improved visualization of and access to the airway [1].

Limited studies suggest that the left lateral decubitus (LLD) positioning may result in higher intubation success rates than the other ground-level techniques. Adnet et al. compared the LLD intubating position versus kneeling with the patient (mannequin) supine on the ground, finding that the LLD position afforded better glottic exposure [2]. A follow-up study of EMS ground level intubations by Adnet et al. again studied LLD positioning versus kneeling in real EMS patients as opposed to mannequins [3]. During this study, they found that provider incidence of laryngoscopic difficulty was lower in the LLD position: 11.1% versus 26.9% for the

Emergency Medical Services: Clinical Practice and Systems Oversight, Second Edition. Volume 1: Clinical Aspects of EMS.
Edited by David C. Cone, Jane H. Brice, Theodore R. Delbridge, and J. Brent Myers.
© 2015 US Government. Published 2015 by John Wiley & Sons, Inc. Companion Website: www.wiley.com/go/cone\naemsp

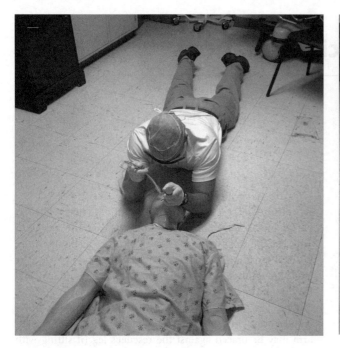

Figure 4.1 Prone intubation.

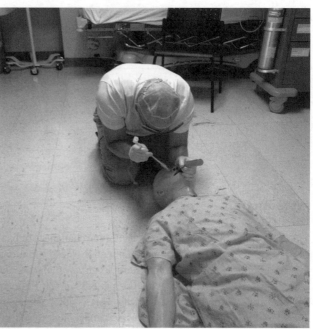

Figure 4.3 Kneeling intubation.

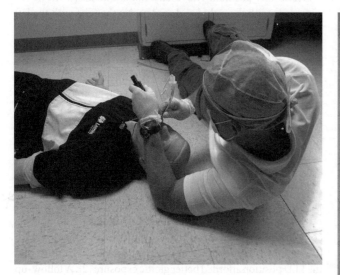

Figure 4.2 Left lateral decubitus intubating position.

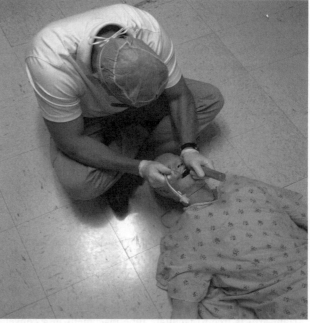

Figure 4.4 Sitting intubation.

kneeling group. They also found that there were a higher number of intubation attempts in the kneeling group than the LLD position. This research group postulated that LLD was a better position than kneeling for three reasons: the operator has better visual alignment with the larynx in the LLD position, the left forearm acts as a lever during exposure which minimizes operator effort, and the right arm is completely free during the procedure for tube placement and suctioning [3].

The rescuer's ability to visualize the glottis during ground-level intubation may be altered. Video laryngoscopy has been proposed as an adjunct for facilitating ground-level intubation. Komatsu et al. evaluated the Airway Scope™ (Pentax) and Macintosh laryngoscope for tracheal intubation in patients

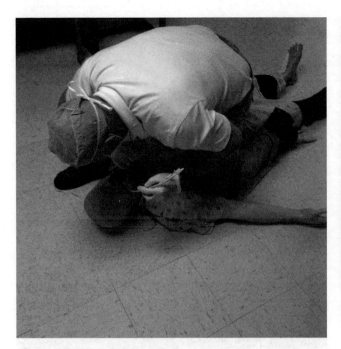

Figure 4.5 Straddle intubation.

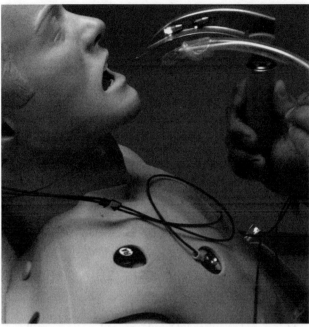

Figure 4.6 Face-to-face "tomahawk" intubation position.

lying on the ground [4]. While both the Airway Scope and Macintosh blade had high intubation success rates (98% and 100%, respectively), time to intubation was 17 seconds faster with the Airway Scope.

Face-to-face intubation

A patient may require intubation while positioned upright; for example, when entrapped in a car. One described approach is to perform ETI while directly facing the patient. With this technique, the operator holds the laryngoscope with the right hand, inserting the laryngoscope blade in an inverted fashion ("tomahawk" or "ice axe" approach) and passing the tracheal tube with the left hand (Figure 4.6).

In a mannequin study, Wetsch et al. studied face-to-face intubation comparing five types of video laryngoscopes and traditional Macintosh laryngoscopy in a simulated model of an entrapped motor vehicle victim [5]. Interestingly, their findings noted that the fastest time to intubation was with traditional Macintosh laryngoscopy, although the video laryngoscopes provide a better view of the glottis. Of the five video layngoscopes studied, the authors did note a shorter time to intubation with the two devices that had tube guides (Airtraq™ and Ambu Pentax™) than the non-guided scopes.

Amathieu et al. also examined face-to-face mannequin intubation times with the LMA Fastrach™, Glidescope™, and Airtraq laryngoscopes [6]. Time to intubation was shorter, intubation success rate was higher, and perceived intubation difficulty was lower with the Airtraq. Silverton et al. compared glottic views during face-to-face Glidescope laryngoscopy and fiberoptic intubation. They noted the Glidescope could be used to obtain adequate intubation visualization in live humans [7].

When face-to-face intubation is the only available option, the provider should assess whether immediate airway intervention or patient extrication is most appropriate. The estimated time of extraction combined with patient condition may influence the decision-making process. High-flow oxygen devices and supraglottic airways may provide suitable alternatives in these situations.

Intubating under low light conditions

Optimal lighting is important in airway management. Increased ambient lighting allows for better gear preparation and procedure execution. EMS practitioners may need to perform airway management in suboptimal lighting conditions such as at night, while conducting military operations, in a confined space rescue, or in indoor areas with poor lighting. There are two major lighting considerations in prehospital airway management: the light illuminating the patient environment, and illumination of the airway.

Simple interventions can significantly improve available lighting. Could a family member or colleague turn on additional lights? At the site of an accident, can portable lighting be provided to illuminate the scene? In some cases, a flashlight or headlamp may provide vital additional illumination.

A common pitfall of intubation is equipment failure resulting in suboptimal airway illumination; for example, broken laryngoscope bulbs, dead laryngoscope batteries, or damaged airway equipment. Regular equipment checks and the use of protective carrying cases are essential aspects of practice. Spare bulbs and batteries should always be part of the standard airway kit. Simple maneuvers such as rotating batteries on a regular basis might have a big effect on airway illumination.

Studies have identified that there is variation in light output among different laryngoscopes. Levitan et al. studied the light output of curved laryngoscope handles at 19 emergency departments in the Philadelphia area [8]. The median luminance varied widely from 11 lux to 5,627 lux (lux is the SI unit of illuminance equal to one lumen per square meter). Factors that may influence illumination brightness include bulbs/laryngoscope type (fiberoptic versus regular), condition of batteries, and equipment condition (e.g. multiple sterilizations potentially causing damage to light output).

Moore et al. examined the influence of laryngoscope illumination grade upon time to successful mannequin intubation [9]. Intubations were conducted on mannequins with three clinically plausible intensities of light: high (600 lux), medium (200 lux), and low (50 lux). At perceived suboptimal intubation lighting conditions (50 lux), there was no difference in time to intubation on mannequins in this study. Scholz et al. studied minimum and optimum light output of Macintosh size 3 blades in mannequins and again noted that providers could see the larynx at very low light levels [10]. The minimal acceptable lighting depending on bulb type was found to be anywhere from 9 to 34 lux. It was hypothesized that straightforward, low-complexity intubations may be possible at very low light conditions, as the airway operator is familiar with anatomy and other visual clues that will lead to a successful intubation. Difficult airways may require increased lighting to identify anatomical landmarks.

If conditions are such that achieving sufficient lighting to facilitate laryngoscopy is not possible, then at least three options exist. Digital intubation may be accomplished using solely tactile feedback. If available, intubation may be achieved using a lighted stylet. Finally, supraglottic airway insertion requires no illumination of the airway. See Volume 1, Chapter 3 for additional discussion of these techniques.

Minimizing airway management equipment

The standard prehospital intubation kit contains a range of equipment and may take up considerable space. For example, it might include a laryngoscope handle, multiple blades, multiple sizes of tracheal tubes, stylets, syringes, tape, a capnometer, and spare batteries and bulbs. There are situations where minimizing the airway management pack might be

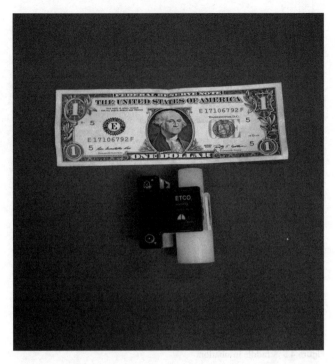

Figure 4.7 Small continuous battery-powered end-tidal CO_2 device. Smith Medical BCI Capnocheck.

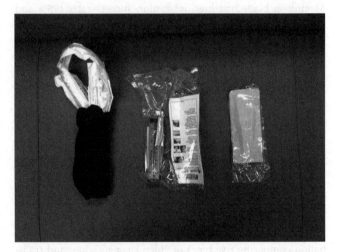

Figure 4.8 An example of a condensed airway pack with a laryngoscope roll (added ET tube and bougie), supraglottic airway, and a cricothyroidotomy kit. (North American Rescue, King LT, H+H)

necessary. For example, a wilderness or tactical mission requires smaller, compact equipment kits [11]. Over the past three decades there have been major advances in miniaturizing medical devices, offering new options for portability, including, for example, portable versions of continuous quantitative end-tidal CO_2 devices (Figure 4.7), suction devices, and video laryngoscopes.

An example of a condensed airway management kit is shown in Figure 4.8.

- Condensed primary airway kit
- Difficult airway device (gum elastic bougie and/or supraglottic device)
- Condensed surgical airway kit
- "Turkey baster" suction (not pictured)
- Small bag-valve-mask (not pictured)

It may be possible to select gear with multiple uses. For instance, a 14 gauge IV catheter may be bent and used as a cricothyroidotomy hook. Along the same lines, one might secure the endotracheal tube with tape rather than a commercial endotracheal tube holder.

Telemedicine-assisted airway management

The field of telemedicine has experienced a tremendous amount of development in the past decade. Applications for providing remote care have been seen in many disciplines including maritime, combat, and concierge medicine. Telemedicine may potentially play a role in prehospital airway management.

Sakles et al. describe tele-intubation assistance for remote hospital and prehospital intubations [12]. In their tele-intubation set-up, ambulances were fitted with wireless modules allowing monitoring of intubations from a distance of 500 feet from the ambulance. Rescuers used a modified video laryngoscope capable of transmitting images back to the telemedicine center. Sibert et al. conducted a feasibility study demonstrating remote assistance of intubation [13]. In this project, mannequin intubation footage was transmitted from the back of an ambulance to a physician in a remote monitoring station. A third study by Mosier et al. used readily available smartphone technology (Apple Facetime™, TangoMe™, Skype™) to facilitate tele-intubation [14].

It is important to recognize that while telemedicine may potentially aid airway management decision making, it cannot replace the actual motor or dexterous actions of airway management. The primary benefit of tele-intubation is to facilitate the airway decision-making process. For example, a remote advisor may guide the decision to intubate (or not intubate) an apneic victim of a drug overdose. This same remote observer may also coach the rescuer through performance of airway procedures. With the advent of new and inexpensive transmission devices such as smartphones, application of this airway assistance paradigm might be closer than we think.

Airway management in the tactical setting

Since 11 September 2001, continuous combat operations in both Iraq and Afghanistan have added greatly to our knowledge base regarding tactical medicine and tactical airway management [15]. Concurrently, there has been growth in the field of tactical EMS (TEMS) as the current wars have demonstrated the utility of specialized tactical medical care. Events in the United States due to active shooters and bombers have also demonstrated the need for specialized providers in tactical medicine [16,17].

Providing airway management during combat or tactical operations

Current Tactical Combat Casualty Care (TCCC) guidelines offer medical interventions based on three phases of care: care under fire, tactical field care, and tactical evacuation care [18]. The Tactical Emergency Casualty Care (TECC) guidelines, the civilian equivalent of TCCC, similarly specify three phases: direct threat care, indirect threat care, and evacuation care [19]. In both guidelines, the range of potential airway management techniques increases in scope as the threat from the enemy diminishes. Sophisticated airway techniques are usually not in the best interest of safety for the provider, the tactical team, or the patient in the highest threat environments.

The highest threat environments in both sets of guidelines include the TCCC care under fire phase or TECC direct threat care phase. In both of these situations, the tactical medical team is taking direct fire/under direct threat. The goal in this phase of care is to accomplish the mission while minimizing casualties, usually accomplished by suppressing or neutralizing the threat. TCCC recommends that airway management be generally deferred until the tactical field care phase. TECC provides similar guidance during direct threat care, including placing or directing the casualty to be placed in a position to protect the airway if tactically feasible.

The next phases of care in TCCC/TECC are tactical field care and indirect threat care. At this stage, direct engagement has ceased, and the provider and patient have been able to move to safe cover. Here more attention can generally be afforded to airway management. Both guidelines advocate for simple airway maneuvers in the field to include chin lift/jaw thrust, nasopharyngeal airway placement, and placement of the casualty in the recovery position for unconscious casualties without airway obstruction. For those patients with airway obstruction or impending airway obstruction, all of the above techniques are useful, including sitting the patient up to allow blood and secretions to drain. If unsuccessful, the military recommends quick transition to surgical cricothyroidotomy. TECC recommends the same, with considerations for oral or nasotracheal intubation and placement of supraglottic airway devices.

In the evacuation phase of field care, the threat has diminished and the provider and patient are normally on their way to higher levels of care via an air, ground, or sea platform. Airway management interventions at this point more closely mirror the normal prehospital environment with more extensive options available to the provider. TCCC and TECC recommend expanding options, including supraglottic airway placement, endotracheal intubation, and surgical cricothyroidotomy.

Larsen et al. compared endotracheal intubation, digital intubation, and use of the King LT™ airway device in a simulated tactical setting [20]. They compared the times to successful ventilation, numbers of attempts to successful intubation, and heights of presentation of the participants above a barricade used to simulate concealment. Important points from this study are that the choice of airway management technique can affect the exposure of the tactical provider above cover or concealment and time to first ventilation was relatively quick for both King LT and standard intubation (59.7 seconds for King LT, 63.3 seconds for endotracheal intubation). The time to ventilation was longer for digital intubation (125.4 seconds) and there was greater risk due to exposure over the barricade (23.5 inches above the barricade for digital intubation versus 17.7 inches for King LT placement).

Tactical operations may occur under low light or near-blackout conditions. Savoy et al. examined endotracheal intubation in ambient light and in the dark with night vision goggles. Providers were able to intubate using the goggles, but were noted to have much longer times to intubation than with typical ambient light [21].

Surgical airways in the tactical setting

United States military personnel often proceed directly to surgical airway placement due to complex facial injuries or the need to expedite care during various tactical scenarios [22]. A study of 72 battlefield prehospital criothyroidotomies by Mabry et al. noted a success rate of 68%, with a 21% rate of miscannulating the trachea [23]. Combat medics performed most of these procedures. Patients undergoing cricothyroidotomy had a high mortality rate at 66%. The authors recommend that tactical EMS providers should be well versed in surgical airway techniques [24].

In a study of Israeli defense forces, Katzenell et al. noted that intubation success rates fall with each subsequent attempt [25]. Therefore rescuers should determine thresholds for abandoning initial intubation efforts in favor of surgical airway placement.

Conclusion

Emergency medical services providers may need to manage the airway in unusual prehospital situations. Important considerations include the following.

- **Ground-level intubation**. Many different intubation positions are described for ground-level intubation. Left lateral decubitus positioning may prove the best approach in this situation.
- **Face-to-face intubation**. The "tomahawk" approach may be viable in this situation.
- **Low light intubation**. Optimizing available ambient light may help to facilitate intubation in low light conditions.
- **Minimize field equipment**. A minimal airway management kit may be necessary. New miniaturized technology affords options for minimizing the airway kit.

- **Telemedicine assistance**. Remote airway management guidance may be possible with new telemedicine technology.
- **Tactical airway management**. Airway management is best deferred until the intensity of the threat has decreased. Operational constraints may force the operator to consider early surgical airway.

Acknowledgments

Special thanks to Scott Poynter, CRNA, for assistance with the photos.

References

1 Pinchalk M, Roth R, Paris P, Hostler D. Comparison of times to intubate a simulated trauma patient in two positions. *Prehospl Emerg Care* 2003;7(2):252–7.

2 Adnet F, Lapostolle F, Borron S, Hennequin B, Leclercq G, Fleury M. Optimization of glottic exposure during intubation of a patient lying supine on the ground. *Am J Emerg Med* 1997;15(6):555–7.

3 Adnet G, Cydulka R, Lapandry C. Emergency tracheal intubation of patients lying supine on the ground: influence of operator body position. *Can J Anesth* 1998;45(3):266–9.

4 Komatsu R, Kamata K, Sessler D, Ozaki M. Airway scope and Macintosh laryngoscope for tracheal intubation in patients lying on the ground. *Anesth Analg* 2010;111(2):427–431.

5 Wetsch W, Carlitscheck M, Spelten O, et al. Success rates and endotracheal tube insertion times of experienced emergency physicians using five video laryngoscopes: a randomised trial in a simulated trapped car accident victim. *Eur J Anaesthesiol* 2011;28(12):850–8.

6 Amathieu R, Sudrial J, Abdi W, et al. Simulating face to face tracheal intubation of a trapped patient: a randomized comparision of the LMA Fastrach, the Glidescope, and the Airtraq laryngoscope. *Br J Anaesth* 2011;108(1):140–5.

7 Silverton N, Youngquist S, Mallin M, et al. Glidescope versus flexible fiber optic for awake upright laryngoscopy. *Ann Emerg Med* 2012;59(3):159–64.

8 Levitan R, Kelly J, Kinkle W, Fasano C. Light intensity of curved l aryngoscope blades in Philadelphia emergency departments. *Ann Emerg Med* 2007;50(3):253–7.

9 Moore S, Dwyer D, Arendts G. Laryngoscope illumination grade does not influence time to successful mannequin inutbation. *Emerg Med Australas* 2009;21:131–5.

10 Scholz A, Farnum N, Wilkes A, Hampson M, Hall J. Minimum and optimum light output of Macintosh size 3 laryngoscopy blades: a mannequin study. *Anaesthesia* 2007;62:163–8.

11 Melsom MA Farrar MD, Volkers RC. Battle casualties. *Ann Roy Coll Surg Engl* 1975;56(6):289–303.

12 Sakles J, Mosier J, Hadeed G, Hudson M, Valenzuela T, Latifi R. Telemedicine and telepresence for prehospital and remote hospital tracheal intubation using a Glidescope videolaryngoscope: a model for tele-intubation. *Telemed J E Health* 2011;17(3):185–8.

13 Sibert K, Ricci M, Caputo M, et al. The feasibility of using ultrasound and video laryngoscopy in a Mobile telemedicine consult. *Teleme E Health* 2008;14(3):266–72.

14 Mosier J, Joseph B, Sakles J. Telebation: next generation telemedicine in remote airway management using current wireles technologies. *Telemed E Health* 2013;19(2):95–8.

15 Butler F, Blackbourne L. Battlefield trauma care then and now: a decade of tactical combat casualty care. *J Trauma Acute Care Surg* 2012;73(6):S395–402.

16 Jacobs L, McSwain N, Rotondo M, et al. Improving survival from active shooter events: the Hartford Consensus. *J Trauma Acute Care Surg* 2013;74(6):1399–1400.

17 Carterson E, Carty M, Weaver M, Holt E. Boston bombings: a surgical view of lessons learned from combat casualty care and the applicability to Boston's terrorist attack. *J Craniofac Surg* 2013; 24(4):1061–7.

18 Tactical Combat Casualty Care Guidelines. Available at: www. usaisr.amedd.army.mil/assets/pdfs/TCCC_Guidelines_140602.pdf

19 Committee for Tactical Emergency Casualty Care (C-TECC). Availabe at: http://c-tecc.org/images/content/TECC_Guidelines_May_2013_update.pdf

20 Larsen M, Guyette F, Suyama J. Comparision of three airway management techniques in a simulated tactical setting. *Prehosp Emerg Care* 2010;14:510–14.

21 Savoy B, Dickinson E, Shofer F, McCans J, Mechem CC. Effect of night vision goggles on performance of advanced life support skills by emergency personnel. *Mil Med* 2006;171:280–2.

22 Mabry R, Edens J, Pearse L. et al Fatal airway injuries during Operation Enduring Freedom and Operation Iraqi Freedom. *Prehosp Emerg Care* 2010;14(2):272–7.

23 Mabry R, Frankfurt A. An analysis of battlefield cricothyroidotomy in Iraq and Afghanistan. *J Spec Oper Med* 2012;12:17–23.

24 Bennett B, Cailteux-Zevallos B, Kotora J. Cricothyroidotomy bottom-up training review: battlefield lessons learned. *Mil Med* 2011;176:1311–19.

25 Katzenell U, Lipsky A, Abramovich A, et al. Prehospital intubation success rates among Israel Defense Forces providers: epidemiologic analysis and effect on doctrine. *J Trauma Acute Care Surg* 2013;75:S178–83.

SECTION II

Breathing

CHAPTER 5

Respiratory distress

Jason Oost and Mohamud Daya

Introduction

Respiratory distress is the second most common chief complaint after minor trauma, making up 13% of adult EMS calls [1]. It is both challenging and rewarding for the EMS provider. Diagnosis depends on often subtle and overlapping signs and symptoms. While incorrect management is potentially detrimental, with correct diagnosis comes the potential for life-saving intervention and rapid improvement. The landmark Ontario Prehospital Advanced Life Support study demonstrated a significant survival benefit in respiratory distress when interventions including nebulized beta-agonists, sublingual nitroglycerin, intubation, and intravenous medications and fluids were added to the EMS systems of the included cities [2].

Prehospital assessment and diagnosis

The approach to the dyspneic patient must always begin with a focus on immediate threats to survival, such as airway obstruction. Once this has been dealt with, provisional causes can be considered so as to guide specific therapy. Accurate diagnosis of the cause of dyspnea in prehospital settings remains difficult. Studies have shown that paramedics are able to determine the etiology of dyspnea with only moderate accuracy. In one of the more positive retrospective studies, a prehospital diagnosis of cardiac, pulmonary, or other as the cause of "difficulty breathing" agreed with that of the emergency department (ED) diagnosis 81% of the time [3]. However, Jaronik et al. studied 144 patients given furosemide in the field and noted that it was given appropriately only 58% of the time to patients with a subsequent diagnosis of congestive heart failure or an elevated B-type natriuretic peptide (BNP) level. It was given inappropriately 42% of the time, and for diagnoses in which it was potentially harmful 17% of the time [4]. Almost one-quarter of patients who received furosemide from EMS in this study subsequently required IV fluid therapy in the hospital [4]. Therefore, prehospital treatment must carefully find a balance between disease severity, diagnostic certainty, and the likelihood of harm.

Much of the assessment of disease severity comes from general observation of the patient supplemented by physical examination and close monitoring of vital signs, cardiac rhythm, pulse oximetry (SpO_2), and end-tidal carbon dioxide ($EtCO_2$) levels. Some of the useful questions that can be asked by a medical oversight physician over the radio or phone include how many words the patient can speak at a time, whether there is associated diaphoresis, and if the patient appears to be fatiguing. If the initial assessment reveals the possibility of impending respiratory failure, appropriate supplemental ventilation should be considered, including the use of non-invasive positive pressure ventilation (NIPPV) or bag-valve-mask (BVM) ventilation in conjunction with oral/nasopharyngeal airways, supraglottic devices, or endotracheal intubation (ETI). An important early task is to question the family/caregivers and gather available paperwork regarding the patient's wishes for life-sustaining treatment or end-of-life care.

Once disease severity and the immediate needs have been addressed, the next step is to attempt to categorize the underlying cause. The four most common categories for respiratory distress are upper airway obstruction, small airway obstruction including chronic obstructive pulmonary disease (COPD) and asthma, acute cardiogenic pulmonary edema (ACPE), and pneumonia. In addition, there are a host of other medical conditions that can cause subjective dyspnea and/or objective impairment of oxygenation and ventilation (Box 5.1).

Acute coronary syndrome is an important consideration among these disparate causes of shortness of breath. It can present as cardiogenic shock with ACPE but can also cause subjective dyspnea without severe impairment of cardiac function. Dyspnea associated with acute coronary syndrome may not be accompanied by chest discomfort and is more common in women, older individuals, and those with diabetes [5,6]. Dysrhythmias can also cause dyspnea and are readily diagnosed by cardiac monitoring.

Emergency Medical Services: Clinical Practice and Systems Oversight, Second Edition. Volume 1: Clinical Aspects of EMS.
Edited by David C. Cone, Jane H. Brice, Theodore R. Delbridge, and J. Brent Myers.
© 2015 NAEMSP. Published 2015 by John Wiley & Sons, Inc. Companion Website: www.wiley.com\go\cone\naemsp

---

Box 5.1 Common causes of respiratory distress in the EMS setting

Pneumonia
Acute decompensated heart failure/acute cardiogenic
  pulmonary edema
Pulmonary embolus
Acute coronary syndrome (ST-segment elevated myocardial infarction,
  non-ST-segment elevated myocardial infarction, unstable angina)
Pneumothorax
Metabolic acidosis with attempted compensation (e.g. septic shock)
Toxic ingestions (e.g. salicylates)
Pleural effusion
Pulmonary hypertension
Upper airway obstruction
Interstitial pulmonary fibrosis
Asthma
Chronic obstructive pulmonary disease
Fever
Physiological dyspnea of pregnancy
Bronchitis
Psychiatric, hyperventilation, panic attack
Arrhythmias, especially atrial fibrillation
Abdominal distension, obesity
Italics = Very common

Box 5.2 History and exam findings by disease state

Asthma
Dyspnea with prolonged expiratory phase, tripoding position when severe, decreased breath sounds when very severe to diffuse wheezing, chest tightness

Chronic obstructive pulmonary disease
Cough, increased or change in sputum production, dyspnea with prolonged expiratory phase, tripoding position when severe, decreased breath sounds when very severe to diffuse wheezing, barrel chest appearance

Acute decompensated heart failure with volume overload
Jugular venous distention, S3 or S4 heart sounds, pulmonary wheezing, pulmonary crackles (rales), lower extremity edema, sacral edema, weight gain with normal or elevated blood pressure

Acute decompensated heart failure with low cardiac output state
Cool skin from peripheral vasoconstriction and low blood pressure

Pneumonia
Unilateral decreased breath sounds, focal wheezing, unilateral or bilateral crackles (rales), fever, normotensive to hypotensive

Pneumothorax
Pleuritic chest pain, unilateral decreased breath sounds, jugular venous distension, hypotension and hypoxia with tension physiology

Pulmonary embolism with infarction
Dyspnea, pleuritic chest pain, hemoptysis, possibly decreased oxygen saturations

Pulmonary embolism with saddle embolism
Syncope, hypoxemia, jugular venous distension, acute right heart strain on ECG, dilated right ventricle on portable echocardiogram

---

If time and the patient's condition allow, a 12-lead electrocardiogram (ECG) may be useful in guiding treatment and destination decisions for the dyspneic patient. Severe sepsis can also present with respiratory distress due to increased oxygen consumption. Toxic exposures can cause respiratory distress either through direct irritation of the respiratory tract or secondarily by central nervous system impairment of respiratory function. Tachypnea and subjective dyspnea may also be compensatory for an underlying metabolic acidosis as with diabetic ketoacidosis or salicylate toxicity. If these acidotic patients require ETI and mechanical ventilation, it is important to continue to hyperventilate them to maintain their preexisting respiratory compensation for the underlying metabolic acidosis. This can be facilitated through the use of continuous EtCO$_2$ monitoring. Neuromuscular diseases such as myasthenia gravis and Guillain–Barré syndrome are rare causes of inadequate ventilation and respiratory failure. Although a diagnosis of exclusion, shortness of breath is also a common manifestation of anxiety disorders, panic attacks, and psychogenic hyperventilation. Having a patient breathe into and out of a paper bag, which is sometimes done by the uninformed for hyperventilation, actually decreases inspired oxygen and has no place in EMS.

Although auscultation of breath sounds is an important part of the physical examination for respiratory distress, there can be much overlap in the cause of any one particular finding. Thus breath sounds must be interpreted in the context of the rest of the focused exam. For example, a common mistake is to equate "crackles" with an ACPE exacerbation and "wheezing" with asthma, although both findings can be found in either disease process. Examination should also include a careful auscultation of heart sounds as well as palpation and inspection of the neck for jugular venous distension (JVD), chest for retractions and injury, lower back for sacral edema, and extremities for edema or evidence of deep vein thrombosis (DVT) (Box 5.2).

The physical exam may be enhanced through the use of ultrasound of the chest in the patient with acute respiratory distress. Ultrasound is now commonly used in the ED for evaluation of pneumothorax, pleural effusion, pericardial effusion, large pulmonary embolism, cardiac function and volume status.

General treatment

As with most potential threats to life, initial therapy should begin with supplemental oxygen, application of monitoring devices, and often IV access. With standard use of SpO$_2$ monitoring, growing information suggests that oxygen therapy should be carefully titrated to a goal between 93% and 96% in patients with general respiratory distress, and to a goal of 88–92% in patients with known COPD [7,8]. A recent randomized controlled prehospital trial by Austin et al. showed decreased mortality among patients who were treated with a titrated oxygen regimen versus those treated with uncontrolled high flow oxygen. Mortality was reduced 58% in patients with any respiratory distress and 78% in patients with known COPD with the titration strategy [7].

Inhaled bronchodilators, including short-acting inhaled beta$_2$-agonists (SABAs) and anticholinergics, are commonly included in protocols for respiratory distress of unclear etiology. Although there is usually little downside to their use, especially if a component of bronchospasm is suspected, SABAs can be potentially harmful in those with ACPE, acute coronary syndrome, and cardiac arrhythmias due to their chronotropic, inotropic, and vasoactive effects on the cardiovascular system. A review of the Acute Decompensated Heart Failure National Registry Emergency Module (ADHERE) database by Singer et al. revealed that 21% of patients ultimately diagnosed with acute decompensated heart failure (ADHF) exacerbation received SABA treatments by EMS or in the ED [9]. The authors also reported an association between bronchodilator use and a subsequent need for IV vasodilators and ETI. It is important to note, however, that no mortality difference was found between patients who did or did not receive SABAs. In addition, patients with combined ADHF and COPD were not studied separately. Fisher et al. reported six cases of acute myocardial infarction precipitated by bronchodilators [10].

Unfortunately, the relationship between cardiac manifestations and bronchodilator use is poorly understood and these cases likely reflect publication bias. SABAs are known to decrease serum potassium concentration by approximately 0.5 meq/L, which could precipitate hypokalemia-associated dysrhythmias. In addition, SABAs may temporarily worsen hypoxemia by increasing the ventilation/perfusion mismatch. Inhaled anticholinergics, such as ipratropium, are not absorbed systemically and have no cardiovascular toxicity. But in the final analysis and in the absence of well-designed trials to better guide the empirical use of bronchodilators in undifferentiated respiratory distress, it seems to make physiological sense to continue to include them in EMS protocols or at the discretion of a medical oversight physician.

Two forms of NIPPV have become standard for treatment of several forms of respiratory distress [11]. A mask is used to deliver ventilation support either at a constant pressure (CPAP) or with a higher pressure during inspiration (BiPAP). The use of NIPPV in the prehospital setting has become accepted as an early intervention, and studies of its use in this setting have demonstrated decreased mortality, reduced intubation rates, shorter intensive care unit (ICU) lengths of stay, and improved vital signs [11,12]. Although NIPPV has been most studied in COPD and ACPE, a recent systematic review and metaanalysis supports its use in all forms of undifferentiated acute respiratory failure [11]. NIPPV may also permit administration of a lower concentration of inspired oxygen, thereby decreasing the potential deleterious effects of hyperoxia [13]. It is important that prehospital providers understand the limitations of this intervention, including patient factors that are specific contraindications to its use. NIPPV is inappropriate for patients who require immediate ETI such as those who are unable to protect their airways, have altered mentation, or cannot tolerate the pressure mask. The patient must have an acceptable respiratory drive prior to application of NIPPV.

Advanced airway management with supraglottic airways or ETI is the final common pathway for most individuals with severe respiratory distress who have failed to respond to the above-mentioned strategies (see Volume 1, Chapters 2–4).

Asthma

Asthma is a chronic inflammatory lung disorder characterized by acute attacks of airway hyperresponsiveness with reversible obstruction. Precipitating factors include upper respiratory tract infections, exposure to allergens, high pollution indices, and failure to use preventive and maintenance therapies. The disease affects more than 22 million individuals in the United States [14]. Although there are hallmark features of an acute exacerbation, assessment of asthma exacerbations can be challenging and potentially misleading (see Box 5.2). For example, absence of wheezing may indicate either severely restricted airflow or clinical improvement following appropriate treatment. A multicomponent guide can be helpful in assessing severity and monitoring the effectiveness of treatment of asthma [14] (Table 5.1).

Oxygen should be provided to relieve hypoxemia and titrated to a SpO_2 of 93–96% [7]. The initial drug of choice for treatment is a SABA, which acts by relaxing bronchial smooth muscle and increasing mucociliary clearance. Nebulization is the preferred route of administration in the acute setting with either intermittent or continuous delivery. SABAs can also be administered through the use of metered dose inhalers (MDI). The use of subcutaneous epinephrine (a non-selective beta-agonist) has declined with the availability of SABAs, but epinephrine can be

Table 5.1 Asthma severity guide

Parameter	Mild	Moderate	Severe
Shortness of breath	Walking	Talking	At rest
Ability to speak	Full sentences	Phrases	Words
Heart rate	100	100–120	>120
Respiratory rate	Increased	Increased	>30
Lung sounds	End expiratory wheezing	Full expiratory wheezing	Absent or biphasic wheezing
Accessory muscle use	Rare	Common	Always
Mental status	Agitation, variable	Agitated, usually	Agitated to somnolent
ETCO$_2$	20–30	30–40	>40

Source: Guidelines for the Diagnosis and Management of Asthma (EPR-3) 2007. National Heart, Lung, and Blood Institute; National Institutes of Health; US Department of Health and Human Services.

very useful when the patient is critically ill or when the inhaled SABA cannot be delivered effectively. For more severe exacerbations an anticholinergic bronchodilator agent, such as ipratropium, can be added to the SABA.

Patients who fail to respond promptly and completely to inhaled bronchodilators benefit from the administration of systemic corticosteroids. The benefits of prehospital corticosteroid administration have not been proven through randomized controlled clinical trials. Non-randomized observational studies, however, have shown that EMS delivery of corticosteroids is associated with decreased hospital admission rates [15]. It has also been suggested that early use of corticosteroids may enhance the effectiveness of SABAs [16]. Corticosteroid options include prednisone (oral), dexamethasone (oral, IM, IV), and methylprednisolone (IV).

For severe exacerbations that fail to respond to inhaled bronchodilators and systemic corticosteroids, adjunctive therapies, such as IV magnesium sulfate or heliox, if available, should be considered. A meta-analysis of seven randomized controlled trials of magnesium sulfate administered in the ED showed it improved peak expiratory flow rates and reduced hospital admission rates compared with placebo in severe asthma exacerbations [17].

Although NIPPV for acute exacerbations of asthma is traditionally viewed as a last resort due to the fear of worsening air trapping and secondary barotrauma, studies of its use in the ED and ICU settings in children have shown benefit [18,19]. A retrospective study of pediatric patients who were placed on BiPAP and given SABAs in the ED, with initial disposition plans for ICU admission, found that 22% of the patients tolerated BiPAP and were able to be downgraded to ward admission. None required subsequent ICU admission. All of these patients had improved SpO$_2$ levels as well as respiratory rates and there were no BiPAP-related adverse events [19].

If rapid sequence ETI is necessary for an asthma patient, the preferred induction agent is ketamine due to its inherent bronchodilator properties. Once intubated, ventilation should be provided at reduced volumes and rates to prevent air trapping and secondary barotrauma. The inspiratory-to-expiratory (I/E) ratios should be adjusted to provide a prolonged expiratory phase. Permissive hypercarbia is generally well tolerated in these individuals. All NIPPV and intubated asthma patients should be monitored closely for signs of secondary barotrauma, such as tension pneumothorax and pneumomediastinum.

Chronic obstructive pulmonary disease

Chronic obstructive pulmonary disease is a chronic disease characterized by expiratory lung flow obstruction that is only partially reversible. The underlying pathophysiology involves a complex process of chronic inflammation, remodeling of the small airways with destruction of alveoli, and increase in extracellular matrix production. COPD is usually a response to noxious particles and gases including cigarette smoke and environmental pollutants, though genetic factors also play a part [20]. It is the fourth leading cause of death in the United States. COPD patients who continue smoking will eventually require permanent oxygen and/or ventilator assistance. EMS is often called to evaluate a COPD patient during an acute exacerbation of the condition precipitated by respiratory tract infections, exposure to pollutants or allergens, or medication non-compliance. The clinical presentation is similar to asthma (see Box 5.2). COPD patients should receive oxygen with a goal to maintain SpO$_2$ between 88% and 92%, which was associated with reduced mortality by twofold in the study by Austin et al. [7] Impending respiratory failure can be detected by continuous EtCO$_2$ monitoring. Increasing EtCO$_2$ levels indicate a deteriorating condition.

As with asthma, the primary treatments during acute exacerbations are directed toward reversing airway obstruction through the use of SABAs and anticholinergic agents. The latter are much more effective in COPD and should be used early. Corticosteroids and antibiotics are also important adjuvant therapies. Use of NIPPV has become established as a life-saving therapy in the treatment of COPD exacerbations [11,12]. If it is necessary to intubate a COPD patient, appropriate settings for mechanical ventilation include decreased respiratory rates, lower tidal volumes, and increased expiratory phase. As with asthma, these patients must be monitored closely for evidence of secondary barotrauma [21].

Acute decompensated heart failure/acute cardiogenic pulmonary edema

No widely accepted guidelines exist for the treatment of ADHF either in the prehospital or ED setting. One pathway proposed by DiDomenico et al. for the ED bases the initial management strategy on whether the problem appears to be a state of volume overload versus one of inadequate cardiac output, which can often be differentiated on exam [22] (see Box 5.2). If the patient is volume overloaded, positioning in an upright posture is the first step. It allows pleural effusions and edema to localize at the lung bases and venous blood to pool in the lower extremities, thereby reducing cardiac preload. If immediate prehospital pharmacotherapy is required, nitrates are the preferred option. If the patient has poor cardiac output, which is far less common, field treatment is largely supportive, although this category of diagnosis should prompt EMS providers to consider causes such as acute myocardial infarction (MI) as well as hypovolemic, distributive, or obstructive causes for shock. If the cause is truly low output cardiac failure, specific treatment might include the use of inotropic and vasopressor medications such as dobutamine, milrinone and dopamine.

If the patient has volume overload with an adequate or high blood pressure and is in acute distress, nitrates should be administered. Diuretics are rarely indicated in prehospital settings.

Nitroglycerin acts rapidly to dilate veins, allowing blood to distribute to the periphery, thereby decreasing cardiac preload. At higher doses, typically above 30 µg/min intravenously, nitroglycerin also acts as an arterial vasodilator, decreasing cardiac afterload [23]. Sublingual nitroglycerin is 50% bioavailable. A dose of 400 µg given every 5 minutes, with frequent reassessment to ensure maintenance of a systolic blood pressure of at least 100 mmHg, is often effective. However, for patients in extremis in terms of respiratory distress, and with an adequate blood pressure, sublingual nitroglycerin spray can be safely administered more frequently, as often as every 2 minutes in some cases, to rescue the patient from invasive airway intervention and ventilation. Sublingual nitroglycerin also has the advantage of a rapid time to peak effect of 5–15 minutes and duration of action of less than 1 hour. Transdermal nitroglycerin paste is not recommended since its effectiveness is limited by slow absorption, which is further worsened by the presence of decreased skin perfusion during ADHF.

Intravenous access should ideally be obtained before the administration of nitroglycerin, as it has the rare potential to produce hypotension and bradycardia [24]. However, inability to obtain IV access should not preclude or delay its use. Observational studies of nitroglycerin use have shown relatively low rates of serious adverse effects ranging from 0.3% to 3.6% [24]. EMS providers must also remember the potential interaction with all antierectile dysfunction phosphodiesterase-inhibiting drugs (e.g. sildenafil), which are contraindications to the use of nitroglycerin. Notably, however, NIPPV is not a contraindication to concomitant nitroglycerin use.

Loop diuretics, including furosemide, have also been used in the prehospital setting for patients with ADHF, especially those presenting with ACPE. However, intravenously, peak response time is 30 minutes, and this is even more delayed in patients with decreased cardiac output and renal vasoconstriction. The duration of action of furosemide is 2 hours, and up to 6–8 hours in renal failure. Further, because of its effects on plasma electrolytes, which in general are not assessed in most field situations, its use is discouraged. Because furosemide has less of an immediate benefit than nitroglycerin, a long duration of action, and unforeseen potential side-effects, it probably has limited utility in the prehospital setting. Many EMS systems have eliminated its use in favor of nitroglycerin alone.

Morphine, once a staple of therapy for ADHF, has also been largely supplanted by other therapies. A review of the large ADHERE database found a significant association between receiving morphine and death, as well as several other adverse outcomes [25]. One explanation may be that as morphine causes hypotension, it takes away the therapeutic room available for other medications used to reduce preload and afterload. In addition, as a respiratory depressant, morphine may decrease the respiratory drive of an already struggling patient.

Non-invasive positive pressure ventilation is very useful in the immediate treatment of ACPE. Continuous pressure at a level of 5–10 cmH$_2$O improves oxygenation by recruiting atelectatic alveoli and decreasing the work of breathing. The increase in intrathoracic pressure also alters hemodynamics by decreasing the transmural wall tension of the heart [26]. Small EMS case series have demonstrated decreased intubation rates and shorter ICU lengths of stay, although effect on mortality is less clear [27,28]. As mentioned, sublingual nitrate therapy should be continued in conjunction with NIPPV.

An emerging modality for diagnosis of ADHF and ACPE in the ED, which may also be useful in the prehospital setting, is focused ultrasonography. In a prospective prehospital study, Prosen et al. reported that the combined use of NT-prBNP (a marker of cardiac atrial stretch) and chest ultrasound had a sensitivity, specificity, negative predictive value (NPV), and positive predictive value (PPV) of 100% for the diagnosis of ADHF and ACPE [29]. More recently, Neesse et al. reported that the presence of a pleural effusion on the prehospital chest ultrasound appears to be a novel marker for ADHF [30]. Portable chest ultrasonography may therefore hold promise as a tool in the differentiation of COPD and ACPE in the prehospital setting.

Pneumonia and infectious respiratory disease

In general, there are few specific field interventions for patients who are determined to have pulmonary infectious causes of their shortness of breath. Pneumonia treatment guidelines are universally focused on prompt diagnosis and early treatment with antibiotics.

Pneumonia should be considered in patients with cough and/or fever. Specific etiologies of these diseases and issues regarding crew protection are discussed in Chapter 25 of both Volumes 1 and 2. It is important to note that some of these diseases can be highly contagious, and it is recommended that some type of respiratory precaution (e.g. an N95 mask to protect against novel viruses as well as tuberculosis) is maintained when evaluating a respiratory distress patient who is presumed to have an infectious etiology.

Treatment of these patients will typically consist of oxygen, NIPPV if ventilation support is needed to further improve oxygenation, IV fluids if hypotensive, and transport. Patients with known asthma or COPD who have reactive airways in response to the inflammation may also benefit from bronchodilators. Many pneumonia patients may also wheeze from infectious inflammatory processes within the small airways, and hence may respond to inhaled bronchodilators.

Pulmonary embolus

Pulmonary embolus (PE) is another clinical condition that can present with respiratory distress. Classic risk factors for venous thromboembolism (VTE) include the Virchow triad of venous stasis, trauma, and hypercoagulability. There are many risk factors for VTE but the ones that have been clinically validated by Wells criteria and the PERC rule for risk stratification include recent surgery or immobilization of an extremity, malignancy, exogenous estrogen use, and prior DVT [31]. Other notable risk factors include genetic deficiency of anticlotting factors, pregnancy, obesity, and extended travel.

Most PEs are the result of DVTs in the pelvic or lower extremity veins, though a DVT from any location can result in a PE. PE is a challenging clinical diagnosis because the manifestations can be subtle. The most common symptom is dyspnea and the most common clinical signs are tachycardia and tachypnea. The pulmonary exam is usually unremarkable, though examination of the extremities, particularly the legs, may reveal swelling, erythema, and/or pain in a limb with a DVT. With the increased use of peripherally inserted central venous catheters, PEs are also reported more frequently as a result of upper extremity DVTs [32]. Small PEs often present with respiratory distress. Larger emboli that cause lung infarction can present with more severe findings, and those with saddle embolism cause findings suggestive of obstructive shock (see Box 5.2). The latter can be detected by findings such as right axis deviation, right ventricle strain, and right bundle branch block on a 12-lead ECG. Additional useful ECG features are the presence of T-wave inversions in both V_1 and lead III as well as the presence of an S-wave in lead I and a Q wave and inverted T wave in lead III (S1Q3T3) [33]. Acute right ventricular dysfunction can also be visualized using portable cardiac ultrasonography. In some severe cases, the embolus can even be visualized directly within the heart.

Emergency medical services treatment priorities include high-flow oxygen, vascular access, and cardiac monitoring. A fluid bolus is indicated in the patient who presents with a suspected massive PE and perfusion failure. In some patients, the presentation can take the form of a cardiac arrest with a narrow complex pulseless electrical activity (PEA) rhythm. The presence of prearrest respiratory distress, altered mental status, and shock, along with a presenting rhythm of PEA, has been shown to be predictive of PE as a cause of cardiac arrest [34]. Although the use of prehospital thrombolysis in these instances has been reported to be effective in selected cases, a randomized controlled clinical trial failed to show improved outcomes during cardiac arrest when tissue plasminogen activator (t-PA) was administered compared to placebo for patients with refractory PEA [35,36].

Pneumothorax

Spontaneous pneumothorax is an uncommon condition that can present as acute respiratory distress. It is caused by rupture of the alveolar air sacs into the pleural space, followed by variable collapse of the lung. Symptoms include dyspnea as well as pleuritic chest pain. The exam may reveal decreased breath sounds on the affected side. Typically, spontaneous pneumothorax

occurs in male patients who are taller than average with a slim build. There are also secondary causes of spontaneous pneumothorax, most notably COPD. Other underlying causes include tumor, infection, or a connective tissue disorder. Spontaneous pneumothorax rarely progresses to tension pneumothorax. Patients with a suspected simple pneumothorax should be monitored closely for evidence of tension physiology such as worsening respiratory distress, hypoxia, hypotension, JVD, and tracheal deviation, in which case immediate chest needle decompression is indicated. In the future, the clinical diagnosis of pneumothorax will be supplemented by objective evidence through the use of portable chest ultrasound.

Conclusion

Respiratory distress is a very common complaint in the prehospital setting. Initial evaluation should be focused on identifying immediate threats to life and determining needs for an immediate intervention such as NIPPV, BVM ventilation, or ETI. Once this evaluation is completed, efforts should be focused on attempting to determine the provisional underlying cause of the respiratory distress. Respiratory distress may be caused by a primary pulmonary problem, a cardiac problem, an infectious problem, or as part of compensation for another non-pulmonary problem.

A vast number of these patients will remain "undifferentiated" through their EMS and possibly even their ED courses. In general, treatment should include titrated oxygen and monitoring of cardiac rhythm, SpO_2, and $ETCO_2$ while ensuring timely transport. In stable situations, the emphasis should focus on avoiding overtreatment and resisting the urge to give multiple medications in an undirected fashion. However, little harm comes to the patient with an initial trial of inhaled bronchodilator therapy, and nitrates should be considered as first-line therapy in the patient with findings consistent with ADHF or ACPE.

References

1 Maio RF, Garrison HG, Spaite DW, et al. Emergency Medical Services Outcomes Project I (EMSOP I): prioritizing conditions for outcomes research. *Ann Emerg Med* 1999;33:423–32.

2 Stiell IG, Spaite DW, Field B, et al. Advanced life support for out-of-hospital respiratory distress. *N Engl J Med* 2007;356:2156–64.

3 Ackerman R, Waldron RL. Difficulty breathing: agreement of paramedic and emergency physician diagnoses. *Prehosp Emerg Care* 2006;10:77–80.

4 Jaronik J, Mikkelson P, Fales W, Overton DT. Evaluation of prehospital use of furosemide in patients with respiratory distress. *Prehosp Emerg Care* 2006;10:194–7.

5 McSweeney JC, Cody M, O'Sullivan P, Elberson K, Moser DK, Garvin BJ. Women's early warning symptoms of acute myocardial infarction. *Circulation* 2003;108:2619–23.

6 DeVon HA, Penckofer S, Larimer K. The association of diabetes and older age with the absence of chest pain during acute coronary syndromes. *West J Nurs Res* 2008;30:130–44.

7 Austin MA, Wills KE, Blizzard L, Walters EH, Wood-Baker R. Effect of high flow oxygen on mortality in chronic obstructive pulmonary disease patients in prehospital setting: randomised controlled trial. *BMJ* 2010;341:1–8.

8 Cameron L, Pilcher J, Weatherall M, Beasley R, Perrin K. The risk of serious adverse outcomes associated with hypoxaemia and hyperoxaemia in acute exacerbations of COPD. *Postgrad Med J* 2012;88:684–9.

9 Singer AJ, Emerman C, Char DM, et al. Bronchodilator therapy in acute decompensated heart failure patients without a history of chronic obstructive pulmonary disease. *Ann Emerg Med* 2008;51:25–34.

10 Fisher AA, Davis MW, McGill DA. Acute myocardial infarction associated with albuterol. *Ann Pharmacother* 2004;38:2045–9.

11 Williams TA, Finn J, Perkins GD, Jacobs IG. Prehospital continuous positive airway pressure for acute respiratory failure: a systematic review and meta-analysis. *Prehosp Emerg Care* 2013;17:261–73.

12 Aguilar SA, Lee J, Castillo E, et al. Assessment of the addition of prehospital continuous positive airway pressure (CPAP) to an urban emergency medical services (EMS) system in person with severe respiratory distress. *J Emerg Med* 2013;45:210–19.

13 Bledsoe BE, Anderson E, Hodnick R, Johnson L, Johnson S, Dievendorf E. Low-fractional oxygen concentration continuous positive airway pressure is effective in the prehospital setting *Prehosp Emerg Care* 2012;16:217–21·

14 Guidelines for the Diagnosis and Management of Asthma (EPR-3) 2007. Available at: www.nhlbi.nih.gov/guidelines/asthma/index.htm

15 Knapp B, Wood C. The prehospital administration of intravenous methylprednisolone lowers hospital admission rates for moderate to severe asthma. *Prehosp Emerg Care* 2003;7:423–6.

16 Gibbs MA, Camargo CA Jr, Rowe BH, Silverman RA. State of the art: therapeutic controversies in severe acute asthma. *Acad Emerg Med* 2000;7:800–15.

17 Rowe BH, Bretzlaff JA, Bourdon C, Bota GW, Camargo CA Jr. Intravenous magnesium sulfate treatment for acute asthma in the emergency department: a systematic review of the literature. *Ann Emerg Med* 2000;36:181–90.

18 Beers SL, Abramo TJ, Bracken A, Wiebe RA. Bilevel positive airway pressure in the treatment of status asthmaticus in pediatrics. *Am J Emerg Med* 2007;25:6–9.

19 Williams AM, Abramo TJ, Shah MV, et al. Safety and clinical findings of BiPAP utilization in children 20 kg or less for asthma exacerbations. *Int Care Med* 2011;37:1338–43.

20 Chung KF, Adcock IM. Multifaceted mechanisms in COPD: inflammation, immunity, and tissue repair and destruction. *Eur Respir J* 2008;31:1334–56.

21 Celli BR. Update on the management of COPD. *Chest* 2008;133:1451–62.

22 DiDomenico RJ, Park HY, Southworth MR, et al. Guidelines for acute decompensated heart failure treatment. *Ann Pharmacother* 2004;38:649–60.

23 Rogers RL, Feller ED, Gottlieb SS. Acute congestive heart failure in the emergency department. *Cardiol Clin* 2006;24:115–23.

24 Engelberg S, Singer AJ, Moldashel J, Sciammarella J, Thode HC, Henry M. Effects of prehospital nitroglycerin hemodynamics and chest pain intensity. *Prehosp Emerg Care* 2000;4:290–3.

25 Peacock WF, Hollander JE, Diercks DB, Lopatin M, Fonarow G, Emerman CL. Morphine and outcomes in acute decompensated heart failure: an ADHERE analysis. *Emerg Med J* 2008;25:205–9.

26 Naughton MT, Rahman MA, Hara K, Floras JS, Bradley TD. Effect of continuous positive airway pressure on intrathoracic and left ventricular transmural pressures in patients with congestive heart failure. *Circulation* 1995;91:1725–31.

27 Kallio T, Kuisma M, Alaspää A, Rosenberg PH. The use of prehospital continuous positive airway pressure treatment in presumed acute severe pulmonary edema. *Prehosp Emerg Care* 2003;7:209–13.

28 Kosowsky JM, Stephanides SL, Branson RD, Sayre MR. Prehospital use of continuous positive airway pressure (CPAP) for presumed pulmonary edema: a preliminary case series. *Prehosp Emerg Care* 2001;5:190–6.

29 Prosen G, Klemen P, Strnad M, Grmec S. Combination of lung ultrasound (a comet-tail sign) and N-terminal pro-brain natriuretic peptide in differentiating acute heart failure from chronic obstructive pulmonary disease and asthma as cause of acute dyspnea in prehospital setting. *Center Crit Care* 2011;15:1–9.

30 Neesse A, Jerrentrup A, Hoffmann S, et al. Prehospital chest emergency sonography trial in Germany: a prospective study. *Eur J Emerg Med* 2012;19:161–6.

31 Kline JA, Courtney DM, Kabrhel C, et al. Prospective multicenter evaluation of the pulmonary embolism rule-out criteria. *J Thromb Haemost* 2008;6:772–80.

32 Lee JA, Zierler BK, Zierler RE. The risk factors and clinical outcomes of upper extremity deep vein thrombosis. *Vasc Endovasc Surg* 2012;46:139–44.

33 Kosuge M, Kimura K, Ishikawa T, et al. Electrocardiographic differentiation between acute pulmonary embolism and acute coronary syndromes on the basis of negative T waves. *Am J Cardiol* 2007;99:817–21.

34 Courtney DM, Kline JA. Prospective use of a clinical decision rule to identify pulmonary embolism as likely cause of outpatient cardiac arrest. *Resuscitation* 2005;65:57–64.

35 Perrott J, Henneberry RJ, Zed PJ. Thrombolytics for cardiac arrest: case report and systematic review of controlled trials. *Ann Pharmacother* 2010;44:2007–13.

36 Abu-Laban RB, Christenson JM, Innes GD, et al. Tissue plasminogen activator in cardiac arrest with pulseless electrical activity. *N Engl J Med* 2002;346:1522–8.

CHAPTER 6

Oxygenation and ventilation

Vincent N. Mosesso and Angus M. Jameson

Introduction

Oxygenation and ventilation are critical life-sustaining functions, and their evaluation and management are primary components of out-of-hospital care. While these two parameters are related, they are distinct physiological functions that require independent assessment. The focus of this chapter will be on diagnostic aids and management, and EMS physicians and providers must develop and maintain expert physical examination skills for the proper assessment of these important processes. The astute provider will observe for demeanor, mentation, ability to speak, ease and volume of air exchange, work of breathing, upper or lower airway obstruction, pulmonary congestion, and central and peripheral cyanosis. These findings should be considered together with diagnostic test results to determine the status of oxygenation and ventilation in an individual patient, whether intervention is needed, and, if so, which treatment modalities are indicated.

Assessment of oxygenation

Adequate oxygen delivery to body tissues is a necessity for life, and is dependent on both the transfer of oxygen from the alveolar airspace to the blood and sufficient tissue perfusion with oxygenated blood. Oxygenation of the blood is dependent on a number of distinct factors, each of which can be impaired by various pathological processes (Table 6.1). Normal hemoglobin oxygen saturation in peripheral arterial blood is 96–99%. It is important to understand the relation between oxygen saturation and the partial pressure of oxygen. This is depicted by the oxyhemoglobin saturation curve (Figure 6.1). This curve demonstrates that above 90%, the saturation percentage is very insensitive to changes in partial pressure of oxygen between 750 and 760 mmHg. This means that, especially in patients on supplemental oxygen, severe impairment

in oxygen transfer into the blood can occur without major changes in the saturation level. Considered another way, as long as the partial pressure of oxygen in blood is at least 60 mmHg, hemoglobin is able to transport oxygen efficiently to the periphery.

Several tools have been developed that can reliably measure oxygenation of blood in the prehospital environment. Portable devices are available that can measure oxygen content in arterial blood samples (i.e. pO_2). However, because of cost and the need to perform arterial puncture, these devices are typically only used at selected special event venues and by critical care teams. Most commonly, oxygen levels in the field are determined by pulse oximetry (i.e. SpO_2). This simple, non-invasive method reports the percentage of hemoglobin in arteriolar blood that is in a saturated state. It is critically important for prehospital clinicians to understand that standard pulse oximetry does not discriminate between hemoglobin saturated with oxygen and hemoglobin saturated with carbon monoxide (oxyhemoglobin versus carboxyhemoglobin). In cases of carbon monoxide exposure, pulse oximetry will be misleading to the unsuspecting clinician [1]. Fortunately, newer generation devices, cooximeters, are now available and can measure carboxyhemoglobin levels distinct from oxyhemoglobin [2].

Pulse oximetry may also be unreliable in states of low tissue perfusion, such as with shock or local vasoconstriction due to cold temperature. Additionally, as this technology relies on transmission and reflection of light waves, barriers such as fingernail polish or skin disease can interfere with accuracy.

Measurement of tissue oxygenation (StO_2) uses near-infrared light resorption to measure oxygen saturation of blood in the skin and underlying soft tissue. This allows assessment of oxygen delivery to local tissue rather than simply the amount of oxygen circulating in the arterial system. Initial studies are promising, but further research will be needed to determine the most appropriate clinical use of this modality [3].

Emergency Medical Services: Clinical Practice and Systems Oversight, Second Edition. Volume 1: Clinical Aspects of EMS.
Edited by David C. Cone, Jane H. Brice, Theodore R. Delbridge, and J. Brent Myers.
© 2015 NAEMSP. Published 2015 by John Wiley & Sons, Inc. Companion Website: www.wiley.com\go\cone\naemsp

Table 6.1 Conditions that impair oxygen transfer in the lungs

Physiological process	Pathological conditions
Partial pressure of oxygen in inhaled air	Displacement by other gases
Minute ventilation (volume of air inhaled per minute)	External compression of chest
	Muscle weakness (chest wall and/or diaphragm)
	Central nervous system control malfunction
	Decreased lung compliance
	Pneumothorax
	Hemothorax and pleural effusion
Diffusion of oxygen across the alveolar membrane	Pneumonitis
	Alveolar and/or interstitial edema
Perfusion of the alveoli	Decreased cardiac output
	Hypotension
	Shunting

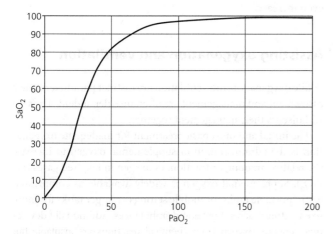

Figure 6.1 Oxygen-hemoglobin dissociation curve.

Assessment of ventilation

Ventilation refers to the volume of air moved in and out of the lungs, and is measured as minute ventilation (volume of air exchanged per minute, which can be estimated by the equation tidal volume × respiratory rate). Normal ventilation ranges from 6 to 7 L/minute. Although hypoventilation can lead to decreased oxygenation and hemoglobin oxygen saturation, ventilatory effectiveness is better evaluated by how well carbon dioxide (CO_2) is being eliminated. Ventilation can be compromised by a number of conditions (Box 6.1), and its assessment is of equal importance to that of oxygenation.

Ventilatory function can be determined directly by measuring the volume of air inhaled or exhaled per minute or indirectly by measuring the CO_2 level in blood or exhaled air. The partial pressure of carbon dioxide (pCO_2) may be measured in either arterial or venous blood samples using portable devices, as both provide similar results. However, just as oxygen content in the blood is usually assessed by non-invasive modalities in the out-of-hospital setting, so too is CO_2. Three types of devices are currently

Box 6.1   Conditions that impair ventilation

Airway obstruction
  Upper
  Lower (asthma, chronic obstructive pulmonary disease)
Muscle weakness (may be neurological)
Pleural effusion (large)
Pneumothorax
Sucking chest wound
Diaphragmatic malfunction (e.g. rupture, paralysis)
Pleuritic pain
Medications and recreational substances
  Opioids
  Sedatives
  Oxygen (in patients with hypoxic drive)

Box 6.2   Factors that affect EtCO$_2$

True decrease in blood $PaCO_2$
  • Hyperventilation (primary or secondary)
  • Shock/cardiac arrest (with constant ventilation)
  • Hypothermia /decreased metabolism
True increase in blood $PaCO_2$
  • Hypoventilation
  • Return of circulation after cardiac arrest
  • Improved perfusion after severe shock
  • Tourniquet release
  • Administration of sodium bicarbonate
  • Fever/increased metabolism
  • Thyroid storm
Increased gap between blood $PaCO_2$ and $EtCO_2$
  • Severe hypoventilation
  • Increased alveolar dead space
  • Decreased perfusion
  • Disconnected or clogged tubing

in use to detect and measure the presence and level of CO_2 in exhaled air, which serves as a surrogate for the level of CO_2 in blood. The simplest, but least useful, are semi-quantitative colorimetric devices that use litmus paper to detect the acid generated by absorption of CO_2 from exhaled air. These devices are compromised by prolonged exposure to air and by contamination from acidic gastric secretions. They may not be able to detect the extremely low levels of CO_2 generated by patients in cardiac arrest. For these reasons and due to the increasing availability of devices that can measure and continuously monitor exhaled CO_2, colorimetric devices are being used less often than quantitative devices.

Capnometry uses light absorption to measure the level of CO_2 in exhaled air. Clinically the level at the end of exhalation is the most useful value and is referred to as end-tidal CO_2 ($EtCO_2$). This measurement reflects the CO_2 content in alveolar gas and therefore in the pulmonary venous blood returning to the left heart. The $EtCO_2$ level is typically about 5 mmHg lower than the actual pCO_2 level in the blood due to alveolar dead space, but various clinical conditions can widen this gap. Continuous waveform capnography provides additional information on the frequency and flow rate of inhalation and exhalation by displaying a graphic depiction of measured expired CO_2 versus time. Field providers should have a good understanding of the interpretation of $EtCO_2$ values as well as waveform morphology as they both are altered by a variety of clinical conditions and may provide diagnostic information to EMS clinicians [4] (Box 6.2).

As a monitor of respiratory function, capnography is superior to pulse oximetry because it changes nearly immediately with ventilation. On the other hand, hypoxia may be delayed by the body's reserve and the shape of the hemoglobin oxygen dissociation curve as discussed above. When capnography waveform analysis is included, a near real-time assessment is possible and EMS clinicians may identify inadequacy of ventilation or the presence of various respiratory disease states, and they may glean information about circulatory and metabolic function as well.

When $EtCO_2$ values rise above normal ranges (35–40 mmHg), impaired ventilation is easily detected. When combined with waveform analysis, respiratory effort may also be monitored as to rate and depth of breathing. When respiratory rate or respiratory depth has become inadequate and $EtCO_2$ values rise, clinicians can initiate or augment respiratory support prior to the development of hypoxia. In the prehospital environment, this application of waveform capnography is especially useful in monitoring respiratory status following the administration of opiate analgesics, benzodiazepines, and other medications capable of producing respiratory depression (Figure 6.2).

Obstructive respiratory physiology is the most often described diagnosis made upon $EtCO_2$ waveform analysis. Both chronic obstructive pulmonary disease (COPD) and asthma fall into this category, and the waveform produced will be similar. The classic description of this waveform is the "shark fin" morphology consisting of a shallower upward sloping of the initial rise of the $EtCO_2$ wave (Figure 6.2a). This represents a slower

rate of exhalation and may be thought of as conceptually similar to the FEV_1 measurement of the pulmonary function test. This slower exhalation is precipitated by collapse or partial occlusion of bronchioles in emphysema and chronic bronchitis and spasm in acute asthma attacks. As the reactive airway physiology is relieved with bronchodilation, the initial upward segment will become more vertical. In more severe cases, the numeric value of the $EtCO_2$ will also rise, heralding respiratory insufficiency, and should lead the clinician to consider ventilatory support measures.

Although less commonly employed, $EtCO_2$ and waveform analysis may also be useful in assessment of metabolic derangements such as diabetic ketoacidosis and aspirin overdose. These conditions cause a respiratory compensation to a metabolic acidosis and will present with hyperventilation, typically with a decreasing level of $EtCO_2$. But, potentially due to markedly high CO_2 production, the $EtCO_2$ level may not decrease or it may even increase.

Assisting oxygenation and ventilation

While oxygenation and ventilation are distinct parameters, their assessment and management are often interdependent. Thus we will discuss their management together.

The initial and most basic treatment for inadequate oxygenation is the administration of supplemental oxygen to increase the relative amount, or fraction, of oxygen in inspired gases (i.e. FiO_2). Supplemental oxygen is widely available as compressed gas in portable tanks for mobile settings or larger tanks for more fixed settings such as homes and ambulances. Additionally, devices that generate oxygen from chemical reactions are available but typically provide short duration of flow. Oxygen concentrators are often used in the outpatient setting by persons with chronic

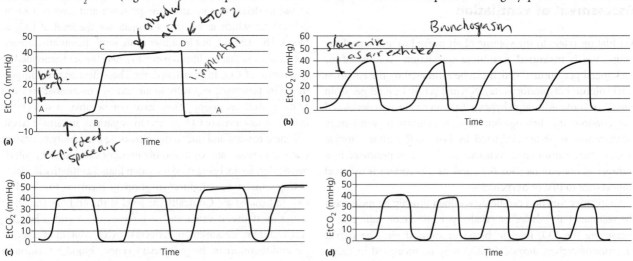

Figure 6.2 Capnography waveforms. (a) Normal waveform. Point A is beginning of expiration. A-B is expiration of dead space air. B-C shows rapid rise in level of CO_2 as air from lungs is exhaled. C-D is the plateau phase representing primarily alveolar air. D represents the value used for determination of $EtCO_2$. D-A represents inspiration. (b) Effect of bronchospasm. Note the slower rise in the CO_2 level leading to the so-called shark fin waveform. (c) Hypoventilation. (d) Hyperventilation.

hypoxemia. Fixed venues may have plumbed systems from central oxygen storage tanks.

Oxygen should be provided to all patients with respiratory distress, with any clinical markers of respiratory compromise (e.g. altered mental status), or with measured inadequate oxygenation or ventilation. There is an increasing trend toward more selective application of oxygen with the growing recognition of oxygen toxicity. Newer recommendations suggest administering supplemental oxygen only if the oxygen saturation is <94%. Unnecessarily elevating the pO_2 above normal levels may in fact be harmful to patients experiencing neurological or cardiac insults associated with ischemic damage [5].

Patients with underlying pulmonary disease, such as COPD and interstitial fibrosis, may have oxygen saturations below 94% on a chronic basis. A subset of these patients will also have chronically high pCO_2 levels (hypercapnia), which lead to dependence on a hypoxic drive for ventilatory control and stimulation. Providing supplemental oxygen, especially at high flow rates, may contribute to respiratory depression and potentially produce apnea [6]. Providers must carefully assess and monitor these patients, administering oxygen if needed and being prepared to assist ventilation.

Supplemental oxygen can be administered through various devices that deliver different ranges of oxygen concentration (Table 6.2). Most EMS systems carry the nasal cannula and non-rebreather face mask, allowing clinicians to choose either a higher or lower amount of FiO_2 supplementation. When supplemental oxygen itself does not lead to adequate oxygenation of blood, non-invasive positive pressure ventilation (NIPPV) can be beneficial to supplement ventilatory function in addition to providing increased FiO_2. This modality is most effective in patients with pulmonary edema, causing poor oxygen diffusion between alveolar air and pulmonary capillary blood. But, it is also useful for patients with other conditions, including asthma, COPD, and pulmonary hypertension. NIPPV is described in more detail below.

While hypoxemia in the setting of adequate ventilation can be treated with supplemental oxygen and augmentation of ventilatory function, inadequate ventilation requires immediate intervention. The provider must rapidly determine the likely cause (see Box 6.1) of the patient's ventilatory insufficiency and determine if it can be quickly corrected. Examples of this would be removal of upper airway obstruction, administration of bronchodilators for bronchospasm, sealing of sucking chest wounds, administration of naloxone for opioid overdose, and needle decompression of tension pneumothorax. Some conditions

cannot be immediately alleviated, particularly in the prehospital setting, such as muscle weakness from Guillain–Barré syndrome or severe physical fatigue, vital capacity reduction from a large pleural effusion, and non-reversible drug toxicity. In other cases, medical interventions may not be sufficiently effective immediately, such as for acute pulmonary edema or severe asthma. Whenever ventilation is compromised and cannot be immediately alleviated, mechanical ventilatory support must be provided. This can be accomplished non-invasively or invasively, through a device placed in the airway.

Non-invasive positive pressure support

Patients who are awake, protecting their airway, have respiratory drive, and can cooperate may be given ventilatory support with non-invasive modalities that provide positive airway pressure. These include continuous positive airway pressure (CPAP), which delivers constant pressure above that of the atmosphere throughout the ventilation cycle, and bilevel positive airway pressure (BiPAP), which delivers different pressures during the inspiratory and expiratory phases. Portable devices for the delivery of CPAP in the prehospital setting are generally of three types. Two of these require a high-pressure (50 psi) oxygen source. One continuously delivers oxygen under pressure to a mask with a pop-off valve that opens when the desired pressure is reached. The other uses a controller that essentially acts as a demand valve, adjusting flow to maintain the desired pressure. The third type of device uses oxygen flow from a standard regulator and a Venturi valve to create a virtual valve resulting in elevated pressure. Usually treatment is started at 5–10 cmH_2O and increased as needed to a maximum of 20 cmH_2O. Prehospital devices generally deliver near 100% FiO_2, while more advanced devices allow FiO_2 to be titrated. BiPAP is generally only available to EMS personnel who carry full-function mechanical ventilators, and so is not widely used in the prehospital setting.

Non-invasive positive pressure ventilation has been shown to improve oxygen delivery, likely due to the hydrostatic pressure effects of increasing the gas diffusion gradient, promoting displacement of fluid in the alveoli back into the capillary bed, and stenting open small bronchioles (which do not have cartilaginous walls), thereby increasing both the volume of air exchanged and the number of alveoli ventilated. NIPPV also decreases the work of breathing in these patients. The ultimate clinical effects are that patients will often have improved oxygenation, improved ventilation, marked improvement in respiratory distress, and a significantly lower likelihood of needing intubation and mechanical ventilation [7].

Bag-mask ventilation

Patients with marked respiratory failure may need more intensive ventilatory support. This is true for patients with inadequate ventilatory effort and those with depressed mental status who cannot protect their airways. Immediate assistance should be provided for these patients using a bag-mask (also known as bag-valve-mask) device to either assist spontaneous ventilations

Table 6.2 Devices for delivery of supplemental oxygen

Device name	O_2 flow rate (L/min)	FiO_2 (approximate %)
Nasal cannula	1–6	24–44
Simple face mask	5–12	35–55
Partial rebreather mask	8–15	35–60
Non-rebreather mask	8–15	60–95
Venturi mask	4–15	24–50
Tracheostomy mask	10–15	35–60

or provide full mechanical ventilation. Proper positioning (head and neck tilt, sniffing position), mechanical airway opening (jaw thrust or modified jaw thrust), and placement of a nasal or oral airway can markedly improve airflow. High-flow oxygen should flow into the bag device, preferably with a reservoir bag. Using this device can be difficult for a single provider, using one hand to seal the mask and the other to squeeze the bag. Whenever possible, a two-person technique should be used, with one provider using both hands and a jaw thrust maneuver to make a firm seal around the mask and open the airway, while the other provider squeezes the bag.

Providers must be cognisant of the volume and rate when assisting ventilation. Patients who are severely hypoxic or hypercarbic may initially require a period of hyperventilation, as do those with severe metabolic acidosis such as diabetic ketoacidosis or sepsis. However, absent such conditions, unnecessary hyperventilation will have detrimental effects, including decreased cerebral perfusion, venous return, and cardiac output, and metabolic impairment from respiratory alkalosis. Capnography can facilitate awareness of $EtCO_2$ levels, but this information must then be interpreted based on the clinical situation.

Mechanical ventilation

While bag-mask ventilation can be an effective and life-saving initial measure, it is difficult to maintain effectiveness in the longer term, especially in a moving vehicle. Additionally, it provides no protection from aspiration of stomach contents, blood, or other secretions. When adequately trained personnel are available, a more definitive airway should be sought in patients who have marked depression of consciousness, inability to protect their airway, or who require full mechanical ventilatory support to maintain oxygenation and ventilation. Usually this will entail placement of either an endotracheal tube or supraglottic advanced airway device (see Volume 1, Chapters 2–4). Patients can then be ventilated either manually (i.e. with a bag device) or with a portable mechanical ventilator. There are many models and types of mechanical ventilators and the decision on which to use should be based on local EMS system and patient characteristics.

Management of mechanical ventilators is a complex topic and a comprehensive tutorial is beyond the scope of this text. However, a basic understanding of the modes, settings, and troubleshooting of mechanical ventilators is important. Mechanical ventilators are typically used in the prehospital setting by air medical services and by ground critical care teams during interfacility transports. EMS providers may also encounter patients who are chronically on ventilators in residential or long-term care settings.

Modes of ventilation

There are three common modes of mechanical ventilation: assist control (AC), synchronized intermittent mandatory ventilation (SIMV), and pressure support (PS). The key to understanding these modes is recognizing that the time of the respiratory cycle (i.e. respiratory rate), tidal volume, flow rate, and pressure developed in the airways are all interdependent and affected by the individual patient's airway physiology. In each of these modes, different combinations of these variables are controlled by the machine, and the patient's respiratory function determines the uncontrolled variables.

In AC mode, the ventilator delivers a set tidal volume with each breath. A default respiratory rate is set but the patient may trigger breaths above that default rate. In AC mode the machine will deliver the full set tidal volume on either a patient-triggered or machine-triggered breath. SIMV is very similar to AC, and, in fact, in patients without spontaneous respiratory effort the two are effectively identical. The major difference is that in SIMV the machine does not deliver the full set tidal volume in response to a patient-triggered breath, but rather allows the patient's effort to determine the volume of the breath. In SIMV mode the ventilator will synchronize ventilator-triggered breaths with patient-triggered breaths, assuring that the set rate is met or exceeded. In both AC and SIMV care must be taken to monitor the airway pressures developed during the respiratory cycle. In contrast, PS mode delivers a set inspiratory pressure above a baseline positive end-expiratory pressure (PEEP) with each patient-triggered breath. The patient's respiratory drive determines the rate and the patient's lung compliance and airway resistance determine the tidal volume developed.

Ventilator settings and troubleshooting

Once the mode of ventilation is selected, prehospital providers will need to set several variables. In AC and SIMV modes, tidal volume (TV), respiratory rate (RR), and PEEP are all determined by the clinician. Tidal volumes are normally chosen to be 6–12 mL/kg of ideal body weight. Tidal volumes closer to 6 mL/kg are felt to be protective against the development of acute respiratory distress syndrome and should be used when possible [8]. Respiratory rates are often set at a default of 12 per minute, but should be adjusted based upon the patient's clinical situation (e.g. increased rate in patients who are dependent upon respiratory compensation of a metabolic acidosis).

Positive end-expiratory pressure may also be applied to assist with oxygenation via mechanisms similar to NIPPV, discussed above, and is often initially set at 5–10 mmHg. In patients with obstructive physiology (e.g. asthma and COPD), care should be taken to maximize expiratory time to avoid incomplete expiration and breath stacking which can lead to increased airway pressures. If air trapping is suspected, excess pressure can be alleviated by disconnecting the endotracheal tube from the ventilator for a few seconds and compressing on the patient's chest.

Peak inspiratory pressure (PIP) represents the maximum pressure developed during the inspiratory phase. Changes in PIP are a common source of ventilator alarms. Low PIP usually indicates a leak in the ventilator circuit. High PIP may represent either an increase in airway resistance (e.g. blocked tube, bronchospasm, secretions) or a decrease in lung compliance (e.g. pulmonary edema, atelectasis, pneumothorax, pleural effusion, hyperinflation). These two states can be distinguished by performing an inspiratory hold test to measure a plateau pressure. This test is performed by pressing the hold button on the ventilator for approximately 5 seconds during inspiration without allowing the patient to exhale. This effectively eliminates the airway resistance from the measured pressure and allows independent assessment of pressure being developed in the lungs with a given tidal volume. This is equivalent to a measurement of lung compliance. If the plateau pressure rises along with PEEP, clinicians should look for correctable causes of decreased lung compliance.

Pneumothorax

Pneumothorax is air in the otherwise "virtual space" between the parietal and visceral pleurae. The volume and pressure of the air in this space determine the clinical effect, which can range from asymptomatic to life-threatening. Early signs and symptoms may be subtle and the condition is often not expected. It is therefore important for EMS clinicians to maintain a high index of suspicion for pneumothorax in a variety of presenting complaints and to be aware of potential predisposing or associated conditions (Box 6.3).

Patients may present with pleuritic pain, sudden onset of a sharp pain, minimal to severe shortness of breath, and hypoxemia. Physical exam findings that should prompt consideration of pneumothorax include decreased or absent unilateral breath sounds, subcutaneous emphysema, and evidence of thoracic trauma. Pulse oximetry may or may not decrease depending on the size of the pneumothorax and the underlying pulmonary function and comorbidities of the individual patient. Similarly, $EtCO_2$ may or may not appreciably change and its interpretation may be further complicated by compensatory hyperventilation or other comorbid conditions. A potentially more sensitive indicator in patients already receiving mechanical ventilation may be decreases in tidal volumes and increases in peak pressures. Ultrasound, if available, can also be used to identify pneumothorax.

The one case in which a pneumothorax definitely should be recognized clinically is a tension pneumothorax. This occurs when the intrathoracic pressure is so great that ventilation and venous return to the heart are obstructed, leading to respiratory distress and shock. Besides unilateral decreased or absent breath sounds and subcutaneous emphysema, tracheal deviation and jugular venous distension may be present, but these should not be relied upon. Tension physiology must be recognized and treated immediately. A radiograph of a tension pneumothorax is considered a marker of suboptimal care (Figure 6.3).

Tension pneumothorax must be treated immediately with needle thoracostomy (needle decompression). To accomplish this, following skin cleansing, a large-bore IV catheter (14 gauge or larger) should be inserted through the anterior chest wall in the second intracostal space at the midclavicular line. When the needle enters the pleural space, a rush of air is often heard. The needle is then removed, leaving the catheter in place. Patients may require decompression with several needle thoracostomies in the prehospital environment as air reaccumulates in the pleural space. Needle decompression may alternatively be accomplished using the same technique at the fourth or fifth intracostal space at the anterior axillary line [9,10]. Some prefer this site because of the decreased likelihood of puncturing vascular structures. In either case, treatment failure is typically due to using too short a needle or the catheter becoming occluded, which requires placement of additional needle(s). The hub of the catheter should either be left open or attached to a Heimlich (one-way) valve. Subsequently, the patient should receive a formal thoracostomy tube placed on suction with water seal. This is often deferred until arrival in the emergency department but may be considered in the prehospital setting if an appropriately trained physician or other advanced provider is available and in the appropriate circumstances.

A patient with a penetrating wound to the chest should have an occlusive dressing applied with watchful monitoring for the

---

Box 6.3   Conditions associated with pneumothorax

Trauma
   Blunt
   Penetrating
Medical
   Acute asthma, especially if cardiac arrest
   Chronic obstructive pulmonary disease or other underlying lung
      disease
   Decompression-associated barotrauma
   Marfan syndrome (or marfanoid habitus)
   Thoracic endometriosis (catamenial)

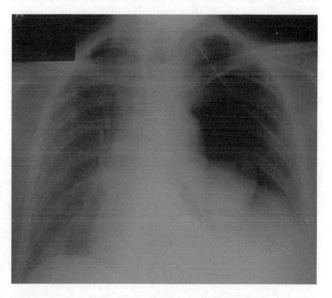

Figure 6.3 Radiograph of tension pneumothorax. Note thoracostomy tube on the left.

development of tension physiology. If tension develops, the dressing should be immediately vented. Some types of occlusive dressings provide one-way air flow (pleural space to environment) to prevent the accumulation of gas in the pleural space that leads to a tension pneumothorax. Alternatively, an occlusive dressing may be left unsealed on one side or corner, which allows it to act like a one-way flap valve.

A frequent concern with the management of patients with pneumothorax is air transport. Boyle's law ($P1 \times V1 = P2 \times V2$) describes that the air in the pleural space will expand with decreasing atmospheric pressure associated with increasing altitude. The EMS provider should be aware that helicopter transport is not typically associated with sufficient altitude to have a significant clinical effect. For example, most medical helicopters fly at 1,000–3,000 feet above the ground. But at 6,000 feet, an altitude sometimes associated with instrument flight conditions (e.g. inclement weather), the increase in size would be about 25% (e.g. $V2 = P1 \times V1/P2 = 760\,mmHg \times 100\,cc/609\,m mHg = 125\,cc$). The clinical effects of such an increase in pneumothorax size are very much patient specific, depending on such things as lung compliance and comorbid conditions. Patients generally should not be flown in fixed-wing aircraft (especially without cabin pressurization) without tube thoracostomy decompression [11].

Conclusion

Oxygenation and ventilation are distinctly different but interrelated physiological processes. In general, adequate oxygenation requires sufficient ventilation to deliver gas to alveolar spaces, where oxygen can then enter pulmonary capillaries for transport to peripheral tissues. Pulse oximetry is a useful tool, except in cases of carbon monoxide poisoning, to help determine the extent of tissue oxygenation. Patients with respiratory distress and/or SpO_2 less than 94% should receive supplemental oxygen. However, use of oxygen should not be indiscriminate.

Ventilation is about gas moving in and out of the lungs. Clearly, it can occur without oxygen, and in that sense is a distinct process. The adequacy of ventilation is generally assessed in terms of minute ventilation. Waveform capnography is a useful tool to both monitor ventilation and evaluate its effectiveness. NIPPV may provide needed support to an awake patient with inadequate ventilation but intact drive. Mechanical ventilation represents the option for maximum ventilatory support tool to deliver the greatest FiO_2. Especially in a dynamic prehospital environment, vigilant monitoring is imperative to promptly identify and address deficiencies in ventilation and oxygenation and complications arising from their treatment.

References

1 Chan ED, Chan MM, Chan MM. Pulse oximetry: understanding its basic principles facilitates appreciation of its limitations. *Respir Med* 2013;107(6):789–99.

2 Barker SJ, Curry J, Redford D, Morgan S. Measurement of carboxyhemoglobin and methemoglobin by pulse oximetry. *Anesthesiology* 2006;105(5):892–7.

3 Sagraves SG, Newell MA, Bard MR, et al. Tissue oxygenation monitoring in the field: a new EMS vital sign. *J Trauma* 2009;67(3):441–3.

4 Kodali BS. Capnography outside the operating rooms. *Anesthesiology* 2013;118:192–201.

5 Berg RA, Hemphill R, Abella BS. Part 5: Adult Basic Life Support: 2010 American Heart Association Guidelines for Cardiopulmonary Resuscitation and Emergency Cardiovascular Care. *Circulation* 2010;122:S695.

6 Austin MA, Wills KE, Blizzard L, et al. Effect of high flow oxygen on mortality in chronic obstructive disease patients in the prehospital setting: randomized controlled trial. *BMJ* 2013;341:c5462.

7 Williams B, Boyle M, Robertson N, Giddings C. When pressure is positive: a literature review of the prehospital use of continuous positive airway pressure. *Prehosp Disaster Med* 2013;28(1):52–60.

8 Acute Respiratory Distress Syndrome Network. Ventilation with lower tidal volumes as compared with traditional tidal volumes for acute lung injury and the acute respiratory distress syndrome. *N Engl J Med* 2000;342:1301–8.

9 Inaba K, Branco B, Eckstein M, et al. Optimal positioning for emergent needle thoracostomy: a cadaver-based study. *J Trauma* 2011;71:1099–103.

10 Sanchez LD, Straszewski S, Saghir A, et al. Anterior versus lateral needle decompression of tension pneumothorax: comparison by computed tomography chest wall measurement. *Acad Emerg Med* 2011;18:1022–6.

11 www.cs.amedd.army.mil/borden/book/ccc/UCLAchp3.pdf

SECTION III

Circulation

CHAPTER 7

Hypotension and shock

Ronald N. Roth, Raymond L. Fowler, and Francis X. Guyette

Introduction

Shock is a life-threatening physiological state characterized by decreased tissue perfusion and end-organ tissue dysfunction, and is a significant predictor for complications including death [1]. The presence of shock must be recognized and therapeutic interventions must be started early to prevent progression. Unfortunately, the identification and treatment of shock in the out-of-hospital setting are fraught with many difficulties and potential pitfalls. Patient assessment is often limited by the challenging out-of-hospital environment and lack of diagnostic and therapeutic options. The tools available for the diagnosis and treatment of shock in the field are limited. Even when shock is properly identified, the most appropriate out-of-hospital management is often unknown or the subject of great debate.

In the out-of-hospital setting, the identification of shock relies primarily on the recognition of signs and symptoms, including tachycardia, poor skin perfusion, and altered mental status. Note that hypotension, arbitrarily defined at a systolic blood pressure of less than 90 mmHg, is not an adequate definition of shock and may not adequately reflect the onset of tissue hypoperfusion [2]. Unfortunately, the early stages of compensated shock, with only subtle alterations in physical findings, are easily overlooked or misinterpreted by out-of-hospital care providers. Physiological changes associated with age, pregnancy, or treatment for medical conditions, such as beta-blockers for hypertension, may also mask or alter the body's compensatory responses. As a result, the patient with severe shock may present with near-normal vital signs.

Pathophysiology

Shock is a complex physiological process defined as the widespread reduction in tissue perfusion leading to cellular and organ dysfunction and death. In the early stages of shock, a series of complex compensatory mechanisms act to preserve critical organ perfusion [3]. In general, the following relationships drive this process.

Blood pressure = Cardiac output × Peripheral vascular resistance
Cardiac output = Heart rate × Stroke volume

Any condition that lowers cardiac output and/or peripheral vascular resistance may decrease blood pressure. Alterations of heart rate (very low or very high) can lower cardiac output and hence blood pressure secondary to decreased cardiac filling. Also, decreasing stroke volume may lower cardiac output with a possible reduction in perfusion, as well. Stroke volume may be reduced by lower circulating blood volume (e.g. hemorrhage or dehydration), by damage to the heart (e.g. myocardial infarction or myocarditis), or by conditions obstructing blood flow through the thorax (e.g. tension pneumothorax, cardiac tamponade, or extensive pulmonary embolism).

To aid in the evaluation and treatment of shock, it is often useful for the physician and EMS personnel to categorize the etiology of the shock condition [4]. Most EMS providers are familiar with the "pump-fluid-pipes" model of the cardiovascular system, with the pump representing the heart, pipes representing the vascular system, and fluid representing the blood [5]. Thus, categorizing shock into four categories may help prehospital providers and EMS physicians organize their assessments and approaches (Table 7.1). Accurate physical assessment is vital for the EMS provider to determine the etiology of the shock state (Box 7.1).

Evaluation

The diagnosis of shock depends on a combination of key historical features and physical findings in the proper clinical setting. For example, tachycardia and hypotension in an elderly patient with fever, cough, and dyspnea may represent pneumonia with septic shock. Hemorrhagic shock should be suspected in a middle-aged man with epigastric pain, hematemesis, melena,

Emergency Medical Services: Clinical Practice and Systems Oversight, Second Edition. Volume 1: Clinical Aspects of EMS.
Edited by David C. Cone, Jane H. Brice, Theodore R. Delbridge, and J. Brent Myers.
© 2015 NAEMSP. Published 2015 by John Wiley & Sons, Inc. Companion Website: www.wiley.com\go\cone\naemsp

Table 7.1 Categories of shock

Type of shock	Disorder	Examples	Comments

Hypovolemic	Decreased intravascular fluid volume	A. External fluid loss
		  1. Hemorrhage
		  2. Gastrointestinal losses
		  3. Renal losses
		  4. Cutaneous loss
		B. Internal fluid loss
		  1. Fractures
		  2. Intestinal obstruction
		  3. Hemothorax
		  4. Hemoperitoneum
		  5. Third spacing
			Hypovolemic shock states, especially hemorrhagic shock, produce flat neck veins, tachycardia, and pallor

Distributive	Increased "pipe" size: peripheral vasodilation	A. Drug or toxin induced B. Spinal cord injury C. Sepsis D. Anaphylaxis E. Hypoxia/anoxia	Distributive shock states usually show flat neck veins, tachycardia, and pallor. Neurogenic shock due to a cervical spinal cord injury tends to show flat neck veins, normal or low pulse rate, and pink skin
Obstruction	Pipe obstruction	A. Pulmonary embolism B. Tension pneumothorax C. Cardiac tamponade D. Severe aortic stenosis E. Venocaval obstruction	Obstructive shock states tend to produce jugular venous distension, tachycardia, and cyanosis
Cardiogenic	"Pump" problems	A. Myocardial infarction B. Arrhythmias C. Cardiomyopathy D. Acute valvular incompetence E. Myocardial contusion F. Myocardial infarction G. Cardiotoxic drugs/poisons	Cardiogenic shock states tend to produce jugular venous distension, tachycardia, and cyanosis

---

Box 7.1 Signs and symptoms of shock

Cardiovascular
- Tachycardia, arrhythmias, hypotension
- Jugular venous distension in obstructive and cardiogenic shock states
- Tracheal deviation away from the affected side in tension pneumothorax

Central nervous system
- Agitation, confusion
- Alterations in level of consciousness
- Coma

Respiratory
- Tachypnea, dyspnea

Skin
- Pallor, diaphoresis
- Cyanosis (in obstructive and cardiogenic shock cases), mottling

---

and hypotension. Hypotension, tachycardia, and an urticarial rash in a victim of a recent bee sting strongly suggest distributive shock secondary to anaphylaxis. Obstructive shock precipitated by a tension pneumothorax should be suspected in a hypotensive trauma patient with unilateral decreased breath sounds and tracheal deviation to the opposite side.

An important problem in the prehospital diagnosis of shock is the frequent inaccuracy of field assessment. For example, Cayten et al. found an error rate of more than 20% for vital signs obtained by emergency medical technicians (EMTs) in a non-emergency setting [6]. The researchers suggest that when critical medical decisions will be based on the data gathered in the field, multiple assessments should be performed.

Emergency medical services providers should look for the signs and symptoms of system-wide reduction in tissue perfusion, such as tachycardia, tachypnea, mental status changes, and cool, clammy skin (see Box 7.1). When available, adjunctive technologies can provide improved recognition and assessment of shock by demonstrating reductions in expired CO_2, hypovolemia, obstruction, or poor contractility on ultrasound, and elevated serum lactate levels.

Vital signs that fall outside of expected ranges must be correlated with the overall clinical presentation. Vital signs have a broad range of normal values and must be interpreted in the context of the individual patient. A petite 45 kg, 16-year-old female with lower abdominal pain with a reported blood pressure of 88 mmHg systolic by palpation may have a ruptured ectopic pregnancy, or may just be at her baseline blood pressure. An elderly patient with significant epistaxis may be hypertensive due to catecholamine release and vasoconstriction despite being relatively volume depleted. Consideration should be given to patient age, comorbid conditions, and medications that may affect the interpretation of vital signs.

In the noisy field environment, providers often measure blood pressure by palpation rather than auscultation. Blood pressure by palpation provides only an estimate of systolic pressure [7]. Without an auscultated diastolic pressure, the pulse pressure (difference between systolic and diastolic pressure) cannot be calculated. A pulse pressure less than 30 mmHg or 25% of the

SBP may provide an early clue to the presence of hypovolemic or obstructive shock. Conversely, a wide pulse pressure may be indicative of distributive shock [3]. Dividing the pulse rate by the systolic pressure typically produces a ratio of approximately 0.5 to 0.8, which is called the "shock index." When that ratio exceeds 1.0, then a shock state may be present [8].

Previously healthy victims of acute hypovolemic shock may maintain relatively normal vital signs with up to 25% blood volume loss [3]. Sympathetic nervous system stimulation with vasoconstriction and increased cardiac contractility may result in a normal blood pressure in the face of decreasing intravascular volume, especially in the pediatric population. In some patients with intraabdominal bleeding (e.g. ruptured abdominal aneurysm, ectopic pregnancy), the pulse may be relatively bradycardic despite significant blood loss [9].

Emergency medical services personnel may equate "normal" vital signs with normal cardiovascular status [5]. The field team may be lulled into a false sense of security initially if the early signs of shock are overlooked, only to be caught off guard when the patient's condition dramatically worsens during transport. Following trends in the vital signs may also help identify shock before patients reach abnormal vital sign triggers. Early recognition and aggressive treatment of shock may prevent progression to the later stages of shock that can result in the death of potentially salvageable patients [10].

Prehospital hypotension may predict in-hospital morbidity and mortality in both trauma and medical patients [11–13]. Jones et al. noted a 30% higher mortality rate for medical patients with prehospital hypotension [11]. Other studies have shown similar findings in trauma patients with prehospital hypotension, even with subsequent normotension in the emergency department [12,13]. Therefore, hospital providers should consider any episode of prehospital hypotension as evidence of significant shock and the presence of a critical illness.

Despite their questionable value, orthostatic vital signs are often evaluated in the emergency department, and occasionally in the field. A positive orthostatic vital sign test for pulse rate would result in a pulse increase of 30 beats per minute after 1 minute of standing [14]. Symptoms of lightheadedness or dizziness are considered a positive test. Occasionally, orthostatic vital signs are performed serendipitously by the patient who refuses treatment while lying down, then stands up to leave the scene, and suffers a syncopal episode. This demonstration of orthostatic hypotension is often helpful in convincing the patient to allow treatment and transport. However, rescuers should not equate absence of orthostatic response with euvolemia.

Capillary refill, an easy test to perform in the field setting, is not a useful test for mild-to-moderate hypovolemia [15]. Moreover, environmental considerations, such as cold temperatures and adverse lighting conditions, also affect the accuracy of this technique for shock assessment. On-scene estimates of blood loss by EMS providers may influence therapeutic interventions, including fluid administration. However, studies suggest that providers are not accurate at estimating spilled blood volumes [16].

Hypoxia is a common manifestation of shock states. Patients in various stages of exsanguination may not have sufficient blood volume to adequately perfuse the body with oxygen. Unfortunately, pulse oximetry alone cannot detect the adequacy of oxygen delivery. Pulse oximetry may fail to detect a pulse when blood flow is reduced [17,18]. Like pulse oximetry, capnography may also serve as an important tool in the evaluation and treatment of shock in the prehospital setting [19–22]. Capnography is the measurement of the exhalation of carbon dioxide from the lungs. Exhaled end-tidal carbon dioxide ($EtCO_2$) levels vary inversely with minute ventilation, providing feedback regarding the effect of changes in ventilatory parameters [23,24]. Additionally, changes in $EtCO_2$ are virtually immediate when the airway is obstructed or the endotracheal tube becomes dislodged [25]. $EtCO_2$ concentration may be influenced by factors other than ventilation. For example, $EtCO_2$ levels are reduced when pulmonary perfusion decreases in shock, cardiac arrest, and pulmonary embolism [26–28]. $EtCO_2$ is most useful as an indicator of perfusion when minute ventilation is held constant (e.g. when mechanical ventilation is applied) [20,26]. Under these conditions, changes in $EtCO_2$ levels reliably indicate changes in pulmonary perfusion. In any patient suffering from a potential shock state, diminished $EtCO_2$ should be a warning of the critical nature of the patient's problem.

Future technologies in the assessment of shock

Use of portable ultrasound in the field can facilitate the recognition of immediately life-threatening causes of shock including intraabdominal hemorrhage, cardiac tamponade, or an abdominal aortic aneurysm. Many EMS agencies, primarily air medical services, have deployed ultrasound for field evaluations, including the focused assessment by sonography in trauma (FAST) examination [29]. Ultimately, the EMS medical director must determine if the cost and time of acquiring equipment, training, and performing the skills translates into improved patient outcomes. The use of field ultrasound has the potential to worsen patient outcome if the procedure delays the time to definitive care, does not influence patient destination or care, or interferes with basic skills (e.g., airway maintenance).

There is growing interest in the use of biomarkers that can be used to identify, monitor, and predict the outcome in shock [30]. Point-of-care testing devices make measurement of biomarkers in the field an attractive option. Elevation of the serum lactate may reflect anaerobic tissue metabolism in acute sepsis and shock [30–32]. In the emergency department, elevated lactate in the setting of infection indicates septic shock and the need for early sepsis therapy. Elevated point-of-care venous lactate is associated with increased mortality risk and the need for resuscitative care in trauma patients. Indeed, recent work by the RESUSCITATION OUTCOMES CONSORTIUM in prehospital trauma research indicates that lactate levels may rise before blood pressure drops, and that an elevated lactate level in the setting of trauma may be a useful predictor of a patient that will require aggressive resuscitation. Serial lactate measurements may indicate the progress of ongoing resuscitation [33].

In summary, although technology may offer future value, the current evaluation of the potential shock victim in the out-of-hospital setting is challenging due both to limited assessment capability in this environment as well as fewer diagnostic tools. Both the provider and the medical oversight physician must be cautioned on placing too much emphasis on a single set of vital signs or a limited assessment.

General approach to shock

All treatment approaches to shock must include the following basic principles.

1 Perform the initial assessment.
2 Deal with issues identified in the initial assessment such as airway, breathing, and circulation issues, including active external bleeding.
3 Determine need for early definitive care.
   • Hemorrhage control and volume resuscitation
   • Needle thoracostomy
   • Electrical therapy for dysrhythmia
   • Invasive airway management
4 Maintain adequate oxygen saturation ($SaO_2 > 94\%$).
5 Ensure adequate ventilation without hyperventilating.
6 Monitor vital signs, ECG, oxygen saturation, capnography, and lactate (if available).
7 Prevent additional injury or exacerbation of existing medical conditions.
8 Protect the patient from the environment.
9 Determine the etiology of the shock state, and treat accordingly.
10 Notify and transport to an appropriate facility.

Often the etiology of the patient's shock state and the initial management options are clear from the history. For example, the out-of-hospital treatment of a young, previously healthy college student with hypotension secondary to severe vomiting and diarrhea includes IV fluids. The treatment of cardiogenic shock in an unresponsive elderly patient with ventricular tachycardia (VT) requires prompt cardioversion. Occasionally, the primary problem may be strongly suspected but not readily diagnosable or treatable in the field (e.g. pulmonary embolism). Less frequent, but most difficult to manage, is the patient in shock without an obvious cause. With the understanding of the limited treatment options in the out-of-hospital setting (primarily fluids, inotropic agents, and vasopressors), field treatment may be individualized for the four categories of shock: hypovolemic, distributive, obstructive, and cardiogenic.

Hypovolemic shock

Hypovolemic shock is the result of significant loss of intravascular volume resulting in hypotension. The many etiologies of hypovolemic shock include external fluid loss and shifting of fluids from the vascular system to a non-vascular body compartment. The treatment of hypotension and shock caused by hypovolemia is relatively straightforward. External bleeding should be controlled. Fluid replacement via vascular access is the mainstay of treatment. Unfortunately, the ideal fluid for the resuscitation of hypovolemic shock and the amount of fluids that should be provided remains controversial [34–46].

Distributive shock

Distributive shock, characterized by a decrease in systemic vascular resistance, is associated with abnormal distribution of microvascular blood flow [47]. Causes of distributive shock include sepsis, anaphylaxis, medication overdose, and acute neurological injury. The treatment of distributive shock involves the combination of vasoactive medications, which constrict the dilated vasculature, and fluids, which fill the expanded vascular tree. Commonly used vasoactive medications in the out-of-hospital setting for distributive shock include epinephrine, norepinephrine, and dopamine. Although epinephrine is easily administered via several routes (e.g. intramuscular, intravenous bolus or infusion), the drug has significant side-effects. Norepinephrine infusions are associated with a lower incidence of cardiac dysrhythmias than either dopamine or epinephrine [48]. In addition, recent studies of cardiogenic shock suggest increased mortality associated with dopamine [49]. However, continuous infusions may be difficult to maintain without special infusion pumps.

Obstructive shock

Obstructive causes of shock are often difficult to diagnose and treat. If possible, the obstruction should be resolved, such as by decompression of a tension pneumothorax. However, when the primary problem cannot be treated successfully in the field (e.g. massive pulmonary embolus or cardiac tamponade), intravenous fluids may be helpful in increasing preload and temporarily improving the condition.

Cardiogenic shock

Causes of cardiogenic shock include arrhythmias, valvular heart disease, cardiotoxic agents, and myocardial infarction. As a result, cardiogenic shock requires individualized treatment. Cardiogenic shock from severe dysrhythmias should be treated with appropriate electrical or pharmacological therapy. "Pump failure" is often difficult to diagnosis and to treat without invasive monitoring. Adult patients without obvious pulmonary edema may benefit from fluid challenges of approximately 200–300 mL of crystalloid. An improvement in the patient's condition suggests that enhancing preload would be beneficial. A worsening of the patient's condition with a modest fluid challenge, or the presence of obvious pulmonary edema on initial evaluation, suggests that fluid therapy would not be helpful. In such settings, treatment with inotropic agents or pressors, such as dobutamine or norepinephrine, would be more appropriate. Intravenous infusions are often difficult to manage in the field without an infusion pump and must be monitored closely.

The causes of cardiogenic shock also can include beta-blocker and calcium channel blocker toxicity. These agents block sympathomimetic receptors, impairing the body's normal compensatory responses. These patients present with profound bradycardia and shock, often refractory to sympathomimetic treatment and fluid challenges due to the receptor blockade. Alternative therapies may include IV glucagon or calcium, which facilitates heart rate stimulation and vasoconstriction through alternative cellular receptors, and which many EMS agencies carry for the treatment of hypoglycemia.

Shock of unclear etiology

In a few disconcerting situations, the primary etiology for the patient's shock state may be difficult to determine. The primary treatment decision is whether or not to give fluids. In hypovolemic, distributive, and obstructive shock, fluids are an appropriate initial treatment for hypotension, given the important caveats mentioned above regarding that in the setting of uncontrolled hemorrhage, indiscriminate administration of large volumes of IV fluids may not improve patient outcome. Some cases of cardiogenic shock will respond to fluids. However, fluids should not be given to patients in cardiogenic shock with pulmonary edema. Fluids are also not appropriate when cardiogenic shock has been precipitated by a treatable arrhythmia. Response to fluid challenges (where appropriate) should dictate whether additional fluid challenges should be given or whether a trial of a sympathomimetic agent should be used.

Occasionally, shock will be refractory to initial attempts at resuscitation. This may reflect the need for definitive care in the hospital (e.g., thoracotomy, laparotomy). If, after vigorous field treatment, the patient remains hypotensive, other etiologies for the hypotension must be considered, including adrenal suppression, hypothyroidism, or toxidromes. In some cases patients with profound acidosis will not respond to vasopressors or inotropes, as their receptors are pH dependent. Administration of sodium bicarbonate at 1 mEq/kg may improve perfusion by buffering acidosis and increasing vasopressor activity. Use of vasopressin to supplement other vasopressors may also improve perfusion as it increases systemic vascular resistance even during acidosis. In cases of refractory shock or adrenal suppression, administration of steroids may also be of benefit. Hydrocortisone is ideal for this purpose, as patients may benefit from both mineralocorticoid and glucocorticoid properties. Methylprednisolone is far more widely available in the prehospital environment and may have some limited utility in refractory shock. Patients exposed to potent cellular toxins such as cyanide or hydrogen sulfide may also present with refractory shock, prompting therapy with agent-specific antidotes.

Shock in the pediatric population

The recognition and management of shock in the pediatric population follow the same general principles as in adults, with a few notable exceptions [50]. Children in shock more commonly present with a low cardiac output and a relatively high systemic vascular resistance (SVR). This has been described as "cold shock," as opposed to the low-SVR state or "warm shock" frequently seen in adults. Children presenting in distributive shock usually require more aggressive fluid resuscitation with volumes of 60 cc/kg or more [51]. If children fail to respond to the initial fluid resuscitation, epinephrine is preferred as the first-line vasopressor in order to counter the relatively low cardiac output seen in pediatric shock. Additional support for patients with low SVR and wide pulse pressure may be provided with norepinephrine or vasopressin. Dobutamine may provide inotropic and chronotropic support in patients with very low cardiac output and improve delivery of oxygen to tissues.

Following initial treatment with fluids and vasoactive agents, pediatric patients may also benefit from adjunctive therapies for shock [50]. Early airway management should be considered, as children may use up to 40% of their cardiac output to support the work of breathing. Ketamine is the preferred induction agent as it preserves cardiac output and will not result in the hypotension or adrenal suppression potentially seen with other induction agents. Hydrocortisone should be administered to children with adrenal insufficiency. Transport to an appropriate facility with pediatric critical care should be an important consideration.

Shock interventions

Fluids

The treatment of shock must be customized to the individual EMS agency and geographic location. In the urban setting with short transport times, the victim of a penetrating cardiac wound probably benefits most from hemorrhage control, airway maintenance, and rapid transport to the hospital. IV or IO access could be attempted en route if it will not delay delivery to definitive care [43]. On the other hand, with longer transport times in the rural setting, a similar patient might benefit from carefully titrated crystalloid volume infusion during the transport. Fluid delivery could be initiated while the patient is en route to the hospital, thereby prolonging neither scene time nor time until definitive care [44]. In the patient who presents a difficult IV access problem, IO infusions may be attempted. Placing the IO needle in the humeral head may result in faster infusion rates than the proximal tibia.

The ideal fluid for use in the field would be small in volume, portable, non-allergenic, inexpensive, and would not interfere with clotting factors [34]. Unfortunately, this ideal fluid has yet to be discovered. Isotonic crystalloids are currently the fluid of choice for out-of-hospital resuscitation in the United States [1,35,38,44]. They are inexpensive and widely available but may contribute to dilutional coagulopathy, hyperchloremic acidosis, and hypothermia when given in large volumes.

Whole blood would arguably provide the greatest benefit as a resuscitation fluid in the setting of hemorrhagic shock but is impractical due to issues of cost storage and availability. Use of blood products in the out-of-hospital environment is limited to a few air medical services which carry O-negative blood for administration to victims of hemorrhagic shock. Prehospital administration of plasma and factor concentrates is being investigated [52]. Several centers have studied hypertonic saline, colloids, and artificial blood substitutes as alternatives to isotonic saline [52,53]. Problems with these alternative fluids include high cost; increased risks including allergic reactions, kidney injury, coagulopathy, and hypernatremia; and lack of demonstrated benefit versus isotonic crystalloids [36–38,54,55]. As a result, none of the alternative fluids has gained widespread acceptance.

The optimal volume of fluids to administer in the out-of-hospital setting is not known, especially in the trauma victim with uncontrolled hemorrhage [35,39–46]. Older trauma algorithms indicate the administration of 2 liters IV fluid for all major trauma victims. Evidence suggests, however, that attempts at normalization of blood pressure with a large volume of fluids in the patient with uncontrolled hemorrhagic shock may be deleterious to patient outcome. Complications may include acidosis, dislodgment of blood clots, and dilution of clotting factors [56]. In such a patient, it appears that the best course is to give sufficient crystalloid to maintain a peripheral pulse, pending the delivery of the patient to the appropriate facility [40–42].

Administration of IV fluids is a gold standard treatment that has a long tradition in the care of critically ill patients. The route of IV administration depends on many factors, including the severity of the patient's illness and the available cannulation sites. Extremity veins provide the typical routes of venous access. External jugular veins are also useful sites in many patients. Few EMS systems use central venous access.

The IO route for vascular access has been used for generations. This was a common form of vascular access during World War II, though it became a less popular route in the postwar era with the rising use of IV cannulation. IO access has become so important as a method of vascular access that it is supported by a position statement from the National Association of EMS Physicians [57]. In patients *in extremis* or cases in which peripheral access is not immediately available, IO access may be preferred. Various devices are available, and EMS medical directors must work with their systems to determine the most appropriate device for use by their providers.

Controlling external hemorrhage is essential for maintaining vascular volume. Direct pressure is usually sufficient to control external bleeding. Military and civilian experience suggests that tourniquets should be used early and liberally [58]. An assortment of topical hemostatic materials to be placed directly on the bleeding wound also exists [58–61]. The hemostatic dressing must be applied in conjunction with direct pressure to

be effective. Pelvic binders may compress bleeding pelvic vessels while reducing the internal volume available for hemorrhage into the pelvis.

Tranexaminic acid (TXA) is a lysine derivative which blocks fibrinolysis. It has long been used to control hemorrhage during surgery [2]. In a randomized controlled study, TXA demonstrated an ability to reduce mortality from traumatic hemorrhage if administered within 3 hours of the time of injury [62]. Some prehospital systems are beginning to use TXA to treat hemorrhagic shock. Evidence for its benefit is found in its early administration, with late administration of TXA being associated with worsening outcomes [63].

Ventilation

The patient in shock may require assisted ventilation. Venous return requires a relative negative pressure in the right atrium to ensure return of blood to the heart. Assisted ventilation using any of the typical techniques, such as bag-mask ventilation, endotracheal intubation, or supraglottic devices, results in an increase in airway pressure, raising intrathoracic pressure. Patients in shock from any cause are extremely sensitive to increases in intrathoracic pressure. Studies in a swine hemorrhagic shock model showed that even modest increases in the rate of positive pressure ventilation significantly reduce brain blood flow and oxygenation [64]. EMS personnel must carefully control the rate of assisted positive pressure ventilation in the shock patient, as overventilation is very common. Generally speaking, a one-handed squeeze on the ventilation bag at a rate of approximately once every 8 seconds is reasonable for an adult, producing a minute ventilation of about 5 L/min. Minute ventilation should be adjusted to ensure an $EtCO_2$ between 35 and 45 cmH_2O.

Vasopressor agents

Administration of vasoactive medications may be required to reverse systemic hypoperfusion from distributive or cardiogenic shock. These agents increase cardiac inotropy, chronotropy, and/or vasoconstriction [65]. Although a wide variety of vasoactive agents is available in the hospital, the drugs carried by prehospital services are limited by local, regional, or state-wide protocols or regulations. In general, most services carry epinephrine and dopamine. Dobutamine, norepinephrine, and vasopressin may also be included in the drug armamentarium of some services.

The choice of vasopressor depends on the suspected underlying pathological process and the patient's response to therapy. Unfortunately, in the out-of-hospital setting, the etiology of the shock state is often unclear, and close monitoring of vital signs is difficult. The administration of vasoactive agents in the field is fraught with many other potential pitfalls such as the difficulty of calculating weight-based drug dosages. Rescuers should use calculators or templates or seek direct medical oversight, where an experienced clinician in a more controlled setting can perform important calculations. When available, particularly during interfacility or air medical transport, portable IV infusion pumps should be used to ensure accurate and precise medication administration.

Other drug agents

Other agents used for shock resuscitation include corticosteroids, antibiotics, colloids, inotropic agents, recombinant human activated protein C, and dextran [66,67]. The role of these agents in out-of-hospital shock management remains undefined. It would be reasonable to administer steroids to shock victims with known adrenal insufficiency or chronic steroid use and refractory hypotension.

Controversies

Shock science

The lack of definitive studies on the treatment of shock in the out-of-hospital setting leaves the EMS medical director without clear guidelines for treating these patients. As a result, considerable controversy exists with respect to many areas of the treatment of shock (especially traumatic shock) in the out-of-hospital setting.

The benefit of an out-of-hospital procedure must be weighed against potential risks. A major pitfall associated with shock treatment is that resuscitative interventions may delay definitive care [68]. For victims of myocardial infarction, for example, Pantridge and Geddes demonstrated that some aspects of definitive care, such as defibrillation and arrhythmia management, can and should be delivered in the field [69]. However, for trauma victims with uncontrolled internal hemorrhage, definitive care can only be provided in the hospital. Any field procedure that significantly delays delivery of definitive care must have proven value. For example, pneumatic anti-shock garments (PASG) were implemented in clinical EMS practice without supporting evidence, and then a formal assessment revealed that PASG actually worsened patient outcome in certain circumstances, particularly thoracic injury [70].

Treatment of hemorrhagic shock

Hemorrhage is a common cause of shock in the trauma victim. Field clinical trials have suggested that volume resuscitation before controlling hemorrhage may be detrimental [35,39–42,44,45]. Possible mechanisms for worse outcomes include dislodgement of clot, dilution of clotting factors, decreased oxygen-carrying capacity of the blood, hyperchloremic metabolic acidosis, and exacerbation of bleeding from injured vessels in the thorax or abdomen [40,41,44].

Studies in Houston and San Diego suggest that mortality following traumatic hemorrhage is not influenced by prehospital administration of fluid [40,42]. Survival to hospital discharge rates were not significantly different for patients receiving fluids versus patients not receiving fluids in the field. Both studies were performed in systems with relatively short scene and transport times.

As discussed above, currently field providers in most clinical settings are taught to administer only enough IV or IO fluid replacement to restore a peripheral pulse or to reach a systolic blood pressure of 80–90 mmHg. However, the optimum target blood pressure for these patients remains undefined. Trauma victims with isolated head injuries who receive excess fluids may develop worsened cerebral swelling. In addition, excess fluids may precipitate congestive heart failure in susceptible individuals or lead to impaired immune response following severe injury.

Conversely, the benefit of limited volume resuscitation has been derived from military and urban data with a predominance of penetrating injuries and young, healthy patients. This population may be more tolerant of hypovolemic resuscitation and benefit from relative hypotension while reducing the risk of clot dislodgment. However, patients with blunt injury and limited organ reserve due to comorbid illness or age may be intolerant of hypotensive resuscitation. A multicenter trial evaluating limited crystalloid resuscitation versus standard aggressive resuscitation coordinated by the Resuscitation Outcomes Consortium (ROC) is currently under way [71].

Attempts at establishing intravascular access in critically injured trauma victims may delay time to definitive care, especially in the urban setting [39,56,72–74]. The majority of IV fluid studies have taken place in urban settings primarily with penetrating trauma victims and rapid transport times. The effectiveness of IV fluids for similar patients in the rural and wilderness settings remains undefined. The subject remains controversial, with several studies providing mixed messages [39,56–59,72–76].

Protocol development

A treatment protocol for treating shock in the field should address the following factors.

1 Performing the initial assessment.

2 The definitive or life-saving interventions appropriate for these patients.

3 Access to definitive care without unnecessary prehospital delay.

4 Resources to be used in the field.

5 Skills of the various levels of prehospital care providers in the field.

Protocols developed for the out-of-hospital treatment of shock must consider the heterogeneity of the disease state, the limited assessment and treatment options, and the environment in which the protocols will be applied. Protocols for the inner city may not be appropriate for the rural setting. The level of training and clinical experience of the providers must also be considered. Ideally, medical directors would use evidence-based medical decision making when developing treatment protocols. It is strongly recommended that the EMS medical director draw from best practices for establishing clinical protocols addressing the evaluation and treatment of shock.

Conclusion

Shock must be correlated with the patient's clinical condition, age, size, and present and past medical history. Providers must identify signs of decreased tissue perfusion when assessing for the presence of shock. Treatment modalities for shock are limited in the field, but include bleeding control, fluid administration, inotropic agents, and careful control of assisted ventilation. Although the mainstay of shock treatment is IV fluids, approaches should be individualized for different clinical scenarios. The potential benefits of shock care interventions must be weighed against the potential risks of delaying definitive care.

References

1 Kobayashi L, Constantini TW, Coimbra, R. Hypovolemic shock resuscitation. *Surg Clin North Am* 2012;92:1403–23.

2 Kerby JD, Cusick MV. Prehospital emergency trauma care. *Surg Clin North Am* 2012;92:823–41.

3 American College of Surgeons, Committee on Trauma. Shock. In: *Advanced Trauma Life Support Program for Doctors: Student Manual*, 9th edn. Chicago: American College of Surgeons, 2012.

4 Weil MH. Personal commentary on the diagnosis and treatment of circulatory shock states. *Curr Opin Crit Care* 2004;10(4):246–9.

5 Fowler RL, Pepe PE, Stevens JT. Shock evaluation and management. In: Campbell JE (ed) *International Trauma Life Support for Prehospital Care Providers*, 7th edn. Upper Saddle River, NJ: Prentice Hall, 2012.

6 Cayten CG, Herrmann N, Cole LW, Walsh S. Assessing the validity of EMS data. *JACEP* 1978;11:390–6.

7 Runcie CJ, Reeve W, Reidy J, Dougall JR. A comparison of measurements of blood pressure, heart-rate and oxygenation during inter-hospital transport of the critically ill. *Intensive Care Med* 1990;5:317–22.

8 Rady MY, Smithline HA, Blake H, Nowak R, Rivers E. A comparison of the shock index and conventional vital signs to identify acute, critical illness in the emergency department. *Ann Emerg Med* 1994;24:685–90.

9 Demetriades D, Chan LS, Bhasin P, et al. Relative bradycardia in patients with traumatic hypotension. *J Trauma* 1998;45:534–9.

10 Poloujadoff MP, Lapostolle F, Lockey D, et al. Survival of severely shocked patients who present with absent radial pulse and unrecordable blood pressure in the pre-hospital phase. *Resuscitation* 2006;69(2):185–9.

11 Jones AE, Stiell IG, Nesbitt LP, et al. Nontraumatic out-of-hospital hypotension predicts inhospital mortality. *Ann Emerg Med* 2004;43(1):106–13.

12 Lipsky AM, Gausche-Hill M, Henneman PL, et al. Prehospital hypotension is a predictor of the need for an emergent, therapeutic operation in trauma patients with normal systolic blood pressure in the emergency department. *J Trauma* 2006;61(5):1228–33.

13 Shapiro NI, Kociszewski C, Harrison T, Chang Y, Wedel SK, Thomas SH. Isolated prehospital hypotension after traumatic injuries: a predictor of mortality? *J Emerg Med* 2003;25(2):175–9.

14 Knopp R, Claypool R, Leonardi D. Use of the tilt test in measuring acute blood loss. *Ann Emerg Med* 1980;9(2):72–5.

15 Schriger DL, Baraff LJ. Capillary refill – is it a useful predictor of hypovolemic states? *Ann Emerg Med* 1991;20(6):601–5.

16 Moscati R, Billittier AJ, Marshall B, Fincher M, Jehle D, Braen GR. Blood loss estimation by out-of-hospital emergency care providers. *Prehosp Emerg Care* 1999;3(3):239–42.

17 Kober A, Schubert B, Bertalanffy P, et al. Capnography in non-tracheally intubated emergency patients as an additional tool in pulse oximetry for prehospital monitoring of respiration. *Anesth Analg* 2004;98(1):206–10.

18 Scheller J, Loeb R. Respiratory artifact during pulse oximetry in critically ill patients. *Anesthesiology* 1988;69(4):602–3.

19 Deakin CD, Sado DM, Coats TJ, Davies G. Prehospital end-tidal carbon dioxide concentration and outcome in major trauma. *J Trauma* 2004;57(1):65–8.

20 Dubin A, Murias G, Estenssoro E, et al. End-tidal CO2 pressure determinants during hemorrhagic shock. *Intensive Care Med* 2000;26(11):1619–23.

21 Tyburski JG, Carlin AM, Harvey EH, Steffes C, Wilson RF. End-tidal CO2-arterial CO2 differences: a useful intraoperative mortality marker in trauma surgery. *J Trauma* 2003;55(5):892–6.

22 Wilson RF, Tyburski JG, Kubinec SM, et al. Intraoperative end-tidal carbon dioxide levels and derived calculations correlated with outcome in trauma patients. *J Trauma* 1996;41(4):606–11.

23 Davis DP, Dunford JV, Ochs M, Park K, Hoyt DB. The use of quantitative end-tidal capnometry to avoid inadvertent severe hyperventilation in patients with head injury after paramedic rapid sequence intubation. *J Trauma* 2004;56(4):808–14.

24 Davis DP, Dunford JV, Poste JC, et al. The impact of hypoxia and hyperventilation on outcome after paramedic rapid sequence intubation of severely head-injured patients. *J Trauma* 2004;57(1):1–8.

25 Silvestri S, Ralls GA, Krauss B, et al. The effectiveness of out-of-hospital use of continuous end-tidal carbon dioxide monitoring on the rate of unrecognized misplaced intubation within a regional emergency medical services system. *Ann Emerg Med* 2005;45(5):497–503.

26 Idris AH, Staples ED, O'Brien DJ, et al. Effect of ventilation on acid-base balance and oxygenation in low blood-flow states. *Crit Care Med* 1994;22(11):1827–34.

27 Idris AH, Staples ED, O'Brien DJ, et al. End-tidal carbon dioxide during extremely low cardiac output. *Ann Emerg Med* 1994;23(3):568–72.

28 Kupnik D, Skok P. Capnometry in the prehospital setting: are we using its potential? *Emerg Med J* 2007;24(9):614–17.

29 Plummer D, Heegaard W, Dries D, Reardon R, Pippert G, Frascone RJ. Ultrasound in HEMS: its role in differentiating shock states. *Air Med J* 2003;22(2):33–6.

30 Mtaweh H, Trakas EV, Su E, Carcillo JA, Aneja RK. Advances in monitoring and managing shock. *Pediatr Clin North Am* 2013;60(3):641–54.

31 Nguyen HB, Rivers EP, Knoblich BP, et al. Early lactate clearance is associated with improved outcome in severe sepsis and septic shock. *Crit Care Med* 2004;32(8):1637–42.

32 Lactate Portable Blood Analyzers. Available at: www.lactate.com

33 Guyette F, Suffoletto B, Castillo JL, Quintero J, Callaway C, Puyana JC. Prehospital serum lactate as a predictor of outcomes in trauma patients: a retrospective observational study. *J Trauma* 2011;70(4):782–6.

34 Moranville MP, Mieure KD, Santayana EM. Evaluation and management of shock states: Hypovolemic, distributive, and cardiogenic shock. *J Pharm Pract* 2011;24(1):44–60.

35 Stern SA, Dronen SC, Birrer P, Wang X. Effect of blood pressure on hemorrhage volume and survival in a near-fatal hemorrhage model incorporating a vascular injury. *Ann Emerg Med* 1993;22(2):155–63.

36 Alderson P, Bunn F, Lefebvre C, et al. Human albumin solution for fluid resuscitation and volume expansion in critically ill patients. *Cochrane Database Syst Rev* 2002;1:CD001208.

37 Finfer S, Bellomo R, Boyce N, et al. A comparison of albumin and saline for fluid resuscitation in the intensive care unit. *N Engl J Med* 2004;350(22):2247–56.

38 SAFE Study Investigators, Australian and New Zealand Intensive Care Society Clinical Trials Group, Australian Red Cross Blood Service, et al. Saline or albumin patients with traumatic brain injury. *N Engl J Med* 2007;357(9):874–84.

39 Bickell WH, Wall MJ Jr, Pepe PE, et al. Immediate versus delayed fluid resuscitation for hypotensive patients with penetrating torso injuries. *N Engl J Med* 1994;331(17):1105–9.

40 Kaweski SM, Sise MJ, Virgilio RW. The effect of prehospital fluids on survival in trauma patients. *J Trauma* 1990;30(10):1215–18.

41 Kowalenko T, Stern S, Dronen S, Wang X. Improved outcome with hypotensive resuscitation of uncontrolled hemorrhagic shock in a swine model. *J Trauma* 1992;33(3):349–53.

42 Martin RR, Bickell WH, Pepe PE, Burch JM, Mattox KL. Prospective evaluation of preoperative fluid resuscitation in hypotensive patients with penetrating truncal injury: a preliminary report. *J Trauma* 1992;33(3):354–61.

43 O'Connor RE, Domeier RM. An evaluation of the pneumatic anti-shock garment (PASG) in various clinical settings. *Prehosp Emerg Care* 1997;1(1):36–44.

44 Pepe PE, Eckstein M. Reappraising the prehospital care of the patient with major trauma. *Emerg Med Clin North Am* 1998;16(1):1–15.

45 Silbergleit R, Satz W, McNamara RM, Lee DC, Schoffstall JM. Effect of permissive hypotension in continuous uncontrolled intra-abdominal hemorrhage. *Acad Emerg Med* 1996;3(10):922–6.

46 Smith JP, Bodai BI, Hill AS, Frey CF. Prehospital stabilization of critically injured patients: a failed concept. *J Trauma* 1985;25(1):65–70.

47 Elbers PW, Ince C. Mechanisms of critical illness – classifying microcirculatory flow abnormalities in distributive shock. *Crit Care* 2006;10(4):221.

48 Patel GP, Grahe JS, Sperry M, et al. Efficacy and safety of dopamine versus norepinephrine in the management of septic shock. *Shock* 2010;33(4):375–80.

49 De Backer D, Biston P, Devriendt J, et al. Comparison of dopamine and norepinephrine in the treatment of shock. *N Engl J Med* 2010;362(9):779–89.

50 Aneja R, Carcillo J. Differences between adult and pediatric septic shock. *Minerva Anestesiol* 2011;77(10):986–92.

51 Kissoon N, Orr RA, Carcillo JA. Updated American College of Critical Care Medicine – pediatric advanced life support guidelines for management of pediatric and neonatal septic shock: relevance to the emergency care clinician. *Pediatr Emerg Care* 2010;26(11):867–9.

52 Prehospital use of plasma for traumatic hemorrhage. (PUPTH), 2011. Funding Opportunity Number W81WXWH–11PUPTH–IAA.

53 Vassar MJ, Fischer RP, O'Brien PE, et al. A multicenter trial for resuscitation of injured patients with 7.5% sodium chloride. The effect of added dextran 70. The Multicenter Group for the Study of Hypertonic Saline in Trauma Patients. *Arch Surg* 1993;128(9):1003–11.

54 Bickell WH, Bruttig SP, Millnamow GA, O'Benar J, Wade CE. Use of hypertonic saline/dextran versus lactated Ringer's solution as a resuscitation fluid after uncontrolled aortic hemorrhage in anesthetized swine. *Ann Emerg Med* 1992;21(9):1077–85.

55 Bulger EM, May S, Brasel KJ, et al. Out-of-hospital hypertonic resuscitation following severe traumatic brain injury: a randomized controlled trial. *JAMA.* 2010;304(13):1455–64.

56 Bickell WH, Wall MJ Jr, Pepe PE, et al. Immediate vs. delayed fluid resuscitation for hypotensive patients with penetrating torso injuries. *N Engl J Med* 1994;331(17):1105–9.

57 Fowler R, Gallagher JV, Isaacs SM, Ossman E, Pepe P, Wayne M. The role of intraosseous vascular access in the out-of-hospital environment (resource document to NAEMSP position statement). *Prehosp Emerg Care* 2007;11(1):63–6.

58 Fox CJ, Starnes BW. Vascular surgery on the modern battlefield. *Surg Clin North Am* 2007;87(5):1193–211.

59 Mabry R, McManus JG. Prehospital advances in the management of severe penetrating trauma. *Crit Care Med* 2008;36(7):S258–66.

60 Alam HB, Uy GB, Miller D, et al. Comparative analysis of hemostatic agents in a swine model of lethal groin injury. *J Trauma* 2003;54(6):1077–82.

61 Achneck HE, Sileshi B, Jamiolkowski RM, Albaia DM, Shapiro ML, Lawson JH. A comprehensive review of topical hemostatic agents: efficacy and recommendations for use. *Ann Surg* 2010;251:217–28.

62 CRASH-2 Collaborators, Shakur H, Roberts I, et al. Effects of tranexamic acid on death, vascular occlusive events, and blood transfusion in trauma patients with significant haemorrhage (CRASH-2): a randomised, placebo-controlled trial. *Lancet* 2010;376(9734):23–32.

63 CRASH-2 Collaborators, Roberts I, Shakur H, et al. The importance of early treatment with tranexamic acid in bleeding trauma patients: an exploratory analysis of the CRASH-2 randomised controlled trial. *Lancet* 2011;377(9771):1096–101.

64 64.Yannopoulos D, Tang W, Roussos C, Aufderheide TP, Idris AH, Lurie KG. Reducing ventilation frequency during cardiopulmonary resuscitation in a porcine model of cardiac arrest. *Respir Care* 2005;50(5):628–35.

65 Neumar RW, Otto CW, Link MS, et al. Part 8: adult advanced cardiovascular life support: 2010 American Heart Association guidelines for cardiopulmonary resuscitation and emergency cardiovascular care. *Circulation* 2010;122:S729–67.

66 Sprung CL, Annane D, Keh D, et al. Hydrocortisone therapy for patients with septic shock. *N Engl J Med* 2008;358(2):111–24.

67 Dellinger RP, Levy MM, Carlet JM, et al. The Surviving Sepsis Campaign: international guidelines for management of severe sepsis and septic shock: 2008. *Crit Care Med* 2008;36(1):296–327.

68 Bickell WH. Are victims of injury sometimes victimized by attempts at fluid resuscitation? *Ann Emerg Med* 1993;22(2):225–6.

69 Pantridge JF, Geddes JS. A mobile intensive-care unit in the management of myocardial infarction. *Lancet* 1967;2(7510):271–3.

70 Mattox KL, Bickell W, Pepe PE, Burch J, Feliciano D. Prospective MAST study in 911 patients. *J Trauma* 1989;29(8):1104–11.

71 Resuscitation Outcomes Consortium. Available at: https://roc.uwctc.org/tiki/tiki-index.php?page=roc-public-home

72 Henderson RA, Thomson DP, Bahrs BA, Norman MP. Unnecessary intravenous access in the emergency setting. *Prehosp Emerg Care* 1998;2(4):312–16.

73 Sampalis JS, Tamim H, Denis R, et al. Ineffectiveness of on-site intravenous lines: is prehospital time the culprit? *J Trauma* 1997;43(4):608–15.

74 Seamon MJ, Fisher CA, Gaughan J, et al. Prehospital procedures before emergency department thoracotomy: "scoop and run" saves lives. *J Trauma* 2007;63(1):113–20.

75 Jacobs LM, Sinclair A, Beiser A, d'Agostino RB. Prehospital advanced life support: benefits in trauma. *J Trauma* 1984;24(1):8–13.

76 O'Gorman M, Trabulsy P, Pilcher DB. Zero-time prehospital I.V. *J Trauma* 1989;29(1):84–6.

CHAPTER 8
Vascular access

Jocelyn M. De Guzman, Bryan B. Kitch, and Jeffrey D. Ferguson

Introduction

While discussions continue concerning the utility of obtaining prehospital vascular access, the skill remains a standard taught to EMS providers. Methods of access include peripheral and central intravenous (IV) catheterization and intraosseous (IO) access, depending on the local scope of practice and the qualifications of prehospital personnel. The medications and fluids administered through these various routes depend on local EMS protocol and the practices of the EMS medical director. Those specifics are beyond the scope of this chapter, but are discussed elsewhere in this text.

Benefits

Similar to its benefit in the emergency department (ED) or any other acute care setting, vascular access provides an avenue for medical intervention by the EMS provider. Early prehospital initiation of treatment for cardiac arrest, cardiac arrhythmia, and sepsis has been shown to be beneficial for patients [1–3]. For the more stable yet ill or distressed patient, the initiation of an IV or IO for symptomatic treatment of nausea, pain, or dehydration can help the continuum of care that will likely progress in the ED. Treatment of potentially reversible conditions like hypoglycemia and narcotic overdose in the prehospital setting can prevent deterioration of the patient's condition and potentially negate the need for transport. Vascular access also facilitates advanced care such as rapid sequence intubation and the administration of vasopressors and thrombolytics.

Risks

Obtaining vascular access involves inherent risks to the provider, including blood exposure and needlestick injury. Whether it is attempted at the scene or in transit, the prehospital environment is often characterized by poor lighting, limited space, or movement in the rear of an ambulance. This offers less than ideal conditions in which to handle lancets, IV and IO needles, and other sharps. A combative and/or confused patient can add to the difficulty. Transmission of HIV, hepatitis B, and hepatitis C remains a constant threat to the EMS provider, with the risks of infection following needlestick injury estimated at 0.3%, 6–30%, and 1.8%, respectively [4]. Consistent use of universal precautions is imperative to reduce the likelihood of occupational exposures. Potential risks to the patient include bleeding, damage to adjacent structures, infection, and thrombosis and will be discussed later.

Establishing an IV is often part of EMS protocols. In many cases, protocols allow for EMS provider assessment and judgment regarding whether or not an IV is necessary. One study revealed that while over 50% of the patients who arrived at an ED via EMS had IVs in place, almost 80% of those IVs were not used in the prehospital setting. The tendency to err on the side of caution to avoid punitive measures from perceived undertreatment seemed to contribute to the discrepancy [5]. Another study similarly found that protocols seemed to drive the decision to start an IV as opposed to an actual need for administration of medicines or fluids [6]. Medical oversight is indicated to continually evaluate the appropriateness of "precautionary" IVs in the contexts of potential risks and costs to the system and to patients.

Several studies in the trauma setting have unveiled a lack of significant benefit regarding prehospital vascular access. The classic EMS mantra of "two large-bore IVs" for trauma patients has been muted by concern for increased on-scene times and delay of transport to definitive medical care. Nevertheless, two studies have shown high success rates when IVs were attempted in transit without delaying transport [7,8]. However, a literature review by the Eastern Association for the Surgery of Trauma resulted in a set of practice management guidelines that found no demonstrable benefit from prehospital IV placement or IV fluid administration for either penetrating or blunt injury patients [9].

Emergency Medical Services: Clinical Practice and Systems Oversight, Second Edition. Volume 1: Clinical Aspects of EMS.
Edited by David C. Cone, Jane H. Brice, Theodore R. Delbridge, and J. Brent Myers.

Recent research in the field of trauma resuscitation suggests that routine administration of IV fluids may have no benefit and in fact can be harmful in the prehospital setting [10,11]. Another study endorsed "scoop and run" transport for EMS as it found that each prehospital procedure before ED thoracotomy led to a reduction in the odds of survival [12].

Peripheral IV access

History
Early records document the use of feather quills and animal bladders for intravenous therapies with animal-to-human transfusions. These were later replaced by hollow steel needles with rubber tubing leading to glass bottles. The evolution to over-the-needle plastic catheters has been focused on operator safety and patient comfort [13].

Flow rate through the catheter is based on Poiseuille's law, dealing with pressure and resistance. The pertinent determinants of the equation include the radius of the catheter and the catheter length. Flow is directly proportional to the radius to the 4th power (r^4), and inversely proportional to catheter length. As such, a large-gauge, short IV catheter can profoundly improve the potential flow rate over a smaller gauge, longer catheter.

Typical locations for peripheral IV access include the antecubital fossa, veins in the forearm and dorsum of the hand and foot, external jugular vein, and scalp veins.

Technique (Video Clip 8.1)
1. Preparation
When the decision to pursue vascular access is made, the preparation for the procedure is just as imperative as the skill itself. Temptations for speed in the prehospital setting, assumptions regarding the patient's health, or other neglectful behavior deviating from the practice of universal precautions can result in occupational exposure. When possible, wash hands prior to putting on gloves.

Prepare the equipment (Figure 8.1). You will need an IV start kit (if available) or you can assemble your own (tourniquet, alcohol wipe or other cleaner, tape or a commercially available adhesive device). Select an IV needle with catheter (Figure 8.2), saline lock, saline flush, and/or IV fluids. Check the IV catheter for integrity.

Prepare the patient for the procedure. When appropriate, discuss with the patient the reason for the procedure along with risks and benefits. Unless a true emergency exists or the patient is not able to make his/her own decisions, verbal consent should be obtained.

2. Site selection
Position the patient's extremity to help straighten the desired vein. Apply the tourniquet proximal to the targeted area (Figure 8.3). When possible, look distally first to allow additional proximal attempts on the same extremity, if necessary. Once the tourniquet is applied, you can have the patient pump his/her fist open and closed several times to help the vasculature become engorged. Feel for a soft, spongy, non-pulsatile vessel.

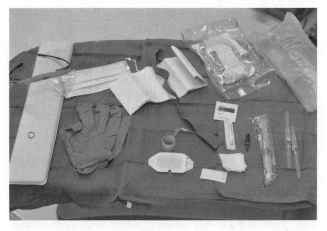

Figure 8.1 IV starting equipment.

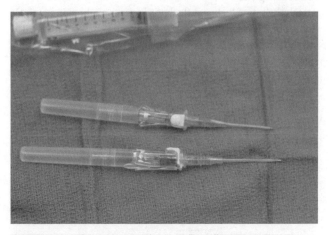

Figure 8.2 18 and 20 gauge IV catheters with needles.

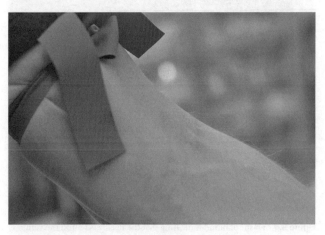

Figure 8.3 Position of tourniquet proximal to target vein.

3. Clean the site

Use an alcohol pad, betadine, chlorhexadine, or a similar anti-septic product to clean the proposed IV site. Allow the area to dry.

4. Insertion of the IV

Hold the skin taut with one hand while inserting the needle with your dominant hand. Approach the vessel as shallow as possible (less than 30° angle to the skin) with the bevel of the needle facing up or away from the patient. Once you feel a "pop" and/or see a flash of blood in the reservoir of the IV needle, advance the needle slightly further and slowly slide the catheter over the needle, cannulating the vessel with the plastic catheter while not moving the needle itself (Figure 8.4).

5. Removing the needle

Hold firm pressure over the tip of the cannulated plastic catheter while you withdraw the needle from the hub of the catheter. If applicable, push the button to retract the needle to its safe position and move the needle to a safe area. The needle needs to be disposed of in a sharps container as soon as the IV is secured.

6. Securing the IV

Attach the saline lock and flush the lock with saline or attach IV fluid tubing directly to the hub of the catheter. Secure the catheter hub with tape or a commercial securing device. Check for signs of infiltration (i.e. localized swelling, inability to flush catheter, pain).

External jugular vein access has a similar technique. The needle is inserted in a caudad direction, but no tourniquet is used. Instead, the index finger of the non-dominant hand can be used to apply gentle pressure to the external jugular vein just above the clavicle to facilitate venous engorgement. Care should be taken to avoid placing a needle puncture too low in the neck (i.e. at or immediately above the clavicle) to avoid lung injury. Blind attempts when the external jugular vein is not readily apparent are not advised due to potential for serious injury to surrounding structures (Figure 8.5).

Contraindications to intravenous access relate mainly to site selection. Sites with burns, cellulitis, trauma, and other conditions that compromise the integrity of the overlying skin should be avoided. Extremities on the side of a recent mastectomy or lymphatic chain removal, those that contain known thromboses, and those that contain permanent modifications for dialysis access should be used only when all other options have been exhausted. Special consideration must be given to patients with known bleeding disorders and those who are taking medications that may alter coagulation, as ensuring ease of compressibility becomes an important factor to limit excessive bleeding from cannulation attempts.

Maintenance of vascular access in the prehospital setting may often prove difficult as perspiration, mud, dirt, and water reduce the effectiveness of tape and adhesive dressings used to secure the catheter. Combative or confused patients can also intentionally or unintentionally dislodge their IV access during transport and may require additional verbal instruction and reminders along with extra padding/support to maintain the line. Gauze wraps, elastic bandages, and arm boards are just a few examples of adjuncts used to protect and optimally position venous access.

Intraosseous access

Intraosseous devices function to access the intramedullary vessels found in the bone marrow of spongy bone that lead to the central circulation of the body. The IO needle, embedded in the bony structure, is protected by the non-collapsible periosteum, solving any problems with patency that may be encountered with IVs during vasoconstriction and low-flow states found in sepsis and cardiac arrest.

Intraosseous access is currently attainable with manual, impact-driven, and powered drill methods. The gauge and length of some of the commercially available products will vary for the

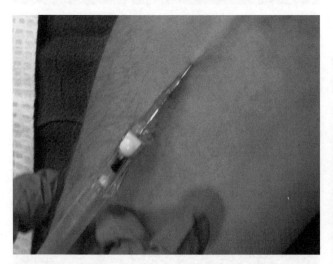

Figure 8.4 "Flash" of blood indicating that the needle is within the vein's lumen and the catheter should be advanced over the needle.

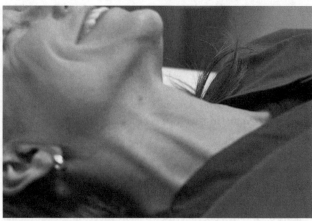

Figure 8.5 External jugular vein.

adult and pediatric patient. The commonly available EZ-IO™ uses a 15 mm long needle for children under 39 kg while 25 mm and 45 mm lengths are available for patients 40 kg or greater; all are 15 gauge. The sites of insertion vary by manufacturer recommendations but locations may include the proximal tibia, distal tibia, proximal humerus, and sternum. Contraindications to IO access are generally site specific and include infection of the overlying skin, fracture at or above the IO site, vascular compromise, and previous surgery or significant deformity of the bone. Previous sternotomy, suspected sternal fracture, and CPR with chest compressions exclude use of sternal IO access. Potential complications include osteomyelitis, fat emboli, fracture, growth plate injury, compartment syndrome, infection, and extravasation resulting in local tissue injury and swelling [14–16].

Drinker and Lund in the 1920s were the first to use IO vascular access in the sternum of animal models, demonstrating that the fluid given did indeed reach intravascular circulation. Josefson followed in 1934, reporting the first IO use in humans. Soon after, in the 1940s, the first use of the IO was documented in the pediatric population. While its use with military personnel during World War II was advocated when IV access was delayed or difficult, the development of the over-the-needle PVC IV catheter by Massa in the 1950s temporarily curtailed use of the IO. The reemergence of the IO in the 1980s in the Pediatric Advanced Life Support and Advanced Pediatric Life Support courses supported its use after failed IV attempts. More recent guidelines from the American Heart Association advocate for the use of IOs as first-line access in pediatric emergencies and as first alternative in adult cardiac arrest, including in out-of-hospital settings [13–15,17].

Several recent studies have shown the success of obtaining vascular access through IOs after failed or difficult attempts at IV access. IO vascular access has demonstrated high first-attempt success rates and overall success rates of 90% and greater in adults and children [16]. The advantages of the commercially available battery-powered driver used in the study included its short learning curve, ability to easily penetrate thick cortical bone given its power source, and rapid drug delivery into the systemic circulation [18]. IO access has been proven to be as quick and effective as IV access [19]. In patients with inaccessible peripheral veins, IO access is faster and more successful than central IV lines [20].

Most medications given through the peripheral IV can be given through an IO, with bioequivalence proven between the two routes [21]. IO has been shown to have clinically comparable times to peak drug concentration compared to central IV access [17].

Wilderness, tactical, disaster, and other specialty EMS groups may encounter situations requiring early consideration of the use of the IO for vascular access. Austere conditions, limited access to an entrapped patient, or cumbersome gear and clothing of both patient and provider can obstruct efforts to initiate peripheral IV access. One study showed significantly shorter times to IO access compared to IV access in providers wearing chemical, biological, radiological, and nuclear (CBRN) protective equipment [22]. IO access is recommended during any resuscitation when IV access is not readily attainable [15].

Technique (Video Clip 8.2)

1. Preparation

Wash hands, don the appropriate personal protective equipment (PPE), and prepare the equipment (Figure 8.6).

2. Idenitify the landmarks and site

- *Humeral head* – keep the arm adducted with the palm pronated. Palpate the proximal humerus and locate the greater tuberosity, which will be the site of insertion.
- *Proximal tibia* – identify the tibial tuberosity. The site of insertion should be two finger breadths below and just medial to this landmark.
- *Distal tibia* – abduct and externally rotate the hip. Palpate the flat portion of bone just proximal to the medial malleolus.

3. Clean the site

Cleanse the targeted area with alcohol prep, betadine, chlorhexidine, or other antiseptic. Allow the site to dry.

4. Insert the IO

Insert the IO needle into the skin overlying the desired location until bone is reached. Insert the needle through the cortex into the marrow either manually or per device-specific instructions. The needle should be relatively stable and freestanding in the bone if inserted appropriately.

5. Assess IO patency

Remove the trocar and dispose of it in a sharps container. Attach a syringe or IO-specific tubing and assess for patency of the IO. Monitor the extremity for extravasation. Attach IV fluids if indicated; use a pressure bag or manually push fluids via syringe to achieve desired infusion rates.

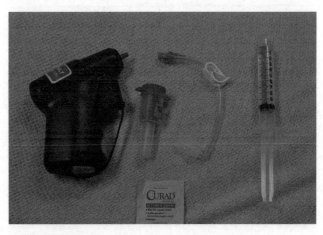

Figure 8.6 Intraosseous equipment.

6. Secure the IO

Stabilize the IO in place with gauze and tape or a commercially available device.

In a non-urgent setting, lidocaine or other anesthetic drugs may be injected into the area of the proposed IO and infused with the fluids to reduce pain and discomfort.

Central intravenous access

Prehospital central venous access is a procedure sometimes performed by advanced-level paramedics, nurses, and EMS physicians. Usually in the form of a large 8.5 French single-lumen catheter, the route provides rapid access to the central venous circulation and a route for rapid fluid resuscitation. Central venous access may be the preferable option when attempts at peripheral and IO lines have failed and/or are contraindicated, but its use in the prehospital arena is sparsely reported (Figure 8.7). Central venous line placement by air medical transport teams has been reported [21,23]. Similarly, one report documented the performance of 115 prehospital central lines placed by field response EMS physicians over a 3-year period [24]. Critical care teams are often responsible for maintenance of these lines during interfacility transport, so familiarity with this form of vascular access is important.

The internal jugular (IJ), subclavian, and femoral veins are options for central venous access. Traumatic injuries above the diaphragm often dictate a femoral location. Attempts at access in the IJ and subclavian veins have a risk of pneumothorax, which should be considered if the patient acutely decompensates during the procedure. Placement of a central line, especially in the upper body, often causes an interruption of CPR efforts [20]. Risks of bleeding from venous or inadvertent arterial puncture, infection, thrombosis, and nerve damage also exist [18]. The prehospital environment makes it nearly impossible to preserve sterile technique. Given that these lines are performed as "code" lines under emergency, semi-sterile

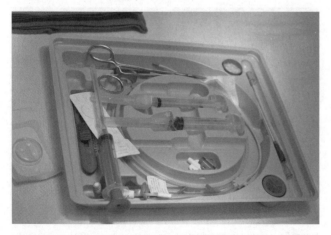

Figure 8.7 Central venous catheter kit.

(similar to a peripheral IV line) conditions, it should be expected that the line would be removed and another one placed if the patient survives to the ED.

Special considerations

Accessing dialysis catheters and indwelling catheters

In the prehospital setting, dialysis catheters, infusion ports, and other long-term artificial structures should not be considered as first-line options for gaining vascular access. The health of these difficult access patients often depends on frequent IV access and medication administration; improper utilization of these routes may result in serious consequences. Alternative forms of vascular access or medication routes should be considered. In the case that the EMS provider must access these types of catheters, special attention must be paid to sterile technique and the specific proper method for accessing each individualized access point.

System medical directors may provide training and protocols for specific patient populations that may include accessing such devices earlier in the treatment algorithm.

Pediatric considerations

The pain and anxiety in the pediatric patient associated with vascular access is often a difficult matter to address in the prehospital setting. The need for rapid vascular access in a critically ill child along with varying transport times does not typically allow for some of the pharmacological options for relieving the pain of IV insertion that are available in the ED and hospital setting. Various commercially available creams, gels, and patches often require from several minutes up to an hour of application time for effectiveness. Local infiltration of lidocaine with either a small-gauge needle or needle-free system such as the J-Tip provides quicker anesthetic delivery but requires a second, often psychologically traumatizing needle puncture or startling noise due to pressurized CO_2. Often, if the child is stable enough to consider the use of these pain-reducing interventions, vascular access can be deferred until arrival to the hospital.

Medical oversight and training for pediatric patient care should focus on helping the EMS provider distinguish the stable transport from the critically ill patient who would benefit from early vascular access [25]. Additionally, attempts at IV access in young children are infrequent and often difficult. Training may be needed to improve technical skills and confidence to increase success [26].

The future: ultrasound-guided IV access

In ED care, ultrasound technology has become a useful tool to improve the success of IV access. Previously, patients who could not be cannulated by more traditional methods were often subject to more invasive procedures such as cut-downs or central lines, posing an increased level of risk. The growing widespread availability of ultrasound technology augments the ability of providers to obtain IV access in a less invasive fashion. While detailed instruction is beyond the scope of this text, ultrasound techniques can be used in a static fashion to identify the location of a suitable vein when one cannot be seen or palpated. The vein is then accessed by the usual techniques. Alternatively, a dynamic approach is often used, wherein the provider uses ultrasound to visualize the needle tip and subsequently the catheter entering the vein, confirming placement. The materials and methods are largely similar to standard peripheral access techniques, with the exception of the need for an ultrasound machine, gel, and longer length catheters for accessing deeper veins.

Multiple studies have been performed analyzing the efficacy, speed, patency, and complications of ultrasound IV access. Across several inpatient and ED environments, ultrasound-guided peripheral access shows trends towards being a comparable or preferable modality with regard to risk of failure, number of attempts, and procedure time [27]. There is clear demonstration of reduction of central line use when ultrasound is available to facilitate peripheral IV placement [28]. Success of ultrasound peripheral IV attempts was non-inferior to the external jugular approach in those who failed traditional attempts [29].

With regard to prehospital use of this technology, there are limited data and several barriers to implementation. Ultrasound machines remain expensive, and despite advances in miniaturization, most devices require a non-trivial amount of physical space. Hand-held ultrasound devices have been produced in recent years and may allow for feasibility studies of EMS-initiated ultrasound-facilitated IV access. As other applications for ultrasound are studied and implemented for prehospital use, the ability to gain vascular access may be an added benefit of the technology, even if not purchased for that primary purpose. As several other modalities are equivalent to if not faster than ultrasound-guided peripheral IV placement, this technology may find a greater stronghold in systems permissive of longer on-scene times or for long-distance/critical care transport.

Conclusion

Vascular access is commonly pursued as part of prehospital emergency care. In some cases it is to facilitate administration of needed medications or resuscitative fluids. In other cases IVs are placed as a precaution in case such measures are eventually needed. Many IVs are not used prior to arrival at an ED. It is important for EMS clinicians to possess the necessary skills and equipment to initiate vascular access under myriad conditions. Further, this is an area that is appropriate for monitoring and evaluating from a quality improvement perspective, including both decision-making and technical skill domains.

References

1 Seymour CW, Cooke CR, Hebert PL, Rea TD. Intravenous access during out-of-hospital emergency care of noninjured patients: a population-based outcome study. *Ann Emerg Med* 2012;59(4): 296–303.

2 Band RA, Gaieski DF, Hylton JH, Shofer FS, Goyal M, Meisel ZF. Arriving by emergency medical services improves time to treatment endpoints for patients with severe sepsis or septic shock. *Acad Emerg Med* 2011;18(9):934–40.

3 Rittenberger JC, Bost JE, Menegazzi JJ. Time to give the first medication during resuscitation in out-of-hospital cardiac arrest. *Resuscitation* 2006;70(2):201–6.

4 Harris SA, Nicolai LA. Occupational exposures in emergency medical service providers and knowledge of and compliance with universal precautions. *Am J Infect Control* 2010;38(2):86–94.

5 Kuzma K, Sporer KA, Michael GE, Youngblood GM. When are prehospital intravenous catheters used for treatment? *J Emerg Med* 2009;36(4):357–62.

6 Stratton SJ. Rethinking out-of-hospital intravenous access. *Ann Emerg Med* 2012;59(4):304–6.

7 Jones SE, Nesper TP, Alcouloumre E. Prehospital intravenous line placement: a prospective study. *Ann Emerg Med* 1989;18(3):244–6.

8 Slovis CM, Herr EW, Londorf D, Little TD, Alexander BR, Guthmann RJ. Success rates for initiation of intravenous therapy en route by prehospital care providers. *Am J Emerg Med* 1990;8(4):305–7.

9 Cotton BA, Jerome R, Collier BR, et al. Guidelines for prehospital fluid resuscitation in the injured patient. *J Trauma* 2009;67(2): 389–402.

10 Bickell WH, Wall MJ Jr, Pepe PE, et al. Immediate versus delayed fluid resuscitation for hypotensive patients with penetrating torso injuries. *N Engl J Med* 1994;331(17):1105–9.

11 Haut ER, Kalish BT, Cotton BA, et al. Prehospital intravenous fluid administration is associated with higher mortality in trauma patients: a National Trauma Data Bank analysis. *Ann Surg* 2011; 253(2):371–7.

12 Seamon MJ, Fisher CA, Gaughan J, et al. Prehospital procedures before emergency department thoracotomy: "scoop and run" saves lives. *J Trauma* 2007;63(1):113–20.

13 Rivera A, Strauss K, van Zundert A, Mortier E. The history of peripheral intravenous catheters: how little plastic tubes revolutionized medicine. *Acta Anaesthesiol Belg* 2005;56(3):271.

14 Fowler R, Gallagher JV, Isaacs SM, Ossman E, Pepe P, Wayne M. The role of intraosseous vascular access in the out-of-hospital environment (resource document to NAEMSP position statement). *Prehosp Emerg Care* 2007;11(1):63–6.

15 Weiser G, Hoffmann Y, Galbraith R, Shavit I. Current advances in intraosseous infusion – a systematic review. *Resuscitation* 2012; 83(1):20–6.

16 Santos D, Carron PN, Yersin B, Pasquier M. EZ-IO((R)) intraosseous device implementation in a pre-hospital emergency service: a prospective study and review of the literature. *Resuscitation* 2013;84(4):440–5.

17 Hoskins SL. Pharmacokinetics of intraosseous and central venous drug delivery during cardiopulmonary resuscitation. *Resuscitation* 2012;83(1):107–12.

18 Gazin N, Auger H, Jabre P, et al. Efficacy and safety of the EZ-IO™ intraosseous device: out-of-hospital implementation of a management algorithm for difficult vascular access. *Resuscitation* 2011;82(1):126–9.

19 Reades R, Studnek JR, Garrett JS, Vandeventer S, Blackwell T. Comparison of first-attempt success between tibial and humeral intraosseous insertions during out-of-hospital cardiac arrest. *Prehosp Emerg Care* 2011;15(2):278–81.

20 Leidel BA, Kirchhoff C, Bogner V, Braunstein V, Biberthaler P, Kanz K. Comparison of intraosseous versus central venous vascular access in adults under resuscitation in the emergency department with inaccessible peripheral veins. *Resuscitation* 2012;83(1):40–5.

21 Von Hoff DD, Kuhn JG, Burris HA III, Miller LJ. Does intraosseous equal intravenous? A pharmacokinetic study. *Am J Emerg Med* 2008;26(1):31–8.

22 Lamhaut L, Dagron C, Apriotesei R, et al. Comparison of intravenous and intraosseous access by pre-hospital medical emergency personnel with and without CBRN protective equipment. *Resuscitation* 2010;81(1):65–8.

23 Davis DP, Ramanujam P. Central venous access by air medical personnel. *Prehosp Emerg Care* 2007;11(2):204–6.

24 Martin-Gill C, Roth RN, Mosesso VN. Resident field response in an emergency medicine prehospital care rotation. *Prehosp Emerg Care* 2010;14(3):370–6.

25 Zempsky WT. Pharmacologic approaches for reducing venous access pain in children. *Pediatrics* 2008;122 Suppl 3:S140–53.

26 Myers LA, Arteaga GM, Kolb LJ, Lohse CM, Russi CS. Prehospital peripheral intravenous vascular access success rates in children. *Prehosp Emerg Care* 2013;17(4):425–8.

27 Heinrichs J, Fritze Z, Vandermeer B, Klassen T, Curtis S. Ultrasonographically guided peripheral intravenous cannulation of children and adults: a systematic review and meta-analysis. *Ann Emerg Med* 2013;61(4):444–54.

28 Shokoohi H, Boniface K, McCarthy M, et al. Ultrasound-guided peripheral intravenous access program is associated with a marked reduction in central venous catheter use in noncritically ill emergency department patients. *Ann Emerg Med* 2013;61(2): 198–203.

29 Costantino TG, Kirtz JF, Satz WA. Ultrasound-guided peripheral venous access vs. the external jugular vein as the initial approach to the patient with difficult vascular access. *J Emerg Med* 2010; 39(4):462–7.

SECTION IV

Medical Problems

CHAPTER 9

The challenge of the undifferentiated patient

Andrew Travers and Ronald D. Stewart

Introduction: the call-taking process

When a patient calls 9-1-1 and speaks with a medical communications officer, the complex process of provision of care has been initiated. This first point of medical contact, the interaction between the patient and communication officer, can influence every subsequent experience of the patient during his or her prehospital and even in-hospital care. Consequently, it is essential for the communication officer to initiate and optimize the patient for the subsequent paramedic–patient contact; the paramedic in turn optimizes the patient for contact with the local emergency department (ED) or other destination.

Although many consider that the 9-1-1 medical communications center is involved only in resource allocation such as dispatching ambulances, it also has a pivotal role in the provision of patient care [1]. The accurate identification of the chief complaint by the communications officer serves as an adjunct to the field personnel by allowing them to incrementally build on the dispatch "diagnosis" and initiate the appropriate therapy. If the communications officer incorrectly identifies the chief complaint, this may result in ineffective or inappropriate prehospital therapies, and even worse, it may introduce systematic biases that affect provision of patient care from the paramedic–patient contact onward [2,3]. (For simplicity, the term *paramedic* will be used in this chapter, though the principles apply to all provider types including EMS physicians.)

For example, during the initial steps in the communicator–patient interview, if the chief complaint includes scene safety (e.g. drowning or electrocution case), the dispatcher decides on the protocol that best addresses the issues [3,4]. If the chief complaint involves trauma, then the dispatcher decides on the protocol that best addresses the mechanism of injury (e.g. fall, traffic accident). When the chief complaint appears to be medical in nature, the dispatcher chooses the protocol that best fits the patient's foremost symptom, with the priority symptoms taking precedence. Regardless of which call is assessed, the subsequent dispatch information can influence the thought processes of the responding paramedics and potentially influence how the paramedics approach the patient [5]. For example, in the case of drowning or electrocution calls, the paramedics are preparing themselves for this type of call, essentially reviewing in their minds the protocols and procedures to use when approaching the patient. For all calls, the EMS personnel consider their previous experiences to determine how to proceed with the call when they initiate their own first medical contact.

En route to the patient

Just as emergency physicians do when they pick up a medical chart, view the chief complaint, and begin their approach to the patient with some element of preconceived notions based on the recorded chief complaint, so do field personnel when they are approaching the patient after being dispatched with some form of dispatch code. This can be beneficial to the paramedic in that it may immediately confer some sense that the patient has no high-priority symptoms, thereby requiring the paramedic to delve further into the reason for the EMS call. It can also be detrimental for the paramedic, in that it may mislead him or her into assuming that no priority symptoms are present when in reality one or more may be present. It may also be detrimental for the patient because it may mislead the paramedic into minimizing and/or underestimating the patient's symptoms, which could result in inaccurate or ineffective use of protocols. This may also pose an increased risk to the patient if the paramedic has a negative interaction with the patient, leading to mistrust, and in some cases, no transport to hospital [5].

Emergency medical services personnel must compile a massive amount of information in a relatively short period of time. They must incorporate this information with their prehospital clinical skills and baseline knowledge in their clinical decision making, which is necessary to diagnose and treat patients effectively. Similar to emergency physicians, paramedics have become very fast in their decision-making processes, using strategies of

Emergency Medical Services: Clinical Practice and Systems Oversight, Second Edition. Volume 1: Clinical Aspects of EMS.
Edited by David C. Cone, Jane H. Brice, Theodore R. Delbridge, and J. Brent Myers.

both efficiency and thoroughness. Paramedics have also developed certain rules of thumb, shortcuts, and abbreviated thinking to make fast, efficient, and accurate decisions, or what clinical decision experts term *heuristics* [6]. Various ethnographic and descriptive studies exploring medical errors, adverse events, and near misses in EMS have shown that paramedic decision making is a predominant factor influencing patient safety in EMS [7,8].

When paramedics are interacting with a patient, there is clinical reasoning related to both the line of medical inquiry, such as the history, physical examination, and diagnostic tests, and the clinical decision making (i.e. the cognitive process of using data to evaluate, diagnose, and treat the patient) [9]. Clinical reasoning is a tremendously complex process and is under intense ongoing investigation. There is no single model of clinical decision making that adequately relates to the very complex environment that exists in the emergency setting. Rather, there are several models or strategies that individuals use in clinical decision making or cognitive performance including:

- pattern recognition or skill based (e.g. making a diagnosis immediately on entering the room, which is frequently unconscious, automatic, and based on years of experience)
- rule based (e.g. Advanced Cardiac Life Support algorithms)
- hypothetical deductive or knowledge based (considered the highest level of deduction; a clinician generates a hypothesis and uses existing and new knowledge to find an answer) [6,10].

Some experts describe a fourth model of a naturalistic or event-driven process of decision making (i.e. treating the patient first and then making the diagnosis) [6]. Interestingly, how and where paramedics make decisions and the density of decision making of paramedics in the patient journey are postulated to differ from those of other health care providers, and are under ongoing research [11].

History taking

It is essential that regardless of the dispatch determinant, the EMS crew approaches each patient in the same manner [2,5]. Field personnel should acquire a history in an unbiased manner by using effective communication strategies. A balance of both subjective and open-ended questions (e.g. Can you describe your pain for me?) and objective and close-ended questions (e.g. Is the pain sharp?) should be used. In fact, throughout all disciplines of health care, traditional dictums state that effective history taking can lead to an accurate diagnosis in the majority of cases.

Three possible outcomes can result from the history taking from a patient dispatched with an undifferentiated dispatch code. First, the paramedic may identify a prehospital diagnosis related to one of the 27 chief complaint conditions listed amongst the non-priority symptoms in the Medical Priority Dispatch System algorithms [4]. It is important that the paramedic does not trivialize the patient's needs in the absence of priority symptoms, as each patient defines his or her own

emergency. Second, the paramedic may establish a prehospital diagnosis that is accurate but not one of the 27 chief complaint conditions. In these situations, the crew members must coordinate their prehospital care knowledge to effectively care for the patient's needs. Third, perhaps the most frustrating for the crew, the paramedics may be unable to identify the specific chief complaint. This last outcome may be the first indication that the patient truly has an undifferentiated condition. At this point, it is important for the crew members to truly optimize the provider–patient interaction, while minimizing the time to treatment and time to transport.

The following strategies can be used to improve diagnostic accuracy during the history taking [6,10].

- Collect information to confirm or exclude life-threatening conditions first, then focus on the most likely diagnosis.
- Reaffirm that there are no high-priority symptoms present that could be affecting the patient's ability to render accurate answers, such as hypoglycemia or receptive and expressive aphasia with stroke.
- Ensure that the patient is oriented to person, place, and time, and that there is no underlying cognitive impairment due to drug ingestion, delirium, dementia, etc.
- When feasible, sit at the patient's bedside to collect a thorough history.
- Use adjuncts to facilitate the history taking (e.g. drawing diagrams or using other visual aids).
- Optimize communications so that the patient clearly understands the language and questions (e.g. asking simple questions).
- Obtain collateral information from the next of kin, friends, or bystanders.
- Allow a few moments of uninterrupted time to mentally process each patient.
- Generate "most life-threatening" and "most likely" diagnostic hypotheses.
- Mentally process one patient at a time.
- Avoid decision making when overly stressed or angry; take time out, regroup, and reevaluate the decision.
- Move on to physical examination to augment the history that has been elicited.

Physical examination

Sir William Osler taught that what was not found in a history was aided by completing an appropriate physical examination, and specifically that the history provided 90% of the diagnosis, that physical examination provided 9%, and that diagnostic tests contributed the remaining 1% of diagnostic certainty.

In the situation of the patient who remains undifferentiated despite optimizing the history, it is paramount that the paramedic perform a thorough and complete physical examination [5]. This begins with ensuring that a complete set of vital signs is taken and recorded. The following strategies can be used to improve the diagnostic accuracy during the physical examination process [5,6,10].

- Ensure a complete and uninterrupted physical examination or secondary survey.
- Clarify the history while conducting the physical examination.
- Perform an environmental scan of the patient's physical surroundings to complement the history (e.g. general surroundings, state of disarray, etc.).
- Have a structured and simple differential diagnosis or impression, based on the presenting history and physical information currently available (e.g. an altered level of consciousness can be broken down into structural, metabolic, and toxicological etiologies).

Adjuncts to the history and physical examination: prehospital diagnostic tests

In the case of the diagnostically undifferentiated patient, paramedics should use appropriate prehospital diagnostic tests to facilitate the working diagnosis. This would include such tests as the fingerstick glucose assessment and a prehospital 12-lead ECG. The following strategies can also be used to improve the clinical decision making for use of diagnostic tests [6,10].

- Employ any readily available decision-making algorithms or decision rules. A classic example is the Ottawa Ankle Rules that help emergency physicians in deciding on ordering ankle x-rays for injured patients. Although there are very few clinical guidelines in practice for the out-of-hospital setting, with the increasing body of evidence, these will increase in the future.
- Use existing prehospital protocols for specific therapeutic decisions whenever possible.
- Use only those tests that will affect the disposition or treatment of the patient by confirming or excluding the disease hypothesis at hand.

The truly undifferentiated patient

The patient who remains truly undifferentiated after the aforementioned maneuvers requires the same degree and level of care as those patients who have clear prehospital diagnoses. To further facilitate the care of the patient, it is important to advocate for the patient and relay the paramedic's concerns to the receiving facility. The hospital in turn can then continue to optimize the patient interaction to identify and meet patient needs.

Transition of care to the receiving facility

Just as the transition of care from the dispatcher to the paramedic occurs, there is also a transition of care between the paramedic and the hospital ED. It is of tremendous importance that this hand-off process maintains and facilitates the conti-

nuity of patient care and does not jeopardize patient safety. Many if not all EDs experience the difficult situation of ED overcrowding and long turnaround times for EMS staff. When a paramedic crew brings in a patient with no priority symptoms and no identifiable chief complaint, this may lead to confrontation between the charge nurse or physician and the paramedics. Moreover, this may lead to the receiving ED triaging the patient to the waiting room or to a lower triage score than is actually required. If the patient is truly deemed to be undifferentiated, then the paramedic must clearly state this to the receiving ED and elaborate on what has been done to optimize the history and physical exam, and provide insight and recommendations for next steps.

Consequences of an undifferentiated patient

There may be absolutely no significant consequences to either the patient or the EMS crew when the patient is undifferentiated. The patient may have an uneventful transport and ED stay. The main frustration is that both the paramedic crew and the patient are left with perhaps an unsatisfactory health care transaction. However, it is also possible that these patients may be subject to increased medical error and potentially compromised patient safety due to undifferentiated diagnoses.

Error in all aspects of medicine has become an international issue with recent publications of the Institute of Medicine report *To Err is Human* [12], and several large retrospective studies (the Harvard Medical Practice Study [13], the Colorado-Utah Study [14], and the Quality in Australian Healthcare study [15]). In the Institute of Medicine report, error is defined as the "failure of a planned action to be completed as intended or the use of a wrong plan to achieve an aim [12]." All these retrospective studies, which evaluated patients admitted from the ED, found surprisingly high rates of medical errors, many of them originating in the ED, and most of them preventable. There have been no large prospective studies describing error in the ED or the prehospital environment. Also there have been no reported associations between undifferentiated patients and the risk of medical error.

There are several ways of classifying clinical errors, which in turn provide a means of reducing or preventing these errors [6,10]. A common way is to have errors classified based on the models of cognitive performance or clinical decision making: skill-based errors (generally known as slips, or a failure in the execution of an action sequence, and lapses, or a failure of execution when the action was not the intended action), rule-based errors (mistakes such as the wrong rule is chosen due to misperception of situation or misapplication of rule), and knowledge-based errors (mistakes such as the lack or misapplication of knowledge or misinterpretation of knowledge) [10]. An alternative approach is to categorize errors into procedural errors (i.e. IV starts, intubations, and such), cognitive errors (any error in the course of diagnosis, management, and disposition of patients), and affective errors (emotional state of the medic unduly influences the clinical decision-making process) [10].

An alternative method of categorizing error is to overlay it on top of the clinical decision sequence of events that occurs when a patient is seen. For example, the progress of a patient through the ED or the ambulance is driven by multiple decisions underlying the sequence of patient assessment, diagnosis, treatment, and disposition. Many experts feel that the largest weighing or pivotal feature in this sequence is the diagnosis and its associate clinical decision making. There are three commonly described sources of diagnostic error: no-fault, system, and cognitive errors. No-fault errors can be related to a variety of factors focused mainly on the patient. This would include situations in which the history is atypical or undifferentiated; patients who are confusing, inaccurate, uncooperative, or non-compliant; and patients who misrepresent their conditions. System diagnostic errors result from a large variety of error-producing conditions (multiple interruptions, stress loads, busy shifts, etc.), equipment failure, and organizational failures. Cognitive diagnostic errors, as the preceding discussion reflects, are any of the errors related to line of medical inquiry.

Diagnostic error, such as misdiagnosis, can thus result in an incorrect choice of therapy, failure to use an indicated diagnostic test, misinterpretation of test results, and failure to act on abnormal results, which in turn may lead to patient harm in the form of incorrect treatment protocols, incorrect destination choices, and risks of no transfer.

Strategies for minimizing errors in clinical reasoning

Paramedics can limit errors in their clinical reasoning by recognizing the potential biases that may be present and incorporating certain strategies or heuristics. The science and evidence around heuristics, clinical decision making, and reasoning are in relative infancy and require prehospital care providers to extrapolate from the current and evolving evidence regarding the heuristics of decision making in medicine and emergency medicine. These may include the following [6].

- Many experts will avoid using a previous diagnosis to influence their diagnosis – perform your own history, conduct a physical exam, employ strategic diagnostic tests, and with your clinical knowledge formulate your own diagnosis and management plan.
- Minimize the influence of personal or external biases (e.g. an overzealous partner or other health care provider) on your clinical decision making.
- Check for critical items in the past medical history and/or risk factors for serious disease.
- Pay particular attention to the vital signs of the patient.
- Avoid premature closure if the diagnosis is uncertain or undifferentiated.
- Be careful of high-risk environments and times, such as high-volume and high-acuity times of day, and personal and emotional fatigue.

- Be careful of high-risk patients – refusal of care, abusive/hostile/violent patients, confrontational and annoying patients, and those with drug etiology or psychiatric disease.
- Be careful of situations in which the presumptive diagnosis does not match the history, physical exam, or diagnostic test results. Go back to your assessment of the patient and reformulate a working plan.

Conclusion

Although some may consider the undifferentiated patient a difficult or frustrating patient to manage in the prehospital setting, others may consider that they are a complex yet challenging patient population to manage. It is paramount that paramedics recognize the importance of clinical reasoning related to both the line of medical inquiry, such as conducting an effective and efficient history, physical examination, and diagnostic testing, and tempering this with their clinical decision making (i.e. the cognitive process of using data to evaluate, diagnose, and treat the patient). Because there is no single model of clinical decision making that adequately relates to the very complex environment that exists in the ED or the out-of-hospital environment, paramedics must be familiar with the various ways in which they can cognitively evaluate, diagnose, and treat the patient. By recognizing effective strategies to optimize collecting a history, conducting a physical exam, and using diagnostic tests, they will reduce and prevent medical error, leading to improved patient safety.

References

1 Lilja GP, Swor RA. Emergency medical services. In: Tintinalli J, Kelen GD, Stapczynski JS (eds) *Emergency Medicine: A Comprehensive Study Guide,* 6th edn. New York: McGraw-Hill, 2004, pp.1–6.

2 Clawson JL. Emergency medical dispatch. In: Kuehl AE (ed) *Prehospital Systems and Medical Oversight*, 3rd edn. Dubuque, IA: Kendall Hunt Publishing Company, 2002, pp.172–208.

3 Clawson JL. Priority dispatch response. In: Kuehl AE (ed) *Prehospital Systems and Medical Oversight*, 3rd edn. Dubuque, IA: Kendall Hunt Publishing Company, 2002, pp.208–22.

4 National Academy QA Guide V 11.3. Medical Priority Dispatch System. Indianapolis, IN: Priority Press, 2006, p.26.

5 Paturas JL. The EMS call. In: Pons PP, Cason D (eds) *Paramedic Field Care: A Complaint Based Approach.* St Louis, MO: Mosby Year Book, 1997, pp.29–33.

6 Chapman DM, Char DM, Aubin CD. Clinical decision making. In: Marx JA, Hockberger RS, Walls RM (eds) *Rosen's Emergency Medicine: Concepts and Clinical Practice*, 5th edn. St Louis, MO: Mosby, 2002, pp.107–15.

7 Fairbanks RJ, Crittenden CN, O'Gara KG, et al. Emergency medical services provider perceptions of the nature of adverse events and near misses in out-of-hospital care: an ethnographic view. *Acad Emerg Med* 2008;15:633–40.

8 Atack L, Maher J. Emergency medical and health providers' perceptions of key issues in prehospital patient safety. *Prehosp Emerg Care* 2010;14:95–102.

9 Kovacs G, Croskerry P. Clinical decision making: an emergency medicine perspective. *Acad Emerg Med* 1999;6:947–52.

10 Hobgood C, Croskerry P, Wears RL. Hevia A. Patient safety in emergency medicine. In: Tintinalli J, Kelen GD, Stapczynski JS (eds) *Emergency Medicine: A Comprehensive Study Guide*, 6th edn. New York: McGraw-Hill, 2004, pp.1912–18.

11 Jensen JL, Croskerry P, Travers AH. Consensus on paramedic clinical decisions during high-acuity emergency calls: results of a Canadian Delphi study. *CJEM* 2011;13(5):310–18.

12 Kohn LT, Corrigan JM, Donaldson MS (eds). *To Err is Human.* Washington, DC: Institute of Medicine, National Academy Press, 2000.

13 Brennan TA, Leape LL, Laird NM, et al. Incidence of adverse events and negligence in hospitalized patients: results of the Harvard Medical Practice Study. *N Engl J Med* 1991;324:370.

14 Thomas EJ, Studdert DM, Burstin HR, et al. Incidence and types of adverse events and negligent care in Utah and Colorado. *Med Care* 2000;38:261.

15 Wilson RM, Harrison BT, Gibberd RW, et al. An analysis of the causes of adverse events from the Quality in Australian Health Care Study. *Med J Aust* 1999;170:411.

CHAPTER 10
Altered mental status

Mark R. Quale and Jefferson G. Williams

Introduction

The patient presenting with altered mental status (AMS), also referred to as altered level of consciousness or ALOC, in the prehospital setting is one of the most common encounters in EMS. Many etiologies of AMS have the potential to cause significant morbidity and mortality. It is essential that proper care be initiated in the field, along with the early consideration of a broad differential diagnosis. Often, treatment must begin before the etiology of AMS is established. In most instances, this treatment should be instituted in conjunction with attempts to determine the underlying cause. The main challenge of a prehospital patient with undifferentiated AMS is to rapidly identify and treat potentially reversible problems in the field in order to prevent added morbidity from the complications of a prolonged condition.

Evaluation

The differential diagnosis for AMS is extensive and complex. Although the definitive treatment for many of these causes may fall outside the scope of practice of the EMS provider or the duration of the prehospital contact, he/she and the EMS physician should focus on identifying and managing conditions that may be effectively treated in the field. A brief on-scene interval and expeditious transport are required for time-critical causes of AMS (e.g. stroke, trauma) if these are identified. A simple and frequently used mnemonic for the potential causes of AMS is AEIOU TIPPS (Box 10.1).

Once scene safety is assured, EMS personnel of all levels should assess the ABCs, check vital signs, and immediately address life-threatening conditions. Once the ABCs are adequately addressed, additional history, physical examination, and field findings may prove useful in developing an appropriate treatment plan.

As the situation permits, EMS personnel should systematically obtain as much information about the patient as possible from the scene. Because the patient often cannot provide an adequate history, field personnel should seek additional information from alternative sources, such as bystanders, family, and physical surroundings. Important questions include the patient's baseline health and past medical history, the rapidity of the onset of the symptoms, and any complaints voiced or signs exhibited by the patient. One particularly useful question is whether or not the patient ever had a complete loss of consciousness or seizure-like activity.

Emergency medical services personnel should search common locations such as bathrooms, medicine cabinets, bedrooms, nightstands, and kitchens for clues about underlying illnesses or possible ingestion. A medical alert bracelet or necklace should be sought. Other household members with similar signs and symptoms, or the presence of multiple patients with altered mental status, or the presence of sick or deceased pets may point to a toxic environmental exposure such as carbon monoxide (CO) poisoning.

If a drug overdose or poisoning is suspected, EMS personnel should gather further pertinent information, including the route of exposure, the type of substance involved, and the time and amount of exposure. In the majority of cases, overdoses will occur by ingestion. If the exact amount of exposure or ingestion is not known, personnel should try to establish the maximum possible quantity. They should also note any actions taken by the patient or bystanders, including the administration of any "antidotes." Empty pill containers, liquor bottles, syringes, and other drug paraphernalia can greatly facilitate later treatment decisions.

One important route of ingestion that is not always considered is "huffing" or the use of chemical vapor to achieve AMS. Data from the 2012 Monitoring the Future Study [1] show that, while inhalant abuse has declined as prescription drug abuse has climbed, inhalants are still easy "legal" drugs to obtain for young teens, with inhalant use declining as age increases. With any inhalant there is a risk of sudden sniffing death caused by an irregular heart rhythm leading to heart failure. Suffocation,

Emergency Medical Services: Clinical Practice and Systems Oversight, Second Edition. Volume 1: Clinical Aspects of EMS.
Edited by David C. Cone, Jane H. Brice, Theodore R. Delbridge, and J. Brent Myers.
© 2015 NAEMSP. Published 2015 by John Wiley & Sons, Inc. Companion Website: www.wiley.com/go/cone\naemsp

<table>
<tr><td>

Box 10.1 Mnemonic for causes of altered mental status

A Alcohol
E Epilepsy, Electrolytes, Encephalopathy
I Insulin (hypoglycemia)
O Oxygen (hypoxia), Overdose
U Uremia
T Trauma, Temperature
I Infection
P Poisons
P Psychiatric
S Shock, Stroke, Space-occupying lesion

</td></tr>
</table>

asphyxiation, and aspiration are also risks inherent to this form of substance abuse.

Regarding the physical examination, the first task is to determine the degree of the AMS. Unfortunately, a variety of inexact terms are commonly used to describe AMS. Descriptive terms such as *stuporous, comatose, semi-comatose, obtunded, confused,* and *delirious* are poorly defined and may lead to different interpretations by bystanders, EMS providers, and hospital-based physicians. In general, it is best for the level of consciousness to be described on the basis of the response that the patient makes to a given stimulus. Field providers can use the simple mnemonic AVPU.

A = the patient is **A**lert
V = the patient responds only to loud **V**erbal stimuli
P = the patient responds only to **P**ainful stimuli
U = the patient is **U**nconscious

Emergency medical services personnel may also use the Glasgow Coma Scale (GCS) (see Volume 1, Chapter 30). A study done with paramedics scoring videotaped patients with AMS confirmed that paramedics can determine GCS scores that correlate well with those of emergency physicians [2].

The directed and focused physical exam and secondary survey can aid in determining the cause of AMS.

Head

The head should be examined for any obvious signs of trauma, such as scalp and facial lacerations, abrasions, and contusions. The pupils should be observed for symmetry and light reactivity. If they demonstrate bilateral mydriasis this may indicate cerebral hypoxia or a toxicological etiology (anticholinergics, sympathomimetics, selective serotonin reuptake inhibitors, etc.). Miosis is often due to opioid overdose. However, clonidine, antipsychotics, organophosphates, sedative-hypnotics, and pontine stroke may also cause miosis. Unequal pupils may be found as a normal variant, but they could also indicate impending herniation from trauma or a spontaneous intracranial hemorrhage. Any odor on the patient's breath (acetone, bitter almonds, ethanol, or volatile agent) should be noted. The tongue should be checked for bleeding, which may indicate seizure activity.

Neck

Any upper airway stridor should be documented, and plans to care for a partially or soon-to-be obstructed airway must take precedence. Should signs of possible acute trauma be found in a patient with AMS, the cervical spine should be evaluated and EMS personnel should maintain cervical spine precautions in keeping with protocols.

Chest

The respiratory rate, pattern, and depth should be noted. Again, any outward signs of trauma should be identified.

Abdomen

A patient with AMS who presents with a rigid, distended, or tender abdomen may be having an intraabdominal catastrophe. Pregnancy and its complications (eclampsia, HELLP syndrome, ectopic pregnancy) should be considered in females of childbearing age, especially if the patient appears gravid. In these situations, EMS protocols or direct medical oversight should provide the option for the patient to be transported to a medical facility capable of caring for acute surgical patients or pregnancy-related complications.

Neurological

In addition to pupillary findings, any focal neurological signs suggesting stroke or increased intracranial pressure, such as extremity flaccidity or Cushing's triad, should be noted and recorded as a baseline for possible progression. Altered speech patterns may also be elicited with the aid of bystanders. EMS personnel should screen for stroke using an established stroke scale, such as the Cincinnati Prehospital Stroke Scale, Los Angeles Prehospital Stroke Screen, or the Melbourne Ambulance Stroke Screen [3–5].

Skin

The skin may be used to determine temperature, which may be increased in infection or heat illness and decreased in cold exposure, dehydration, or alcohol or barbiturate overdose. Rashes potentially indicating infection or allergic reaction should be noted. Track marks consistent with needle injections and narcotic overdose should be checked for. Signs of a previous suicide attempt, such as healed wrist scars, may be apparent. The undifferentiated patient should be log-rolled and examined head to toe for occult puncture wounds or other subtle findings.

Management

The focus of a care protocol for the patient with AMS is to secure the ABCs and rapidly identify and treat reversible conditions. Appropriate basic life support measures, such as basic airway management and spinal precautions, should be instituted before any attempt is made to gather a complete history or perform a detailed physical examination.

Airway

For the majority of AMS patients, the first priority is to establish and maintain an adequate airway. If the patient is apneic or hypoventilating, respirations should be assisted by bag-valve-mask (BVM). Advanced airway placement may be considered if BVM ventilation is not effective, but the majority of patients can be managed with airway adjuncts, enough hands, and basic maneuvers. For the patient with adequate respirations, a nasal or oropharyngeal airway with oxygen via a non-rebreather mask may be appropriate. Continuous positive airway pressure (CPAP) may be of great assistance in the patient with adequate respiratory drive but shallow or ineffective ventilation, who may be hypercapneic. End-tidal CO_2 monitoring can assist the prehospital provider in both diagnosing and managing the patient with elevated pCO_2 as a cause for AMS. Should the patient become agitated or not tolerate CPAP, manual supportive airway measures such as BVM may be required. If no contraindication exists (particularly the need for spinal immobilization), the lateral decubitus position may be advantageous for airway protection in many AMS patients. For additional information on airway management, see Volume 1, Chapters 2 and 3.

Vital signs

Once the airway is secured, the next step is to accurately measure and frequently reassess the patient's pulse, blood pressure, pulse oximetry, end-tidal CO_2, and cardiac rhythm. Identification of fever or hypothermia may prove helpful in determining the etiology for AMS. A serious mistake is the failure to recognize shock or cardiac dysrhythmia. Many of the newest generation cardiac monitors also have the ability to measure carbon monoxide and methemoglobin levels via cooximetry. Should vital signs taken automatically via the cardiac monitor be incongruent with the rest of the clinical picture, take them manually (e.g. blood pressure measurement via a manual cuff) to ensure accuracy.

Glucose evaluation and administration

After vital signs have been addressed, the next step in most EMS protocols calls for the measurement of serum glucose and/or drawing other blood samples for point-of-care testing, usually done concurrently with establishment of IV access. Although the defined level for hypoglycemia varies from system to system, many use a level of less than or equal to 70 mg/dL when accompanied by appropriate signs and symptoms of hypoglycemia. This method of testing then treating is generally preferable to the blind administration of exogenous glucose to all patients with AMS. Only 25% of patients with AMS are hypoglycemic. The common assumption that an ampule of dextrose 50% in water "won't hurt anyone" has been refuted [6]. Exogenous dextrose may result in skin necrosis after inadvertent extravasation or subcutaneous infiltration, variable elevations in the serum glucose level, hyperosmolality, hyperkalemia, and potentially a worsened neurological outcome in patients with focal or global cerebral or myocardial ischemia [7,8]. Worsened neurological outcome is the greatest point of concern and the current consensus is that the blind administration of exogenous glucose may be harmful [7]. However, after administration of dextrose to the known hypoglycemic patient, an improvement in mental status is usually seen within 5 minutes. The average increase in serum glucose level following one ampule of dextrose is approximately 150 mg/dL [9].

Emergency medical services personnel may have difficulty establishing IV access in patients with hypoglycemia. In these cases the use of intramuscular glucagon has been shown to be safe and effective [10]. Some patients without glycogen stores will not respond adequately to glucagon. The mean time to response to glucagon is approximately 6–9 minutes, with an increase in glucose level of about 100 mg/dL [10]. Because of the risk of aspiration, EMS personnel must exercise care when using oral glucose solutions in patients with AMS. In general, if IV access is difficult or prolonged in the critically ill patient, placement of an intraosseous (IO) line is an alternative route for IV therapies, including dextrose administration.

Naloxone

If vital signs have been obtained and shock and/or hypoglycemia are being managed, another common early step in the evaluation and management of AMS is to consider toxic ingestion or overdose. With the rise in prescription drug abuse [2], including opiates, the next step in many protocols is to consider administration of an opiate antagonist, as opiate overdose is a potentially reversible cause of life-threatening AMS in the prehospital setting.

Naloxone is the current opiate antagonist of choice in the acute care setting. Naloxone is generally safe, with very few serious side-effects, the most common being precipitation of withdrawal. Many EMS physicians advocate a low-dose administration protocol (0.4 mg initially, titrated to respiratory improvement), which may reverse the life-threatening respiratory depression of opiate overdose without precipitating the violent "emergence" from opioid sedation that occasionally accompanies full and rapid reversal. However, failure to give an appropriate amount of an opioid antagonist is a potential pitfall. The synthetic and semi-synthetic opioids, as well as illicit heroin use, especially in the naïve user, may require very large doses of naloxone for reversal. Thus, frequent titration with repeated small doses of naloxone and close monitoring are recommended.

In cases in which opioid overdose is suspected, ventilation should be supported with a BVM while waiting for the onset of naloxone. Given the effectiveness of prehospital naloxone, early advanced airway management is contraindicated in the opiate overdose patient. Naloxone can be given by the IM, IN, IV, and IO routes, all of which have been shown to be similarly effective in the prehospital setting [11,12]. Given the comparable efficacy of the intranasal route, IN naloxone may be the initial route of choice, reducing the risk of a needlestick incident [13]. Also, IN naloxone provides a way for BLS providers and even laypersons to deliver a potentially life-saving medicine to those suffering from opioid overdose [14,15]. In all cases, it is extremely important that the prehospital care provider observe and record any response by the patient to the administered medication, as this will greatly facilitate the management by subsequent medical personnel.

Other "reversal" agents: use of flumazenil

Given the prevalence of benzodiazepine use and abuse, it is tempting to consider flumazenil, a benzodiazepine antagonist, for the obtunded patient with history of benzodiazepine overdose. However, the use of flumazenil in patients who have also ingested seizure-inducing medications (e.g. tricyclic antidepressants) or in those chronically prescribed benzodiazepines may result in seizures [16]. These seizures may be refractory to benzodiazepine treatment because of blockade of the benzodiazepine receptor; death from flumazenil-induced seizures has been reported [17]. Due to these considerations and because benzodiazepine toxicity is generally managed well with supportive care alone, most medical directors and medical toxicologists do not advocate the use of flumazenil in the field [17].

Challenges with the AMS patient

There is probably no patient category that can be more challenging than those presenting with AMS. The large differential diagnosis, combined with the lack of direct pertinent information due to the inability of the patient to give a history, contribute to significant potentials for error. In addition, the prehospital provider on the scene with an AMS patient with a broad differential must rapidly either rule in or rule out time-sensitive conditions that require rapid transport rather than further on-scene management.

For example, a patient who meets trauma criteria should have a short scene time and rapid transport to a trauma specialty center. Trauma, particularly of the head and neck, is always a possibility for patients with AMS. Although AMS (decreased GCS) is a criterion for specialty transport to a trauma center [18], a patient with AMS and otherwise minimal signs of trauma may have another competing or underlying etiology for his or her AMS.

A major challenge with AMS patients is that they can be easily triaged into the AMS "not otherwise specified" protocol, while actually having a definable process. In addition to trauma patients, those with ST-segment elevated myocardial infarction (STEMI) and stroke require rapid recognition and transport. Dysrythmia and/or hypotension associated with inferior MI may present with AMS as the predominant sign, and stroke patients who are non-verbal or who have isolated slurred speech may be classified first as AMS. Indeed, the various forms of shock all may present with AMS, yet must be treated differently. Keeping a broad differential diagnosis throughout the prehospital encounter, and avoiding "tunnel vision" even while proceeding down a treatment pathway, are essential to preventing errors or delaying definitive care in the AMS patient.

Furthermore, patients with AMS may have multiple ongoing causes for their altered level of consciousness that should be addressed in the prehospital environment. For example, it is tempting to assume that a patient with seizures, who may be actively seizing or postictal, has an underlying seizure disorder. However, seizures may be caused by cardiac arrest (ventricular fibrillation), hypoxia, hypoglycemia, trauma, intracranial hemorrhage, stroke, infection and drug overdose and withdrawal, all etiologies which can separately contribute to the patient's AMS.

Altered mental status patients with any of multiple etiologies may also be physically aggressive or combative, presenting a challenge as well as a risk to EMS providers. Patients with traumatic head injuries, those under the influence of either prescription or illicit drugs or alcohol, and those with medical emergencies such as hypoglycemia, postictal state, decompensated psychiatric disorders, and many others may be violent. The experienced EMS provider will recognize that these patients may have combative altered mental status due to an underlying medical condition, but that does not lessen the risks of physical harm to the patient or the provider. Care should be taken to ensure both crew and patient safety with potentially combative patients, and early involvement of law enforcement in these cases may be warranted.

In addition, even experienced medical personnel may not be able to immediately differentiate between patients who are simply altered, due to hypoglycemia for example, and relatively easily calmed and treated, and those who are suffering from emergency life-threatening situations such as excited delirium syndrome [19]. Therefore, after immediate attempts at verbal redirection fail, EMS providers may need to assist law enforcement with the application of physical restraints, always with concurrent chemical restraint, in order to assess, treat, and possibly resuscitate these critically ill patients. For additional information on managing the combative patient, refer to Volume 1, Chapter 59.

One group that deserves special mention is those AMS patients who are diagnosed as being "just drunk." EMS personnel, including field physicians, often focus on the presumption of alcohol intoxication without considering other potential conditions causing AMS in the patient who abuses alcohol. The alcoholic is also prone to myriad medical and traumatic problems, including liver disease, diabetes, hypoglycemia, electrolyte imbalances, and an increased propensity for intracranial hemorrhage (Box 10.2). The intoxicated patient should always have a rapid, but thorough, evaluation for trauma and other acute conditions.

Refusal of care after resolution of altered mental status: treatment for hypoglycemia or opiate overdose

Despite the broad differential diagnosis, EMS providers will "fix" many patients with AMS on the scene, especially those with relatively straightforward, isolated conditions such as hypoglycemia or opiate overdose. One of the greatest challenges with these patients is determining who has a single,

> **Box 10.2** Causes of altered mental status in alcoholics
>
> - Intoxication
> - Electrolyte abnormalities
> - Hypothermia
> - Hypoxia
> - Infection/sepsis
> - Liver disease
>   - Hepatic encephalopathy
>   - Coagulation disorders
>   - Hypoglycemia
> - Overdose/intoxication
> - Seizures
> - Trauma
> - Withdrawal

self-limited process that has been fixed and that is unlikely to recur, and therefore may be safe to not be transported to the ED or otherwise refuse care, and who requires further treatment or extended observation and therefore should be transported to the ED. Many hypoglycemic patients who have improvement in mental status with field treatment will refuse further medical care and transport. This practice has been shown to be generally safe if certain criteria are met [20,21]. Many EMS systems have "treat and release" protocols for resolved hypoglycemia. In general, some common proposed criteria for safe treatment and non-transport are as follows.

- History of insulin-dependent diabetes mellitus, and/or the patient is not taking long-acting oral hypoglycemics.
- Posttreatment blood glucose level greater than 80–100 mg/dL.
- Return of normal mental status within a short time of dextrose administration.
- Ability to tolerate food and liquid by mouth, and/or the patient must eat a meal in the presence of EMS.
- A responsible adult is present to assist the patient as needed, especially in case of recurrent hypoglycemia.
- Absence of complicating factors (e.g. chest pain, arrhythmias, dyspnea, seizures, alcohol intoxication, chronic renal failure requiring dialysis, or focal neurological signs/symptoms).

It is always important for the EMS provider to determine whether the patient is taking a long-acting oral hypoglycemic agent. Despite any immediate improvement, in the absence of a plan for in-home medical care and close glucose monitoring, all patients taking these medications should be transported to the emergency department for further evaluation and extended observation due to the prolonged half-life of their medications and high likelihood of relapsing hypoglycemia.

A similar controversy may arise for narcotic overdose patients successfully treated with naloxone. These individuals may feel well and wish to refuse transport to the emergency department. Because of the relatively short half-life of naloxone, there is concern that these patients may later develop the recurrence of symptoms.

Experience in EMS systems that have been fully reversing opioid overdose and allowing transport refusals would suggest the actual risk of clinically significant resedation is small [22,23]. Some EMS systems have protocols that allow uncomplicated narcotic overdose patients to refuse transport, often after consenting to an additional dose of naloxone prior to the end of the EMS encounter [24]. In general, some common proposed criteria for safe treatment and non-transport of resolved narcotic overdose include the following.

- Isolated IV heroin use, and/or the patient has not overdosed on any oral or long-acting opioids.
- The patient was not in cardiac arrest and naloxone was used only for the treatment of AMS/respiratory depression.
- A relatively small dose of naloxone, perhaps ≤2 mg, was required to return the patient to normal mental status.
- The patient consents to receiving an additional naloxone dose and/or has naloxone available to be readministered if necessary.
- A responsible adult is present to assist the patient as needed.

Conclusion and EMS protocol recommendations

The EMS physician, and all prehospital providers, must always approach the prehospital management of the patient with AMS in a systematic fashion and with a great deal of care. A broad differential diagnosis must be considered and maintained throughout the patient encounter. Ongoing evaluation must occur even while treatment steps are accomplished. Attention must be given to supporting the patient's vital functions and to reversing those disorders that can be treated in the field.

Basic Life Support protocols for patients with AMS should focus on the evaluation and treatment of airway and breathing problems, while assuring spinal stabilization when indicated. For the patient who is alert and able to take oral glucose, this treatment could be considered within the basic provider's scope of practice, depending on state or regional protocols.

Advanced Life Support practitioners may provide fluid resuscitation, IV dextrose to known diabetics with hypoglycemia, naloxone via one of multiple possible routes to suspected opioid overdoses, and many other medications to treat the suspected underlying cause of AMS. The advanced provider's greatest tool, however, is perhaps his or her advanced training and ability to maintain a high degree of suspicion for multiple possible contributors to a patient's AMS. The appropriate EMS protocol for AMS is one that prioritizes rapid and thorough assessment and management of vital signs, allows for the correction of conditions that are reversible in the field, and branches to consider other protocols based on the likely underlying cause(s) of AMS.

Acknowledgment

A special thank you and recognition to Dr Paul W. Beck who authored the previous edition of this chapter.

References

1 Johnston LD, O'Malley PM, Bachman JG, Schulenberg JE. *Monitoring the Future. National Results on Drug Use*: 2012 Overview, Key Findings on Adolescent Drug Use. Ann Arbor, MI: Institute for Social Research, University of Michigan, 2013.

2 Menegazzi JJ, Davis EA, Sucov AN, Paris PM. Reliability of the Glasgow Coma Scale when used by emergency physicians and paramedics. *J Trauma* 1993;34(1):46–8.

3 Kothari RU, Pancioli A, Liu T, Brott T, Broderick J. Cincinnati Prehospital Stroke Scale: reproducibility and validity. *Ann Emerg Med* 1999;33(4):373–8.

4 Kidwell CS, Starkman S, Eckstein M, Weems K, Saver JL. Identifying stroke in the field. Prospective validation of the Los Angeles prehospital stroke screen (LAPSS). *Stroke* 2000;31(1):71–6.

5 Bray JE, Martin J, Cooper G, Barger B, Bernard S, Bladin C. Paramedic identification of stroke: community validation of the Melbourne ambulance stroke screen. *Cerebrovasc Dis* 2005;20(1):28–33.

6 Browning RG, Olson DW, Stueven HA, Mateer JR. 50% dextrose: antidote or toxin? *Ann Emerg Med* 1990;19(6):683–7.

7 Pulsinelli WA, Levy DE, Sigsbee B, Scherer P, Plum F. Increased damage after ischemic stroke in patients with hyperglycemia with or without established diabetes mellitus. *Am J Med* 1983;74(4): 540–4.

8 Longstreth WT Jr, Inui TS. High blood glucose level on hospital admission and poor neurological recovery after cardiac arrest. *Ann Neurol* 1984;15(1):59–63.

9 Collier A, Steedman DJ, Patrick AW, et al. Comparison of intravenous glucagon and dextrose in treatment of severe hypoglycemia in an accident and emergency department. *Diabetes Care* 1987;10(6):712–15.

10 Vukmir RB, Paris PM, Yealy DM. Glucagon: prehospital therapy for hypoglycemia. *Ann Emerg Med* 1991;20(4):375–9.

11 Kelly AM, Kerr D, Dietze P, Patrick I, Walker T, Koutsogiannis Z. Randomised trial of intranasal versus intramuscular naloxone in prehospital treatment for suspected opioid overdose. *Med J Aust* 2005;182(1):24–7.

12 Ashton H, Hassan Z. Best evidence topic report. Intranasal naloxone in suspected opioid overdose. *Emerg Med J* 2006;23(3):221–3.

13 Barton ED, Colwell CB, Wolfe T, et al. Efficacy of intranasal naloxone as a needleless alternative for treatment of opioid overdose in the prehospital setting. *J Emerg Med* 2005;29(3):265–71.

14 Maxwell S, Bigg D, Stanczykiewicz K, Carlberg-Racich S. Prescribing naloxone to actively injecting heroin users: a program to reduce heroin overdose deaths. *J Addict Dis* 2006;25(3):89–96.

15 Belz D, Lieb J, Rea T, Eisenberg MS. Naloxone use in a tiered-response emergency medical services system. *Prehosp Emerg Care* 2006;10(4):468–71.

16 Haverkos GP, DiSalvo RP, Imhoff TE. Fatal seizures after flumazenil administration in a patient with mixed overdose. *Ann Pharmacother* 1994;28(12):1347–9.

17 Weinbroum AA, Flaishon R, Sorkine P, Szold O, Rudick V. A risk-benefit assessment of flumazenil in the management of benzodiazepine overdose. *Drug Saf* 1997;17(3):181–96.

18 Sasser SM, Hunt RC, Faul M, et al. Guidelines for field triage of injured patients: recommendations of the National Expert Panel on Field Triage, 2011. *MMWR Recomm Rep* 2012;61(RR-1):1–20.

19 Vilke GM, DeBard ML, Chan TC, et al. Excited Delirium Syndrome (EXDS): defining based on a review of the literature. *J Emerg Med* 2012;43(5):897–905.

20 Anderson S, Hogskilde PD, Wetterslev J, Bredgaard M, Moller JT, Dahl JB. Appropriateness of leaving emergency medical service treated hypoglycemic patients at home: a retrospective study. *Acta Anaesthesiol Scand* 2002;46(4):464–8.

21 Thompson R, Wolford R. Development and evaluation of criteria allowing paramedics to treat and release patients presenting with hypoglycemia: a retrospective study. *Prehosp Disast Med* 1991;6: 309–13.

22 Vilke GM, Sloane C, Smith AM, Chan TC. Assessment for deaths in out-of-hospital heroin overdose patients treated with naloxone who refuse transport. *Acad Emerg Med* 2003;10(8):893–6.

23 Wampler DA, Molina DK, McManus J, Laws P, Manifold CA. No deaths associated with patient refusal of transport after naloxone-reversed opioid overdose. *Prehosp Emerg Care* 2011;15(3): 320–4.

24 Myers JB, Williams JG. Personal communication. *Wake County EMS System Standards and Practice 2013: Protocol 38: Overdose/ Toxic Ingestion.*

CHAPTER 11

Cardiac arrest systems of care

Bryan McNally, Paul M. Middleton, and Marcus Ong

Introduction

The original motivations for the development of EMS were to improve the care of patients suffering from major trauma and out-of-hospital cardiac arrest (OHCA). Physicians and resuscitation researchers often focus on patient-level perspectives of cardiac arrest care (e.g. specific drug agents or treatment algorithms). However, the most important factors determining OHCA survival involve the systems of community care.

The recognition that sudden cardiac arrest (SCA) survival depended on the time intervals from collapse to initiation of cardiopulmonary resuscitation (CPR) and to defibrillation spurred extensive EMS and public safety efforts to achieve faster response and earlier defibrillation. These efforts included the use of fire fighters and police officers as first responders, training EMTs to perform defibrillation, and strategic deployment of ALS units (systems status management). However, there were (and remain) inherent logistical limits to first responder speed.

The development of the automated external defibrillator (AED) led to the concept of public access defibrillation (PAD) [1]. The AED highlighted the critical importance of immediate bystander action in the management of cardiac arrest. Every EMS medical director, manager, and provider must recognize the importance of this principle. EMS responders and hospital staff have less impact on OHCA survival than bystander CPR and AED use [2]. OHCA survival when bystander CPR and AED are used may be as high as 33–50% [3–5].

The effect of bystander CPR or bystander AED happening early on in the chain of survival is described in Table 11.1. The data are from the Cardiac Arrest Registry to Enhance Survival (CARES) Program and are specific to those patients who have a witnessed OHCA and are found in a shockable rhythm.

Optimal OHCA survival depends on a comprehensive community-based approach that includes collecting essential OHCA outcome data as part of a continuous quality improvement program to improve care. In 2004 only 13 of the 50 largest cities in

the US collected meaningful OHCA outcomes. Today 45 of these communities collect OHCA outcome data [6]. Programs like CARES (https://mycares.net) and the Pan Asian Resuscitation Outcomes Study (PAROS) (www.scri.edu.sg/index.php/networks-paros) provide communities with the necessary tools to collect OHCA data in an ongoing efficient manner, allowing for benchmarking and gauging effectiveness in a real-world environment [4,7,8]. In King County, Washington, the Resuscitation Academy was created to help communities develop local quality assurance programs through a 3-day fellowship program designed specifically for EMS providers, administrators. and medical directors (www.resuscitationacademy.com/).

Implementation of this community systems-based approach is as important a role for EMS agencies as is training and preparing for their own direct patient care. This chapter provides an overview of the system-level considerations in cardiac arrest resuscitation and care. The other components of clinical cardiac arrest care are discussed in Volume 1, Chapter 12.

Epidemiology of cardiac arrest

The annual incidence of SCA in the United States is estimated at between 166,000 and 450,000 cases [5,9,10]. The reported incidence varies with the source of the data and definitions used. Precise epidemiological information is limited because the Centers for Disease Control and Prevention (CDC) does not consider OHCA a reportable disease [11].

Many cardiac arrests are due to ventricular fibrillation (VF) or ventricular tachycardia, but the proportion in a shockable rhythm on EMS arrival varies with the time from collapse to initial assessment. Studies based on hospitalized patients report a shockable rhythm in about 75% of cases, whereas EMS studies report figures ranging from 24% to 60% [4,12–17]. EMS data suggest that the rate of out-of-hospital VF/ ventricular tachycardia (VT) may be decreasing, but the overall incidence of OHCA is not

Emergency Medical Services: Clinical Practice and Systems Oversight, Second Edition. Volume 1: Clinical Aspects of EMS.
Edited by David C. Cone, Jane H. Brice, Theodore R. Delbridge, and J. Brent Myers.
© 2015 NAEMSP. Published 2015 by John Wiley & Sons, Inc. Companion Website: www.wiley.com\go\cone\naemsp

Table 11.1 Number and percentage of persons who experience and those who survive a bystander-witnessed out-of-hospital cardiac arrest and are found in a shockable rhythm, by clinical characteristics, United States, 2005–2010

Characteristic	Experience		Survive	
	No.	(%)	No.	(%)
Who first initiated CPR?				
Bystander	2,076	49.0	696	33.5
9-1-1 responder	2,164	51.0	580	26.8
Total	**4,240**	**100**	**1,276**	**30.1**
Who first applied AED/monitor?				
Bystander	376	8.9	188	50.0
9-1-1 responder	3,867	91.1	1,090	28.2
Total	**4,243**	**100**	**1,278**	**30.1**

CARES 2005–2012

[18–21]. However, studies with rhythms recorded by on-site defibrillators continue to identify VF/VT as the most common initial rhythm. VF/VT was the presenting rhythm in 61% of arrests in the Casino trial and 59% of the patients in the PAD trial [22,23].

The average survival to hospital discharge after OHCA is estimated to be between 5% and 10%,[4,24–27] but reported OHCA survival rates also vary widely. There are likely several reasons for this, including differing denominators, varying definitions of survival, and possibly true regional differences [24]. In the Resuscitation Outcomes Consortium composed of nine communities in North America, a five-fold difference in survival was found between sites [28]. Survival rates are highest in patients in whom the collapse is witnessed and the presenting rhythm is shockable. CARES data in 2012 (see Table 11.1) revealed a 37% survival rate for this subset of patients, which increased to 50% with use of an on-site defibrillator. Survival is lowest for unwitnessed and asystolic arrests.

Elements of a community cardiac arrest care system

The key elements of a community cardiac arrest care system include the following.
- Early recognition and calling for help.
- 9-1-1 dispatching and provision of bystander CPR instructions
- Bystander CPR
- PAD
- First responder BLS care, including defibrillation
- ALS care
- Postarrest care
- Participation in an OHCA registry and local quality improvement program

Emergency medical services directly provide only two elements of this chain. Thus, community-oriented approaches are essential in facilitating improved cardiac arrest survival. EMS medical directors and agencies cannot successfully care for victims of OHCA in isolation. They must work with the community to optimize all elements of care and should serve leadership roles in this effort.

Bystander recognition of arrest and calling for help

The most important first steps in cardiac arrest care are recognition of the event and summoning help. These actions require widespread public awareness of the existence of OHCA, how to recognize OHCA, and the importance of immediate action.

The methods for teaching laypersons the recognition of OHCA have evolved over recent years. Many studies have described the difficulty of and delays caused by laypersons attempting to feel for a pulse [29]. One showed that even trained EMTs were inaccurate in detecting the presence or absence of a pulse in patients undergoing cardiac bypass during open heart surgery [30]. Thus, current American Heart Association (AHA) guidelines advise that bystanders should call 9-1-1 and begin treatment for OHCA if the person has no movement and no regular breathing. Bystanders must not mistake agonal gasps for normal breathing [31].

Emergency medical dispatch (EMD) is essential in cardiac arrest care. Dispatch centers must quickly and accurately recognize potential cardiac arrest calls and promptly dispatch appropriate first responder and EMS units. Providing prearrival instructions for bystander CPR and AED use is another important EMD role. Dispatcher instruction in CPR improves the likelihood of the caller performing CPR [32]. The details and requirements for emergency dispatching systems are discussed in Volume 2, Chapter 10.

Bystander cardiopulmonary resuscitation

Bystander CPR refers to CPR performed by someone who was already present at or passing by the location of the patient. This contrasts with CPR performed by dispatched emergency responders. Bystanders have the earliest opportunity to provide CPR to the cardiac arrest victim. Multiple studies have demonstrated the survival benefit of bystander CPR as well as the increase in mortality with delays in CPR delivery [33,34].EMS medical directors and agencies should monitor and optimize the rate of bystander CPR in their communities [35]. Prior efforts have included community education about OHCA and the importance of CPR, increasing access to training, and teaching CPR in schools to develop a culture of bystander assistance.

When callers do not know CPR, the dispatcher should provide real-time instructions over the phone. Most current EMD protocols detail specific CPR instructions [36]. Growing evidence suggests that properly performed chest compressions are more important than ventilations [37–39]. Most emergency dispatch protocols now favor providing instructions only for chest compressions.

The AHA recommends that bystanders not trained in CPR and those trained but not confident or willing to perform ventilations should perform chest compression-only CPR until a defibrillator is ready for use (Class IIa) [37]. Unrecognized fatigue is common after just 1–2 minutes, so bystanders providing chest compressions should switch frequently [40].

Public access defibrillation

The most important cardiac arrest interventions for patients in VF or VT are early chest compressions and defibrillation. Although 70–80% of VF can be successfully converted to a perfusing rhythm if shocked within 3 minutes of VF onset, this success rate deteriorates rapidly with each additional minute [41]. Survival decreases 7–10% for each minute that passes before defibrillation [34] (Figure 11.1).

Automated external defibrillators provide lay bystanders with the ability to deliver rescue shocks. These devices were first used clinically in 1979 to recognize and deliver rescue shocks for VF and rapid VT [42]. AEDs are automated and simple to use with visual and audible instructions for operating the defibrillator and initiating CPR. They are relatively inexpensive and extremely safe; modern AEDs do not allow delivery of inappropriate shocks [43]. Most are equipped with memory modules that can record the entire resuscitation event, including continuous ECG and audio recording.

Defibrillators with CPR feedback use accelerometers embedded within chest defibrillation pads to measure depth and rate of compression, or use variations in chest impedance to reflect chest wall movements [44,45]. These devices are able to give verbal as well as visual prompts to cue the rescuer to speed up, slow down, or increase the depth of compressions or ventilations [46]. Such devices have been shown to improve the quality of CPR for out-of-hospital [47] as well as in-hospital cardiac arrest [46].

A variety of AED models are now available, ranging in sophistication and ruggedness. Some models are designed for minimally trained lay bystanders, and are available for consumer purchase without physician prescription.

There is strong scientific evidence confirming the efficacy of early first responder, bystander, and public access defibrillation. A trial which trained security personnel in casinos to recognize OHCA, start CPR, and use on-site AEDs achieved 53% survival from VF, and among patients shocked within 3 minutes survival was 74% [23]. AEDs have also been successfully used on aircraft and in the airport [48]. In the multicenter PAD trial, 993 high-risk locations were randomized to deploy or not deploy on-site AEDs. A response plan with identification and training of on-site responders was implemented at all sites. Survival was double at AED sites compared to non-AED sites [22]. Other reports also describe successful PAD programs [49].

One successful real-world example is Japan, where public access defibrillators have rapidly become more available since 2004 [50,51]. The cumulative number of public access defibrillators (excluding medical facilities and EMS institutions) increased from 9,906 in 2005 to 297,095 in 2011 [52]. From 2005 to 2007, the proportion of bystander-witnessed VF/VT arrests who received public access defibrillation increased from 1.2% (45/3841) to 6.2% (274/4402) [50]. The latest data show that over 40% of cardiac arrests in public places like train

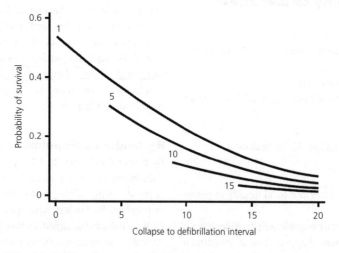

Figure 11.1 Relation of collapse to CPR and defibrillation to survival: simplified model. Graphical representation of simplified (includes collapse to CPR and collapse to defibrillation only) predictive model of survival after witnessed, out-of-hospital cardiac arrest due to VF. Each curve represents change in probability of survival as delay (minutes) to defibrillation increases for a given collapse-to-CPR interval (minutes). Source: Valenzuela TD. *Circulation* 1997;96:3308–13. Reproduced with permission of Lippincott, Williams and Wilkins.

stations and sports facilities received shocks with public access defibrillators.

The observation that a majority of OHCA events occur in residential settings raised interest in home deployment of AEDs. This concept was evaluated in a large, multicenter, international trial of anterior wall myocardial infarction survivors who were not candidates for implantable cardiac defibrillators [53]. A related innovation is the wearable cardioverter-defibrillator, which combines a long-term ECG monitoring system with an AED [54].

Locations at high risk can be identified using public health surveillance tools such as registries that collect standardized data on OHCA. Cardiac arrest locations can be analyzed using geographic information systems and spatial epidemiology methods to identify and target high-risk neighborhoods within a community [55,56]. These should have emergency preparedness and response plans that include AED deployment [57–59]. These areas may include airports, fitness centers, large workplaces, arenas and convention centers, and even jails. AED deployment and response plans should include registration with dispatch centers, development of a notification system to alert on-site responders, selection and training of responders, and deployment of appropriate AED and other rescue equipment. Equipment maintenance, annual response plan review, and quality improvement incident reviews are essential components of an effective PAD program. Smartphone apps are also available which can show the location of the nearest AED during an emergency. These can be integrated into local response systems.

There is an important opportunity for local EMS agencies and medical directors to assist public and private sites with implementing PAD programs. Several websites and publications provide detailed suggestions for PAD program development [60–72].

First responder and Basic Life Support care

Before the advent of PAD, medical directors sought ways to shorten the delays to initial defibrillation.One solution was to equip first responders with AEDs because these individuals could often reach a cardiac arrest victim faster than an ALS ambulance. The first important report of this concept involved firefighterfirst responders in King County, Washington, in 1989 [73]. Police first responders in Rochester, Minnesota, and suburban areas near Pittsburgh, Pennsylvania, also successfully used AEDs [19,74,75]. These programs demonstrated benefit even if the first responders arrived only 2 minutes before EMS. Cardiac arrest survival was 50% in Rochester, Minnesota, after introducing a police AED program [75,76]. The use of motorcycles in urban settings to reduce response time has also been described [77].

The OPALS study specifically evaluated the effect of optimizing time to defibrillation by BLS responders, with a goal of having a defibrillator-equipped vehicle on scene within 8 minutes of 9-1-1 call receipt in 90% of calls. Increasing the proportion of responses that met the 8-minute standard from 77% to 92% improved survival to hospital discharge from 3.9% to 5.2% [78]. A subsequent analysis found that increasing time to defibrillation was associated with decreased survival [1] (Figure 11.2). These observations further underscored the greater importance of bystander action in facilitating additional survival.

Performing high-quality, continuous chest compressions is another important role for first responders. There is increasing evidence of the role of high-quality chest compressions in improving defibrillation success [79–81]. Research indicates that the quality of CPR is vitally important [54,80], especially rate, depth, and reducing prolonged interruption of chest compressions, as interruptions result in less cycle time and lower coronary perfusion pressures [74–77]. Use of multiple first

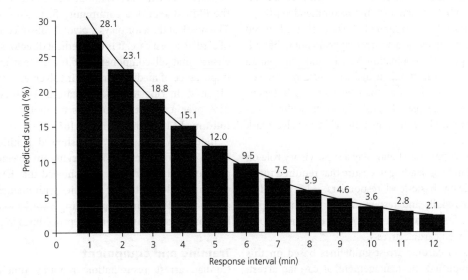

Figure 11.2 Predicted survival versus defibrillation response interval. Source: De Maio VJ. *Ann Emerg Med* 2003;42:242–50. Reproduced with permission from Elsevier.

responders (teams of four or more) to allow for closely supervised BLS has also been advocated as "high-performance CPR." Also, use of mechanical CPR has been recommended, especially if transport with ongoing CPR is needed, for example in BLS ambulance systems [78].

Advanced Life Support care

Although traditionally viewed as the cornerstone of cardiac arrest care, the limited effectiveness of traditional ALS interventions in cardiac arrest is increasingly being shown. In the OPALS study, which added ALS care to previously optimized first responder defibrillation, ALS care did not further improve cardiac arrest survival [2]. In other words, early CPR and defibrillation had greater effects on cardiac arrest survival than advanced airway management or drug administration.

In the systematic and comprehensive evidence review undertaken for the production of the International Liaison Committee on Resuscitation (ILCOR) guidelines in 2010, many ALS interventions previously accepted as routine were found to be supported by little good-quality evidence. ILCOR Consensus on Science authors stated that there were no data to support the routine use of any specific approach to airway management during cardiac arrest, and elaborated on concerns that extended attempts to insert an endotracheal tube may lead to harmful interruption of chest compressions [82].

They concluded that there was insufficient evidence to define the optimal timing of advanced airway placement during cardiac arrest, and also stated that supraglottic airway devices may be considered by health care professionals trained in their use as an alternative to bag-valve-mask ventilation during CPR. Cricoid pressure was not recommended for use in cardiac arrest, whereas waveform capnography was. A lack of evidence supporting many ALS pharmacological interventions was emphasized, including vasopressors, atropine, steroids, fibrinolytics, and fluids during cardiac arrest, with placebo-controlled trials being called for; calcium and sodium bicarbonate were not recommended [82].

Since 2010, studies have continued to show that advanced airway management during cardiac arrest appears not to benefit patients. A prospective, population-based study in Japan involving 650,000 out-of-hospital cardiac arrest patients showed that any type of advanced airway management was independently associated with decreased odds of neurologically favorable survival compared with conventional bag-valve-mask ventilation [83].

If dispatched, ALS personnel may play a supervisory role on scene, taking part in team leading to ensure that required interventions are made by basic-level responders. ALS providers also have advanced skills and resources that may be helpful in select scenarios (e.g. treating a tension pneumothorax or a hyperkalemia-induced cardiac arrest).

Recent changes in cardiac arrest guidelines based on this evidence have simplified the management of cardiac arrest, highlighting the preeminence of BLS measures such as immediate bystander chest compressions, and the use of AEDs by bystanders whether or not previously trained, with ALS interventions being delayed until later in the course of the patient journey.

Of interest is that interventions considered to be most beneficial in the postresuscitation care phase, such as the induction of therapeutic hypothermia, have increasingly been trialled in the prehospital phase of cardiac arrest. It has been shown that prehospital cooling can be carried out safely and efficaciously [84–86]; however, survival benefit has not yet been convincingly demonstrated [87].

Postresuscitation care

Postresuscitation care and in-hospital postarrest therapies are an important factor affecting OHCA survival and subsequent functional outcome [79]. Significant morbidity and mortality after OHCA are due to cerebral and cardiac dysfunction in what has been termed the "postcardiac arrest syndrome" [80]. Despite initial coma after OHCA, subsequent neurological recovery can be influenced by in-hospital postarrest treatments [81,87,88].

Despite these advances, many medical centers do not provide standardized postarrest care [89] for reasons including a sense of futility, staffing, cost, expertise, and resources [90–93]. This is despite published recommendations on postarrest care including implementation and barriers to implementation and guidelines for cardiac resuscitation systems of care [94,95].

Regionalized postresuscitation care has been proposed, with "cardiac arrest centers" equipped and staffed to provide guideline-based therapies such as targeted temperature management, 24-7 postcardiac arrest percutaneous coronary intervention, and extracorporeal membrane oxygenation (ECMO). An example of a state-wide regionalized system of postarrest care was implemented in Arizona in 2007 [96].

Role of the medical director

Stewart commented, "Without dedicated medical leadership, the EMS system of a community flirts with mediocrity" [97]. The medical director plays a pivotal role in community systems of cardiac arrest care. It is the medical director's responsibility to ensure that all components of the system are in place. The importance of medical director involvement cannot be overemphasized. In Houston, the increase in VF survival from 0% to 21% over a 5-year period was attributed to the hiring of a full-time EMS medical director [65].

Indeed, Williams et al. [98] showed significant variation in EMS scope of practice with varying involvement of a medical director, and Greer et al. [99] showed that EMS agencies with paid medical directors or agencies with medical director interaction with EMTs in the preceding 4 weeks were more likely to have prehospital cardiovascular procedures in place.

Training and equipment

Cardiac arrest resuscitation requires timely and accurate execution of interventions. Because of the multitude of simultaneous tasks, cardiac arrest resuscitation requires a carefully coordinated team effort, potentially between rescuers from different agencies. EMS personnel should regularly train for cardiac arrest situations to determine the most efficient ways to carry out protocols. When possible, such training should involve the first responders who may also respond to these incidents. Recent studies of medical emergency team training in simulation settings demonstrate the importance of teamwork and assigned roles [100,101].

One systematic review described a lack of well-designed studies examining the retention of adult ALS knowledge and skills in health care providers [102] but commented that the available evidence suggests that ALS knowledge and skills decay by 6 months to 1 year after training, with skills decaying faster than knowledge. Simulation has been shown to be superior in the development and maintenance of skills in cardiac arrest management, and another large systematic review [103] showed that non-simulation intervention, learner satisfaction, and process skill outcomes favored simulation over non-simulation teaching, and commented that simulation-based training for resuscitation is highly effective, particularly if employing strategies such as team/group dynamics, distraction, and integrated feedback.

Team training, particularly using simulation, is potentially even more important since the 2010 ILCOR and American Heart Association guideline changes to cardiac arrest processes, as cardiac arrest management involves strategies such as charging while chest compressions are continuing, which despite having been shown to be highly effective in decreasing non-CPR periods, causes anxiety among providers about injury due to defibrillation. Another recent study [104] showed that charging during compressions was underutilized but was associated with minimal risk to patients or rescuers.

Emergency medical services personnel must possess the equipment necessary to carry out cardiac arrest resuscitation. Key resuscitation equipment includes monitor-defibrillators, airway management tools, vascular access equipment, and appropriate medications. Cardiac monitors that record and provide real-time chest compression feedback are preferable, as are monitors that are able to use dynamic filtering to remove compression artifact and reveal underlying rhythms, although it must be remembered that accelerometer-based compression feedback devices overestimate chest compression depth when performed on soft surfaces [105].

In addition to intubation equipment, airway management tools should include capnography and alternative airway devices such as the Combitube™, King LT airway™, or iGel™. In addition to standard IV catheters, EMS crews should also carry rapid-access vascular tools such as intraosseous devices. Medical directors should provide regular training on the use of all equipment to ensure that personnel can operate them efficiently. Even in busy systems, many personnel may not perform these various skills or use specific equipment for months at a time.

Optimizing system design

Medical directors should play a key role in developing the system design for cardiac arrest care. One potential intervention is to optimize the positioning of EMS and other resources to match areas with the most cardiac arrests. Geographic mapping systems can play an important role, illustrating not only the distribution of cardiac arrest cases throughout a community but also variables such as the preferred placement of AEDs [106,107]. The OPALS study reduced cardiac arrest response and defibrillation times by moving first responders closer to areas with many cardiac arrests.

Some have touted the advantages of system status management, a formal system of continuously redeploying units based on current and anticipated use [108]. Others suggest that skill dilution occurs with too many ALS personnel; these experts recommend using fewer ALS personnel in a tiered response fashion [108,109]. A Scottish study [110] reported on an initiative to more fully formalize the roles of senior EMS personnel, who are known to be able to contribute characteristics essential to high-quality resuscitation including non-technical skills such as resuscitation team leadership, communication, and clinical decision making in a second tier, expert paramedic response to OHCA.

Hospital liaison

There is growing awareness of the importance of postresuscitation care, which formally constitutes the final link in the chain of survival [111]. Care initiated in the field may prove fruitless if not continued in the hospital. The medical director should work closely with receiving hospitals to ensure continuity in cardiac arrest care, and targeted interventions and care algorithms initiated in the field should be continued in the hospital. For example, when determining the receiving hospital facility, EMS agencies that induce hypothermia after cardiac arrest in unconscious survivors should consider if the receiving facility will continue this therapy [112–116]. Studies are currently being performed which use a system-based approach in an attempt to integrate therapies which may have synergistic effects, and which are likely to show codependence in outcome. These are typified by the CHEER study, which aims to treat cardiac arrest patients with mechanical chest compressions and cool them to 33 °C in the prehospital setting, place them on ECMO at the hospital, transport them to the interventional cardiac catheter laboratory for angioplasty, then maintain hypothermia for 24 hours [117].

Davis et al. demonstrated that diverting postarrest patients past the closest available hospital to a tertiary care center did not worsen outcomes [118]. Future work should consider if regionalization of care and transfer of these patients to specialty facilities improves outcomes as it does for victims of major trauma [119–122]. Regional systems of care have improved both provider experience and patient outcomes, for those with ST-elevation myocardial infarction and with life-threatening traumatic injury. A Japanese cardiac arrest registry of 10,000 OHCA patients transported to critical cardiac care hospitals showed improved 1-month survival compared with those patients transported to hospitals without specialized cardiac facilities [123]. Compared with historical controls, survival to hospital discharge in the Take Heart America Program [124], a regionalized system of cardiac arrest care in Minnesota, improved from 8.5% to 19%, driven by a dramatic improvement in survival after admission to intensive care from 24% to 51%. This program is based on optimization of prehospital care including EMS and community training, while establishing transport and treatment protocols with three dedicated cardiac arrest centers providing therapeutic hypothermia, interventional coronary artery evaluation and treatment, and electrophysiological evaluation. However, a similar relationship between survival or neurological outcome and presence of a coronary catheterization laboratory or the volume of patients received was not seen in an analysis from CARES data [125].

Quality improvement program

A prerequisite for improving cardiac arrest resuscitation quality is the collection of performance and quality data. Medical directors should implement quality inspection and assurance programs to ensure the delivery of high-quality cardiac arrest care. Commonly collected cardiac arrest quality data include treatment time intervals such as call to dispatch, dispatch to scene arrival, arrival to patient side, and call to first defibrillation. Another important measure is CPR performance. Monitors now permit the medical director to evaluate the depth, rate, and interruptions of chest compressions delivered throughout the entire episode [126,127].

The Utstein style for reporting of cardiac arrest data attempts to provide some common denominators for comparing resuscitation rates among various systems [128]. EMS services should adopt standardized data collection methods that allow for uniform reporting and benchmarking capability.

Conclusion

Improving survival from OHCA requires a comprehensive community systems approach. No single component, including EMS, can improve cardiac arrest survival independently. EMS agencies must assume a leadership role in promoting, developing, and implementing this systems-based approach.

References

1 De Maio VJ, Stiell IG, Wells GA, Spaite DW. Optimal defibrillation response intervals for maximum out-of-hospital cardiac arrest survival rates. *Ann Emerg Med* 2003;42(2):242–50.

2 Stiell IG, Wells GA, Field B, et al. Advanced cardiac life support in out-of-hospital cardiac arrest. *N Engl J Med* 2004;351(7):647–56.

3 Weisfeldt M. Bystanders save lives with CPR and automated external defibrillators. In: *American Heart Scientific Sessions*, Orlando, FL, 2007.

4 McNally B, Robb R, Mehta M, et al. Out-of-hospital cardiac arrest surveillance – Cardiac Arrest Registry to Enhance Survival (CARES), United States, October 1, 2005–December 31, 2010. *MMWR Surveill Summ* 2011;60(8):1–19.

5 2001 Heart and Stroke Statistical Update. Dallas, TX: American Heart Association, 2000.

6 Davis R. Six minutes to live or die. *USA Today*, May 20, 2005. Available at: http://usatoday30.usatoday.com/news/nation/ems-day1-cover.htm

7 McNally B, Stokes A, Crouch A, Kellermann AL, CARES Surveillance Group. CARES – Cardiac Arrest Registry to Enhance Survival. *Ann Emerg Med* 2009;54(5):674–83.

8 Ong ME, Shin SD, Tanaka H, et al. Pan-Asian Resuscitation Outcomes Study (PAROS): rationale, methodology, and implementation. *Acad Emerg Med* 2011;18(8):890–7.

9 Rosamund W, Flegal K, Furie K, et al. Heart disease and stroke statistics – 2008 update: a report from the American Heart Association Statistics Committee and Stroke Statistics Subcommittee. *Circulation* 2008;117(4):e25–146.

10 Zheng ZJ, Croft JB, Giles WH, Mensah GA. Sudden cardiac death in the United States, 1989 to 1998. *Circulation* 2001;104(18): 2158–63.

11 Nichol G, Rumsfeld J, Eigel B, et al. Essential features of designating out-of-hospital cardiac arrest as a reportable event. A scientific statement from the American Heart Association Emergency Cardiovascular Care Committee; Council on Cardiopulmonary, Perioperative, and Critical Care; Council on Cardiovascular Nursing; Council on Clinical Cardiology; and Quality of Care and Outcomes Research Interdisciplinary Working Group. *Circulation* 2008;117(17):2299–308.

12 Callaway CW, Hostler D, Doshi AA, et al. Usefulness of vasopressin administered with epinephrine during out-of-hospital cardiac arrest. *Am J Cardiol* 2006;98(10):1316–21.

13 Eisenberg MS, Horwood BT, Cummins RO, Reynolds-Haertle R, Hearne TR. Cardiac arrest and resuscitation: a tale of 29 cities. *Ann Emerg Med* 1990;19(2):179–86.

14 Mitchell RG, Guly UM, Rainer TH, Robertson CE. Paramedic activities, drug administration and survival from out of hospital cardiac arrest. *Resuscitation* 2000;43(2):95–100.

15 Mosesso VN Jr, Davis EA, Auble TE, Paris PM, Yealy DM. Use of automated external defibrillators by police officers for treatment of out-of-hospital cardiac arrest. *Ann Emerg Med* 1998;32(2):200–7.

16 Schaffer WA, Cobb LA. Recurrent ventricular fibrillation and modes of death in survivors of out-of-hospital ventricular fibrillation. *N Engl J Med* 1975;293(6):259–62.

17 Yusuf S, Venkatesh G, Teo KK. Critical review of the approaches to the prevention of sudden death. *Am J Cardiol* 1993;72(16):51F–8F.

18 Bunch TJ, White RD, Friedman PA, Kottke TE, Wu LA, Packer DL. Trends in treated ventricular fibrillation out-of-hospital cardiac arrest: a 17-year population-based study. *Heart Rhythm* 2004;1(3):255–9.

19 Cobb LA, Fahrenbruch CE, Olsufka M, Copass MK. Changing incidence of out-of-hospital ventricular fibrillation, 1980–2000. *JAMA* 2002;288(23):3008–13.

20 Polentini MS, Pirrallo RG, McGill W. The changing incidence of ventricular fibrillation in Milwaukee, Wisconsin (1992–2002). *Prehosp Emerg Care* 2006;10(1):52–60.

21 Youngquist ST, Kaji AH, Niemann JT. Beta-blocker use and the changing epidemiology of out-of-hospital cardiac arrest rhythms. *Resuscitation* 2008;76(3):376–80.

22 Hallstrom AP, Ornato JP, Weisfeldt M, et al. Public-access defibrillation and survival after out-of-hospital cardiac arrest. *N Engl J Med* 2004;351(7):637–46.

23 Valenzuela TD, Roe DJ, Nichol G, Clark LL, Spaite DW, Hardman RG. Outcomes of rapid defibrillation by security officers after cardiac arrest in casinos. *N Engl J Med* 2000;343(17):1206–9.

24 Cummins RO, Chamberlain DA, Abramson NS, et al. Recommended guidelines for uniform reporting of data from out-of-hospital cardiac arrest: the Utstein Style. Task Force of the American Heart Association, the European Resuscitation Council, the Heart and Stroke Foundation of Canada, and the Australian Resuscitation Council. *Circulation* 1991;84(2):960–75.

25 Nichol G, Stiell IG, Hebert P, Wells GA, Vandemheen K, Laupacis A. What is the quality of life for survivors of cardiac arrest? A prospective study. *Acad Emerg Med* 1999;6(2):95–102.

26 Nichol G, Stiell IG, Laupacis A, Pham B, De Maio VJ, Wells GA. A cumulative meta-analysis of the effectiveness of defibrillator-capable emergency medical services for victims of out-of-hospital cardiac arrest. *Ann Emerg Med* 1999;34(4 Pt 1):517–25.

27 Callaway CW. Improving neurologic outcomes after out-of-hospital cardiac arrest. *Prehosp Emerg Care* 1997;1(1):45–57.

28 Nichol G, Thomas E, Callaway CW, et al. Regional variation in out-of-hospital cardiac arrest incidence and outcome. *JAMA* 2008; 300(12):1423–31.

29 Bahr J, Klingler H, Panzer W, Rode H, Kettler D. Skills of lay people in checking the carotid pulse. *Resuscitation* 1997;35(1):23–6.

30 Eberle B, Dick WF, Schneider T, Wisser G, Doetsch S, Tzanova I. Checking the carotid pulse check: diagnostic accuracy of first responders in patients with and without a pulse. *Resuscitation* 1996; 33(2):107–16.

31 ECC Committee, Subcommittees and Task Forces of the American Heart Association. 2005 American Heart Association Guidelines for Cardio-pulmonary Resuscitation and Emergency Cardiovascular Care. *Circulation* 2005;112(24 Suppl):IV1–203.

32 Vaillancourt C, Verma A, Trickett J, et al. Evaluating the effectiveness of dispatch-assisted cardiopulmonary resuscitation instructions. *Acad Emerg Med* 2007;14(10):877–83.

33 Larsen MP, Eisenberg MS, Cummins RO, Hallstrom AP. Predicting survival from out-of-hospital cardiac arrest: a graphic model. *Ann Emerg Med* 1993;22(11):1652–8.

34 Valenzuela TD, Roe DJ, Cretin S, Spaite DW, Larsen MP. Estimating effectiveness of cardiac arrest interventions: a logistic regression survival model. *Circulation* 1997;96(10):3308–13.

35 Sasson C, Meischke H, Abella BS, et al. increasing cardiopulmonary resuscitation provision in communities with low bystander cardiopulmonary resuscitation rates a science advisory from the American Heart Association for healthcare providers, policymakers, public health departments, and community leaders. *Circulation* 2013;127:1342–50.

36 Lerner EB, Rea TD, Bobrow BJ, et al., for the American Heart Association Emergency Cardiovascular Care Committee and the Council on Cardiopulmonary, Critical Care, Perioperative and Resuscitation. Emergency medical service dispatch cardiopulmonary resuscitation prearrival instructions to improve survival from out-of-hospital cardiac arrest: a scientific statement from the American Heart Association. *Circulation* 2012;125:1–8.

37 Sayre MR, Berg RA, Cave DM, Page RL, Potts J, White RD. Hands-only (compression-only) cardiopulmonary resuscitation: a call to action for bystander response to adults who experience out-of-hospital sudden cardiac arrest: a science advisory for the public from the American Heart Association Emergency Cardiovascular Care Committee. *Circulation* 2008;117(16):2162–7.

38 Hupfl M, Selig H, Nagele P. Chest-compression-only versus standard cardiopulmonary resuscitation: a meta-analysis. *Lancet* 2010;376(9752):1552–7.

39 Bobrow BJ, Spaite DW, Berg RA, et al. Chest compression-only CPR by lay rescuers and survival from out-of-hospital cardiac arrest. *JAMA* 2010;304(13):1447–54.

40 Hallstrom A, Cobb L, Johnson E, Copass M. Cardiopulmonary resuscitation by chest compression alone or with mouth-to-mouth ventilation. *N Engl J Med* 2000;342(21):1546–53.

41 Weaver WD, Cobb LA, Hallstrom AP, Fahrenbruch C, Copass MK, Ray R. Factors influencing survival after out-of-hospital cardiac arrest. *J Am Coll Cardiol* 1986;7(4):752–7.

42 Diack AW, Welborn WS, Rullman RG, Walter CW, Wayne MA. An automatic cardiac resuscitator for emergency treatment of cardiac arrest. *Med Instrum* 1979;13(2):78–83.

43 Marenco JP, Wang PJ, Link MS, Homoud MK, Estes NA 3rd. Improving survival from sudden cardiac arrest: the role of the automated external defibrillator. *JAMA* 2001;285(9):1193–200.

44 Abella BS, Alvarado JP, Myklebust H, et al. Quality of cardiopulmonary resuscitation during in-hospital cardiac arrest. *JAMA* 2005;293(3):305–10.

45 Wik L, Kramer-Johansen J, Myklebust H, et al. Quality of cardiopulmonary resuscitation during out-of-hospital cardiac arrest. *JAMA* 2005;293(3):299–304.

46 Abella BS, Edelson DP, Kim S, et al. CPR quality improvement during in-hospital cardiac arrest using a real-time audiovisual feedback system. *Resuscitation* 2007;73(1):54–61.

47 Kramer-Johansen J, Myklebust H, Wik L, et al. Quality of out-of-hospital cardiopulmonary resuscitation with real time automated feedback: a prospective interventional study. *Resuscitation* 2006; 71(3):283–92.

48 Page RL, Joglar JA, Kowal RC, et al. Use of automated external defibrillators by a U.S. airline. *N Engl J Med* 2000;343(17):1210–16.

49 Caffrey SL, Willoughby PJ, Pepe PE, Becker LB. Public use of automated external defibrillators. *N Engl J Med* 2002;347(16): 1242–7.

50 Kitamura T, Iwami T, Kawamura T, et al. Nationwide public-access defibrillation in Japan. *N Engl J Med* 2010;362(11):994–1004.

51 Mitamura H. Public access defibrillation: advances from Japan. *Nat Clin Pract Cardiovasc Med* 2008;5(11):690–2.

52 Report on a study on social system development to improve survival from emergency cardiovascular disease using automated external defibrillator (Marukawa's report) (in Japanese).Available at: http://aed-hyogo.sakura.ne.jp/wpm/archivepdf/23/2_11a.pdf

53 Bardy GH, Lee KL, Mark DB, et al. Home use of automated external defibrillators for sudden cardiac arrest. *N Engl J Med* 2008; 258(17):1793–804.

54 Klein HU, Goldenberg I, Moss AJ. Risk stratification for implantable cardioverter defibrillator therapy: the role of the wearable cardioverter-defibrillator. *Eur Heart J* 2013;34(29):2230–42.

55 Sasson C, Meischke H, Abella BS, et al. Increasing cardiopulmonary resuscitation provision in communities with low bystander cardiopulmonary resuscitation rates: a science advisory from the American Heart Association for healthcare providers, policymakers, public health departments, and community leaders. *Circulation* 2013;127(12):1342–50.

56 Ong ME, Tan EH, Yan X, et al. An observational study describing the geographic-time distribution of cardiac arrests in Singapore: what is the utility of geographic information systems for planning public access defibrillation? (PADS Phase I). *Resuscitation* 2008;76:388–96.

57 Becker L, Eisenberg M, Fahrenbruch C, Cobb L. Public locations of cardiac arrest. Implications for public access defibrillation. *Circulation* 1998;97(21):2106–9.

58 Frank RL, Rausch MA, Menegazzi JJ, Rickens M. The locations of nonresidential out-of-hospital cardiac arrests in the City of Pittsburgh over a three-year period: implications for automated external defibrillator placement. *Prehosp Emerg Care* 2001;5(3):247–51.

59 Reed DB, Birnbaum A, Brown LH, et al. Location of cardiac arrests in the public access defibrillation trial. *Prehosp Emerg Care* 2006; 10(1):61–76.

60 Automated External Defibrillation Implementation Guide. Dallas, TX: American Heart Association. Available at: www.heart.org/idc/groups/heart-public/@wcm/@ecc/documents/downloadable/ucm_438703.pdf

61 Early Defibrillation Program Policies and Procedures. AED Brands, Kennesaw, GA. Available at: www.aedbrands.com/AED-Program-Policies-and-Procedures.pdf

62 AED Program Implementation Guide. Medtronic Physio-Control, Redmond, WA. Available at: www.physio-control.com/uploaded Files/learning/pad/AED_Program_Implementation_ Guide_3201991-001.pdf

63 AED Implementation Guide. Lifesaving Society, Toronto, Ontario, Canada. Available at: www.lifesavingsociety.com/media/81836/98aedimplementationguidejan2012.pdf

64 Weaver WD, Hill D, Fahrenbruch CE, et al. Use of the automatic external defibrillator in the management of out-of-hospital cardiac arrest. *N Engl J Med* 1988;319(11):661–6.

65 Davis EA, Mosesso VN Jr. Performance of police first responders in utilizing automated external defibrillation on victims of sudden cardiac arrest. *Prehosp Emerg Care* 1998;2(2):101–7.

66 White RD, Asplin BR, Bugliosi TF, Hankins DG. High discharge survival rate after out-of-hospital ventricular fibrillation with rapid defibrillation by police and paramedics. *Ann Emerg Med* 1996; 28(5):480–5.

67 White RD, Hankins DG, Bugliosi TF. Seven years' experience with early defibrillation by police and paramedics in an emergency medical services system. *Resuscitation* 1998;39(3):145–51.

68 Ong MEH, Chan YH, Anantharaman V. Improved response times with motorcycle based Fast Response Paramedics. *SGH Proceedings* 2003;12:114–19.

69 Stiell IG, Wells GA, Field BJ, et al. Improved out-of-hospital cardiac arrest survival through the inexpensive optimization of an existing defibrillation program: OPALS study phase II. *JAMA* 1999;281(13):1175–81.

70 Wilk L, Hansen TB, Fylling F, et al. Delaying defibrillation to give basic cardiopulmonary resuscitation to patients with out-of-hospital ventricular fibrillation: a randomized trial. *JAMA* 2003;289(11):1389–95.

71 Cobb LA, Fahrenbruch CE, Walsh TR, et al. Influence of cardiopulmonary resuscitation prior to defibrillation in patients with out-of-hospital ventricular fibrillation. *JAMA* 1999;281(13):1182–8.

72 Weisfeldt ML, Becker LB. Resuscitation after cardiac arrest: a 3-phase time-sensitive model. *JAMA* 2002;288(23):3035–8.

73 Olasveengen TM, Wik L, Steen PA. Quality of cardiopulmonary resuscitation before and during transport in out-of-hospital cardiac arrest. *Resuscitation* 2008;76:185–90.

74 Hostler D, Guimond G, Callaway C. A comparison of CPR delivery with various compression-to-ventilation ratios during two-rescuer CPR. *Resuscitation* 2005;65(3):325–8.

75 Kern KB, Hilwig RW, Berg RA, Sanders AB, Ewy GA. Importance of continuous chest compressions during cardiopulmonary resuscitation: improved outcome during a simulated single lay-rescuer scenario. *Circulation* 2002;105(5):645–9.

76 Berg RA, Kern KB, Sanders AB, Otto CW, Hilwig RW, Ewy GA. Bystander cardiopulmonary resuscitation. Is ventilation necessary? *Circulation* 1993;88(4 Pt 1):1907–15.

77 Yu T, Weil MH, Tang W, et al. Adverse outcomes of interrupted precordial compression during automated defibrillation. *Circulation* 2002;106(3):368–72.

78 Ong MEH, Shin SD, Soon SS, et al. Recommendations on ambulance cardiopulmonary resuscitation in basic life support systems. *Prehosp Emerg Care* 2013;17(4):491–500.

79 Nichol G, Thomas E, Callaway CW, et al. Regional variation in out-of-hospital cardiac arrest incidence and outcome. *JAMA* 2008; 300(12):1423–31.

80 Negovsky VA. Postresuscitation disease. *Crit Care Med* 1988; 16(10):942–6.

81 Herlitz J, Castren M, Friberg H, et al. Post resuscitation care: what are the therapeutic alternatives and what do we know? *Resuscitation* 2006;69(1):15–22.

82 Morrison LJ, Deakin CD, Morley PT, et al. Part 8: Advanced life support: 2010 International Consensus on Cardiopulmonary Resuscitation and Emergency Cardiovascular Care Science with Treatment Recommendations. *Circulation* 2010;122(16 Suppl 2): S345–421.

83 Hasegawa K, Hiraide A, Chang Y, Brown DFM. Association of prehospital advanced airway management with neurologic outcome and survival in patients with out-of-hospital cardiac arrest. *JAMA* 2013;309(3):257–66.

84 Virkkunen I, Yli-Hankala A, Silfvast T. Induction of therapeutic hypothermia after cardiac arrest in prehospital patients using ice-cold Ringer's solution: a pilot study. *Resuscitation* 2004; 62:299–302.

85 Castrén M, Nordberg P, Svensson L, et al. Intra-arrest trans-nasal evaporative cooling: a randomized, prehospital, multi-center study (PRINCE: Pre-ROSC IntraNasal cooling effectiveness). *Circulation* 2010;122(7):729–36.

86 Bernard SA, Smith K, Cameron P, et al. Induction of therapeutic hypothermia by paramedics after resuscitation from out-of-hospital ventricular fibrillation cardiac arrest: a randomized controlled trial. *Circulation* 2010;122:737–42.

87 Engdahl J, Abrahamsson P, Bang A, Lindqvist J, Karlsson T, Herlitz J. Is hospital care of major importance for outcome after out-of-hospital cardiac arrest? Experience acquired from patients with out-of-hospital cardiac arrest resuscitated by the same Emergency Medical Service and admitted to one of two hospitals over a 16-year period in the municipality of Goteborg. *Resuscitation* 2000; 43(3):201–11.

88 Langhelle A, Tyvold SS, Lexow K, Hapnes SA, Sunde K, Steen PA. In-hospital factors associated with improved outcome after out-of-hospital cardiac arrest. A comparison between four regions in Norway. *Resuscitation* 2003;56(3):247–63.

89 Merchant RM, Soar J, Skrifvars MB, et al. Therapeutic hypothermia utilization among physicians after resuscitation from cardiac arrest. *Crit Care Med* 2006;34(7):1935–40.

90 Peberdy MA, Ornato JP. Post-resuscitation care: is it the missing link in the Chain of Survival? *Resuscitation* 2005;64(2):135–7.

91 Peberdy MA, Kaye W, Ornato JP, et al. Cardiopulmonary resuscitation of adults in the hospital: a report of 14720 cardiac arrests from the National Registry of Cardiopulmonary Resuscitation. *Resuscitation* 2003;58(3):297–308.

92 Edgren E, Hedstrand U, Kelsey S, Sutton-Tyrrell K, Safar P. Assessment of neurological prognosis in comatose survivors of cardiac arrest. BRCT I Study Group. Lancet 1994;343(8905):1055–9.

93 Langhelle A, Nolan J, Herlitz J, et al. Recommended guidelines for reviewing, reporting, and conducting research on post-resuscitation care: the Utstein style. *Resuscitation* 2005;66(3):271–83.

94 Neumar RW, Nolan JP, Adrie C, et al. Post-cardiac arrest syndrome: epidemiology, pathophysiology, treatment, and prognostication. *Circulation* 2008;118(23):2452–83.

95 Nichol G, Aufderheide TP, Eigel B, et al. Regional systems of care for out-of-hospital cardiac arrest: a policy statement from the American Heart Association. *Circulation* 2010;121(5):709–29.

96 Geyer BC, Striegel T, Spaite DW, et al. Abstract P36: Statewide network of cardiac arrest centers improves survival from out of hospital cardiac arrest. *Circulation* 2009;120(18_MeetingAbstracts):S1448–9.

97 Stewart RD. Medical direction in emergency medical services: the role of the physician. *Emerg Med Clin North Am* 1987;5(1):119–32.

98 Williams I, Valderrama AL, Bolton P, et al. Factors associated with emergency medical services scope of practice for acute cardiovascular events. *Prehosp Emerg Care* 2012;16:189–97.

99 Greer S, Williams I, Valderrama AL, Bolton P, Patterson DG, Zhang Z. EMS medical direction and prehospital practices for acute cardiovascular events. *Prehosp Emerg Care* 2013;17:38–45.

100 De Vries W, van Alem AP, de Vos R, van Oostrom J, Koster RW. Trained first-responders with an automated external defibrillator: how do they perform in real resuscitation attempts? *Resuscitation* 2005;64(2):157–61.

101 DeVita MA, Schaefer J, Lutz J, Wang H, Dongilli T. Improving medical emergency team (MET) performance using a novel curriculum and a computerized human patient simulator. *Qual Saf Health Care* 2005;14(5):326–31.

102 Yang CW, Yen ZS, McGowan JE, et al. A systematic review of retention of adult advanced life support knowledge and skills in healthcare providers. *Resuscitation* 2012;83(9):1055–60.

103 Mundell WC, Kennedy CC, Szostek JH, Cook DA. Simulation technology for resuscitation training: a systematic review and meta-analysis. *Resuscitation* 2013;84(9):1174–83.

104 Edelson DP, Robertson-Dick BJ, Yuen TC, et al. Safety and efficacy of defibrillator charging during ongoing chest compressions: a multi-center study. *Resuscitation* 2010;81(11):1521–6.

105 Perkins GD, Kocierz L, Smith SCL, McCulloch RA, Davies RP. Compression feedback devices over estimate chest compression depth when performed on a bed. *Resuscitation* 2009;80(1):79–82.

106 Ong MEH, Tan EH, Yan X, et al. An observational study describing the geographic-time distribution of cardiac arrests in Singapore: what is the utility of geographic information systems for planning public access defibrillation? (PADS Phase I). *Resuscitation* 2008;76(3):388–96.

107 Sakai T, Iwami T, Kitamura T, et al. Effectiveness of the new 'Mobile AED Map' to find and retrieve an AED: a randomised controlled trial. *Resuscitation* 2011;82(1):69–73.

108 Stout J, Pepe PE, Mosesso VN Jr. All-advanced life support vs tiered-response ambulance systems. *Prehosp Emerg Care* 2000;4(1):1–6.

109 Persse DE, Key CB, Bradley RN, Miller CC, Dhingra A. Cardiac arrest survival as a function of ambulance deployment strategy in a large urban emergency medical services system. *Resuscitation* 2003;59(1):97–104.

110 Clarke S, Lyon RM, Short S, Crookston C, Clegg GR. A specialist, second-tier response to out-of-hospital cardiac arrest: setting up TOPCAT2. *Emerg Med J* 2013 Jan 30. [Epub ahead of print]

111 Chain of survival. Dallas, TX: American Heart Association. Available at: www.heart.org/HEARTORG/CPRAndECC/WhatisCPR/ECCIntro/ Chain-of-Survival_UCM_307516_Article.jsp

112 Abella BS, Rhee JW, Huang KN, Vanden Hoek TL, Becker LB. Induced hypothermia is underused after resuscitation from cardiac arrest: a current practice survey. *Resuscitation* 2005;64(2):181–6.

113 Laver SR, Padkin A, Atalla A, Nolan JP. Therapeutic hypothermia after cardiac arrest: a survey of practice in intensive care units in the United Kingdom. *Anaesthesia* 2006;61(9):873–7.

114 Merchant RM, Soar J, Skrifvars MB, et al. Therapeutic hypothermia utilization among physicians after resuscitation from cardiac arrest. *Crit Care Med* 2006;34(7):1935–40.

115 Oksanen T, Pettila V, Hynynen M, Varpula T. Therapeutic hypothermia after cardiac arrest: implementation and outcome in Finnish intensive care units. *Acta Anaesthesiol Scand* 2007;51(7):866–71.

116 Wolfrum S, Radke PW, Pischon T, Willich SN, Schunkert H, Kurowski V. Mild therapeutic hypothermia after cardiac arrest – a nationwide survey on the implementation of the ILCOR guidelines in German intensive care units. *Resuscitation* 2007;72(2):207–13.

117 Refractory out-of-hospital cardiac arrest treated with mechanical CPR, hypothermia, ECMO and early reperfusion (CHEER). Available at: http://clinicaltrials.gov/ct2/show/NCT01186614

118 Davis DP, Fisher R, Aguilar S, et al. The feasibility of a regional cardiac arrest receiving system. *Resuscitation* 2007;74(1):44–51.

119 Mann NC, Mullins RJ, Hedges JR, Rowland D, Arthur M, Zechnich AD. Mortality among seriously injured patients treated in remote rural trauma centers before and after implementation of a statewide trauma system. *Med Care* 2001;39(7):643–53.

120 Newgard CD, McConnell KJ, Hedges JR, Mullins RJ. The benefit of higher level of care transfer of injured patients from nontertiary hospital emergency departments. *J Trauma* 2007; 63(5):965–71.

121 Sampalis JS, Denis R, Frechette P, Brown R, Fleiszer D, Mulder D. Direct transport to tertiary trauma centers versus transfer from lower level facilities: impact on mortality and morbidity among patients with major trauma. *J Trauma* 1997;43(2):288–95.

122 Sampalis JS, Denis R, Lavoie A, et al. Trauma care regionalization: a process-outcome evaluation. *J Trauma* 1999;46(4):565–79.

123 Kajino K, Iwami T, Daya M, et al. Impact of transport to critical care medical centers on outcomes after out-of-hospital cardiac arrest. *Resuscitation* 2010;81:549–54.

124 Lick CJ, Aufderheide TP, Niskanen RA, et al. Take heart America: a comprehensive, community-wide, systems-based approach to the treatment of cardiac arrest. *Crit Care Med* 2011;39:26–33.

125 Cudnik MT, Sasson C, Rea TD, et al. Increasing hospital volume is not associated with improved survival in out of hospital cardiac arrest of cardiac etiology. *Resuscitation* 2012;83:862–8.

126 Wik L, Kramer-Johansen J, Myklebust H, et al. Quality of cardiopulmonary resuscitation during out-of-hospital cardiac arrest. *JAMA* 2005;293(3):299–304.

127 Abella BS, Alvarado JP, Myklebust H, et al. Quality of cardiopulmonary resuscitation during in-hospital cardiac arrest. *JAMA* 2005;293(3):305–10.

128 Recommended guidelines for uniform reporting of data from out-of-hospital cardiac arrest: the 'Utstein style'. Prepared by a Task Force of Representatives from the European Resuscitation Council, American Heart Association, Heart and Stroke Foundation of Canada, Australian Resuscitation Council. *Resuscitation* 1991; 22(1):1–26.

CHAPTER 12

Cardiac arrest: clinical management

Jon C. Rittenberger and Vincent N. Mosesso, Jr

Introduction

Although detailed algorithms and consensus guidelines exist for management of cardiac arrest, often referred to as Basic Life Support (BLS) and Advanced Cardiac Life Support (ACLS), there are unique practical and scientific considerations that may affect the execution of resuscitation efforts in the out-of-hospital setting. EMS medical directors and field personnel including EMS physicians must be aware of these factors when developing protocols for prehospital resuscitation. They must also understand the scientific basis for and the controversies surrounding recommended resuscitation actions.

This chapter reviews scientific and practical considerations for carrying out BLS and ACLS in the prehospital setting. For specific treatment algorithms, the reader is referred to the American Heart Association (AHA) Emergency Cardiac Care (ECC) guidelines [1].

Specific interventions

Chest compressions

Chest compressions are essential in cardiac arrest resuscitation. Paradis demonstrated that only chest compressions generate coronary perfusion pressure (CPP) and that a CPP of at least 20 mmHg is important for achieving return of spontaneous circulation (ROSC) [2]. Multiple studies highlight the role of early chest compressions in survival from cardiac arrest [3–6].

The most recent BLS and ACLS guidelines emphasize the delivery of continuous chest compressions with as few interruptions as possible [1]. Kern et al. demonstrated that several consecutive chest compressions are necessary to generate adequate CPP [7]. CPP drops off immediately when chest compressions are discontinued [8]. The proportion of resuscitation time without chest compressions, termed *hands-off time* or *no-flow fraction*, is inversely associated with cardiac arrest

survival [9]. Compression depth, rate, and full recoil are also critical characteristics for effectiveness.

Prior work highlighted the often substandard CPR performed by prehospital and in-hospital providers. In a series of prehospital cardiac arrests in Europe, Wik et al. showed that chest compressions were delivered on average only half of the time while the patient was in arrest and that most compressions were too shallow [10]. Abella et al. found similar observations in an in-hospital series [11].

Delivering chest compressions during cardiac arrest resuscitation poses practical challenges. The treating EMS team must provide continuous chest compressions with as few interruptions as possible and must ensure high-quality chest compressions with adequate depth, rate, and recoil. To achieve these chest compression goals, additional rescuers should be dispatched to provide assistance at cardiac arrests. Team members providing chest compressions should rotate frequently, ideally every 1–2 minutes [1].

Several cardiac monitors use a compression paddle or other technology to measure the depth and rate of chest compressions [10,11]. These monitors are able to provide real-time audio and/ or visual feedback, indicating to the rescuer whether or not to increase the depth or rate of compressions. Preliminary data suggest improved clinical chest compression performance through the use of feedback systems [12].

Various mechanical devices for automating chest compressions are now available. The Thumper (Michigan Instruments, Grand Rapids, MI) has been used for approximately 40 years and provides chest compressions using a pneumatic piston [13]. The Autopulse Resuscitation System (Zoll Corporation, Chelmsford, MA) facilitates chest compressions using a circumferential load-distributing band [14,15]. The Lund University Cardiopulmonary Assist Device (LUCAS) (Lund, Sweden) provides active compression and decompression through a pneumatic piston attached to a suction cup on the chest [16]. Use of mechanical compression devices is fairly widespread in Europe and is growing in the United States.

Emergency Medical Services: Clinical Practice and Systems Oversight, Second Edition. Volume 1: Clinical Aspects of EMS.
Edited by David C. Cone, Jane H. Brice, Theodore R. Delbridge, and J. Brent Myers.
© 2015 NAEMSP. Published 2015 by John Wiley & Sons, Inc. Companion Website: www.wiley.com\go\cone\naemsp

The scientific data evaluating the effectiveness of these devices remain inconclusive. One urban EMS agency evaluated the Autopulse in a before/after fashion and found increases in both ROSC and survival [14]. However, a larger, multicenter, randomized controlled trial demonstrated worsened outcomes with the intervention [15]. The authors attributed this observation to potential delays in CPR required to place and activate the device. The LUCAS device was effective in a small study of 100 patients, but its benefit was only noted in those who received it within 15 minutes from the ambulance call [16]. Additional innovations and trials are sure to follow. It is important to note that each device requires time to place on the patient, during which no compressions occur. Any protocol that incorporates the use of mechanical devices must stress the importance of continuing manual compressions as much as possible until the device starts; some experts suggest withholding use of mechanical devices during the initial resuscitation effort.

Defibrillation

Defibrillation of ventricular fibrillation or ventricular tachycardia (VF/VT) is the most effective intervention for resuscitation from cardiac arrest. Ideally, automated external defibrillators (AEDs) are present at the site of the arrest for use by willing trained or untrained bystanders, perhaps at the prompting of the 9-1-1 call-taker. All medical first responders and BLS providers, including all BLS ambulances, should be equipped with AEDs. Most ALS personnel deliver shocks by manually operating a cardiac monitor-defibrillator after determining the patient has a shockable rhythm. Although many devices are configured with both hand-held paddles and cables for "hands-off" self-adhesive pads, use of the pads is believed to be safer, particularly in the uncontrolled field setting.

An important technical consideration is the type of electrical waveform delivered by the defibrillator [17]. Older defibrillators use monophasic electrical current. In this mode, the device delivers electrical current in a single direction only. To compensate for increased impedance (electrical resistance), older protocols specified escalating energy levels for each successive rescue shock. Now that shocks are given one at a time, each shock should be at maximum energy output, typically 360 J. Although most current defibrillators are biphasic, some EMS systems may still use monophasic defibrillators.

In a biphasic defibrillator, electrical current flows first in one direction, then in the opposite direction. This modality theoretically purges excess electrical charge from the heart. Biphasic defibrillators measure the impedance across the chest and adjust the voltage and/or duration of current appropriately. Different models also alter the pattern of delivered current, most often using a rectilinear or truncated exponential waveform. Compared with monophasic defibrillators, biphasic defibrillators demonstrate higher rescue shock success at lower energy levels and have been associated with increased rates of ROSC [18].

Energy levels for biphasic defibrillators should be based on manufacturer recommendations because each model has different waveform and delivery characteristics that affect shock efficacy. Although some manufacturers endorse non-escalating low-energy shocks (150 J), recent data suggest that higher energy biphasic shocks may increase rescue shock success without impairing cardiac function [19].

Another consideration is the interface between BLS and ALS defibrillation equipment. Some AEDs can be converted to manual mode by ALS personnel. This feature is an important logistical consideration because switching from the BLS AED to the ALS defibrillator may incur delays. Some brands use the same defibrillation pads on BLS and ALS models, allowing providers to simply unplug the connector from one device and plug into the other. The EMS physician should be aware that the AED "analyze and shock" algorithm may add 49–59 seconds of hands-off time [20]. This is an important consideration when ALS rescuers care for a patient with an AED attached. One method of minimizing hands-off time is to continue chest compressions until just before defibrillation. Recent data have suggested that continuing chest compressions during defibrillation may be feasible [21]. Others have demonstrated that standard examination gloves may be insufficient protection from electrical shock during external defibrillation [22]. Balancing safety and minimizing hands-off time remains an active area of research.

A current scientific controversy is whether initial defibrillation should precede or follow an initial course of chest compressions. Prior AHA ECC algorithms specified rescue shocks first for VF, regardless of arrest duration [23]. However, several factors support performing initial chest compressions before rescue shocks, including the prolonged duration of most out-of-hospital arrests before treatment is initiated, which leads to the depletion of myocardial high-energy phosphates, cellular damage resulting from accumulated free radicals, and the development of severe acidosis [24,25]. Theoretically, a period of chest compressions may perfuse the heart and reduce the severity of these anomalies, better preparing the heart for defibrillation.

However, a recent randomized clinical trial between chest compressions before rhythm analysis and immediate rhythm analysis showed no difference in the rate of good neurological outcome between groups (19.4% in early analysis versus 18.5% in chest compressions before analysis cohorts) [26]. Two clinical studies have demonstrated improved outcomes in prolonged (>4 minutes) VF arrests when chest compressions were delivered before defibrillation [27,28]. Current ACLS guidelines recommend immediate defibrillation in witnessed arrests but delivering chest compressions for about 2 minutes before rhythm analysis in unwitnessed arrests [1].

Airway management

For many years airway management received emphasis in cardiac arrest care, and ALS rescuers placed high priority on endotracheal intubation (ETI) of cardiac arrest patients. However, the results of several studies question the wisdom of intubation during out-of-hospital cardiac arrest resuscitation. Some of the adverse events noted were tube misplacement, tube dislodgment, multiple laryngoscopy efforts, and failed ETI efforts [29–32]. Aufderheide et al. found that inadvertent hyperventilation often occurs after ETI, raising intrathoracic pressure and compromising CPP [33]. Perhaps most important is the frequent and often prolonged interruption of chest compressions [34].

The application of these findings to EMS practice poses important challenges. Although bag-valve-mask ventilation is theoretically adequate for resuscitation, the technique is difficult to execute in the prehospital setting, in which providers may need to deliver ventilations with the patient situated on the floor, in the back of a moving ambulance, or on a moving stretcher [35]. Most EMS agencies still perform ETI for cardiac arrest, but many try to limit the number and duration of ETI attempts [32]. Capnography should be used to verify endotracheal tube placement [36]. Although dependent on the quality of chest compressions, capnography waveforms in low-flow states are still useful for ensuring endotracheal tube position.

Another emerging approach to cardiac arrest airway management is to use supraglottic airways (such as the King LT®) instead of ETI. These devices are inserted blindly into the airway without the need for direct laryngoscopy, and can typically be placed very quickly without pausing compressions (see Volume 1, Chapter 3). Several EMS agencies have chosen this approach, reasoning that they cannot perform traditional ETI without compromising chest compressions [37]. Retrospective studies have conflicting results. In a review of out-of-hospital cardiac arrests in Japan between 2005 and 2008, there was no difference in the rate of good neurological outcome in patients receiving endotracheal intubation rather than supraglottic airways (odds ratio (OR) 0.71; 95% confidence interval (CI) 0.39, 1.30) [38]. A subanalysis of the ROC PRIMED trial demonstrated a higher rate of survival with good functional status in patients receiving endotracheal intubation rather than supraglottic airway placement (OR 1.40; 95% CI 1.04, 1.89) during the resuscitation [37].

Ventilation

Another important consideration is the role of ventilation during chest compressions. Recent data question the need for ventilation with bystander CPR in patients with short-duration VF [7,39–43]. The theoretical bases for this approach include:

- the distractions posed by multiple interventions
- the subsequent reduction in number of chest compressions
- the adverse effect of hyperventilation on CPP
- bystander reluctance to perform mouth-to-mouth ventilation [33, 44–46].

Although "no ventilation" has practical value for bystander care, it is not clear how or if these principles should be applied to EMS care. There is some evidence that prearrival instruction for compression-only CPR by dispatchers results in delivery of earlier and more chest compressions, but not an increase in survival [47,48]. Some EMS systems have adopted protocols making active ventilation optional during the initial resuscitation, instead

placing an oral airway and oxygen mask until sufficient rescuers are on scene. This allows the first-arriving crew to focus on compressions and defibrillation.

Considerable scientific data have highlighted the importance of controlled ventilation during resuscitation. Aufderheide et al. demonstrated in cardiac arrests that hyperventilation increases intrathoracic pressure, resulting in decreased preload and CPP [33]. They also showed that inadvertent hyperventilation occurs frequently during resuscitation efforts, despite specific training to avoid this phenomenon. Ventilation during cardiac arrest should consist of tidal volumes of 500–600 mL at a respiratory rate of 8–10 breaths/min.

The impedance threshold device (ITD) is a ventilation adjunct that may be attached to either a face mask or an endotracheal tube and contains a one-way valve that permits exhalation during the downstroke of chest compression but prevents passive inhalation during the upstroke of chest compression. As a result, the ITD generates increased negative intrathoracic pressure during chest recoil, increasing cardiac preload and CPP. While preclinical and small trial data were favorable, a large randomized trial of the ITD versus sham device yielded similar rates of survival with good neurological outcome between groups (ITD 5.8% versus sham device 6.0%; p=0.71) [49–54].

Medications

Although numerous medications may be used during treatment of cardiac arrest, the primary agents are vasopressors (e.g. epinephrine and vasopressin) and antiarrhythmics (e.g. lidocaine and amiodarone). ACLS algorithms provide specific guidelines for the use and doses of these agents [1].

No drug has demonstrated improved outcomes following cardiac arrest in humans [55–58]. The continued use of these drugs is based on tradition, theory, and animal research, and the selection of specific agents in each class is largely a matter of individual choice. EMS physicians must be aware that the only medications evaluated by randomized clinical trials are epinephrine, amiodarone, vasopressin, and magnesium [56,59,60]. Current ACLS guidelines downplay the use of these medications in favor of quality CPR performance [1].

Vasopressors serve two intended purposes in cardiac arrest: vasoconstriction, and exerting positive inotropy and chronotropy. Alpha-agonists increase peripheral resistance, shunting blood flow to the brain and heart. Beta-agonists increase inotropy and chronotropy. In the clinical context, these agents should help to sustain coronary and cerebral perfusion before restoration of pulses. AHA guidelines suggest administering 1 mg of IV epinephrine every 3–5 minutes and provide an option to substitute one dose with 40 units of vasopressin [1].

Compelling animal data indicate increased ROSC with the early delivery of epinephrine or vasopressin [61–64]. Although several small clinical series have reported increases in ROSC and survival to admission for patients treated with vasopressin, a randomized trial comparing vasopressin with epinephrine versus epinephrine alone did not demonstrate additional benefit from vasopressin use [59,65–67]. Two randomized controlled trials have shown no improvement in survival to discharge, but have shown increased rates of ROSC [68,69].

With the use of vasopressors, there is a trade-off between increased coronary perfusion and reduced cerebral perfusion (possibly via increased cerebral vasoconstriction). A once-popular ACLS approach was the use of high-dose epinephrine (5–7 mg IV) [55]. Although clinical trials using high-dose epinephrine demonstrated increased rates of ROSC, this did not translate into survival to discharge [55].

Antiarrhythmics are commonly used in cases of VT/VF cardiac arrest and may increase the likelihood of conversion to a perfusing rhythm. Lidocaine and amiodarone are currently recommended antiarrhythmics for shock-refractory VF; both have Class IIb recommendations (conflicting evidence) [1]. One randomized controlled trial of amiodarone demonstrated an increase in ROSC, but not improved survival to hospital discharge [60]. An important point for use in critical situations, especially with limited resources such as the out-of-hospital setting, is that amiodarone is logistically more difficult to administer than lidocaine, requiring the medication to be dispensed from glass vials. ACLS guidelines indicate that amiodarone has a stronger supporting evidence base than lidocaine, as there have been no studies evaluating lidocaine [1]. EMS physicians may choose between an IV bolus of 300 mg of amiodarone or 1–1.5 mg/kg of lidocaine for patients suffering pulseless VT/VF. A randomized, controlled trial evaluating amiodarone, lidocaine, and placebo is currently enrolling and might help to clarify this issue (ClinicalTrials.gov, identifier NCT01401647).

Epidemiological studies suggest that pulseless electrical activity (PEA) and asystole are increasingly common in out-of-hospital cardiac arrests [70–73]. Atropine is a vagolytic and reverses cholinergic-mediated decreases in heart rate, blood pressure (BP), and vascular resistance [1]. Although traditionally it has been used in PEA or asystolic cardiac arrest, the limited available research does not suggest any benefit, and this drug is no longer recommended for routine use. Epinephrine should be administered, and potentially treatable causes (the 5 Hs and 5 Ts of ACLS) considered (Box 12.1).

Box 12.1 The potentially treatable Hs and Ts of cardiac arrest

Hs:
Hypovolemia
Hypoxia
Hyper-/hypokalemia
Hydrogen ion (acidosis)
Hypothermia
Ts:
Toxins
Tamponade (cardiac)
Tension pneumothorax
Thrombosis (coronary)
Thrombosis (massive pulmonary)

An additional drug worth comment is sodium bicarbonate. For years, sodium bicarbonate was administered routinely during cardiac arrest to reverse the metabolic acidosis of cardiac arrest, and hopefully increase the effectiveness of vasopressors and antiarrhythmics. In formal trials, this drug did not improve survival [74]. Sodium bicarbonate may be reasonable in scenarios of suspected hyperkalemic arrest (such as individuals with known renal failure) and in prolonged resuscitations with adequate ventilation. Calcium (chloride or gluconate), however, is the most effective medication in cases of severe hyperkalemia affecting cardiac conduction.

Additional therapies

Cardiac arrest represents the ultimate scenario of cardiovascular collapse. Consequently, cardiopulmonary bypass or extracorporeal life support (ECLS) may represent one potential solution. In tightly defined populations, ECLS combined with early angiography and hypothermia therapy has yielded good neurological outcomes in a significant proportion of patients [75–77]. In a study which used ECLS only after standard therapy failed, the rate of good neurological outcome was small [78]. Optimal selection of patients for this therapy will require early mobilization of resources given the association between prolonged arrest and poor neurological outcomes [79].

Principles of management

Resuscitation protocols

Cardiac arrest care interventions are time-critical. Thus, protocols should allow EMS personnel to initiate resuscitation immediately. Non-physician providers should provide initial cardiac arrest care using standing orders, as there is inadequate time to consult with the direct medical oversight physician for detailed guidance. The protocols should detail interventions for the various ECG rhythms likely to be encountered: VF, VT, PEA, and asystole. Protocols should provide convenient reference to medication dosages, mixtures, and administration rates. Other practical information should also be included, such as criteria for termination of resuscitation. Many systems use current AHA ACLS algorithms as the basis for cardiac arrest protocols [1].

Emergency medical services personnel should be encouraged to contact the direct medical oversight physician for additional direction after initial successful or unsuccessful resuscitative efforts, as well as for unusual or complicated situations. Due to the time-sensitive nature of cardiac arrest and the often chaotic resuscitation scene, radio or phone interactions with the EMS personnel must be short, directed, and relevant. The physician must understand that detailed medical history or preceding symptoms are usually not known and are largely (although not entirely) irrelevant to the acute resuscitation phase of the patient's care. EMS personnel may seek medical oversight physician direction for more complex interventions and situations, such as initiating a dopamine infusion or external pacing. Direct medical oversight physicians must be prepared to provide adequate direction for these less common situations.

High-performance CPR: the pit crew approach

Based on the emerging concepts described above, an appreciation has developed for the importance of doing CPR in a very high-quality and precise manner and for providing the other components of resuscitation in a more timely and more measured way. Achieving these goals requires a team of providers working together in a carefully choreographed approach. Some have suggested that personnel at a cardiac arrest scene should function like a racing pit crew, each very skilled, with a specific task or tasks, and working in a synchronized manner.

This concept also emphasizes and includes practice sessions on high-quality performance: assuring continuous chest compressions with proper depth, rate, and recoil, changing compressors (quickly) every 100–200 compressions, and integrating defibrillation such as charging the defibrillator with 20 or so compressions left in the cycle so the operator can quickly assess the rhythm and push to shock as soon as the compressor is off the chest. The first two responders should position themselves on each side of the chest, and while one (EMS1) starts compressions, the other (EMS2) applies the defibrillation pads and turns on the monitor. As EMS1 finishes the first round of compressions, the rhythm is analyzed. If a shockable rhythm is found, EMS2 can defibrillate and then begin chest compressions. Meanwhile, EMS1 is relieved of compressing (for 1 minute), and he or she should insert an oral airway and place an O_2 mask (or ventilate with a bag-valve-mask). When EMS2 is relieved for his or her minute break, he or she looks for IV or IO access and administers epinephrine (or vasopressin, based on system protocol as established by the medical director). The rhythm should be checked every 200 compressions or every 2 minutes. As more personnel arrive, attention can be paid to ventilation and placement of an advanced airway (endotracheal intubation or supraglottic airway). Finally the team leader should reassess all ongoing therapies, monitor function, and consider potentially treatable specific conditions.

Care during this initial 10–20 minutes of resuscitation should all occur at the location where the patient was found, or an area as close as possible. Efforts to "package the patient" or to begin to transfer the patient to the ambulance compromise all resuscitation efforts, not just the quality of chest compressions. Moving the patient to the ambulance or transporting immediately, except for some very rare situations, is not beneficial.

Withholding resuscitation

In the past, EMS personnel initiated resuscitative efforts regardless of the family's or patient's wishes or a written do not resuscitate (DNR) order. This practice was fueled by the belief that EMS personnel could follow only the orders of an EMS medical oversight physician, not those of an independent physician, such as the patient's own primary care physician or oncologist. Also, EMS personnel feared medicolegal repercussions if they did not initiate resuscitation. Fortunately, current practices take a more progressive approach, recognizing the importance of patient autonomy, the futility of initiating or pursuing resuscitation in select cases, and the unwarranted risks of futile resuscitation.

The primary EMS situations involving non-initiation of resuscitation efforts include the following.

- The patient has a DNR order and should not receive resuscitative efforts.
- The patient has clear signs of irreversible death (such as rigor mortis) and should not receive resuscitative efforts.

Emergency medical services agencies should have protocols and policies reflecting these situations. Personnel should receive education in the ethical principle of patient autonomy and the local regulations regarding patient directives. In each situation, consultation with the direct medical oversight physician is appropriate.

Do not resuscitate status

Do not resuscitate is a specific physician order. This differs from living wills or advance directives that merely outline the patient's general wishes regarding life-sustaining interventions. The most common EMS scenarios involving cardiac arrest patients with DNR orders include nursing home or assisted living facilities. Patients with known terminal conditions may also have DNR orders but may live in private residences or hospice facilities.

Bystanders or caregivers may summon 9-1-1 despite the presence of a DNR order. This may occur because of lack of knowledge of the patient's status, uncertainty about the patient's condition, panic, or simply the caregiver's wish to have an independent person confirm death. EMS personnel should not be surprised by these situations. Prompt consultation with the direct medical oversight physician may be appropriate in these situations.

A recent initiative, Physician Orders for Life-Sustaining Treatment (POLST) is an effort to provide a uniform DNR order sheet transcending prehospital, hospital, and long-term care settings. A number of states are enacting legislation for this program. The specific operational details must be implemented prospectively to avoid confusion and misunderstanding at the patient's side.

Dead on arrival

Non-initiation of resuscitation may be appropriate in certain situations when lividity, rigor mortis, decomposition, and other signs of obvious death are present. Protocols should specify when EMS personnel should and should not initiate resuscitation. These guidelines should address special circumstances, such as hypothermia and trauma, in addition to medical arrests. Consultation with the direct medical oversight physician is prudent in unclear situations.

Protocols should also detail specific tasks that EMS personnel must carry out after non-initiation of resuscitation, including notification of police, the coroner, or the medical examiner. EMS providers should also receive training in providing emotional support to family and bystanders.

Termination of resuscitation

Traditionally, in many areas EMS crews transported all cardiac arrest victims to the hospital, continuing resuscitative efforts en route. However, there is growing awareness that cardiac arrest patients who are not responding to initial treatment will likely not receive additional benefit from transport to the hospital [80]. Therefore, many EMS agencies now have protocols for terminating resuscitation efforts in the field.

Several studies have evaluated the prediction of futility by BLS providers [81–85]. The Verbeek/Morrison rule indicates termination of resuscitation in patients with an unwitnessed arrest after three periods of CPR, three AED analyses without shock recommendation, and no ROSC [85].

Patients who receive appropriate initial ACLS (including airway management and IV access) and who remain in asystole or PEA for greater than 20–30 minutes of resuscitative efforts without return of pulses are unlikely to be resuscitated [83,85]. ACLS guidelines support cessation of efforts in these patients without transport to the hospital [1,80,82,84]. Consultation with the direct medical oversight physician may be appropriate in these cases. Non-transport after termination of efforts applies only to patients with sustained pulselessness from suspected cardiac etiologies. This approach does *not* apply to patients with drug overdoses, hypothermic arrest, or other special situations.

The decision to terminate resuscitation or transport to the hospital involves important social and ethical concerns. Although some express concern that cessation of resuscitative efforts at the scene may be poorly accepted, two studies suggest that non-transport is well accepted and often preferred if proper counseling and explanation are given to bystanders and family members [86,87]. Nonetheless, there may be circumstances in which transport to the hospital may be prudent (e.g. cardiac arrests occurring in public locations, unexpected death in the very young, and situations with extremely distraught or unaccepting family members). Paramedics are often uncomfortable terminating resuscitation in children [88]. Direct medical oversight physician input may prove helpful in these situations.

As resuscitation strategies and postarrest care continue to improve, the accepted criteria for termination of resuscitation will have to be reevaluated. See Volume 1, Chapter 65 for additional information on termination of resuscitation.

Postarrest care

A common misconception is that the resuscitation ends after restoration of pulses. In fact, the body is in an extremely tenuous state in the immediate postarrest period. Without proper support, cardiac arrest may recur. In essence, the restoration of pulses represents the *beginning* of postarrest care.

The goals of postarrest care are to maintain hemodynamic stability, preserve the brain, and correct metabolic derangements. The salient elements of postarrest care include:

- vasopressor titration
- therapeutic hypothermia
- appropriate cardiac catheterization
- sedation
- glucose and electrolyte management.

The most important EMS consideration is vasopressor support after ROSC. Animal models of cardiac arrest predictably develop cardiovascular collapse shortly after ROSC [89]. This hemodynamic instability may result from myocardial stunning as well as the waning effect of epinephrine [90–93]. These patients frequently require vasopressor support. Because of the likely need for vasopressor support, it is reasonable to prepare a dopamine, norepinephrine, or epinephrine infusion immediately after achieving ROSC. Rescuers need to anticipate cardiovascular collapse. If they wait for collapse to occur, the patient will deteriorate before rescue therapy can be initiated.

Coronary artery disease is common in this population, and is independent of the primary arrest rhythm [94]. Early coronary angiography is strongly supported in guideline statements and has been associated with improved outcomes following ROSC [94,95]. Consequently, 12-lead ECG analysis is indicated in the patient successfully resuscitated from cardiac arrest. Patients with a history consistent with acute coronary syndrome or obvious ECG changes should be transported to a percutaneous coronary intervention center and receive prompt coronary angiography.

The induction of mild hypothermia for brain preservation has demonstrated significant improvement in neurological outcome in comatose patients following cardiac arrest [96,97]. Hypothermia is believed to decrease cerebral metabolism, reduce free radical production, and impose direct protective effects on neural and cardiac tissue [98–102].

In the Hypothermia After Cardiac Arrest (HACA) study, comatose survivors of VF/VT cardiac arrest were randomized to a goal temperature of 32–34°C for 24 hours or normal care and normothermia [96]. The investigators noted that 55% of patients receiving hypothermia enjoyed a good outcome (defined as a Cerebral Performance Category 1 [Good Recovery] or 2 [Moderate Disability]) compared with 39% of normothermic patients. In the Bernard study, patients were randomized to a goal temperature of 33°C for 12 hours or normal care and normothermia [97]. Further, 49% of the hypothermic patients enjoyed a good outcome (defined as discharge home or to acute rehabilitation), compared with 26% of the normothermic patients.

Therapeutic hypothermia has an AHA Class I recommendation for comatose survivors of out-of-hospital VT/VF cardiac arrest and a Class IIb recommendation for other rhythms or in-hospital cardiac arrests [103]. Recent evidence suggests that controlling temperature between 32–36°C results in similar outcomes in the out-of-hospital VF/VT population [104].

Early prehospital induction of hypothermia is empirically appealing and supported by animal studies. Kim et al. have demonstrated that induction of hypothermia during the prehospital phase is feasible [105,106]. The Bernard trial initiated cooling in the ambulance while en route to the hospital [97]. Perhaps the most compelling reason for starting hypothermia in the field is that hospital personnel often fail to initiate the therapy [107–111]. Initiation of hypothermia by EMS personnel may remind or compel hospital caregivers to continue this intervention.

Induction of hypothermia is relatively simple, does not require specialized techniques, and can be initiated in the prehospital setting. Kim et al. noted that rapid infusion of 1–2 L of cold (4°C) saline resulted in a 1° drop in patient temperature in the first 30 minutes [105]. Bernard et al. used surface cooling with skin exposure and ice packs, an approach that is slower but complementary [97]. Moore et al. demonstrated that healthy volunteers could achieve a 1° temperature drop with infusion of 30 mL/kg of cold saline during a 30-minute infusion [112]. The initial temperature in many postarrest patients is approximately 35–35.5°C [113]. Therefore, practitioners may potentially reach the target temperature with only a 1° reduction in body temperature. In the largest randomized controlled trial to date, prehospital cooling was not associated with a higher rate of good neurological outcome than the hospital-initiated group (risk ratio 0.90; 95% CI 0.70, 1.17) [114]. In addition, recent data demonstrate that rapid infusion of saline in the prehospital arena is associated with pulmonary edema [115]. To date, intraarrest hypothermia has not yielded additional survival benefit [116]. Nasogastric, bladder, and endovascular cooling are other viable options in the hospital, but they are impractical in the prehospital setting.

Most importantly, the receiving medical facility must continue hypothermia therapy for it to be effective. The EMS physician should ensure that a patient cooled in the prehospital arena is transported to a facility that can continue this therapy. Although the ultimate target temperature is 32–34°C, this goal may require several hours with concomitant sedation and pharmacological paralysis.

The other elements of postarrest care do not need to be initiated in the field. However, the postarrest patient is critically ill and frequently requires the care of multiple specialists who may not be available at all hospital facilities [110,117–120]. The management of the postarrest patient is a low-frequency, resource-intensive event requiring regimented, multidisciplinary strategies to optimize outcome [118,120]. One retrospective study has demonstrated that the risk of rearrest during prolonged air medical transport is low, but critical events such as hypotension or hypoxemia were encountered in 23% of patients [121]. Because many hospitals cannot provide these services at all hours, some systems have regionalized the care of postarrest patients [122]. EMS medical directors should consider developing policy regarding the proper destination for postarrest patients in their systems.

Conclusion

Successful resuscitation of patients from out-of-hospital cardiac arrest requires a comprehensive system of care. Prehospital care providers face many practical and logistical challenges in this setting, but intense, expert resuscitation efforts can improve the bleak rate of survival from this condition. Prompt initiation and continuous performance of high-quality chest compressions, timely defibrillation, avoidance of hyperventilation, and appropriate postarrest care are the keys to successful outcomes.

References

1 Morrison LJ, Deakin CD, Morley PT, et al. Part 8: Advanced life support: 2010 international consensus on cardiopulmonary resuscitation and emergency cardiovascular care science with treatment recommendations. *Circulation* 2010;122:S345–421.

2 Paradis NA, Martin GB, Rivers EP, et al. *JAMA* 1990;263(8):1106–13.

3 Callaham M, Madsen CD. Relationship of timeliness of paramedic advanced life support interventions to outcome in out-of-hospital cardiac arrest treated by first responders with defibrillators. *Ann Emerg Med* 1996;27(5):638–48.

4 Spaite DW, Hanlon T, Criss EA, et al. Prehospital cardiac arrest: the impact of witnessed collapse and bystander CPR in a metropolitan EMS system with short response times. *Ann Emerg Med* 1990;19(11):1264–9.

5 Stiell IG, Wells GA, DeMaio VJ, et al. Modifiable factors associated with improved cardiac arrest survival in a multicenter basic life support/defibrillation system: OPALS Study Phase I results. Ontario Prehospital Advanced Life Support. *Ann Emerg Med* 1999;33(1): 44–50.

6 Wik L, Steen PA, Bircher NG. Quality of bystander cardiopulmonary resuscitation influences outcome after prehospital cardiac arrest. *Resuscitation* 1994;28(3):195–203.

7 Kern KB, Hilwig RW, Berg RA, Sanders AB, Ewy GA. Importance of continuous chest compressions during cardiopulmonary resuscitation: improved outcome during a simulated single lay-rescuer scenario. *Circulation* 2002;105(5):645–9.

8 Berg RA, Sanders AB, Kern KB, et al. Adverse hemodynamic effects of interrupting chest compressions for rescue breathing during cardiopulmonary resuscitation for ventricular fibrillation cardiac arrest. *Circulation* 2001;104(20):2465–70.

9 Christenson J, Andrusiek D, Everson-Stewart SP, et al. Chest compression fraction determine survival in patients with out-of-hospital ventricular fibrillation. *Circulation* 2009;120(13):1241–7.

10 Wik L, Kramer-Johansen J, Myklebust H, et al. Quality of cardiopulmonary resuscitation during out-of-hospital cardiac arrest. *JAMA* 2005;293(3):299–304.

11 Abella BS, Alvarado JP, Myklebust H, et al. Quality of cardiopulmonary resuscitation during in-hospital cardiac arrest. *JAMA* 2005;293(3):305–10.

12 Kramer-Johansen J, Myklebust H, Wik L, et al. Quality of out-of-hospital cardiopulmonary resuscitation with real time automated feedback: a prospective interventional study. *Resuscitation* 2006; 71(3):283–92.

13 Ward KR, Menegazzi JJ, Zelenak RR, Sullivan RJ, McSwain NE Jr. A comparison of chest compressions between mechanical and manual CPR by monitoring end-tidal PCO2 during human cardiac arrest. *Ann Emerg Med* 1993;22(4):669–74.

14 Ong MEH, Ornato JP, Edwards DP, et al. Use of an automated, load-distributing band chest compression device for out-of-hospital cardiac arrest resuscitation. *JAMA* 2006;295(22): 2629–37.

15 Hallstrom A, Rea TD, Sayre MR, et al. Manual chest compression vs use of an automated chest compression device during resuscitation following out-of-hospital cardiac arrest: a randomized trial. *JAMA* 2006;295(22):2620–8.

16 Steen S, Sjoberg T, Olsson P, Young M. Treatment of out-of-hospital cardiac arrest with LUCAS, a new device for automatic mechanical compression and active decompression resuscitation. *Resuscitation* 2005;67(1):25–30.

17 Cummins RO, Hazinski MF, Kerber RE, et al. Low-energy biphasic waveform defibrillation: evidence-based review applied to emergency cardiovascular care guidelines: a statement for healthcare professionals from the American Heart Association Committee on Emergency Cardiovascular Care and the Subcommittees on Basic Life Support, Advanced Cardiac Life Support, and Pediatric Resuscitation. *Circulation* 1998;97(16):1654–67.

18 Hess EP, Atkinson EJ, White RD. Increased prevalence of sustained return of spontaneous circulation following transition to biphasic waveform defibrillation. *Resuscitation* 2008;77(1):39–45.

19 Stiell IG, Walker RG, Nesbitt LP, et al. BIPHASIC Trial: a randomized comparison of fixed lower versus escalating higher energy levels for defibrillation in out-of-hospital cardiac arrest. *Circulation* 2007;115(12):1511–17.

20 Van Alem AP, Sanou BT, Koster RW. Interruption of cardiopulmonary resuscitation with the use of the automated external defibrillator in out-of-hospital cardiac arrest. *Ann Emerg Med* 2003;42(4):449–57.

21 Lloyd MS, Heeke B, Walter PF, Langberg JJ. Hands-on defibrillation: an analysis of external current flow through rescuers in direct contact with patients during biphasic external defibrillation. *Circulation* 2008;117(19):2510–4.

22 Petley GW, Deakin CD. Do clinical examination gloves provide adequate electrical insulation for safe hands-on defibrillation? II: Material integrity following exposure to defibrillation waveforms. *Resuscitation* 2013;84(7):900–3.

23 Part 1: Introduction to the International Guidelines 2000 for CPR and ECC: a consensus on science. *Circulation* 2000;102(8 Suppl):I1–11.

24 Kern KB, Garewal HS, Sanders AB, et al. Depletion of myocardial adenosine triphosphate during prolonged untreated ventricular fibrillation: effect on defibrillation success. *Resuscitation* 1990; 20(3):221–9.

25 Maldonado FA, Weil MH, Tang W, et al. Myocardial hypercarbic acidosis reduces cardiac resuscitability. *Anesthesiology* 1993;78(2):343–52.

26 Stiell IG, Nichol G, Leroux BG, et al. Early versus later rhythm analysis in patients with out-of-hospital cardiac arrest. *N Engl J Med* 2011;365(9):787–97.

27 Cobb LA, Fahrenbruch CE, Walsh TR, et al. Influence of cardiopulmonary resuscitation prior to defibrillation in patients with out-of-hospital ventricular fibrillation. *JAMA* 1999;281(13):1182–8.

28 Wik L, Hansen TB, Fylling F, et al. Delaying defibrillation to give basic cardiopulmonary resuscitation to patients with out-of-hospital ventricular fibrillation: a randomized trial. *JAMA* 2003;289(11):1389–95.

29 Katz SH, Falk JL. Misplaced endotracheal tubes by paramedics in an urban emergency medical services system. *Ann Emerg Med* 2001;37(1):32–7.

30 Wang HE, Kupas DF, Paris PM, Bates RR, Yealy DM. Preliminary experience with a prospective, multi-centered evaluation of out-of-hospital endotracheal intubation. *Resuscitation* 2003;58(1):49–58.

31 Wang HE, Lave JR, Sirio CA, Yealy DM. Paramedic intubation errors: isolated events or symptoms of larger problems? *Health Aff (Millwood)* 2006;25(2):501–9.

32 Wang HE, Yealy DM. Out-of-hospital endotracheal intubation: where are we? *Ann Emerg Med* 2006;47(6):532–41.

33 Aufderheide TP, Sigurdsson G, Pirrallo RG, et al. Hyperventilation-induced hypotension during cardiopulmonary resuscitation. *Circulation* 2004;109(16):1960–5.

34 Abo BN, Hostler D, Wang HE. Does the type of out-of-hospital airway interfere with other cardiopulmonary resuscitation tasks? *Resuscitation* 2007;72(2):234–9.

35 Kim JA, Vogel D, Guimond G, Hostler D, Wang HE, Menegazzi JJ. A randomized, controlled comparison of cardiopulmonary resuscitation performed on the floor and on a moving ambulance stretcher. *Prehosp Emerg Care* 2006;10(1):68–70.

36 Silvestri S, Ralls GA, Krauss B, et al. The effectiveness of out-of-hospital use of continuous end-tidal carbon dioxide monitoring on the rate of unrecognized misplaced intubation within a regional emergency medical services system. *Ann Emerg Med* 2005;45(5):497–503.

37 Wang HE, Szydio D, Stouffer JA, et al. Endotracheal intubation versus supraglottic airway insertion in out-of-hospital cardiac arrest. *Resuscitation* 2012;83(9):1061–6.

38 Kajino K, Iwami T, Kitamura T, et al. Comparison of supraglottic airway versus endotracheal intubation for the pre-hospital treatment of out-of-hospital cardiac arrest. *Crit Care* 2011;15(5):R236.

39 Berg RA, Kern KB, Hilwig RW, Ewy GA. Assisted ventilation during 'bystander' CPR in a swine acute myocardial infarction model does not improve outcome. *Circulation* 1997;96(12):4364–71.

40 Berg RA, Kern KB, Sanders AB, Otto CW, Hilwig RW, Ewy GA. Bystander cardiopulmonary resuscitation. Is ventilation necessary? *Circulation* 1993;88(4 Pt 1):1907–15.

41 Ewy GA, Zuercher M, Hilwig RW, et al. Improved neurological outcome with continuous chest compressions compared with 30:2 compressions-to-ventilations cardiopulmonary resuscitation in a realistic swine model of out-of-hospital cardiac arrest. *Circulation* 2007;116(22):2525–30.

42 Hallstrom A, Cobb L, Johnson E, Copass M. Cardiopulmonary resuscitation by chest compression alone or with mouth-to-mouth ventilation. *N Engl J Med* 2000;342(21):1546–53.

43 Kern KB, Hilwig RW, Berg RA, Ewy GA. Efficacy of chest compression-only BLS CPR in the presence of an occluded airway. *Resuscitation* 1998;39(3):179–88.

44 Hostler D, Rittenberger JC, Roth R, Callaway CW. Increased chest compression to ventilation ratio improves delivery of CPR. *Resuscitation* 2007;74(3):446–52.

45 Paradis NA, Martin GB, Goetting MG, et al. Simultaneous aortic, jugular bulb, and right atrial pressures during cardiopulmonary resuscitation in humans. Insights into mechanisms. *Circulation* 1989;80(2):361–8.

46 Rittenberger JC, Guimond G, Platt TE, Hostler D. Quality of BLS decreases with increasing resuscitation complexity. *Resuscitation* 2006;68(3):365–9.

47 Williams JG, Brice JH, DeMaio VJ, Jalbuena T. A simulation trial of traditional dispatcher-assisted CPR versus compression-only dispatcher-assisted CPR. *Prehosp Emerg Care* 2006;10(2):247–53.

48 Rea TD, Fahrenbruch C, Culley L, et al. CPR with chest compression alone or with rescue breathing. *N Engl J Med* 2010:363: 423–33.

49 Lurie KG, Voelckel WG, Zielinski T, et al. Improving standard cardiopulmonary resuscitation with an inspiratory impedance threshold valve in a procine model of cardiac arrest. *Anesth Analg* 2001;93(3):649–55.

50 Lurie KG, Zielinski T, McKnite S, Aufderheide T, Voelckel W. Use of an inspiratory impedance valve improves neurologically intact survival in a porcine model of ventricular fibrillation. *Circulation* 2002;105(1):124–9.

51 Plaisance P, Lurie KG, Payen D. Inspiratory impedance during active compression-decompression cardiopulmonary resuscitation: a randomized evaluation in patients in cardiac arrest. *Circulation* 2000;101(9):989–94.

52 Aufderheide TP, Pirrallo RG, Provo TA, Lurie KG. Clinical evaluation of an inspiratory impedance threshold device during standard cardiopulmonary resuscitation in patients with out-of-hospital cardiac arrest. *Crit Care Med* 2005;33(4):734–40.

53 Thayne RC, Thomas DC, Neville JD, Van Dellen A. Use of an impedance threshold device improves short-term outcomes following out-of-hospital cardiac arrest. *Resuscitation* 2005;67(1):103–8.

54 Aufderheide TP, Nichol G, Rea TD, et al. A trial of an impedance threshold device in out-of-hospital cardiac arrest. *N Engl J Med* 2011;365(9):798–806.

55 Callaham M, Madsen CD, Barton CW, Saunders CE, Pointer J. A randomized clinical trial of high-dose epinephrine and norepinephrine vs standard-dose epinephrine in prehospital cardiac arrest. *JAMA* 1992;268(19):2667–72.

56 Fatovich DM, Prentice DA, Dobb GJ. Magnesium in cardiac arrest (the MAGIC trial). *Resuscitation* 1997;35(3): 237–41.

57 Stiell IG, Wells GA, Field B, et al. Advanced cardiac life support in out-of-hospital cardiac arrest. *N Engl J Med* 2004;351(7):647–56.

58 Wang HE, Min A, Hostler D, Chang CC, Callaway CW. Differential effects of out-of-hospital interventions on short- and long-term survival after cardiopulmonary arrest. *Resuscitation* 2005;67(1): 69–74.

59 Callaway CW, Hostler D, Doshi AA, et al. Usefulness of vasopressin administered with epinephrine during out-of-hospital cardiac arrest. *Am J Cardiol* 2006;98(10):1316–21.

60 Kudenchuk PJ, Cobb LA, Copass MK, et al. Amiodarone for resuscitation after out-of-hospital cardiac arrest due to ventricular fibrillation. *N Engl J Med* 1999;341(12):871–8.

61 Cammarata G, Weil MH, Sun S, Tang W, Wang J, Huang L. Beta1-adrenergic blockade during cardiopulmonary resuscitation improves survival. *Crit Care Med* 2004;32(9 Suppl):S440–3.

62 Niemann JT, Cairns CB, Sharma J, Lewis RJ. Treatment of prolonged ventricular fibrillation. Immediate countershock versus high-dose epinephrine and CPR preceding countershock. *Circulation* 1992;85(1):281–7.

63 Prengel AW, Linstedt U, Zenz M, Wenzel V. Effects of combined administration of vasopressin, epinephrine, and norepinephrine during cardiopulmonary resuscitation in pigs. *Crit Care Med* 2005;33(11):2587–91.

64 Seaberg DC, Menegazzi JJ, Check B, MacLeod BA, Yealy DM. Use of a cardiocerebral-protective drug cocktail prior to countershock in a porcine model of prolonged ventricular fibrillation. *Resuscitation* 2001;51(3):301–8.

65 Grmec S, Mally S. Vasopressin improves outcome in out-of-hospital cardiopulmonary resuscitation of ventricular fibrillation and pulseless ventricular tachycardia: a observational cohort study. *Crit Care* 2006;10(1):R13.

66 Guyette FX, Guimond GE, Hostler D, Callaway CW. Vasopressin administered with epinephrine is associated with a return of a pulse in out-of-hospital cardiac arrest. *Resuscitation* 2004;63(3):277–82.

67 Mally S, Jelatancev A, Grmec S. Effects of epinephrine and vasopressin on end-tidal carbon dioxide tension and mean arterial blood pressure in out-of-hospital cardiopulmonary resuscitation: an observational study. *Crit Care* 2007;11(2):R39.

68 Jacobs IG, Finn JC, Jelinek GA, Oxer HF, Thompson PL. Effect of adrenaline on survival in out-of-hospital cardiac arrest: a randomized double blind placebo-controlled trial. *Resuscitation* 2011;82(9):1138–43.

69 Olasveengen TV, Sunde K, Brungborg Wik L. Intravenous drug administration during out-of-hospital cardiac arrest. *JAMA* 2009;302(20):2222–9.

70 Bunch TJ, White RD, Friedman PA, Kottke TE, Wu LA, Packer DL. Trends in treated ventricular fibrillation out-of-hospital cardiac arrest: a 17-year population-based study. *Heart Rhythm* 2004;1(3): 255–9.

71 Cobb LA, Fahrenbruch CE, Olsufka M, Copass MK. Changing incidence of out-of-hospital ventricular fibrillation, 1980–2000. *JAMA* 2002;288(23):3008–13.

72 Polentini MS, Pirrallo RG, McGill W. The changing incidence of ventricular fibrillation in Milwaukee, Wisconsin (1992–2002). *Prehosp Emerg Care* 2006;10(1):52–60.

73 Youngquist ST, Kaji AH, Niemann JT. Beta-blocker use and the changing epidemiology of out-of-hospital cardiac arrest rhythms. *Resuscitation* 2008;76(3):376–80.

74 Bar-Joseph G, Abramson NS, Kelsey SF, Mashiach T, Craig MT, Safar P. Improved resuscitation outcome in emergency medical systems with increased usage of sodium bicarbonate during cardiopulmonary resuscitation. *Acta Anaesthesiol Scand* 2005; 49(1):6–15.

75 Nagao K, Kikushima K, Watanabe K, et al. Early induction of hypothermia during cardiac arrest improves neurological outcomes in patients with out-of-hospital cardiac arrest who undergo emergency cardiopulmonary bypass and percutaneous coronary intervention. *Circu J* 2010;74:77–85.

76 Nagao K, Nayashi N, Kanmatsuse K, et al. Cardiopulmonary cerebral resuscitation using emergency cardiopulmonary bypass, coronary reperfusion therapy and mild hypothermia in patients with cardiac arrest outside the hospital. *J Am Coll Cardiol* 2000; 36:776–83.

77 Bellezzo JM, Shinar Z, Davis DP, et al. Emergency physician-initiated extracorporeal cardiopulmonary resuscitation. *Resuscitation* 2012;83:966–70.

78 Le Guen M, Nicolas-Robin A, Carreira S, et al. Extracorporeal life support following out-of-hospital refractory cardiac arrest. *Crit Care* 2011;15:R29.

79 Reynolds JC, Frisch A, Rittenberger JC, Callaway CW. Duration of resuscitation efforts and functional outcome after out-of-hospital cardiac arrest: when should we change to novel therapies? *Circulation* 2013;128(23):2488–94.

80 Gray WA, Capone RJ, Most AS. Unsuccessful emergency medical resuscitation – are continued efforts in the emergency department justified? *N Engl J Med* 1991;325(20):1393–8.

81 Ong MEH, Jaffey J, Stiell I, Nesbitt L. Comparison of termination-of-resuscitation guidelines for basic life support: defibrillator providers in out-of-hospital cardiac arrest. *Ann Emerg Med* 2006; 47(4):337–43.

82 Bonnin MJ, Pepe PE, Kimball KT, Clark PS Jr. Distinct criteria for termination of resuscitation in the out-of-hospital setting. *JAMA* 1993;270(12):1457–62.

83 Cone DC, Bailey ED, Spackman AB. The safety of a field termination-of-resuscitation protocol. *Prehosp Emerg Care* 2005;9(3):276–81.

84 Kellermann AL. Criteria for dead-on-arrivals, prehospital termination of CPR, and do-not-resuscitate orders. *Ann Emerg Med* 1993;22(1):47–51.

85 Morrison LJ, Visentin LM, Kiss A, et al. Validation of a rule for termination of resuscitation in out-of-hospital cardiac arrest. *N Engl J Med* 2006;355(5):478–87.

86 Delbridge TR, Fosnocht DE, Garrison HG, Auble TE. Field termination of unsuccessful out-of-hospital cardiac arrest resuscitation: acceptance by family members. *Ann Emerg Med* 1996;27(5):649–54.

87 Schmidt TA, Harrahill MA. Family response to death in the field. *Ann Emerg Med* 1993;22:918.

88 Hall WL II, Myers JH, Pepe PE, Larkin GL, Sirbaugh PE, Persse DE. The perspective of paramedics about on-scene termination of resuscitation efforts for pediatric patients. *Resuscitation* 2004;60(2):175–87.

89 Ramiro R, Menegazzi JJ, Wang HE, Callaway CW. Post-resuscitation hemodynamics and relationship to duration of ventricular fibrillation. *Prehosp Emerg Care* 2004;8(1):81.

90 Adrie C, Adib-Conquy M, Laurent I, et al. Successful cardiopulmonary resuscitation after cardiac arrest as a "sepsis-like" syndrome. *Circulation* 2002;106(5):562–8.

91 Kern KB, Hilwig RW, Rhee KH, Berg RA. Myocardial dysfunction after resuscitation from cardiac arrest: an example of global myocardial stunning. *J Am Coll Cardiol* 1996;28(1):232–40.

92 Tennyson H, Kern KB, Hilwig RW, Berg RA, Ewy GA. Treatment of post resuscitation myocardial dysfunction: aortic counterpulsation versus dobutamine. *Resuscitation* 2002;54(1):69–75.

93 Vasquez A, Kern KB, Hilwig RW, Heidenreich J, Berg RA, Ewy GA. Optimal dosing of dobutamine for treating post-resuscitation left ventricular dysfunction. *Resuscitation* 2004;61(2):199–207.

94 Reynolds JC, Callaway CW, El Khoudary SR, Moore CG, Alvarez RJ, Rittenberger JC. Coronary angiography predicts improved outcome following cardiac arrest: propensity-adjusted analysis. *J Intens Care Med* 2009;24(3):179–86.

95 Dumas F, Cariou A, Manzo-Silberman S, et al. Immediate percutaneous coronary intervention is associated with better survival after out-of-hospital cardiac arrest: insights from the PROCAT (Parisian Region Out of hospital Cardiac ArresT) registry. *Circ Cardiovasc Interv* 2010;3(3):200–7.

96 Hypothermia after Cardiac Arrest Study Group. Mild therapeutic hypothermia to improve the neurologic outcome after cardiac arrest. *N Engl J Med* 2002;346(8):549–56.

97 Bernard SA, Gray TW, Buist MD, et al. Treatment of comatose survivors of out-of-hospital cardiac arrest with induced hypothermia. *N Engl J Med* 2002;346(8):557–63.

98 Dempsey RJ, Combs DJ, Maley ME, Cowen DE, Roy MW, Donaldson DL. Moderate hypothermia reduces postischemic edema development and leukotriene production. *Neurosurgery* 1987;21(2):177–81.

99 Kramer RS, Sanders AP, Lesage AM, Woodhall B, Sealy WC. The effect profound hypothermia on preservation of cerebral ATP content during circulatory arrest. *J Thorac Cardiovasc Surg* 1968; 56(5):699–709.

100 Natale JA, D'Alecy LG. Protection from cerebral ischemia by brain cooling without reduced lactate accumulation in dogs. *Stroke* 1989;20(6):770–7.

101 Sterz F, Leonov Y, Safar P, et al. Multifocal cerebral blood flow by Xe-CT and global cerebral metabolism after prolonged cardiac arrest in dogs. Reperfusion with open-chest CPR or cardiopulmonary bypass. *Resuscitation* 1992;24(1):27–47.

102 Mezrow CK, Sadeghi AM, Gandsas A, et al. Cerebral blood flow and metabolism in hypothermic circulatory arrest. *Ann Thorac Surg* 1992;54(4):609–15.

103 Peberdy MA, Callaway CW, Neumar RW, et al. Part 9: Post-cardiac arrest care: 2010 American Heart Association guidelines for cardiopulmonary resuscitation and emergency cardiovascular care. *Circulation* 2010;122:S768–86.

104 Nielsen N, Wetterslev J, Cronberg T, et al. Targeted temperature management at 33C versus 36C after cardiac arrest. *N Engl J Med* 2013;369:2197–206.

105 Kim F, Olsufka M, Longstreth WT Jr, et al. Pilot randomized clinical trial of prehospital induction of mild hypothermia in out-of-hospital cardiac arrest patients with a rapid infusion of 4 degrees C normal saline. *Circulation* 2007;115(24):3064–70.

106 Virkkunen I, Yli-Hankala A, Silfvast T. Induction of therapeutic hypothermia after cardiac arrest in prehospital patients using ice-cold Ringer's solution: a pilot study. *Resuscitation* 2004;62(3): 299–302.

107 Abella BS, Rhee JW, Huang KN, Vanden Hoek TL, Becker LB. Induced hypothermia is underused after resuscitation from cardiac arrest: a current practice survey. *Resuscitation* 2005;64(2):181–6.

108 Laver SR, Padkin A, Atalla A, Nolan JP. Therapeutic hypothermia after cardiac arrest: a survey of practice in intensive care units in the United Kingdom. *Anaesthesia* 2006;61(9):873–7.

109 Merchant RM, Soar J, Skrifvars MB, et al. Therapeutic hypothermia utilization among physicians after resuscitation from cardiac arrest. *Crit Care Med* 2006;34(7):1935–40.

110 Oksanen T, Pettila V, Hynynen M, Varpula T. Therapeutic hypothermia after cardiac arrest: implementation and outcome in Finnish intensive care units. *Acta Anaesthesiol Scand* 2007;51(7):866–71.

111 Wolfrum S, Radke PW, Pischon T, Willich SN, Schunkert H, Kurowski V. Mild therapeutic hypothermia after cardiac arrest – a nationwide survey on the implementation of the ILCOR guidelines in German intensive care units. *Resuscitation* 2007;72(2):207–13.

112 Moore TM, Callaway CW, Hostler D. Core temperature cooling in healthy volunteers after rapid intravenous infusion of cold and room temperature saline solution. *Ann Emerg Med* 2008;51(2):153–9.

113 Callaway CW, Tadler SC, Katz LM, Lipinski CL, Brader E. Feasibility of external cranial cooling during out-of-hospital cardiac arrest. *Resuscitation* 2002;52(2):159–65.

114 Bernard SA, Smith K, Cameron P, et al. *Circulation* 2010;122: 737–42.

115 Kim F, Nichol G, Maynard C, et al. Effect of prehospital induction of mild hypothermia on survival and neurological status among adults with cardiac arrest: a randomized clinical trial. *JAMA* 2014;311(1):45–52.

116 Castren M, Nordberg P, Svensson L, et al. Intra-arrest transnasal evaporative cooling: a randomized, prehospital, multicenter study (PRINCE: Pre-ROSC IntraNasal Cooling Effectiveness). *Circulation* 2010;122(7):729–36.

117 Langhelle A, Tyvold SS, Lexow K, Hapnes SA, Sunde K, Steen PA. In-hospital factors associated with improved outcome after

out-of-hospital cardiac arrest. A comparison between four regions in Norway. *Resuscitation* 2003;56(3):247–63.

118 Sunde K, Pytte M, Jacobsen D, et al. Implementation of a standardised treatment protocol for post resuscitation care after out-of-hospital cardiac arrest. *Resuscitation* 2007;73(1):29–39.

119 Rittenberger JC, Guyette FX, Tisherman SA, DeVita MA, Alvarez RJ, Callaway CW. Outcomes of a hospital-wide plan to improve care of comatose survivors of cardiac arrest. *Resuscitation* 2008;79(2):198–204.

120 Werling M, Thoren AB, Axelsson C, Herlitz J. Treatment and outcome in post-resuscitation care after out-of-hospital cardiac arrest when a modern therapeutic approach was introduced. *Resuscitation* 2007;73(1):40–5.

121 Hartke A, Mumma BE, Rittenberger JC, Callaway CW, Guyette FX. Incidence of re-arrest and critical events during prolonged transport of post-cardiac arrest patients. *Resuscitation* 2010;81:938–42.

122 Davis DP, Fisher R, Aguilar S, et al. The feasibility of a regional cardiac arrest receiving system. *Resuscitation* 2007;74(1):44–51.

CHAPTER 13

Chest pain and acute coronary syndrome

Joseph P. Ornato, Michael R. Sayre, and James I. Syrett

Introduction

In the United States, someone experiences a myocardial infarction every 26 seconds, and alarmingly the disease claims one life each minute [1]. Acute myocardial infarction (AMI) accounts for almost five times as many deaths in the United States as are attributed to unintentional injuries, which has major implications for EMS systems [2]. About half of those who suffer acute myocardial infarctions are transported to the hospital by EMS, and many more patients call EMS for help because they are experiencing chest pain [3].

The prehospital management of chest pain has improved with better clinical examination, earlier administration of effective medications, and the broad use of 12-lead ECGs to detect acute coronary syndromes (ACS) and myocardial infarction more accurately before arrival in the emergency department (ED) [4]. Because more rapid reperfusion during acute myocardial infarction improves heart function and patient survival, EMS and health care systems have focused on developing strategies to identify chest pain patients with myocardial infarction quickly and to provide effective treatment while transporting them directly to definitive care [5–7].

The goals of management for patients with chest pain include rapid identification of patients with ACS, relief of their symptoms, and transport to an appropriate hospital. This chapter will cover the assessment and treatment of patients with a chief complaint of chest pain and will focus on the scientific basis for prehospital medical care of those patients. It will also review common conditions that can cause chest pain.

General approach

When evaluating a patient with a complaint of chest pain, EMS professionals should begin by assessing the patient's stability and then obtain a basic clinical history and examination. Early in the assessment, an EMS provider should apply a cardiac monitor to rapidly identify dysrhythmias, perform a diagnostic 12-lead ECG, and administer specific treatment depending on the results of the initial evaluation. Because only a small minority of the patients with chest pain actually have ACS, maintaining vigilance in this assessment and diagnostic routine can be difficult [8].

Complete accuracy in the diagnosis of chest pain is not always possible in any setting, not even in the hospital [9]. The prehospital provider should not expect to diagnose a patient with a complaint of chest pain definitively. A careful history can lead the provider to a correct "category" of diagnosis much of the time. As a general approach, the patient should be treated as if he or she has the most likely serious illness consistent with the signs and symptoms.

Discomfort due to cardiac ischemia is usually, but not always, substernal and may radiate to the shoulder, either arm, both arms, upper abdomen, back, or jaw [9,10]. Other symptoms such as nausea and diaphoresis are commonly present but do not predict the presence or absence of ACS accurately. Cardiac disease is most often seen beginning in middle-aged men and older women. However, even younger adults under the age of 40 with no cardiac risk factors and a normal ECG have a 1–2% risk of ACS [11]. Taking a focused history using the "PQRST method" can be helpful (Box 13.1).

There are many causes of chest pain and their incidence changes depending on the characteristics of the population being studied. Patients calling on EMS are more likely to have acute myocardial infarction or other serious causes of chest pain than are patients in the general emergency department (ED) population [3]. Although the majority of this chapter focuses on the management of an ACS, other causes of chest pain are present more commonly.

Role of emergency medical dispatch

Prehospital care of the patient with a complaint of chest pain begins at emergency medical dispatch. Identification of patients suspected to have ACS allows an EMS system to send

Emergency Medical Services: Clinical Practice and Systems Oversight, Second Edition. Volume 1: Clinical Aspects of EMS.
Edited by David C. Cone, Jane H. Brice, Theodore R. Delbridge, and J. Brent Myers.
© 2015 NAEMSP. Published 2015 by John Wiley & Sons, Inc. Companion Website: www.wiley.com\go\cone\naemsp

advanced-level providers to the patient. Many EMS systems with both basic and advanced-level ambulances use a trained emergency medical call taker who asks the caller a series of questions to determine the nature of the emergency and the likelihood that advanced-level care will be needed (see Volume 2, Chapter 10).

A retrospective cohort study from England took a rigorous approach to determining the accuracy of one set of dispatcher questions in identifying patients with ACS [12]. About 8% of calls at the "9-9-9" center were classified as "chest pain." Subsequent chart review at the hospital identified all patients with the ultimate diagnosis of ACS and found that this represented only 0.6% of all 9-9-9 patients. About 80% of the ACS patients were classified correctly as chest pain at the dispatch level. Another 7% were classified in a variety of other categories that still received a paramedic level response (e.g. severe respiratory distress). Sensitivity of the dispatch system for detecting ACS was 71% and specificity was 93%. However, a great deal of overtriage occurred, and the positive predictive value of the dispatch system for detecting ACS was only 6%. Additional refinement of the dispatch question sequence to reduce overtriage seems possible. The emergency dispatch question sequence for stroke performs much better, with a positive predictive value of 42% and a similar sensitivity to ACS at 83% [13].

The American Heart Association (AHA) and American College of Cardiology (ACC) recommend that emergency medical dispatchers prompt patients with non-traumatic chest pain to take aspirin if they have no contraindications while awaiting EMS arrival [14,15]. This recommendation is based on extrapolation from data showing that patients who take aspirin before hospital arrival are less likely to die and that the practice is likely quite safe [16].

The 12-lead electrocardiogram

The 12-lead ECG remains the quickest method of detecting myocardial ischemia or infarction. Although ECGs have been used to diagnose ACS since 1932, the technology has now advanced to the point that a prehospital ECG can be done quickly and accurately and can be sent wirelessly to the receiving hospital at a relatively low cost. Additional benefit can be gained by having the prehospital ECG become the first of a series of ECGs, increasing the sensitivity of diagnosis of coronary syndromes [17].

Performing a prehospital ECG on a patient exhibiting signs and symptoms of ACS is a Class I AHA/ACC recommendation [14,15]. This recommendation is based on evidence demonstrating that, despite at most slightly increased time spent on scene for patients receiving ECGs, the time to definitive treatment for ST-elevation myocardial infarction (STEMI) with fibrinolysis or percutaneous coronary intervention (PCI) is shortened overall, with a significant reduction in mortality [18].

Prehospital electrocardiogram: interpretation

With the ease of obtaining a prehospital 12-lead ECG comes the need for its accurate interpretation. Precise interpretations can influence decisions to transport patients to more appropriate but more distant facilities, as well as immediate management strategies on hospital arrival. A 12-lead ECG is required to diagnose STEMI and can often provide evidence that ACS is present.

Currently three methods of out-of-hospital ECG interpretation exist: computer algorithms integrated into the ECG machine, direct interpretation by paramedics, or wireless transmission of the ECG to a physician for interpretation. One, two, or all three can be used in a given EMS system.

All prehospital 12-lead ECG machines contain computer programs that will interpret the ECG, and the machines can be configured to print the interpretation on the ECG. If this technology is sufficiently sensitive and specific for STEMI, the EMS professionals would theoretically not require education in interpretation, which would allow EMS systems to use advanced- and basic-level providers to acquire 12-lead ECGs. Additional benefits of using the computer's interpretation include avoidance of the technical issues and cost of establishing base stations dedicated to receiving incoming ECGs, as well as the provision of consistent interpretation that does not depend on the variable skills and experience of EMS providers. Many prehospital 12-lead ECG systems use computerized interpretation systems which have high specificity, but the computer interpretation alone can miss up to 20% of true STEMI events [19].

Despite the high specificity, many emergency physicians and cardiologists do not place enough trust in the computer interpretation alone to routinely activate the cardiac catheterization PCI team that can provide rapid reperfusion treatment for a STEMI patient [20]. EMS provider interpretation is another option. More extensive training is required, and interpretation accuracy can be affected by both experience and interest in the subject matter [21]. Although several studies have shown that trained paramedics can accurately interpret the presence of STEMI, experience also plays an important role [22–24]. Having a paramedic identify and report "tombstones" on the 12-lead is a powerful motivator for action by experienced physicians.

> **Box 13.2** The most common prehospital causes of ST-segment elevation
>
> - ST-segment elevation acute myocardial infarction
> - Early repolarization
> - Left bundle branch block
> - Acute pericarditis

The third method of interpretation is by transmission of the acquired ECG to a base station for interpretation by a physician. This method has generally been used as the gold standard when comparing other methods of interpretation, and its accuracy has been shown to be slightly better than other methods. It relies both on the availability of the interpreting physician and on an infrastructure that allows reliable transmission of the ECG.

In one observational cohort study, positive predictive value of prehospital 12-lead ECGs was improved by transmitting them to emergency physicians compared with interpretation solely by paramedics [24]. In some cases automated systems have been developed that allow simultaneous transmission of the 12-lead ECG to the receiving ED and to an invasive cardiologist on call [25]. These systems have the potential to decrease treatment times further because both the ED staff and the PCI team are activated early.

The AHA guidelines state that the ECG may be transmitted for remote interpretation by a physician or screened for STEMI by properly trained paramedics, with or without the assistance of computer interpretation [14]. Advance notification should be provided to the receiving hospital for patients identified as having STEMI. Implementation of 12-lead ECG diagnostic programs with concurrent medically directed quality assurance is recommended.

No diagnostic test is perfect, and the 12-lead ECG is no exception. There are a number of conditions other than acute myocardial infarction that can cause ST-segment elevation, such as left bundle branch block and hyperkalemia [26] (Box 13.2). Some of the differences between STEMI and the mimics of acute ST-segment elevation are subtle and missed easily.

Medications

Several medications are important for EMS management of the patient with chest pain. Providing the chest pain patient with medication for relief of pain whenever safe and feasible and regardless of the etiology of the pain is fundamental. Treatment of pain reduces anxiety in addition to relieving the patient's discomfort. For ACS patients, treatment of pain can reduce catecholamine levels and thus improve the balance between oxygen demand and supply for ischemic cardiac muscle.

Oxygen

Despite its historical use, the evidence review leading up to the 2010 AHA guidelines did not find sufficient evidence to recommend the routine use of oxygen therapy in patients with uncomplicated AMI or ACS who have no signs of hypoxemia or heart failure [14]. The guidelines do, however, recommend oxygen administration if the patient is dyspneic, or has an arterial oxyhemoglobin saturation <94%, signs of heart failure, or shock.

Aspirin

Aspirin is inexpensive, readily available, and has been shown to benefit patients having myocardial infarction or other ACS. The ISIS-2 study established that the absolute benefit of aspirin administration for myocardial infarction patients results in 26 fewer deaths per 1,000 patients treated, with the maximum benefit occurring in the first 4 hours [27]. Prehospital administration of aspirin is safe [28] and may improve outcome [29,30], and should be given as soon as possible to patients with suspected ACS unless contraindicated [14,15].

Varying doses of aspirin have been proposed, but for ACS the most widely used dose is four 81 mg baby aspirin tablets. These tablets are well tolerated, easy to swallow, and more rapidly absorbed than other preparations [31]. Rectal preparations (300 mg) should be considered in patients unable to swallow. Acceptable contraindications to aspirin administration include definitive aspirin allergy or a history of active gastrointestinal bleeding.

Nitroglycerin

Nitroglycerin is a time-honored treatment to relieve chest pain due to angina by decreasing myocardial oxygen demand and increasing collateral blood flow to ischemic areas of the heart. Somewhat surprisingly, nitroglycerin is not effective at reducing STEMI patient mortality [32], nor is the response, or lack thereof, to nitroglycerin administration an accurate diagnostic test to determine whether cardiac ischemia is the underlying cause of a patient's chest pain [33]. For example, because it relaxes smooth muscle, nitroglycerin may also relieve pain in patients with esophageal spasm.

Nitroglycerin can be administered as sublingual tablets or an oral spray. The usual dose of either method of delivery is 0.4 mg. Although up to three doses can be given at an interval of 5 minutes between doses, current AHA/ACC recommendations for self-administered patient use of nitroglycerin is for them to call EMS if chest pain is not improved 5 minutes after only a single dose of nitroglycerin to avoid a 15–20-minute delay before activating the EMS system among STEMI patients [14,15].

Nitroglycerin should be avoided in several groups of patients with chest pain. Patients who have used phosphodiesterase inhibitors and then take nitrates can have profound, refractory hypotension. Nitrates generally should be avoided for 24 hours following sildenafil or vardenafil use, and for 48 hours following tadalafil use.

Patients with right ventricular infarction are dependent on right ventricular filling pressure to maintain cardiac output and a normal systolic blood pressure. If the patient has a systolic blood pressure below 100 mmHg or a heart rate below 60 beats per minute, nitroglycerin should be avoided until a 12-lead ECG, including right-sided leads, documents the absence of a right ventricular infarction. Nitroglycerin should also be avoided in patients who already have systolic blood pressures <90 mmHg or heart rates <50 or >100 beats per minute.

Morphine sulfate

A large retrospective case series of hospitalized patients with non-ST segment elevation ACS found that patients who received morphine had a higher mortality than those who did not [34]. It is unclear whether this was a causal effect or simply indicated that those who required morphine may have had more severe disease. The AHA/ACC treatment guidelines for patients with unstable angina or non-ST-elevation MI (NSTEMI) reduce the strength of recommendation for morphine from Class I to Class IIa for patients with NSTEMI [35]. The 2013 AHA/ACC STEMI guidelines give morphine a Class I recommendation in STEMI patients because those patients are going to have reperfusion therapy [15]. The recommended dose of morphine in the patient with chest pain is 2–4 mg intravenously with increments of 2–8 mg intravenously repeated at 5–15-minute intervals when pain is not adequately controlled with nitroglycerin.

Beta-blockers

Older guidelines recommended IV beta-blocker (typically metoprolol) administration early in the course of acute myocardial infarction because of data suggesting reduced rates of reinfarction and recurrent ischemia when patients received both fibrinolytics and IV beta-blockers. A large placebo-controlled randomized trial showed that the effect of beta-blockers in reducing arrhythmic events is equally offset by an increase in development of cardiogenic shock, and survival is similar regardless of early administration of intravenous beta-blockers [36]. Current AHA/ACC recommendations for administration of intravenous beta-blockers in the setting of STEMI are limited to patients who are hypertensive or have ongoing ischemia with no contraindications to their use [15]. On balance, the guidelines suggest that the need for prehospital administration of beta-blockers to patients with STEMI is limited.

Prehospital fibrinolysis

Since fibrinolytics were introduced to emergency cardiac care in the mid-1980s, some have proposed initiating these drugs in the prehospital setting. Several studies published in the early 1990s showed that the strategy was feasible [37] and that it could decrease mortality from STEMI in settings that had relatively long EMS response and/or transport time intervals [38]. Additional studies reinforced the original findings, and a metaanalysis of pooled results from six randomized trials enrolling more than 6,000 subjects concluded that prehospital initiation of fibrinolytics decreased all-cause mortality by shortening initiation of treatment by 58 minutes [39].

Few systems in the United States have implemented prehospital fibrinolysis, although additional research has continued to show time savings over in-hospital treatment. In Europe, particularly where there are often physician-staffed ambulances, prehospital fibrinolysis is used more frequently.

A primary reason why prehospital fibrinolysis is not used regularly in the United States has been a shift in favor of primary PCI for treatment of STEMI. In a prospective observational cohort study of 26,205 consecutive patients with STEMI in Sweden, representing about 95% of the population of STEMI patients in the country, those who were treated with primary PCI had lower 30-day mortality than those treated with fibrinolytics in the hospital (4.9% versus 11.4%) [40]. Primary PCI patients also had lower mortality than those treated with prehospital fibrinolytics (4.9% versus 7.6%).

Several large clinical trials have examined the strategy of transferring patients to a PCI-capable institution from a local hospital compared with administration of fibrinolytics at the local hospital [41,42]. A metaanalysis of six large studies involving 3,750 patients showed that timely transfer for primary PCI strategy is superior in reducing rates of reinfarction, stroke, and the combined end-point criteria of death, reinfarction, or stroke [29].

For situations in which transfer directly to a center capable of primary PCI is not possible in a timely fashion, a strategy of prehospital or non-PCI hospital-based fibrinolysis is reasonable. The available science suggests that the drugs can be safely administered by full-time paramedics or EMS physicians in the field. The EMS system should have a medical director with experience in STEMI management and a well-organized quality assurance program.

Systems of care for ST-elevation myocardial infarction

The EMS system plays a key role in shortening the process of caring for patients with STEMI. Patients who are transported by EMS have shorter treatment intervals than those of patients who arrive at the hospital by other means [43]. Patients can be encouraged to use EMS appropriately. A community intervention to shorten the time interval from symptom onset to ED arrival was shown to increase the proportion of ACS patients who used EMS for transport to the ED [44].

Prehospital notification and field cardiac catheterization laboratory activation

A key benefit of a prehospital 12-lead ECG is notification of the receiving facility of an impending STEMI patient's arrival. Shortening door-to-balloon time by 30 minutes reduces in-hospital mortality from STEMI by about 1% [45]. Implementation of a prehospital 12-lead ECG program with prehospital notification shortened door-to-balloon times by about 60 minutes in San Diego [46]. In an evaluation of a large patient registry, prehospital notification with ED activation of the catheterization team before patient arrival at the hospital shortened door-to-balloon time by about 15 minutes [47].

Occasional false-positive activation of the PCI team is a necessary byproduct of an aggressive field approach to alerting hospitals about patients with suspected STEMI. One report suggests that up to 15–20% of team activations may not result in any intervention [48]. The rate of false-positive activations depends on the pretest probability of finding a STEMI. If EMS providers perform 12-lead ECGs broadly (e.g. everyone over the age of 30 with any of the following characteristics: chest pain, shortness of breath, abdominal pain, diabetes, or cardiac history), such that the prevalence of actual STEMI is between 0.5% and 5%, then the positive predictive value of a "STEMI-positive" prehospital 12-lead ECG may be around 50% [49]. Such a system would result in more false-positive than true-positive activations of the PCI team.

When patients have a reasonable likelihood of STEMI based on their clinical presentations and 12-lead ECG findings, prehospital cardiac catheterization PCI team activation has consistently been shown to shorten time to definitive treatment of STEMI patients considerably. For example, Nestler et al. showed that prehospital activation of the catheterization laboratory reduced the median door-to-balloon times from 59 to 32 minutes [50]. Cone et al. found that field activation of the catheterization laboratory was associated with 37 and 35 minute shorter door-to-balloon times than ED activation for walk-in STEMI patients or STEMI patients arriving by EMS without field activation, respectively [51]. In addition, field activation of the catheterization laboratory was associated with better compliance with 90-minute STEMI treatment benchmarks. Finally, Horvath et al. found similar reduction in the door-to-balloon times (44 versus 57 minutes) in EMS-transported STEMI patients who had prehospital activation of the cardiac catheterization laboratory compared to those who had the laboratory activated after ED arrival [52].

In summary, field activation of the cardiac catheterization laboratory when a prehospital ECG shows evidence of STEMI is strongly supported by published data. EMS systems should work with their PCI-capable hospitals to establish cardiac catheterization laboratory prehospital STEMI activation protocols and quality improvement monitoring.

Emergency medical services transport

Despite the benefits of EMS for chest pain patients, many patients misinterpret their symptoms, delay calling EMS, or use personal transportation to go to the hospital. Public education campaigns attempted to date have not shortened the overall time interval from symptom onset to hospital arrival, but they have increased the proportion of ACS patients who use EMS [53].

Destination protocols

Almost 80% of the adult population of the United States lives within 60 driving minutes of a PCI-capable center [54]. Of those patients whose closest hospital is not capable of PCI, 74% require additional transport time less than 30 minutes to reach a PCI-capable institution.

Therefore, several urban communities have developed protocols to encourage EMS to transport STEMI patients directly to hospitals with 24/7 capability to perform PCI. In Ottawa, a STEMI bypass protocol for EMS was implemented in May 2005 [55]. Paramedics performed a 12-lead ECG, and if STEMI was identified in a hemodynamically stable patient, the patient was transported directly to the region's single cardiac center catheterization lab with prehospital notification of the impending arrival of the STEMI patient, often bypassing one of the four other EDs in the city. The median first door-to-balloon time was 69 minutes for patients brought to the catheterization lab directly by EMS, compared with 123 minutes for those needing interhospital transfer. In The Netherlands, prehospital identification of patients with STEMI and transport to a PCI-capable center bypassing other EDs was associated with improved left ventricular function [56].

Some systems are directing EMS to take STEMI patients directly to the heart catheterization lab, bypassing the ED. The strategy reduces door-to-balloon time up to 60 minutes [57]. In more rural settings without available PCI centers, coordinated programs with regional STEMI receiving centers can achieve remarkable door-to-balloon times, even when measuring from the first door (i.e. the door of the rural ED). Two reports from Minnesota show that excellent treatment times can be achieved. In the Minneapolis area, the median first door-to-balloon time was 95 minutes if the referring hospital was less than 60 miles from the PCI center and 120 minutes if the referring hospital was further away [58]. In the Mayo Clinic STEMI system, patients were transferred from 28 regional hospitals up to 150 miles away from the PCI center. The median first door-to-balloon time for the transferred patients was 116 minutes [59].

Air medical evacuation of ST-elevation myocardial infarction patients

A key to a successful regional STEMI system is ready access to air medical transport. Rapid transport of the patient by highly skilled teams in medical helicopters can save significant time from the first door to balloon. Some air medical programs are working closely with referring hospitals and ground EMS systems to dispatch helicopters before arrival of a STEMI patient at a referring hospital [60].

Expanding the role of Basic Life Support providers

Many prearrival 9-1-1 instructions already direct callers to take aspirin if they have chest pain. Allowing BLS providers to administer aspirin, if not contraindicated, and if permitted by EMS laws and regulations, seems the next logical step. One reason stated for the lack of aspirin administration to eligible

ACS patients is the inability of BLS providers to administer it based on local protocols or regulations [61].

Basic Life Support providers can be taught to acquire and transmit 12-lead ECGs. This approach may be particularly beneficial in rural areas, with scant ALS coverage and long transport times to definitive care. Using the 12-lead ECG to triage STEMI patients to air transport from the scene may lead to improved cardiac care in rural areas and more efficient use of available resources [62].

Other common causes of chest discomfort

Although most of the available prehospital interventions for chest pain are focused on the identification and treatment of ischemic cardiac disease, the majority of EMS chest pain patients will have other causes for their symptoms, some of which are also immediate threats to life (Box 13.3). A chest pain protocol should focus on treatments that may benefit the ACS/STEMI patient while considering the effects of these treatments on other causes of chest pain.

Aortic dissection

Acute aortic dissection classically causes sudden pain in the chest, sometimes radiating to the back. The dissection is caused by a tear in the intimal lining of the aorta with entry of high-pressure blood into the wall of the aorta. The dissection propagates distally and sometimes also proximally. If the dissection extends around the origin of a peripheral artery, then that vessel can be partially or completely occluded, creating a >15–20 mmHg difference in blood pressures between both patient arms. If the origin of a carotid or vertebral artery is occluded, then the patient may develop neurological signs suggesting a stroke. Occlusion of a spinal artery off the aorta can cause acute paralysis of both legs. Most patients with dissection have long-standing hypertension, but the problem can occur in younger patients with other conditions such as Marfan syndrome.

In the majority of cases of aortic dissection, the 12-lead ECG will be abnormal, but will not show ST-segment elevation unless the origin of a coronary artery is occluded by the dissection [63]. Without imaging capability that exists in the hospital, EMS providers may suspect, but cannot identify, aortic dissection definitively [64,65]. If aortic dissection is suspected, morphine can be used for pain control but aspirin should be avoided since patients with acute aortic syndrome who receive

antithrombotic agents such as aspirin or fibrinolytics are more likely to bleed [66].

Pericarditis

Individuals with pericarditis may present to EMS with ST-segment elevation on an ECG that looks similar to an extensive myocardial infarction. Administration of fibrinolytics in this condition may be fatal because these patients can bleed into the pericardial sac, resulting in pericardial tamponade. Aspirin administration is somewhat less concerning because antiinflammatory medications are part of the recommended treatment.

Pneumothorax

A pneumothorax may cause chest pain, shortness of breath, hypoxia, and diaphoresis. Clinical signs may point more to this diagnosis than to acute myocardial infarction. EMS systems should have a separate protocol for management of a pneumothorax. Oxygen and morphine may help the patient. Nitroglycerin should be avoided because it can cause hypotension by further decreasing venous return if the patient is developing a tension pneumothorax. If a developing tension pneumothorax is evident, needle decompression is required.

Pulmonary embolism

Pulmonary embolism is a great masquerader because its symptoms may be similar to those of other causes of chest pain and shortness of breath. Its presentation can easily be confused with myocardial infarction or anxiety. Treatment should focus on maximizing oxygenation to the patient. If pulmonary embolism is suspected, nitroglycerin should be avoided because it can cause significant hypotension. Administration of fibrinolytics may potentially benefit the patient, but it is preferable to delay administration until the patient has reached a hospital and undergone a definitive diagnostic imaging study.

Esophageal perforation

A patient with a perforated esophagus may present with chest pain. A careful and focused history and examination will often help differentiate this condition from other causes of chest pain. Nitroglycerin should be avoided because it may cause significant hypotension, and fibrinolytics are contraindicated because of the need for immediate surgery.

Conclusion

Quality prehospital care of patients with chest pain can relieve discomfort and improve outcome. EMS systems should have the capability to perform prehospital 12-lead ECGs and regional protocols should focus on delivering patients with STEMI to PCI centers promptly. Prehospital activation of the cardiac catheterization laboratory is highly effective at shortening the time to definitive reperfusion treatment and should be encouraged.

Box 13.3 Causes of chest discomfort that are immediate life threats

- Acute coronary syndrome
- Pericardial tamponade
- Pulmonary embolism
- Tension pneumothorax
- Thoracic aortic dissection

References

1 Go AS, Mozaffarian D, Roger VL, et al. Heart disease and stroke statistics – 2013 update: a report from the American Heart Association. *Circulation* 2013;127:e6–e245.

2 CDC. Leading Causes of Death. 2005. Available at: www.cdc.gov/nchs/data/nvsr/nvsr56/nvsr56_10.pdf

3 Canto JG, Zalenski RJ, Ornato JP, et al. Use of emergency medical services in acute myocardial infarction and subsequent quality of care: observations from the National Registry of Myocardial Infarction 2. *Circulation* 2002;106:3018–23.

4 Brainard AH, Raynovich W, Tandberg D, Bedrick EJ. The prehospital 12-lead electrocardiogram's effect on time to initiation of reperfusion therapy: a systematic review and meta-analysis of existing literature. *Am J Emerg Med* 2005;23:351–6.

5 Jollis JG, Al-Khalidi HR, Monk L, et al. Expansion of a regional ST-segment-elevation myocardial infarction system to an entire state. *Circulation* 2012;126:189–95.

6 Jollis JG, Granger CB, Henry TD, et al. Systems of care for ST-segment-elevation myocardial infarction: a report From the American Heart Association's Mission: Lifeline. *Circ Cardiovasc Qual Outcomes* 2012;5:423–8.

7 Jollis JG, Roettig ML, Aluko AO, et al. Implementation of a statewide system for coronary reperfusion for ST-segment elevation myocardial infarction. *JAMA* 2007;298:2371–80.

8 Kohn MA, Kwan E, Gupta M, Tabas JA. Prevalence of acute myocardial infarction and other serious diagnoses in patients presenting to an urban emergency department with chest pain. *J Emerg Med* 2005;29:383–90.

9 Goodacre S, Locker T, Morris F, Campbell S. How useful are clinical features in the diagnosis of acute, undifferentiated chest pain? *Acad Emerg Med* 2002;9:203–8.

10 Goodacre SW, Angelini K, Arnold J, Revill S, Morris F. Clinical predictors of acute coronary syndromes in patients with undifferentiated chest pain. *QJM* 2003;96:893–8.

11 Marsan RJ Jr, Shaver KJ, Sease KL, Shofer FS, Sites FD, Hollander JE. Evaluation of a clinical decision rule for young adult patients with chest pain. *Acad Emerg Med* 2005;12:26–31.

12 Deakin CD, Sherwood DM, Smith A, Cassidy M. Does telephone triage of emergency (999) calls using Advanced Medical Priority Dispatch (AMPDS) with Department of Health (DH) call prioritisation effectively identify patients with an acute coronary syndrome? An audit of 42,657 emergency calls to Hampshire Ambulance Service NHS Trust. *Emerg Med J* 2006;23:232–5.

13 Ramanujam P, Guluma KZ, Castillo EM, et al. Accuracy of stroke recognition by emergency medical dispatchers and paramedics – San Diego experience. *Prehosp Emerg Care* 2008;12:307–13.

14 O'Connor RE, Brady W, Brooks SC, et al. Part 10: acute coronary syndromes: 2010 American Heart Association Guidelines for Cardiopulmonary Resuscitation and Emergency Cardiovascular Care. *Circulation* 2010;122:S787-817.

15 O'Gara PT, Kushner FG, Ascheim DD, et al. 2013 ACCF/AHA guideline for the management of ST-elevation myocardial infarction: executive summary: a report of the American College of Cardiology Foundation/American Heart Association Task Force on Practice Guidelines. *J Am Coll Cardiol* 2013;61:485–510.

16 Eisenberg MJ, Topal EJ. Prehospital administration of aspirin in patients with unstable angina and acute myocardial infarction. *Arch Intern Med* 1996;156:1506–10.

17 Kudenchuk PJ, Maynard C, Cobb LA, et al. Utility of the prehospital electrocardiogram in diagnosing acute coronary syndromes: the Myocardial Infarction Triage and Intervention (MITI) Project. *J Am Coll Cardiol* 1998;32:17–27.

18 Morrison LJ, Brooks S, Sawadsky B, McDonald A, Verbeek PR. Prehospital 12-lead electrocardiography impact on acute myocardial infarction treatment times and mortality: a systematic review. *Acad Emerg Med* 2006;13:84–9.

19 Massel D, Dawdy JA, Melendez LJ. Strict reliance on a computer algorithm or measurable ST segment criteria may lead to errors in thrombolytic therapy eligibility. *Am Heart J* 2000;140:221–6.

20 Swor R, Hegerberg S, McHugh-McNally A, Goldstein M, McEachin CC. Prehospital 12-lead ECG: efficacy or effectiveness? *Prehosp Emerg Care* 2006;10:374–7.

21 Berger JS, Eisen L, Nozad V, et al. Competency in electrocardiogram interpretation among internal medicine and emergency medicine residents. *Am J Med* 2005;118:873–80.

22 Whitbread M, Leah V, Bell T, Coats TJ. Recognition of ST elevation by paramedics. *Emerg Med J* 2002;19:66–7.

23 Feldman JA, Brinsfield K, Bernard S, White D, Maciejko T. Real-time paramedic compared with blinded physician identification of ST-segment elevation myocardial infarction: results of an observational study. *Am J Emerg Med* 2005;23:443–8.

24 Davis DP, Graydon C, Stein R, et al. The positive predictive value of paramedic versus emergency physician interpretation of the prehospital 12-lead electrocardiogram. *Prehosp Emerg Care* 2007;11:399–402.

25 Dhruva VN, Abdelhadi SI, Anis A, et al. ST-Segment Analysis Using Wireless Technology in Acute Myocardial Infarction (STAT-MI) trial. *J Am Coll Cardiol* 2007;50:509–13.

26 Wang K, Asinger RW, Marriott HJ. ST-segment elevation in conditions other than acute myocardial infarction. *N Engl J Med* 2003;349:2128–35.

27 ISIS-2 Investigators. Randomised trial of intravenous streptokinase, oral aspirin, both, or neither among 17,187 cases of suspected acute myocardial infarction: ISIS-2. ISIS-2 (Second International Study of Infarct Survival) Collaborative Group. *Lancet* 1988;2:349–60.

28 Quan D, LoVecchio F, Clark B, Gallagher JV 3rd. Prehospital use of aspirin rarely is associated with adverse events. *Prehosp Disaster Med* 2004;19:362–5.

29 Barbash I, Freimark D, Gottlieb S, et al. Outcome of myocardial infarction in patients treated with aspirin is enhanced by pre-hospital administration. *Cardiology* 2002;98:141–7.

30 Freimark D, Matetzky S, Leor J, et al. Timing of aspirin administration as a determinant of survival of patients with acute myocardial infarction treated with thrombolysis. *Am J Cardiol* 2002;89:381–5.

31 Cox D, Maree AO, Dooley M, Conroy R, Byrne MF, Fitzgerald DJ. Effect of enteric coating on antiplatelet activity of low-dose aspirin in healthy volunteers. *Stroke* 2006;37:2153–8.

32 GISSI-3 Investigators. GISSI-3: effects of lisinopril and transdermal glyceryl trinitrate singly and together on 6-week mortality and ventricular function after acute myocardial infarction. Gruppo Italiano per lo Studio della Sopravvivenza nell'infarto Miocardico. *Lancet* 1994;343:1115–22.

33 Henrikson CA, Howell EE, Bush DE, et al. Chest pain relief by nitroglycerin does not predict active coronary artery disease. *Ann Intern Med* 2003;139:979–86.

34 Meine TJ, Roe MT, Chen AY, et al. Association of intravenous morphine use and outcomes in acute coronary syndromes: results from the CRUSADE Quality Improvement Initiative. *Am Heart J* 2005;149:1043–9.

35 Antman EM, Hand M, Armstrong PW, et al. 2007 Focused Update of the ACC/AHA 2004 Guidelines for the Management of Patients With ST-Elevation Myocardial Infarction: a report of the American College of Cardiology/American Heart Association Task Force on Practice Guidelines: developed in collaboration With the Canadian Cardiovascular Society endorsed by the American Academy of Family Physicians: 2007 Writing Group to Review New Evidence and Update the ACC/AHA 2004 Guidelines for the Management of Patients With ST-Elevation Myocardial Infarction, Writing on Behalf of the 2004 Writing Committee. *Circulation* 2008;117: 296–329.

36 Chen ZM, Pan HC, Chen YP, et al. Early intravenous then oral metoprolol in 45,852 patients with acute myocardial infarction: randomised placebo-controlled trial. *Lancet* 2005;366:1622–32.

37 Weaver WD, Cerqueira M, Hallstrom AP, et al. Prehospital-initiated vs hospital-initiated thrombolytic therapy. The Myocardial Infarction Triage and Intervention Trial. *JAMA* 1993;270:1211–16.

38 European Myocardial Infarction Project Group. Prehospital thrombolytic therapy in patients with suspected acute myocardial infarction. *N Engl J Med* 1993;329:383–9.

39 Morrison LJ, Verbeek PR, McDonald AC, Sawadsky BV, Cook DJ. Mortality and prehospital thrombolysis for acute myocardial infarction: A meta-analysis. *JAMA* 2000;283:2686–92.

40 Stenestrand U, Lindback J, Wallentin L. Long-term outcome of primary percutaneous coronary intervention vs prehospital and in-hospital thrombolysis for patients with ST-elevation myocardial infarction. *JAMA* 2006;296:1749–56.

41 Widimsky P, Budesinsky T, Vorac D, et al. Long distance transport for primary angioplasty vs immediate thrombolysis in acute myocardial infarction. Final results of the randomized national multicentre trial – PRAGUE-2. *Eur Heart J* 2003;24:94–104.

42 Busk M, Maeng M, Rasmussen K, et al. The Danish multicentre randomized study of fibrinolytic therapy vs. primary angioplasty in acute myocardial infarction (the DANAMI-2 trial): outcome after 3 years follow-up. *Eur Heart J* 2008;29:1259–66.

43 Swor R, Anderson W, Jackson R, Wilson A. Effects of EMS transportation on time to diagnosis and treatment of acute myocardial infarction in the emergency department. *Prehosp Disaster Med* 1994;9:160–4.

44 Luepker RV, Raczynski JM, Osganian S, et al. Effect of a community intervention on patient delay and emergency medical service use in acute coronary heart disease: the Rapid Early Action for Coronary Treatment (REACT) trial. *JAMA* 2000;284:60–7.

45 McNamara RL, Wang Y, Herrin J, et al. Effect of door-to-balloon time on mortality in patients with ST-segment elevation myocardial infarction. *J Am Coll Cardiol* 2006;47:2180–6.

46 Brown JP, Mahmud E, Dunford JV, Ben-Yehuda O. Effect of prehospital 12-lead electrocardiogram on activation of the cardiac catheterization laboratory and door-to-balloon time in ST-segment elevation acute myocardial infarction. *Am J Cardiol* 2008;101: 158–61.

47 Bradley EH, Herrin J, Wang Y, et al. Strategies for reducing the door-to-balloon time in acute myocardial infarction. *N Engl J Med* 2006;355:2308–20.

48 Larson DM, Menssen KM, Sharkey SW, et al. "False-positive" cardiac catheterization laboratory activation among patients with suspected ST-segment elevation myocardial infarction. *JAMA* 2007;298:2754–60.

49 Youngquist ST, Kaji AH, Lipsky AM, Koenig WJ, Niemann JT. A Bayesian sensitivity analysis of out-of-hospital 12-lead electrocardiograms: implications for regionalization of cardiac care. *Acad Emerg Med* 2007;14:1165–71.

50 Nestler DM, White RD, Rihal CS, et al. Impact of prehospital electrocardiogram protocol and immediate catheterization team activation for patients with ST-elevation-myocardial infarction. *Circ Cardiovasc Qual Outcomes* 2011;4:640–6.

51 Cone DC, Lee CH, van Gelder C. EMS activation of the cardiac catheterization laboratory is associated with process improvements in the care of myocardial infarction patients. *Prehosp Emerg Care* 2013;17:293–8.

52 Horvath SA, Xu K, Nwanyanwu F, et al. Impact of the prehospital activation strategy in patients with ST-elevation myocardial infarction undergoing primary percutaneous revascularization: a single center community hospital experience. *Crit Pathw Cardiol* 2012;11:186–92.

53 Osganian SK, Zapka JG, Feldman HA, et al. Use of emergency medical services for suspected acute cardiac ischemia among demographic and clinical patient subgroups: the REACT trial. Rapid Early Action for Coronary Treatment. *Prehosp Emerg Care* 2002;6:175–85.

54 Nallamothu BK, Bates ER, Wang Y, Bradley EH, Krumholz HM. Driving times and distances to hospitals with percutaneous coronary intervention in the United States: implications for prehospital triage of patients with ST-elevation myocardial infarction. *Circulation* 2006;113:1189–95.

55 Le May MR, So DY, Dionne R, et al. A citywide protocol for primary PCI in ST-segment elevation myocardial infarction. *N Engl J Med* 2008;358:231–40.

56 Van't Hof AW, Rasoul S, van de Wetering H, et al. Feasibility and benefit of prehospital diagnosis, triage, and therapy by paramedics only in patients who are candidates for primary angioplasty for acute myocardial infarction. *Am Heart J* 2006;151: 1255 e1–5.

57 Dorsch MF, Greenwood JP, Priestley C, et al. Direct ambulance admission to the cardiac catheterization laboratory significantly reduces door-to-balloon times in primary percutaneous coronary intervention. *Am Heart J* 2008;155:1054–8.

58 Henry TD, Sharkey SW, Burke MN, et al. A regional system to provide timely access to percutaneous coronary intervention for ST-elevation myocardial infarction. *Circulation* 2007;116: 721–8.

59 Ting HH, Rihal CS, Gersh BJ, et al. Regional systems of care to optimize timeliness of reperfusion therapy for ST-elevation myocardial infarction: the Mayo Clinic STEMI Protocol. *Circulation* 2007;116:729–36.

60 Thomas SH, Kociszewski C, Hyde RJ, Brennan PJ, Wedel SK. Prehospital electrocardiogram and early helicopter dispatch to expedite interfacility transfer for percutaneous coronary intervention. *Crit Pathw Cardiol* 2006;5:155–9.

61 Hooker EA, Benoit T, Price TG. Reasons prehospital personnel do not administer aspirin to all patients complaining of chest pain. *Prehosp Disaster Med* 2006;21:101–3.

62 Provo TA, Frascone RJ. 12-lead electrocardiograms during basic life support care. *Prehosp Emerg Care* 2004;8:212–16.

63 Biagini E, Lofiego C, Ferlito M, et al. Frequency, determinants, and clinical relevance of acute coronary syndrome-like electrocardiographic findings in patients with acute aortic syndrome. *Am J Cardiol* 2007;100:1013–19.

64 Johnson TR, Nikolaou K, Wintersperger BJ, et al. ECG-gated 64-MDCT angiography in the differential diagnosis of acute chest pain. *Am J Roentgenol* 2007;188:76–82.

65 Shiga T, Wajima Z, Apfel CC, Inoue T, Ohe Y. Diagnostic accuracy of transesophageal echocardiography, helical computed tomography, and magnetic resonance imaging for suspected thoracic aortic dissection: systematic review and meta-analysis. *Arch Intern Med* 2006;166:1350–6.

66 Hansen MS, Nogareda GJ, Hutchison SJ. Frequency of and inappropriate treatment of misdiagnosis of acute aortic dissection. *Am J Cardiol* 2007;99:852–6.

CHAPTER 14

Cardiac dysrhythmias

Christian C. Knutsen and Donald M. Yealy

Introduction

Emergency medical services physicians often use the same approach in the field and the hospital to provide patient care, even though the goals in each area differ. The care of patients with dysrhythmias before hospital arrival focuses on treating all life-threatening or imminently life-threatening rhythm changes within minutes. In the emergency department (ED) and in the hospital, the same need exists but more time is available to identify other non-lethal rhythms and deliver definitive long-term treatment.

This chapter discusses a pragmatic method of providing medical oversight for non-arrest dysrhythmias. The most important field observations and actions will be highlighted to help simplify the approach when giving direct medical oversight, creating written protocols, or providing direct patient care. We offer a "low-tech" approach to the problems, emphasizing simple tools including a brief history, physical examination, and standard 3- or 12-lead field ECG. Similarly, we focus on interventions that are effective and easily provided in the out-of-hospital setting. In general, the approach offered is consistent with the 2010 American Heart Association (AHA) Advanced Cardiac Life Support (ACLS) guidelines, although we highlight areas where simplified or alternative approaches exist.

Evaluation

Three basic sources of information are available during the assessment of field dysrhythmias: patient history, physical examination, and the ECG. Rarely will any one of these suffice in guiding treatment. Rather, all three considered together guide care [1,2]. Four steps can be used to manage patients with dysrhythmias in the field. Treatment decisions often can be made before completing all steps, allowing an economy of effort.

Step 1: identify symptoms and how they relate to the rhythm

Two groups of patients present with dysrhythmias: asymptomatic patients with incidental rhythm changes and patients with symptomatic rhythm changes. Incidental dysrhythmias may relate to the symptoms, but are the result and not the cause of another problem, and they do not worsen the immediate outcome. Patients with incidental dysrhythmias or who are asymptomatic rarely require field rhythm-directed treatment. Those with incidental dysrhythmias typically require treatment of any underlying acute condition (e.g. analgesia for pain or fluids for hypovolemia).

A 67-year-old male patient with a history of "extra heart beats" transported for an isolated ankle injury displays a sinus tachycardia (from pain) and occasional premature ventricular complexes, but no other symptoms or abnormalities on physical examination. He requires splinting and analgesia, not antidysrhythmics. This should not be confused with dysrhythmias with symptoms, such as tachycardia or bradycardia associated with chest pain, weakness, breathing difficulties, or syncope.

Step 2: identify stable and unstable patients

Because asymptomatic or incidental dysrhythmias usually require no direct treatment, the prehospital focus shifts to those dysrhythmias associated with symptoms. These patients are classified based on the severity of symptoms as either stable or unstable. Although many patients have symptoms attributable to the change from a "normal" rhythm, most tolerate these well and are stable. However, unstable patients are likely to suffer harm or deteriorate. Providers and EMS physicians must identify these unstable patients and rapidly intervene.

Unstable patients have signs and symptoms of inadequate end-organ perfusion due to the rhythm disturbance [2]. A few brief historical questions and physical examination steps must be rapidly completed to identify these patients early in their evaluation.

Emergency Medical Services: Clinical Practice and Systems Oversight, Second Edition. Volume 1: Clinical Aspects of EMS.
Edited by David C. Cone, Jane H. Brice, Theodore R. Delbridge, and J. Brent Myers.
© 2015 NAEMSP. Published 2015 by John Wiley & Sons, Inc. Companion Website: www.wiley.com\go\cone\naemsp

- Hypotension – often arbitrarily defined as a systolic blood pressure below 90 mmHg, though any departure of more than 15% from a known baseline may be functional hypotension.
- Cardiac dysfunction – seen as chest pain, shortness of breath, or rales (signifying inadequate myocardial perfusion or function).
- Altered consciousness – from mild agitation or somnolence to obtundation or coma (signifying central nervous system [CNS] hypoperfusion).

Delayed capillary refill and lowered skin temperature can indicate poor perfusion; the subjective nature of these observations and multiple other potential causes limit their use in the field.

Assessing instability is usually a continuum, not an "all-or-nothing" phenomenon. Either a single severe sign or symptom or multiple mild findings is diagnostic of an unstable rhythm. A single mildly abnormal finding suggests "borderline" stability. The blood pressure is the simplest method of assessing circulatory adequacy, but it alone may be insufficient in accurately classifying patients. A patient with a systolic blood pressure of 60 mmHg is always unstable. Another patient with a blood pressure of 90 mmHg systolic, rales, and a depressed sensorium is also unstable. If awake and with no rales, chest pain, or other symptoms, the patient with a systolic blood pressure of 90 mmHg occupies a borderline position due to the singular mild finding. Similarly, agitation suggests mild CNS hypoperfusion and borderline stability, whereas coma is associated with more profound derangement and instability.

In the absence of clear evidence of instability, each patient can receive a more complete evaluation, although the total prehospital time interval should not be prolonged. Unstable patients need rapid therapy, usually with electrical interventions such as external countershock or pacing. Symptomatic but stable or borderline unstable patients can be initially treated with pharmacological agents, with electrical devices nearby in case of deterioration. The more extreme the sign or symptom of instability (e.g. coma versus mild anxiety), the more intensive the initial treatment should be.

Step 3: classify the electrocardiogram findings

After assessing stability, the field providers need to categorize the ECG. Using a traditional approach of separating dysrhythmias into dozens of categories is tempting. In the field evaluation, a simpler scheme should be used based on the assessment of stability and three ECG features: QRS complex rate, regularity, and duration.

Electrocardiogram interpretation is performed in two ways: by medical oversight physicians receiving transmitted tracings, or independently by the field personnel. Transmitted tracings are occasionally hampered by technical problems which can obscure salient features. Field providers can learn the basics of ECG interpretation to identify common and lethal rhythms. However, some errors are common. For example, misclassification of QRS duration and rate occurs in up to 20–30% of tachycardias [3]. Protocols and medical oversight decisions must assume that the potential for misclassification exists and attempt to minimize attendant adverse outcomes. The strategies outlined herein apply to both field and transmitted interpretation. In all steps, ECG interpretation must be done from a printed strip and not "guesstimated" from the monitor screen.

Rate

Initially, the rate should be classified as fast (>120/minute), slow (<60/minute), or normal/near normal (60–120/minute) based on the frequency of QRS complexes over 6 seconds multiplied by 10. After the estimation of rate, sinus P-waves should be sought in those patients with normal or fast rates. Sinus P-waves always precede the QRS complexes and have a consistent appearance and relationship (i.e. distance) to the QRS complexes.

As a simple rule, all unstable patients with non-sinus fast rhythms (no discernible P-waves and QRS rate >120/minute) deserve immediate synchronized countershock with 100 J. Often, lower energy levels can convert specific rhythms, such as supraventricular tachycardia (SVT) or atrial flutter, but little benefit is gained by attempting to make fine distinctions in these unstable patients. Although changes in heart rate that fall into the normal range can cause symptoms, these are usually of little importance in the field management.

Biphasic waveform defibrillators are increasingly common among EMS services. In general, lower energy biphasic waveform shocks are equally or more effective than monophasic shocks [4]. However, no outcome benefit to biphasic waveforms has yet been demonstrated [5]. In addition, the ideal energy for first-shock biphasic waveform defibrillation is uncertain [4]. The defibrillator manufacturer's recommended energy levels for cardioversion and defibrillation should be used.

Patients with slow dysrhythmias only require classification of their stability. All other details (e.g. P-wave characteristics, type I or II second-degree block, junctional versus ventricular escape) add little value in prehospital management. Slow stable dysrhythmias need no intervention besides continued monitoring for deterioration. Slow unstable dysrhythmias require external pacing (preferred) or atropine (0.5–1 mg IV in adults, repeated up to 2–3 mg total). Transcutaneous pacing is best started as early as possible to maximize the potential for mechanical or clinical capture and restoration of perfusion [6,7]. Also, do not delay pacing in unstable patients to administer atropine. Conversely, concerns of clinical deterioration after atropine are unwarranted when the correct dose is given to those with symptomatic bradycardia, though there may be no response.

Internal, implanted pacemakers should prevent bradycardias, but they may malfunction. When a patient has pacer spikes on the ECG and is still bradycardic, the pacemaker is not working properly and the patient should be treated in the same fashion previously described with atropine or external pacing. The pacer pads should be kept 10 cm or more away from the internal pacemaker pouch. Trying to evaluate the pacemaker in the field is impossible and should await hospital evaluation (see Volume 1, Chapter 15).

Bradycardias resulting from beta-blocker or calcium channel blocker overdoses may be refractory to atropine. In these cases, glucagon (1–3 mg IV) may improve the heart rate. Again, drug administration should not delay transcutaneous pacing.

Previously, isoproterenol was a second-line therapy for atropine-resistant bradycardias. With the availability of external pacemakers in the field and the poor clinical effectiveness of isoproterenol, this treatment is not currently recommended. In adults, a pressor medication (e.g. dopamine) infusion and a fluid bolus should be administered if transcutaneous pacing has normalized the heart rate but hypotension persists.

Regularity and duration

In contrast to bradycardia, if the ventricular rate is fast, the regularity and duration of the QRS complexes should be assessed. Regularity is divided into two categories: mostly or completely regular, and chaotic (i.e. "irregularly irregular" without any pattern). Chaotic rhythms are usually due to atrial fibrillation, irrespective of the appearance of the baseline or QRS duration. Other less common causes include multifocal atrial tachycardia and frequent extrasystoles (i.e. atrial, ventricular, or junctional).

To simplify the process of measuring duration and assessing regularity, EMS personnel should run an ECG strip. From this, they or the medical oversight physician can measure in "small boxes" how wide the QRS duration is and look for irregularity. Each small box represents 0.04 seconds at normal paper speed. Having providers seek out "How many small boxes wide is the QRS complex?" will limit mathematic or conversion errors. Similarly, evaluating printed strips also helps detect irregularity, which may be difficult to appreciate on a monitor screen if the ventricular rate is greater than 150/minute. In these cases, close tracking on a 6-second ECG strip may help detect chaos and identify atrial fibrillation.

Those rhythms with a QRS duration of less than three small boxes (0.12 seconds) are narrow-complex dysrhythmias. Conversely, any rhythm with a QRS duration of greater than three small boxes is a wide-complex dysrhythmia. Nearly all narrow complex rhythms originate from atrial or nodal (i.e. supraventricular) sources. Wide complex rhythms can originate from a ventricular or a supraventricular source. In the latter situation, some abnormality in ventricular conduction is responsible for the prolonged QRS duration. In the field, attempts to separate the myriad causes of wide-complex tachydysrhythmias (WCTs) rarely alter therapy and are unnecessary. Treatment should be based on the clinical stability of the patient, basic history, and the simple ECG characteristics previously defined.

Unstable tachydysrhythmias

Aside from sinus tachycardia, all unstable patients with a WCT or a narrow-complex tachydysrhythmia (NCT) deserve countershock(s), irrespective of the exact source, ventricular or supraventricular. The QRS duration will help dictate care after countershock, but does not fundamentally drive the initial care in unstable patients with a tachydysrhythmia.

The initial energy level used to treat tachycardias is based on the QRS pattern. If the QRS pattern is regular or nearly regular in any unstable patient with a tachydysrhythmia and a palpable pulse, synchronized cardioversion with 100 J should be used, followed by step-wise energy increases to 200 J with a biphasic device or 360 J with a monophasic device, if necessary. Some rhythms may require less energy, but attempts to carefully titrate this life-saving therapy in unstable patients is of little practical benefit. Synchronized countershock is recommended to avoid post-countershock ventricular fibrillation (VF). However, sensing problems often make reliable identification of the QRS complex needed for synchronization impossible. We recommend an unsynchronized shock promptly if any sensing problem occurs. Any patient without pulses and/or an irregular tachydysrhythmia should be immediately given a high-energy unsynchronized countershock.

Patients with internal pacemakers or automatic implantable cardioverter defibrillators (AICDs) are still at risk of cardiac dysrhythmias. Although meant to cardiovert dysrhythmias, AICDs do not always convert these rhythms, and sometimes these devices deliver shocks inappropriately. If a patient has an unstable tachydysrhythmia and the AICD is not firing or is ineffective, externally cardiovert as previously recommended, with pads in the anterior-posterior configuration and 10 cm away from the internal device pouch. Postconversion care with medical therapy will be unaffected.

If an AICD is repeatedly firing absent a ventricular dysrhythmia (wide complexes), a magnet over the device may inactivate the shock mechanism, simplifying patient care and improving patient comfort (see Volume 1, Chapter 15). However, given the rarity of this event, the EMS director should weigh deployment of magnets and training for all providers versus likely benefits. Prompt transfer to the ED is wise in many settings.

If countershock fails in an unstable patient with a WCT, give either amiodarone (5 mg/kg) or lidocaine (1–2 mg/kg) as a bolus and repeat the countershock. The ALIVE trial [8] and recent AHA guidelines [1] recommend amiodarone as the first-line agent in unstable and especially pulseless WCT. Lidocaine is still the easiest to deliver quickly, but is considered a second-line agent due to variable success in terminating ventricular tachycardia (VT) [1].

If the QRS complexes are chaotic, the most common diagnosis is atrial fibrillation. When chaos and a QRS duration of more than three small boxes appear together, atrial fibrillation with altered conduction is the diagnosis. All unstable fast chaotic rhythms should be cardioverted with 50–100 J unsynchronized initially, and titrated up as needed. No post-countershock medications are needed.

One practical point: if regularity versus irregularity cannot be established during assessment of a patient with an unstable

WCT or NCT, 100 J is an appropriate starting energy level for countershock. Similarly, if simplicity of treatment protocols is sought, 100 J is reasonable for all unstable non-sinus tachycardias, because the extra energy delivered to the rapid atrial fibrillation patient is unlikely to cause harm or worsen discomfort compared to 50 J.

Step 4: focus actions to evaluate stable but symptomatic and borderline patients

Up to this point, little specific history and only a few basic physical examination and ECG reading skills have been required. This is intentional, so as not to "clutter" the field evaluation of those who need it the most (i.e. the unstable patient) or do not need it at all (i.e. the asymptomatic patient). The remaining patients are those with symptoms, albeit none clearly identifying instability. Here, a few questions and actions can help to deliver the appropriate prehospital care.

History

The field teams should focus on cardiac-related previous problems in stable patients. For example, a patient who presents with new-onset WCT with a history of previous myocardial infarction is much more likely to have ventricular tachycardia than a supraventricular rhythm with abnormal conduction. Similarly, one with a history of a previous dysrhythmia who presents with similar symptoms again is likely to have recurrence rather than a new dysrhythmia. Neither of these clinical rules is infallible, but this information can help guide therapy. Other points are also helpful. For instance, a patient with a history of poorly controlled hypertension presenting with a lowered but "normal" blood pressure suggests a dramatic change, prompting more intensive treatment.

History can influence the dosing of field agents. Subjects with liver or heart failure, and those aged 65 years and older, should receive lower lidocaine infusions or follow-up boluses. Those patients with renal failure are at risk for hyperkalemia and rhythm changes. The current medications can provide a clue to any previous conditions or guide field drug therapy. A patient treated with digoxin or a beta-blocker plus warfarin for palpitations may have atrial fibrillation. Finally, although rare, a brief search for drug allergies or intolerances ("Has any heart drug been bad for you?") may help avoid a complication. The key is to take a focused history, looking for information regarding heart disease and other specific conditions.

Physical examination

In addition to a search for signs of instability, some manipulations can help when assessing and managing tachycardias. Specifically, actions that alter atrioventricular node conduction ("vagal maneuvers") can help terminate or uncover a specific dysrhythmia [2,9]. In a patient less than 50 years old, carotid body massage can be attempted. This procedure is often restricted or prohibited in the field because of poorly documented concerns about embolization. The Valsalva action can be used with massage in young patients or as the sole maneuver in those over 50 years old. Other maneuvers, including ocular and rectal massage, ice packs or cold-water dunking, and rapid inflation of pneumatic antishock garments, are not recommended.

Stable narrow-complex tachydysrhythmias

In patients who are symptomatic but stable or who have one borderline symptom of instability (e.g. dizzy or anxious with a low blood pressure), certain actions are indicated. Patients with a regular NCT between 120 and 140 per minute are likely to have a sinus tachycardia and require no antidysrhythmic treatment. Stable patients with a regular NCT at a rate of 140 per minute or greater should have vagal stimulating maneuvers performed to terminate the rhythm. Sometimes, this maneuver uncovers sinus P-waves, clarifying the sinus or atrial etiology. When P-waves are seen, treatment is directed at the cause, not the rhythm.

Those with minor symptoms (e.g. isolated subjective dizziness or palpitations) do not require field treatment beyond vagal maneuvers. For those with more prominent symptoms during a regular NCT at 140 per minute or greater, give adenosine (6–12 mg as a rapid IV bolus followed with a flush) [1–3,8]. The smaller initial dose (6 mg) is effective about 60% of the time, and it should be repeated within 2 minutes at the higher dose if no effect is seen. If adenosine causes slowing followed by a return to tachycardia, repeat or larger doses will not help. The cause is a non-reentrant source, often an atrial rhythm, possibly atrial tachycardia, fibrillation, or flutter.

Adenosine is effective in 85–90% of patients with regular NCT. The drug has a duration of effect of 20 seconds or less, and recurrence of an NCT may occur in 10–58% of cases. It is common for patients to complain of transient chest pain, flushing, or dyspnea during adenosine treatment. Some patients may experience bradycardia or asystole after adenosine. Usually, this lasts only seconds, but it may require temporary external pacing if prolonged. Contrary to popular belief, adenosine can occasionally terminate VT, although the majority of such patients are unaffected [10].

Verapamil (2.5–5 mg IV initially followed by 5–10 mg in 15 minutes if unsuccessful) and diltiazem (0.15 mg/kg initially, followed by 0.20–0.25 mg/kg in 15 minutes if unsuccessful) will terminate 85–90% of regular NCT [11,12]. However, both can cause hypotension and congestive heart failure, though diltiazem is alleged to have slightly lower rates of this in equipotent doses. Because of these disadvantages, many prefer to use adenosine in the field. Whenever giving adenosine, verapamil, or diltiazem in the field, it must be absolutely clear that the QRS duration is less than three small boxes (0.12 seconds). This will help avoid the hemodynamic collapse that can occur with these drugs in VT or atrial fibrillation with an accessory pathway. Most patients tolerate the transient effects of adenosine, often "fooling" providers into thinking no harm is possible if given in error. The potential harm is real, albeit much less frequent than with calcium channel blockers. If hypotension occurs after IV verapamil or diltiazem in the absence of bradycardia, treatment with saline infusions, IV calcium salts (5–10 mL of a 10% calcium chloride solution) or catecholamines (i.e. dopamine or epinephrine) should be given.

Many WCTs are erroneously classified in the field as narrow (up to 20% of cases). Therefore, many medical oversight physicians prefer adenosine to treat all regular and symptomatic NCT, avoiding the risks associated with giving a calcium channel blocker to a patient with WCT. For those patients with chaotic NCT, atrial fibrillation is the likely rhythm. If mildly symptomatic and stable, no field treatment is required. An example is an elderly patient with an irregular NCT at a rate of 130/minute complaining of weakness. Although rapid atrial fibrillation may contribute to the symptoms, no field treatment is needed in the absence of other clear signs or symptoms of decompensation. Those with instability deserve immediate countershock with 50–100 J. If transport is prolonged and the patient has either borderline symptoms or a rate of 140–180/minute, metoprolol (5–10 mg intravenously) or diltiazem (0.15–0.25 mg/kg intravenously) will control the ventricular rate in 85–90% cases of rapid atrial fibrillation [10,11].

One pitfall in the treatment of stable NCT must be highlighted. When the ventricular rate is greater than 220/minute, the risk of decompensation rises and the ability to detect irregularity is limited [2]. Therefore, all adults with a very fast regular NCT (heart rate >220/minute) should be either cardioverted with 100 J or treated with adenosine and prepared for cardioversion. If the rate rises to greater than 250/minute, cardioversion is the best choice given the risk of deterioration. Irregular NCT greater than 220/minute deserves countershock promptly as previously noted (50–100 J).

Stable wide-complex tachydysrhythmias

Wide-complex tachydysrhythmias can be due to VT or a SVT with abnormal conduction. Until proven otherwise, field providers should assume any new WCT is due to VT. Hospital data suggest that about two-thirds of patients with new WCT have VT. With a history of previous myocardial infarction, the frequency of VT increases to 90%. Although it is possible to assemble evidence to detect supraventricular rhythms from a detailed examination and 12-lead ECG, these data are not easily obtainable in the field. Thus, actions in managing WCT should either treat or cause no harm in VT.

All unstable patients with WCT should be cardioverted with 100 J, with escalating energy doses if needed. When stable or borderline, a few simple measures can help stratify patients. It is always an option to observe this group, intervening only if conditions worsen.

If P-waves precede each QRS complex during a stable WCT with a rate of 140/minute or less, a supraventricular source is likely, especially sinus or atrial tachycardia, although VT is a remote possibility. Treatment focuses on correcting any potential causes (e.g. pain, hypovolemia, or hypoxemia) and observation. Irregular QRS complexes suggest atrial fibrillation or multifocal atrial tachycardia. Neither requires field rhythm-directed therapy in stable patients, although other actions (e.g. oxygen, bronchodilators) may be needed.

When no clear P-QRS relationship exists, differentiating between SVT and VT is difficult during a WCT. The following key features help decide a clinical course of action.

- A patient with new-onset WCT and a history of previous myocardial infarction or VT very likely will have VT.
- VT will often not slow during vagal maneuvers. Therefore, slowing of a WCT during these efforts suggests SVT. However, the absence of change does not diagnose VT.
- Most VT does not respond to adenosine, whereas SVT usually slows or terminates. Conversely, lidocaine has little effect on most SVT and will terminate 75–85% of VT.
- VT is usually regular and rarely seen at a rate of greater than 220/minute. Any chaotic WCT should be considered atrial fibrillation with abnormal conduction. When a chaotic WCT at a rate of greater than 220/minute occurs, atrial fibrillation from Wolff–Parkinson–White syndrome is present. This rhythm is prone to deteriorate.

From these clinical observations, the following scheme can be used in approaching the stable or borderline (one minor sign or symptom of instability alone) patient with a WCT.

- All stable patients with regular WCT at a rate of 120–220/minute should receive vagal maneuvers. Those who slow but then elevate again should receive adenosine (6–12 mg IV). If no slowing with vagal maneuvers occurs, one of three paths should be taken.
  - Young (age <50 years) previously healthy patients with stable (or borderline) regular WCT that slows with vagal maneuvers should receive adenosine. If this fails or there is no response to vagal maneuvers, or if the patient has had prior VT or prior MI, assume VT and give amiodarone (5 mg/kg IV over 5 minutes) or possibly lidocaine (1.0–1.5 mg/kg IV up to 3 mg/kg). The AHA has emphasized the role of amiodarone over lidocaine despite limited direct comparisons. If lidocaine converts the rhythm, repeat boluses at 5–10 minutes of 0.5 mg/kg should be given during transport to prevent recurrence. Continuous infusions after lidocaine loading are generally impractical in the field unless prolonged transport times are likely and infusion pumps are available.
  - Because of the risk of deterioration, any patient with WCT at a rate of greater than 220/minute deserves countershock with 100 J, irrespective of symptoms.
  - Patients with a chaotic WCT usually have atrial fibrillation with altered conduction. If stable with a heart rate of less than 200/minute, they deserve close observation and expeditious transport. If the rate elevates to 220/minute or higher, immediate countershock with 100 J is indicated.

Other agents are available but have a limited role in the field. Procainamide (50–100 mg IV every 1–2 minutes up to a maximum of 15–18 mg/kg or until side-effects occur) treats both VT and SVT but is difficult to give in the field.

Controversies

Rhythm strip versus monitor interpretation

Besides clearly abnormal rhythms (e.g. obvious VT or severe bradycardia), ECG interpretation should be taken from a tracing and not from the monitor screen. It is tempting to avoid printing strips, but misclassifications may result from a "screen look." Strips are valuable in the ED evaluation, documenting conditions before and after field treatment, which helps unravel the causes in certain dysrhythmias. At least two leads should be sampled.

Synchronization and sedation during countershock

When possible, delivering a countershock synchronized with the intrinsic QRS complexes is preferred. Synchronization helps avoid depolarization during the vulnerable phases of repolarization, theoretically decreasing the risk of post-countershock VF. During most dysrhythmias, the defibrillator unit senses the underlying QRS pattern and delivers the shock at the appropriate time. When the rhythm is extremely fast or irregular or the QRS complexes are markedly abnormal (i.e. very wide or small), sensing is difficult. In these cases, an unsynchronized countershock is appropriate. Electrophysiological data do not support the notion that this will increase the likelihood of VF. If post-countershock VF occurs, repeat countershock is usually successful in restoring an organized rhythm.

The usual controversy surrounding field countershock is the awake unstable patient. Medical oversight must clearly communicate the need for this unpleasant but life-saving intervention for appropriate patients. Sedation with a benzodiazepine before countershock may improve patient comfort. However, countershock should not be delayed in unstable patients while awaiting clinical sedation.

Prophylactic lidocaine for premature ventricular contractions

In the past, lidocaine was given for all patients with suspected acute coronary ischemia and any evidence of ventricular ectopy. Research clearly details that most patients do not benefit from this medication and some may be harmed [12–14].

If the premature ventricular contractions (PVCs) are asymptomatic or trivial, there is no proven benefit from treatment. PVCs associated with more pronounced symptoms should receive an antidysrhythmic, usually lidocaine. Although oft-cited lists of ominous ECG "warning" signs exist (e.g. multiform, >6/minute, couplets, R-on-T, or runs of PVCs), treatment of these and other asymptomatic PVCs does not confer any benefit. Do not use prophylactic lidocaine for all patients with chest pain. Lidocaine may reduce the risk of VF but will increase the risk of asystole.

Pediatric dysrhythmias

When evaluating pediatric tachycardias, a crucial difference compared with adults must be stressed. Children under the age of 5 years can sustain a sinus tachycardia at much higher rates (up to 225/minute) in response to physiological stresses. Therefore, a search for hypovolemia, hypercarbia, and hypoxemia is mandatory in stable children with NCT before drug therapy is used. A volume challenge with 10–20 mL/kg of saline IV is useful before other therapies. Although some guidelines make a distinction between energy levels when performing synchronized versus unsynchronized countershock, the use of this distinction is dubious. To keep treatments simple but effective, unstable children deserve countershock with 2 J/kg. Antidysrhythmic principles are otherwise similar to those outlined previously, with agents given in the appropriate weight-based doses. Pediatric non-cardiac arrest bradycardias are also usually secondary to another cause, often respiratory distress or hypoxia. When symptomatic, these rhythms are treated primarily with epinephrine and airway maneuvers and rarely need transcutaneous pacing or atropine (0.02 mg/kg/dose).

Torsades de pointes

This rare dysrhythmia classically presents with paroxysms of syncope and polymorphic "twisting" of the QRS complexes (Figure 14.1). Torsades de pointes (TdP) in adults is usually "pause dependent," flourishing when intrinsic heart rate drops below 80–100/minute. A variety of antidysrhythmics (essentially all aside from lidocaine and calcium channel or beta-adrenergic blocking agents), antihistamines, antimicrobials, and psychoactive drugs, along with metabolic disorders, can precipitate TdP. Field treatment consists of countershock when unstable and transcutaneous pacing or

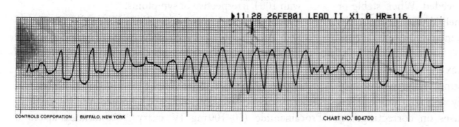

11:28 26FEB01 LEAD II X1.0 HR=116

CONTROLS CORPORATION | BUFFALO, NEW YORK   CHART NO. 804700

Figure 14.1 The classic one-lead ECG appearance (lead II here) of torsades de pointes. Note the shifting of the QRS complex axis and appearance.

isoproterenol (titrated to a heart rate >120/minute). Magnesium sulfate, 2 g as a rapid IV bolus, is also suggested for those who fail countershock.

A more practical problem is mistaking VT or VF for TdP. VT or VF often display some changes in QRS complex appearance. Field providers may mistake these variations for the classic, but rare, QRS twisting. If recurrent polymorphic VT occurs in a patient with one or more of the aforementioned risks, treatment should be started. Otherwise, orders and protocols should focus on the treatment of common VT.

Rhythm disturbances in renal failure patients

This group often falls prey to metabolic derangements that alter rhythms, in addition to having high rates of underlying heart disease. Hyperkalemia is a common complication of renal failure that can cause a bradycardia or a wide complex rhythm, although the latter is usually not above a rate of 100–120/minute and often much slower. Treatment should include IV calcium (10 mL of 10% of $CaCl_2$), sodium bicarbonate (1–2 ampules intravenously), nebulized albuterol, and insulin plus glucose. The last three interventions rapidly (but temporarily) shift potassium into the cells and should be part of protocols for any renal failure patient with new-onset symptomatic bradycardia or a wide-complex rhythm. Because of the risk of hypoglycemia, insulin and glucose infusions in the field are best done under medical oversight supervision rather than by protocol. Lidocaine can cause asystole in the presence of hyperkalemia. The role of other agents, including amiodarone, is unknown in the rare event of hyperkalemia and new-onset WCT [15]. If a rhythm-specific intervention is needed in unstable patients with suspected hyperkalemia, electricity (pacing for slow, countershock for fast rates) is a safe choice.

Protocols

When developing protocols, focus on the simple data and steps. For example, both the bradycardia and tachycardia protocols should start with a division between "stable/no symptoms" and "symptomatic and unstable or borderline." Those in the "stable/no symptoms" category should be observed, expeditiously transported, and monitored, with precautionary IV insertion and oxygen. As a corollary, unstable patients with bradycardia or tachycardia should receive prompt electrical therapy (pacing or countershock), airway support, monitoring, and IV insertion occurring either in tandem with or after electrical therapy. Remind the providers to save rhythm strips and to give sedation if possible, but not to withhold life-saving treatment trying to "get a good strip" or titrating sedation. Unless the signs of instability are subtle, medical oversight contact should follow the initial treatment of unstable patients.

For patients who are symptomatic without signs of instability, EMS personnel should assess a rhythm strip first. In the tachycardia protocols, three questions should be asked: rate, QRS duration in small boxes, and regularity. Narrow-complex tachycardias that are regular deserve either vagal maneuvers (carotid massage and/or Valsalva) or adenosine. Those patients with irregular narrow-complex rhythms deserve calcium channel blocker therapy if symptomatic but stable. Patients with wide-complex regular rhythms who are stable or borderline should receive lidocaine or amiodarone, and countershock if these medications fail or deterioration occurs. Finally, those with irregular WCTs should be transported without therapy unless unstable, in which case, they should be treated with countershock.

Conclusion

Prehospital dysrhythmia evaluation must be tailored to the time restraints, physical limitations, and outcome needs that are specific to the field setting. Decision trees should be simple and effective, focusing on treating patients, and not rhythms per se. Protocols must identify and treat all unstable patients. Those without symptoms or with trivial symptoms do not require rhythm-directed therapies. For symptomatic but stable patients, a few key steps should be taken to help manage each case.

References

1 American Heart Association. Part 8: Adult Advanced Cardiovascular Life Support. *Circulation* 2010;122:S729–S767.

2 Yealy DM, Delbridge TR. Dysrhythmias. In: Marx JA, et al (eds) *Emergency Medicine: Concepts and Clinical Practice*, 6th edn. St Louis, MO: C.V. Mosby, 2005.

3 McCabe J, Menegazzi JJ, Adhar G, Paris PM. Intravenous adenosine in the prehospital treatment of supraventricular tachycardia. *Ann Emerg Med* 1992;21(4):358–61.

4 American Heart Association. Part 6: Electrical Therapies: Automated External Defibrillators, Defibrillation, Cardioversion, and Pacing. *Circulation* 2010;112:S706–S719.

5 Tanabe S, Yasunaga H, Ogawa T, et al. Comparison of outcomes after use of biphasic or monophasic defibrillators among out-of-hospital cardiac arrest patients. *Circ Cardiovasc Qual Outcomes* 2012;5:689–96.

6 Hedges JR, Syverud SA, Dalsey WC, et al. Prehospital trial of emergency transcutaneous pacing. *Circulation* 1987;76:1337–40.

7 Paris PM, Stewart RD, Kaplan RM, Whipkey R. Transcutaneous pacing for bradyasystolic cardiac arrest in prehospital care. *Ann Emerg Med* 1985;14(4):320–3.

8 Dorian P, Case D, Schwartz B, et al. Amiodarone as compared with lidocaine for shock-resistant ventricular fibrillation. *N Engl J Med* 2002;346(12):884–90.

9 Wrenn K. Management strategies in wide QRS complex tachycardia. *Am J Emerg Med* 1991;9(6):592–7.

10 Wilber DJ, Baerman J, Olshansky B, et al. Adenosine sensitive ventricular tachycardia: clinical characteristics and response to catheter ablation. *Circulation* 1993;87(1):126–34.

11 O'Toole KS, Heller MB, Menegazzi JJ, Paris PM. Intravenous verapamil in the treatment of paroxysmal supraventricular tachycardia. *Ann Emerg Med* 1990;19(3):279–85.

12 Wang HE, O'Connor RE, Megargel RE, et al. The use of diltiazem for treating rapid atrial fibrillation in the out-of-hospital setting. *Ann Emerg Med* 2001;37(1):38–45.

13 Hine LK, Laird N, Hewitt P, Chalmers TC. Meta-analytic evidence against prophylactic use of lidocaine in acute myocardial infarction. *Arch Intern Med* 1989;149(12):2694–8.

14 Cardiac Arrhythmia Suppression Trial (CAST) Investigators. Preliminary report: effect of encainide and flecainide on mortality in a randomized trial of arrhythmia suppression after myocardial infarction. *N Engl J Med* 1989;321(6):406–12.

15 McLean SA, Paul ID, Spector PS. Lidocaine-induced conduction disturbance in patients with systemic hyperkalemia. *Ann Emerg Med* 2000;36(6):626–7.

CHAPTER 15

Cardiac procedures and managing technology

T.J. Doyle

Intraaortic balloon pump

The intraaortic balloon pump (IABP) is a mechanical device used in the stabilization of an acutely ill cardiac diseased patient. The EMS physician or critical care transport team will most commonly encounter the device during a patient transfer from a facility with limited or unavailable cardiac surgery capabilities to a tertiary care center. The role of the IABP is to provide cardiac stabilization until definitive care can be obtained. Goals of IABP therapy include decreasing cardiac afterload, augmenting diastolic perfusion pressure, and increasing coronary artery perfusion [1]. These efforts help to improve cardiac output that can in turn improve tissue perfusion. The decrease in afterload reduces the workload on the heart, and the improved coronary artery circulation can increase oxygen supply to the myocardium.

Indications for IABPs most commonly encountered by EMS physicians are acute myocardial infarction, cardiogenic shock, ventricular aneurysm, left ventricular failure, valve or papillary muscle rupture, or a combination of these factors [2]. The patient is most commonly found in a catheterization lab, operating room, or coronary intensive care unit.

The IABP catheter is placed via an incision in the lower extremity, inserted in the femoral artery, and then advanced into the thoracic aorta. The balloon should be placed 1–2 cm distal to the beginning of the subclavian artery, and must be above the branches of the renal arteries. If the balloon is not placed correctly, occlusion of coronary, subclavian, or renal arteries could occur [1]. On a chest x-ray, the tip of the catheter should be visible between the second and third intercostal spaces. When inflated, the balloon should not completely occlude the aortic lumen, as this can damage the aortic wall and blood components [1]. Most devices have different sized balloons for patients based on weight or height. It is important to ensure the appropriate balloon volume is being used.

Absolute contraindications for an IABP include aortic dissection, abdominal aortic aneurysm, and aortic valve incompetence. Relative contraindications include bleeding disorders and atherosclerosis [1].

A patient with an IABP who requires interfacility transportation must be attended to by a specially trained team. In some cases, critical care paramedics, nurses, or physicians are trained to address IABP complications. Otherwise, it is vital that the transport team include a perfusionist or biomedical engineer.

Intraaortic balloon pump function is critically dependent on timing. The balloon is cycled in conjunction with the cardiac cycle. It is important to remember that the balloon is inflated during diastole and deflated just prior to systole. While the balloon is inflated, blood is pushed both back toward the heart, as well as further down the aorta. The result is increased blood flow to coronary and carotid arteries, and increased systemic perfusion. The balloon is deflated very rapidly, and this rapid loss of volume reduces the pressure in the aorta. The result is that the left ventricle does not contract as hard as it would otherwise. Cardiac workload and myocardial oxygen demands are reduced. If the timing is not correct, these advantages are lost, and further harm to the patient may occur [1].

The IABP can use several different triggers for the inflation and deflation cycle. The most common modalities use the ECG or the arterial pressure waveform as a trigger. The IABP may also have an internal trigger in the event of cardiac arrest. Using arterial pressure as a trigger requires the patient to have an arterial catheter placed and connected to the balloon pump. Some IABP devices may have specialized fiberoptic connectors to measure arterial pressures. It is important to note that once a fiberoptic connector is placed and zeroed, it cannot be removed and connected to a different transport IABP. Another trigger modality needs to be used, such as ECG. Most devices have an "automatic" trigger mode, where the pump automatically switches between trigger modes if needed. An example would be a switch between ECG and arterial pressure modes if the ECG signal is lost. Most modern pumps can also compensate for arrhythmias such as atrial fibrillation and pacing modes [1].

With the trigger mode established, attention should focus on timing. Most patients are transported with a 1:1 frequency, where each cardiac cycle is assisted. In order to assess timing, it may be helpful to place the device in a 1:2 frequency to get a

Emergency Medical Services: Clinical Practice and Systems Oversight, Second Edition. Volume 1: Clinical Aspects of EMS.
Edited by David C. Cone, Jane H. Brice, Theodore R. Delbridge, and J. Brent Myers.
© 2015 NAEMSP. Published 2015 by John Wiley & Sons, Inc. Companion Website: www.wiley.com\go\cone\naemsp

better picture of the arterial pressure waveform landmarks. For transport, the operator should ensure that the balloon is set to inflate at the dicrotic notch, and to deflate during the next isovolumetric contraction (IVC) phase. The dicrotic notch phase on the arterial pressure waveform represents aortic valve closure and diastole. Once the timing is correct, the device can be placed back into a 1:1 frequency and put in the "automatic" mode if available [1]. Potential complications include limb ischemia, compartment syndrome, aortic dissection, bleeding, thrombocytopenia and red blood cell destruction, gas embolus, infection, and cardiac decompensation from incorrect timing [1].

Special care must be taken when transferring a patient from one brand of IABP to another to enable transport. There may be a difference in the balloon size, and an adapter may be needed to connect a "Brand D" catheter to a "Brand A" IABP. The balloon size should be noted and adjusted on the pump if necessary.

On arrival to a patient's side, the transport team should examine the patient paying particular attention to the insertion site, as well as to the distal extremity. The insertion site should be examined for bleeding or protruding balloon. The catheter tubing should be examined for any blood or blood flecks. The distal extremity should be examined for ischemia. Catheter tubing should be examined for kinking. Any positive findings noted above should delay the transport until the situation can be corrected. Fresh ECG leads should be applied to the patient. The referring hospital balloon pump should not be disconnected or shut off until the transport pump is connected and tested. The transport balloon pump should be plugged into an outlet during this time and not run on battery power. The pump should also be plugged into an aircraft or ambulance power inverter during transport. Pure battery operation should be used only to transport the patient from the vehicle to his or her hospital destination.

Special circumstances

In the event of cardiac arrest, the IABP will lose all trigger modes, give a "trigger arrest" alarm, and then stop counterpulsation. If left unchanged, this could result in a thrombus formation. When cardiopulmonary resuscitation (CPR) is initiated, the IABP should be switched to "arterial trigger." Effective CPR should allow for the IABP to function off the arterial pressures. In the event that arterial pressures are not sufficient, the IABP should be switched to an "internal trigger." This last resort trigger provides asynchronous counterpulsation and will help prevent clot formation. "Internal trigger" mode should be stopped if there is a return of circulation and the ECG or arterial pressure mode is restarted [2].

In the event of IABP failure during transport, a large Luer-Lok syringe should be attached to the quick connector to aspirate the balloon for blood. If no blood is found, use air to inflate the balloon to the volume capacity of the balloon. Then quickly aspirate the air and deflate the balloon. Repeat 4–5 times every 5–10 minutes until the pump is repaired or replaced [1].

Ventricular assist device

Ventricular assist devices (VAD) are surgically implanted pumps that are intended to assist one or both ventricles of the heart to pump when disease has diminished the heart's native ability to do so. They are most often placed in patients with severe congestive heart failure. Devices include left ventricular assist devices (LVAD), right ventricular assist devices (RVAD), and biventricular assist devices (BIVAD). The most commonly placed device is the LVAD. The LVAD will have a cannula placed in the apex of the left ventricle with blood flow to the pump and a cannula placed into the ascending aorta with blood flow from the pump. Thus the device assists the ventricle in moving blood through the circulatory system [2].

Ventricular assist devices were first developed in the 1960s and the technology progressed during the 1970s and 1980s. Advances made them more portable, but the patient was still confined to the hospital. In the 1990s fully portable devices were developed that, for the first time, allowed VAD patients to be discharged from the hospital [3,4]. The devices are most commonly used as a bridge to cardiac transplantation, but they also may be used as a bridge to a reversible cardiac condition, or as a permanent therapy. There are two types of VAD patients: those with non-portable VADs, who would require critical care transport with a perfusionist, and those with portable VADs who may be living at home or in an assisted living facility. It is the second group of patients who are potentially encountered by EMS.

Currently, there are four generations of VADs with features that can vary based on the generation and the particular device (Box 15.1). First-generation devices mimic the pumping action

---

Box 15.1 Generations of Left Ventricular-Assist Devices

First Generation
  Berlin Heart ECXOR (Berlin Heart AG)
  HeartMate XVE (Thoratec)
  Novacor LVAS (World Heart Corp.)
  Thoratec PVAD (Thoratec)
Second Generation
  HeartMate II (Thoratec)
  Jarvik 2000 (Jarvik Heart)
  MicroMed DeBakey VAD (MicroMed Cardiovascular)
Third Generation
  Berlin Heart INCOR (Berlin Heart AG)
  CentriMag (Levitronix)
  CorAide (Cleveland Clinic Foundation)
  DuraHeart LVAS (Terumo Somerset, USA)
  HeartMate III (Thoratec)
  HeartQuest (WorldHeart)
  HVAD Pump (HeartWare)
  Levacor (World Heart Corp.)
  VentrAssist (formerly Ventracor)
Fourth Generation
  MAGNEVAD (Gold Medical Technologies)
  Heart Assist 5 (MicroMed Cardiovascular)

Source: Mechem CC. *Prehosp Emerg Care* 2013;17(2):223–9.
Reproduced with permission

of the left ventricle via the use of diaphragms or pusher plates that cause blood to be sucked into the left ventricle and expelled into the aorta. This mechanism results in pulsatile blood flow. The patient will have a pulse and blood pressure that can be measured [4]. The pumps are powered by electricity and can be either electromechanical or pneumatic. Electromechanical pumps use an electromagnetic pusher plate to drive the blood, whereas pneumatic devices use air pressure to move the blood. Both devices require electrical power to function. Pneumatic devices may come with a hand pump in case of device failure [3].

Second-generation LVADs have continuous-flow rotary pumps. If the device only assists with the work of the left ventricle, the underlying function may result in a palpable pulse. If the LVAD is fully replacing the function of the ventricle, there may not be a palpable pulse. As with other technology advances, these devices offer advantages in size, ease of implantation, and durability. The number of moving parts has been reduced to one: the impeller. Second-generation LVADs are subdivided into devices with axial pumps and those with radial (centrifugal) pumps [3] (Figure 15.1).

Axial pumps use a corkscrew and the Archimedes principle against gravity. The inflow and outflow pumps are in line with the impeller, resulting in a smaller size pump. In contrast, centrifugal pumps have the inflow and outflow cannulas at right angles to the flow. Right angles allow for less suction, which can decrease the risk of the ventricle collapsing around the inflow cannula or distortion of the interventricular septum. Both can result in right ventricular failure [3]. One study found 58% survival rates for continuous-flow devices versus 24% for pulsatile flow devices. They also have a lower rate of complications. As continuous-flow pumps are valveless, there is an increased risk of blood flow back into the aorta if the pump stops [5].

Third-generation LVADs represent a further technology step forward. They can use continuous-flow, axial flow, or centrifugal pumps. The impeller is suspended by magnets and driven by electromagnets. This results in no contact between the impeller and the sides of the pump. Benefits include less trauma to blood components and less thrombus formation. The devices are also quieter and can last longer [3].

Fourth-generation LVADs, currently in testing and trials, are exploring further advances in technology, including wireless monitoring and elimination of the driveline. This would remove the cabling from the pump, which must travel through the skin in order to connect to the power source. As driveline infections are a major source of LVAD complications, driveline removal could result in significantly less morbidity [3].

The results of these advances are devices that allow the patient to leave the hospital and function either at home or in an assisted living facility. Prior to discharge, the patient and family are given extensive training on the operation and maintenance of the device, and how to troubleshoot problems and alarms. The patient is followed by a hospital team, and is given written instructions for EMS providers, which outline the device, emergency interventions, and hospital contact information [6].

Left ventricular assist device complications

Left ventricular assist device complications can be divided into two categories: device problems and patient problems. The most common problems consist of neurological events, bleeding, and cardiac arrhythmias. Neurological events include acute strokes and transient ischemic attacks. Thrombotic and hemorrhagic events can occur. The incidence of stroke has been reported ranging from 8% to 25%. The risk is increased for patients with stroke histories and those who have had device-related infections [3].

The most commonly experienced forms of bleeding include epistaxis, gastrointestinal bleeding, and hematoma formation. Bleeding can result from trauma to blood components, from acquired von Willebrand disease, or from iatrogenic anticoagulation [7]. Most patients are given anticoagulants and/or antiplatelet drugs to reduce the risk of thrombus formation [3,8]. LVAD patients are also at increased risk of arrhythmias. Patients may have atrial fibrillation, often as a result of underlying disease. The LVAD will provide left ventricle support, but the loss of atrial "kick" may affect right ventricular function. LVAD patients may also suffer from ventricular arrhythmias. These arrhythmias may result from underlying disease, from irritation of the myocardium by the device, or from ventricular

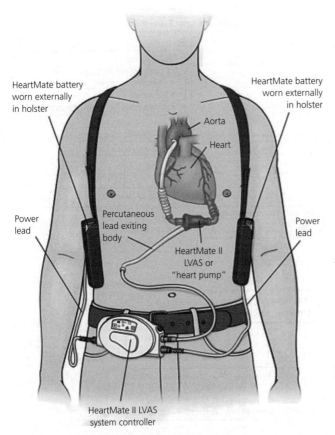

HeartMate battery worn externally in holster

HeartMate battery worn externally in holster

Aorta

Heart

Power lead

Percutaneous lead exiting body

Power lead

HeartMate II LVAS or "heart pump"

HeartMate II LVAS system controller

Figure 15.1 HeartMate II left ventricular assist device (LVAD). LVAS, left ventricular assist system. Source: Thoratec Corporation. Reproduced with permission of the Thoratec Corporation.

collapse or septal deviation from excessive pump function. Some patients may require an implanted cardioverter-defibrillator (ICD) [3,8].

Infection is the most common complication, with infection rates ranging from 18% to 59% among LVAD patients. Infection is second only to heart failure as a cause of mortality in these patients. Infections can present at the surgical site, the driveline, the pump pocket, or the pump itself in the form of endocarditis [3,9].

Device-specific problems can manifest as device failure (fortunately rare) or from battery or cable connection issues. Suction events can occur when there is not enough volume in the left ventricle to support the speed of the pump. This causes the intake cannula to collapse and subsequent ventricular arrhythmias [3]. LVADs in place for a long time can become dislodged, resulting in incomplete left ventricle emptying , right ventricular failure, and arrhythmias. LVAD placement may also result in thrombosis [10]. The patient might then suffer symptoms ranging from dyspnea to cardiogenic shock [11] (Box 15.2).

Prehospital encounters

Balloon pump patients are not routinely encountered by EMS providers except during critical care interfacility transports. In contrast, a patient with a portable LVAD could be at home, have an event, and summon EMS. It is beneficial for EMS services to be aware of LVAD patients in their service area, and have device information and contact information accessible. Hospital policies may dictate that a perfusionist or pump technician be sent to the scene to evaluate the device in the event of a problem. This situation then could result in a delay in patient transport while the perfusionist is in transit. If the patient is having a medical issue not related to the device, a medical oversight decision may need to be made regarding transport. For example, a portable LVAD patient is having an acute stroke or gastrointestinal (GI) bleed, and no LVAD issues. The perfusionist can arrive in 45 minutes. The patient can be transported

by helicopter to the tertiary care center in 15 minutes. The crew is not familiar with the LVAD. The medical oversight physician will need to weigh the risks of delay to care in waiting for the perfusionist versus the risk of an LVAD complication during the 15-minute flight.

The LVAD patient in distress might be having an issue with the device, an exacerbation of the underlying cardiac disease, or an unrelated medical event. The intial EMS assessment should be to determine if the issue is LVAD related or not (Figure 15.2). If the event does not seem to be LVAD related, then local protocols and/or medical oversight should be consulted for further guidance. The next step would be to determine the type of LVAD involved. The patient and caregiver should have device information available. This information should include whether the patient can receive electrical therapy, and whether or not CPR can be performed. Obviously, these questions need immediate answers [3].

Emergency medical services personnel must determine if the device provides pulsatile or continuous flow. A patient with a pulsatile flow device should have a palpable pulse and blood pressure. Pulsatile pump LVAD failure requires the use of a hand pump to continue flow. A patient with a continuous-flow device will have no detectable pulse. A functioning pump should make a humming sound on auscultation [3].

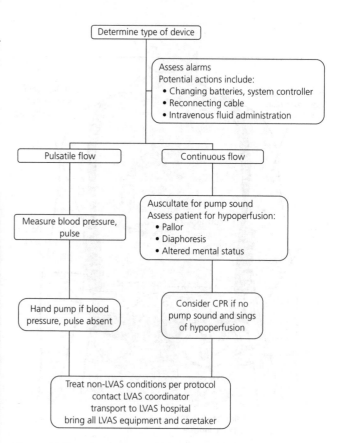

Figure 15.2 Emergency assessment of a patient with a left ventricular assist system (LVAS). CPR, cardiopulmonary resuscitation.

Box 15.2 Complications Encountered in Left Ventricular-Assist Device Patients

Infection
  Bleeding
  Stroke/transient ischemic attack
  Hemolysis
  Arrhythmias
  Volume overload
  Dehydration
  Hypertension
  Hypotension
  Cardiac tamponade
  Recurrence of heart failure
  New right ventricular failure
  Aortic insufficiency

Source: Mechem CC. *Prehosp Emerg Care* 2013;17(2):223–9. Reproduced with permission

In the event of device malfunction, the LVAD should generate a series of auditory and visual alarms. These alarms will be device and manufacturer specific. The patient, caregiver, and device literature should be used to determine alarm causes. Power alarms may be triggered by low voltage in the batteries, necessitating battery changes, or, in the case of a pulsatile device power failure, hand pumping. Low-flow pump alarms most likely result from hypovolemia, which would indicate the need for IV fluids or blood products. Other alarms may indicate cable disconnections which will require troubleshooting. Transport should not be delayed to perform these interventions [3].

As with all patients, the initial assessment should consist of airway, breathing, and circulatory assessments. Patients with continuous-flow devices may not have reliable pulse oximetry readings due to low pulse pressures. Furthermore, a continuous-flow device will not produce a palpable pulse or a measureable blood pressure. The EMS provider will need to then use other signs to assess perfusion, such as pale skin, diaphoresis, or mental status changes. The patient should be placed on a cardiac monitor and a 12-lead ECG should be performed if possible. Patients showing signs and symptoms of another illness, such as stroke, should be assessed in the usual fashion, regardless of the assist device. LVAD patients should also be exposed to examine for cable disconnections. The driveline skin site should not be routinely examined unless absolutely necessary, due to risk of infection. Clothes should not be cut with shears as there is risk of cutting the cables with disastrous results. For the same reasons the patient should be moved carefully to prevent dislodgment [3].

Patients with evidence of hemodynamic compromise and/or hypoperfusion should have large-bore IV access, and be volume resuscitated. Vasopressors are not generally a good initial therapy, as many problems are volume related, and vasopressors will increase afterload, which can worsen pump flow [3].

Arrhythmias should only be treated if they are symptomatic. An LVAD patient with full left ventricle support may be able to tolerate ventricular tachycardia or fibrillation. If the arrhythmia requires treatment, the usual therapies can be used for rate control and rhythm conversion. The patient can also receive electrical therapy [3]. Defibrillator pads should not be placed over the device. Some devices may require that the system controller cables be disconnected prior to defibrillation to prevent damage to the electronics. The patient should also be examined for the presence of an ICD, which would provide the appropriate treatment [12].

The decision on when to perform CPR can be a major conundrum in treating these patients. Knowledge of the device type and function is crucial. First-generation LVADs with pulsatile flow should not get chest compressions. Instead, the hand pump should be used. Second-generation and later continuous-flow devices will not have a hand pump. Chest compressions carry the risk that they may dislodge the device, resulting in exsanguination and death. On the other hand, if the LVAD is not pumping, the underlying left ventricle will not have the ability to maintain perfusion of organ systems. Patient survival is not likely. Lack of compressions may also result in a thrombus formation in the pump, resulting in obstruction to pump flow and potential downstream embolic events. EMS awareness of the patient's advance directives regarding resuscitation may be important, as these patients have chronic severe disease and may wish to not be resuscitated [3].

Ideally, device information, patient wishes and treatment plans, and contact information should be prepared prior to initial discharge from the hospital. In the event of an EMS contact with a patient who is hypoperfused and has a non-functioning pump, an attempt may be made to contact the LVAD coordinator for further recommendations. If the coordinator cannot be reached, and the patient is to be resuscitated, compressions should be started and transport initiated [3].

The LVAD patient should be transported to the hospital that placed the device. These hospitals are usually tertiary care centers, and should be capable of managing not only LVAD complications but also other issues such as stroke or GI bleeding. If there are distance issues, air medical transport should be considered. This can shorten time and also provide critical care services. Regardless of transport mode, the LVAD patient should be transported with all device equipment, batteries, controllers, documentation, and caregivers (if possible).

Implanted cardiac devices

Emergency medical services personnel may also encounter patients in the field with implanted cardiac devices, such as pacemakers and ICDs. The approach to a patient with an implantable device who is suffering from a medical condition is to determine if the problem lies with the device or the underlying medical condition.

Pacemakers

Cardiac pacemakers are implanted devices used in patients suffering from bradyarrhythmias. If the patient's intrinsic rhythm falls below a set target, the pacemaker will provide an electrical stimulus to the myocardium. There are a variety of pacemaker manufacturers and pacing modes, depending on the needs of the patient. The device will be palpable within the patient's chest wall.

Pacing modes

Pacemakers are designated with a five-letter code; the first three letters are referred to most often [14]. The first letter indicates the chamber paced, the second letter indicates the chamber sensed, and the third letter the response after sensing [13].

AOO	Atrial pace; no sense, no inhibitions
AAI	Atrial pace; atrial sense, inhibited by atrial beat
VOO	Ventricular pace; no sense, no inhibitions

VVI	Ventricular pace; ventricular sense, inhibited by ventricular beat
DOO	Dual chamber pace; no sense, no inhibitions
DVI	Dual chamber pace; ventricular sense, inhibited by ventricular beat
DDD	Dual chamber pace; dual chamber sense, inhibited by either chamber

The EMS physician who responds to a pacemaker patient with a clinical issue first needs to determine if the device is the problem. Vital signs and cardiac monitoring are the best tools to identify the problem. The first determinant is the heart rate. If the patient is markedly bradycardic, the pacemaker should be presumed to have failed. The patient will require hemodynamic support, which may include external cardiac pacing. If external pacing is indicated, care should be taken to not cover the implanted device with the external pads. If the patient is tachycardic, the physician will need to determine if the pacer is firing inappropriately, or if there is another medical cause. The presence of pacer spikes prior to every tachycardic beat is the best indicator of a pacer issue.

The next step is to determine what therapy is needed. Optimally, the patient can be transported to a facility where the implanted device can be interrogated by an electrophysiologist, preferably at the hospital where the device was implanted. If the patient's clinical condition requires more urgent intervention, a special magnet can be placed to suspend inappropriate pacing. The magnet will *not* turn the pacer off, rather it will trigger the device to pace at an asynchronous (fixed) rate depending on the device and manufacturer [15]. A DDD pacemaker will pace at DOO, a VVI device will pace at VOO, and an AII device will pace at AOO [15]. Magnet therapy is only effective when the magnet is on the skin over the pacemaker. In the event that magnet therapy is ineffective, it is theoretically possible to cut the pacer wires, but this would be difficult in the field, may permanently damage the device, and should only be performed as a last resort.

Implantable cardioverter-defibrillators

Implantable cardioverter-defibrillators are a first-line therapy for many patients at risk for sudden cardiac death. ICDs are usually implanted in the left infraclavicular region and are typically palpable. All patients with the device get an ID card that notes the manufacturer and device model. ICDs have four main functions:
- sensing atrial and ventricular signals
- classification of those signals into programmable heart rate zones
- administration of electrical therapy to terminate ventricular tachycardia or ventricular fibrillation
- pacing for bradycardia and/or cardiac resynchronization therapy (equivalent to a standard pacemaker) [16].

If ventricular fibrillation or ventricular tachycardia is detected, high-energy shocks of 1–40 J can be delivered [16]. Although this is less energy than external defibrillation or cardioversion, the shock can be painful to the patient.

The EMS physician will most likely encounter one of three possible scenarios in an ICD patient who is suffering from an ICD-related cardiac event. The first is device failure in the event of a ventricular arrhythmia. The second is an appropriately functioning device in the setting of a ventricular arrhythmia. The third possibility is the ICD delivering shocks inappropriately in the absence of a ventricular arrhythmia. The first step in all cases is assessment of mental status, vital signs, and cardiac monitoring. If the patient has an unstable ventricular arrhythmia and the ICD does not fire, it should be assumed the device is non-functional and ACLS protocols should be followed. If external defibrillation is needed, the defibrillator pads should not be placed over the implanted device.

If the patient has a ventricular rhythm and the ICD is giving appropriate shocks, care should be focused on additional treatment of the arrhythmia, as well as rapid transport to the hospital. The patient may benefit from analgesia and possibly sedation in the event of multiple shocks. External electrical therapy should not be needed.

In the third scenario, the ICD is giving inappropriate shocks in the absence of a ventricular arrhythmia. As with pacemaker malfunctions, ideally the device can be interrogated by an electrophysiologist at the receiving hospital. If the patient's condition requires emergency intervention to stop inappropriate shocks, a special magnet can be placed over the device. The magnet will suspend detection of ventricular fibrillation and ventricular tachycardia and should stop the shocks. The magnet will not stop the pacemaker function of the ICD, nor place the pacer in asynchronous (fixed) mode [16]. In the event of magnet placement, cardiac monitoring is required because the ICD will no longer be able to sense nor shock arrhythmias. Magnet therapy is only effective while the magnet is secured to the skin over the device. It may also be prudent to apply external defibrillator pads during transport. As with a pacemaker, cutting the lead wires of an ICD will most likely permanently damage the device, is difficult to perform in the field, and is not recommended short of a dire last resort.

Pericardiocentesis

Pericardiocentesis may be indicated in the ACLS algorithm for pulseless electrical activity (PEA) in the event of cardiac arrest. If the PEA is the result of cardiac tamponade, pericardiocentesis may reverse the condition. The prehospital provider should use the subxiphoid approach, inserting a needle to the left of the xiphoid and aiming at the left shoulder at a shallow angle. An 18 gauge spinal needle or 3" IV catheter may be used. Aspiration of blood that does not clot indicates removal from the pericardial space, as opposed to intraventricular blood. This procedure is more difficult to perform in the prehospital environment where ultrasound guidance is typically less available. It should be used as a final resort when all other therapies have failed [17].

Conclusion

Only critical care teams with extensive additional training should attempt to transport patients with IABPs, unless they are accompanied by a perfusionist. Such patients are not generally encountered by the EMS system except to facilitate interfacility transportation. Careful attention must be paid when transitioning a patient from one pump to another, and proper timing of inflation is crucial.

Patients in the community with VADs are growing in prevalence. Preplanning for potential emergencies, including awareness by the EMS system, is an important aspect of ensuring an appropriate response when complications or unrelated medical events arise. A coordinated exchange of information between the VAD hospital team and surrounding EMS agencies is key to the safe and effective treatment and transfer of these patients. Depending on the brand and type of VAD, the patient may or may not have a palpable pulse or blood pressure. Most pump flow alarms occur because of low volume and require volume resuscitation. Vasopressors in these patients may do more harm than good.

The prehospital provider may also encounter patients with implanted cardiac devices. Assessment of these patients will determine if the clinical condition is due to a device malfunction or not. While not routinely carried or used by EMS personnel, the EMS physician may want to have access to a special magnet used to turn off an ICD, or reset a pacemaker to asynchronous pacing.

References

1 Anon. *An Introduction to Intra-Aortic Balloon Pumping.* Reading, PA: Arrow International, 2005.

2 York-Clark D, Stocking J, Johnson J. Mechanically assisted cardiovascular transport. In: *Flight and Ground Transport Nursing Core Curriculum.* Denver, CO: Air and Surface Transport Nurses Association, 2006, pp.205–10.

3 Mecham CC. Prehospital assessment and management of patients with ventricular assist devices. *Prehosp Emerg Care* 2013;17:223–9.

4 Myers TJ, Dasse K, Macris M, et al. Use of a left ventricular assist device in an outpatient setting. *ASAIO J* 2001;47:590–5.

5 Fukamachi K, Smedira N. Smaller safer, totally implantable LVADs: fact or fantasy? *Am Coll Cardiol Curr J Rev* 2005;14:40–2.

6 Hoshi H, Shinshi T, Takatani S. Third-generation blood pumps with mechanical non-contact magnetic bearings. *Artif Organ* 2006; 30:324–8.

7 Geisen U, Heilmann C, Beyersdorf F, et al. Non-surgical bleeding in patients with ventricular assist devices could be explained by acquired von willebrand disease. *Eur J Cardiothorac Surg* 2008; 33:679–84.

8 Kato TS, Schulze P, Yang J, et al. Pre-operative and post-operative risk factors associated with neurologic complications in patients with advanced heart failure supported by a left ventricular assist device. *J Heart Lung Transplant* 2012;31:1–8.

9 Califano S, Pagani F, Malani P. Left ventricular assist device associated infections. *Infect Dis Clin North Am* 2012;26:77–87.

10 Kiernan MS, Pham D, DeNofrio D, Kapur N. Management of HeartWare left ventricular assist device thrombosis using intracavitary thrombolytics. *J Thorac Cardiovasc Surg* 2011;142:712–14.

11 Felix SE, Martina J, Kirkels J, et al. Continuous flow left ventricular assist device support in patients with advanced heart failure: points of interest for daily management. *Eur J Heart Fail* 2012;14:351–6.

12 Boyle A. Arrhythmias in patients with ventricular assist devices. *Curr Opin Cardiol* 2012;27:13–18.

13 Pacemakers: Nomenclature. Available at: www.unc.edu/~rup/old/ RP_Anesthesia/Basics/Pacers/html

14 Wallace A. Pacemakers for Anesthesiologists Made Incredibly Simple. Available at: www.cardiacengineering.com/pacemakers-wallace.pdf

15 Jacob S, Panaich S, Maheshwari R,et al. Clinical applications of magnets on cardiac rhythm management devices. *Europace* 2011;13(9):1222–30.

16 Stevenson W, Chaitman B, Ellenbogen K, et al. Clinical assessment and management of patients with implanted cardioverter-defibrillators presenting to non-electrophysiologists. *Circulation* 2004;110: 3866–9.

17 Thomson D, Cooney D. Procedures. In: Krohmer JR, Sahni R, Schwartz B, Wang HE (eds) *Emergency Medical Services: Clinical Practice and Systems Oversight, Volume 1, Clinical Aspects of Prehospital Medicine.* Lenexa, KS: National Association of EMS Physicians, 2009.

CHAPTER 16

Abdominal pain

Jeffrey D. Ferguson and Jennifer Monroe

Introduction

Patients with abdominal complaints who activate the EMS system can be among the most challenging. Their histories may be non-specific and their exams and vital signs may be unreliable with regard to the etiology or severity of their illnesses. Vital signs are frequently abnormal in critically ill patients. However, normal vital signs do not preclude the presence of a life-threatening illness. Certain populations with abdominal pain commonly encountered by EMS personnel may deserve special attention, including the elderly, women of child-bearing age, children, post-bariatric surgery patients, and immunocompromised patients. Finally, many significant extraabdominal conditions can present with mostly abdominal complaints.

Abdominal pain is the most frequent chief complaint in the emergency department, accounting for 8% of total visits [1]. A recent survey from the Centers for Disease Control found that the chief complaint of non-traumatic abdominal pain increased by 37% between 1999 and 2008 [2]. It is also one of the most common reasons to call EMS. At least one in 20 EMS calls is for abdominal complaints [3]. Thus, EMS providers encounter patients with abdominal pain on a regular basis, but options for patient assessment and management are limited.

Approach to the patient with abdominal pain

Assessment and management of abdominal pain patients in the prehospital setting are difficult for a variety of reasons. The following objectives apply.
- The initial priority must be to recognize patients with abnormal vital signs and provide hemodynamic support.
- Consider life-threatening conditions that can present with abdominal complaints (Box 16.1).
- Recognize high-risk patient populations, including the elderly, children, women of child-bearing age, and patients who are immunocompromised (e.g. HIV patients, cancer patients, transplant patients, others receiving immunosuppressive agents).
- Be aware of extraabdominal and systemic illnesses that can present with abdominal pain, including acute myocardial infarction, pneumonia, and diabetic ketoacidosis (Box 16.2).

Anatomy and physiology considerations

The lungs, pleural cavity, and base of the heart are all in close proximity to the abdominal cavity and can be involved in conditions that can be perceived as abdominal pain. During development, the abdominal organs protrude into the peritoneal cavity and become enveloped with a layer of peritoneal lining, the visceral peritoneum. The outer surface of the peritoneal cavity is the parietal peritoneum. The peritoneal cavity allows for normal movement and sliding of the abdominal organs and provides a source of protection to the abdominal contents. The peritoneum provides a potential space for air, blood, or other fluids in pathological conditions. Some structures, such as the kidneys, ureters, pancreas, aorta, and portions of the duodenum, lie in the retroperitoneum. This area contains less sensory innervation, accounting for decreased pain perception and localization of pathological conditions involving these structures.

The abdomen is traditionally divided into four quadrants by vertical and horizontal lines through the umbilicus. Use of the quadrant description not only provides common terminology, but is also an important determinant in the development of a differential diagnosis of abdominal complaints (Box 16.3).

The etiologies of abdominal pain can be described as mechanical, inflammatory, or ischemic in nature. Mechanical etiologies include distension of a hollow organ (e.g. stomach, intestine, gallbladder, ureter) or stretching of the capsule of a solid organ (e.g. liver, spleen, kidney). Inflammatory causes include immune processes such as Crohn's disease or ulcerative colitis and infection like appendicitis or diverticulitis. Ischemic pain may result from thrombotic or embolic disease of the vascular bed of abdominal organs or anatomic torsion (e.g. testicle or ovary).

Emergency Medical Services: Clinical Practice and Systems Oversight, Second Edition. Volume 1: Clinical Aspects of EMS.
Edited by David C. Cone, Jane H. Brice, Theodore R. Delbridge, and J. Brent Myers.
© 2015 NAEMSP. Published 2015 by John Wiley & Sons, Inc. Companion Website: www.wiley.com/go/cone/naemsp

Box 16.1 Life-threatening conditions causing abdominal pain

Abdominal aortic aneurysm (ruptured)
Acute myocardial infarction
Aortic dissection
Bowel obstruction/perforation
Diabetic ketoacidosis
Ectopic pregnancy (ruptured)
Envenomation (e.g. black widow spider bite)
Mesenteric ischemia
Pancreatitis
Peritonitis
Poisoning/overdose (e.g.iron tablets)
Tuboovarian abscess

Box 16.2 Systemic causes of abdominal pain

Acute myocardial infarction
Acute intermittent porphyria
Black widow envenomation
Diabetic ketoacidosis
Familial Mediterranean fever
Glaucoma
Heavy metal poisoning
Hereditary angioedema
Hyperthyroidism
Poisoning/overdose (iron, others)
Pneumonia
Streptococcal pharyngitis
Sickle cell vasoocclusive crisis
Shingles (Zoster herpeticus)
Uremia
Vasculitis

Box 16.3 Etiologies of abdominal pain by anatomical location

Right upper quadrant	Left upper quadrant
Cholelithiasis/cholecystitis	Pancreatitis
Acute hepatitis	Renal colic
Acute pancreatitis	Gastric ulcer
Renal colic	Gastritis
Duodenal ulcer	Splenic enlargement/infarction
Right lower lobe pneumonia	Left lower lobe pneumonia
Myocardial infarction	Myocardial infarction
Right lower quadrant	**Left lower quadrant**
Acute appendicitis	Sigmoid diverticulosis
Cecal diverticulitis	Colitis (i.e. inflammatory bowel disease)
Colitis (inflammatory bowel disease)	
Renal colic	Renal colic
Abdominal aortic aneurysm	Abdominal aortic aneurysm
Inguinal hernia	Inguinal hernia
Testicular/ovarian torsion	Testicular/ovarian torsion
Ectopic pregnancy	Ectopic pregnancy
Pelvic inflammatory disease	Pelvic inflammatory disease
Ovarian cyst	Ovarian cyst
Endometriosis	Endometriosis

Table 16.1 Common sites of referred abdominal pain

Etiology	Region of perceived pain
Biliary colic/cholecystitis	Right scapula
Renal colic	Testicle, labia, inguinal region
Pancreatitis	Midback
Gastric or bowel perforation	Shoulder
Ruptured ectopic pregnancy	Shoulder
Rectal or prostate disorder	Lower back

The perception of these pathological states may cause different types of pain: visceral, somatic, or referred pain. Luminal or capsular distension will typically produce visceral pain by stimulation of nerves surrounding a hollow or solid organ. Because the innervation of organs is sparse and multisegmented, this pain is usually dull and poorly localized. When caused by an obstructive process, the pain is typically intermittent or colicky. Distension of a solid organ tends to produce more constant pain (e.g. hydronephrosis, hepatitis). Visceral pain is typically associated with other autonomic phenomena such as anorexia, nausea, and vomiting.

Somatic abdominal pain typically results from irritation of the parietal peritoneum from infection or inflammation. The pathological process stimulates peripheral nerves and the pain tends to be more intense and distinct than visceral pain. The evolution of acute appendicitis demonstrates both visceral and somatic pain. Early obstruction and distension of the appendix generate dull, poorly localized pain around the umbilicus. As inflammation progresses, the parietal peritoneum becomes involved and the pain becomes localized to the right lower quadrant.

A third type of pain is referred pain; pain at a site not directly involved with the disease process. Visceral and somatic nerves from different areas converge at the spinal cord, allowing for misinterpretation of location by the brain. An example is irritation of the diaphragm by blood in the peritoneal cavity as might be seen following a ruptured ectopic pregnancy. This is perceived as shoulder pain because both the diaphragm and the skin near the shoulder share the C4 sensory level. Other common sites of referred pain are shown in Table 16.1.

Many systemic diseases may present with abdominal pain as the primary complaint. Some common examples of these conditions are listed in Box 16.2.

History and physical examination

An organized assessment must be applied to any patient with a presenting complaint of abdominal pain. High priority must be given to life-threatening conditions (see Box 16.1). A careful

Box 16.4 OPQRST questions in abdominal pain

Onset: When did your pain begin?

Palliation/provocation: What were you doing when your pain started? What makes your pain better or worse? If you have taken anything for the pain, has it changed your symptoms? Are you more comfortable in a certain position?

Quality: Can you describe what your pain feels like?

Radiation: Do you feel pain anywhere else? Does the pain move to any other place?

Severity: How bad is your pain on a scale from 1 to 10, if 10 is the worst pain you can imagine?

Timing: Since it started, has your pain changed in quality, severity, or location?

history will yield an appropriate list of potential etiologies in most patients. This list can be additionally refined using the abdominal quadrant as an indicator of the source of the complaint (see Box 16.3).

Useful historical data may be obtained directly from the patient or from a parent or other care provider. Emphasizing a SAMPLE history is encouraged. The OPQRST mnemonic (Box 16.4) highlights important questions regarding signs and symptoms. Ask the patient about allergies prior to medication administration and consider anaphylactic reactions as a source of abdominal discomfort. EMS providers should be encouraged to bring all medications with the patient. Particular attention should be paid to cardiac, diabetic, steroidal, and immunosuppressive agents. Medications such as beta-blockers, antiinflammatory agents, and over-the-counter medications can affect the patient's response to infection and inflammation. The past medical history may provide clues to the underlying condition. This history should include information about previous episodes of similar pain, diagnosis, and management. The patient should be questioned about his/her last oral intake and menstrual period. Finally, the events leading up to the current illness and EMS activation should be elicited.

The patient's general appearance should be assessed. Seasoned EMS providers develop an immediate impression of those who are "sick." A patient who limits his or her movement due to abdominal pain may have peritonitis as opposed to one who cannot find a position of comfort (e.g. kidney stones or aneurysmal pain).

The focus of the physical examination should be to identify potentially life-threatening conditions. Assessment and monitoring of vital signs are crucial. Indications of shock, including hypotension, tachycardia, narrow pulse pressure, and tachypnea, should be recognized. A hypotensive patient should be presumed to have a serious medical condition requiring immediate intervention. The patient's temperature should also be evaluated, recalling that both fever and hypothermia may indicate significant disease such as sepsis.

A careful examination of the heart and lungs should be completed. Abnormal or diminished lung sounds may indicate pneumonia or pleural effusion, which may present as ipsilateral upper abdominal pain. Cardiac auscultation may detect murmurs or gallop rhythms, which may be associated with an acute myocardial infarction or heart failure which may present with vague abdominal pain or gastrointestinal (GI) symptoms as the chief complaint.

Prehospital providers should be taught to perform a brief, directed examination of the abdomen. Inspection of the abdomen should be performed to detect distension, skin lesions, or bruising. The presence of therapeutic appliances such as feeding tubes, dialysis access ports, ostomies, and urinary catheters should be observed as well as their perceived functional status and condition of the surrounding tissue. Auscultation of bowel sounds is neither accurate nor productive in the out-of-hospital setting. Similarly, percussion does not yield any important findings in these patients.

Palpation should first be performed in the areas away from the region of discomfort. The area of pain should be assessed last with gradually increased pressure to allow some qualification of the level of discomfort (e.g. pain with mild palpation). Specific findings such as Murphy's sign (right upper quadrant tenderness with deep inspiration), Rovsing's sign (right lower quadrant tenderness with left-sided palpation), obturator sign (right lower quadrant pain elicited by external hip rotation of right hip), and psoas sign (right lower quadrant pain with right hip extension) are neither sensitive nor specific for gallbladder disease or appendicitis. Percussion of the patient's heel while the leg is fully extended may be more effective than depressing and releasing the abdominal wall to detect rebound tenderness. Deep palpation to detect a pulsatile mass in the abdomen is discouraged due to its low yield and theoretical potential for exacerbating the patient's condition if an aortic aneurysm is present.

Management

Management of the patient with abdominal pain begins with attention to the patient's airway, ventilation, and hemodynamic stability. Patients in profound shock may benefit from a secure airway and positive pressure ventilation. Vascular access is critical for fluid and medication administration. If the patient has experienced significant fluid loss or has evidence of shock, two large-bore IVs should be established. If IV access is difficult or unobtainable, intraosseous access may be indicated. Resuscitation with crystalloid solution (normal saline or Ringer's lactate) is generally indicated for prehospital resuscitation. Vasopressors such as norepinephrine may be indicated if septic shock from an abdominal source is suspected and the mean arterial pressure is below 65 mmHg despite adequate volume resuscitation. While such medications are often not available to prehospital EMS personnel, they may be available to EMS physicians or to personnel providing an interfacility transport for more advanced care.

Any patient with hemodynamic compromise should have continuous cardiac monitoring; the same may be true for all patients over 50 years of age. A 12-lead ECG should be obtained and interpreted to rule out acute myocardial infarction in patients with cardiac risk factors such as age, diabetes, or hypertension. Continuous pulse oximetry should be used in critically ill patients or those with suspected pulmonary etiologies. Supplemental oxygen should be administered to patients with respiratory distress or measured hypoxia.

There are reports describing the use of ultrasound in the prehospital setting. New ultrasound technology is lightweight, provides high-quality resolution, and can withstand a wider range of environmental conditions. Paramedics are being trained in the Focused Assessment Sonography in Trauma (FAST) exam as well as abdominal aortic ultrasound to evaluate for aneurysm [4,5]. Investigations of the value of prehospital ultrasound are still under way. It shows promise as it potentially provides earlier information regarding the patient's condition, leading to more informed triage decisions, reduced time to diagnosis, and sooner appropriate treatment. See Volume 1, Chapter 69 for additional information.

Another novel advance in prehospital care is point-of-care lactic acid testing. Several studies have evaluated lactic acid measurement in the trauma patient. However, there are also uses for prehospital measurement of lactic acid in the medical patient with abdominal pain. Elevation in prehospital lactate has been linked to mortality and may provide information superior to that of the patient's vital signs in detecting occult shock, facilitating resuscitation at an earlier stage in patient care [6,7].

The prehospital administration of opioid analgesics to the patient with abdominal pain remains a controversial practice. Early surgical literature emphasized the loss of diagnostic accuracy with the use of morphine in the patient with undiagnosed abdominal pain [8]. However, this was in an age of few laboratory and radiological diagnostic aids [9,10]. Since then, the practice of administering opioid analgesics has found widespread support in the literature [11–13]. Yet there remains theoretical concern about the loss of diagnostic acumen in medicated patients, as well as continued lack of evidence of effect on the overall outcome of such patients [14–16]. Analgesics are commonly employed in the care of patients with abdominal pain in both the emergency department (ED) [17] and prehospital environments [3]. The best recommendation for emergency care personnel is to provide small IV doses of opioid analgesics in patients with abdominal pain, titrating the dose with the expectation of reducing, but perhaps not eliminating, the patient's pain.

Additional mention should be made in regard to the resuscitation of patients with abdominal pain and suspected or known intraabdominal hemorrhage, such as ruptured aortic aneurysm or ruptured ectopic pregnancy. Attempts to restore normotensive states may not be possible in the prehospital environment and may, in fact, be harmful. These conclusions are drawn from animal [18,19] and clinical studies [20] of hemorrhagic shock that demonstrate that some level of "permissive hypotension" may improve outcomes. Recent animal research showed no

difference among organ perfusion, cardiac output, and lactic acid levels between permissive hypotension and normotensive resuscitation groups. It defined permissive hypotension as 60% of baseline mean arterial pressure [21].

Urinary catheters serve as both a source and management of some abdominal pain. Their presence and functionality should be included in the examination of the patient. Patients with both indwelling urethral and suprapubic catheters are at risk for urinary tract infections, mechanical obstruction, or catheter displacement. EMS providers may be trained to place urinary catheters, observing sterile technique, to relieve bladder distension. They should be educated that patients with recent urethral procedures or bleeding from the urethral meatus should not be catheterized due to risk of urethral injury.

Disposition

Based on the previous discussions, one can assume that it would be difficult for EMS personnel to identify patients who do not require transport and to make the somewhat related decision regarding the need for medical evaluation in an ED. It is possible that a patient may not require EMS transport but may still require medical evaluation. The accuracy of such decisions has been addressed by several authors. Dunne [22] compared the assessment by EMS personnel with physician evaluation of the need for transport. The sensitivity of EMS judgment of the need for transport was 22.1%, with a specificity of 80.5%. The presence of abdominal pain was found to be highly associated with the need for transport as judged by the physicians. On the other hand, Kennedy [23] found an overtriage rate of 84% for the need for ALS services in patients with abdominal pain. Gratton [24] found a low but clinically significant undertriage rate of 11%. Other authors have confirmed significant undertriage rates for a variety of medical conditions by EMS providers [25–27]. These studies reaffirm the need to exercise due caution in approaching transport decisions in patients with abdominal complaints.

Special populations

There are certain populations who represent a particular risk for a poor outcome and require a cautious approach.

Elderly patients

In 2010, there were 40 million people aged 65 and over in the US, accounting for 13% of the population. By 2030 the number is projected to represent nearly 20% of the total US population [28]. This population represents high-volume users of the EMS system [29]. Compared with younger patients, geriatric patients have higher mortality when admitted to a hospital with abdominal pain and a higher rate of surgical intervention [30,31]. One-third of elderly patients who present with abdominal pain require surgery, compared with 10% for other adult patients [32].

The higher mortality rate in geriatric patients is due to several factors. Elderly patients delay seeking medical care for abdominal complaints and will often present later in their disease processes than younger patients. They tend to have more vague symptoms, which can make the evaluation difficult. The elderly have a decreased perception of abdominal pain [33]. Because of this, many elderly patients with significant underlying pathology are misdiagnosed with benign conditions.

Use of medications such as beta-blockers, non-steroidal anti-inflammatory drugs (NSAIDs), pain medications, anticoagulants, and steroids is more common in this population. In addition, other physiological responses including fever, immune responsiveness, rebound tenderness, and laboratory abnormalities may not be as prominent in the older patient. Complex medical problems predispose this population to certain conditions, such as abdominal aortic aneurysm and mesenteric ischemia.

Common diagnoses found in the geriatric population with abdominal pain include diverticulitis, diverticulosis, small bowel obstruction, volvulus, malignancy, perforated viscus, urinary tract infection, appendicitis, and biliary tract disease. This list is not exhaustive. As mentioned previously, cardiac or pulmonary pathology can also present in a similar manner, and must be entertained based on the patient's history and physical exam. Additional historical information about abdominal pain as related to food intake, vomiting and/or diarrhea, melena or bright red blood per rectum, previous abdominal surgeries, fever, sick contacts, and other areas of pain should be elicited. Focus on the cardiac, pulmonary, and abdominal components of the physical exam. Cardiac and pulse oximetry monitoring is recommended.

Women of child-bearing age

Women of child-bearing age represent a particular challenge because the number of problems that cause abdominal pain in this population must be expanded to include conditions involving the pelvic organs. Specifically, ectopic pregnancy, ovarian torsion, ruptured ovarian cyst, and tuboovarian abscess (TOA) as a consequence of pelvic inflammatory disease (PID) are significant causes of pain in this population. The difficulty in establishing the diagnosis lies in the fact that neither pelvic examination nor pregnancy testing is routinely available in the prehospital setting. Many patients do not know they are pregnant, and the physical exam is not reliable in establishing the diagnosis of pregnancy.

Ectopic pregnancy is one of the leading causes of pregnancy-related deaths in women. Hemorrhagic shock from a ruptured ectopic pregnancy should be considered in any woman of appropriate age with hypotension and abdominal pain. A past history of PID, known tubal pregnancy, prior tubal surgery, or intrauterine device use increases the likelihood of ectopic pregnancy.

Pelvic pain caused by ovarian torsion tends to be sudden in onset in reproductive-age women. It is typically described as sharp and knife-like. Right-sided torsion is more common. The signs and symptoms of a ruptured ovarian cyst are difficult to distinguish from torsion. TOA occurs in approximately 1–4% of patients with PID [34]. The pain is more insidious in onset and rupture of the abscess causes signs of peritonitis. Rupture of a TOA carries a mortality of approximately 10% [35].

Pediatrics

Pediatric patients present a challenge to EMS providers for a variety of reasons. As a rule, pediatric patients are not high-volume users of the EMS system. In addition, infants and children may be unable to describe their symptoms, which is particularly problematic given the importance of historical data in establishing a cause. It is important to discuss the history of the patient's symptoms and the reason why EMS was called with a parent or guardian familiar with the situation. Non-specific findings such as irritability, inability to be consoled, and poor feeding may be the only signs of an abdominal problem in the very young. Vomiting, oral intake, urine output, last bowel movement, fevers, sick contacts, and vaccination status are useful points from the history. The birth history is important when treating a neonate. Questions that should be asked include whether the pregnancy was at term at the time of birth, did the mother receive prenatal care, were there any complications during the delivery, did the patient require an extended hospital stay after the birth, or have there been any subsequent hospitalizations since birth for any reason.

Vital signs can be difficult to interpret in the pediatric population due to age-related variations and the tremendous physiological reserve that these patients possess. The examination can be compromised by the patient's fear of pain and of the unfamiliar examiner. Finally, abdominal pain is a particularly common complaint in many extraabdominal conditions, as discussed above [36].

Age is a key factor in the evaluation of abdominal pain in the pediatric patient. For patients up to 1 year old, some of the considerations include infantile colic, Hirschsprung disease, necrotizing enterocolitis, intussusception, pyloric stenosis, volvulus, and incarcerated hernia. Bilious vomiting accompanying abdominal pain in an infant is particularly concerning, often indicating an acute surgical problem. Between 2 and 5 years old, consider testicular torsion, Henoch–Schönlein purpura (HSP), intussusception, and appendicitis. Older children between 5 years and adolescence can have inflammatory bowel disease, testicular torsion, HSP, and pharyngitis. This is not an all-encompassing list, but more of a differential with which to start when obtaining the history.

On initial presentation, it may be difficult for EMS providers to distinguish a benign condition in children from a true surgical emergency. Up to one-third of pediatric patients admitted to the ED fail to have diagnoses at the time of discharge [37], and a significant number of ED discharge diagnoses may be incorrect [36]. Extrapolating such information to prehospital conditions makes it apparent that there should be a low threshold for transporting pediatric patients with abdominal pain.

Immunocompromised patients

Many patients are considered relatively immunocompromised due to their underlying medical states. Examples include the elderly, cancer patients undergoing treatment, malnourished patients, diabetics, patients with end-stage renal disease, patients on certain medications (e.g. chronic steroids and many medications for diseases such as rheumatoid arthritis and irritable bowel disease) and those with HIV infection but adequate CD4 counts. As a result of their underlying conditions, these patients have depressed inflammatory responses and tend to present later in their courses.

Of greater concern are patients who are more profoundly immunocompromised, often based on treatments they receive for their underlying conditions. Examples include AIDS patients with low CD4 counts, transplant patients on chronic immunosuppressive medications, leukopenic cancer patients on chemotherapy, and patients with other conditions requiring immune-modulating medications such as inflammatory bowel disease or rheumatoid arthritis. These patients present with an expanded list of serious conditions leading to abdominal complaints, including neutropenic enterocolitis (typhlitis), graft- versus-host disease, cytomegalovirus perforation, and tuberculous peritonitis [38]. Important questions to ask include history of fevers, vomiting and/or diarrhea, recent changes in medication regimen (including non-compliance due to financial or other logistical barriers), and any prior similar episodes. Transplant patients should have the date and location of their surgery noted. EMS protocols or direct medical oversight should provide the option for such patients to be transported to specialty centers capable of managing their potentially complex conditions. Because immunocompromised patients present late in their courses, their mortality tends to be high.

Obesity and bariatric surgery patients

Statistics from 2010 estimate that over 35% of US adults are obese [39], a condition with known links to increased rates of diabetes and heart disease. Obesity may also be linked to an increase in abdominal complaints including dyspepsia, irritable bowel syndrome, and constipation, [40] as well as abdominal wall hernias which predispose patients to bowel obstructions. The care of the obese patient may be hindered by an unreliable physical exam as well as equipment which is not suited for the patient's size.

Not surprisingly, the rate of bariatric surgery has increased dramatically in recent years. The rate of hospital admission of patients after bariatric surgery is 20% during the first postoperative year and increases to 40% within 3 years [41]. Recognized complications include ulceration and bleeding, perforation, and mechanical obstruction. The EMS professional should be aware of the increased rate of these conditions in this patient population.

Conclusion

Patients with abdominal pain can present a significant challenge to prehospital care providers. An approach that emphasizes immediate consideration of life-threatening abdominal and extraabdominal conditions is imperative. The patient's history and the location of the pain are the primary determinants of the differential diagnosis. Stabilization of ABCs and restoring hemodynamic stability remain the primary focus of patient management. Controversies in the use of pain medication in patients with abdominal pain and appropriate fluid resuscitation in the face of acute hemorrhage exist. Specific attention to high-risk populations, including the elderly, women of reproductive age, children, immunocompromised, and bariatric patients, must be exercised.

References

1 National Hospital Ambulatory Medical Care Survey: 2010 Emergency Department Summary Tables. Available at: www.cdc.gov/nchs/data/ahcd/nhamcs_emergency/2010_ed_web_tables.pdf
2 Bhuiya FA, Pitts SR, McCaig LF. Emergency department visits for chest pain and abdominal pain: United States, 1999–2008. *NCHS Data Brief* 2010;(43):1–8.
3 Pointer JE, Harlan K. Impact of liberalization of protocols for the use of morphine sulfate in an urban emergency medical services system. *Prehosp Emerg Care* 2005;9(4):377–81.
4 Nelson BP, Chason K. Use of ultrasound by emergency medical services: a review. *Int J Emerg Med* 2008;1(4):253–9.
5 Heegaard W, Hildebrandt D, Spear D, Chason K, Nelson B, Ho J. Prehospital ultrasound by paramedics: results of field trial. *Acad Emerg Med* 2010;17(6):624–30.
6 Jansen TC, van Bommel J, Mulder PG, Rommes JH, Schieveld SJ, Bakker J. The prognostic value of blood lactate levels relative to that of vital signs in the prehospital setting: a pilot study. *Crit Care* 2008;12(6):R160.
7 Van Beest PA, Mulder PJ, Oetomo SB, van den Broek B, Kuiper MA, Spronk PE. Measurement of lactate in a prehospital setting is related to outcome. *Eur J Emerg Med* 2009;16(6):318–22.
8 Cope Z. *The Early Diagnosis of the Acute Abdomen.* New York: Oxford University Press, 1921.
9 Rosen MP, Sands DZ, Longmaid HE III, Reynolds KF, Wagner M, Raptopoulos V. Impact of abdominal CT on the management of patients presenting to the emergency department with acute abdominal pain. *Am J Roentgenol* 2000;174(5):1391–6.
10 Esses D, Birnbaum A, Bijur P, Shah S, Gleyzer A, Gallagher EJ. Ability of CT to alter decision making in elderly patients with acute abdominal pain. *Am J Emerg Med* 2004;22(4):270–2.
11 Gallagher E, Esses D, Lee C, Lahn M, Bijur PE. Randomized clinical trial of morphine in acute abdominal pain. *Ann Emerg Med* 2006;48(2):150–60.
12 Mahadevan M, Graff L. Prospective randomized study of analgesic use for ED patients with right lower quadrant pain. *Am J Emerg Med* 2000;18(7):753–6.
13 Wolfe JM, Smithline HA, Phipen S, Montano G, Garb JL, Fiallo V. Does morphine change the physical examination in patients with acute appendicitis? *Am J Emerg Med* 2004;22(4):280–5.

14 Nissman SA, Kaplan LJ, Mann BD. Critically reappraising the literature driven practice of analgesia administration for acute abdominal pain in the emergency room prior to surgical evaluation. *Am J Surg* 2003;185(4):291–6.

15 Thomas SH, Silen W. Effect on diagnostic efficiency of analgesia for undifferentiated abdominal pain. *Br J Surg* 2003;90(1):5–9.

16 Lee JS, Stiell IG, Wells GA, Elder BR, Vandemheen K, Shapiro S. Adverse outcomes and opioid analgesic administration in acute abdominal pain. *Acad Emerg Med* 2000;7(9):980–7.

17 Neighbor ML, Baird CH, Kohn MA. Changing opioid use for right lower quadrant abdominal pain in the emergency department. *Acad Emerg Med* 2005;12(12):1216–20.

18 Sindlinger JF, Soucy DM, Greene SP, Barber AE, Illner H, Shires GT. The effects of isotonic saline volume resuscitation in uncontrolled hemorrhage. *Surg Gynecol Obstet* 1993;177(6):545–50.

19 Hachimi-Idrissi S, Yang X, Nguyen DN, Huyghens L. Combination of therapeutic mild hypothermia and delayed fluid resuscitation improved survival after uncontrolled haemorrhagic shock in mechanically ventilated rats. *Resuscitation* 2004;62(3):303–10.

20 Bickell WH, Wall MJ, Pepe PE, et al. Immediate versus delayed fluid resuscitation for hypotensive patients with penetrating torso injuries. *N Engl J Med* 1994;331(17):1105–9.

21 Schmidt BM, Rezende-Neto JB, Andrade MV, et al. Permissive hypotension does not reduce regional organ perfusion compared to normotensive resuscitation: animal study with fluorescent microspheres. *World J Emerg Surg* 2012;7(Suppl 1):S9.

22 Dunne RB, Compton S, Welch RD, Zalenski RJ, Bock BF. Prehospital onsite triaging. *Prehosp Emerg Care* 2003;7(1):85–8.

23 Kennedy JD, Sweeney TA, Roberts D, O'Connor RE. Effectiveness of a medical priority dispatch protocol for abdominal pain. *Prehosp Emerg Care* 2003;7(1):89–93.

24 Gratton MC, Ellison SR, Hunt J, Ma OJ. Prospective determination of medical necessity for ambulance transport by paramedics. *Prehosp Emerg Care* 2003;7(4):466–9.

25 Pointer JE, Levitz MA, Young JC, Promes SB, Messana BJ, Adèr ME. Can paramedics using guidelines accurately triage patients? *Ann Emerg Med* 2001; 38(3):268–77.

26 Schmidt TA, Atcheson R, Foderiuk C, et al. Hospital follow-up of patients categorized as not needing an ambulance using a set of emergency medical technician protocols. *Prehosp Emerg Care* 2001;5(4):366–70.

27 Silvestri S, Rothrock SG, Kennedy D, Ladde J, Bryant M, Pagane J. Can paramedics accurately identify patients who do not require emergency care? *Prehosp Emerg Care* 2002;6(4):387–90.

28 National Institutes of Health, National Institute on Aging. *Older Americans 2012: Key Indicators of Well-Being*. Available at: www.agingstats.gov

29 Rucker DW, Edwards RA, Burstin HR, O'Neil AC, Brennan TA. Patient specific predictors of ambulance use. *Ann Emerg Med* 1997;29(4):484–91.

30 De Dombal PT. Acute abdominal pain in the elderly. *J Clin Gastroenterol* 1994;19(4):331–5.

31 Bugliosi TM, Meloy TD, Vukov LF. Acute abdominal pain in the elderly. *Ann Emerg Med* 1990;19(12):1383–6.

32 Laurell H, Hansson LE, Gunnarsson U. Acute abdominal pain among elderly patients. *Gerontology* 2006;52(6):339–44.

33 Cooper GS, Shlaes DM, Salata RA. Intraabdominal infection: differences in presentation and outcome between younger patients and the elderly. *Clin Infect Dis* 1994;19(1):146–8.

34 Roberts W, Dockery JL. Management of tuboovarian abscess due to pelvic inflammatory disease. *South Med J* 1984;77(7):860–3.

35 Krivak TC, Cooksey C, Propst AM. Tuboovarian abscess: diagnosis, medical and surgical managment. *Comp Ther* 2004; 30(2):93–100.

36 Scholer SJ, Pituch K, Orr DP, Dittus RS. Clinical outcomes of children with acute abdominal pain. *Pediatrics* 1996;98(4 Pt 1):680–5.

37 D'Agostino J. Common abdominal emergencies in children. *Emerg Med Clin North Am* 2002;20(1):139–53.

38 Scott-Conner CEH, Fabrega AJ. Gastrointestinal problems in immunocompromised host: a review for surgeons. *Surg Endoscopy* 1996;10(10):959–64.

39 Ogden CL, Carroll MD, Kit BK, Flegal KM. Prevalence of obesity in the United States, 2009–2010. *NCHS Data Brief* 2012;(82):1–8.

40 Ho W, Spiegel BMR. The relationship between obesity and functional gastrointestinal disorders: causation, association, or neither? *Gastroenterol Hepatol* 2008;4(8):572–8.

41 Zingmond DS, McGory ML, Ko CY. Hospitalization before and after gastric bypass surgery. *JAMA* 2005;294:1918–24.

CHAPTER 17

Submersion injuries/drowning

Robert Lowe

Epidemiology

Drowning remains a leading cause of unintentional death and unintentional injury [1]. The Centers for Disease Control (CDC) place the incidence of non-fatal drowning at between 4,000 and 7,000 cases per year [1–5]. Fatalities range from 3,200 and 6,000 cases per year [1,4,5]. The incidence of non-fatal drownings ranges from one to four times that of fatal drownings [3]. Over 50% of all non-fatal drownings require hospitalization [1].

Drowning and near drowning are the second most common unintentional injuries for ages 1–4 and 15–19 [2,6]. In infants less than 1 year old, most drownings occur in the bathtub [7]. For children less than 4 years old, most drownings occur in private pools. For age greater than 15 years the predominant drowning locations include natural water settings such as beaches and lakes [8]. Fatalities are higher for victims less than 4 years old. Compared with females, males have twice the rate of non-fatal and five times the rate of fatal drowning [1]. Over half of adolescent and adult drownings involve alcohol or illicit substance use [8,9]. Approximately 35% of persons who drown under the age of 20 are classified as accomplished swimmers [10]. Preexisting medical conditions may play a role as well, as noted in children with seizures having a four-fold increase in risk compared to the general population [3].

Drowning accidents involving children commonly result from lapses in adult supervision. In the majority of child drownings, the child was under the care of one or both parents and was "out of sight" for less than 5 minutes [9]. While surveyed pool owners favor cardiopulmonary resuscitation (CPR) requirements, less than half of these households actually have a CPR-qualified individual. Of pool owners favoring isolation fencing around pools, only one-third had their pool fenced. The risk of drowning or near drowning is 3–4 times higher in unfenced than fenced pools [5].

Epidemiological and public health data highlight the role of education, planning, and other community-level interventions in drowning prevention. Estimates of preventable drowning deaths are as high as 80% [3]. Many EMS systems participate in drowning prevention efforts, such as education and water safety programs.

Pathophysiology of drowning

Drowning is commonly defined as suffocation and death as the result of submersion in a liquid environment [5,9,10]. Historically, two types of drowning have been described, wet and dry. "Wet drowning" is the aspiration of material such as water, sand, vomitus, etc [11–13]. This material can lead to pulmonary edema, pneumonitis, and surfactant dysfunction, impairing gas exchange. "Dry drowning" involves minimal aspiration; the inhaled liquid triggers laryngospasm, resulting in suffocation. Experts have questioned the mechanisms and clinical significance of this differentiation. Some postulate that decreasing level of consciousness and increasing hypoxia will eventual break any "spasm," allowing liquid to enter the lungs [9,14]. Submersion describes the airway opening beneath the surface of the liquid medium–air interface, while immersion is the splashing of liquid in or about the airway.

Classically, drowning begins as a period of panic and struggle, but in a minority of cases (for example, cervical trauma or seizure), this initial phase may not be present [9,12]. Death from drowning ultimately results from suffocation, tissue hypoxia, and cardiac arrest. Successful resuscitation after a drowning-induced cardiac arrest is rare.

Historically, drowning education materials have emphasized differences in fresh-water and salt-water drowning, citing the theoretical electrolyte and fluid shifts occurring with each situation. However, current practice downplays the importance of these differences [5,11]. Some consideration of the water contaminants may be clinically important in the hospital setting, and the EMS insight into those scene variables may be helpful to hospital staff.

Cerebral hypoxia plays a significant role in the functional recovery of the victim. Many drowning survivors suffer some permanent neurological damage, with up to 10% suffering severe lasting effects [13,15]. The duration of hypoxia is correlated with sub-mersion time and is an important determinant of recovery [11,13]. Another important consideration is the neuroprotective effect of hypothermia. The medical literature and the lay press are replete

Emergency Medical Services: Clinical Practice and Systems Oversight, Second Edition. Volume 1: Clinical Aspects of EMS.
Edited by David C. Cone, Jane H. Brice, Theodore R. Delbridge, and J. Brent Myers.
© 2015 NAEMSP. Published 2015 by John Wiley & Sons, Inc. Companion Website: www.wiley.com\go\cone\naemsp

with examples of survival after lengthy submersion in frigid or near freezing water. Cold-water submersion does not guarantee survival but may play a significant role in management decisions during and after the resuscitation [11,16].

The term "secondary drowning" typically refers to patients who survive the submersion injury for some period of time, yet later develop respiratory failure and death attributed to the original submersion event [5]. This deterioration may occur from hours to days later [8,13]. While the term "drowning-related death" has been proposed to describe deaths occurring more than 24 hours after a submersion, this definition is not widely used [10].

"Near drowning" is defined as immediate survival after a submersion event [13]. While most of these individuals may survive, many will deteriorate. The definition has some variability among authors and published sources, with some including asphyxia or loss of consciousness in the definition [5,9,10]. There remain ongoing efforts to better formalize definitions, including the use of the term "drowning" (defined as a process resulting in primary respiratory impairment from submersion and immersion in a liquid medium) to classify all events regardless of outcome as drowning [3]. To date, this has not been widely accepted in medicine or by the lay public. The remainder of this chapter will distinguish drowning (death) from near drowning.

Clinical management

Dispatch life support

Emergency dispatchers should provide dispatch life support, including standard respiratory and/or cardiopulmonary arrest instructions. Minimizing delays in delivering instructions is essential. DeNicola showed that 42% of children drowning in home swimming pools were rescued by bystanders but did not have CPR initiated until EMS personnel arrived [5]. The use of an automated external defibrillator (AED) is appropriate and should be included when such a device is available. A less clear area is whether dispatchers should direct callers to rescue drowning victims. All water rescues involve risk and may potentially result in additional victims.

Scene and crowd control

The first step in successful drowning management is rapid extraction of the victim from the water. Scene safety is paramount, especially in natural water and moving water scenarios. Rescuers not specifically trained in water rescue should not attempt extraction or rescue in moving water.

Crowd control and prevention of secondary victims are essential. Drownings are dramatic events. Depending on the setting (public pool, hotel pool, natural water setting), a large number of bystanders may be present. Bystanders acting as rescuers may inadvertently become secondary victims, especially in natural water settings or in large groups with several non-swimmers. Rescuers should liberally request and utilize crowd control resources.

Management of the drowning victim in cardiac arrest

The most dramatic clinical presentation of drowning is cardiopulmonary arrest. Rescuers should initiate standard BLS, ACLS, and Pediatric Advanced Life Support (PALS) protocols on drowning victims in cardiac arrest. CPR should begin as soon as practical, with some advocating initiation of CPR while the victim is still in the water [10]. Airway management should begin immediately with bag-valve-mask (BVM) ventilation [16]. Typically extrication from the water should not be delayed for more definitive airway management. Once extricated from the water, additional airway procedures consistent with cardiac arrest protocols may be considered. Rescuers should anticipate vomiting, which may occur in up to 86% of drowning victims receiving rescue breathing and chest compressions [16,17]. Maneuvers to clear water from the lungs, such as laying the patient prone and lifting the arms behind the back toward the head, are not necessary and should not be performed [5,8,12,16].

Cardiac arrest treatment algorithms do not require modification for drowning victims. While experts have historically emphasized minimizing movement in the severely hypothermic patient to avoid precipitating ventricular dysrhythmias, this recommendation seems to be based more on theory and conjecture than data. Advanced airway management is appropriate in services and personnel competent in the skill. Airway management while in the water is fraught with difficulty and risk of aspiration and delay of CPR initiation. While each scene may pose a unique risk–benefit analysis around patient access and timely egress, typically anything more than basic maneuvers should be deferred to accomplish rapid extrication and initiation of full resuscitation efforts. In the severely hypothermic patient, advanced airway placement may allow for warmed, humidified ventilation. Vascular access and drug therapy should follow standard resuscitation protocols.

Some experts have raised concerns that medications may reach toxic levels in the circulation due to decreased metabolism in the severely hypothermic patient [16]. However, little scientific evidence distinguishes drug metabolism in hypothermic versus normothermic cardiac arrest patients. Despite this concern, most guidelines recommend minor alterations of cardiac arrest protocols for patients with hypothermia [16]. Specifically, in moderate hypothermia (30–34°C), rescuers may increase the time interval between intravenous medications. Rescuers should also perform active external rewarming for moderate-to-severe hypothermia. For severe hypothermia (<30°C), current ACLS guidelines recommend providing a single defibrillation attempt and withholding intravenous medications until the core temperature is >30°C [18]. The determination of an accurate core temperature in the field setting is difficult, and rescuers should base their actions on the best available clinical information.

Management of near drownings

By definition, the near drowning patient has vital signs. Near drownings may include patients who never lost vital signs, and those successfully resuscitated. Airway management, hemodynamic stabilization, and transport are the mainstays of treatment. These individuals may be apneic, hypotensive, or hypothermic and should receive appropriate resuscitative interventions. Near drowning victims have strong potential for pulmonary injury and should receive emergency department evaluation. Over half of near drowning victims ultimately require hospital admission. Near drowning victims should be transported and evaluated, as initial presentation can progress rapidly, and refusals should be strongly discouraged [5,10].

Field management should focus on management and evaluation of oxygenation. Monitoring of pulse oximetry, cardiac rhythms, vital signs, and overall neurological status is warranted. Monitoring of end-tidal CO_2 may also be helpful. Continuous positive airway pressure (CPAP) in the conscious breathing patient is being increasingly advocated [10,14]. Rapid deterioration in ventilation, oxygenation, or ability to protect the airway may require more aggressive airway management techniques consistent with medical respiratory distress protocols. Secondary aspiration from vomiting is a risk in the declining near drowning victim. Intravenous access should be established in most near drownings. Consideration should be given to potential concurrent trauma. Victims may have had concurrent medical conditions that triggered the event, such as hypoglycemia, seizures and cardiac dysrhythmias. These should be addressed and treated appropriately.

Management of concurrent trauma

Many drownings occur concurrently with other major trauma. For example, an individual may sustain a cervical or spinal cord injury after diving into shallow water. Swimmers in lakes have sustained traumatic brain injuries or penetrating trauma after being struck by motor boats.

The most important consideration in drowning victims is the potential for cervical spine injury. Hwang et al. [4] identified seven cervical spinal injuries in 143 pediatric drowning and near drowning patients transported to a pediatric trauma center. Watson et al. identified 11 cervical spine injuries in 2,244 drowning victims [18]. All patients in each series were identified with mechanisms of injury suggestive of trauma (diving, high-impact, or assault).

Emergency medical services rescuers should consider cervical spine injuries in all diving, high-impact (e.g. dive from a height), white water, and submersion injuries. However, the rescuers must weigh the risks and benefits of cervical immobilization. For example, cervical immobilization may be dangerous and difficult in swift water rescues [18]. Current American Heart Association guidelines state "... routine stabilization of the cervical spine is not necessary unless the circumstances leading to the submersion episode indicate that trauma is likely ..." Drowning circumstances potentially linked to cervical injury include a history of diving, water slide use, concern for alcohol intoxication, or physical signs of injury [16]. The decision to initiate spine immobilization while in the water is a risk–benefit decision for the patient and rescue team. An absence of identified risk for cervical injury precludes the need for spine immobilization in or out of the water. Swimming pools in particular may be a more appropriate setting for floating backboards or baskets and application of cervical collars without undue risk to the patient or the rescue team. Swift water environments may require a more limited cervical spine control maneuver and rapid extrication to the water's edge prior to application of rigid collars and boards. In all events, if secondary concerns for cervical injury are discovered by examination or history, cervical protection measures should be instituted.

Rewarming of drowning victims

Rewarming is appropriate for severely hypothermic patients. Initial thermal management begins with removal of the patient from the offending environment. The patient should be removed from the water. The resuscitation effort should continue in a warmed environment. EMS rescuers should prewarm the ambulance if possible. To prevent further heat loss, the patient's wet clothing should be removed.

Additional rewarming techniques are commonly classified as active external rewarming and active internal rewarming. Active external rewarming includes the use of warm packs, warm water packs, forced air, thermal blankets, warmed O_2, and warmed IV infusions. Care should be taken to avoid secondary thermal injury from warm packs against the native skin. Concern for a paradoxical drop in the core temperature due to vasodilation of the peripheral vasculature during rewarming has been postulated. Careful hemodynamic monitoring should be instituted [16].

Active internal rewarming includes the use of peritoneal lavage with warmed fluids, esophageal tubes for rewarming, chest lavage with warm fluids via chest tubes, and the cardiac bypass or extracorporeal circulation; these measures are typically not carried out in the prehospital environment.

Traditionally, most experts argued for rewarming by whatever means available and to do so aggressively during the resuscitation. The old adage "A victim is not dead until warm and dead" may require reconsideration. Mounting evidence has shown that induced hypothermia after return of spontaneous circulation may impart some neurological benefit for ventricular fibrillation arrest and possibly other arrhythmias. It would seem logical that a drowning victim may benefit from induced or continued hypothermia [3,10]. Additionally, ACLS guidelines now target core temperature to 32–34 °C with return of spontaneous circulation in cardiac arrest due to accidental hypothermia [16]. In the absence of specific drowning data, and the success of prehospital hypothermia in general cardiac arrest, the historic practice of aggressive rewarming is being questioned. Some in medicine are specifically calling for abandoning the practice altogether [14].

Destination decisions

Patients in cardiac arrest should be transported to the nearest emergency facility. Patients with perfusing rhythms may benefit from transport to a specialized facility (for example, trauma or pediatric center), provided that the additional transport time is limited. While many victims have concurrent trauma, it is not clear whether transport to a trauma center is warranted for all drownings.

Grief reactions

Drownings are unexpected events in typically young and healthy patients. Relatives and bystanders may express significant grief from these events. After the incident, attention should be paid to possible grief reactions in rescue personnel so that appropriate referral or interventions can be implemented.

References

1 CDC. Nonfatal and fatal drownings in recreational water settings – United States 2001–2002. *MMWR* 2004;53(21):447–52.

2 CDC. Injury Prevention and Control: Data & Statistics, 2000-2007 drowning data. Available at: www.cdc.gov/injury/wisqars/facts.html

3 Meyer RJ, Theodorou AA, Berg RA. Childhood drowning. *Pediatr Rev* 2006;27(5):163–9.

4 Hwang V, Shofer FS, Durbin DR, Baren JM. Prevalence of traumatic injuries in drowning and near drowning in children and adolescents. *Arch Pediatr Adolesc Med* 2003;157:50.

5 DeNicola LK, Falk JL, Swanson ME, Gayle MO, Kissoon N. Submersion injuries in children and adults. *Crit Care Clin* 1997; 13(3):477–502.

6 *10 Leading Causes of Death by Age Group, United States – 2004.* Bethesda, MD: Office of Statistics and Programming, National Center for Injury Prevention and Control, CDC.

7 Brenner RA, Trumble AC, Smith GS, Kessler EP, Overpeck MD. Where children drown, United States 1995. *Pediatrics* 2001;108:85–9.

8 Olshaker JS. Submersion. *Emerg Med Clin North Am* 2004;22:357–67.

9 Moon RE, Long RJ. Drowning and near-drowning. *Emerg Med* 2002;14(4):377–86.

10 Layton AJ, Modell JH. Drowning: update 2009. *Anesthesiology* 2009;110:1390–401.

11 Gheen KM. Near drowning and cold water submersion. *Semin Pediatr Surg* 2001;10:26.

12 Ibsen LM, Koch T. Submersion and asphyxial injury. *Crit Care Med* 2002;30(11):S402–8.

13 Burfor AE, Ryan LM, Stone BJ, Hirshon JM, Klein BL. Drowning and near-drowning in children and adolescents: a succinct review for emergency physicians and nurses. *Pediatr Emerg Care* 2005;21(9): 610–11.

14 Tropjian AA, Berg RA, Joost JL, et al. Brain resuscitation in the drowning victim. *Neurocrit Care* 2012;17:441–67.

15 Quan L. Near-drowning. *Pediatr Rev* 1999;20:255–60.

16 Vanden Hoek TL, Morrison LJ, Shuster M, et al. Part 12.11: Drowning. Part 12: Cardiac Arrest in Special Situations 2010 American Heart Association Guidelines for Cardiopulmonary Resuscitation and Emergency Cardiovascular Care. *Circulation* 2010;122:S829–61.

17 Manolios N, Mackie I. Drowning and near-drowning on Australian beaches patrolled by life-savers: a 10-year study, 1973–1983. *Med J Aust* 1988;148:165–71.

18 Watson RS, Cummings P, Quan L, Bratton S, Weiss NS. Cervical spine injuries among submersion victims. *J Trauma* 2001;51:658–62.

CHAPTER 18

Choking

Gregory H. Gilbert

Introduction

Choking emergencies are important in EMS because of their time-sensitive nature. Victims of choking can rapidly progress from airway obstruction to loss of consciousness and cardiac arrest. Bystanders must act quickly to resolve true choking episodes. EMS personnel will likely arrive on scene several minutes after the onset of choking. Therefore, they must be prepared to manage a patient in the advanced stages of crisis. Choking is an emergency that must be solved on scene; there is limited value in bringing an unresolved choking victim to the emergency department for definitive treatment.

Pathophysiology and epidemiology

Choking results from obstruction of the trachea by a foreign object. It is the nature of the so-called "café coronary" that occurs during or shortly after a meal [1]. Although most choking episodes are associated with food, non-edible objects may also cause airway occlusion; particularly, children may inadvertently aspirate coins, toys, or other objects. Choking can occur with liquids as well as solid substances.

Although most obstructions occur in the hypopharynx, a small foreign body may lodge in either bronchus, causing selective obstruction of a lung or lung segment. Because the right bronchus travels more directly off the trachea, most selective obstructions involve the right lung.

Choking may be classified as partial or complete. A complete obstruction impairs the ability to breathe, to talk, and to cough and is an immediate life threat. A partial obstruction results in incomplete occlusion of the airway. In these instances the individual may still be able to breathe, talk, or cough. A complete occlusion generally mandates immediate intervention (such as the Heimlich maneuver, or direct laryngoscopy if ALS personnel are present). Other less invasive maneuvers may be appropriate in individuals with partial obstruction. However, in instances of partial obstruction with compromised air exchange, cyanosis, or loss of consciousness, the rescuer must approach the case as though it involves a complete airway obstruction [1].

The incidence of choking varies with age. Children younger than 1 year of age are most likely to choke, with food and liquids causing most of these episodes. Toddlers aged 1–4 years tend to choke on non-food items such as coins or latex balloons. Choking is less common in those aged 4–9 years and often occurs from gum and candy [2,3].

Choking incidence rises again at age 60 years from concurrent conditions impairing coordinated swallowing (e.g. Alzheimer dementia, stroke, drinking alcohol, seizure, or Parkinson disease) [4]. A prior choking episode significantly increases the chances of future choking.

Patient assessment

Because complete or partial airway obstruction may rapidly lead to cardiopulmonary arrest, expeditious recognition of choking is essential. Ideally, bystanders will recognize and immediately treat choking victims. Delay of recognition and treatment until EMS arrival will likely result in clinical deterioration. Patients suffering from complete airway obstruction usually present with classic signs, including aphonia, hands to the throat, and hyperemia of the face. Other more serious signs include altered mental status, cyanosis, and unconsciousness. Many conscious choking victims will exhibit the universal choking sign (hands crossed over the throat) and will nod in affirmation to the question, "Are you choking?" [5]

Partial airway obstruction may be more difficult to assess, especially in pediatric patients. These individuals may still have partial speaking ability. In many cases, the victim may exhibit paroxysmal coughing, drooling, stridor, or poor feeding. Common conditions mimicking foreign body aspiration include pneumonia, asthma, croup, and reactive airway disease [6,7]. An esophageal foreign body may also cause or mimic airway obstruction. Vital signs, pulse oximetry, and other diagnostic tools are not typically useful in establishing the severity

Emergency Medical Services: Clinical Practice and Systems Oversight, Second Edition. Volume 1: Clinical Aspects of EMS.
Edited by David C. Cone, Jane H. Brice, Theodore R. Delbridge, and J. Brent Myers.

of a choking episode. In one series, 2% of admitted adult choking patients had normal prehospital vital signs [8].

Clinical management

The clinical course and subsequent deterioration due to choking progress rapidly. In ideal circumstances, bystanders should resolve the airway obstruction, because even the most prompt EMS agencies will not arrive in time to perform needed interventions.

Patients presenting with complete airway obstruction should receive the Heimlich maneuver [9]. In the classic Heimlich procedure, the rescuer positions himself behind the sitting or standing patient, placing his arms around the chest at the level of the epigastrium. The rescuer places one fist against the epigastrium, using the other hand to apply quick upwards thrusts. The rescuer repeats the process until the obstruction clears.

For the unconscious patient, current ACLS guidelines recommend performing standard cardiopulmonary resuscitation (CPR) chest compressions [5]. The only caveat is that when giving breaths, rescuers should look inside the mouth to visualize and remove any foreign bodies. Abdominal compressions and blind finger sweeps are no longer recommended for unconscious persons [5,6].

For infants less than 1 year of age, the rescuer typically positions the victim with the head downward, alternating back blows with chest compressions. Bulb suction, visualized finger sweeps, and back blows often work well without the need for chest compressions [5,6,10].

Emergency medical services personnel responding to a choking emergency must be prepared to manage the advanced stages of crisis, and must act quickly on arriving at the scene. Bystanders may have failed to recognize that the patient is choking, leading emergency medical dispatchers to miscategorize the call as a condition other than choking (e.g. respiratory distress, chest pain, or unconscious person) due to inaccurate or incomplete information from the 9-1-1 caller. Bystanders may have already made unsuccessful attempts to clear the obstruction with the Heimlich maneuver. The patient may be unconscious or in cardiac arrest.

On confirming the presence of complete airway obstruction, rescuers should perform the Heimlich maneuver or chest compressions. In cases of partial airway obstruction, rescuers should monitor for signs of cyanosis, inadequate breathing, or unconsciousness, signifying the need to immediately provide the Heimlich maneuver or chest compressions. If the Heimlich maneuver does not resolve the obstruction, ALS personnel may attempt to directly visualize the airway with a laryngoscope, making efforts to remove visualized foreign bodies using Magill forceps. Foreign bodies below the vocal cords may be more problematic. Anecdotal reports suggest using a rigid suction catheter in these situations. Although data in this area are lacking, intubation is risky in these cases and may further lodge the foreign body. As a last resort, rescuers may consider performing cricothyroidotomy or transtracheal jet ventilation (TTJV). This approach will only work if the surgical airway is placed below the foreign body. There are anecdotal reports of high-pressure TTJV to eject entrapped foreign bodies. However, there are no organized reports of choking management using cricothyroidotomy or TTJV.

For patients with partial airway obstruction, there are additional management options. The patient should be encouraged to cough and expel the object. High-flow supplemental oxygen may be appropriate, although the sensation of the mask may make the patient feel uncomfortable, aggravating the situation. If the patient is able to adequately move air, it may be acceptable (and even preferable) to carefully transport the patient to the hospital for definitive care. In these cases, close monitoring of vital signs, oxygen saturation, respiratory effort, and level of consciousness are prudent. Monitoring of end-tidal carbon dioxide may also help to reveal early clinical deterioration, though research data on this are lacking. EMS personnel should provide advance notification to the receiving facility so that the emergency department can prepare its equipment and summon appropriate personnel. Because this is an airway emergency, it typically makes the most sense to go to the nearest hospital. At the receiving hospital, the patient may require urgent sedation, direct or video laryngoscopy, or surgical airway intervention by an emergency physician, otolaryngologist, gastroenterologist, anesthesiologist, or surgeon. Many emergency departments have a "difficult airway" algorithm that involves summoning various specialists to the emergency department to provide assistance in these situations.

Many choking victims refuse EMS care and/or transport. In general, however, it is recommended that patients who have their choking resolved before EMS arrival or by EMS providers be transported to the hospital for further evaluation to ensure that no complications have occurred [5,8,9,11]. This recommendation is based primarily on case reports of laryngospasm, pulmonary edema, anoxic brain injury, and retained foreign body occurring after choking episodes. In addition, there are case reports of damaged internal organs following abdominal and chest thrusts [12]. A patient who persists in refusing transport should be made aware of these possible risks. Informed refusal should be obtained by field personnel following system protocols.

As a final consideration, an anaphylactic reaction may masquerade as an upper airway obstruction, especially if the patient has recently eaten nuts [13]. If the history and presentation are suggestive of this situation, rescuers should consider therapy with epinephrine and antihistamines.

Medical oversight considerations

Deterioration after complete airway obstruction occurs so rapidly that direct medical oversight by phone or radio likely provides only limited value. In cases of partial obstruction, direct medical oversight may provide useful guidance regarding management and receiving hospital options. The most important consideration is to educate EMS personnel to recognize signs and symptoms of partial and complete obstruction. As bystander intervention is essential in treating choking, EMS community outreach and education efforts are equally important.

Emergency medical services physician presence at the scene may potentially play a role in selected complicated choking cases. Patients with partial airway obstructions may prove tenuous and difficult to manage, requiring a fine balance between supportive care and skilled airway intervention. An on-scene EMS physician may facilitate selection of optimal treatment strategies. In the event of complete airway obstruction unresolved by basic techniques, an on-scene EMS physician may be best qualified to perform advanced airway interventions, such as direct or video laryngoscopy and foreign body removal, rapid sequence intubation, or cricothyroidotomy. In all cases, the EMS physician's value will be greatest if he/she is present at the earliest stages of the event, before complete airway obstruction or anoxic injury.

Controversies

The most important controversies in choking management are the use of back blows and chest thrusts. The Heimlich Institute opposes both of these techniques. The American Heart Association (AHA) recommends these interventions if the Heimlich maneuver fails and the American Red Cross (ARC) also advocates for both [5,6,11]. The AHA and the ARC recommend chest thrusts instead of the Heimlich maneuver for unconscious, pregnant, and obese patients and for children less than 1 year of age.

Critics note that back blows can cause the object to lodge deeper and waste valuable time better spent performing the Heimlich maneuver. In a recent study, the Heimlich maneuver was 86.5% effective at removing an obstruction [8]. Back blows may prove effective in children less than 5 years of age [10]. Chest thrusts are associated with significantly higher morbidity and mortality than the Heimlich maneuver and should probably be reserved for the most serious choking victims [14].

Conclusion

Advanced Cardiac Life Support- and PALS-trained public and EMS providers have improved choking survival rates beyond 95% [5,15]. Expeditious recognition and treatment of choking

are essential and should ideally be accomplished by bystanders. EMS personnel arriving on the scene should be prepared to manage a significantly deteriorated patient. Patients with partial airway obstructions may tolerate supportive care and rapid transport to the hospital. All choking victims should receive transport to the hospital for evaluation.

References

1 Jacob B, Wiedbrauck C, Lamprecht J, Bonte W. Laryngologic aspects of bolus asphyxiation-bolus death. *Dysphagia* 1992;7:31–5.

2 Centers for Disease Control Nonfatal choking-related episodes among children — United States, 2001. *MMWR* 2002;51:945–8.

3 American Academy of Pediatrics Policy Statement. Prevention of choking among children. *Pediatrics* 2010;125:601–7.

4 Ekberg O, Feinberg M. Clinical and demographic data in 75 patients with near-fatal choking episodes. *Dysphagia* 1992;7:205–8.

5 Berg RA, Hemphill R, Abella BS, et al. 2010 American Heart Association Guidelines for Cardiopulmonary Resuscitation and Emergency Cardiovascular Care Science Part 5: Adult Basic Life Support. *Circulation* 2010;122:S685–S705.

6 Berg DB, Schexnayder SM, Chameides L, et al. 2010 American Heart Association Guidelines for Cardiopulmonary Resuscitation and Emergency Cardiovascular Care Science Part 13: Pediatric Basic Life Support. *Circulation* 2010;122:S862–S875.

7 Franzese CB, Schweinfurth JM. Delayed diagnosis of a pediatric airway foreign body: case report and review of the literature. *Ear Nose Throat J* 2002;81:655–6.

8 Soroudi A, Shipp HE, Stepanski BM, et al. Adult foreign body airway obstruction in the prehospital setting. *Prehosp Emerg Care* 2007;11:25–9.

9 Heimlich HJ. A life-saving maneuver to prevent food-choking. *JAMA* 1975;234:398–401.

10 Vilke GM, Smith AM, Ray LU, Steen PJ, Murrin PA, Chan TC. Airway obstruction in children aged less than 5 years: the prehospital experience. *Prehosp Emerg Care* 2004;8:196–9.

11 Heimlich HJ, Patrick EA. The Heimlich maneuver: best technique for saving any choking victim's life. *Postgrad Med* 1990; 87:38–48,53.

12 Fearing NM, Harrison PB. Complications of the Heimlich maneuver: case report and literature review. *J Trauma* 2002;53: 978–9.

13 Nguyen AD, Gern JE. Food allergy masquerading as foreign body obstruction. *Ann Allergy Asthma Immunol* 2003;90:271–2.

14 Hashimoto Y, Moriya F, Furumiya J. Forensic aspects of complications resulting from cardiopulmonary resuscitation. *Leg Med (Tokyo)* 2007;9:94–9.

15 Baker TW, King W, Soto W, Asher C, Stolfi A, Rowin ME. The efficacy of pediatric advanced life support training in emergency medical service providers. *Pediatr Emerg Care* 2009;8:508–12.

CHAPTER 19

Syncope

David J. Schoenwetter

Introduction

Syncope is defined as a "loss of consciousness and postural tone caused by diminished cerebral blood flow [1]." Also, by definition, the condition must be self-corrected so as to cause a return to normal state of consciousness. Syncope is a common complaint in both the emergency department (ED) and in prehospital medicine and is the sixth leading cause of hospital admission in people over the age of 65 [2,3]. Of course, estimates are limited by the accuracy of determining true syncope versus other transient causes of loss of consciousness. Transient loss of consciousness has a cumulative lifetime incidence of approximately 35% [4].

Pathophysiology

It is important to understand the multiple etiologies that lead to the final pathway of a transient loss of consciousness. Any process that results in a loss of consciousness must affect both cerebral hemispheres simultaneously or involve the reticular activating system in the brainstem. In the case of syncope, the pathological process is transient, resulting from a loss of needed substrate to the brain (be it oxygen or other nutrients) that corrects without external therapeutic intervention (such as the administration of IV dextrose). Typically, the impairment of substrate delivery is caused in part by upright posture. Thus, assuming a supine position after consciousness is lost improves substrate delivery and typically leads to spontaneous recovery.

As with any disease process, classification of etiology aids in diagnosis, treatment, and prognosis for patients. Understanding the patient's prognosis helps in ensuring a safe disposition. Unfortunately, the classification schemes for etiologies of syncope are broad, vary by author, are to some degree subjective, and frequently overlap. For the purpose of this discussion, syncope will be classified into four broad categories: cardiac, neurological, vascular (or reflex mediated), and idiopathic (Table 19.1).

Cardiac syncope is due to a transient lack of adequate cardiac output, causing inadequate cerebral perfusion and subsequent loss of consciousness. Dysrhythmia is a common cardiac etiology and is one of great clinical importance. The most common dysrhythmia associated with syncope is transient ventricular tachycardia (VT). These occurrences are seen most frequently in patients with histories of congestive heart failure and low ejection fraction and portend a poor prognosis (1-year mortality up to 40%). Other culprit dysrhythmias include severe sinus bradycardia or transient high-grade heart blocks, supraventricular tachycardias, sick sinus syndrome, and atrial fibrillation with rapid ventricular response. As a rule, all of the aforementioned dysrhythmias must be paroxysmal in nature to cause a syncope episode, because there must be a return of cerebral perfusion for the patient to regain consciousness.

Other cardiac causes of syncope include restrictive cardiomyopathies, valvular heart disease (especially severe aortic stenosis and mitral regurgitation), pulmonary embolus, and, rarely, cardiac ischemia (although syncope from such is most likely dysrhythmia related). Although these pathologies can cause transient reductions in cardiac output sufficient to create a syncopal episode, their overall occurrence is rare. One population of young patients who have dangerous syncope is those with congenital prolonged QT syndrome. This is why it is important to check a rhythm strip on every syncope patient.

Reflex-mediated syncope is the most common cause and (barring secondary trauma, as from a subsequent fall or automobile collision) poses the best prognosis. Although listed as 35% here, some studies have attributed up to 58% of syncope to this etiology [5]. Reflex-mediated syncope occurs when the body has an inappropriate autonomic response to a change in posture. Under normal circumstances, when a person moves from recumbent to upright, a significant amount of blood (300–800 mL) will pool in the lower extremities [6]. In response, the sympathetic nervous system causes peripheral vasoconstriction, stimulates increased cardiac contractility, and increases the heart rate. These processes counteract the transient

Emergency Medical Services: Clinical Practice and Systems Oversight, Second Edition. Volume 1: Clinical Aspects of EMS.
Edited by David C. Cone, Jane H. Brice, Theodore R. Delbridge, and J. Brent Myers.

Table 19.1 Classification of syncope

Cardiac (~20%)	Neurological (~10%)	Reflex mediated (~35%)	Idiopathic (~35%)
Dysrhythmia	Migraine	Vasovagal	
Ventricular fibrillation	Subclavian steal	Orthostatic	
Ventricular tachycardia	Transient ischemia	Hyperventilation	
Supraventricular tachycardia	Subarachnoid hemorrhage	Carotid sinus syndrome	
Atrial fibrillation with	Psychogenic		
rapid ventricular response			
Outflow obstruction			
Aortic stenosis			
Atrial myxoma			
Mitral stenosis			
Restrictive cardiomyopathy			
Pericardial tamponade			
Cardiac ischemia			
Pulmonary embolism			
Aortic dissection			
Congenital heart disease			
Congenital prolonged			
QT syndrome			

"distributive shock" experienced by the central nervous system, thus preventing syncope.

For patients experiencing reflex-mediated syncope, there is an inappropriate reflexive stimulation of the parasympathetic nervous system that overshadows the appropriate sympathetic response. These patients experience hypotension, with or without bradycardia. The resultant lack of cerebral perfusion results in a syncopal episode.

Neurogenic syncope, as a pure cause of transient loss of consciousness, is actually a rare event. Many of the neurological events that result in syncope have poorly explained mechanisms. Additionally, many neurological events that involve a loss of consciousness are incorrectly labeled as syncope. It is important to note, however, that some neurological causes of syncope represent serious pathological processes, such as subarachnoid hemorrhage and transient ischemic attack. It is rare that such diseases manifest as syncopal episodes, but caution must be exercised if these diagnoses are considered.

Assessment

The first task in assessing and managing syncope, in both the prehospital and ED settings, is to separate syncope from the other potential reasons for a loss of consciousness. First, any non-transient loss of consciousness, by definition, is not syncope. A patient who has a loss of consciousness from hypoglycemia, requires IV dextrose, and then awakens to a normal level of consciousness has not had a syncopal episode. Likewise, if the patient has a complex, non-motor seizure and then recovers from a postictal state to a normal mental status, this too is not syncope. However, for the EMS provider, all of these might be dispatched as "altered mental status," "unconscious," or "syncope," depending on a number of variables, including the quality of information exchanged between the caller and call-taker. This can incorrectly prejudice providers to presume or discount syncope as the diagnosis.

As with all medical problems, proper assessment and evaluation begin with an appropriately focused history and physical examination. Although 85–90% of all patient pathology can be determined by history and physical exam, these are even more important in the case of syncope. There are very few diagnostic tests that will aid in determining the cause of a syncopal episode or in ascertaining syncope as the problem versus another malady. If one takes a diagnosis such as appendicitis, we know that it can be determined clinically almost 90% of the time, but also can be "confirmed" by computed tomography (CT) scanning, by surgical findings, or by the pathology results. However, in the case of a syncopal episode, there are few laboratory or other diagnostic studies that will aid significantly in the diagnosis.

History is the most important information in the case of syncope. For patients in the prehospital setting, the history obtained by EMS providers is pivotal to the patient's evaluation. Because true syncope involves a loss of consciousness, there will be details of the event that patients will not be able to provide. Frequently these patients arrive alone to the ED, and the emergency physician has no opportunity to interview others who may have witnessed the episode. Therefore, maximizing history obtained at the scene and relaying this to the ED staff is pivotal to accurate diagnosis and treatment.

It is important to ask the patient what he or she can remember before the event. No recollection at all is of particular importance. If the patient felt no prodromal symptoms at all, and then had a period of unconsciousness, this is particularly concerning for cardiac causes of syncope. Chest pain, palpitations, and shortness of breath are other symptoms that can be associated with dysrhythmia or other cardiac pathology. Abdominal pain, nausea, or lightheadedness frequently precede reflex-mediated syncope. Always attempt to ascertain the last thing the patient remembers before the event, as well as the first thing he or she can remember after regaining consciousness.

In the case of a true syncopal event, the patient will not be able to convey information about happenings during his or her period of unconsciousness. Bystander interview is paramount, and, as mentioned previously, EMS personnel may be the only medical providers able to obtain this vital information. Did the bystanders notice anything before the patient lost consciousness? Was there any seizure activity noted (tonic/clonic, focal, etc.)? Were there any periods of apnea noted? Bystander history is also imperative for determining the length of the unresponsive period. Unfortunately, this time interval will frequently be overestimated due to the anxiety provoked in bystanders seeing someone unresponsive. Still, careful and compassionate interviews by EMS personnel can frequently elicit valuable references to attempt to establish a time course. Was the patient unconscious for the entire 9-1-1 phone call? How long before EMS arrival did the patient regain consciousness?

Finally, prehospital providers must obtain the bystanders' history of events as the patient regained consciousness. Did the patient's mental status improve rapidly or was there a period of confusion? Did the patient have any complaints on awakening that he or she cannot recall now? Did the patient appear hot or cold, sweaty, or pale? If the bystanders took the patient's pulse, what was the rate and quality?

Beyond the history of present illness, EMS providers must also obtain other pertinent medical history. Chronic health problems (especially cardiac, vascular, or neurological problems) need to be documented because they are important risk factors in syncope. A complete medication list (as always) must be obtained because many medications can predispose a patient to syncope. Additionally, medications can frequently point to other causes of loss of consciousness that are not syncopal episodes, such as seizures or hypoglycemia. Last oral intake should be ascertained to determine if the patient is at risk for hypoglycemia and to see if there are any confounders to the mental status examination, such as drugs or alcohol.

A focused physical examination is always important for any complete patient assessment. Vital signs, skin condition, heart, lung, and abdominal examination, and a thorough neurological examination are essential. Many recommend checking orthostatic vital signs, at least lying and sitting (for fear of patient trauma if there is a fall when standing). However, there are many confounders to positive or negative orthostatic vital signs and even much debate over what are the appropriate and inappropriate changes [6]. But if the patient becomes symptomatic with changes in position, this is important to note.

It is important to remember that, at the time of EMS assessment, the physical examination may be completely normal. Vital signs may be within normal limits, and the remainder of the examination may be unremarkable. Unfortunately, this does not preclude the existence of serious pathology. Cardiac syncope in particular is likely to present with a normal physical examination, despite being potentially lethal.

Consistent with most prehospital encounters, diagnostic testing is of limited value. A glucometer reading should be obtained, despite the fact that glucose abnormalities rarely cause transient loss of consciousness. A prehospital 12-lead ECG is indicated because this may help to risk-stratify the patient's potential syncopal etiology. According to the 2009 European Society of Cardiology (ESC) guidelines, the following ECG findings are considered diagnostic for syncope due to a dysrhythmia [7].

- Persistent sinus bradycardia <40 bpm
- Repetitive sinoatrial blocks or sinus pauses >3 seconds
- Mobitz II – second-degree heart block
- Third-degree heart block
- Alternating left and right bundle branch blocks
- Ventricular tachycardia
- Rapid paroxysmal supraventricular tachycardia
- Automatic implantable cardioverter defibrillator or pacer dysfunction

It is important to note, however, that a normal 12-lead ECG does not preclude life-threatening causes of syncope, as the event has usually passed at the time of EMS assessment. As in the ED, it is hoped that future research can determine which patients are at risk for a life-threatening cause of syncope.

Differential diagnosis

One of the most important steps in evaluating syncope is to ensure the event was truly a syncopal episode and not a loss or alteration of consciousness attributable to some other pathology. The most common pathology confused with syncope is seizures. Both clearly involve a loss of consciousness, and other findings classically associated with seizures can occur with true syncopal episodes. Incontinence is rare in syncope but does occur. Also, shortly following a syncopal episode, a patient may experience myoclonic jerks that can be confused with seizure. The most important distinguishing feature is the postictal period. Generalized seizure patients typically have postictal phases lasting minutes, whereas the return to normal mentation after a syncopal episode rarely exceeds 30 seconds.

Pseudosyncope is a psychiatric condition in which there is no actual loss of consciousness, and a syncopal episode is fabricated for whatever psychiatric reason exists. This condition is separate from psychogenic syncope, which involves a true syncopal episode (with an actual loss of consciousness) that is caused by a psychiatric stimulus (severe emotional distress, pain, other psychiatric condition). Frequently, it will be difficult to separate these in the prehospital environment. Confronting the patient regarding presumed pseudosyncope will frequently destroy the therapeutic relationship in an uncontrolled environment, and therefore should be discouraged.

Two other rare conditions that may be confused with syncope are narcolepsy and cataplexy. Narcolepsy is a condition in which patients have profound daytime sleepiness such that they may suddenly fall asleep in the middle of the day. This will rarely occur so suddenly, however, as to result in a loss in postural tone. Cataplexy however, is defined as a sudden, uncontrolled loss of postural tone, and to witnesses this may appear as a syncope episode. However, patients with true cataplexy will not lose consciousness.

Many of the other presentations that are commonly confused with syncope are readily identifiable by health care providers once they assess the patient and situation. Pathologies such as hypoglycemia, stroke, cardiac failure, hypoxia, anaphylaxis, and the like should be readily identifiable by EMS physicians and other providers performing the history and physical examination.

Treatment

For most cases of true syncope in the prehospital environment, immediate treatment needs are minimal. Unless witnessed by prehospital personnel, the event has almost by definition resolved on EMS arrival. As always, each patient requires a careful, thorough, but focused history and physical examination. Each patient should also receive cardiac monitoring to evaluate for dysrhythmia. The value of IV access is debatable, unless the suspicion for a cardiac dysrhythmia (which may recur and require IV medication) is high. Glucose testing is indicated. Although ischemia is rare, a 12-lead ECG should be performed by EMS.

Disposition

Experience shows that determining patient disposition after EMS contact can be complicated, time consuming, and fraught with medical and legal hazards. This is particularly true for patients who, at the time of EMS assessment, are not having any complaints or lack an obvious acute pathology that requires intervention. Unfortunately, patients experiencing syncope frequently fall into this category. Usually, by the time of EMS arrival, the patient has regained consciousness and his or her mental status has returned to baseline. Even patients with potentially life-threatening causes of syncope, such as dysrhythmia, may have no complaints or physical examination findings during prehospital assessment.

So what should we do with these patients? In the vast majority of EMS systems, the only two choices are to transport the patient or obtain an informed refusal of care and transport. It is rare that syncope patients require specialty referral centers, especially if they are asymptomatic at time of EMS arrival. Usually, the rare causes of syncope that may require specialty referral (e.g. myocardial infarction,

subarachnoid hemorrhage, and trauma after syncope) do not present asymptomatically. Therefore, for patients who agree to transport to the ED for evaluation, the closest facility is usually appropriate.

For the patient refusing transport, EMS personnel must decide if the patient has adequately displayed decision-making capacity, including full understanding of risks, benefits, and alternatives. The explanation of the risks is perhaps the most important issue when considering the syncopal patient's capacity to refuse transport. It is imperative that the prehospital personnel have a clear understanding of the pathologies previously mentioned and can correlate those with the patient's presentation. The level of training of the prehospital personnel (EMT, paramedic, nurse, or physician) will alter the ability to determine possible pathologies, the understanding of these, and the risk of not receiving evaluation in the ED.

The prehospital environment presents a complicated and dynamic practice arena, even more so than the ED. Due to this, it is impossible to cover all possibilities regarding patient presentation and disposition. In the end, it is up to the prehospital provider to ensure that the patient's final disposition is safe and in his or her best interest. Although the patient's right to make decisions regarding his or her health care must be respected, it is equally important that all patients fully understand the potential risks associated with their conditions, and the evaluation and treatment options that exist.

Conclusion

Syncope is a transient loss of consciousness with a spontaneous return to a normal, baseline mental status. It is a common complaint in both the prehospital and ED settings. Although the exact etiology of syncope is frequently not ascertained, careful history and physical examination can determine the cause for the majority of those patients who can be diagnosed. Certain diagnoses, especially cardiac dysrhythmias, can be potentially life threatening and require proper evaluation and observation. Safe disposition of the patient requires a careful evaluation in the prehospital setting, and appropriate explanation to those who frequently have no symptoms at the time of evaluation.

References

1 *Stedman's Medical Dictionary*, 27th edn. Baltimore, MD: Williams and Wilkins, 2000, p.1745.
2 Kenny RA, O'Shea D, Walker HF. Impact of a dedicated syncope and falls facility for older adults on emergency beds. *Age Ageing* 2002;31(4):272–5.
3 Thijs RD, Wieling W, Kaufmann H, van Dijk JG. Defining and classifying syncope. *Clin Auton Res* 2004;14(suppl 1):4–8.

4 Ganzeboom KS, Mairuhu G, Reitsma J, et al. Lifetime cumulative incidence of syncope in the general population: a study of 549 Dutch subjects aged 35–60 years. *J Cardiovasc Electrophysiol* 2006;17(11):1172–6.

5 5.Olshansky B. Evaluation of syncope in adults. *UpToDate* 2012; Jun 15.

6 Morag R. Syncope. Available at: http://emedicine.medscape.com/article/811669-overview

7 Task Force for the Diagnosis and Management of Syncope, European Society of Cardiology (ESC), European Heart Rhythm Association (EHRA), Heart Failure Association (HFA), Heart Rhythm Society (HRS), Moya A, Sutton R, Ammirati F, et al. Guidelines for the diagnosis and management of syncope (version 2009). *Eur Heart J* 2009;30(21):2631.

Further reading

Blok BK. Syncope. In: Tintinalli JE, Kelen GD, Stapczynski JS (eds) *Emergency Medicine, A Comprehensive Study Guide*, 5th edn. New York: McGraw Hill, 2000, pp.352–6.

Daroff RB, Martin JB. Faintness, syncope, dizziness and vertigo. In: Fauci AS, Braunwald E, Isselbacher KJ, et al (eds) *Harrison's Principles of Internal Medicine*, 14th edn. New York: McGraw-Hill, 1998.

Henry GL, Jagoda A, Little N, Pellegrino TR (eds) Syncope. In: *Neurologic Emergencies, A Symptom-oriented Approach*, 2nd edn. New York: McGraw-Hill, 2004, pp.283–94.

Koziol-McLain J, Lowenstein SR, Fuller B. Orthostatic vital signs in emergency department patients. *Ann Emerg Med* 1991;20(6): 606–10.

CHAPTER 20

Seizures

J. Stephen Huff

Introduction

Generalized convulsive seizures are frightening to observe and often result in EMS calls. Provoked seizures represent symptoms of an acute underlying medical or neurological condition. Seizures often occur without clear etiology or provocation. Epilepsy, sometimes referred to as a seizure disorder, is defined by recurrent unprovoked seizures.

It is estimated that between 1% and 2% of emergency department (ED) visits are for seizure-related complaints, with many of these patients using EMS systems. Most receive advanced-level care [1]. In one study, seizures accounted for almost 12% of pediatric EMS transports [2].

One study showed that seizures were a common cause of repeated ambulance use [3]. Every community has a cadre of patients with poorly controlled seizures or alcohol-related seizures who use EMS frequently. This familiar group of frequent users may lead to a casual indifference to all patients with seizures. Physicians and providers must recall that seizures at some level are the symptom of some central nervous system (CNS) dysfunction and initiate appropriate management steps to terminate seizures to lessen morbidity.

Pathophysiology

The concept of a seizure threshold suggests that everyone has the capacity to experience seizures at some level of individual physiological stress. The precipitating events may be electrolyte abnormalities, medications, medication withdrawal, toxins, hypoxia, CNS infections, systemic infections, trauma, or even sleep deprivation. A fundamental distinction in management is to determine whether a seizure results from some identifiable cause or if it is unprovoked. When seizures are secondary to some other condition, they are termed *symptomatic seizures* or *provoked seizures*. Unprovoked seizures occur without an identifiable cause. Again, epilepsy is defined by episodes of unprovoked seizures.

At a cellular level, seizures are thought to originate in the cerebral cortex or thalamus. Lesions of the brainstem, deep white matter, and cerebellum are not epileptogenic. Seizures result from excitation of susceptible groups of cerebral neurons, with progressively larger groups of neurons developing synchronous discharges. Clinical signs and symptoms follow when a critical mass of neurons is reached [4]. At a biochemical level, there is a disturbance in the balance of cellular excitation and inhibition. Glutamate is the most common excitatory neurotransmitter and acts at the n-methyl-D-asparate (NMDA) receptor. Current theory is that failure of inhibition mediated by the neurotransmitter gamma-aminobutyric acid (GABA) system leads to prolongation of most seizure types. The neurotransmitter receptor sites are thought to be the sites of action of the antiepileptic drugs.

With frequent or persistent seizure activity, physiological changes of hypoxia, acidosis, hyperthermia, hypotension, and reduced cerebral perfusion may occur. At one time these were thought to be the cause of neuronal injury. However, many different avenues of investigation have suggested that injury follows prolonged excessive neuronal discharges even if systemic pathophysiological factors are controlled [4]. Some experimental evidence suggests that neurotransmitter receptors may change in sensitivity or quantity with prolonged seizures; potentially effectiveness of medications might change as seizure duration persists [5,6].

Differential diagnosis

There is a differential diagnosis for seizures since a number of clinical conditions may simulate generalized convulsions (Box 20.1). Syncope is a frequent consideration in the differential diagnosis. Loss of consciousness is abrupt in syncope and occasionally the brief myoclonic jerks that accompany the faint are a source of confusion. "Convulsive syncope" results from the cerebral hypoperfusion during the syncopal event. Investigations and treatments should be directed toward the cause of syncope [7].

Emergency Medical Services: Clinical Practice and Systems Oversight, Second Edition. Volume 1: Clinical Aspects of EMS.
Edited by David C. Cone, Jane H. Brice, Theodore R. Delbridge, and J. Brent Myers.
© 2015 NAEMSP. Published 2015 by John Wiley & Sons, Inc. Companion Website: www.wiley.com\go\cone\naemsp

A person suffering a blow to the head may have a brief episode of extremity stiffening at the time of impact that understandably may be confused with seizure activity. These events clinically resemble brief abnormal extensor posturing, though myoclonic and tonic-clonic movements are also described. Return to consciousness following these events is usually prompt. These "convulsive concussions" are not associated with injury or neurological sequelae and do not predict future seizures [8,9]. Posttraumatic epilepsy may occur after head trauma but is associated with more severe head injuries. These seizures are typical in appearance and associated with a postictal confusional state.

In any series of stroke patients, seizures and postictal states are a significant source of diagnostic confusion [10,11]. Seizure patients may have postictal weakness or confusion that mimics some stroke symptoms. Subarachnoid hemorrhage may cause fragmentary or repetitive extensor posturing that at times is confused with seizures [12,13].

Non-epileptic seizures, also known as pseudoseizures, psychogenic, or hysterical seizures, often result in diagnostic uncertainty. Simply stated, the patient appears to be having a seizure but subsequent observations prove that the apparent convulsion does not follow from the excessive neuronal discharges that characterize epileptic seizures. The usual descriptions of non-epileptic seizures include side-to-side head movements, out-of-phase limb movements, and pelvic thrusting [14]. However, other reports indicate that simple unresponsiveness without motor movements is a frequent presentation [15].

Classification of seizure types

In theory, almost any behavior or experience may result from the abnormal synchronous discharges of groups of neurons. Motor movements, sensory experiences, or abnormal behaviors may all represent seizures [16]. Patterns are seen that allow a categorization of seizures (Box 20.2) [17]. Modern classification schemes are based on video electroencephalogram (EEG) correlations, but at times seizure-type classification may be made from direct patient observation.

A fundamental distinction is whether the seizure is of partial onset or generalized onset. This distinction may be important clinically because partial-onset seizures may imply focal or structural CNS abnormalities and because different medications are effective in different seizure types. In partial-onset seizures, clinical information indicates that seizure onset is limited to one part of the brain. Partial seizures may be further divided into simple partial seizures, complex partial seizures, and partial seizures that secondarily become generalized.

In a simple partial seizure, the patient remains at normal consciousness. Partial seizures with sensory symptoms include some patients with episodic paresthesias. Special sensory symptoms delineate seizures with gustatory, olfactory, or auditory components. The term *complex* implies that consciousness is clouded. Symptoms of these patients are often altered mental status with confusion and simple repetitive motor movements such as lip smacking or picking at clothes. Sometimes prolonged confusional states occur with complex partial seizures, one of the types of non-convulsive status epilepticus [18].

Generalized-onset seizures imply that the cerebral cortex is bilaterally involved at seizure onset. This often requires EEG evaluation for definitive diagnosis. The types of generalized seizures are listed in Box 20.2. Some seizure types are typical enough in appearance that they can be classified by observation alone. Partial-onset seizures with secondary generalization are the most common type of generalized seizure in adults. An example of a partial-onset seizure with secondary generalization would be a patient with onset of finger twitching, progression of movements to the arm and face, and then a subsequent generalized convulsive seizure. However, often this secondary generalization occurs too rapidly to be appreciated by witnesses or in the field.

A few words concerning terminology are in order. *Convulsion* refers to the motor movements associated with a seizure. *Tonic* refers to the stiffening of the extremities seen in convulsions. *Clonic* is the rhythmic, synchronized movements of the extremities. Some patients experience an *aura*, which is the initial subjective perception of a seizure. *Grand mal* is generally used in a manner to be synonymous with a generalized convulsion. *Petit mal*, however, is so frequently misused by patients and physicians that perhaps that term is best not used. Correctly used, it is synonymous with absence seizures, a generalized-onset seizure that has a characteristic EEG three-cycle-per-second pattern. In common usage, however, petit mal is corrupted by association with the word petite, meaning "small," so that fragments of seizures or partial seizures are incorrectly labeled petit mal seizures.

Symptomatic seizures

A basic point in assessment and management is whether a seizure is secondary to some medical condition, such as electrolyte abnormalities, toxins, hypoxia, CNS infections, systemic infections, or trauma. EMS plays a key role in gathering historical information to identify likely seizure causes and initiating therapy. A few causes of symptomatic seizures warrant particular comment.

Alcohol withdrawal seizure is a type of symptomatic seizure that usually occurs within 48 hours of cessation of drinking [19]. Usually alcohol withdrawal seizures are single and brief, but up to 30% of patients have recurrent seizures in the ED [20,21]. Studies of patients with status epilepticus show that in a significant proportion, the seizures are alcohol related [22].

Many different toxins may cause seizures [23,24]. Sympathomimetics, including cocaine, are perhaps the most frequently encountered. Other toxins that may cause seizures include antidepressants, antihistamines, salicylates, and anticholinergics. Isoniazid, used to treat tuberculosis, deserves specific mention because the mechanism of action of the drug requires a specific antidote: pyridoxine (vitamin B_6) [25].

Seizures in association with advanced pregnancy or in the postpartum patient may represent eclampsia. Hypertension is present. Treatment involves magnesium sulfate and possibly benzodiazepines.

Febrile seizures

Febrile seizures are one of the most common seizure types encountered in emergency practice, in both the field and the ED. Definitions in the literature vary, but a seizure associated with fever in children aged 6 months to 5 years without evidence of intracranial infection or other definite cause of seizure is an accepted definition. The age-delineated definition acknowledges the sensitivity of the maturing brain to fever [26]. Excluded are febrile-associated seizures in patients who have experienced afebrile seizures. Peak incidence is at 18 months. Other events that may simulate seizures in this age group include rigors, breath-holding spells, apneic episodes, and anoxic seizures. History is key in sorting out these events.

Many febrile seizures occur early in the course of the underlying illness and may be the presenting symptom of the illness.

The magnitude and peak of the fever are likely to be more important than the rate of increase in provoking seizures. Antipyretics have not been shown to be effective in reducing the risk of febrile seizures [26].

Febrile seizures are often divided into simple and complex types. A simple febrile seizure is a generalized tonic-clonic convulsion without focal signs lasting less than 10 minutes, resolving spontaneously, and not recurring within 24 hours. Complex febrile seizures fall outside this definition due to focal signs during the seizures, seizure duration, or recurrence.

By definition, a simple febrile seizure will likely have ceased by arrival of EMS, unless the response interval is very short. Recurrent or prolonged seizures exclude this diagnosis and point to a complex febrile seizure or another cause for the seizure. EMS and other sources of history are important in eliciting a history of irritability, decreased feeding, or abnormal consciousness that might suggest an underlying CNS infection. Most children experiencing febrile seizures recover within 30 minutes. Postictal alteration of consciousness persisting more than 60 minutes has been suggested as a risk factor for a complicating medical condition [27].

Status epilepticus

Ongoing seizures or status epilepticus may occur in any seizure type and terminology may be confusing (Box 20.3). Generalized convulsive status epilepticus represents a true emergency condition because the ongoing electrical seizure activity is itself injurious to the brain. In late or decompensated status epilepticus, there may be a dissociation between the ongoing electrical seizure activity and motor convulsions [28,29]. In other types of status epilepticus, such as the non-convulsive status seen in prolonged absence seizures, the link between prolonged electrical activity and neuronal injury is not established.

Morbidity in generalized convulsive status epilepticus is related to the duration of the seizures and, importantly, to any underlying medical causes of the seizures. Modern definitions of generalized convulsive status epilepticus use a period as short

---

Box 20.3 Proposed terminology: status epilepticus

Non-convulsive status epilepticus
    Complex partial status epilepticus
    Absence status epilepticus
Generalized convulsive status epilepticus
    Generalized convulsive status epilepticus, overt
    Generalized convulsive status epilepticus, subtle
Simple partial status epilepticus with motor symptoms
Other enduring seizure types

Note: Confusion exists in the terminology. Non-convulsive status epilepticus has been used in the past to encompass such diverse seizure types as partial complex status epilepticus, absence status epilepticus, and epileptic confusional states, as well as generalized convulsive status epilepticus that has evolved a dissociation of the motor convulsions and ongoing electrical activity.

Box 20.4 Differential diagnosis of generalized convulsive status epilepticus

Non-epileptic seizures (pseudoseizures)
Repetitive abnormal posturing
Tetanus
Neuroleptic malignant syndrome
Rigors
Myoclonic jerks
Tremors
Involuntary movements including hemiballismus

Box 20.5 Prehospital approach to patient with generalized seizures

If convulsion is recurrent or ongoing:
Assess ABCs: oxygen supplementation, adjunctive airway if necessary
Protect patient from harm: protect head, move away from hard objects
Rapid glucose determination or dextrose administration
Benzodiazepine administration IM or IV
Intravenous access

as 5 minutes of continuous seizures to define the status and indicate the need to initiate treatment to terminate the seizures [30]. The other component of the definition is generalized seizures without recovery to full consciousness between seizures. There is a differential diagnosis for generalized convulsive status epilepticus (Box 20.4).

EMS evaluation and response

The most appropriate system response to a patient with seizures is not known because presentations vary greatly. Many patients experience a brief event that has terminated by time of EMS arrival . Other patients may be convulsing at the time of EMS arrival and require ALS interventions. Often a patient with a history of seizures requests not to be transported. Usual system protocols should be followed for patient non-transport with the caveat that the patient is awake, alert, and judged to be capable of making decisions. Ideally, there should be a companion present for assistance should the seizures reoccur.

A brief period of observation and examination should be performed after EMS arrival. Establish unresponsiveness as a survey for trauma is undertaken. Note if there is resistance to eye opening because most patients with seizures will have open eyes. Forced eye closure may suggest non-epileptic seizures.

Safety issues include protection by moving the patient away from any hard or sharp objects that might be struck during convulsive movements. If the teeth are clenched, they should not be pried open. However, if chewing movements are continuing and the tongue is being lacerated, an adjunctive airway device, such as an oropharyngeal airway, may be gently placed between the teeth to prevent further injury.

Following a generalized seizure, the patient is often somnolent and snoring respirations are present that will typically resolve with placement of a nasopharyngeal airway. Oxygen supplementation by mask is recommended. Assessment for airway integrity proceeds as usual but with the expectation that the patient will become more responsive as the postictal state resolves. IV access is recommended if the patient is not fully awake.

Hypoglycemia is common and may cause seizures. Perform rapid glucose determination if possible; consider dextrose administration in diabetics or if hypoglycemia is suspected. In some systems thiamine is available and should be administered if the possibility of malnutrition is present.

History should be obtained if possible. Key factors include a history of epilepsy, current medications, substance abuse, medical conditions, or trauma. A description of the event should be obtained from witnesses, including a description of any prodromal symptoms.

Physical examination includes a survey for injury. Some physical examination findings suggest seizures. Tongue biting on the lateral portion of the tongue suggests convulsions, although absence of tongue biting has no diagnostic value [31]. Incontinence suggests a generalized seizure.

If the patient is still convulsing at the time of EMS arrival, status epilepticus may be presumed to be present, again unless the response interval is very short [30,32]. Seizure duration of greater than 5 minutes or recurrent seizures without regaining consciousness between convulsions are the modern definition of status epilepticus. Initial stabilization steps and preparation for medication administration should proceed (Box 20.5).

Pharmacological interventions

Pharmacological interventions by EMS will often be limited to benzodiazepines, with the exception of some EMS physician units and critical care transport units. Boxes 20.6 and 20.7 summarize dose recommendations.

Generally speaking, IV administration of benzodiazepines has been the standard because of rapid therapeutic drug levels, but a variety of reports substantiates the effectiveness of intramuscular, rectal, nasal, and buccal administration of different agents. Benzodiazepines are well tolerated, with the primary side-effects of sedation and respiratory depression. The respiratory depression seems to be related to time to peak serum concentration. Somewhat paradoxically, the IV route may offer the quickest time to peak concentrations but at a risk of greater respiratory depression.

The use of alternative routes is particularly attractive in the pediatric population. Intraosseous administration should be an effective route of administration but is little studied in seizure patients. Rectal administration of benzodiazepines (particularly diazepam) for status epilepticus in children has been reported for years [33]. Studied dosages are 0.5 mg/kg administered using a syringe and a soft catheter. Correction should be made for

> **Box 20.6** Initial benzodiazepine dosing for generalized convulsive status epilepticus in adults
>
> Lorazepam (Ativan) 0.1–0.15 mg/kg IV over 1–2 minutes (repeat once if no response after 5 minutes – maximum dose 8 mg)
> OR
> Midazolam (Versed) 10 mg IV or IM
> OR
> Diazepam (Valium) 0.2 mg/kg at 5 mg/min (max. 20 mg)

> **Box 20.7** Initial benzodiazepine dosing for generalized convulsive status epilepticus in children
>
> Lorazepam (Ativan) 0.1–0.15 mg/kg IV over 2–5 minutes or IM to maximum dose of 8 mg
> OR
> Midazolam (Versed) 0.2 mg/kg IV or IM to maximum of 10 mg
> OR
> Diazepam (Valium) 0.2–0.3 mg/kg IV over 2–5 minutes (max. 10 mg) or 0.5 mg/kg per rectum
>
> Note: See text for details of alternative dosing regimens. Respiratory depression is the most serious side-effect and is likely related to rate of administration.

volume left in the catheter. A second dose of 0.25 mg/kg may be administered if needed. Peak levels are thought to be reached within 10 minutes. A Food and Drug Administration (FDA)-approved preparation, Diastat, is available [34].

Nasal administration of benzodiazepines (usually midazolam) has been reported in small case series [35]. Ease of use was the focus in studies comparing nasal midazolam with IV diazepam [36]. Time to seizure cessation was comparable. Another report compared intranasal administration of midazolam using an atomizer device with rectal diazepam and found better seizure control and fewer respiratory complications in the group treated with intranasal midazolam [37].

Buccal midazolam has been studied for seizure control in children in the ED, in comparison with rectal diazepam, and has been found to be as effective or more effective without increased risk of respiratory depression [38,39]. Dosages administered were 0.25 mg/kg [39] or 0.5 mg/kg with adjustments by age with a 10 mg maximum dosage for children age 10 or older [38]. As with many of the therapies discussed here, this is off-label usage. Buccal midazolam is advocated by some as a choice for initial management of prolonged seizures in children, although issues of dosing (range 0.2–0.5 mg/kg) remain and further study is desirable [40,41].

Intramuscular (IM) administration of a benzodiazepine is possible with midazolam, which has solubility characteristics favorable for absorption [42]. IM administration is rapid and aspiration is not a concern. Increased use of midazolam intramuscularly has been noted in some systems [43]. In one small series of children with seizures, comparing treatment with IM midazolam with IV diazepam, the former was found to be an effective alternative.

Part of the efficacy was thought to be from the rapid administration possible by the IM route without waiting for IV access to be established [44]. The recently published RAMPART study established the safety and efficacy of IM midazolam compared to IV lorazepam when administered for prehospital status epilepticus [45]. This large, randomized, double-blind trial administered midazolam intramuscularly using a preloaded autoinjector. Advantages of the intramuscular route included more rapid drug administration. Dosages of midazolam were 10 mg IM for adults and children estimated to weigh more than 40 kg; for children estimated to weigh 13–40 kg, the dosage was 5 mg midazolam IM. Adverse events were similar in both groups.

Intravenous administration of midazolam was found to be more effective than IM administration in one prehospital study, with minimal risk of respiratory depression in both groups [46].

Seizure-associated trauma

In many EMS systems, full spinal immobilization is standard for patients who have experienced seizures. There appears to be very limited evidence to support this practice, although trauma from seizures has been reported in case reports, case series, and retrospective reviews.

Seizures uncommonly cause fractures and dislocations. Some uncommon orthopedic injuries, such as bilateral posterior dislocation of the shoulder, fracture-dislocation of the shoulder, or fracture-dislocation of the hip, suggest a generalized convulsion as the etiology. Bilateral hip fractures have been reported [47]. These cases are notable for their rarity.

Only very rare cases of cervical fractures from uncomplicated seizures are reported. There is one description of an odontoid fracture following an epileptic seizure [48]. One retrospective study of over 1,600 transports for uncomplicated seizures (i.e. age greater than 5 years, no associated major trauma, afebrile) found no spinal fractures. Transport charges and nursing charges were increased in this group of patients. The authors raise the question of the need for full spinal precautions in patients sustaining uncomplicated seizures [49]. Compression fractures of the thoracic vertebrae were reported in a patient taking steroids [50].

There is one report of a higher risk of cervical spinal cord injuries in patients with refractory epilepsy attributed to seizure-related falls. This residential facility for patients with refractory epilepsy reported four instances of spinal cord injuries in its patient population over 10 years, which they extrapolated to be a 30-fold to 40-fold risk increase [51].

Retrospective chart reviews of patients with seizures have also identified patients with intracranial hematomas resulting from falls associated with seizures. The authors advocate early investigation in patients with head injury due to seizures and caution that decreases in level of consciousness or focal neurological deficits in seizure patients should only cautiously be interpreted as postictal until traumatic hematomas have been excluded [52]. This review was from a neurosurgical service and undoubtedly incorporates significant ascertainment bias.

Given the paucity of reports of significant trauma following uncomplicated seizures, routine immobilization in all cases does not seem warranted, although caregivers should keep in mind that unusual injuries may exist.

Continuing management

Continued patient management in the ED is informed by what occurred in the field. If the patient's condition does not evolve to an alert state, the degree of unresponsiveness should be continuously monitored as evaluation proceeds along the pattern of primary survey, resuscitation, secondary survey, and definitive care steps. Information from EMS personnel regarding level of alertness in the field is helpful. Should the need for a definitive airway be established, rapid sequence intubation (RSI) is performed in the usual manner, and this is a field option for some paramedics and EMS physicians. Concerns for possible increased intracranial pressure, if suspected from history or physical examination, may prompt consideration for lidocaine administration as part of RSI, although this remains controversial. Most induction agents have some anticonvulsant properties and use of benzodiazepines would seem prudent, although data are lacking to support these actions. The use of short-acting paralytic agents, if necessary, should proceed in the usual manner [53]. There are only rare case reports in medically complex seizure patients of complications from succinylcholine [54]. Longer-acting neuromuscular blockade should be avoided, however, unless EEG monitoring can be established, because of concerns that seizure activity may be disguised by neuromuscular paralysis.

Somnolent patients should be observed and monitored. The postictal state is not well defined, but the possibility of ongoing subclinical seizure activity, complex medical issues, or trauma should be considered if a seizure patient is not starting to become alert within approximately 30 minutes.

Refractory generalized convulsive status epilepticus

Detailed management of status epilepticus is beyond the scope of this chapter. Benzodiazepines are the mainstay of initial therapy whatever the seizure type or cause, and lorazepam is the recommended initial drug. Most reviews recommend doses in adults of 4–8 mg. The possibility that the seizures are precipitated by an acute medical condition should be kept in mind and subsequently investigated.

Recommendations for second-line drug lack strong evidence and most reviews and guidelines recommend one of several drugs including phenytoin or fosphenytoin, valproate, levetiracetam, or propofol [55–60]. While these agents are not generally available in typical EMS environments, they may be found in critical care transport situations and physician response teams. There is a trend in recent guidelines to deemphasize barbiturates in favor of levetiracetam or propofol for generalized convulsive status epilepticus that fails to respond to optimal benzodiazepine administration.

Refractory status epilepticus may be defined as generalized seizures that persist through administration of optimal benzodiazepines and a second-line drug, historically a phenytoin. There are no prospective, randomized trials to guide third-line therapy [59]. Anecdotal reports and recommendations list a variety of agents, including high-dose phenytoin [57], lidocaine [61–64], etomidate [65], ketamine [66,67], midazolam [68,69], propofol [69–73], and valproic acid [74–76]. Because lidocaine is ubiquitously carried on ALS units, it may be a rational choice in systems with prolonged transport times. Definitive airway management and blood pressure support will be needed with the use of many of these agents.

Conclusion

Seizures are one of the most common conditions resulting in EMS activation. In many cases, the patient is recovering consciousness at the time of EMS arrival, and little if any care is needed. However, generalized convulsive status epilepticus represents an emergency with early interventions potentially limiting morbidity. After brief diagnostic intervention to confirm seizures, early treatment of persistent or recurrent generalized convulsions with benzodiazepines is indicated. A variety of treatment options is available for route of administration and drug choices. Persistent convulsions will require additional ALS interventions.

References

1 Huff JS, Morris DL, Kothari RU, Gibbs MA, Emergency Medicine Seizure Study Group. Emergency department management of patients with seizures: a multicenter study. *Acad Emerg Med* 2001; 8(6):622–8.

2 Richard J, Osmond MH, Nesbitt L, Stiell IG. Management and outcomes of pediatric patients transported by emergency medical services in a Canadian prehospital system. *CJEM* 2006;8(1):6–12.

3 Brokaw J, Olson L, Fullerton L, Tandberg D, Skiar D. Repeated ambulance use by patients with acute alcohol intoxication, seizure disorder, and respiratory illness. *Am J Emerg Med* 1998;16(2):141–4.

4 Fountain NB, Lothman EW. Pathophysiology of status epilepticus. *J Clin Neurophysiol* 1995;12(4):326–42.

5 Kapur J, Macdonald RL. Rapid seizure-induced reduction of benzodiazepine and Zn2+ sensitivity of hippocampal dentate granule cell GABAA receptors. *J Neurosci* 1997;17(19):7532–40.

6 Goodkin HP, Yeh JL, Kapur J. Status epilepticus increases the intracellular accumulation of GABAA receptors. *J Neurosci* 2005; 25(23):5511–20.

7 Lin JT, Ziegler DK, Lai CW, Bayer W. Convulsive syncope in blood donors. *Ann Neurol* 1982;11(5):525–8.

8 McCrory PR, Berkovic SF. Concussive convulsions. Incidence in sport and treatment recommendations. *Sports Med* 1998;25(2):131–6.

9 Perron AD, Brady WJ, Huff JS. Concussive convulsions: emergency department assessment and management of a frequently misunderstood entity. *Acad Emerg Med* 2001;8(3):296–8.

10 Huff JS. Stroke mimics and chameleons. *Emerg Med Clin North Am* 2002;20(3):583–95.

11 Hand PJ, Kwan J, Lindley RI, Dennis MS, Wardlaw JM. Distinguishing between stroke and mimic at the bedside: the brain attack study. *Stroke* 2006;37(3):769–75.

12 Haines SJ. Decerebrate posturing misinterpreted as seizure activity. *Am J Emerg Med* 1988;6(2):173–7.

13 Huff JS, Perron AD. Onset seizures independently predict poor outcome after subarachnoid hemorrhage. *Neurology* 2001;56(10):1423–4.

14 Jagoda A, Riggio S. Psychogenic convulsive seizures. *Am J Emerg Med* 1993;11(6):626–32.

15 Leis AA, Ross MA, Summers AK. Psychogenic seizures: ictal characteristics and diagnostic pitfalls. *Neurology* 1992;42(1):95–9.

16 Mosewich RK, So EL. A clinical approach to the classification of seizures and epileptic syndromes. *Mayo Clin Proc* 1996;71(4):405–14.

17 Engel J Jr. Report of the ILAE classification core group. *Epilepsia* 2006;47(9):1558–68.

18 Kaplan PW. Nonconvulsive status epilepticus in the emergency room. *Epilepsia* 1996;37(7):643–50.

19 McKeon A, Frye MA, Delanty N. The alcohol withdrawal syndrome. *J Neurol Neurosurg Psychiatry* 2008;79(8):854–62.

20 Rathlev NK, D'Onofrio G, Fish SS, et al. The lack of efficacy of phenytoin in the prevention of recurrent alcohol-related seizures. *Ann Emerg Med* 1994;23(3):513–18.

21 D'Onofrio G, Rathlev NK, Ulrich AS, Fish SS, Freedland ES. Lorazepam for the prevention of recurrent seizures related to alcohol. *N Engl J Med* 1999;340(12):915–19.

22 Alldredge BK, Lowenstein DH. Status epilepticus related to alcohol abuse. *Epilepsia* 1993;34(6):1033–7.

23 Olson KR, Kearney TE, Dyer JE, Benowitz NL, Blanc PD. Seizures associated with poisoning and drug overdose. *Am J Emerg Med* 1993;11(6):565–8.

24 Wills B, Erickson T. Drug- and toxin-associated seizures. *Med Clin North Am* 2005;89(6):1297–321.

25 Wason S, Lacouture PG, Lovejoy FH Jr. Single high-dose pyridoxine treatment for isoniazid overdose. *JAMA* 1981;246(10):1102–4.

26 Waruiru C, Appleton R. Febrile seizures: an update. *Arch Dis Child* 2004;89(8):751–6.

27 Allen JE, Ferrie CD, Livingston JH, Feltbower RG. Recovery of consciousness after epileptic seizures in children. *Arch Dis Child* 2007;92(1):39–42.

28 Treiman DM, Meyers PD, Walton NY, et al. A comparison of four treatments for generalized convulsive status epilepticus. Veterans Affairs Status Epilepticus Cooperative Study Group. *N Engl J Med* 1998;339(12):792–8.

29 Treiman DM. Treatment of convulsive status epilepticus. *Int Rev Neurobiol* 2007;81:273–85.

30 Lowenstein DH, Bleck T, Macdonald RL. It's time to revise the definition of status epilepticus. *Epilepsia* 1999;40(1):120–2.

31 Benbadis SR, Wolgamuth BR, Goren H, Brener S, Fouad-Tarazi F. Value of tongue biting in the diagnosis of seizures. *Arch Intern Med* 1995;155(21):2346–9.

32 Lowenstein DH, Alldredge BK, Allen F, et al. The prehospital treatment of status epilepticus (PHTSE) study: design and methodology. *Control Clin Trials* 2001;22(3):290–309.

33 Albano A, Reisdorff EJ, Wiegenstein JG. Rectal diazepam in pediatric status epilepticus. *Am J Emerg Med* 1989;7(2):168–72.

34 Pellock JM. Safety of Diastat, a rectal gel formulation of diazepam for acute seizure treatment. *Drug Saf* 2004;27(6):383–92.

35 O'Regan ME, Brown JK, Clarke M. Nasal rather than rectal benzodiazepines in the management of acute childhood seizures? *Dev Med Child Neurol* 1996;38(11):1037–45.

36 Mahmoudian T, Zadeh MM. Comparison of intranasal midazolam with intravenous diazepam for treating acute seizures in children. *Epilepsy Behav* 2004;5(2):253–5.

37 Holsti M, Sill BL, Firth SD, Filloux FM, Joyce SM, Furnival RA. Prehospital intranasal midazolam for the treatment of pediatric seizures. *Pediatr Emerg Care* 2007;23(3):148–53.

38 McIntyre J, Robertson S, Norris E, et al. Safety and efficacy of buccal midazolam versus rectal diazepam for emergency treatment of seizures in children: a randomised controlled trial. *Lancet* 2005; 366(9481):205–10.

39 Baysun S, Aydin OF, Atmaca E, Gürer YK. A comparison of buccal midazolam and rectal diazepam for the acute treatment of seizures. *Clin Pediatr (Phila)* 2005;44(9):771–6.

40 Wiznitzer M. Buccal midazolam for seizures. *Lancet* 2005;366 (9481):182–3.

41 Wiznitzer M. Buccal midazolam is effective for acute treatment of seizures. *J Pediatr* 2006;148(1):143.

42 Towne AR, DeLorenzo RJ. Use of intramuscular midazolam for status epilepticus. *J Emerg Med* 1999;17(2):323–8.

43 Warden CR, Frederick C. Midazolam and diazepam for pediatric seizures in the prehospital setting. *Prehosp Emerg Care* 2006;10(4):463–7.

44 Chamberlain JM, Altieri MA, Futterman C, Young GM, Ochsenschlager DW, Waisman Y. A prospective, randomized study comparing intramuscular midazolam with intravenous diazepam for the treatment of seizures in children. *Pediatr Emerg Care* 1997; 13(2):92–4.

45 Silbergleit R, Durkalski V, Lowenstein D, et al. Intramuscular versus intravenous therapy for prehospital status epilepticus. *N Engl J Med* 2012;366(7):591–600.

46 Vilke GM, Sharieff GQ, Marino A, Gerhart AE, Chan TC. Midazolam for the treatment of out-of-hospital pediatric seizures. *Prehosp Emerg Care* 2002;6(2):215–17.

47 Ribacoba-Montero R, Salas-Puig J. Simultaneous bilateral fractures of the hip following a grand mal seizure. An unusual complication. *Seizure* 1997;6(5):403–4.

48 Torreggiani WC, Lyburn ID, Harris AC, Nicolaou S. Odontoid fracture following an epileptic seizure. *Australas Radiol* 2001;45(3):359–61.

49 McArthur CL III, Rooke CT. Are spinal precautions necessary in all seizure patients? *Am J Emerg Med* 1995;13(5):512–13.

50 Gnanalingham K, Macanovic M, Joshi S, Afshar F, Yeh J. Nontraumatic compression fractures of the thoracic spine following a seizure – treatment by percutaneous kyphoplasty. *Minim Invasive Neurosurg* 2004;47(4):256–7.

51 Kruitbosch JM, Schouten EJ, Tan IY, Veendrick-Meekes MJ, de Vocht JW. Cervical spinal cord injuries in patients with refractory epilepsy. *Seizure* 2006;15(8):633–6.

52 Zwimpfer TJ, Brown J, Sullivan I, Moulton RJ. Head injuries due to falls caused by seizures: a group at high risk for traumatic intracranial hematomas. *J Neurosurg* 1997;86(3):433–7.

53 Walls RM, Sagarin MJ. Status epilepticus. *N Engl J Med* 1998;339(6):409.

54 Verma A, Bedlack RS, Radtke RA, VanLandingham KE, Erwin CW. Succinylcholine induced hyperkalemia and cardiac arrest death related to an EEG study. *J Clin Neurophysiol* 1999;16(1):46–50.

55 Lowenstein DH, Alldredge B. Managing status epilepticus. *Lancet* 1990;336(8728):1451.

56 Lowenstein DH. The management of refractory status epilepticus: an update. *Epilepsia* 2006;47 (Suppl 1):35–40.

57 Treatment of convulsive status epilepticus. Recommendations of the Epilepsy Foundation of America's Working Group on Status Epilepticus. *JAMA* 1993;270(7):854–9.

58 ACEP Clinical Policies Committee, Clinical Policies Subcommittee on Seizures. Clinical policy: critical issues in the evaluation and management of adult patients presenting to the emergency department with seizures. *Ann Emerg Med* 2004;43(5):605–25.

59 Huff JS. Seizures and status epilepticus in adults. Part II. *Emerg Med Reports* 2007;28(23):281–92.

60 Brophy GM, Bell R, Claassen J, et al. Guidelines for the evaluation and management of status epilepticus. *Neurocrit Care* 2012;17(1):3–23.

61 Aggarwal P, Wali JP. Lidocaine in refractory status epilepticus: a forgotten drug in the emergency department. *Am J Emerg Med* 1993;11(3):243–4.

62 Pascual J, Sedano MJ, Polo JM, Berciano J. Intravenous lidocaine for status epilepticus. *Epilepsia* 1988;29(5):584–9.

63 Hamano S, Sugiyama N, Yamashita S, et al. Intravenous lidocaine for status epilepticus during childhood. *Dev Med Child Neurol* 2006;48(3):220–2.

64 Walker IA, Slovis CM. Lidocaine in the treatment of status epilepticus. *Acad Emerg Med* 1997;4(9):918–22.

65 Yeoman P, Hutchinson A, Byrne A, Smith J, Durham S. Etomidate infusions for the control of refractory status epilepticus. *Intensive Care Med* 1989;15(4):255–9.

66 Sheth RD, Gidal BE. Refractory status epilepticus: response to ketamine. *Neurology* 1998;51(6):1765–6.

67 Nathan BR, Smith TL, Bleck T. The use of ketamine in the treatment of refractory status epilepticus (abstract). *Neurology* 2002;58 (Suppl 3):A197.

68 Fountain NB, Adams RE. Midazolam treatment of acute and refractory status epilepticus. *Clin Neuropharmacol* 1999;22 (5):261–7.

69 Prasad A, Worrall BB, Bertram EH, Bleck TP. Propofol and midazolam in the treatment of refractory status epilepticus. *Epilepsia* 2001;42(3):380–6.

70 Stecker MM, Kramer TH, Raps EC, O'Meeghan R, Dulaney E, Skaar DJ. Treatment of refractory status epilepticus with propofol: clinical and pharmacokinetic findings. *Epilepsia* 1998;39(1):18–26.

71 Rossetti AO, Reichhart MD, Schaller MD, Despland PA, Bogousslavsky J. Propofol treatment of refractory status epilepticus: a study of 31 episodes. *Epilepsia* 2004;45(7):757–63.

72 Schor NF, Riviello JJ Jr. Treatment with propofol: the new status quo for status epilepticus? *Neurology* 2005;65(4):506–7.

73 Parviainen I, Uusaro A, Kälviäinen R, Mervaala E, Ruokonen E. Propofol in the treatment of refractory status epilepticus. *Intensive Care Med* 2006;32(7):1075–9.

74 Rossetti AO, Bromfield EB. Efficacy of rapid IV administration of valproic acid for status epilepticus. *Neurology* 2005;65(3): 500–1.

75 Wheless JW, Vazquez BR, Kanner AM, Ramsay RE, Morton L, Pellock JM. Rapid infusion with valproate sodium is well tolerated in patients with epilepsy. *Neurology* 2004;63(8):1507–8.

76 Peters CN, Pohlmann-Eden B. Intravenous valproate as an innovative therapy in seizure emergency situations including status epilepticus – experience in 102 adult patients. *Seizure* 2005; 14(3):164–9.

CHAPTER 21

Stroke

Todd J. Crocco, Allison Tadros, and Stephen M. Davis

Introduction

The concepts of "time is muscle" for myocardial infarction (MI) patients and "the golden hour" for trauma patients are familiar. Until the mid-1990s, the treatment of stroke was focused on rehabilitation, because there were limited treatment options available. There was no urgency. Thankfully, that is no longer the case. With timely treatment, many stroke patients can return to baseline neurological functioning.

The EMS system plays a vital role in the sequence of events that gets eligible stroke patients to available interventions that will change their outcomes. In addition to EMS providers' knowledge and skills at identifying strokes and facilitating patients' access to timely care, they can participate with other health care colleagues to help improve general public awareness of stroke, its symptoms, and the importance of seeking help early. Early diagnosis, within a narrow window of opportunity, helps to keep treatment options available, including possible administration of fibrinolytics or mechanical clot retrieval. Thus, appropriate triage to a facility that can provide these treatments is essential.

Overview of stroke

Stroke is now the fourth leading cause of death in the United States, and it remains the leading cause of adult disability. According to the American Heart Association (AHA), approximately 795,000 people in the United States will suffer strokes each year, with 610,000 being first attacks [1].

In broad terms, strokes are classified as either hemorrhagic or ischemic. Greater than 80% percent of strokes are ischemic, but it is difficult to differentiate between these two subtypes in the prehospital setting. Radiographic imaging in a hospital setting is required. An ischemic stroke is caused by either *in situ* thrombus formation from atherosclerosis or an embolic event (usually from the heart or large vessels) that leads to occlusion of a cerebral blood vessel and subsequent interruption of blood flow

and oxygen supply to an area of the brain. For example, one of the contributing causes of embolic strokes is atrial fibrillation, leading to embolization of a clot from the heart.

Spontaneous intracranial hemorrhage (ICH) may result from several underlying diseases. Hypertension and arteriovenous malformations are two such predisposing conditions. Patients taking warfarin or with brain tumors are also at risk. Patients with ICH sometimes have more dramatic presentations accompanied by nausea and vomiting, headache, or a sudden decrease in level of consciousness. These are the result of the nature of the insult, where the hemorrhage acts to increase intracerebral pressure. Pupillary changes and motor deficits will be dependent on the location and extent of the bleeding. For example, bleeding into the pontine area of the brainstem will result in pinpoint pupils due to the interruption of sympathetic tracts [2].

Patients with ICH may deteriorate rapidly and require airway support as the hemorrhage expands. The mass effect of an expanding hematoma may also cause contralateral motor deficits, ECG abnormalities, and incidental dysrhythmias.

When occlusion of a vessel occurs, there is a central area or "core" of ischemia in that region of the brain. However, there can also be a surrounding area that has decreased blood supply with the potential to recover without permanent damage. This area surrounding the central area of ischemia is referred to as the "ischemic penumbra." Whether or not the ischemic penumbra can be salvaged depends on the severity and duration of ischemia. If possible, it is important to restore blood flow to this penumbra to decrease the morbidity and mortality of a stroke. In addition to the aspects of stroke related to blood supply, there are several chemical responses that occur on a cellular level that affect brain function. These include the release of excitatory amino acids, alterations in calcium release, and free radical formation. Inflammatory responses and alterations in chemical function affect the penumbra and its ability to recover [3].

When neurological deficits consistent with a stroke occur but resolve spontaneously, this is referred to as a transient ischemic attack (TIA). A TIA, according to the National Institute of Neurological Disorders and Stroke (NINDS), is a

Emergency Medical Services: Clinical Practice and Systems Oversight, Second Edition. Volume 1: Clinical Aspects of EMS.
Edited by David C. Cone, Jane H. Brice, Theodore R. Delbridge, and J. Brent Myers.
© 2015 NAEMSP. Published 2015 by John Wiley & Sons, Inc. Companion Website: www.wiley.com\go\cone\naemsp

focal neurological deficit lasting only a few minutes [4]. TIAs had been previously defined as a neurological deficit that resolved within 24 hours. In fact, most TIAs resolve within 60 minutes and many do so within half an hour. People who experience TIAs have a 10–20% risk of stroke in the subsequent 90 days, and half will occur within the next 24–48 hours [5]. TIAs should be considered very serious events that require prompt diagnostic evaluations.

Dispatcher guidelines and call prioritization

As the first contact for the EMS systems, an emergency medical dispatcher has the opportunity to influence the expediency (or delay) of stroke patient care and ultimate arrival at an appropriate ED. In one review of recorded calls to 9-1-1, dispatchers were able to identify and correctly categorize the call as "stroke" only 31–52% of the time. It was also noted in this study that when the caller used the word "stroke," this was highly predictive of an actual stroke. The study concluded that dispatcher recognition of stroke could be improved if key words such as stroke, difficulty communicating, weakness or falling, and facial droop were communicated to the dispatcher by the caller [6]. Another study found that, even when the caller used the word "stroke," the call was dispatched as a stroke only 48% of the time, and only 41% were dispatched as high priority [7]. The symptoms most frequently reported by callers were speech problems (26%) followed by extremity weakness (22%). Interestingly, "fall" was stated as the primary problem in 21%. Symptoms such as vertigo or sensory impairment were mentioned much less frequently [8].

Use of a modified stroke scale may help dispatchers identify potential stroke victims and ensure appropriate prioritization of calls. The goal is to facilitate patient arrival at an ED as soon as possible to allow imaging studies and treatment to occur within a narrow window of opportunity. After sending appropriate resources, the dispatcher should provide instructions to the caller. In addition to providing dispatch life support, dispatchers can help expedite the time EMS personnel will spend on the scene by preparing the caller for certain important questions.

These include past medical history, a complete list of medications, and, most importantly, when the patient was last known to be at his or her neurological baseline. These factors will be crucial for EMS personnel who can then begin to make decisions about the patient's eligibility for various interventions at specific receiving facilities. EMS dispatchers should use the guidelines set forth by the AHA and American Stroke Association (ASA). The use of modified stroke assessment tools and software that meet the AHA/ASA standards can help correctly identify stroke patients. All emergency medical dispatchers should complete an emergency medical dispatch course and be certified [9] (see Volume 2, Chapter 10).

EMS personnel on the scene

It is imperative that EMS providers be familiar not only with the signs and symptoms of stroke, but also with currently available therapeutic protocols. Case-based education following the guidelines of the AHA can lead to significant improvement in prehospital personnel knowledge of stroke signs and symptoms. The 2010 AHA guidelines for CPR and emergency cardiovascular care should be followed [10]. The Cincinnati Prehospital Stroke Scale (CPSS) and the Los Angeles Prehospital Stroke Scale (LAPSS) are both validated tools that can increase the sensitivity for identification of stroke [11–13]. The Melbourne Ambulance Stroke Screen (MASS) is a hybrid of the two and is also credible for prehospital stroke assessment [13,14] (Tables 21.1 and 21.2).

While prehospital stroke scales are valuable tools to help identify potential stroke victims, there are also a number of stroke imposters that should be considered (Box 21.1). Not all will be easily differentiated in the field. However, hypoglycemia can manifest with focal neurological findings. Thus, all potential stroke patients should have point-of-care glucose testing, and hypoglycemia should be treated. Additional historical features may help to determine the nature of some problems that subsequently appear similar to strokes. For example, preceding seizure activity might indicate Todd paralysis or increase the probability of ICH. Accompanying symptoms of migraine

Table 21.1 The Cincinnati Prehospital Stroke Scale

Evaluate the following	Result
Facial droop (ask the patient to smile showing teeth)	Normal: No asymmetry
	Abnormal: One side of the face droops
Arm drift (with eyes closed, have the patient hold arms in front of body, palms up, for 10 seconds)	Normal: Able to hold arms out at 90°; both arms stay up or fall together
	Abnormal: One arm drifts downward
Abnormal speech (ask the patient to say a simple sentence, for example, "It is sunny today")	Normal: No slurring
	Abnormal: Slurs words or uses words that make no sense

Source: Kothari RU. *Ann Emerg Med* 1999;33:373–7. Reproduced with permission of Elsevier.

Table 21.2 Los Angeles Prehospital Stroke Scale

Criteria	Results		
Over age 45	Yes	Unknown	
No history of seizures	Yes	Unknown	
Symptoms less than 24 hours	Yes	Unknown	
Patient's baseline function is *not* bedridden or confined to a wheelchair	Yes	Unknown	
Blood glucose between 60 and 400	Yes	No	
Examination for asymmetry			
Facial droop	Normal	Right	Left
Grip strength	Normal	Weak/none	
Arm strength (by downward drift)	Normal	Drifts down	Falls rapidly
Examination finding unilateral?	Yes	No	

If exam findings are positive and answers are "yes" then LAPSS screening criteria are met and stroke is suspected. Source: Kidwell C. *Stroke* 2000; 31: 71–6. Reproduced with permission of Wolters Kluwer Health.

Box 21.1 Mimics of stroke

Bell palsy
Complex migraine
Conversion disorders
Encephalopathy
Hypoglycemia
Labyrinthitis
Ménière disease
Postictal (Todd) paralysis
Ramsay–Hunt syndrome

---

might indicate a complex migraine. In any case, expediency is important, but so is history that EMS providers may be in the best position to gather quickly.

There are some immediately relevant points with regard to the medical history of a potential stroke victim. Examples of important pieces of information include any recent trauma or use of warfarin, clopidogrel, or aspirin. Because potential witnesses frequently do not arrive at the hospital with the patient, attempting to determine the inclusion and exclusion criteria for thrombolytic therapy before hospital arrival can be very helpful (Box 21.2). However, this should not delay transport, with one caveat. Finding out from family members or others at the scene when the patient was last at his baseline neurological function is imperative.

Prehospital treatment of stroke

Initial attention should be directed, as always, to airway, breathing, and circulation issues to ensure a stable patient notwithstanding the new neurological deficit. A stroke scale should be completed as it will add a degree of objectivity to the description of exam findings that can be conveyed to medical personnel later in the sequence of care. If possible, an IV cannula may be inserted to facilitate acquisition of blood for point-of-care testing and subsequent laboratory tests.

Box 21.2 Inclusion and exclusion criteria for intravenous tPA [24]

Inclusion criteria

Ischemic stroke onset within 4.5 h of drug administration
Measurable deficit on NIH Stroke Scale examination
Head CT does not show hemorrhage or non-stroke cause of deficit
Patient's age is >18 years

Exclusion criteria

Minor or rapidly improving symptoms
Seizure at onset of stroke
Major surgery within 14 days
Prior stroke or serious head trauma with past 3 months
Known history of intracranial hemorrhage
Sustained blood pressure >185/110 mmHg
Aggressive treatment necessary to lower blood pressure
Symptoms suggestive of subarachnoid hemorrhage
Gastrointestinal or genitourinary hemorrhage in last 21 days
Arterial puncture at a non-compressible site within 7 days
Heparin administration within 48 h with elevated aPTT
Prothrombin time >15 s
Platelet count <100,000 uL
Serum glucose <50 mg/dL or >400 mg/dL

Relative contraindications

Large stroke with NIH Stroke Scale score >22
CT shows evidence of large MCA territory infarction (sulcal effacement or blurring of gray-white junction in greater than one-third of MCA territory)

Relative contraindications for the 3-to 4.5-hour treatment window

History of prior stroke and diabetes mellitus
NIH Stroke Scale >25
Oral anticoagulant use regardless of INR
Age >80 years

Source: Miller 2012.[24] Reproduced with permission of Springer. INR, international normalized ratio; MCA, middle cerebral artery; NIH, National Institutes of Health; aPTT, activated partial thromboplastin time; t-PA, tissue plasminogen activator.

In general, dextrose-containing solutions should be avoided unless treating hypoglycemia. Hyperglycemia is associated with delays in recanalization of the occluded vessel [15]. Hypoxia should be treated to decrease further insult to the already ischemic brain. However, indiscriminate administration of high-flow oxygen has not proven to be of any benefit. The current evidence indicates that maintaining normal oxygen saturation levels (i.e. treating hypoxia) is the best recommendation [16]. Supplemental oxygen should only be used to achieve oxygen saturations of 94% [10].

Stroke patients are at risk for arrhythmias due to the increase in catecholamine release. Therefore, continuous cardiac monitoring is recommended [16,17]. Most stroke patients will not experience arrhythmias that require treatment unless they have a concomitant illness, but this is always a consideration (see

Volume 1, Chapter 14). Acute myocardial infarction and stroke may also present simultaneously. It is important to consider concomitant disorders and prioritize care.

Blood pressure control among stroke patients is an area of controversy and active investigation. Perfusion to the ischemic brain following a stroke is dependent on arterial blood pressure to maintain cerebral perfusion. Thus, hypotension or a relatively low blood pressure for a patient with chronic hypertension could theoretically adversely affect necessary cerebral perfusion to at-risk areas (e.g. penumbra). In fact, many patients experience hypertension immediately after a stroke, and studies have indicated that hypertension usually resolves spontaneously within a few hours. Yet, systolic blood pressure greater than 185 mmHg has been associated with increased risk of ICH among patients who subsequently receive fibrinolytic therapy. Blood pressure control is also postulated to be helpful in reducing hematoma expansion among ICH patients. Thus, too little blood pressure is not good, but neither is too much blood pressure. In general, blood pressure management is best deferred until the patient is in a more controlled environment, such as an ED, where invasive monitoring is possible. If there are compelling reasons to lower a patient's blood pressure in the field, such as coexisting pulmonary edema, for example, great care must be taken not to overcorrect. A suitable initial target is a 10% reduction of systolic blood pressure, but not lower than 150 mmHg.

Some literature suggests that placing the patient supine may increase cerebral perfusion, but this also increases intracranial pressure, and this remains an area of uncertainty and investigation. Obviously, supine positioning is not advised in a patient who has clinical evidence of elevated intracranial pressure. As always, the risk of aspiration must be considered as well [16].

Ultimately, the goals for prehospital care of the possible stroke patient include rapid evaluation, stabilization as necessary, neurological examination, and expedited transport to a hospital capable of caring for a stroke patient [18]. Early communication to the destination hospital is important. Studies have shown that such notification gives time for the stroke team to arrive in the ED and decreases the time from ED door to computed tomography (CT) scans and increased rates of IV tissue plasminogen activator (tPA) administration [19,20].

Treatment options and the importance of time

Pioneers in the 1940s and 1950s contemplated the use of fibrinolytics for the treatment of stroke, and in 1958 Sussman and Fitch reported the first use of thrombolytics to treat acute ischemic stroke. However, early studies using either streptokinase (SK) or urokinase (UK) resulted in high incidences of ICH. Therefore, these therapeutic agents were abandoned for the treatment of stroke until the 1970s, when advanced imaging technology could rule out the possibility of ICH prior to thrombolytic administration and allow for a more definitive

diagnosis of ischemic stroke. Unfortunately, high rates of ICH secondary to SK treatment persisted in later trials, and ultimately led to the early termination of the Multicenter Acute Stroke Trial-Italy (MAST-I) and Multicenter Acute Stroke Trial-Europe (MAST-E) in the mid-1990s, as well as the abandonment of SK as a viable ischemic stroke treatment option [21].

Around the same time as the MAST-E trial, several trials of tPA, which was thought to have a better risk–benefit profile compared to other thrombolytics, were conducted that failed to demonstrate favorable outcomes. However, it was felt that the use of tPA held promise if the correct dose and the right population of patients were selected [21]. The NINDS trial demonstrated improved functional outcomes at 3 months as measured by the National Institutes of Health Stroke Scale (NIHSS) score, the modified Rankin score, and other neurological assessment tools in highly selected ischemic stroke patients treated within 3 hours of symptom onset [22]. Patients treated with tPA were 30% more likely to have minimal to no disability at 3 months compared with patients treated with placebo (absolute benefit of 12%; number needed to treat (NNT) = 8), which was found to persist at 12 months [22,23]. Based upon these findings, in 1996 the Food and Drug Administration (FDA) approved the use of intravenous tPA for the treatment of acute ischemic stroke within 3 hours of the onset of symptoms [21].

Recently, evidence has emerged supporting the extension of the 3-hour treatment window to 4.5 hours. The European Cooperative Acute Stroke Study (ECASS III) randomized patients to tPA or placebo within 4.5 hours of symptom onset and found that patients receiving tPA were significantly more likely to have a favorable outcome (52.4% versus 45.2%; NNT = 14) [24].

As important, among patients who present within the treatment time windows for tPA, those treated sooner have much better odds of having a good outcome. Specifically, patients treated up to 90 minutes from symptom onset have an odds ratio (OR) of having improved functional outcomes of 2.6 (NNT = 4.5) compared to an OR of 1.6 (NNT = 9) for those treated between 91 and 180 minutes and an OR of 1.3 (NNT = 14.1) for those treated between 181 and 270 minutes [24].

Intraarterial tPA and devices for mechanical clot extraction are two other options for stroke patients who fall outside the 4.5-hour window or who have not substantially improved after IV tPA therapy [24].

The decision to use intraarterial tPA is determined by angiographic imaging and requires an interventional neuroradiologist with specific expertise. The PROACT II (Prolyse in Acute Cerebral Thromboembolism) study evaluated the safety and efficacy of this procedure using prourokinase injected into middle cerebral artery occlusions. The study results indicated that there was a significant improvement in outcome (measured as independent function at 90 days) in

40% of patients in the treated group compared with 25% of patients in the placebo group [25].

There are currently several mechanical clot extraction devices approved by the FDA for use in acute ischemic stroke up to 8 hours after symptom onset, including MERCI, Penumbra, SWIFT (Solitare), and TREVO 2 [26]. Rates of successful recanalization with these devices range from 46% using the MERCI device to 85% using the TREVO 2 device. Following a similar trend, good neurological outcomes at 90 days were seen in 28% of patients treated with the MERCI system and 40% of patients treated with the TREVO 2 system. Overall, 90 day mortality ranged from 17% to 44% [26].

A large-scale trial (IMS-III) comparing endovascular therapy in patients who failed to improve after receiving a reduced dose of tPA within 3 hours of symptom onset was halted early due to futility. Good functional outcomes at 90 days did not differ between the endovascular group (40.8%) and the IV tPA alone group (38.7%). It has been suggested that combining advanced imaging with these devices may lead to optimal patient selection and better functional outcomes. However, the MR RESCUE trial failed to demonstrate a favorable benefit in patients selected for treatment who had an ischemic penumbra as defined by a magnetic resonance diffusion-perfusion mismatch. There are a number of factors that may have affected these negative trials that suggest the need for continuing research to elucidate the best implementation of these devices in practice [26].

All of these treatments have potentially devastating complications, the most noteworthy being intracranial bleeding. Also, these interventions have several exclusion criteria that must be considered in the selection of patients but which are beyond the scope of this chapter. Nonetheless, it is important that EMS personnel have at least a general understanding of available stroke treatments, as well as the rationale for accurate and rapid identification of the stroke victim. Box 21.3 describes the current AHA/ASA time-to-treatment goals related to IV tPA. Ideally, the time window from ED arrival to drug administration should not exceed 60 minutes [10].

Box 21.3 Time interval goals for fibrinolytic therapy

Arrival at the ED via EMS as soon as safely possible
Assessment by stroke team or emergency physician within 10 minutes
Completion of CT scan within 25 minutes
CT scan interpretation within 25 minutes
Administration of fibrinolytic (tPA) within 60 minutes of arrival to ED
    and within 3 hours of symptom onset

Adapted from: American Heart Association. *Advanced Cardiovascular Life Support Provider Manual*, 2006, pp.103–17. American Heart Association. Part 9: Adult stroke. *Circulation* 2005;112 (22): IV-111–IV-120. Reproduced with permission of Wolters Kluwer Health.

Role of the EMS system in promoting early patient arrival

Given the narrow time windows of opportunity associated with the various interventional stroke therapies and the clearly demonstrated benefit of earlier treatment, EMS is a critical link to ensuring that patients arrive as soon as possible to a facility capable of treating stroke. Numerous studies have shown that stroke patients accessing the EMS system have a significantly greater chance of arriving earlier to a hospital for treatment, which in turn can promote higher thrombolytic treatment rates [27–30]. More specifically, the California Acute Stroke Prototype Registry (CASPR) collected data from several California hospitals to identify factors that resulted in delayed presentation for treatment. This study indicated that if patients experiencing stroke symptoms (that did not occur overnight) had called EMS immediately, the percentage eligible for tPA would have increased from 4.3% to 28.6% [31]. Furthermore, one randomized trial examining the effect of an intervention comprising a prehospital stroke assessment tool, an ambulance protocol for hospital bypass for potential thrombolysis-eligible patients, and prehospital notification of the acute stroke team demonstrated a significant increase in thrombolytic administration. In this study, the time from symptom onset to ED arrival decreased from 150 minutes to 90 minutes, and the proportion of patients receiving tPA increased from 4.7% to 21.4% after the intervention, with 43% of patients having minimal to no disability at 3 months [32].

Importance of transport to an appropriate facility

Rapid stabilization and transport of the stroke patient by EMS is only one important aspect of the critical role of EMS in stroke treatment and care. Equally important is a robust knowledge of the stroke treatment capabilities among area hospitals. Health care facilities that are not stroke centers may be able to administer tPA, but often lack the capability to perform more invasive techniques such as intraarterial tPA administration or mechanical clot retrieval [25,33]. These procedures require an interventional neuroradiologist trained in these techniques. In addition, the personnel treating strokes must be available quickly and trained in the evaluation of stroke.

The staffing of EDs throughout the country still varies widely, as does the relative stroke experience of practitioners. Designation as a primary stroke center by the Joint Commission indicates that a hospital has been evaluated and found to be in compliance with the specific guidelines as set forth by the Joint Commission [34,35] (Box 21.4). More recently, the Joint Commission has begun the process of certifying hospitals as comprehensive stroke center if they meet specific criteria [36,37] (Box 21.5). Such designation

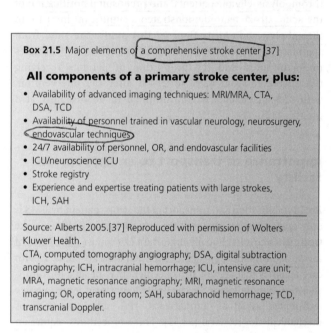

Box 21.4 Major elements of a primary stroke center [35]

Patient care elements

Acute stroke team
Written care protocols
Emergency medical services
Emergency department
Stroke unit
Neurosurgical services
Imaging services: brain, cerebral vasculature, cardiac
Laboratory services
Rehabilitation services

Administrative/support elements

Institutional commitment and support
Primary stroke center director, reimbursement for call
Stroke registry with outcomes and QI components
Educational programs: public and professional
Support certification process
Participation in stroke system of care

Source: Alberts 2011.[35] Reproduced with permission of Wolters
Kluwer Health.

Box 21.5 Major elements of a comprehensive stroke center [37]

All components of a primary stroke center, plus:

- Availability of advanced imaging techniques: MRI/MRA, CTA,
  DSA, TCD
- Availability of personnel trained in vascular neurology, neurosurgery,
  endovascular techniques
- 24/7 availability of personnel, OR, and endovascular facilities
- ICU/neuroscience ICU
- Stroke registry
- Experience and expertise treating patients with large strokes,
  ICH, SAH

Source: Alberts 2005.[37] Reproduced with permission of Wolters
Kluwer Health.
CTA, computed tomography angiography; DSA, digital subtraction
angiography; ICH, intracranial hemorrhage; ICU, intensive care unit;
MRA, magnetic resonance angiography; MRI, magnetic resonance
imaging; OR, operating room; SAH, subarachnoid hemorrhage; TCD,
transcranial Doppler.

indicates those hospitals are uniquely equipped and staffed to
treat the most complex stroke cases. Additionally, the creation
of guidelines for becoming an acute stroke ready hospital is
currently in process.

However, early presentation for treatment ultimately depends
upon the ability of the public to recognize the signs and symptoms of stroke and appropriately access the EMS system. EMS
personnel play an important role in promoting community education regarding the signs and symptoms of stroke and accessing the EMS system.

Protocols

Each community must evaluate its own resources and the
population it serves to develop protocols for the treatment of
stroke. This should be done in conjunction with the local and
regional health care facilities. It should be determined whether
the local community hospital is capable of managing acute stroke
victims. Hospital transport destinations should be predeter-
mined based on time and distance variables. In addition, air
medical transport may be considered, including direct air medical evacuation of stroke patients from the scene. Air medical
transport may be an appropriate option if the ground EMS transport time is expected to exceed an hour, and the air medical crew
could arrive at a stroke center in time to have appropriate evaluation and treatment within the therapeutic window. In making
such a decision, it is important to consider all the elements of air
medical response that consume time, including flight time, time
to prepare the patient, and time to load and unload. It is easy to
overestimate the potential time savings, otherwise.

The cost-effectiveness of the helicopter will vary at every
setting but must be considered in the formation of any protocol.
One study estimated the cost per additional good outcome at 3
months for acute stroke patients transported by helicopter to a
tertiary care center for thrombolytic therapy to be $35,000, or
$6,100 per quality-adjusted life year (QALY). Published stan-
dards consider $200,000 per additional good outcome and
$50,000 per QALY to be the limit at which benefits are worth the
related costs [38]. Therefore, this study would indicate that air
medical transport is a cost-effective procedure, although more
research is needed. The medical oversight physician must be
familiar with the logistics of air medical transport to ensure the
appropriate use of this resource.

Air medical transport of stroke patients in rural areas may
facilitate access to thrombolytic treatment. A recent study
looked at access of rural communities to stroke care. It found
that stroke protocols that included the administration of tPA
were present in only 31 of 125 facilities. Almost 40% of ischemic
stroke patients transported by helicopter in this program were
treated with thrombolytic therapy [39]. It seems clear that the
role of medical helicopter transport as part of regional systems
of care is expanding [40].

Controversies

The administration of tPA has potentially serious side-effects,
yet these can be minimized by strict adherence to the protocols
set forth by the NINDS trial. Protocol violations have been associated with increased rates of ICH. A study of community hospitals found that in 50 patients who received tPA for acute
ischemic stroke, NINDS protocol violations had occurred in the
treatment of eight patients. It has been determined in other
studies that strict protocol adherence can yield patient outcomes
similar to those reported for patients in the NINDS study. The

best outcomes occur when practitioners are knowledgeable in the treatment of acute stroke, and there is absolute compliance to the protocol [41].

The NINDS trial itself has been criticized and the results questioned. One criticism is that patients treated with tPA had less severe stroke scores than the placebo group, which altered the measured outcome. After further analysis, it was determined that the difference in the stroke severity did not account for the differences [42]. Though this is still somewhat debated, it is the general consensus and the recommendation of the AHA/ASA that tPA be given in the setting of acute ischemic stroke when it can be performed by personnel trained in the care of acute stroke and without protocol violations [10].

Conclusion

It is the responsibility of EMS physicians, nurses, and other EMS personnel to work together to develop a stroke system of care that maximizes the use of local resources. This can be accomplished by referring to the current strategies promoted by the ASA. An active public education effort is essential to ensure prompt activation of the EMS system. Ongoing education of EMS personnel in the recognition of stroke and the use of a stroke assessment tool such as the CPSS or LAPSS help stroke victims gain access to therapy in a timely manner [11,12]. Stroke centers with comprehensive protocols and therapies, technical capabilities, and experienced physicians are the ideal destinations for stroke patients. Through a collaborative effort between health care professionals in the prehospital and in-hospital settings, improved access to acute stroke therapies and interventions can result in improved patient morbidity and mortality from the devastating effects of stroke.

References

1 Go AS, Mozaffarian D, Roger VL, et al. Executive summary: heart disease and stroke statistics – 2013 update: a report from the American Heart Association. *Circulation* 2013;127(1):143–52.

2 Marx J. *Rosen's Emergency Medicine Concepts and Clinical Practice*, 6th edn. Philadelphia: Mosby, 2006.

3 Van der Worp HB, van Gijn J. Clinical Practice.Acute ischemic stroke. *N Engl J Med* 2007;357(6):572–9.

4 National Institute of Neurological Disorders and Stroke. Available at: www.ninds.nih.gov/disorders/tia/tia.htm

5 Albers W, Caplan L, Easton D, et al. Transient ischemic attack – proposal for a new definition. *N Engl J Med* 2002;347(21):1713–14.

6 Reginella RL, Crocco T, Tadros A, Shackleford A, Davis SM. Predictors of stroke during 9-1-1 calls: Opportunities for improving EMS response. *Prehosp Emerg Care* 2006;10(3):369–73.

7 Porteous GH, Corry MD, Smith W. Emergency medical services dispatcher identification of stroke and transient ischemic attacks. *Prehosp Emerg Care* 1999;3(3):211–16.

8 Handschu R, Poppe R, Rauss J, Neundörfer B, Erbguth F. Emergency calls in acute stroke. *Stroke* 2003;34(4):1005–9.

9 Acker JE III, Pancioli AM, Crocco TJ, et al. Implementation strategies for emergency medical services within stroke systems of care; a policy statement from the American heart Association/ American Stroke Association expert panel on emergency medical services systems and stroke council. *Stroke* 2007;38(11):3097–115.

10 Jauch EC, Cucchiara B, Adeoye O, et al. Part 11: adult stroke: 2010 American Heart Association Guidelines for Cardiopulmonary Resuscitation and Emergency Cardiovascular Care. *Circulation* 2010;122(18 Suppl 3):S818–28.

11 Kothari RU, Pancioli A, Liu T, Brott T, Broderick J. Cincinnati prehospital stroke scale: reproducibility and validity. *Ann Emerg Med* 1999;33(4):373–7.

12 Kidwell C, Starkman S, Eckstein M, Weems K, Saver JL. Identifying stroke in the field Prospective validation of the Los Angeles prehospital stroke screen (LAPSS). *Stroke* 2000;31(1):71–6.

13 Bray JE, Martin J, Cooper G, Barger B, Bernard S, Bladin C. Paramedic identification of stroke: community validation of the Melbourne ambulance stroke screen. *Cerebrovasc Dis* 2005; 20(1):28–33.

14 Bray J, Martin J, Cooper G, Barger B, Bernard S, Bladin C. An interventional study to improve paramedic diagnosis of stroke. *Prehosp Emerg Care* 2005;9(3):297–302.

15 Ribo M, Molina C, Montaner J, et al. Acute hyperglycemia state is associated with lower tPA induced recanalization rates in stroke patients. *Stroke* 2005;36(8):1705–9.

16 Millin M, Gullett T, Daya M. EMS management of acute stroke out of hospital treatment and stroke system development. *Prehosp Emerg Care* 2007;11(3):318–25.

17 American Heart Association. *Advanced Cardiovascular Life Support Provider Manual*. Dallas, TX: American Heart Association, 2006.

18 Jauch EC, Saver JL, Adams HP Jr, et al. Guidelines for the early management of patients with acute ischemic stroke: a guideline for healthcare professionals from the American Heart Association/ American Stroke Association. *Stroke*. 2013;44(3):870–947.

19 McKinney JS, Mylavarapu K, Lane J, Roberts V, Ohman-Strickland P, Merlin MA. Hospital prenotification of stroke patients by emergency medical services improves stroke time targets. *J Stroke Cerebrovasc Dis* 2013;22:113–18.

20 Patel MD, Rose KM, O'Brien EC, Rosamond WD. Prehospital notification by emergency medical services reduces delays in stroke evaluation: findings from the North Carolina stroke care collaborative. *Stroke* 2011;42:2263–8.

21 Röther J, Ford GA, Thijs VN. Thrombolytics in acute ischaemic stroke: historical perspective and future opportunities. *Cerebrovasc Dis* 2013;35(4):313–19.

22 National Institute of Neurological Disorders and Stroke rt-PA Stroke Study Group. Tissue plasminogen activator for acute ischemic stroke. *N Engl J Med* 1995;333(24):1581–7.

23 Kwiatkowski TG, Libman RB, Frankel M, et al. Effects of tissue plasminogen activator for acute ischemic stroke at one year. National Institute of Neurological Disorders and Stroke Recombinant Tissue Plasminogen Activator Stroke Study Group. *N Engl J Med* 1999;340(23):1781–7.

24 Miller J, Hartwell C, Lewandowski C. Stroke treatment using intravenous and intra-arterial tissue plasminogen activator. *Curr Treat Options Cardiovasc Med* 2012;14(3):273–83.

25 Lewandowski C, Barsan W. Treatment of acute ischemic stroke. *Ann Emerg Med* 2001;37(2):202–16.

26 Cohen JE, Leker RR, Rabinstein A. New strategies for endovascular recanalization of acute ischemic stroke. *Neurol Clin* 2013;31(3):705–19.

27 Rossnagel K, Jungehülsing GJ, Nolte CH, et al. Out-of-hospital delays in patients with acute stroke. *Ann Emerg Med* 2004;44(5):476–83.

28 Maestroni A, Mandelli C, Manganaro D, et al. Factors influencing delay in presentation for acute stroke in an emergency department in Milan,Italy. *Emerg Med J* 2008;25(6):340–5.

29 Wester P, Rådberg J, Lundgren B, Peltonen M. Factors associated with delayed admission to hospital and in-hospital delays in acute stroke and TIA: a prospective, multicenter study. Seek- Medical-Attention-in-Time Study Group. *Stroke*. 1999;30(1):40–8.

30 Derex L, Adeleine P, Nighoghossian N, Honnorat J, Trouillas P. Factors influencing early admission in a French stroke unit. *Stroke* 2002;33(1):153–9.

31 California Acute Stroke Pilot Registry (CASPR) Investigators. Prioritizing interventions to improve rates of thrombolysis for ischemic stroke. *Neurology* 2005;64(4):654–9.

32 Quain DA, Parsons MW, Loudfoot AR, et al. Improving access to acute stroke therapies: a controlled trial of organised pre-hospital and emergency care. *Med J Aust* 2008;189(8):429–33.

33 Smith W, Sung G, Starkman S, et al. Safety and efficacy of mechanical embolectomy in acute ischemic stroke results of the MERCI trial. *Stroke* 2005:36(7);1432–40.

34 Joint Commission on Hospital Accreditation of Healthcare Organizations. Advanced Certification for Primary Stroke Centers. Available at: www.jointcommission.org/certification/primary_stroke_centers.aspx

35 Alberts MJ, Latchaw RE, Jagoda A, et al. Revised and updated recommendations for the establishment of primary stroke centers: a summary statement from the brain attack coalition. *Stroke* 2011;42(9):2651–65.

36 Joint Commission on Hospital Accreditation of Healthcare Organizations. Advanced Certification for Comprehensive Stroke Centers. Available at: www.jointcommission.org/certification/advanced_certification_comprehensive_stroke_centers.aspx

37 Alberts MJ, Latchaw RE, Selman WR, et al. Recommendations for comprehensive stroke centers: a consensus statement from the Brain Attack Coalition. *Stroke* 2005;36(7):1597–616.

38 Silbergleit R, Scott PA, Lowell MJ. Cost-effectiveness of helicopter transport of stroke patients for thrombolysis. *Acad Emerg Med* 2003;10(9):966–72.

39 Silliman SL, Quinn B, Huggett V, Merino JG. Use of a field-to-stroke center helicopter transport program to extend thrombolytic therapy to rural residents. *Stroke* 2003;34(3):729–33.

40 Thomas SH, Kociszewski C, Schwamm LH, Wedel SK. The evolving role of helicopter emergency medical services in the transfer of stroke patients to specialized centers. *Prehosp Emerg Care* 2002;6(2):210–14.

41 Lopez-Yunez A, Bruno A, Williams L, Yilmaz E, Zurrú C, Biller J. Protocol violations in community based rTPA stroke treatment are associated with symptomatic intracerebral hemorrhage. *Stroke* 2001;32(1):12–16.

42 Magid D, Naviaux N, Wears R. Stroking the data: re-analysis of the NINDS trial. *Ann Emerg Med* 2005;45(4):385–7.

CHAPTER 22

Allergic reactions

Debra G. Perina and Douglas R. Gallo

Introduction

Potential allergic reactions and their sequelae are common complaints encountered in the EMS system. Allergic reactions can be triggered by many agents, such as foods, medications, topical products, and limitless environmental exposures including arthropod stings. Severity can vary from local reactions and discomfort to life-threatening systemic anaphylaxis. EMS physicians and other providers must be able to rapidly recognize the manifestations of allergic reactions and begin to provide prehospital treatment that can be life-saving.

Physiology of allergic reactions

Allergic reactions are hypersensitivity reactions resulting from the exposure to an allergen [1]. In milder forms they may result in localized edema and pruritus. Systemic reactions can also be mild, resulting in a more widespread rash that can be pruritic. In their most severe form, allergic reactions progress to anaphylaxis with multisystem and potentially life-threatening manifestations that include respiratory failure, circulatory collapse, and shock.

There are four types of hypersensitivity reactions (Box 22.1). Type I accounts for most cases of anaphylaxis. Type II reactions are typically seen in the setting of blood transfusions, drug reactions, and cases of idiopathic thrombocytopenic purpura. Type III reactions are responsible for serum sickness, reactions to tetanus toxoid, and poststreptococcal glomerulonephritis. Type IV reactions are T-cell-mediated and delayed hypersensitivity responses which do not cause anaphylaxis.

Urticaria, or hives, is an often-encountered symptom and physical sign of an acute allergic reaction. Although the potential etiologies of urticaria are numerous, the temporal link to a likely allergen can often be made upon consideration of recent exposures. For example, the patient might have recently started a new medication, been stung by an insect, or eaten a certain food. Urticaria, itself, is not particularly concerning. However,

its potential as an indicator of a reaction in the evolution of systemic effects should not go unrecognized.

Allergic reactions that present as urticaria can progress to angioedema that results in facial or tongue swelling. Subsequently, airway obstruction might develop precipitously with obvious consequences. Angioedema also often occurs without other apparent manifestations of an allergic reaction. One of the more common causes is angiotensin-converting enzyme inhibitors. The patient may have been taking the medication for some time before such a reaction occurs, which can be confusing to some who assume that a reaction would have occurred earlier if the patient was going to exhibit one. Hereditary angioedema, on the other hand, does not represent a response to a specific allergen, but it deserves mention because of its similar presentation to allergic reactions and other forms of angioedema. Hereditary angioedema is an autosomal dominant genetic disorder caused by a defect in the complement pathway that results in either a low C1 esterase level or a high level of dysfunctional C1 esterase. Symptoms can include pruritus, urticaria, wheezing, facial and tongue swelling, dizziness, hypotension, syncope, and gastrointestinal distress [2].

At the severe end of the allergic reaction spectrum is anaphylaxis. Anaphylaxis can be variable in presentation and is defined by rapid progression to multiple system involvement (Box 22.2). In general, the incidence of anaphylaxis is increasing. The most common triggers are insect stings and food ingestions, particularly nuts. Food ingestions are particularly concerning and most often the most severe. The faster a reaction develops after exposure to an allergen, the more likely it is to be severe and life-threatening.

Causative agents

Almost anything can be a potential allergen (Box 22.3). Common agents include medications, foods and food additives, latex, arthropod bites and stings, mold, radiographic contrast media, and certain marine envenomations [1] (see Volume 1, Chapter 38). Some insect bites or stings, such as those of millipedes, caterpillars,

Emergency Medical Services: Clinical Practice and Systems Oversight, Second Edition. Volume 1: Clinical Aspects of EMS.
Edited by David C. Cone, Jane H. Brice, Theodore R. Delbridge, and J. Brent Myers.
© 2015 NAEMSP. Published 2015 by John Wiley & Sons, Inc. Companion Website: www.wiley.com\go\cone\naemsp

Box 22.1 Types of hypersensitivity reactions and anaphylaxis production

Type I Immediate(IgE or IgG) – most common
Type II Cytotoxic complement cascade (IgG or IgM)-Yes
Type III Immune complex (IgG or IgM)-Yes
Type IV Delayed T-cell-No anaphylaxis

Box 22.2 Definition of anaphylaxis

Acute cutaneous and/or mucosal involvement after antigen exposure
plus:
- Respiratory compromise
  - Bronchospasm
  - Stridor
  - Hypoxia
- Cardiovascular compromise
  - Hypotension
  - Collapse
- Persistent gastrointestinal symptoms
  - Vomiting
  - Crampy abdominal pain

Box 22.3 Common causes of allergic reactions

Medications
Antibiotics
  Penicillin, vancomycin, trimethoprim-sulfamethoxazole
Angiotensin-converting enzyme inhibitors
Aspirin
Non-steroidal antiinflammatory drugs
Radiographic iodine-based dyes
Skin creams, cosmetics
Human/animal proteins
Vaccines
Transfusions
Foods
Peanuts/nuts
Eggs
Wheat, soybeans
Shellfish
Additives
Red dye sulfites
Stings/bites
Insects
- Hornets/wasps
- Fire ants
- Scorpion
- Caterpillars
- Kissing bugs
- Centipedes, millipedes
- Arachnids
- Ticks
Vertebrates (lizards, Gila monster)
Marine bites (sea nettle, man-o-war, jellyfish)
Mammals (rats/mice, gerbils, hamsters)
Environmental exposures
Mold
Latex
Pollen
Perfumes

and centipedes, most often cause only pain and local skin reactions such as blistering [3,4]. Certain species of caterpillars have venom-filled hair and spines that can cause systemic reactions, including anaphylaxis, within 2 hours of the sting [3]. Bites from kissing bugs are painless and usually occur during sleep. Most often, this results in localized swelling at the bite site, but can progress to systemic reactions [5]. There are also occasional rare reports of anaphylaxis from the bites of horse flies, deer flies, rats, and mice.

Hymenoptera account for the majority of severe allergic responses and anaphylaxis related to insect bites. There are three families of Hymenoptera: bees (honeybees and bumble-bees), vespids (yellow jackets, hornets, and wasps), and stinging ants (fire ants). Since fire ants are in the Hymenoptera order, the venom in fire ant bites is similar to that of bees and hornets, so that a patient allergic to bee stings will also display an allergic reaction to a fire ant bite [6]. Africanized honeybees ("killer bees") are an aggressive hybrid of the honeybee and have the same venom, but they sting repeatedly, thus increasing the risk of a severe reaction [7]. Approximately 1% of children and 3% of adults have reportedly had severe systemic allergic reactions to Hymenoptera venom [8]. Anaphylaxis can occur with a first-time exposure. Insect stings are the only allergen for which specific immunotherapy currently exists. This is most likely due to the prevalence and severity of such responses in humans [9].

Assessment and general approach

The first step in EMS response to calls regarding allergic reactions and/or bites and stings is to ensure that the scene is safe. No rescue or treatment can occur if providers fall victim to the same process that is affecting the patient. Next, EMS providers should determine how the patient was stung or what activity was occurring before the allergic reaction. This will help the provider determine if there is any special treatment needed and the potential for development of a severe reaction or anaphylaxis. EMS personnel should take all proper equipment, including life support, emergency drugs, and monitoring equipment with them when initially approaching the patient. Failure to do so may delay necessary treatment and result in further physiological decompensation of the patient.

Patient assessment should be done rapidly, first ensuring a patent airway. The patient should be queried about subjective shortness of breath or dysphagia, and the provider should note if the patient's voice is hoarse. The EMS provider should listen to breath sounds, assessing for stridor or wheezing. Facial, tongue, uvula, or orbital swelling should be noted. A full set of vital signs should be obtained. The patient should be evacuated from the scene as soon as feasible to prevent further contact with the allergen. Continuous patient reassessment should center on ensuring a patent airway and monitoring vital signs. Any patient with a significant allergic reaction or potential for deterioration during transport should have at least one large-bore IV line started with normal saline. The patient should be transported expediently to the closest most appropriate facility, depending on availability of local resources and other factors such as distance, weather, and terrain.

Prehospital treatment

If the patient is wheezing or in respiratory distress, 100% oxygen should be given with a non-rebreather mask. A large-bore IV with normal saline should be started and a fluid bolus given of at least 500 mL for an adult and 10 mL/kg for a child. If the patient was stung, any wounds should be inspected for retained stingers. If discovered, removal should be accomplished by scraping across the sting with a rigid thin object, such as an identification badge or credit card, to dislodge the stinger. Forceps or other squeezing devices should not be used because they may inadvertently disrupt the venom sac and release more venom into the patient. Local wound care with cool compresses and gauze covering should be applied. If there is the possibility of injected venom, the patient should be kept still and the affected extremity should be kept dependent, below the level of the heart, to slow the spread of venom [10,11].

If there is only a local isolated reaction, patient comfort and pain relief are all that is necessary. However, if the patient has a systemic allergic response, there is an immediate need for additional medications. Several medications are useful in this setting, and their use will depend on the severity of the patient's symptoms, vital signs, and past medical history. Before administering any medication, the provider should ensure that the patient has no medication allergies. The provider should also determine if the patient has taken any of his or her own medication (e.g. epinephrine autoinjector, oral diphenhydramine, or other oral antihistamine) before EMS arrival that may be masking the severity of the reaction or affect any of the medications EMS will administer. If the patient has his or her own autoinjector, EMS personnel of all training levels may assist with administration. Research has demonstrated that epinephrine autoinjectors can be used safely by EMTs in the treatment of anaphylaxis in the field [12].

Antihistamines are by far the most commonly used class of medication. Antihistamines block the action of histamine at H_1 receptors, but do not decrease histamine release. Diphenhydramine is the most common medication in this class and can be given orally, intravenously, intraosseously, or intramuscularly in a typical dose of 25–50 mg for adults, depending on their weight and the severity of the reaction. Research suggests that H_2 blockers have a synergistic action when used in conjunction with diphenhydramine, blocking both H_1 and H_2 cellular histamine receptors [13]. Both famotidine and ranitidine are useful H_2 blockers, but cimetidine is not recommended due to its

multiple drug interactions. Adult doses are IV famotidine 20 mg or IV ranitidine 50 mg. Corticosteroids, either orally or intravenously, may also be useful to prevent return of symptoms once other medications are metabolized. Peak onset of action of corticosteroids is 2–4 hours. Nebulized beta-agonists, such as albuterol, can be used for patients with persistent bronchospasm. Nebulized ipratropium bromide may also be used in conjunction with albuterol but should not be used alone. Although both the multidose inhaler and the nasal spray formulations of ipratropium contain an ingredient that may cause an allergic reaction in patients with known peanut allergies (soy lecithin, used to keep the medication in suspension), the nebulized formulation typically used by EMS and emergency departments lacks this ingredient [2]. All of the aforementioned drugs may also be used in children, but, as with any pediatric medication, dosages must be calculated based on the child's weight (Table 22.1).

Local allergic reactions can progress from one body system to anaphylaxis involving several systems, including skin, respiratory, and circulatory. If untreated, this can progress to anaphylactic shock with circulatory collapse and hypotension. Epinephrine is the first-line medication for a patient with anaphylaxis. Delaying its administration has been associated with poor outcomes. However, epinephrine should be used with caution in patients older than 50 years, those with known coronary artery disease, or in cases with life-threatening tachydysrhythmias. Infrequently, myocardial ischemia and infarction can be precipitated and have been reported [14]. Two different concentrations of epinephrine may be used, and the provider must be attentive to use the proper dosage and formulation when administering it. In adults, 0.3 mL of epinephrine 1:1000 solution can be given subcutaneously or intramuscularly except when the patient is on the verge of cardiovascular collapse. The intramuscular route at the lateral thigh is preferred. This route produces higher peak plasma concentrations in less time than subcutaneous injection or intramuscular injection in the deltoid [15]. Faster absorption from intramuscular injection in the thigh is thought to be due to the increased vascularity of the vastus lateralis muscle [5].

If the patient is hemodynamically unstable, 1 mL of epinephrine 1:10,000 mixed with 10 mL of normal saline can be given slowly by IV or intraosseous push over 5–10 minutes. Caution is advised. On the one hand, epinephrine given intravenously to a

Table 22.1 Pediatric allergic reaction treatment drug dosages

Drug	Weight-based dose
Epinephrine	1:1000 IM (0.3 mL maximum)
	1 mL of 1:10,000 mixed with 10 mL NS
	0.5 mL of 1:1000 in 2.5 mL NS nebulized
Diphenhydramine	1 mg/kg IM/IV/IO/PO (max. 50 mg)
Methylprednisolone	1–2 mg/kg
Famotidine	0.5 mg/kg to max. of 20 mg IV/IO
Ranitidine	2–4 mg/kg to max. of 50 mg IV/IO

IM, intramuscularly; IO, intraosseously; NS, normal saline; PO, by mouth.

patient who is not in cardiac arrest can be risky, resulting in hypertension or myocardial ischemia. On the other hand, it can be life-saving and should not be delayed in the case of a hemo-dynamically unstable or "crashing" patient. Epinephrine may also be nebulized by placing 0.5 mL of 1:1000 solution in 2.5 mL of normal saline.

If the patient is hypotensive, rapid fluid resuscitation with 1–2 liters of normal saline (20–40 mL/kg in children) is indicated in addition to the aforementioned medications. Patients often will become intermittently hypotensive and require multiple fluid boluses and additional medications, so frequent monitoring of vital signs is imperative. At least two large-bore IV lines are desirable.

Localized angioedema is treated as an allergic reaction with antihistamines and steroids, along with epinephrine in severe cases. However, little actual benefit or significant improvement has been shown with these medications. As with medication-induced angioedema, hereditary angioedema is generally not responsive to antihistamines, steroids, or epinephrine, although they are routinely administered [5]. The mainstay of treatment is supportive, with early consideration for intubation if there is airway compromise.

Emergency medical services personnel should anticipate that any airway intervention for a patient with an allergic reaction or angioedema is going to be especially difficult. The edema can extend to the glottic and subglottic regions and not be externally visible. The only clue the provider might have is that the patient's voice is hoarse or different from normal. Oral-pharyngeal, glottis, and subglottic edema can obscure anatomical landmarks and decrease airway caliber that alter the effective sizes of airway tools. If bronchospasm is present, ventilation before and between intubation attempts may be difficult, adding pressure for expedient success. Thus, it is imperative that the provider is prepared for a difficult airway with airway skills, adjuncts, and emergency rescue devices and techniques, such as cricothyrotomy, especially if rapid sequence intubation (RSI) is also being performed [16].

Special considerations

Several points may be helpful to remember when responding to allergic reactions in the field. In general, stinging insects, especially Hymenoptera, can cause systemic allergic reactions and anaphylaxis, but these reactions are rare with biting insects [17]. There is a greater chance of a systemic reaction with multiple stings. One should remember that the clinical presentation may be quite varied and the history may be vague. Patients may have significant symptoms yet not be able to recall exposure to a specific allergen. In cases such as these, interventions necessary for stabilization should take priority over identification of the culprit allergen. In cases of true anaphylaxis, the axiom "stabilize first, diagnose later" should be followed. After emergency interventions are completed, care should be taken to frequently

reassess the patient and document pertinent findings, which may be the first clue that an allergic reaction is present if the patient does not relate an exposure or inciting event. Symptoms can be exacerbated by fear, exercise, alcohol intake, heat exposure, or underlying cardiovascular disease. The provider should be careful not to become complacent or attribute clinical signs and symptoms solely to these conditions because allergic reactions can progress insidiously.

Anaphylaxis to stings can occur abruptly years after the first exposure, even without intervening stings. Furthermore, approximately 20% of patients exhibit biphasic anaphylaxis responses where the initial symptoms resolve and there is a symptom-free period before the onset of the late phase reaction 4–6 hours after the initial symptoms began. The symptoms of the late reaction can be markedly different from those of the initial reaction, and can be life-threatening even if those of the initial reaction were not. It is nearly impossible to predict which patients will exhibit this biphasic response. This could result in repeat EMS calls for allergic reactions featuring substantially different symptoms, particularly if a patient refuses transport or is seen and discharged from an ED before the late phase reaction occurs.

If the patient experiencing a severe allergic reaction or anaphylaxis routinely takes beta-blocker medications, the action of epinephrine may be blunted. Glucagon may be given in 1 mg increments by any parenteral route to overcome the effects of beta-blockade. Cutaneous symptoms are the most common clinical response in both adults and children. Hypotension is uncommon in children, but it has been reported in up to 60% of adults [18]. Patients will sometimes complain of a prodrome of chest pain or shortness of breath before development of a more generalized severe allergic reaction.

Emergency medical services providers should have a high index of suspicion on calls with these complaints to ensure that there was no contact with an allergen that may have caused these symptoms. For instance, allergy-producing contrast media are frequently given in free-standing imaging centers. Consider the possibility of allergic reactions and anaphylaxis when responding to calls of shortness of breath or chest pain at these sorts of facilities [19]. Anaphylaxis should be one of the etiologies considered when responding to cardiac arrests in outdoor areas, such as golf courses, because the patient may have been stung before the cardiac arrest.

Although bites from a Gila monster are infrequent, if it is still attached to the patient, the provider should remove it by prying its jaws apart with a stick or metal object, holding a flame under the lizard's chin, or submerging it in cold water [20]. Obviously, care should be taken to avoid additional bites to the patient or the providers.

To determine the most appropriate destination facility for allergic reaction patients, it helps to consider the etiology of the reaction and the availability of certain subspecialties, such as otolaryngology, anesthesia, critical care, toxicology, and so on, which may be necessary to definitively treat the reaction. Transportation time should also be considered. If the patient is unstable or is likely to become unstable during an extended transport time to an appropriate facility, then air medical evacuation should be considered. Transport to the closest available facility for stabilization followed by transfer of the patient to a higher level of care is also an option, and will depend on the availability of air medical services, the distance to the closest facility, weather, traffic, terrain and other conditions which must be factored in when making destination decisions.

Conclusion

Allergic reactions and anaphylaxis are frequently seen in the prehospital environment. EMS providers should be alert to the potential for rapid progression of allergic reactions and be prepared to support the patient hemodynamically and provide appropriate airway management. All patients should be provided with oxygen, IV fluid administration, and continuous monitoring during transport. Providers should be familiar with the common medications and the dosages used to treat allergic reactions. Antihistamines and epinephrine are the mainstays of treatment. In cases of generalized allergic reactions and anaphylaxis, epinephrine administration should not be delayed. Transport to an appropriate hospital should occur as soon as feasible.

References

1 Ewan PW. Anaphylaxis. *BMJ* 1998;316:1442.
2 Kemp SF. Current concepts in pathophysiology, diagnosis, and management of anaphylaxis. *Immunol Allergy Clin North Am* 2001;21:611–34.
3 Norris RL. Caterpillar envenomations. Available at: http://emedicine.medscape.com
4 Norris RL. Millipede envenomations. Available at: http://emedicine.medscape.com
5 Schneir AB,Clark RF. Bites and stings. In: *Tintinalli's Emergency Medicine: A Comprehensive Study Guide,* 7th edn. New York: McGraw-Hill, 2011, pp.1344–54.
6 deSchazo RD, Butcher BT, Banks WA. Reactions to the stings of the imported fire ant. *N Engl J Med* 1990;323:462.
7 Klotz JH, Klotz SA, Pinnas JL. Animal bites and stings with anaphylactic potential. *J Emerg Med* 2009;36(2):148–56.
8 Yates AB, Moffitt JE, deShazo RD. Anaphylaxis to arthropod bites and stings. *Immunol Allergy Clin North Am* 2001;21:635–51.
9 Graft DF. Insect sting allergy. *Med Clin North Am* 2006;90:211–32.
10 Pinnas JL. Allergic reactions to insect stings. In: *Conn's Current Therapy.* Philadelphia: W.B. Saunders, 2001, pp.797–9.
11 Rowe BH, Geata T. Anaphylaxis, acute allergic reactions and angioedema. In: *Tintinalli's Emergency Medicine: A Comprehensive Study Guide,* 7th edn. New York: McGraw-Hill, 2011, pp.177–81
12 Gold MS, Sainsbury R. First aid anaphylaxis management in children who were prescribed an epinephrine autoinjector device (EpiPen). *J Allergy Clin Immunol* 2000;106:171.
13 Lin RY, Curry A, Pesola GR, et al. Improved outcomes in patients with acute allergic syndromes who are treated with combined H1 and H2 antagonists. *Ann Emerg Med* 2000;36:462–8.
14 Anchor J, Settipane R. Appropriate use of epinephrine in anaphylaxis. *Am J Emerg Med* 2004;22(6):488–90.
15 Estelle F, Simons R, Gu X, et al. Epinephrine absorption in adults: intramuscular versus subcutaneous injection. *J Allergy Clin Immunol* 2001;108:871–3.
16 Tran TP, Muelleman RL. Allergy, hypersensitivity, angioedema and anaphylaxis. In: *Rosen's Emergency Medicine Concepts and Clinical Practice,* 8th edn, vol 2. Philadelphia: Elsevier, 2014, pp.1543–57.
17 Golden DB. Insect sting anaphylaxis. *Immunol Allergy Clin North Am* 2007;27(2):261–6.
18 Moffitt JE, Golden DB, Reisman RE, et al. Stinging insect hypersensitivity: a practice parameter update. *J Allergy Clin Immunol* 2004;114:869.
19 Pumphrey RS. Lessons for management of anaphylaxis from a study of fatal reactions. *Clin Exp Allergy* 2000;30:1144.
20 Piacentine J, Curry SC, Ryan PJ. Life-threatening anaphylaxis following Gila monster bite. *Ann Emerg Med* 1986;15(8):959–61.

CHAPTER 23

Diabetic emergencies

José G. Cabañas, Jorge L. Falcon-Chevere, and Jane H. Brice

Introduction

Diabetes is a commonly encountered disease in the out-of-hospital environment. Characterized by defective insulin production and use, diabetes is the most common endocrine disorder, and hypoglycemia is the most common endocrine emergency [1].

Several types of diabetes are recognized. Type 1 diabetes occurs when the pancreatic beta cells are destroyed, which removes the body's only insulin-producing mechanism. Typically occurring in children and adolescents, type 1 diabetes accounts for 5–10% of all cases of diabetes. These individuals require exogenous insulin administration to survive. Type 2 diabetes is more common, responsible for 90–95% of all diabetes diagnoses. Rather than a defect of insulin production, type 2 diabetes is characterized by insulin resistance at the cellular level and gradual failure of pancreatic production of insulin. Type 2 diabetes is a disease predominantly in older adults and is associated with physical inactivity, obesity, and a history of gestational diabetes, a form of glucose intolerance found among pregnant women. Typically resolving after delivery of the infant, the individual who was diagnosed with gestational diabetes carries a 35–60% chance of developing diabetes over the next 5–10 years [2]. Diabetes remains a major cause of coronary heart disease and stroke, and it is the seventh leading cause of death in the United States.

Diabetes is a chronic disease that, at present, has no cure. In 2011, it was estimated that 25.8 million persons in the United States suffered from diabetes. This represents 8.3% of the total US population. Of these 25.8 million, 18.8 million are persons with a known diagnosis of diabetes, and the remaining 7 million have unrecognized and untreated diabetes. It is also estimated that 51 million people aged 40–74 years have impaired glucose tolerance, impaired fasting glucose, or both [2]. Diabetes occurs more frequently in certain populations, including African Americans, Hispanics, and Native Americans.

One-and-a-half million new cases of diabetes are diagnosed each year, and diabetes-related visits to US emergency departments (EDs) totaled 20.2 million between 1997 and 2007 [2,3]. Additionally, there were approximately 5 million ED visits for hypoglycemia between 1992 and 2005, with 25% of these visits resulting in admission to hospital. In the same interval, there were approximately 750,000 ED visits for diabetic ketoacidosis (DKA), with 87% admitted predominantly to intensive care settings [4,5].

The cost of diabetes in the United States is staggering. An estimated $174 billion is spent annually for direct and indirect medical costs. This is in addition to lost work opportunities and disability, summing to an estimated $58 billion per year [2].

Diabetic emergencies account for 3–4% of EMS call volume. The majority of EMS responses for diabetic emergencies are for hypoglycemia [1]. The consequences of both hypoglycemia and hyperglycemia are dire. Therefore, it is imperative that appropriate care is started in the field to decrease morbidity and mortality. EMS physicians and medical directors must have adequate clinical operating guidelines to appropriately manage these patients in the prehospital setting. This chapter addresses the most common diabetic conditions prehospital providers will encounter.

Prehospital assessment

General approach

The initial evaluation of a diabetic emergency starts with the emergency medical dispatcher when 9-1-1 is called. Crucial information may be obtained through the telephone while the response unit is dispatched. Treatment may begin with prearrival instructions. Medical oversight is crucial to ensure quality within the dispatcher's interrogation protocols and that prearrival instructions are appropriately given (see Volume 2, Chapter 10).

Once responders arrive, scene safety is a priority, given that patients experiencing diabetic emergencies have altered mental

Emergency Medical Services: Clinical Practice and Systems Oversight, Second Edition. Volume 1: Clinical Aspects of EMS.
Edited by David C. Cone, Jane H. Brice, Theodore R. Delbridge, and J. Brent Myers.

Box 23.1 Key elements in the prehospital assessment of diabetic emergencies

I Evaluation of ABCs and level of consciousness
  A ABCs (airway, breathing, circulation)
  B AVPU scale (alert, verbal, painful, unresponsive)
  C Vital signs
  D Glucose check
II History
  A Past medical history, diabetes mellitus?
  B Recent illness or injury
  C Pregnancy
  D Precipitating factors
  E Medications
III Physical examination
  A General impression
  B Focused examination

status and may act in unpredictable ways. Although most diabetic patients may call for an ambulance for a specific diabetic condition, such as hypoglycemia, many patients will have non-specific complaints such as nausea, vomiting, dizziness, or abdominal pain, requiring the responders to gather information to determine the cause of the illness.

The initial patient evaluation is the same as any other case in the prehospital setting (Box 23.1). In the instance of diabetic emergencies, history taking is important because it provides pertinent information that may alter treatment, particularly in patients with altered mental status. Key history elements in the assessment of a patient with altered mental status should include the following:
- medical history, especially history of diabetes
- medications
- onset of symptoms
- complete set of vital signs
- measurement of glucose.

Other considerations

The possibility of intentional overdose in the hypoglycemic, depressed patient, and of inadvertent overdose in the elderly or confused patient should be considered. Attention should be paid to the type of insulin or medication the patient is taking. The use of long-acting insulin formulations may require close monitoring of the patient by a responsible adult at home or continuous monitoring and additional treatment at the hospital. Patients on certain oral hypoglycemic agents should be transported to the hospital because they have a higher risk of recurrent hypoglycemia and, by extension, increased morbidity. Hyperglycemia should prompt prehospital personnel to think about infectious sources such as urinary tract infection or pneumonia, especially in an elderly or debilitated patient. Acute medical illnesses, such as myocardial infarction, stroke, or pancreatitis, can also cause hyperglycemia in the diabetic patient. Recent cocaine use or poor compliance with medication can also be causes of hyperglycemia, all of which should be considered by prehospital personnel.

Measurement of glucose

Current EMS practice embraces the prehospital measurement of plasma glucose using glucometers. In past decades, dextrose was empirically given to all patients with altered mental status without first measuring plasma glucose. Investigators found that few patients benefited from such empiric treatment, and a few patients were harmed, as in the case of stroke [6,7]. Glucometer use by prehospital personnel has been found to be safe and accurate [8,9]. It is important to note that the glucose strips must be stored in temperature-controlled sections of the ambulance so they provide reliable readings [10]. The prehospital measurement of plasma glucose is now considered a standard practice in EMS.

Prehospital treatment

Hypoglycemia

Diabetic management emphasizes tight glycemic control to prevent long-term complications, such as heart disease and blindness. This strategy, however, may lead to adverse consequences, such as the development of hypoglycemia. Hypoglycemia, usually defined as a serum glucose concentration less than 70 mg/dL (3.8 mmol/L), is the most common endocrine emergency [7]. Estimates are that persons with diabetes suffer mild (self-treated) hypoglycemic events 1–2 times per week and that 30% of persons with diabetes suffer severe hypoglycemic events annually [11–14].

Symptomatic hypoglycemia requires intervention to prevent organ compromise. Several treatment options exist for the prehospital environment, including oral glucose, IV dextrose, or intramuscular (IM) glucagon. Oral glucose may be used in alert patients with intact swallowing mechanisms. For patients with decreased level of consciousness or concern for aspiration, IV administration of 50% dextrose has been the standard for many years. One study found that the administration of 50 mL of 50% dextrose raised blood glucose by an average of 166 mg/dL, but the response varied widely among patients, from an increase of 37 mg/dL to 370 mg/dL [15]. In the unconscious patient, IV glucose administration provides a rapid onset of action (2–5 minutes). There are, however, several reports in the literature of tissue injury secondary to extravasation, which can cause significant complications, including skin and soft tissue injury, compartment syndrome, and loss of limb [16,17].

In a controlled clinical trial, Moore and Woollard found no difference in time to regain consciousness in hypoglycemic patients when comparing the administration of 10% dextrose versus 50% dextrose. In their cohort of 51 patients, 25 patients received a 10% dextrose solution and 26 received a 50% dextrose solution. Both groups had a median recovery time of 8 minutes. Patients in the 10% dextrose group received a median of 15 g less glucose than the 50% dextrose group to achieve the same response. Additionally, patients in the 10% dextrose group were less likely to have high glucose levels after treatment.

Patients occasionally had difficulty bringing their glucose levels back into a normal range after treatment with 50% dextrose [18].

For patients in whom IV access cannot be achieved in a timely manner, the administration of glucagon provides a means of rescue. However, in alcoholic or malnourished patients with depleted glycogen storage, it is less likely to be beneficial. Recovery time may be significantly longer with glucagon than with dextrose. These response times are dependent on the severity of hypoglycemia and have been shown to be anywhere from 8 to 21 minutes. Although most sources describe glucagon as an IM drug, it has also been used successfully subcutaneously and intranasally [19–23]. Intranasal (IN) glucagon has been shown to have comparable efficacy to IM or SC glucagon. Hvidberg showed that both intramuscular and intranasal glucagon elevated glucose levels, but the response was faster in those treated via the IM route [22]. Sibley et al. described the case of a diabetic hypoglycemic patient who was successfully treated with IN glucagon in the prehospital setting without further side-effects or complications [23]. Intraosseous (IO) access is another potential route to provide 50% dextrose for critically ill hypoglycemic patients without IV access. However, this should be reserved for extreme clinical circumstances given that IO insertion poses a risk for infection or poor wound healing in diabetic patients.

Hyperglycemia

Hyperglycemia is defined as blood glucose levels greater than 200 mg/dL (11.1 mmol/L). An elevated glucose level alone does not represent a medical emergency. Markedly elevated glucose and hyperglycemia in the setting of DKA are urgent medical problems that should be recognized and treated accordingly.

Diabetic ketoacidosis mortality rates range from 9% to 14% [24]. EMS providers will encounter this condition predominantly in type 1 diabetics, but it may also rarely occur in type 2 diabetics. Usually these patients are dependent on daily insulin therapy to maintain glycemic control. DKA may be precipitated by certain metabolic stressors such as infectious processes, myocardial infarction, pregnancy, and trauma, especially if they interrupt the insulin regimen. Patients present with non-specific signs and symptoms that can include fatigue, tachypnea, altered sensorium, abdominal pain, nausea, vomiting, polydipsia, and polyuria. They may also present with severe dehydration and may be hypotensive. EMS providers should be trained to recognize and suspect such an emergency.

There has been no research dedicated to the out-of-hospital treatment of DKA patients. However, most of the treatment modalities in emergency medicine for DKA can apply in the out-of-hospital setting. The most important intervention is to recognize the emergency and start treatment without delay. IV fluid resuscitation should be initiated to restore volume depletion. These patients should be closely monitored. There is no role for insulin therapy in the prehospital setting. An important caveat relates to pediatric patients, for whom there is a risk of life-threatening cerebral edema with rapid volume repletion. For them, insulin (at the hospital) plays a more critical early role, and initial resuscitation should only be intended to reverse appearance of shock or hypotension. Additional correction of a fluid deficit should occur over 24–48 hours.

Patients with hyperglycemia may also present in a non-ketotic hyperosmolar state (NKHS). NKHS is a serious diabetic emergency that carries a mortality rate between 10% and 50% [24]. Providers may not be able to differentiate DKA from NKHS. However, they may be able to suspect it from the patient's history. NKHS is more common in patients with type 2 diabetes and is triggered by the same stressors that elicit DKA. Patients in NKHS will present with marked volume depletion, necessitating the initiation of intravenous fluid resuscitation without delay. Prehospital providers should promptly establish support according to their scope of practice and clinical operating guidelines. Directing field treatment should be targeted to hemodynamic stabilization first. Supportive measures consist of oxygen, cardiac monitoring, and IV isotonic fluids through two peripheral lines. Fluid boluses should be given with constant reassessment of vital signs.

Pediatric considerations

Approximately one in every 400–600 children and adolescents has type 1 diabetes [2]. The age of presentation has a bimodal distribution that peaks at 4–6 years of age and 10–14 years of age. This requires that prehospital providers be alert for hyperglycemia in children who present with volume depletion, weight loss, polydipsia, and polyuria, as this may be the patient's first presentation of diabetes. In addition, hypoglycemia should be suspected and glucose should be measured in any pediatric patient who is actively seizing, has altered mental status, or has volume depletion secondary to illness or gastroenteritis. In one study of children requiring resuscitation in an ED, 18% were found to be hypoglycemic, requiring administration of dextrose [25].

The prehospital management of pediatric hypoglycemia mirrors that of treatment in the adult. The recognition of hypoglycemia followed by administration of dextrose is important. Dextrose in children and infants is diluted to 25% (from the 50% given to adults) because dextrose is irritating to vascular structures. The current literature regarding the efficacy of 10% dextrose in the field may allow EMS systems to carry a single concentration of dextrose [18]. Table 23.1 provides guidance for treating hypoglycemia in pediatric patients using $D_{10}W$ solution. Hyperglycemia is treated with fluid resuscitation as appropriate, given the patient's vital signs, with attention to the issue of potential cerebral edema discussed above.

Pregnancy

Prehospital providers may occasionally encounter derangements of glucose levels in pregnant patients. Insulin resistance is raised during pregnancy. Approximately 7% of pregnant women in the United States develop gestational diabetes [26].

Table 23.1 Pediatric dextrose administration. Courtesy of the Office of the Medical Director, Austin/Travis County EMS System.

Pediatric Dextrose Administration							
				Dose 1.0 gram/kg			
			Concentration is 1 gram/10mL in 250mL bag sterile water (D10W)				
			Must use volume control device (IV Burette) for Infusion				
			Titrate to patient's condition and response				
Patient weight	3kg	5kg	7kg	9kg	11kg	13kg	15kg	17kg
Grams Dextrose	3	5	7	9	11	13	15	17
mL D10w	30 mL	50 mL	70 mL	90 mL	110 mL	130 mL	150 mL	170 mL
Patient weight	19kg	21kg	23kg	25kg	27kg	30kg	33kg	35kg
Grams Dextrose	19	21	23	25	25	25	25	25
mL D10w	190 mL	210 mL	230 mL	250 mL	250 mL	250 mL	250 mL	250mL

The current practice is to intensively manage glucose in the pregnant patient to avoid complications such as macrosomia or intrauterine fetal death. Because of this very tight glucose control, it is not uncommon for pregnant patients to experience hypoglycemia. Alternatively, given the emphasis on tight glycemic control, hyperglycemia is rare, with the exception of the non-compliant or undiagnosed patient. Treatment of hypoglycemia and hyperglycemia in the pregnant patient is no different from that in the non-pregnant patient [27,28].

Medication overdose

Intentional insulin overdose has been reported with some frequency in the literature. Persistent or refractory hypoglycemia should prompt the prehospital providers to consider the possibility of overdose, whether intentional or unintentional. Treatment should be aimed at restoring glucose levels to a normal range, continued monitoring of glucose levels, and transport to an ED for continued monitoring and care. Recurrent hypoglycemia has been reported for 2–3 days in patients with massive overdoses [29–31].

Disposition

The disposition of diabetic prehospital patients with successfully corrected hypoglycemia has been controversial. The concern for adverse outcomes, recurrent hypoglycemia, poor access to care, and possible litigation has fueled the discussion. Currently, it is estimated that between 34% and 69% of hypoglycemic patients may refuse transport after paramedic contact. Several studies have found that the practice of releasing treated hypoglycemic patients appears to be safe [1,32–36].

A study of the reasons for EMS non-transport after a 9-1-1 call demonstrated that diabetic calls account for approximately 9% of non-transports. Previous studies had reported diabetes accounting for 2–7% of non-transports [37]. Studies examining the safety of allowing patients to refuse care have shown that

Box 23.2 Key elements for safe discharge after treatment for hypoglycemia

1 History of insulin-dependent diabetes mellitus
2 Return of normal mental state within 10 minutes of dextrose administration
3 Pretreatment blood glucose less than 80 mg/dL
4 Posttreatment blood glucose greater than 80 mg/dL
5 Ability to tolerate food by mouth
6 Absence of comorbid conditions or complicating factors
7 The patient has follow-up with a primary care physician
8 No use of sulfonylurea medications
9 Normal vital signs after treatment
10 Patient understands discharge instructions
11 Patient has a responsible adult to monitor him/her

those who refuse transport are no more likely than transported patients to experience recurrence of hypoglycemia or to require later care. Thus, these studies have derived a set of reasonable guidelines for refusal of care instructions. Patients should be able to eat, have a responsible adult who will remain with them, and not have any condition that would predispose the patient to a repeat episode, such as persistent vomiting. Additionally, the patient should be given written instructions directing follow-up with a physician [1,32,38]. Research has shown that patients prefer a permanent protocol that allows the discharge of hypoglycemic patients without admission to the ED [36]. It is clear that EMS systems should develop specific guidelines for patient refusal after hypoglycemia treatment. The most important elements for these prehospital guidelines are summarized in Box 23.2.

Protocols

Emergency medical services protocols should clearly provide appropriate assessment and treatment guidelines. When hypoglycemia is encountered, treatment protocols should include administration of dextrose in some form ($D_{50}W$, $D_{25}W$, or $D_{10}W$)

if IV access can be obtained, or the administration of glucagon when IV access cannot be obtained. Policies concerning treat-and-release protocols or transport refusal in patients successfully treated in the field should be very clear and well understood by all personnel. A strong quality assurance program is necessary to monitor compliance with clinical standards and identify opportunities for improvement and education. It is highly recommended that patients who are not transported to the hospital for whatever reason be audited and reviewed by the EMS medical director. Symptomatic hyperglycemia mandates administration of IV fluid and transport to a hospital.

Conclusion

Diabetes mellitus is a highly prevalent chronic disease among the US population, responsible for large expenditures of health care dollars. Diabetic emergencies are commonly encountered by EMS providers in the prehospital setting. Of these emergencies, hypoglycemia is the most common. It is imperative for providers to be adequately prepared and trained to manage such conditions. The primary evaluation starts with the 9-1-1 dispatcher, who may be able to gather crucial medical information. Providers should be prepared to manage the ABCs and start treatment without delay. Patients should be assessed for the need for transport and, if required, transported to the most appropriate medical facility capable of managing their problems.

References

1 Cain E, Ackroyd-Stolarz S, Alexiadia P, Murray D. Prehospital hypoglycemia: the safety of not transporting treated patients. *Prehosp Emerg Care* 2003;7(4):458–65.

2 Centers for Disease Control and Prevention. *National Diabetes Fact Sheet: General Information and National Estimates on Diabetes in the United States*, 2011. Available at: www.cdc.gov/diabetes/pubs/pdf/ndfs_2011.pdf

3 Menchine MD, Wiechmann W, Peters AL, Arora S. Trends in diabetes-related visits to US EDs from 1997 to 2007. *Am J Emerg Med* 2012;30(5):754–8.

4 Ginde AA, Lieberman RM, Pallin DJ, Camargo CA Jr. Emergency department visits for hypoglycemia: epidemiology, patient education and outcomes [abstract]. *Ann Emerg Med* 2007;50 (suppl):S54.

5 Ginde AA, Pelletier AJ, Camargo CA Jr. National study of U.S. emergency department visits with diabetic ketoacidosis, 1993–2003. *Diabetes Care* 2006;29(9):2117–19.

6 Hoffman JR, Schriger DL, Votey SR, Luo JS. The empiric use of hypertonic dextrose in patients with altered mental status: a reappraisal. *Ann Emerg Med* 1992;21(1):20–4.

7 Browning RG, Olson DW, Stueven HA, Mateer JR. 50% dextrose: antidote or toxin. *Ann Emerg Med* 1990;19(60):113–17.

8 Jones JL, Ray VG, Gough JE, Garrison HG, Whitley TW. Determination of prehospital blood glucose: a prospective, controlled study. *J Emerg Med* 1992;10(6):679–82.

9 Lavery RF, Allegra JR, Cody RP, Zacharias D, Schreck DM. A prospective evaluation of glucose reagent teststrips in the prehospital setting. *Am J Emerg Med* 1991;9(4):304–8.

10 Herr RD. Effect of time and storage conditions of Chemstrip bG on estimating blood glucose aboard ambulances. *J Int Fed Clin Chem* 1992;4(2):71–5.

11 Pramming S, Thorsteinsson B, Bendtson I, Binder C. Symptomatic hypoglycemia in 411 type 1 diabetic patients. *Diabet Med* 1991; 8(3):217–22.

12 Pramming S, Pedersen-Bjergaard U, Heller SP, et al. Severe hypoglycemia in unselected patients with type 1 diabetes: a cross-sectional multicenter survey (Abstract). *Diabetologica* 2000;43(Suppl 1):A194.

13 MacLeod KM, Hepburn DA, Frier BM. Frequency and morbidity of severe hypoglycemia in insulin-treated diabetic patients. *Diabet Med* 1993;10(3):238–45.

14 Ter Braak EWMT, Appleman AMMF, van de Laak MF, Stolk RP, van Haeften TW, Erkelens DW. Clinical characteristics of type 1 diabetic patients with and without severe hypoglycemia. *Diabetes Care* 2000;23(10):1467–71.

15 Adler, PM. Serum glucose changes after administration of 50% dextrose solutions. *Am J Emerg Med* 1986;4(6):504–6.

16 DeLorenzo RA, Vista JP. Another hazard of hypertonic dextrose. *Am J Emerg Med* 1994;12(2):262–3.

17 Lawson SL, Brady W, Mahmoud A. Identification of highly concentrated dextrose solution (50% dextrose) extravasation and treatment – a clinical report. *Am J Emerg Med* 2013;31(5):886.e3–5.

18 Moore C, Woollard M. Dextrose 10% or 50% in the treatment of hypoglycaemia out of hospital? A randomized controlled trial. *Emerg Med J* 2005;22(7):512–15.

19 Vukmir RB, Paris PM, Yealy DM. Glucagon: prehospital therapy for hypoglycemia. *Ann Emerg Med* 1991;20(4):375–9.

20 Carstens S, Sprehn M. Prehospital treatment of severe hypoglycemia: a comparison of intramuscular glucagon and intravenous glucose. *Prehosp Dis Med* 1998;13(2):114–25.

21 Vermeulen MJ, Klompas M, Ray JG, Mazza C, Morrison LJ. Subcutaneous glucagon may be better than oral glucose for prehospital treatment of symptomatic hypoglycemia. *Diabetes Care* 2003; 26(8):2472–3.

22 Hvidberg A, Djurup R, Hilsted J. Glucose recovery after intranasal glucagon during hypoglycemia in man. *Eur J Clin Pharmacol* 1994; 46:15–17.

23 Sibley T, Jacobsen R, Salomone J. Successful administration of intranasal glucagon in the out-of-hospital environment. *Prehosp Emerg Care* 2013;17(1):98–102.

24 Fishbein H, Palumbo PJ. Acute metabolic complications in diabetes. In: National Diabetes Data Group of the National Institute of Diabetes and Digestive and Kidney Diseases, National Institutes of Health. *Diabetes in America*, 2nd edn. Bethesda, MD: National Diabetes Data Group, 1995. Available at: diabetes.niddk.nih.gov/dm/pubs/america/pdf/chapter13.pdf

25 Losek JD. Hypoglycemia and the ABC'S (Sugar) of pediatric resuscitation. *Ann Emerg Med* 2000;35(1):43–6.

26 Reece EA. Perspectives on obesity, pregnancy and birth outcomes in the United States: the scope of the problem. *Am J Obstet Gynecol* 2008;198(1):23–7.

27 Rosenn BM, Miodovnik M, Holcberg C, Khoury JC, Siddiqi TA. Hypoglycemia: the price of intensive insulin therapy for pregnant women with insulin dependent diabetes mellitus. *Obstet Gynecol* 1995;85(3):417–22.

28 Gabbe SG, Carlenter LB, Garrison EA. New strategies for glucose control in patients with type 1 and type 2 diabetes mellitus in pregnancy. *Clin Obstet Gynecol* 2007;50(4):1014–24.

29 Shibutani Y, Ogawa C. Suicidal insulin overdose in a type 1 diabetic patient: relation of serum insulin concentrations to the duration of hypoglycemia. *J Diabetes Complications* 2000;14(1):60–2.

30 Roberge RJ, Martin TG, Delbridge TR. Intentional massive insulin overdose: recognition and management. *Ann Emerg Med* 1993; 22(2):228–34.

31 Fuller ET, Miller MA, Kaylor DW, Janke C. Lantus over-dose: case presentation and management options. *J Emerg Med* 2009; 36(1):26–9.

32 Mechem CC, Kreshak AA, Barger J, Shofer FS. The short-term outcome of hypoglycemic patients who refuse ambulance transport after out-of-hospital therapy. *Acad Emerg Med* 1998;5(8):768–72.

33 Carter AJ, Keane PS, Dreyer JF. Transport refusal by hypoglycemic patients after on-scene intravenous dextrose. *Acad Emerg Med* 2002;9(8):855–7.

34 Thompson RH, Wolford RW. Development and evaluation of criteria allowing paramedics to treat and release patients with hypoglycemia: a retrospective study. *Prehosp Disaster Med* 1991; 6(3):309–13.

35 Mattila EM, Kuisma MJ, Sund KP, Voipio-Pulkki. Out-of- hospital hypoglycaemia is safely and cost-effectively treated by paramedics. *Eur J Emerg Med* 2004;11(2):70–4.

36 Lerner EB, Billittier AJ 4th, Lance DR, Janicke DM, Teuscher JA. Can paramedics safely treat and discharge hypoglycemic patients in the field? *Am J Emerg Med* 2003;21(2):115–20.

37 Moss ST, Chan TC, Buchanan J, Dunford JV, Vilke GM. Outcome study of prehospital patients signed out against medical advice by field paramedics. *Ann Emerg Med* 1998;31(2):247–50.

38 Socransky SJ, Pirrallo RG, Rubin JM. Out-of-hospital treatment of hypoglycemia: refusal of transport and patient outcome. *Acad Emerg Med* 1998;5(11):1080–5.

CHAPTER 24
Renal failure and dialysis

Bryan B. Kitch and Jocelyn M. De Guzman

Introduction

Renal failure in its various forms represents a spectrum of disease with profound implications for patient management. With differing etiologies for both acute and chronic forms of the disease, patients may present with a wide variety of complaints that directly relate to their renal function. This chapter will discuss the array of disorders including acute, chronic, and end-stage renal disease, the complications thereof, and treatments most pertinent to the emergency prehospital care provider.

Definitions and pathophysiology

The kidney functions through a series of both microscopic and macroscopic elements that serve to filter blood. In doing so, the renal system manages fluid balance, processes waste, and removes complex compounds from the body. It also affects blood electrolytes and pH.

The smallest functional unit of the kidney is the nephron, where blood filters through the glomerulus and into a system of tubules. Through microscopic transporters and diffusion gradients, electrolytes and other compounds are shifted to and from the blood and filtrate. The resultant fluid at the distal end of the nephron leaves the body as urine [1].

Structurally, the nephrons' tubules combine into larger structures forming the renal calyces, which then form the ureter, exiting at the renal hilum near the artery and vein. A single artery delivers blood flow from the body for filtration while the renal vein returns filtered, deoxygenated blood back to the central circulation. The ureter carries the urine to the bladder for storage. Damage to any of the aforementioned structures can result in renal dysfunction and/or failure.

Together, the two kidneys receive about 20% of the cardiac output [1]. Renal function is largely defined by the estimated glomerular filtration rate (eGFR), which is an objective measure of the kidney's ability to filter blood. It is by convention measured in $mL/min/1.73\,m^2$ (body surface area). eGFR is directly related to renal function, and the lower the eGFR, the more severe the renal impairment.

Acute kidney injury

Acute kidney injury (AKI), formerly known as acute renal failure, is defined as the rapid loss of the kidney's excretory function and is typically diagnosed by the accumulation of urea and creatinine or decreased urine output [2]. According to the Acute Kidney Injury Network recommendations, AKI is defined as an increase in serum creatinine by ≥0.3 mg/dL within 48 hours, increase in serum creatinine to ≥1.5 times baseline within the prior 7 days, or urine volume <0.5 mL/kg/h for 6 hours [3].

The causes of AKI are often designated by the location at which the pathophysiology occurs. Prerenal causes of failure refer to a disease process affecting the kidney before the renal artery enters the kidney. Postrenal causes are those that occur after the collection system forms. Intrarenal causes are those affecting the microscopic and macroscopic structures of the kidney, directly.

Acute causes of renal failure occurring before the kidney result from systemic processes that decrease blood flow to the organ. Systemic hypotension and shock states are easily recognized. Reduction of blood flow to the kidney can result in injury. Operating through a similar pathway, dehydration (especially in the elderly with limited reserve) can also lead to renal damage. Additionally, low-flow states, as found in decompensated heart failure, can lead to AKI. In many other disease conditions, renal dysfunction is a key marker of end-organ damage and carries a higher rate of morbidity and mortality [4].

Pathology occurring after the collection system of the kidney can result in postrenal or obstructive kidney disease. Obstruction causes backflow of urine into the kidney, increasing the hydrostatic pressure within the tubules, thus hindering filtration of fluids and excretion of compounds. Any lesion obstructing the flow of urine, from the tip of the urethra to the renal calyx, can cause postrenal failure. One of the more common causes in this category is urolithiasis. Lesions within the bladder causing delayed or impaired emptying as well as

Emergency Medical Services: Clinical Practice and Systems Oversight, Second Edition. Volume 1: Clinical Aspects of EMS.
Edited by David C. Cone, Jane H. Brice, Theodore R. Delbridge, and J. Brent Myers.
© 2015 NAEMSP. Published 2015 by John Wiley & Sons, Inc. Companion Website: www.wiley.com\go\cone\naemsp

strictures or compression of the urethra can cause similar pathology. In a patient with a history of hematuria, clot formation in the bladder can result in obstruction and renal failure. Regardless of the cause, treatment of these conditions revolves around identification and relief of urinary tract obstruction.

Causes of injury that are neither prerenal nor postrenal make up the spectrum of acute intrinsic causes of renal failure. The multitude of etiologies of this category includes processes affecting the blood vessels, nephron, glomerulus, tubules, and the interstitium of the kidney. The most common cause of intrinsic renal failure is acute tubular necrosis [5]. A variety of medications such as non-steroidal antiinflammatory drugs, certain antibiotics, and intravenous contrast dye are commonly implicated in causing intrinsic renal failure. Special care must be taken by the EMS and the emergency department providers to avoid nephrotoxic drugs in patients with suspected renal failure.

Rhabdomyolysis is caused by muscle breakdown and release of intracellular material including myoglobin, leading to renal damage. In adults, alcohol and drug intoxication, trauma, prolonged immobility, excessive strenuous activity, toxic ingestions, and infections can lead to this syndrome. Symptoms include weakness, myalgia, mental status change, and darkened urine. The mainstay of treatment is resuscitation with a potassium-free crystalloid IV fluid, and often admission for treatment of metabolic abnormalities.

Chronic kidney disease

Chronic kidney disease (CKD) is based on the presence of kidney damage or renal dysfunction with eGFR <60 for greater than 3 months duration [6]. The majority of CKD is a result of intrarenal disease.

Chronic kidney disease is broken into categories of dysfunction with the ultimate being termed end-stage renal disease (ESRD). CKD usually follows an irreversible and progressive course that requires early detection, lifestyle modification, and medications to slow down progression to kidney failure.

Epidemiology

As of 2011, approximately 616,000 people in the United States are being treated for ESRD with hemodialysis, a functional renal transplant, or peritoneal dialysis [7]. This represents one in 526 Americans, and one in 2,800 will be newly diagnosed each year. Forty-four percent of newly diagnosed ESRD patients have a history of diabetes and 28% have a history of hypertension, common problems encountered by EMS personnel. African Americans have an incidence of ESRD 3.4 times higher than Caucasians. The annual costs for treating ESRD in the US is more than $49.3 billion, and it takes more than 7.2% of the US Medicare budget [8].

Treatment of renal disease

Depending on the degree of renal dysfunction, definitive management involves measures to temporize and protect the remaining renal capabilities, and/or renal replacement through dialysis or transplantation. Patients with kidney disease are often advised to eat a certain diet, optimized for the decreased excretion abilities of their kidney. Foods are often low in protein, phosphorus, calcium, and potassium. Consideration of supplementation with vitamin D, vitamin C, and iron is suggested [9]. Oral medications can be taken by patients to assist with binding bloodstream chemicals and excreting them through the gastrointestinal (GI) tract, compensating for impaired renal function. Such medications are typically phosphate binders, which exist as multiple drug classes, often calcium salts. Newer agents are entering the market which seek to provide the same therapeutic advantage without risk of supplying extra exogenous calcium [10].

Dialysis refers to a process by which fluids and chemicals are removed from the body. The system uses a variety of membranes and fluids of different concentrations for diffusion and osmosis, extracting unwanted substances into the dialysate, effectively removing them from the circulation. Hemodialysis uses an external machine to filter the patient's blood, rapidly removing fluid and solutes. This requires specialized high-volume IV access to the patient with either a catheter or a surgical vascular device. The patient typically requires three sessions of dialysis a week, averaging 3–4 hours per session. Home hemodialysis is also possible for a selected patient population. In peritoneal dialysis (PD), the patient's own abdominal contents serve as the membrane rather than those of an external machine. The patient has a permanent catheter through the abdominal wall. Fluid is delivered into the abdomen, allowed to dwell for a period of time, and then extracted by a machine. The fluids infused into the abdominal cavity are specially calibrated to allow for removal of electrolytes and excess body fluid. Typically, the patient will require several exchanges of fluid to reach goal. This is either performed with an automated process during sleep, or can be performed with several extraction/replacements of fluid spaced out throughout the day [11].

An alternative to dialysis in the ESRD patient is renal transplantation. A successful transplant can allow a dialysis-dependent patient to live a nearly normal lifestyle without the need for multiple weekly visits for renal replacement therapy. With this therapeutic option comes a variety of specialized concerns regarding the patient's care.

Typically, the patient's new kidney is implanted in the abdominal cavity or pelvis. This has implications for any patient complaining of abdominal pain. A renal cause must be considered. Furthermore, the kidney is not protected in its usual location in the retroperitoneum. The physical exam and focused history after trauma should be mindful of this anatomical difference, although outcomes and injury patterns may not be greater than in the non-transplant patient [12].

Kidney transplant patients continue to receive immunosuppressive medication to avoid rejection. These patients may not mount a fever with infection and are at risk for atypical and opportunistic infections. Many vague and mild symptoms may be a concerning sign for infection and should warrant careful evaluation. A thorough medication history can alert the provider to the presence of immunosuppression. Similarly, noncompliance with the regimen should lower the threshold for a rejection evaluation.

Complications of renal disease

Many of the complications of renal failure are more likely to be found in those with no remaining renal function. While possible in the acute renal failure patient, those known to be dialysis dependent more often present to the EMS provider with one of the following acute complications of chronic disease.

Fluid status
As one of the primary roles of the kidney is regulating fluid balance, those with impaired or absent renal function may present with derangement of their fluid status. In the healthy patient, the kidney filters 180 liters of blood, producing almost 2 liters of extra water and waste products excreted in the form of urine daily [1]. Without the ability to excrete this extra fluid, patients with renal disease may rapidly become fluid overloaded.

Much like a patient with congestive heart failure, patients may present in respiratory distress. They may report weight gain, which combined with dyspnea may suggest a state of fluid overload to the provider.

Congestive heart failure is a similar condition to the fluid overload in renal disease. Given the comorbid cardiac disease in this population, dyspnea and pulmonary edema may result from either pump failure from a primary cardiac etiology or excretion failure from the poor renal function. Additionally, the ESRD patient may enter a state of high-output heart failure due to the presence of an AV fistula. The inability to clear waste products can also result in a uremic cardiomyopathy.

Diagnosis and treatment of fluid overload in this patient population overlap with the heart failure cohort. In the acutely ill patient, management is similar, with use of oxygen and nitrates. Non-invasive positive pressure ventilation or intubation and ventilation may be required for worsening respiratory failure. Field or bedside echocardiogram can provide information regarding the nature of cardiac contractility or pericardial effusion from uremia. Ultimately, dialysis may be required to offload the fluid burden and allow for return to baseline hemodynamic and pulmonary function [7].

Electrolytes
The kidney plays a dominant role in regulation of serum electrolyte levels. Renal failure can cause life-threatening imbalances in this chemistry. Medications and diet in the renal patient must be considered for their effects on the patient's impaired electrolyte regulation.

Potassium
Perhaps the most well-known and feared complication of renal failure is hyperkalemia. The healthy kidney excretes 95% of the daily potassium intake [13]. Fatal arrhythmias are most likely to occur with serum levels over 9 mEq/L [14]. Of note, the patient with CKD can often tolerate higher levels of potassium than the healthy individual and has lower rates of mortality for any given serum potassium level [15]. In contrast to other electrolytes, the patient with hyperkalemia may not voice any specific complaints. The ECG is often used as a screening test for electrolyte disturbance, but it has overall poor sensitivity and specificity (Figure 24.1). ECG tracing changes that may be seen in hyperkalemia are listed in Box 24.1. While it is an easy and noninvasive test, the provider must not exclusively rely on an ECG for evaluation of the patient [14]. Specific management of hyperkalemia will be addressed later in the chapter.

Magnesium
Like potassium, the kidney functions to excrete magnesium from the body. A kidney that is impaired by acute or chronic kidney disease can lose its ability to conserve magnesium, while ESRD implies loss of ability to excrete magnesium. Thus, hypomagnesemia can occur in kidney disease and hypermagnesemia in ESRD. The patient with a magnesium disturbance may have an arrhythmia or ECG disturbance, often related to QT interval changes. Classically, patients with low magnesium have increased reflexes and weakness, while hypermagnesemia is associated with hyporeflexia. Mental status changes and respiratory depression may also occur.

Phosphate
The kidneys are very effective at eliminating phosphate from the body. Profoundly elevated phosphate levels are relatively unique to the dialysis patient. When phosphate circulates in excess levels in the bloodstream, it can bind and precipitate with calcium, causing symptoms of hypocalcemia such as weakness, increased reflexes, and neurological disturbances. The calcium-phosphate complex can deposit in cardiac tissue, leading to arrhythmia and death.

Pericarditis
Inflammation of the pericardium with or without effusion is a known complication in the dialysis patient. While uremia predisposes the patient to pericarditis, more classic etiologies such as infections are also possible.

A patient with uremic pericarditis may present with chest pain that can be positional in nature and there may be a friction rub on exam. Classic ECG findings may not be present as the inflammatory cells associated with non-infectious uremic pericarditis do not penetrate the myocardium. Cardiac tamponade is a realistic possibility and should be considered in the hypotensive ESRD patient.

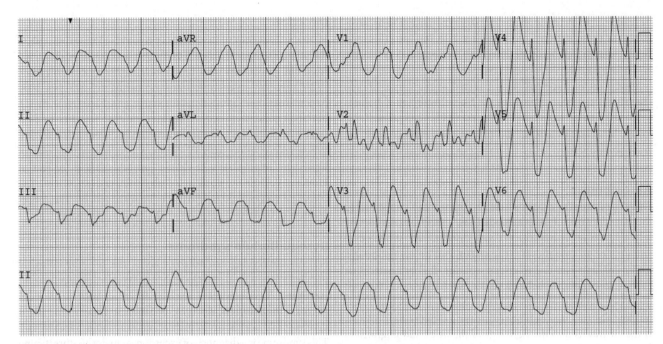

Figure 24.1 ECG of a patient with hyperkalemia. Note wide complex tachycardia and development of sine wave.

Box 24.1 ECG changes in hyperkalemia	
Peaked T-waves	Slow atrial fibrillation
PR prolongation	Sine wave
Wide unusual QRS complexes	Asystole
Conduction blocks	Ventricular fibrillation
Bradycardia	Wide complex pulseless electrical activity

Cardiovascular disease

A direct relationship exists between the degree of renal dysfunction and the risk of coronary artery disease (CAD). While both kidney disease and heart disease have similar causal factors, unique properties of the renal patient's physiology also impose higher cardiac risk. Such factors as inflammation, oxidative stress, uremia, and metabolic abnormalities contribute to higher CAD incidence and mortality. Diagnosis of cardiac disease can be more difficult in this patient population. Typical ECG findings of ischemia may be subtle due to underlying left ventricular hypertrophic morphologies on the tracing.

Stroke is also more common in the renal disease patient than the general population. The risk is increased in patients with more advanced CKD, and even higher rates of stroke exist in the first year after dialysis begins. Both hemodialysis and peritoneal dialysis carry elevated stroke risks, although incidence may be slightly lower for the latter [16].

Anemia

Patients with kidney disease are often anemic. Their red blood cell counts tend to be low, with hemoglobin usually less than 10 g/dL upon starting dialysis [8]. The cause is multifactorial and includes renal undersecretion of erythropoietin, a hormone responsible for red blood cell production [17].

Infection

Patients, especially those on dialysis, have an increased risk for infection, with greater associated morbidity. Those with indwelling devices for dialysis access have an obvious source for contamination and seeding with bacteria. All patients possess a degree of immunodeficiency, partially caused by uremia but also related to nutrition and direct dysfunction of white blood cells [18]. Sepsis is a common manifestation of bacterial infections.

Complications of hemodialysis

Hypotension

Hypotension is common, occurring in 10–50% of patients [17]. Often, this is a direct result of fluid shifts from the dialysis procedure. At times, there may be calibration issues and the patient has an overzealous removal of fluid, leaving him or her intravascularly depleted. Additionally, medications and temperature shifts commonly found in the dialysis circuit, combined with the patient's baseline autonomic irritability, contribute to high rates of decreased blood pressure [17]. However, care must be taken not to attribute all postdialysis hypotension to hypovolemia, as these patients are at higher risk for infection and sepsis, cardiac tamponade, bleeding, myocardial ischemia, and heart failure.

Treatment of hypotension is directed at the cause. Should dialysis-related hypovolemia be the likely insult, small boluses (250–500 mL) of isotonic IV fluid should be considered, followed by reassessment of the patient for response and any respiratory distress.

Air embolism

Since the patient's vascular circuit is violated and connected to the outside world during hemodialysis, concern exists for the introduction of air into the patient's bloodstream. While small amounts of air into the vascular system can be asymptomatic, larger amounts can cause serious sequelae. It is estimated that 3–5 mL/kg of air is the lethal dose [19]. Should air travel through the vasculature toward the brain, it can cause cerebral blood outflow obstruction, leading to increasing intracranial pressure. If the air travels into the right side of the heart and migrates to the lung, it can act as a pulmonary embolism and cause hemodynamic instability. In rare cases, a heart defect could allow air to pass from the right-sided circulation into the arterial flow to the body, leading to stroke or myocardial infarction as an arterial gas embolism.

Management of the patient with air embolism requires hemodynamic support, high-flow oxygen, and prevention of further air aspiration. In the rapidly deteriorating patient, there is a role for aspiration of air from the right ventricle. Positioning an affected patient in the left lateral recumbent position (right heart up) may help to stabilize trapped air in the right heart, stopping further embolization. Hyperbaric oxygen has been established as a treatment modality for this disease process in the patient stable enough for therapy [19].

Bleeding

Patients undergoing hemodialysis have a high-capacity vascular structure accessed multiple times weekly, leading to increased risk of bleeding. Grafts and fistulas have high rates of blood flow and pressure compared to peripheral veins. Aneurysms are rare but can occur, and may catastrophically rupture, causing exsanguination [18]. More common is persistent bleeding after dialysis from the needle insertion site. The patient's underlying platelet dysfunction contributes to difficulty in obtaining hemostasis. Typically, oozing of blood after dialysis will respond to firm pressure for extended periods of time. Immediate use of topical hemostatic compounds can be useful. Failing this, life-saving measures to stop bleeding may need to be implemented, including suturing the wound or applying a proximal tourniquet. Damage control measures such as these may result in permanent damage or loss of the patient's dialysis access and should be considered only in critical situations.

Infection

With the frequency of vascular access comes an increased risk of infection. The specific classes of dialysis access will be discussed later, but all patients with ESRD have higher risk of infection. With vascular access infections occurring in 103 per 1000 patient-years and admissions for sepsis and bacteremia in 116 per 1000 patient-years, the provider must be mindful to consider evaluation for and early treatment of severe infection [8]. When resuscitation with IV fluids is needed on the basis of sepsis and hypotension, it should not be withheld for fear of inducing volume overload in a dialysis-dependent patient. The consequences of fluid overload can be managed, but the consequences of underresuscitation might be more permanent.

Dysequilibrium syndrome

Patients undergoing hemodialysis are at risk for a neurological manifestation of fluid and electrolyte shifts called dysequilibrium syndrome. This syndrome may be severe enough to produce altered consciousness, seizures, or coma, although typically it involves mild symptoms of malaise, nausea, and headaches [20]. This syndrome is a diagnosis of exclusion, as many life-threatening entities can cause similar symptoms. Thus, the renal patient with new onset of these features requires prompt evaluation. Treatment is similar to that of cerebral edema with consideration of IV hypertonic therapy and termination of dialysis.

Medication concerns

Many pharmacological agents existing today have interactions with the renal system. Frequently, dose adjustments are required in the renal disease patient. As a corollary, dialysis can remove some medications from the circulation, leading to decreased efficacy. Depending on medication timing and properties, patients may have subtherapeutic or supratherapeutic drug levels if prescriptions are not tailored appropriately.

Complications of peritoneal dialysis

While electrolyte disturbances can occur, they are typically not as severe as in patients on hemodialysis. As the patient's dialysis exchange occurs over a longer period of time, there is less gradient with the dialysate, and thus electrolyte shifts are of a smaller magnitude.

The most common complication in peritoneal dialysis (PD) is peritonitis, with a hospitalization rate of 85 per 1000 patient-years [8]. The indwelling abdominal catheter used is a nidus for infection. Patients with peritonitis may complain of abdominal pain or non-specific symptoms of nausea, fatigue, or fever. They may range from being asymptomatic to frankly septic, with guarding of the abdomen and hypotension. One clue to peritonitis is a change in the fluid coming from the catheter during a fluid exchange.

The fluid used for dialysis in PD often contains high amounts of glucose, drawing water out of the body. In rare cases, patients can absorb the glucose and present with a hyperglycemic, hyperosmolar state and critical illness from the same [21].

Peritoneal dialysis patients have the highest rate of admission for any infection, with 558 cases per 1000 patient-years in 2010. The rate of admission for peritonitis is 85 per 1000 patient-years, and for peritoneal catheter infections it is 152 infections per 1000 patient-years [8].

Special considerations

The missed dialysis patient

Non-compliance with dialysis is known to occur about 33% of the time, with some studies indicating 50% of patients not following some portion of their dialysis instructions [22]. Younger patients and smokers consistently are found to have higher rates of compliance issues [22,23]. As these patients require dialysis to sustain life, the patient who has missed a session (or several) is at higher risk for deterioration.

When a patient who admits to having missed dialysis sessions presents to the EMS provider, the more likely pathophysiology and required treatments can be inferred. Should the patient present in respiratory distress, the potential for fluid overload exists, and management can be multimodal. Non-invasive positive pressure ventilation can be implemented in the awake patient, using continuous positive airway pressure (CPAP)/bilevel positive airway pressure (BiPAP) to improve oxygenation [24]. Consideration of nitroglycerin or other vasodilators is an option, facilitating fluid shifts by increasing venous capacitance. In the setting of uncomplicated fluid overload from dialysis non-compliance, the patient should be hypertensive and tolerate nitrates well [24]. Should the patient be exhibiting signs of cardiogenic shock, consideration of pericardial tamponade should ensue.

Diuretics such as furosemide can be used in the renal disease patient, provided he or she makes urine. Careful assessment of the patient's volume status should be made, as giving diuretics to an intravascularly depleted patient can worsen renal function. In the euvolemic or hypervolemic patient, higher than average doses of diuretic will be needed to overcome renal dysfunction [25].

The hyperkalemic patient

Dialysis-dependent patients are already at risk for hyperkalemia; those who miss one or more regular sessions are at much greater risk. If the patient presents with arrhythmia, hypotension, or obvious ECG changes, empiric management of hyperkalemia is warranted.

Intravenous calcium is administered for the purpose of stabilizing the cardiac membrane. This therapy has a duration of action of 30–60 minutes, which may necessitate the need for redosing depending on transport times [13].

Ampules of sodium bicarbonate given as slow IV push can help to alkalinize the blood and promote the shift of potassium intracellularly. This also can be administered as an infusion of a bicarbonate solution with concentration 150 mmol/L (typically 3 ampules in a liter of D5W), being mindful of the potential for fluid overload [13].

Albuterol can be given in the usual fashion to also shift potassium out of the plasma. It is easily administered to the patient and has the advantage of being non-invasive. However, the onset of action is not immediate and tachyarrhythmia is a possible consequence [13].

Regardless of the medication(s) used in the field, the ESRD patient with hyperkalemia will require definitive management, as these therapies serve only to either prevent arrhythmia or temporarily shift potassium from the serum. The total body potassium does not decrease with these methods. Consequently, if management is performed in this regard, it must be well communicated to the next patient care providers, as serum potassium assays may be falsely reassuring.

Vascular access

All hemodialysis patients require specialized vascular devices to allow for rapid infusion and removal of blood. These devices must be able to support over 350 mL/min of blood flow, with some patients achieving rates of 600–1200 mL/min [26]. A variety of devices are commonly used today.

Nephrologists often prefer that the patient's dialysis access not be used except in extreme emergency (e.g. cardiac arrest resuscitation). Patients are advised to avoid use of blood pressure cuffs, tourniquets, and venepuncture distal to their devices, and will typically convey this concern to EMS personnel [18].

Arteriovenous fistula

A surgically created connection between an artery and a vein, usually the brachial or radial artery to the cephalic vein. It takes over 4 weeks (and often more than 8 weeks depending on local practices) to mature and be ready to use. A patient may have a fistula created and be in the process of maturation while using a different device for dialysis.

Arteriovenous graft

Similar to a fistula, the artery and the vein are connected by way of a synthetic device. It is more prone to complication than the fistula [27].

Tunneled catheter

A large IV catheter that accesses a central vein, usually the internal jugular [28]. Prior to entering the vein, the catheter is run through the skin and soft tissue from a different site. In doing so, this can reduce infection and need for frequent dressing changes [29]. These catheters are often held in place by balloons and other securing devices. This method has the advantage that it is immediately available for use once inserted. Compared to other long-term methods of venous access, the catheter has the highest rates of complication and mortality [28].

Non-tunneled catheter

A large-bore IV in a central vein with two ports. Usually used as a temporary measure as a bridge to a different device [30].

Complications of vascular devices

The hemodialysis access site is effectively a large vascular structure that undergoes multiple punctures a week in a patient with underlying hemodynamic, hematological, and immunological compromise. Screening for complication and failure can occur through a careful evaluation and history.

Thrombosis of the device may be reported by the patient or staff who find they were unable to obtain blood flow during a dialysis session. In the case of the AV fistula, one should palpate and auscultate the site for presence of a thrill and bruit indicating proper function [30]. Interventional procedures to remove thrombosis from the device may cause migration of the clot, leading to pulmonary embolism. This should be considered in the acutely short of breath dialysis patient status post device manipulation.

Hemorrhage is easily recognized on physical exam and usually results from delayed hemostasis after hemodialysis. Development and rupture of an aneurysm is rare and requires prompt surgical evaluation. Immediate management of bleeding from the dialysis access site involves direct and constant pressure on the epicenter of the bleed. As there are higher pressures in this location than at typical cutaneous bleeds, one must be mindful to not allow thick loose gauze dressings to absorb and mask ongoing bleeding. Specialized clamp devices exist to deliver hands-free pressure to the bleed. A low-cost solution exists by using a glass spherical marble on the puncture site and tightly wrapped gauze forming a pressure dressing.

The ill-appearing ESRD patient may be suffering from bloodstream infection, possibly related to the access device. Inspection of the skin overlying a fistula or graft or around the entry point of a catheter may provide valuable clues.

Fluid resuscitation

Administration of fluids to the renal patient should be performed with careful consideration of cardiopulmonary reserve. This does not mean that necessary fluids should be withheld, for example when resuscitating a septic patient. Rather, clinicians should be aware that standard 1 L bags of isotonic fluids may represent too much of a bolus volume without an intervening assessment. Patients should receive serial smaller aliquots of IV fluids, delivered rapidly, with frequent reassessments to assess ongoing needs. The EMS provider should clearly communicate fluid volumes administered to the ED staff.

Cardiac or respiratory arrest

Specific consideration of the patient's electrolyte status must be made. A hyperkalemic cardiac arrest is a realistic possibility in the dialysis patient. While not routinely used in algorithms for resuscitation, sodium bicarbonate could be considered for empiric shift of potassium [31]. Calcium chloride or gluconate should also be considered.

Should the renal patient require rapid sequence intubation for airway management, the choice of neuromuscular blockade agent needs to take into account potassium levels and the well-documented hyperkalemic effects of succinylcholine. In other words, unless the serum potassium level is known, succinylcholine is best avoided.

EMS pearls

Focused history

When the EMS provider encounters a dialysis patient, a set of focused questions from the patient and any family/medical staff present can greatly assist in their hospital care.

- **Dialysis schedule.** Knowing what days of the week the patient has dialysis, as well as the day of their last session, is useful.
- **Length of sessions.** Attempt to determine how many hours each dialysis session is, as well as if the patient is completing the full length each time, with attention to the last session.
- **Weights.** Patients should have a known "dry weight," which is the ideal euvolemic weight of the patient. Additionally, knowing the patient's current weight can greatly help with fluid status assessment. The patient may also be able to state how much weight/fluid is removed with each dialysis.
- **Vitals.** Dialysis patients may have abnormal vitals at their baseline and if so, careful documentation of their normal heart rate and blood pressure is important.

Destination selection

Should a patient with ESRD require transport, it may be necessary to choose a destination hospital that can care for his or her needs. Even if the patient is not presenting to EMS for a dialysis-related complaint, should he/she require hospital admission, he/she will eventually need renal replacement therapy. The higher incidence of CAD and stroke may necessitate specialty care more often than the otherwise healthy non-dialysis patient. Local protocols may be beneficial to facilitate triage to the appropriate facility.

Resource preplanning

The individual in the community who is dialysis dependent requires unique resources for his or her survival. Under normal conditions the patient likely has established mechanisms for obtaining transportation and treatment, but this system can be disrupted in the case of disaster. The local emergency management agency should work alongside medical directors and the dialysis providers to develop contingency plans appropriate for the local environment. Other government and local agencies will need to contribute to this planning process, as operation of a hemodialysis machine requires infrastructure that is easily disrupted. Identification and registry of the patients who will require emergency dialysis services in times of need can allow for continued access to life-sustaining care.

Convalescent transportation

Hemodialysis patients in particular have a frequent need for transportation to a medical facility. Patients may require assistance in this regard, relying on non-emergency transportation services. There exists a wide variety in the training level of personnel handling this form of transportation. Providers in this field may become well acquainted with the dialysis patients and be able to recognize subtle changes in their condition which may require diversion to a higher level of care. Protocols should be established to assist these caregivers in the recognition of emergencies in this high-risk population. If the particular transport unit does not possess the capabilities to care for emergency medical conditions, the provider should know the best method of accessing the resources required to do so.

References

1 Rhoades R, Tanner GA. Kidney function. In: Rhoades R, Tanner GA (eds) *Medical Physiology*. Philadelphia: Lippincott Williams & Wilkins, 2003.

2 Bellomo R, Kellum JA, Ronco C. Acute kidney injury. *Lancet* 2012;380(9843):756–66.

3 Khwaja A. KDIGO clinical practice guidelines for acute kidney injury. *Nephron Clin Pract* 2012;120(4):179–84.

4 Ricci Z, Cruz D, Ronco C. The RIFLE criteria and mortality in acute kidney injury: a systematic review. *Kidney Int* 2008;73(5):538–46.

5 Waikar SS, Liu KD, Chertow GM. Diagnosis, epidemiology and outcomes of acute kidney injury. *Clin J Am Soc Nephrol* 2008;3(3):844–61.

6 Levey AS, Coresh J. Chronic kidney disease. *Lancet* 2012;379(9811): 165–80.

7 Herzog CA, Asinger RW, Berger AK, et al. Cardiovascular disease in chronic kidney disease. A clinical update from kidney disease: improving global outcomes (KDIGO). *Kidney Int* 2011;80(6):572–86.

8 2013 USRDS Annual Data Report: *Atlas of End-Stage Renal Disease in the United States*. Available at: www.usrds.org/2013/pdf/v2_00_intro_13.pdf

9 American Diabetic Association. Chronic Kidney Disease Evidence-Based Nutrition Practice Guideline. Chicago, IL: American Diabetic Association, 2010.

10 Coladonato JA. Control of hyperphosphatemia among patients with ESRD. *J Am Soc Nephrol* 2005;16 (Suppl 2):S107–14.

11 National Institute of Diabetes and Digestive and Kidney Diseases. Treatment Methods for Kidney Failure: Peritoneal Dialysis, May 2006. Available at: http://kidney.niddk.nih.gov/KUDiseases/pubs/peritoneal/index.aspx

12 Scalea JR, Menaker J, Meeks AK, et al. Trauma patients with a previous organ transplant: outcomes are better than expected – a retrospective analysis. *J Trauma Acute Care Surg* 2013;74(6): 1498–503.

13 Weisberg LS. Management of severe hyperkalemia. *Crit Care Med* 2008;36(12):3246–51.

14 Montague BT, Ouellette JR, Buller GK. Retrospective review of the frequency of ECG changes in hyperkalemia. *Clin J Am Soc Nephrol* 2008;3(2):324–30.

15 Einhorn LM, Zhan M, Hsu VD, et al. The frequency of hyperkalemia and its significance in chronic kidney disease. *Arch Intern Med* 2009;169(12):1156–62.

16 Murray AM, Seliger S, Lakshminarayan K, Herzog CA, Solid CA. Incidence of stroke before and after dialysis initiation in older patients. *J Am Soc Nephrol* 2013;24(7):1166–73.

17 Venkat A, Kaufmann KR, Venkat K. Care of the end-stage renal disease patient on dialysis in the ED. *Am J Emerg Med* 2006;24(7):847–58.

18 Wolfson AB, Singer I. Hemodialysis-related emergencies – part 1. *J Emerg Med* 1987;5(6):533–43.

19 Mirski MA, Lele AV, Fitzsimmons L, Toung TJ. Diagnosis and treatment of vascular air embolism. *Anesthesiology* 2007;106(1):164–77.

20 Tuchman S, Khademian P, Mistry K. Dialysis disequilibrium syndrome occurring during continuous renal replacement therapy. *Clin Kidney J* 2013. Available at: http://ckj.oxfordjournals.org/content/early/2013/08/12/ckj.sft087.full.pdf+html

21 Boyer J, Gill GN, Epstein FH. Hyperglycemia and hyperosmolality complicating peritoneal dialysis. *Ann Intern Med* 1967;67(3):568–72.

22 Kutner NG, Zhang R, McClellan WM, Cole SA. Psychosocial predictors of non-compliance in haemodialysis and peritoneal dialysis patients. *Nephrol Dial Transplant* 2002;17(1):93–9.

23 Leggat JE, Orzol SM, Hulbert-Shearon TE, et al. Noncompliance in hemodialysis: predictors and survival analysis. *Am J Kidney Dis* 1998;32(1):139–45.

24 Gehm L, Propp DA. Pulmonary edema in the renal failure patient. *Am J Emerg Med* 1989;7(3):336–9.

25 Wilcox CS. New insights into diuretic use in patients with chronic renal disease. *J Am Soc Nephrol* 2002;13(3):798–805.

26 Konner K, Nonnast-Daniel B, Ritz E. The arteriovenous fistula. *J Am Soc Nephrol* 2003;14(6):1669–80.

27 Gibson KD, Gillen DL, Caps MT, Kohler TR, Sherrard DJ, Stehman-Breen CO. Vascular access survival and incidence of revisions: a comparison of prosthetic grafts, simple autogenous fistulas, and venous transposition fistulas from the united states renal data system dialysis morbidity and mortality study. *J Vasc Surg* 2001; 34(4):694–700.

28 Feldman HI, Kobrin S, Wasserstein A. Hemodialysis vascular access morbidity. *J Am Soc Nephrol* 1996;7(4):523–35.

29 O'Grady NP, Alexander M, Dellinger EP, et al. Guidelines for the prevention of intravascular catheter-related infections. The Hospital Infection Control Practices Advisory Committee, Centers for Disease Control and Prevention, U.S. *Pediatrics* 2002;110(5):e51.

30 Beathard GA. Physical examination of the dialysis vascular access. *Semin Dial* 1998;11(4):231–6.

31 Vukmir RB, Bircher N, Safar P. Sodium bicarbonate in cardiac arrest: a reappraisal. *Am J Emerg Med* 1996;14(2):192–206.

CHAPTER 25

Infectious and communicable diseases

Russell D. MacDonald

Introduction

Paramedics are typically the first health care personnel to encounter sudden illnesses or other health care emergencies in the community, placing them at risk of communicable and infectious diseases. The Occupational Safety and Health Administration (OSHA) identifies more than 1.2 million community-based first response personnel, including law enforcement, fire, and EMS personnel, who are at risk for infectious exposure [1]. While infectious and communicable disease preparation may not have previously been a priority in some EMS agencies, the 2003 severe acute respiratory syndrome (SARS) outbreaks made it one. Emergency medical personnel during the onset of the SARS outbreaks in Toronto and Taipei were exposed to or contracted SARS in significant numbers resulting in one paramedic fatality [2,3]. More importantly, the loss of paramedics available for work due to exposure, illness, and quarantine affected the ability to maintain staffing during the outbreak, and highlighted the need for EMS systems to adequately prepare and protect the workforce from potential exposure [4].

Paramedic and patient

An *infectious* disease results from the invasion of a host by disease-producing organisms, such as bacteria, viruses, fungi or parasites. A *communicable* (or contagious) disease is one that can be transmitted from one person to another. Not all infectious diseases are communicable. For example, malaria is a serious infectious disease transmitted to the human bloodstream by a mosquito bite, but malaria is infectious, not communicable. On the other hand, chickenpox is an infectious disease which is also highly communicable because it can be easily transmitted from one person to another.

The mode of transmission is the mechanism by which an agent is transferred to the host. Modes of transmission include contact transmission (direct, indirect, droplet), airborne, vector borne, or common vehicle (food, equipment). Contact transmission is the most common mode of transmission in the EMS setting, and can be effectively prevented using routine practices.

Direct contact transmission occurs when there is direct contact between an infected or colonized individual and a susceptible host. Transmission may occur, for example, by biting, kissing, or sexual contact. Indirect contact occurs when there is passive transfer of an infectious agent to a susceptible host through a contaminated intermediate object. This can occur if contaminated hands, equipment, or surfaces are not washed between patient contacts. Examples of diseases transmitted by direct or indirect contact include human immunodeficiency virus (HIV), hepatitis, and methicillin-resistant *Staphylococcus aureus* (MRSA).

Droplet transmission is a form of contact transmission requiring special attention. It refers to large droplets generated from the respiratory tract of a patient when coughing or sneezing, or during invasive airway procedures (e.g. intubation, suctioning). These droplets are propelled and may be deposited on the mucous membranes of the susceptible host. The droplets may also settle in the immediate environment, and the infectious agents may remain viable for prolonged periods of time to be later transmitted by indirect contact. Examples of diseases transmitted by droplet transmission include meningitis, influenza, rhinovirus, respiratory syncytial virus (RSV), and severe acute respiratory syndrome (SARS).

Airborne transmission refers to the spread of infectious agents to susceptible hosts through the air. In this case, infectious agents are contained in very small droplets which can remain suspended in the air for prolonged periods of time. These agents are dispersed widely by air currents and can be inhaled by a susceptible host located at some distance from the source. Examples of airborne transmission diseases include measles (rubeola), varicella (chickenpox), and tuberculosis.

Vector-borne transmission refers to the spread of infectious agents by means of an insect or animal (the "vector"). Examples of vector-borne illnesses include rabies, where the infected animal is

Emergency Medical Services: Clinical Practice and Systems Oversight, Second Edition. Volume 1: Clinical Aspects of EMS.
Edited by David C. Cone, Jane H. Brice, Theodore R. Delbridge, and J. Brent Myers.
© 2015 NAEMSP. Published 2015 by John Wiley & Sons, Inc. Companion Website: www.wiley.com\go\cone\naemsp

the vector, and West Nile virus or malaria, where infected mosquitos are the vectors. Transmission of vector-borne illness does not occur between emergency personnel and their patients.

Common vehicle transmission refers to the spread of infectious agents by a single contaminated source to multiple hosts. This can result in large outbreaks of disease. Examples of this type of transmission include contaminated water sources (*E. coli*), contaminated food (Salmonella), or contaminated medication, medical equipment, or IV solutions.

General approach and patient assessment

The risk of communicable disease is not as apparent as other physical risks, such as road traffic, power lines, firearms, or chemical agents. EMS personnel must use the same level of suspicion and precaution whenever approaching a patient. The use of routine practices, as a minimum, is necessary for every patient encounter in order to mitigate this risk. All personnel must take appropriate precautions when a patient presents with any signs or symptoms suspected to be due to an infectious or communicable disease. All EMS and first responder agencies must provide appropriate training that enables personnel to identify at-risk patients and use appropriate personal protective equipment (PPE).

The risk assessment begins with information from an EMS dispatch or communication center, prior to making patient contact. Call-taking procedures should include basic screening information to identify potential communicable disease threats and provide this information to all responding personnel. The screening information can identify patients with symptoms of fever, chills, cough, shortness of breath, or diarrhea. The call-taker can also identify if the patient location, such as nursing home, group home or other institutional setting, poses a potential risk to the responding personnel. This information helps responding personnel to determine what precautions are necessary before they make patient contact.

When patient contact is made, personnel can determine if the patient has a potential risk for a communicable disease. A rapid history and physical examination can help raise suspicion. The following screening questions help identify a patient with a communicable disease.

- Do you have a new or worsening cough or shortness of breath?
- Do you have a fever?
- Have you had shakes or chills in the past 24 hours?
- Have you had an abnormal temperature (>38 °C)?
- Have you taken medication for fever?
- Have you recently returned, or been in contact with someone who has recently returned, from a geographic region where an outbreak is underway?

A screening physical examination will also identify obvious signs of a communicable disease. They may include any new symptom of infection (fever, headache, muscle ache, cough, sputum, weight loss, and exposure history), rash, diarrhea, skin lesions, or draining wounds.

Influenza

Influenza classically presents with the abrupt onset of fever, usually 38–40 °C, sore throat, non-productive cough, myalgias, headache, and chills. Influenza is caused by a virus with three subtypes: A, B, and C. Influenza A causes more severe disease and is mainly responsible for pandemics. Influenza A has different subtypes determined by surface antigens H (hemagglutinin) and N (neuraminidase). Influenza B causes more mild disease and mainly affects children. Influenza C rarely causes human illness and has not been associated with epidemics [5].

Influenza transmission occurs primarily through airborne spread when a person coughs or sneezes, but may also occur through direct contact of surfaces contaminated with respiratory secretions. Hand-washing and shielding coughs and sneezes help prevent spread. Influenza is transmissible from one day before symptom onset to about 5 days after symptoms begin and may last up to 10 days in children. Time from infection to development of symptoms is 1–4 days [6].

Influenza has been responsible for at least 31 pandemics in history. The most lethal "Spanish flu" pandemic of 1918–1919 is estimated to have caused 40 million deaths globally with 700,000 of those deaths occurring in the USA in a single year. In this pandemic, deaths occurred mainly in healthy 20–40 year olds, which differs from the usual young children and elderly pattern of mortality and morbidity in the seasonal outbreaks of influenza.

Influenza vaccine is the principal means of preventing influenza morbidity and mortality. The vaccine changes yearly based on the antigenic and genetic composition of circulating strains of influenza A and B found in January to March, when influenza reaches its peak activity. When the vaccine strain is similar to the circulating strain, influenza vaccine is effective in protecting from illness 70–90% of those younger than age 65 who are vaccinated. Among those aged 65 and older, the vaccine is 30–40% effective in preventing illness, 50–60% effective in preventing hospitalization, and up to 80% effective in preventing death. EMS personnel should be immunized annually, typically in October.

Four antiviral drugs are available for preventing and treating influenza in the US. When used for prevention of influenza, they can be 70–90% effective. Antiviral agents should be used as an adjunct to vaccination, but should not replace vaccination. The Centers for Disease Control and Prevention (CDC) recommends influenza antivirals for individuals who have not as yet been vaccinated at the time of exposure, or who have a contraindication to vaccination, and are also at high risk of influenza complications. Also, if an influenza outbreak is caused by a variant strain of influenza not controlled by vaccination, chemoprophylaxis should be considered for health care providers caring for patients at high risk of influenza complications, regardless of their vaccination status. In the setting of an influenza outbreak, EMS systems may opt to restrict duties for EMS providers who are not immunized or who have not yet received prophylactic antiviral therapy in an attempt to prevent spread of the outbreak [5].

Avian influenza

Influenza A virus infects humans and also can be found naturally in birds. Wild birds carry a type of influenza A virus, called avian influenza virus, in their intestines and usually do not get sick from them. However, avian influenza virus can make domesticated birds (including chickens, turkeys, and ducks) quite ill and lead to death.

The avian influenza virus is chiefly found in birds, but infection in humans from contact with infected poultry has been reported since 1996. A particular subtype of avian influenza A virus, H5N1, is highly contagious and deadly among birds. In 1997 in Hong Kong, an outbreak of avian influenza H5N1 occurred not only in poultry but also in 18 humans, six of whom died. In subsequent infections of avian influenza H5N1 in humans, more than half of those infected with the virus have died. In contrast to seasonal influenza, most cases of avian influenza H5N1 have occurred in young adults and healthy children who have come into contact with infected poultry, or surfaces contaminated with H5N1 virus. By the end of 2007, there were 346 documented human infections with influenza H5N1 and 213 deaths (62%). Although transmission of avian influenza H5N1 from human to human is rare, inefficient, and unsustained, there is concern that the H5N1 virus could adapt and acquire the ability for sustained transmission in the human population. If the H5N1 virus could gain the ability to transmit easily from person to person, a global influenza pandemic could occur. A vaccine is now available for H5N1, as a two-dose regimen. It is not currently available or advocated for use in the general population, but is being stockpiled by several countries. The H5N1 virus is resistant to the adamantanes, but likely sensitive to the neuraminidase inhibitors [7].

In April 2009, a novel influenza A (H1N1) virus, similar to but genetically and antigenically distinct from other influenza A (H1N1) viruses, was determined to be the cause of respiratory illnesses that spread across North America and many areas of the world. Influenza morbidity caused by the 2009 pandemic influenza A (H1N1) remained above seasonal baselines throughout spring and summer 2009, and was the first pandemic since 1968. Data from epidemiological studies conducted during the 2009 influenza A (H1N1) pandemic indicate that the risk for influenza complications among adults aged 19–64 years who had 2009 pandemic influenza A (H1N1) was greater than typically occurs for seasonal influenza [8].

Tuberculosis

Tuberculosis is caused by the *Mycobacterium* tuberculosis complex. The majority of active TB is pulmonary (70%), while the remainder is extrapulmonary (30%). Patients with active pulmonary TB will typically present with cough, scant amounts of non-purulent sputum and possibly hemoptysis. Systemic signs such as weight loss, loss of appetite, chills, night sweats, fever, and fatigue may also be present. Clinically, the EMS provider will be unable to distinguish pulmonary TB from other respiratory illnesses. However, certain risk factors may alert the EMS provider to the possibility of tuberculosis: immigration from a high-prevalence country, homelessness, exposure to active pulmonary

TB, silicosis, HIV infection, chronic renal failure, cancer, transplantation, or any other immunosuppressed state [9,10].

Active pulmonary TB is transmitted via droplet nuclei from people with pulmonary tuberculosis during coughing, sneezing, speaking, or singing. Procedures such as intubation or bronchoscopies are high risk for the transmission of TB. Respiratory secretions on a surface rapidly lose the potential for infection. The probability of infection is related to duration of exposure, distance from the case, concentration of bacilli in droplets, ventilation in the room, and the susceptibility of the host exposed. Effective medical therapy eliminates communicability within 2–4 weeks of starting treatment [11].

If transporting a patient who is known to have or suspected of having TB, respiratory precautions should be followed by EMS providers, including use of submicron masks. Patients should cover their mouths when coughing or sneezing, or wear surgical masks. In the event of suspected exposure to a patient with active pulmonary tuberculosis, report the case and the exposure to the EMS system or public health authority. Close contacts should be monitored for the development of active TB symptoms. Two tuberculin skin tests should be performed, based on public health recommendations, on those closely exposed to patients with active TB [12]. Because the incubation period after contact ranges from 2 to 10 weeks, the first test is typically done as soon as possible after exposure, and the second test is typically done 8–12 weeks after the exposure. If the EMS provider or contact develops either active TB with symptoms or latent asymptomatic TB, as diagnosed with a new positive TB skin test, treatment should be offered.

Treatment for latent TB is typically isoniazid (INH) for 6–9 months [13]. This single-drug regimen is 65–80% effective. For active TB, a four-drug regimen is typically used for 2 months: isoniazid, rifampin, pyrazinamide, and ethambutol. This is followed by INH and rifampin for an additional 4 months. Several forms of multidrug-resistant TB and extensively drug-resistant TB have been identified [14]. These forms require an aggressive, multidrug regimen for prolonged periods of time and are dependent on the organism's patterns of drug sensitivity and resistance. In all cases, a physician skilled in management of TB must initiate and monitor treatment and provide suitable follow-up. Public health officials must also be notified [15].

SARS and related coronaviruses

It is difficult to distinguish SARS from other respiratory infections because patients present with symptoms similar to other febrile respiratory illnesses [16,17]. Fever is the most common and earliest symptom of SARS, often accompanied by headache, malaise or myalgia [18]. In patients with SARS, high fever, diarrhea, and vomiting were more common compared to patients with other respiratory illnesses [19]. Cough occurred later in the course of disease and patients were less likely to have rhinorrhea or sore throat compared to other lower respiratory tract illness [20]. Since clinical features alone cannot reliably distinguish SARS from other respiratory illnesses, knowledge of contacts is essential [21]. Contact with known SARS patients, contact with

SARS-affected areas, or linkage to a cluster of pneumonia cases should be obtained in the history [22].

Severe acute respiratory syndrome was first recognized in 2003 after outbreaks occurred in Toronto, Singapore, Vietnam, Taiwan, and China [23]. The illness is caused by a coronavirus. About 11% of those who develop SARS eventually die, usually due to respiratory failure. The case fatality is less than 1% for SARS patients less than age 24 and up to 50% for those age 65 and greater or those with comorbid illness [24].

The coronavirus is found in respiratory secretions, urine, and fecal matter. Transmission is via droplets spread from respiratory secretions, with a high risk of transmission during intubation and procedures which aerosolize respiratory secretions. Transmission can also occur from fecal or urine contamination of surfaces. There have been no confirmed cases of transmission from asymptomatic cases.

If SARS is suspected, EMS providers must use all routine practices and additional precautions [25]. EMS systems may also elect to limit or avoid any procedures that may increase risk to EMS personnel. These include tracheal intubation, deep suctioning, use of non-invasive ventilatory support, administration of nebulized medication, and any other procedure that may aerosolize respiratory secretions. During the SARS outbreaks in Toronto, EMS medical direction modified medical directives such that paramedics did not intubate patients or deliver nebulized therapy in the prehospital setting [26]. Finally, EMS personnel and systems should also notify the receiving facility of a patient suspected of SARS, permitting the staff to have appropriate PPE in place and a suitable isolation room prepared for the patient [27,28].

There have not been any cases of SARS infections since 2004 anywhere in the world. However, a novel coronavirus related to SARS emerged in 2012 to cause a number of fatal infections. This new virus is referred to as Middle East respiratory syndrome coronavirus, or MERS-CoV. As of 9 May 2014, 536 laboratory-confirmed cases have been reported to the World Health Organization [29]. Of those, 145 (27%) were fatal. All diagnosed cases were among people who resided in or traveled from one of four countries, Kingdom of Saudi Arabia, United Arab Emirates, Qatar, or Jordan, within 14 days of their symptom onset, or who had close contact with people who resided in or traveled from those countries. Cases with a history of travel from these countries or contact with travelers from these countries have been identified in residents of France, the United Kingdom, Tunisia, and Italy. Like SARS, this novel coronavirus has spread from ill people to others through close contact. However, the virus has not been shown to spread in a sustained way throughout communities. Two cases were reported in the United States, both of them imported by Americans working as health care providers in Saudi Arabia.

Biological weapons

The CDC categorizes bioterrorism agents as shown in Box 25.1. Certain of these agents are discussed here; additional information about all agents is available via the CDC website

---

Box 25.1 Centers for Disease Control and Prevention categorization of bioterrorism agents (source: www.bt.cdc.gov/agent/agentlist-category.asp)

Category A

High-priority agents include organisms that pose a risk to national security because they:
- can be easily disseminated or transmitted from person to person
- result in high mortality rates and have the potential for major public health impact
- might cause public panic and social disruption; and
- require special action for public health preparedness.

Anthrax (*Bacillus anthracis*)
Botulism (*Clostridium botulinum* toxin)
Plague (*Yersinia pestis*)
Smallpox (variola major)
Tularemia (*Francisella tularensis*)
Viral hemorrhagic fevers (filoviruses, e.g. Ebola, Marburg, and arenaviruses, e.g. Lassa, Machupo)

Category B

Second highest priority agents include those that:
- are moderately easy to disseminate
- result in moderate morbidity rates and low mortality rates; and
- require specific enhancements of CDC's diagnostic capacity and enhanced disease surveillance.

Brucellosis (*Brucella* species)
Epsilon toxin of *Clostridium perfringens*
Food safety threats (e.g. *Salmonella* species, *Escherichia coli* O157:H7, *Shigella*)
Glanders (*Burkholderia mallei*)
Melioidosis (*Burkholderia pseudomallei*)
Psittacosis (*Chlamydia psittaci*)
Q fever (*Coxiella burnetii*)
Ricin toxin from *Ricinus communis* (castor beans)
Staphylococcal enterotoxin B
Typhus fever (*Rickettsia prowazekii*)
Viral encephalitis (alphaviruses, e.g. Venezuelan equine encephalitis, eastern equine encephalitis, western equine encephalitis)
Water safety threats (e.g. *Vibrio cholerae*, *Cryptosporidium parvum*)

Category C

Third highest priority agents include emerging pathogens that could be engineered for mass dissemination in the future because of:
- availability
- ease of production and dissemination
- potential for high morbidity and mortality rates and major health impact
- emerging infectious diseases such as Nipah virus and hantavirus.

(www.bt.cdc.gov/bioterrorism/). Some of the listed agents, such as botulisim toxin and ricin, are not infectious diseases but rather biological toxins.

Anthrax

The symptoms of anthrax are determined by the route of transmission of the bacterium which causes anthrax, *Bacillus anthracis*. There are three forms of anthrax: cutaneous, gastrointestinal, and inhalational [30,31].

Cutaneous anthrax presents as a small, painless, pruritic papule, which progresses to a vesicle which ruptures and erodes, leaving a necrotic ulcer that later gets covered with a black, painless eschar. Pathognomonic features of anthrax include the presence of an eschar, lack of pain, and edema out of proportion to the size of the lesion. Associated symptoms include swelling of adjacent lymph nodes, fever, malaise, and headache. Cutaneous anthrax is caused by *B. anthracis* entering a cut or abrasion in exposed areas of the body such as the face, neck, arms, and hands. The case-fatality rate can be as high as 20% without antibiotic therapy, but 1% with therapy.

Gastrointestinal anthrax presents with more non-specific symptoms. There are two forms: oropharyngeal and intestinal. Oropharyngeal anthrax starts with edematous lesions at the base of the tongue or tonsils that progress to necrotic ulcers with a pseudomembrane. Sore throat, fever, cervical adenopathy, and profound oropharynx edema are associated symptoms. This form of anthrax initially presents with fever, nausea, vomiting, abdominal pain, and tenderness that may progress to hematemesis, bloody diarrhea, and abdominal swelling from hemorrhagic ascites. Gastrointestinal anthrax is caused by consumption of meat contaminated with anthrax. The case-fatality rate of gastrointestinal anthrax is estimated to be 25–60%.

Inhalational anthrax initially causes non-specific symptoms that mimic influenza. These early symptoms are low-grade fever, non-productive cough, malaise, and myalgias. Two to three days later, the patient rapidly progresses to severe dyspnea, profuse sweating, high fever, cyanosis, and shock. Hemorrhagic meningitis occurs in up to half of patients. It is critical that the EMS provider attempt to distinguish any influenza-like illness from anthrax, because of the narrow window of opportunity for successful treatment. Nasal congestion and rhinorrhea are not common with inhalational anthrax, but more common with influenza-like illness. Further, shortness of breath is more common in inhalational anthrax and less common in influenza-like illness. Chest x-ray demonstrates mediastinal widening or pleural effusion. These findings are the most accurate predictors of inhalational anthrax. Inhalational anthrax can be caused by inhalation of spores, commonly seen following intentional release of aerosolized anthrax, or from the processing of materials from infected animals, such as goat hair. The case-fatality rate of inhalational anthrax can be as high as 97% without antibiotics and up to 75% with antibiotics.

Human-to-human transmission of any form of anthrax is rare. A vaccine for anthrax is licensed in the US and is administered in a six-dose schedule with annual boosters thereafter. Vaccination is not currently recommended for emergency first responders or medical personnel. However, it may be indicated for certain military personnel. In cases of deliberate use of anthrax as a biological weapon, first responders should wear a full-face respirator with HEPA filters or a self-contained breathing apparatus, gloves, and splash protection. If clothing is contaminated, it should be removed and placed in plastic bags. Soap and copious amounts of water should be used to decon-

taminate skin, and bleach should be applied for 10–15 minutes in a 1:10 dilution if there is gross contamination. If exposure to aerosolized anthrax occurs, postexposure prophylaxis (PEP) with ciprofloxacin or doxycycline should begin and continue for 60 days. Vaccination for PEP should be administered because of the persistence of anthrax spores in the lungs. Quarantine is not appropriate for persons exposed to anthrax as they are not contagious. Patients suspected of being infected with anthrax and requiring hospitalization should be immediately started on IV antibiotics [32–34].

Botulism

Botulism is caused by a neurotoxin produced by *Clostridium botulinum*, which ultimately leads to a flaccid paralysis. There are four forms of botulism based on site of toxin production: food-borne, wound, intestinal, and inhalational [35].

In food-borne botulism, early symptoms are non-specific gastrointestinal symptoms, and include nausea, vomiting, and diarrhea. This may progress to blurred vision, double vision, dry mouth, and difficulty in swallowing, breathing, and speaking. Descending muscle paralysis occurs, starting with shoulders and progressing to upper arms, lower arms, thighs, and then calves. Respiratory muscle paralysis ultimately leads to death. Food-borne botulism is caused by the ingestion of *Clostridium botulinum* toxin present in contaminated food, or by deliberate contamination as a biological weapon. The case-fatality rate in the USA is 5–10%.

Intestinal botulism is rare and occurs mainly in infants. It causes a striking loss of head control, constipation, loss of appetite, weakness, and an altered cry. Intestinal botulism occurs with ingestion of botulism spores, rather than ingestion of toxin. Spores, which may come from honey, food and dust, germinate in the colon. The case-fatality rate of hospitalized cases is less than 1%.

Wound botulism causes the same symptoms as food-borne botulism. This is rare and is caused by spores entering an open wound from soil or gravel. Inhalational botulism would be the most common form if botulinum toxin were used as a biological weapon. Symptoms would be the same as food-borne botulism, but the incubation period may be longer.

There are no reported cases of person-to-person transmission of botulism. Therefore, EMS providers do not require any special equipment to manage a patient with suspected or known botulism infection. In the case of suspected aerosol exposure to the toxin, clothing should be removed and placed in plastic bags, and the exposed person should shower thoroughly.

Plague

Plague is caused by the bacterium *Yersinia pestis*. Initial signs and symptoms may be non-specific and include fever, chills, sore throat, malaise, and headache. Tender, swollen, warm, and suppurative lymph nodes, mainly in the inguinal area, often follow. Patients infected with the plague may progress to septicemia, meningitis, pneumonia, or shock. Untreated plague has a case-fatality rate of 50–90%. If treated, the death rate is 15%.

Plague is transmitted to humans by bites, scratches, respiratory droplets, or by direct skin contact. Bites from infected rat fleas are the most frequent source of transmission, but bites or scratches from cats may also transmit plague. With deliberate use as a biological weapon, plague bacilli would be transmitted via the aerosolized airborne droplets. Direct contact with tissue or body fluids of a plague-infected sick or dead animal can lead to transmission to humans through a break in the skin [36,37].

For patients with pneumonic plague, strict isolation is indicated with precautions against airborne spread until 48 hours after start of antibiotic therapy. Close contacts of patients infected with pneumonic plague should receive chemoprophylaxis and be placed under surveillance for 7 days. Articles soiled with sputum or purulent discharges should be disinfected.

Yersinia pestis could be used as a potential biological weapon disseminated through aerosol spread and leading to pneumonic plague. Many patients presenting with fever and cough, particularly hemoptysis in a fulminant course with high case-fatality, should raise suspicions for a biological weapon [38–40].

Smallpox

There are two clinical forms of smallpox: variola major and variola minor. Variola major is the more severe form of disease with a case-fatality rate of greater than 30%, while variola minor is less severe form with a case-fatality rate less than 1%. All smallpox begins with a prodrome that lasts 2–4 days. The prodrome starts abruptly and consists of fever, headache, nausea, vomiting, muscle pain, headache, and malaise.

Variola major has four principal clinical presentations: ordinary, modified, flat, and hemorrhagic. Ordinary is the most common, occurring in 90% of cases. Modified is mild. Flat and hemorrhagic forms are uncommon, but usually severe and fatal [41].

In ordinary smallpox, after the prodrome, mucous membrane lesions called enanthem begin in the mouth. This consists of red spots on the tongue and mucosa which enlarge and ulcerate quickly, followed by a rash on the face. The rash then progresses from the proximal extremities to the distal extremities and trunk within 24 hours. The macules progress to papules, vesicles, pustules, and crusts. Crusts later separate leaving depigmented skin and pitted scars. The case-fatality rate for ordinary smallpox is about 30%.

Modified smallpox occurs in previously vaccinated persons. During the prodrome, fever is absent and the illness is less severe. The skin rash is more superficial and progresses quickly, and lesions are less numerous. This form is more easily confused with chickenpox.

Flat smallpox has a more severe prodrome with soft, flat skin lesions that contain little fluid. Most cases are fatal.

Hemorrhagic smallpox consists of a more severe and prolonged prodrome along with extensive bleeding into the skin, mucous membranes, and gastrointestinal tract. The skin rash remains flat and does not progress beyond the vesicular stage. Hemorrhagic smallpox is usually abruptly fatal between the 5th and 7th days of illness. The case-fatality rate for hemorrhagic and flat smallpox is greater than 90%.

Variola minor produces a rash like ordinary smallpox but results in much less severe systemic reactions.

Transmission is via virus inhalation from airborne droplets or fine particle aerosols from the oral, pharyngeal, or nasal mucosa of an infected person, physical contact with an infected person, or with contaminated articles through skin inoculation. EMS personnel should be able to identify the rash due to smallpox, and try to distinguish it from other less virulent diseases, particularly chickenpox. Information to differentiate these illnesses from smallpox is available from the CDC at www.bt.cdc.gov/agent/smallpox/.

The last naturally occurring cases of smallpox were identified in 1977, and in 1980 the World Health Organization declared smallpox officially eradicated from the planet. While there are only two sanctioned repositories of smallpox virus in storage and for research purposes, there may exist virus samples outside these two sanctioned repositories. Any new suspected cases of smallpox are a medical and public health emergency. Strict respiratory and contact isolation of confirmed or suspected smallpox cases must be undertaken.

Medical personnel in contact with suspected or confirmed smallpox cases should be wearing N95 fit-tested masks, and use other standard precautions. All bedding and clothing should be autoclaved or laundered in hot water with bleach.

Tularemia

Tularemia, caused by the bacterium *Francisella tularensis*, has various clinical manifestations related to the route of introduction. All forms have a sudden onset of non-specific influenza-like symptoms, including high fever, cough, sore throat, chills, headache, and generalized body aches. Sometimes nausea, vomiting, and diarrhea may also occur. All forms may lead to sepsis, pneumonia, and meningitis. The clinical forms include ulceroglandular, glandular, oculoglandular, septic, oropharyngeal, and pneumonic [42].

Ulceroglandular tularemia is the most common form. It begins at the skin site of the bite of a tick or fly. A papule appears that becomes pustular and later ulcerates, and finally develops into an eschar. Regional lymph nodes become swollen, painful, and tender and rarely suppurate and discharge purulent material. Glandular tularemia has no skin involvement, only regional lymphadenopathy similar to that which occurs with ulceroglandular disease. Oculoglandular tularemia is caused by the bacillus entering the eye. Conjunctival ulceration occurs followed by regional lymphadenopathy of the cervical and preauricular nodes. Septic tularemia begins with non-specific symptoms of fever, nausea, vomiting, and abdominal pain, eventually leading to confusion, coma, multisystem organ failure, and septic shock.

Oropharyngeal tularemia is caused by consumption of contaminated water or food, leading to exudative pharyngitis which may be accompanied by oral ulceration. Abdominal pain, diarrhea, and vomiting may accompany this type. Regional lymphadenopathy occurs affecting the cervical and retropharyngeal nodes.

Pneumonic tularemia may be caused by lung exposure to an infective aerosol from soil, grain, or hay, or due to deliberate use of an infective aerosol as a bioterrorist attack. The clinical presentation may be cough, pleuritic pain, and rarely dyspnea. Despite the lungs being the primary route of entry, it is not uncommon for tularemic pneumonia to present as non-specific systemic signs without respiratory symptoms, and often a normal chest-x-ray.

Tularemia is transmitted through the skin, mucous membranes, lungs, and gastrointestinal tract. The bacteria pass through the skin by bites, oropharyngeal mucosa, and conjunctiva by contaminated water, or by contaminated blood or tissue while handling carcasses of infected animals. Through the gastrointestinal tract, it is transmitted by ingestion of insufficiently cooked meat of infected animals or by consumption of contaminated water. Finally, tularemia can be transmitted through the lungs by contaminated soil, by handling contaminated furs, or by deliberate aerosolization of the bacterium as a biological weapon. The incubation period is usually 3–5 days but can range from 1 to 14 days.

There is no documented person-to-person transmission of tularemia. Routine precautions are adequate when transporting and caring for patients. The vehicle and equipment, however, must be thoroughly cleaned and decontaminated after patient transport.

Viral hemorrhagic fevers

Viral hemorrhagic fevers are caused by different families of viruses and lead to similar clinical syndromes. In the case of bioterrorist attack, it is essential that first responders are able to recognize the illness associated with the intentional release of the biological agent.

In hemorrhagic fever, the initial signs and symptoms are non-specific and include high fever, headache, muscle aches, and severe fatigue. There may be associated gastrointestinal symptoms of nausea, vomiting, diarrhea, and abdominal pain. Respiratory symptoms of cough and sore throat may also occur. About 5 days after the onset of illness, a truncal maculopapular rash develops in most patients. As the disease progresses, bleeding occurs from internal organs, the mouth, eyes, ears, and from under the skin, which would be evidenced as petechiae and ecchymosis. Shock, coma, seizures, and kidney failure may ensure in severe cases.

Viral hemorrhagic fevers are caused by viruses in four families: arenaviruses, bunyaviruses, flaviviruses, and filoviruses, causing diseases such as Ebola hemorrhagic fever, hantavirus pulmonary syndrome, Lassa fever, Marburg hemorrhagic fever, hemorrhagic fever with renal syndrome, and Crimean-Congo hemorrhagic fever [43]. Transmission occurs when humans have direct contact with infected animals, mainly rodents, or are bitten by a mosquito or tick vector. Once a person has become infected, some viruses can be transmitted from person to person, mainly by close contact with infected people but also indirectly by objects contaminated with infected body fluids.

Transmission of viral hemorrhagic fever mainly occurs in the later stages of illness when the patient suffers vomiting, diarrhea, shock, and hemorrhage. In the case of Ebola virus, there are reports of transmission within a few days of the onset of fever. The incubation period ranges from 2 days to 3 weeks, and no transmission has been documented during the incubation period.

While there is currently no vaccine for viral hemorrhagic fevers, except for yellow fever and Argentine hemorrhagic fever, significant research and clinical trials are underway to develop a vaccine for Ebola. There are also several experimental treatments under development for patients who have contracted Ebola. To prevent infection, contact with rodents and bites from ticks and mosquitos should be prevented. Person-to-person transmission can be prevented by strict adherence to routine precautions. In addition, patients with known or suspected viral hemorrhagic fever must be isolated. While this is not routinely possible in the EMS setting, there exist portable isolation systems that can enhance the ability to isolate patients with active symptoms of viral hemorrhagic fever during prolonged or inter-facility critical care transports. The transport vehicle itself can also serve as an isolation unit, enabling the patient to be isolated from the scene and while in transit.

If personnel are exposed to viral hemorrhagic fever, they should be placed under surveillance for fever. The World Health Organization and CDC have prepared a number of documents specific to viral hemorrhagic fever management and control, with detailed and comprehensive strategies to prevent spread and protect health care workers during an outbreak [44–47]. In 2014, an outbreak of Ebola viral hemorrhagic fever was declared in Guinea, Liberia, Sierra Leone, and Nigeria. As of 16 August 2014, there were 2240 confirmed and suspected cases, and 1229 deaths. Of particular interest was the air medical evacuation of two American health care workers infected with Ebola from Liberia to a hospital in the United States in August 2014. Due to the rapidly evolving nature of this recent Ebola outbreak, the CDC is maintaining up to date information, including methods to prevent disease transmission [48].

Other infections

Chickenpox – varicella zoster virus

Varicella zoster virus (VZV) causes two distinct diseases: chickenpox and "shingles" (herpes zoster). Acute chickenpox is highly contagious and usually runs its course in about a week or two, producing immunity, but VZV is not eliminated from the body. The virus becomes dormant in the sensory ganglia and may reactivate decades later to produce zoster [49]. To decrease the incidence of chickenpox in adults who were never exposed to VZV as a child, routine childhood vaccination began in 1995. The full vaccine regimen (two doses) is 90–100% protective against chickenpox and "virtually 100% effective against severe disease [49]." Serological screening for VZV IgG is indicated for health care professionals who do not have a documented history of chickenpox. VZV is common, so ensuring prehospital employees are immune prior to patient care is important and cost-effective. Only immune health care professionals should care for patients with chickenpox or shingles. If a pregnant EMS provider has a documented history of chickenpox or has positive titers, she is considered immune and can care for patients. Both she and the fetus are protected.

Non-immune adults exposed to either chickenpox or zoster can develop acute chickenpox, complications of which include pneumonia, encephalitis, and death. Non-immune personnel exposed to chickenpox or disseminated zoster must avoid patient contact from 10 days after the exposure (the incubation period) until day 21 [49]. An exposure is defined as a breach of contact precautions (such as localized direct contact with uncovered lesions) and/or breach of airborne precautions (chickenpox or disseminated zoster).

If an unprotected exposure occurs to a non-immune health care professional, unless that person is pregnant or immuno-compromised, the vaccine should be given within 3–5 days. If a pregnant or immunocompromised worker is exposed, varicella zoster immune globulin (VZIG) should be offered up to 96 hours after exposure.

Meningitis – bacterial

Neisseria meningitidis, or meningococcus, is an uncommon nosocomial transmission [50–52] but it is possible to contract the disease from a patient infected with *N. meningitidis* when routine mask use on the patient is not observed. In addition, this disease has a high case-fatality rate (10%) [52]. All health care professionals should understand that preventing transmission of meningococcus requires use of droplet precautions and that it is not an airborne transmitted disease.

Postexposure prophylaxis should be administered when close, unprotected (mask) contact occurs, such as while performing unprotected mouth-to-mouth resuscitation on an infected patient, or if splash/splatter of secretions into mucous membranes occurs (as with suctioning, intubation, vomiting, coughing, or endotracheal tube management) [52]. Simple proximity to the patient does not qualify as close contact, unless the EMS provider was <3 feet from the patient for >8 hours [52]. Because many patients with symptoms consistent with *N. meningitidis* infection are actually infected with viruses or other organisms, PEP should be given only after substantial exposure (as defined above) to a patient with culture- or Gram stain-proven meningococcus.

Patients may be considered infectious for 1 week before the onset of symptoms and for 24 hours after effective treatment

began. Exposed workers may return to duty 24 hours after PEP was begun. There is time to determine if *N. meningitidis* is present before empirically administering prophylaxis to many EMS personnel unnecessarily. PEP for meningococcus should be started within 24 hours (but may be begun up to 10 days) after exposure; options include ceftriaxone 250 mg IM, ciprofloxacin 500 mg PO once, or rifampin 600 mg PO bid for 2 days [52].

The medical director plays an important role in ensuring that prehospital personnel are treated quickly and appropriately when a true exposure to *N. meningitidis* has taken place. Often one of the following situations occurs.

- A crew transports a patient suspected of having meningitis to an ED and calls the infection control officer with concerns about exposure.
- Hospital infection control personnel attempt to contact exposed prehospital personnel involved with treatment/transport of an inpatient now diagnosed with meningococcus.

Usually the infection control officer is directly involved, but the medical director can assist hospital infection control, occupational health service, and ED providers by including prehospital providers in the pool of exposed providers. The designated infection control officer should gather specific information, confirming which (if any) prehospital personnel were close enough to the patient to warrant having them report for evaluation and possible PEP administration.

Routine vaccination is not recommended for any health care worker group, including fire/EMS personnel. However, such personnel may fall into any of the following categories, and if so, they should contact their regular provider or occupational health service to consider vaccination: persons aged 19–55 years who are at increased risk for meningococcal disease, including college freshmen living in dormitories, military recruits, microbiologists routinely exposed to isolates of *N. meningitidis*, travelers to or residents of countries in which *N. meningitidis* meningitis is hyperendemic or epidemic, persons with terminal complement-component deficiencies, and persons with anatomical or functional asplenia [52].

References

1 US Department of Labor, Occupational Safety and Health Administration. *Occupational Exposure to Blood-Borne Pathogens: Precautions for Emergency Responders.* OSHA 3130. Washington DC, 1992.

2 Varia M, Wilson S, Sarwal S, et al. Investigation of nosocomial outbreak of severe acute respiratory syndrome (SARS) in Toronto, Canada. *CMAJ* 2003;169:285–92.

3 Ko PC, Chen WJ, Ha MH, et al. Emergency medical service utilization during an outbreak of severe acute respiratory syndrome (SARS) and the incidence of SARS-associated coronavirus infection among emergency medical technicians. *Acad Emerg Med* 2004;11:903–11.

4 Verbeek PR, McLelland IW, Silverman AC, Burgess RJ. Loss of para-medic availability in an urban emergency medical services system during a severe acute respiratory syndrome outbreak. *Acad Emerg Med* 2004:11:973–78.

5 Centers for Disease Control and Prevention. Seasonal influenza (flu). Available at: www.cdc.gov/flu/

6 Advisory Committee on Immunization Practices. Prevention and control of influenza. Recommendations of the Advisory Committee on Immunization Practices 2008. *MMWR* 2008;57:1–60.

7 Centers for Disease Control and Prevention. Seasonal influenza (flu) treatment – antiviral drugs. Available at: www.cdc.gov/flu/antivirals/index.htm

8 Centers for Disease Control and Prevention. Prevention and control of seasonal influenza with vaccines. Available at: www.cdc.gov/flu/professionals/acip/background.htm

9 Brandli O. The clinical presentation of tuberculosis. *Respiration* 1998;65:97–105.

10 Cohen R, Muzaffar S, Capellan J, Azar H, Chinikamwala M. The validity of classic symptoms and chest radiographic configuration in predicting pulmonary tuberculosis. *Chest* 1996; 109:420–3.

11 American Thoracic Society, Centers for Disease Control, Infectious Diseases Society of America. Treatment of tuberculosis. *MMWR* 2003;52:1–77.

12 Centers for Disease Control and Prevention. Targeted tuberculin skin testing and treatment of latent tuberculosis infection. *MMWR* 2000;49:1–77.

13 Varia M, Wilson S, Sarwal S, et al. Investigation of nosocomial outbreak of severe acute respiratory syndrome (SARS) in Toronto, Canada. *CMAJ* 2003;169(4):285–92.

14 Centers for Disease Control and Prevention. Extensively drug-resistant tuberculosis – United States 1993–2006. *MMWR* 2007; 56(11):250–3.

15 Tuberculosis Committee, Canadian Thoracic Society. *Canadian Tuberculosis Standards*, 5th edn. Ottawa: Canadian Lung Association, 2000.

16 Liu CL, Lu YT, Peng MJ, et al. Clinical and laboratory features of SARS vis-à-vis onset of fever. *Chest* 2004;126:509–17.

17 Chan PK, Tang JW, Hui DS. SARS: clinical presentation, transmission, pathogenesis and treatment options. *Clin Sci* 2006;110: 193–204.

18 Wong WN, Sek AC, Lau RF, et al. Early clinical predictors of SARS in the emergency department. *CJEM* 2004;6:12–21.

19 Chen SY, Su CP, Ma MH, et al. Predictive model of diagnosing probable cases of SARS in febrile patients with exposure risk. *Ann Emerg Med* 2004;43:1–5.

20 Su CP, Chiang WC, Ma MH, et al. Validation of a novel SARS scoring system. *Ann Emerg Med* 2004;43:34–42.

21 Wang TL, Jang TN, Huang CH, et al. Establishing a clinical decision rule of SARS at the Emergency Department. *Ann Emerg Med* 2004;43:17–22.

22 Booth CM, Matukas LM, Tomlinson GA, et al. Clinical features and short-term outcomes of 144 patients with SARS in the greater Toronto area. *JAMA* 2003;289:2801–9.

23 Dwosh H, Hong H, Austgarden D, Herman S, Schabas R. Identification and containment of an outbreak of SARS in a community hospital. *Can Med Assoc J* 2003;168:1415–20.

24 Poutanen SM, Low DE, Henry B, et al. Identification of SARS in Canada. *N Engl J Med* 2003;348:1995–2005.

25 Seto WH, Tsang D, Yung RW, et al. Effectiveness of precautions against droplets and contact in prevention of nosocomial transmission of severe acute respiratory syndrome (SARS). *Lancet* 2003;361:1519–20.

26 Verbeek PR, Schwartz B, Burgess RJ. Should paramedics intubate patients with SARS-like symptoms? *CMAJ* 2003;169: 199–200.

27 Interdisciplinary Respiratory Protection Study Group. Protecting health care workers from SARS and other respiratory pathogens: a review of the infection control literature. *Am J Infect Control* 2005; 33:114–121.

28 Chen MI, Chow AL, Earnest A, Leong HN, Leo YS. Clinical and epidemiological predictors of transmission in Severe Acute Respiratory Syndrome (SARS). *BMC Infect Dis* 2006;6:151.

29 Centers for Disease Control and Prevention. Middle east respiratory syndrome coronavirus (MERS-CoV) summary and literature update – as of 9 May 2014. Avaiable at http://www.who.int/csr/disease/coronavirus_infections/MERS_CoV_Update_09_May_2014.pdf?ua=1. Accessed 22 August, 2014.

30 Inglesby TV, O'Toole T, Henderson DA, et al. Anthrax as a biological weapon, 2002. Update recommendations for management. *JAMA* 2002;287:2236–52.

31 Bell DM, Kozarsky PE, Stephens DS. Clinical issues in the prophylaxis, diagnosis, and treatment of anthrax. *Emerg Infect Dis* 2002; 8:222–5.

32 American Public Health Association. Anthrax. In: Heymann DL (ed) *Control of Communicable Diseases Manual*, 18th edn. Washington, DC: American Public Health Association, 2004.

33 Shadomy SV, Rosenstein NE. Anthrax. In: Wallace RB (ed) *Maxcy-Rosenau-Last Public Health & Preventive Medicine*, 15th edn. New York: McGraw-Hill Medical, 2007.

34 Centers for Disease Control and Prevention. Anthrax. In: Atkinson W, Hamborsky J, McIntyre L, Wolfe S (eds) *Epidemiology and Prevention of Vaccine-Preventable Diseases*, 9th edn. Washington, DC: Public Health Foundation, 2006.

35 American Academy of Pediatrics. Botulism. In: Pickering LK (ed) *Red Book: 2000 Report of the Committee on Infectious Diseases*, 25th edn. Elk Grove Village, IL: American Academy of Pediatrics, 2000.

36 Campbell GL, Dennis DT. Plague and other *Yersinia* infections. In: Harrison RT, Fauci AS (eds) *Harrison's Principles of Internal Medicine*, 14th edn. New York: McGraw-Hill, 1998.

37 Dennis DT, Gage KL. Plague. In: Armstrong D, Cohen J (eds) *Infectious Diseases*, 2nd edn, Vol 2. London: Mosby, 2003.

38 American Public Health Association. Plague (Pestis). In: Heymann DL (ed) *Control of Communicable Diseases Manual*, 18th edn. Washington, DC: American Public Health Association, 2004.

39 Staples JE. Plague. In: Wallace RB (ed) *Maxcy-Rosenau-Last Public Health & Preventive Medicine*, 15th edn. New York: McGraw-Hill Medical, 2007.

40 Centers for Disease Control. Plague. Available at: www.cdc.gov/plague/

41 Centers for Disease Control and Prevention. Overview of smallpox, clinical presentations, and medical care of smallpox patients. Available at: http://emergency.cdc.gov/agent/smallpox/response-plan/files/annex-1-part1of3.pdf

42 Dennis DT, Ingelsby TV, Henderson DA, et al. Tularemia as a biological weapon. Medical and public health management. *JAMA* 2001;285:2763–73.

43 Centers for Disease Control and Prevention. Viral hemorrhagic fevers – fact sheet. Available at: www.cdc.gov/ncidod/dvrd/spb/mnpages/dispages/Fact_Sheets/Viral_Hemorrhagic_Fevers_Fact_Sheet.pdf

44 Centers for Disease Control and Prevention, World Health Organization. Infection control for viral haemorrhagic fevers in the African health care setting. Atlanta, GA: Centers for Disease Control and Prevention, 1998. Available at: www.cdc.gov/vhf/abroad/vhf-manual.html

45 Centers for Disease Control and Prevention. Management of patients with suspected viral hemorrhagic fever. *MMWR* 1988;37 (S–3):1–15.

46 LeDuc JW. Epidemiology of viral hemorrhagic fevers. In: Wallace RB (ed) *Maxcy-Rosenau-Last Public Health & Preventive Medicine*, 15th edn. New York: McGraw-Hill Medical, 2007.

47 Centers for Disease Control and Prevention. Varicella vaccination: information for health care providers. June 4, 2013. Available at: www.cdc.gov/vaccines/vpd-vac/varicella/default-hcp.htm

48 Centers for Disease Control and Prevention. Ebola hemorrhagic fever. Available at http://www.cdc.gov/vhf/ebola/index.html?s_cid=cdc_homepage_feature_001. Accessed 22 August, 2014.

49 Bolyard EA, Tablan OC, Williams WW, Pearson ML, Shapiro CN, Deitchmann SD. Guideline for infection control in health-care personnel, 1998. Hospital Infection Control Practices Advisory Committee. *Infect Control Hosp Epidemiol* 1998;19(6):407–63.

50 Centers for Disease Control and Prevention. Immunization of health-care workers: recommendations of the Advisory Committee on Immunization Practices (ACIP) and the Hospital Infection Control Practices Advisory Committee (HICPAC). *MMWR* 1997;46(RR-18):1–42.

51 Gardner P. Clinical practice: prevention of meningococcal disease. *N Engl J Med* 1006;355(14):1466–73.

52 Centers for Disease Control and Prevention. Prevention and control of meningococcal disease: recommendations of the Advisory Committee on Immunization Practices (ACIP). *MMWR* 2005;54 (RRj07):1–21.

Trauma Problems

CHAPTER 26

Trauma Systems of Care

Jeffrey P. Salomone and Joseph A. Salomone

Introduction

In its broadest sense, a trauma system consists of both an organized approach to managing patients who have suffered acute injury, across the continuum from initial medical care through rehabilitation, as well as injury prevention activities aimed at those at risk of suffering trauma. While the trauma system should be integrated with both public health and emergency management, there is significant overlap between trauma and EMS systems. This chapter will focus primarily on the close interaction between these two systems.

Trauma system organization

Trauma systems are typically organized on a state-wide basis, although some larger counties may have sophisticated systems (e.g. San Diego County, CA). In 1988, West and colleagues described the ideal criteria for a state-wide trauma care system (Box 26.1) [1]. State laws generally delegate the authority for designation of trauma centers to a state agency, such as a department of health, and describe the process by which hospitals may seek designation. Because of their close relationship, most state trauma offices are colocated with the state office of EMS.

While most states utilize the standards promulgated by the American College of Surgeons Committee on Trauma (ACS-COT) [2], some states (e.g. Florida) opt to draft their own trauma center criteria. The term "designation" refers to authorization from a state agency for an institution to represent itself to the public as a trauma center, while "verification" refers to the inspection by a non-biased team of experts (usually from outside the community) who have confirmed that all necessary services and processes are in place to meet the ACS-COT (or equivalent) standards.

In the ideal trauma system, the lead agency would have the authority to designate trauma centers based upon need, rather than simply approving any facility that desires designation in a competitive, free-market approach. Need for additional trauma centers should be based upon the population of a geographic area, the volume of trauma patients encountered, or proximity to other designated centers. Trauma centers that regularly see large numbers of patients are able to maintain readiness so that management becomes a matter of routine practice, while those that fail to see sufficient numbers of injured patients, especially the seriously injured, may find that their personnel struggle to maintain their organizational processes and procedural skills.

Like the trauma centers themselves, performance improvement is a key component of a trauma system. Data collected in trauma registries are pooled on a system-wide basis and analyzed. This information may provide insight for focusing injury prevention activities in addition to opportunities for improvement in system design or the need for education. Over the past few years, the ACS-COT has developed the Trauma Quality Improvement Project (TQIP) which conducts risk-adjusted analysis of outcomes at trauma centers that voluntarily participate. By presenting its data as observed-to-expected ratios, TQIP allows centers to voluntarily benchmark themselves to other centers across the country. When fully implemented, TQIP will allow high-performing trauma centers (low observed-to-expected ratios) to share best practices with lower performing facilities (high observed-to-expected ratios).

Most states have trauma advisory committees composed of individuals who represent stakeholder sectors involved in trauma care in that state. These committees provide oversight and advise the state trauma office on matters related to improvements in their trauma system. These committees often draft or approve a state trauma plan that serves as a strategic blueprint for enhancing the system over a period of time. Often the state trauma advisory committee also assists the state in determining how governmental funding, if available, will be distributed to stakeholders in the trauma system. This funding helps offset the expensive costs of maintaining trauma center readiness and data collection for trauma registries and aids with the uncompensated care delivered by these centers. State funding may also help provide education to individuals who care for trauma patients and may even purchase some needed equipment.

Emergency Medical Services: Clinical Practice and Systems Oversight, Second Edition. Volume 1: Clinical Aspects of EMS.
Edited by David C. Cone, Jane H. Brice, Theodore R. Delbridge, and J. Brent Myers.
© 2015 NAEMSP. Published 2015 by John Wiley & Sons, Inc. Companion Website: www.wiley.com/go/cone\naemsp

Box 26.1 Criteria for state-wide trauma systems

- Legal authority for designation
- Formal process for designation
- Use of American College of Surgeons standards
- Use of non-biased survey teams (from out of area)
- Number of trauma centers based upon population or volume
- Triage criteria that permit direct transport to a trauma center
- Monitoring of system performance
- Full geographic coverage

Trauma care facilities

Trauma centers represent one of the essential components of a trauma system. A trauma center is an institution committed to the care of injured patients across the spectrum of initial resuscitation through rehabilitation, including operative management and critical care. A trauma center is a unique blend of personnel (surgeons and other physician specialists, nurses, and allied health care workers), equipment, and processes (robust ongoing performance improvement program). The various physicians, nurses, therapists, and technologists must work together as a cohesive team, under the direction of the trauma surgeon.

The most widely accepted criteria for trauma center designation are those promulgated by the ACS-COT [2].

- **Level III trauma center**: the "basic" trauma care facility that possesses a 24-hour emergency department staffed by emergency physicians. General surgeons must be immediately available while orthopedic surgeons, plastic surgeons, radiologists, and anesthesia personnel must be on call.
- **Level II trauma center**: capable of managing more complex cases. Trauma surgeons must be available within 15 minutes of the arrival of the most critically injured patients. In addition to the criteria from Level III, a Level II center must include on-call physicians in the following specialties: neurosurgery, hand surgery, obstetrics/gynecology, ophthalmology, oral/maxillofacial surgery, thoracic surgery, and critical care medicine.
- **Level I trauma center**: the highest level trauma center. While medical capabilities are only slightly enhanced over the Level II facility (cardiac surgery with cardiopulmonary bypass capability and microvascular capability for replantation), a Level I center must have operating room personnel who are in-house around the clock as well as a surgically directed critical care service. In addition to providing the most comprehensive trauma care, a Level I facility serves as a regional referral resource. As part of its teaching responsibilities, a Level I center must participate in training of surgical residents and conduct Advanced Trauma Life Support courses. Level I facilities must also have an ongoing research program related to injury.

When first conceived, the system that included only Level I–III facilities was seen as an exclusive system, allowing only hospitals with certain minimal capabilities to participate. In response to this criticism, the ACS-COT added the Level IV trauma facility, which is a smaller hospital with limited capabilities that is viewed as a resuscitation point in a community that lacks Level I– II trauma centers. Following attempts at initial stabilization at a Level IV center, the injured patient would be transferred on to a higher level of care in a more distant location. The Level IV centers allowed for the creation of an inclusive trauma system and the ability to provide full geographic coverage for a regional system.

In additional to trauma centers, other facilities included in the trauma system are specialty hospitals, such as pediatric trauma centers or spinal cord injury facilities, and rehabilitation hospitals. In some communities, patients with isolated spinal cord injuries may be transported directly to an institution dedicated to managing spinal trauma and rehabilitation.

Communications

Communications are a key aspect of both the EMS and trauma systems. Traditional telephone (landline) and cellular phones are used by callers to access public safety answering points via 9-1-1 in order to report trauma victims. After obtaining essential information for EMS response, trained emergency medical dispatchers are capable of providing prearrival instructions of Basic Life Support measures that a lay bystander could provide while EMS is responding, such as direct pressure for hemorrhage control. Dispatchers also gather additional information from callers or first responders about the need for specialized personnel or equipment, such as extrication or hazardous materials experts.

For the most critically injured patients, rapid response and transport should result in a more expeditious arrival of the patient at the trauma center. Radio communications are used both between the dispatch center and the responding/transporting EMS unit, as well as between the EMS unit and the receiving facility. Prompt notification of the trauma center that a seriously injured patient is en route allows the facility to assemble its trauma team in the emergency department prior to patient arrival.

Some recent mass casualty events, such as the terrorist attacks of 11 September 2001, illustrated that many public safety agencies (law enforcement, fire, and EMS) were unable to communicate with each other. Since then, emergency management organizations have focused significant emphasis on increasing interoperability, resulting in enhanced communication between first responders in an effort to improve mass casualty response. Many state trauma and EMS agencies host a website for receiving facilities to post their current status (open versus on diversion, etc.). Some of these web-based systems are robust enough to indicate the number of available beds, permitting a rapid assessment of surge capacity in a disaster.

Emergency response

The greatest overlap between the trauma and EMS systems is seen with emergency response, from dispatch of EMS to patient arrival at the receiving facility. The adage of "getting the right patient to the right place in the right amount of time" truly describes the challenge faced by EMS providers when caring for trauma patients. "Field triage" represents the decision making for selecting which injured patients ("the right patient") require transport to a trauma center ("the right place"). In 2006 and again in 2011, the Centers for Disease Control and Prevention assembled national expert panels to review evidence and revise the field triage algorithm originally developed by the ACS-COT (see Volume 1, Chapter 45) [3].

"The right amount of time" includes decisions regarding both the interventions and time spent at the scene as well as determining the best mode of transport, namely ground EMS versus air medical service. While air medical transport can get an injured patient from a distant scene to a trauma center significantly faster than ground transport, ground transportation may be more expeditious when the patient is located closer to the trauma center (within 10 miles or so), because of the time required to set up a landing zone and power up and power down engines. Trauma surgeons should have input into regional protocols regarding transport modality of injured patients.

Emergency medical services personnel may also be called upon to transport a patient from initial receiving facility (perhaps a non-trauma center) to a trauma center. The care required en route (Basic Life Support versus Advanced Life Support) and need for rapid transfer are the major determinants of whether ground or air transport is utilized. In some jurisdictions, the transferring facility may need to send a nurse along with the patient if the patient requires care that exceeds the scope of practice of the EMS personnel (e.g. in many jurisdictions, an EMS provider may not transfuse blood unless also licensed as a nurse).

All ACS-COT verified trauma centers are required to participate in public and professional education. Several standardized trauma training courses for EMS personnel exist, including Prehospital Trauma Life Support (PHTLS) and International Trauma Life Support (ITLS). Many EMS systems require their personnel to maintain current certification in one of these programs. These courses provide an opportunity for nurses and physicians from trauma centers to share their expertise in managing trauma patients. Some trauma centers provide regularly scheduled case reviews for EMS personnel, offering follow-up on diagnostic procedures and management after arrival at the facility, in combination with reinforcement of basic trauma care principles.

Medical oversight

Medical oversight for EMS is divided into direct and indirect oversight. Direct oversight involves providing instructions to prehospital care providers via radio or telephone. In the early days of Advanced Life Support in the prehospital setting, this form of medical direction was heavily utilized with the thought that close communication between the receiving or base station physician and the EMS providers was essential for quality care in the field. Because of the time involved in contacting a

physician, direct medical oversight may actually be associated with longer prehospital times. As years passed, focus has shifted more toward one form of indirect medical oversight, where EMS providers follow written protocols or treatment guidelines, each focused on a specific condition or chief complaint. Given the staffing of receiving emergency departments, direct oversight is virtually always provided by emergency physicians rather than trauma surgeons.

Another aspect of direct medical oversight involves a physician riding along with EMS personnel to monitor care and providing orders in those circumstances. Unlike emergency physicians who have mandatory rotations in EMS during their residencies, most trauma surgeons have limited exposure to prehospital care, unless they worked as EMS providers before medical school. As a result, trauma surgeons often have a poor understanding of how prehospital care is delivered and the unusual circumstances under which EMS providers must render care. One could argue that it would be beneficial for trauma surgeons to occasionally spend some time in the field observing the assessment and management delivered by both ground and air EMS personnel.

There are significant opportunities for trauma surgeons to participate in indirect medical oversight. In fact, trauma surgeons should have the opportunity to actively participate in the development of, or review and provide input to, written protocols utilized by the EMS providers in their trauma system. As a part of their performance improvement program, trauma centers should review the prehospital care provided to patients transported to their facilities. Most commonly, this is accomplished by review of the patient care reports for the most critical patients or those who died in the emergency department. Feedback should be provided to the transporting EMS agency, either through its performance improvement coordinator or the service medical director. Similarly, some trauma programs invite representatives from EMS services to participate in their monthly performance improvement meetings. Examples of audit filters for evaluating prehospital trauma care are listed in Box 26.2 [4].

Box 26.2 Audit filters for prehospital trauma care [4]

- Lack of adequate airway
- Misplaced endotracheal tube
- Hypoxia (SpO$_2$ <90%) upon patient arrival
- Inability to control external hemorrhage (e.g. no tourniquet applied to an extremity)
- Spinal immobilization performed for penetrating torso trauma
- Scene time >10 minutes for critical patient
- Appropriateness of needle decompression of pleural cavity
- Failure to transport a critically injured patient to the closest appropriate facility

---

Source: Salomone JP, Salomone JA [4]. Reproduced with permission of McGraw-Hill.

Data collection

Data collection is an essential component of the trauma system, and the data are utilized in many ways. All trauma centers are required to maintain trauma registries, databanks of key information regarding the trauma patients managed at their facilities. Data from these institutional trauma centers are then pooled on a system level, either regional or statewide. Many centers also voluntarily submit data to the National Trauma Data Bank (NTDB). In some trauma systems, all hospitals, including those that are not trauma centers, are required to provide information about the injured patients for which they care, as not all injured patients require management at trauma centers. This allows the system to evaluate undertriage of trauma patients, which occurs when patients requiring trauma center capabilities are transported to hospitals that are not trauma centers. The ACS-COT believes a highly functioning trauma system has an undertriage rate of 5% or lower.

Data are the basis of a strong performance improvement project. By collecting data on complications or other issues, a trauma center or system may identify a problem that should be addressed. Such trends pose an opportunity for implementing a process change that is anticipated to result in improved care. In fact, progressive trauma systems have adopted a public health model that consists of three core phases: assessment, policy development, and assurance. In the trauma system, the assessment phase consists of data collection followed by data analysis. Once problems are identified, solutions are proposed and implemented in the policy development phase. Finally, in the assurance phase additional data are collected to confirm that the implemented intervention is producing the desired effect, e.g. lowering complications, etc. These three phases create a never-ending loop of performance improvement wherein the trauma center or system continually strives to provide better and better care.

Research is another important use of the trauma registry. As these registries include increasing numbers of patients, they provide a rich repository of data for retrospective studies comparing different management options and their respective outcomes. Linkages between databases of EMS records to hospital or system trauma registries allow for analysis of the relationship between the EMS system and trauma system. Efforts are currently under way to link the National EMS Information System to the NTDB. This linkage will permit robust analysis of how prehospital interventions and system design affect the outcome of trauma patients.

Emergency management

Emergency management is the discipline that focuses on the care of citizens affected by various disasters. Because there is significant overlap between the issues that arise from many different types of disasters, modern emergency management systems tend to utilize an all-hazards approach rather than developing different responses depending upon the type of the disaster. Because most disasters include some number of injured patients, there needs to be close cooperation and interaction between emergency management and trauma programs, both inside the trauma center as well as on the system level. Trauma centers should have internal strategies that open up extra beds, thereby creating surge capacity in the event of a disaster.

Preplanning is essential for successful disaster response. Along with their colleagues in emergency management, leaders in the trauma program should periodically test their trauma center's readiness by conducting disaster drills. Ideally, drills should be held on different days and shifts to ensure all members are properly prepared. Similarly, trauma systems and their corresponding emergency management agencies should evaluate their system's preparedness through drills that include numerous simulated patients, multiple EMS and first responder agencies, regional emergency management personnel, and multiple facilities. Such drills can uncover potential system weaknesses while emphasizing the need for system coordination and communication.

Injury prevention

Injury prevention represents another aspect of the integration between the public health model and the trauma system. In this model, trauma is viewed as a disease and efforts should be focused on preventing new cases. Trauma registry data, either from the trauma center or the trauma system, are analyzed to determine common causes of injury (e.g. motor vehicle crashes or falls) and at-risk groups (children or the elderly). Interventions aimed at preventing or ameliorating these injuries are conceived and implemented. Further analysis is used to monitor for the effect of these prevention strategies. In some EMS systems, EMS professionals routinely participate in injury prevention activities, such as distribution of car seats and educating parents on their use, or providing evaluations of homes for the elderly looking for conditions that may lead to falls, such as throw rugs or lack of anti-slip mats in bathtubs.

Conclusion

Trauma remains the leading cause of death for individuals between the age of 1 and 44 years. Significant overlap exists between the trauma and EMS systems, community public health, and emergency management. Although these systems each have somewhat different objectives, when these systems coordinate their activities related to injury and the injured patient, great strides can be accomplished toward achieving optimal care of the injured patients on a regional basis.

References

1 West JG, Williams MJ, Trunkey DD, Wolferth CC. Trauma systems: current status–future challenges. *JAMA* 1988;259:3597–600.

2 American College of Surgeons Committee on Trauma. *Resources for Optimal Care of the Injured Patient 2006*. Chicago: American College of Surgeons, 2006.

3 Sasser SM, Hunt RC, Faul M, et al. Guidelines for field triage of injured patients: recommendations of the national expert panel on field triage, 2011. *MMWR* 2012;61:1–20.

4 Salomone JP, Salomone JA. Prehospital care. In: Mattox KL, Moore EE, Feliciano DV (eds) *Trauma*, 7th edn. New York: McGraw-Hill, 2013.

CHAPTER 27

Blunt trauma considerations

Sabina A. Braithwaite and Jeffrey M. Goodloe

Introduction

Trauma is a disease whose severity is largely dictated by time and energy kinematics: *time* to definitive care, including operative intervention when required in a minority of cases, and *energy* mechanically transferred to the body to produce injury. Appropriate integration of out-of-hospital and in-hospital management of trauma can have a major effect on overall patient morbidity and mortality. Studies continue to clarify which out-of-hospital interventions truly benefit the patient and which interventions may actually worsen outcomes or delay more effective care options. Specifics on how mechanisms of injury, injury severity, available resources (including air medical services), provider training level, and specialty centers affect management and outcome of trauma patients have become clearer in recent years. Controversy exists as how to best balance the need for expeditious patient transfer from the out-of-hospital environment to in-hospital definitive assessment-based care with the patient's need for critical or time-sensitive interventions prior to hospital arrival. An ever-enlarging body of experience and scientific study is further defining what management options improve outcomes in specific subpopulations of trauma patients.

In short, trauma is a multifaceted disease that requires a systems-thinking and systems-operating approach, while incorporating new scientific knowledge to provide optimal patient management in the practice of EMS medicine.

Effect on emergency medical services

Proper assessment and management of blunt traumatic injuries are among the core goals for EMS physicians, paramedics, and EMTs. The physical demands encountered while managing the trauma patient can be considerable for EMS providers. Extrication from adverse environments and working in inclement weather are common. The ability to adapt the core trauma evaluation and management concepts to any given situation is paramount.

Emergency medical services system structure elements, including ALS versus BLS, staffing level, and use of air evacuation resources, all contribute to a system's ability to care for the trauma patient. Scientific comparison of different operational models is just beginning to demonstrate which can provide the greatest benefit to specific patient populations [1]. Long-held notions of the superiority of ALS interventions in the field (such as IV access for fluid resuscitation and endotracheal airway management) have been called into question [2]. It may be that severely injured patients (at least in an urban setting) are best served by primary application of the basic skills of hemorrhage control, airway support, and rapid transport to the appropriate level trauma center.

Training for EMS providers

The central concepts for EMS providers caring for trauma patients include the following.

1 Thorough training on a consistent, organized patient assessment algorithm that can be applied to any trauma patient, regardless of injury severity, is foundational. It should provide hierarchical management that focuses on identification and management of life threats, yet incorporates full, sequenced evaluation and integrated management options for actual and potential injuries. Frequent reassessments and ability to integrate information and recognize trends that require urgent intervention are essential.

2 Efficient, appropriate use of local resources (air transport, hazardous materials, specialized rescue) and knowledge of hospital capabilities and destination policies (e.g. trauma center, pediatric trauma center, specialty burn care center) can improve patient outcomes in patients with significant, time-critical injuries. EMS systems should have policies and procedures to identify such patients and promote primary transport to the most appropriate facility. This concept, pioneered by trauma systems, is now being extended effectively to non-trauma disease processes such as acute myocardial

Emergency Medical Services: Clinical Practice and Systems Oversight, Second Edition. Volume 1: Clinical Aspects of EMS.
Edited by David C. Cone, Jane H. Brice, Theodore R. Delbridge, and J. Brent Myers.
© 2015 NAEMSP. Published 2015 by John Wiley & Sons, Inc. Companion Website: www.wiley.com\go\cone\naemsp

infarction and acute stroke (see Volume 1, Chapter 13 and 21). Extrication-related issues that may affect management and timeliness of transport are addressed in Volume 1, Chapter 28.

3 Proper use of spinal motion restriction, splinting, fluid resuscitation, and pain management to limit additional morbidity. Knowing how and when to properly use infrequent invasive procedures such as cricothyrotomy or needle thoracostomy is essential for patient safety and care (see Volume 1, Chapter 3).

4 Universal precautions against blood and body fluid exposure and scene safety training are a vital component of every patient interaction, especially in traumatic injury, where the source of the injury (e.g. a downed power line, broken heavy machinery, or a collapsed building) may pose a serious ongoing threat to rescuers.

Monitoring and reinforcing proper application of these concepts through performance measurement and improvement (see Volume 1, Chapter 72.), together with adequate practice on infrequently used psychomotor skills, are important parts of medical oversight and can have a demonstrated effect on patient morbidity and mortality. Realistic, relevant, integrated assessment and management scenario-based training, potentially including high-fidelity simulation, has been demonstrated to improve skill consistency and retention and may improve providers' ability to translate didactics into clinical performance [3]. Nationally and internationally recognized courses that incorporate these elements exist and span the spectrum of care.

Resuscitation and initial assessment

The mechanism of injury, while not entirely predictive of actual injury sustained, often alerts the astute clinician to potential injuries that may be encountered during the assessment and management of the blunt trauma patient in the field. The importance of integration of local EMS and hospital resources, and tailoring guidelines to optimize patient care within these parameters, cannot be overemphasized. Blunt trauma management differs significantly from penetrating trauma, which is addressed in Volume 1, Chapter 29.

Emergency medical services systems should strive to limit the time from patient contact to departure from the scene to 10 minutes or less in injuries compatible with life threat. Except for control of life-threatening hemorrhage and support of airway and oxygenation/ventilation, all other interventions should take place en route to definitive care.

The primary survey
The goal of the primary survey is to identify and address any immediate life threats while the critical patient is promptly packaged for transport. Assessment can begin before arrival on the scene using dispatch information to prepare anticipated care needs based on patient mechanism of injury, potential notification of additional needed resources, and other local considerations.

Once patient contact is safely made, attention to discovering life threats through an organized approach is essential. Attention to arterial hemorrhage control, establishing and/or maintaining airway patency, correcting oxygenation and/or ventilation failure, and improving shock from blunt trauma are key aspects of the primary survey. In the severely injured patient with possible survival, the only survey to be done on-scene is the primary survey.

Scene photography may help convey aspects of mechanism of injury to the receiving physician as long as patient confidentiality is respected [4]. Event data recorders (automotive "black boxes") will increasingly integrate with EMS to provide objective prearrival information in motor vehicle collisions (MVCs), potentially tailoring data-driven resource allocation based on actual mechanism and patient information. Newer telemedicine applications that allow concurrent assessment by EMS and receiving emergency physicians may facilitate triage and expedite care at the receiving facility for a number of time-sensitive medical complaints, including trauma.

The secondary survey
The secondary survey, like the primary survey, is conducted using an organized, consistent approach. It differs substantially from the primary survey in its detail. The secondary survey is a methodical head-to-toe assessment exam designed to identify many non-life threatening injuries that are easily obscured by visually captivating injury or primary survey life threat discovery. While important for all trauma patients, due to management priorities that are identified in the primary survey and require frequent reassessment, the secondary survey may not be performed until after arrival at the destination trauma center for some patients. Omission of the secondary survey for this reason is not incorrect and in fact, may represent a conscious decision by an astute EMS clinician to focus on immediate life threats identified in the primary survey.

The role of Basic Life Support and Advanced Life Support
Heated scientific debate continues over the value of out-of-hospital ALS in general, and in trauma care interventions specifically. Selection bias as well as significant variability in system elements and capabilities precludes a definite answer from existing literature at this time. Some evidence-based EMS practice recommendations have been extrapolated from the in-hospital literature, and their ability to translate into patient benefit in the out-of-hospital environment has yet to be demonstrated. A large-scale before-and-after study of ALS has cast significant doubt on the use of ALS in trauma [2]. Initiatives that will provide national data collection and evaluation will foster more evidence-based implementation of patient management in the future. As a result, absent evidence to the contrary, EMS has used what are felt to be time-sensitive interventions that have demonstrated efficacy in the ED and other critical care environments.

Constellations of blunt traumatic injury

There are a number of recognized patterns of blunt trauma injury. For example, displaced sternal fractures are associated with a high risk of associated head, spinal, rib, and cardiac injury [5]. The likelihood of intraabdominal injury to motor vehicle occupants increases significantly at speeds greater than 12 mph and exceeds 5% at 20 mph. Extensive abdominal injury evaluation due to mechanism of injury alone appears unwarranted in the absence of associated head, spine, chest, or leg injury [6]. Scapular fractures are commonly associated with rib and lower and upper extremity injury resulting from the high kinetic energy transfer, but not with blunt traumatic aortic injury [7]. Facial fractures due to assault and motor vehicle crashes are associated with intracerebral and pulmonary injuries with a high percentage of these patients requiring intubation during their inpatient course [8]. Obesity (body mass index >30 kg/m [2]) confers a risk for longer hospital and intensive care length of stay, as well as higher mortality in critical blunt trauma patients. Interestingly, head injuries are decreased in this population [9]. Specific recommendations on management of traumatic brain injury and spine injuries are addressed in Volume 1, Chapters 30 and 36, respectively.

Issues in specific patient populations

Blunt trauma in pregnancy

Trauma is a leading cause for maternal mortality [10]. Pregnant trauma patients should be managed with the maxim "what's best for mom is best for baby." Supporting maternal oxygenation and perfusion is most likely to produce a positive outcome for both patients whenever possible.

The most frequent traumatic incidents affecting pregnant patients are MVCs. The majority of fetal deaths are due to MVC, with abruptio placentae and abdominal penetrating trauma as other common causes [11]. A study of hospitalized pregnant trauma patients, 80% of whom were involved in MVCs, showed that predictors for fetal loss included higher injury severity score (ISS), maternal death, lower Glasgow Coma Scale score, abdominal abbreviated injury scale (AIS) score greater than 3, vaginal bleeding, and shock with significant base excess. Morbidity, mortality, and hospital length of stay were not significantly different in pregnant versus non-pregnant matched case controls [12].

One small study showed the overall immediate complication rate to be low, most commonly preterm labor and placental abruption [13]. However, an increase in long-term complications was noted as well, with more severe trauma, multiple gestation, vaginal bleeding, and uterine contractions all being independent risk factors.

Destination choice may be affected by potential fetal viability and immediate need for neonatal specialty care. Estimating potential viability at greater than 24–26 weeks gestation by history or palpation of the uterine fundus above the umbilicus can facilitate this decision-making process [12]. Patients at greater than 20 weeks estimated gestational age should be placed with their left side elevated 15°, or up to 30° of reverse Trendelenburg positioning, to relieve pressure on the great vessels, preventing supine hypotension and subsequent significant loss of preload and cardiac output [14]. Although normal pregnancy-related changes in vital signs can imitate early shock, proactive oxygenation, fluid resuscitation, and monitoring are indicated to minimize risk of uterine hypoperfusion and fetal distress.

Emergency caesarean sections are extremely rare and should be reserved for salvageable infants in selected situations, performed by adequate, trained staff including emergency physicians and obstetricians (see Volume 1, Chapter 45).

Geriatric trauma

With an ever-growing geriatric population, awareness of special considerations is important, particularly in trauma [15]. Geriatric patients are more likely to have intraabdominal injury with concurrent head, leg, or chest injuries, regardless of MVC speed. CDC field triage criteria use age 55 as the break where patient management considerations change to recognize the increased risk of death from trauma after that age (see Volume 1, Chapter 39 for additional information on field trauma triage).

Medical oversight issues in trauma

Among the most important aspects of medical oversight is teaching the ability to effect a prompt and smooth patient transition from scene to hospital. Guidelines for management should be evidence based whenever possible and should take into consideration neighboring regions, hospital practice, and other regional specialty resources. Physician participation in regional and state medical oversight committees helps add clinical practice consistency while taking into consideration specific agency and provider capabilities, which may vary significantly within a locality. Monitoring of current literature and research allows the medical director to modify guidelines in keeping with national trends as tempered by local capabilities. Networking with inpatient physicians (particularly those in critical care, trauma, burns, and pediatrics) helps assure that EMS is focused on similar issues, using complementary technology and practice that will facilitate and expedite optimal patient outcomes both in the hospital and out of the hospital. Such networking will help limit "us versus them" attitudes toward EMS and reinforce that EMS is an equal and essential professional partner in the emergency health care team, dedicated to the same basic principles as the inpatient team.

In the case of trauma care, having specific, agreed-upon regional hospital triage criteria and guidelines on issues such as airway management, fluid resuscitation, medication management, spinal immobilization, and trauma alert categories all facilitate uniformity of in-hospital and out-of-hospital care. Ongoing monitoring of performance on established criteria, such as scene time in high-priority trauma [16], allows for modification of practice and assessment of effect of practice on patient outcomes [17].

Guidelines for out-of-hospital management

Guidelines for management of the trauma patient should be focused on providing necessary interventions, together with rapid transport to the closest appropriate facility. Triage guidelines should also address trauma patients who need different types of specialty care by identifying regional facilities with special capabilities such as pediatric trauma, burn care, hyperbaric therapy, and extremity replantation. Scene time should not be delayed while the provider waits for direct medical oversight.

Air medical transport

Transport of trauma patients by helicopter has become increasingly common in the United States in recent years. Its positive effect on saving the lives of combat casualties in the Korean and Vietnam conflicts, the Gulf War, and now Iraq and Afghanistan is well documented, though its effect on outcomes in specific civilian patient populations is still being studied, Staffing models vary significantly between the US and European systems. As such, use, patient injury severity, and effects on scene internal and mortality are difficult to compare [18].

There is recent concern that air medical transport may not uniformly provide added patient benefit for a number of reasons, including poor triage by field providers [19]. Systems should implement guidelines to appropriately integrate valuable air medical assets into their trauma system, particularly given the cost and potential additional risks to both crew and patient [20,21].

Hospital destination

Patient outcomes are significantly better at trauma centers than at non-trauma centers. Both in-hospital and 1-year adjusted case fatality and relative death risk rates for moderately to severely injured patients are significantly better, typically with a 25% reduction in fatality risk [22]. Studies support the importance of rapid transport to a regional trauma center where definitive care can be rendered [23]. With the exception of safety issues, securing an unstable airway, and absent extrication issues, there is generally no indication for prolonging scene times, particularly in the severely traumatized patient.

It is crucial that the out-of-hospital provider rapidly and accurately identify the subset of trauma patients who may most

benefit from trauma center management. The field triage decision scheme is fully described in Volume 1, Chapter 39. The most current version has shown efficacy and de-emphasizes trauma scoring, relying instead on progressive assessment of patient physiology, injury anatomy, mechanism, and special circumstances to provide trauma center destination guidance.

Provider judgment has been introduced as a factor in decision making for transport to a regional trauma center in the field triage decision scheme. Trauma scores and mechanism of injury should not override provider judgment and divert a patient away from a trauma center [24].

Intriguing new research raises questions on structure of hospital trauma systems. Inclusive systems, in which every facility in a region or state participates to the extent of their capabilities, are compared with exclusive systems, in which a limited number of high-level centers receive the majority of patients. In one study, the odds of triage to a regional trauma center and inpatient mortality were similar in both groups; however, the most inclusive systems were associated with the lowest odds of death [25].

Trauma scoring

Trauma scoring systems were first developed to attempt to quantify severity of injury and guide appropriate triage of patients to trauma centers. A variety of scoring systems exist, but their use is likely greater for research purposes than for patient care in the field [26].

Multiple different scoring systems and permutations have been developed and continue to evolve to assist in predicting injury, need for emergency surgery, and outcomes [27,28]. The Revised Trauma Score (RTS) is one of the more common trauma scoring systems (Table 27.1). It combines the Glasgow Coma Scale score with respiratory rate and systolic blood pressure. Some systems, including the RTS and the ISS as well as derivations such as the survival risk ratio (SRR), have been used to predict patient outcome [29–32]. Each trauma system must determine acceptable levels of overtriage and undertriage and how to best achieve these goals through ongoing quality improvement and surveillance.

Table 27.1 Revised Trauma Score

RR/min	SBP (mmHg)	GCS	RTS points
10–29	>89	13–15	4
>29	76–89	9–12	3
6–9	50–75	6–8	2
1–5	1–40	4–5	1
0	0	3	0

Adapted from Champion [32], with permission from Lippincott, Williams and Wilkins.
GCS, Glasgow Coma Scale; RR, respiratory rate; SBP, systolic blood pressure.

Prevention and other public health issues

Trauma is largely a preventable disease with a tremendous cost to society. Although it affects all age groups, it is particularly devastating to the young and remains the major killer of North Americans under 40 years of age. As part of their role as advocates for their entire community's health status, EMS physicians and systems must play an active role in injury prevention.

Participation in community-based programs to encourage safer behaviors and risk reduction can reduce the number of injured persons. Programs such as helmet use [33], cycle and pool safety, proper use of car seats, and use of seat belts have all helped to reduce the number and severity of injuries. Programs targeting safe storage of firearms, reduction in drunk driving, and home safety assessments for elders can have positive effects on the community and may be led at the local, state, or national level. Local systems are able to tie into these resources without having to commit large amounts of financial and/or personnel support. This also represents an opportunity to put forward a proactive, positive "public face" for the EMS agency involved. The leadership for this effort must involve physician medical oversight. The CDC's Injury and Violence Prevention and Control page (www.cdc.gov/injury) is an excellent resource. See also Volume 2, Chapter 13, for additional information.

References

1 Iirola TT, Laaksonen MI, Vahlberg TJ, Palve HK. Effect of physician-staffed helicopter emergency medical service on blunt trauma patient survival and prehospital care. *Eur J Emerg Med* 2006;13: 335–9.

2 Stiell IG, Nesbitt LP, Pickett W, et al. The OPALS Major Trauma Study: impact of advanced life-support on survival and morbidity. *CMAJ* 2008;178:1141–52.

3 Holcomb JB, Dumire RD, Crommett JW, et al. Evaluation of trauma team performance using an advanced human patient simulator for resuscitation training. *J Trauma* 2002;52:1078–86.

4 Bennett TD, Kaufman R, Schiff M, Mock C, Quan L. Crash analysis of lower extremity injuries in children restrained in forward-facing car seats during front and rear impacts. *J Trauma* 2006;61:592–7.

5 Von Garrel T, Ince A, Junge A, Schnabel M, Bahrs C. The sternal fracture: radiographic analysis of 200 fractures with special reference to concomitant injuries. *J Trauma* 2004;57:837–44.

6 Brasel KJ, Nirula R. What mechanism justifies abdominal evaluation in motor vehicle crashes? *J Trauma* 2005;59:1057–61.

7 Brown CV, Velmahos G, Wang D, Kennedy S, Demetriades D, Rhee P. Association of scapular fractures and blunt thoracic aortic injury: fact or fiction? *Am Surg* 2005;71:54–7.

8 Alvi A, Doherty T, Lewen G. Facial fractures and concomitant injuries in trauma patients. *Laryngoscope* 2003;113:102–6.

9 Brown CVR, Neville AL, Rhee P, Salim A, Velmahos GC, Demetriades D. The impact of obesity on the outcomes of 1,153 critically injured blunt trauma patients. *J Trauma* 2005;59:1048–51.

10 Romero VC, Pearlman M. Maternal Mortality Due to Trauma. *Semin Perinatol* 2012;36:60–7.

11 Mattox KL, Goetzl L. Trauma in pregnancy. *Crit Care Med* 2005;33:S385–9.

12 Shah KH, Simons RK, Holbrook T, Fortlage D, Winchell RJ, Hoyt DB. Trauma in pregnancy: maternal and fetal outcomes. *J Trauma* 1998;45:83–6.

13 Melamed N, Aviram A, Silver M, et al. Pregnancy course and outcome following blunt trauma. *J Matern Fetal Neonatal Med* 2012;25:1612–7.

14 Cusick SS, Tibbles CD. Trauma in pregnancy. *Emerg Med Clin North Am* 2007;25:861–72.

15 Mitra B, Cameron PA. Optimising management of the elderly trauma patient. *Injury* 2012;43:973–5.

16 Eckstein M, Alo K. The effect of a quality improvement program on paramedic on-scene times for patients with penetrating trauma. *Acad Emerg Med* 1999;6:191–5.

17 Gage AM, Traven N, Rivara FP, Jurkovich GJ, Arbabi S. Compliance with Centers for Disease Control and Prevention field triage guidelines in an established trauma system. *J Am Coll Surg* 2012;215:148–54.

18 Ringburg AN, Spanjersberg WR, Frankema SP, Steyerberg EW, Patka P, Schipper IB. Helicopter emergency medical services (HEMS): impact on on-scene times. *J Trauma* 2007;63:258–62.

19 Bledsoe BE, Wesley AK, Eckstein M, Dunne TM, O'Keefe MF. Helicopter scene transport of trauma patients with nonlife-threatening injuries: a meta-analysis. *J Trauma* 2006;60:1257–66.

20 Thomson DP, Thomas SH, 2002–2003 Air Medical Services Committee of the National Association of EMS Physicians. Guidelines for air medical dispatch. *Prehosp Emerg Care* 2003;7:265–71.

21 Floccare DJ, Stuhlmiller DFE, Braithwaite SA, et al. Appropriate and safe utilization of helicopter emergency medical services: a joint position statement with resource document. *Prehosp Emerg Care* 2013;17:521–5.

22 MacKenzie EJ, Rivara FP, Jurkovich GJ, et al. A national evaluation of the effect of trauma-center care on mortality. *N Engl J Med* 2006;354:366–78.

23 Driscoll P, Kent A. The effect of scene time on survival. *Trauma* 1999;1:23–30.

24 Newgard CD, Kampp M, Nelson M, et al. Deciphering the use and predictive value of "emergency medical services provider judgment" in out-of-hospital trauma triage: a multisite, mixed methods assessment. *J Trauma Acute Care Surg* 2012;72(5):1239–48.

25 Utter GH, Maier RV, Rivara FP, Mock C, Jurkovich GJ, Nathens AB. Inclusive trauma systems: do they improve triage or outcomes of the severely injured? *J Trauma* 2006;60:529–35.

26 Gabbe BJ, Cameron PA, Finch CF. Is the revised trauma score still useful? *ANZ J Surg* 2003;73:944–8.

27 Moore L, Lavoie A, LeSage N, et al. Statistical validation of the Revised Trauma Score. *J Trauma* 2006;60:305–11.

28 Moore L, Lavoie A, Abdous B, et al. Unification of the revised trauma score. *J Trauma* 2006;61:718–22.

29 Millham FH, LaMorte WW. Factors associated with mortality in trauma: re-evaluation of the TRISS method using the National Trauma Data Bank. *J Trauma* 2004;56:1090–6.

30 Clarke JR, Ragone AV, Greenwald L. Comparisons of survival predictions using survival risk ratios based on International Classification of Diseases, Ninth Revision and Abbreviated Injury Scale trauma diagnosis codes. *J Trauma* 2005;59:563–7.

31 Hannan EL, Farrell LS. Predicting trauma inpatient mortality in an administrative database: an investigation of survival risk ratios using New York data. *J Trauma* 2007;62:964–8.

32 Champion HR, Sacco WJ, Copes WS, Gann DS, Gennarelli TA, Flanagan ME. A revision of the Trauma Score. *J Trauma* 1989; 29:623–9.

33 Konkin DE, Garraway N, Hameed SM, et al. Population-based analysis of severe injuries from nonmotorized wheeled vehicles. *Am J Surg* 2006;191:615–18.

CHAPTER 28

Motor vehicle crashes

Stewart C. Wang and Carla Kohoyda-Inglis

Introduction

Death by motor vehicle crash/collision (MVC) is currently the fifth leading cause of death for all Americans [1]. The American Automobile Association reported that the economic costs associated with traffic crashes were $299.5 billion, based on 2009 data [2]. Over the past decade, vehicle-related death and injury rates have steadily decreased. In 2002, the occupant fatality rate per 100 million vehicle miles of travel (VMT) was 1.51; from 2010 to 2011 it was 0.98/VMT – a historic low. Despite this improvement in fatality rates, there were still over 5 million MVCs in the US during 2011. These crashes resulted in about 2.2 million injuries and just over 32,000 deaths [3].

Effect on EMS

In the US, someone dies in an MVC every 16 minutes [3]. Moreover, fatal crashes are far outnumbered by crashes with non-fatal but serious injuries requiring urgent medical attention. Therefore, a significant percentage of EMS calls relates to MVCs. While many crashes involve only single vehicles, there may be multiple occupants in that vehicle. In a crash involving more than two vehicles, many more EMS resources may be required. Likewise, if public transportation, such as trains or buses, is involved, the need for those resources is greatly expanded.

The hazards present at the scene of the MVC are many and varied. Continued high-speed traffic flow on freeways represents a significant threat to the safety of the rescue crews. Spilled fuel can result in a fire risk and broken glass and sharp metal edges can also prove hazardous to the unprotected EMS provider. Grounded power lines and hazardous materials being transported on the roadways present additional risks.

Emergency medical services physicians and providers may not have the personal protective gear to operate in such environments. Fire department response is often required to address hazardous issues. Rural or smaller agencies may not have the heavy extrication equipment necessary to access trapped patients. Regardless of whether the EMS system is fire department based, additional resources (e.g. rescue, law enforcement) are often used at the scene of an MVC.

Motor vehicle crash injury biomechanics

During a crash, different parts of an occupant's body are subjected to sudden acceleration or deceleration. Injury results when tissues are disrupted by local concentrations of physical force generated by a crash event. Morbidity and mortality occur when vital organs absorb energy beyond their tolerance. The ability to tolerate physical forces varies considerably from individual to individual. Clinically, it is important to remember that those at either end of the age spectrum (children and the elderly) are particularly sensitive to serious injury due to the reduced ability of their tissues to absorb energy.

Acceleration and deceleration are defined as changes in velocity over time, measured in G forces (the weight of objects in earth's gravitational field). In healthy, non-elderly, adult individuals, the upper end of transient G force that can be tolerated is about 30 G [4]. Both speed and stopping distance contribute to the overall G force experienced during an MVC. Gs increase by the speed squared, while doubling the stopping distance cuts the Gs by half. Automotive safety equipment such as seat belts, airbags, and vehicle deformation (crumple) zones effectively increase the stopping distance for the vehicle occupant during a crash.

Four possible collisions occur during a MVC.

1 The vehicle strikes another object and the crushing of the vehicle's structure absorbs energy. Vehicles with a greater capacity to deform absorb more energy and effectively increase the stopping distance. During this phase occupants continue in motion.

2 A second collision occurs as a passenger strikes the vehicle's interior or restraint system such as seat belt and airbags.

Emergency Medical Services: Clinical Practice and Systems Oversight, Second Edition. Volume 1: Clinical Aspects of EMS.
Edited by David C. Cone, Jane H. Brice, Theodore R. Delbridge, and J. Brent Myers.
© 2015 NAEMSP. Published 2015 by John Wiley & Sons, Inc. Companion Website: www.wiley.com\go\cone\naemsp

3 Internal organs continue in motion until they strike surfaces such as the skull or chest wall.

4 Loose objects and unrestrained occupants can strike the person, resulting in further injury [4].

Poor automotive design, absence of airbags, and lack of seat belt use decrease the stopping distance and thereby increase the G force experienced by a vehicle occupant.

Safety restraints

Inertia causes occupants of a car to be moving at the same speed as the car. In a crash, the car comes to an abrupt halt and the occupants inside continue at the speed the car was traveling until their bodies are stopped by objects such as the windshield, instrument panel, or steering wheel, if they are not wearing seat belts. Stopping an object's momentum requires force acting over a period of time.

A seat belt, anchored to the vehicle, is designed to apply the stopping force to more durable parts of the body over a longer period, allowing the occupant to "ride down" the crash as the vehicle crumple zones crush and absorb the energy, and helps protect the body from serious injuries. In contrast, unrestrained occupants do not get the additional "ride down" time and, at higher speed, hit the vehicle interior with weaker parts of the body, e.g. upper abdomen to steering wheel. The use of three-point seat belts reduces the risk of fatal injury in passenger car occupants by 45% and the risk of moderate-to-critical injury by 50%. The risks are reduced by 60% and 65% respectively for light truck occupants [5].

Airbags spread the force required to stop the occupants over a large part of their bodies, minimizing local concentrations of force that can disrupt tissues and cause injury. The airbag has the space between the passenger and the frontal or side components of a vehicle and a fraction of a second in which to work. Even that tiny amount of space and time is valuable, however, if the system can slow the passenger evenly rather than forcing an abrupt halt to the occupant's motion. The National Highway Traffic Safety Administration estimates that belts alone reduce fatalities by 45%, and when combined with airbags, there is a 50% overall reduction in mortality [5].

Motor vehicle crash types

Even with the most advanced vehicle restraint systems, crash injuries still occur. Injuries are caused by physical forces, and the direction and magnitude of these forces are dependent on the configuration of the crash. Therefore, the type of crash (e.g. frontal, side, rollover) largely determines the injury patterns seen. Properly evaluating the crash scenario will help EMS physicians and providers to predict the most likely injuries they will need to treat. Relaying accurate information about the crash event to the medical team will enable the proper assessment and care of the patient in the emergency department.

Major crash types include planar crashes, rollovers, and a host of unusual crashes. Frontal crashes typically make up about 42% of all crashes; side and rear crashes occur in almost equal numbers, 25% and 22% respectively. While rollovers only make up approximately 9% of all crashes, they tend to be the most highly injurious. Each of these crash types has its own injury patterns and concerns.

Planar crashes

These crashes are characterized by forces occurring in two dimensions, x and y (flat). They include frontal, side, and rear impacts. Additionally, any of these crashes can be further classified as a narrow-impact crash. Typically, this means the vehicle strikes a narrow object, such as a tree or light pole, which then crushes into the vehicle further than would be the case if the vehicle had struck a broad object.

Frontal crashes

Automotive manufacturers have created "crush zones" to deal with this most common type of crash. The front of the vehicle is designed to absorb the energy from the crash and to minimize intrusion of vehicle structure into the occupant compartment. In assessing a crash, it is very important to differentiate between damage to the exterior of the vehicle and intrusion of vehicle structure into the passenger compartment of the vehicle. Significant intrusion of vehicle structure into the interior of the passenger compartment is much more predictive of serious occupant injury than external vehicle damage.

Since the advent of frontal airbags, head and facial injuries have become much less common. While chest injuries such as rib fractures are still quite common, particularly in the elderly, incidences of aortic and heart injuries have substantially decreased. Currently, the most common serious injuries observed in frontal crashes affect these body regions in descending order of frequency.

1 Lower extremities
2 Pelvis
3 Thorax
4 Head
5 Abdomen

Side-impact crashes

Most side-impact crashes involve two vehicles: a "bullet vehicle" that hits the "struck vehicle" in the side. In assessing and describing side-impact occupants, it is important to determine whether they were "near-side" or "far-side" occupants relative to the crash location. Near-side occupants are at greater risk for severe injury. It is also important to remember that side-impact crashes are generally far more dangerous than frontal crashes. Therefore, when arriving at the scene of a side-impact crash, barring extenuating circumstances, medical priority should typically be given to the near-side occupants of the struck vehicle, followed by the far-side occupants, and then the front-seat occupants of the bullet vehicle, and finally the rear-seat occupants of the bullet vehicle.

Side impacts, those that strike the right or left planes of the vehicle, can be further characterized as being L-type (i.e. striking in front of or behind the passenger compartment) or T-type (i.e. striking within the passenger compartment). The T-type side-impact crashes are more dangerous for vehicle occupants than L-type.

Side impacts tend to be more severe as there is less space for "crush zones" and therefore very little way of absorbing energy. Narrow T-type side-impact cases are particularly dangerous for the occupants as there is far greater intrusion into the passenger compartment. There has been an increase in side protection in the form of curtain and seat-mounted airbags but these safety features are far from common in the fleet.

Currently, the most common serious injuries observed in side crashes affect these body regions in decreasing order of frequency.

1 Head
2 Thorax
3 Pelvis
4 Abdomen

Rear crashes

For vehicle occupants this is generally the least dangerous of the planar impacts. The large crush zone in the back of many vehicles tends to absorb much of the energy of the incoming vehicle. In addition, the occupants are protected by their seats.

Rollover crashes

These crashes are characterized by forces occurring in three dimensions: x, y, and z. There is a type of rollover, called an arrested roll, which indicates the roll has been stopped by an object in the crash zone such as a utility pole or tree. Arrested rolls are associated with greater intrusion of vehicle structure into the passenger compartment and a greater risk of injury to the occupants.

Restraint use has a huge effect on injury risk and patterns in rollover crashes. Rollovers are problematic for the occupants as the rotation during the crash event throws them upward and outward. As the roof hits the ground, the occupants dive toward the roof. If the roll continues, occupants may slide out of their seat belts and continue to be thrown around the interior of the vehicle outward toward the side windows. As a result, ejection of the occupant is much more likely in rollovers than other crash types.

Complete or partial ejection of the occupants is associated with the most severe injuries and must be suspected in all rollovers due to the movement experienced by the occupants. Indeed, EMS findings of complete or partial ejection are a field triage criterion. Finding complex lacerations with road debris or "road rash" on any part of the body constitutes "partial ejection." Due to the likelihood of occupant ejection in rollover crashes, it is very important that EMS canvass a large area around the vehicle to detect ejected occupants. In addition, the vehicle damage makes this type of crash hard to assess, adding to the complexity of these cases. Roof intrusion is an important indicator of potential injury in rollover crashes. A rule of thumb is that there is approximately 2 feet of distance between the bottom of the window/top of door panel and the roof. If half of that distance is gone, there has been 12 inches of downward roof intrusion.

The most common serious injuries observed in rollovers affect these body regions in descending order.

1 Thorax
2 Abdomen
3 Head
4 Spine
5 Extremities

Unusual crashes

Further complicating matters are the unusual types of crashes that may occur in real-life situations. These include incompatibility between the vehicles involved in the crash (e.g. an SUV striking a compact car), underride (e.g. a passenger vehicle rear-ending a semitrailer and traveling under the restraining bar), and override (e.g. a semi crashing into a passenger vehicle and driving up and over the back of it).

Incompatibility between vehicles involved in a crash is based on three elements: mass, stiffness, and geometry. In the US, the popularity of SUVs and trucks, with their greater height, stiffness, and weight, has increased the risk of injuries suffered by occupants of the vehicles they strike in a crash. These vehicles are designed to perform heavy-duty functions and consequently they can be dangerous to the occupants of lighter vehicles. In addition, their stiffness makes them less able to protect their own occupants in severe crashes, as they are less able to absorb some of the crash energy.

Incompatible side impacts are especially problematic as they compromise the ability of a struck vehicle's safety systems to properly sense the crash and protect occupants, thus increasing the risk and severity of injuries. The occupants of the more vulnerable vehicle frequently sustain injuries higher in the body, such as the head and chest. These injuries can compromise the ABCs. Rapid response and proper triage are therefore essential.

Ejection can be a problem in these crashes as well. Partial ejection, where part of an occupant's body strikes something outside the vehicle, such as an intruding hood or tree branch, is associated with very high risk of serious injury and thus is a criterion for transport to the highest level of care available.

Any crash may contain elements of several of these types, confounding EMS providers, physicians, and crash investigators.

Crashes involving vulnerable road users

In addition to occupants of vehicles, there are other vulnerable populations sharing the roadways, including pedestrians, pedal cyclists, and motorcyclists [6]. While these numbers are lower than those reported for 2002, all these populations experienced

Table 28.1 Morbidity and mortality for vulnerable road users

2011	Killed	Injured
Pedestrians	4,432	69,000
Pedal cyclists	677	48,000
Motorcyclists	4,612	81,000

more fatalities and injuries in 2011 than 2010 (Table 28.1). These patients tend to be more seriously injured than vehicle occupants as they do not have the protection offered by a motor vehicle.

EMS crash assessment priorities

When approaching the scene of a crash, there are things to look for [7].

- Unrestrained occupant(s)
- Possibly ejected occupants:
  - complex open wounds
  - empty child safety seat
  - broken window or windshield
  - rollover
- Intrusion into the occupant space

The intrusion criterion for high-risk auto crashes is 12 inches at the occupant seating location or 18 inches at any interior site. One key rule of thumb to remember is that a seat is approximately 24" by 24". Therefore, if vehicle structure intrusion is such that only half the normal seat width remains, the occupant seated there is at high risk of serious injury (10% risk of ISS 15+). In addition, the footwell area is approximately 24" by 24" and the lower part of the dashboard is approximately 12" from the front edge of the seat. If a leg is entrapped between the dash and the front of the seat, there has been 12" of intrusion (Figures 28.1, 28.2).

The crash and vehicle information at the scene is essential for properly triaging the patient, and this information can predict the most likely injuries. Properly relaying this information to the medical team will enable the optimum assessment and care of the patient.

Extrication

First responders are well aware that the quicker they remove occupants from a damaged vehicle and get them to treatment, the better the outcome will be. It is imperative that clinical care begins at the scene and is a priority during the extrication process.

Integration of EMS into the incident command structure at an MVC can ensure that clinical care of the patient is not underemphasized during extrication. Whenever safely possible, it is desirable to have an EMS provider (wearing appropriate personal protective equipment) inside the vehicle with the patient while extrication proceeds.

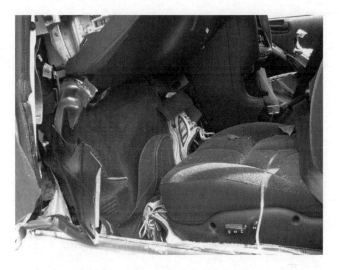

Figure 28.1 View of driver's footwell from the left side. Source: International Center for Automotive Medicine. Reproduced with permission of ICAM.

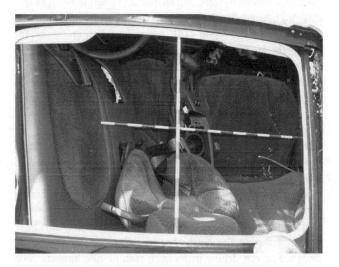

Figure 28.2 View of the driver's seat through the sunroof. Source: International Center for Automotive Medicine. Reproduced with permission of ICAM.

Packaging patients for removal from a motor vehicle typically involves manually stabilizing the cervical spine and then immobilizing the spine with a cervical collar and any one of a variety of spine immobilization devices. When necessary, spine immobilization and patient removal is a personnel-intensive process requiring a team approach.

Field triage

At the scene of any MVC or other event involving traumatic injury, EMS physicians and providers must identify those patients who are at greatest risk for severe injury and then choose the most appropriate facility to which to transport them within the trauma system. This decision process is known as "field triage" and is based on a practice algorithm called a "decision scheme." The first Field Triage Decision Scheme was published by the American College of Surgeons (ACS) in 1986 [8], with subsequent updates in 1990, 1993, 1999, 2006, and 2012 [9]. See Volume 1, Chapter 39 for a detailed discussion of this topic.

Unique motor vehicle crash problems

There are many hazards involved in dealing with MVCs. In many cases, EMS physicians and providers will be watching for traffic and avoiding the usual detritus that comes from a crash, such as broken glass, spilled fuel, and jagged metal pieces. EMS physicians and providers must also be ready to protect themselves from bodily fluids and blood-borne pathogens.

Batteries

Many of the systems in today's vehicle fleet contain electronic control units, which can include controls for airbags, door locks, electronic windows, seats, and telematics. Gasoline-hybrid vehicles also have high-voltage cables, which are identifiable by the use of orange insulation [10]. For this reason, an important initial step for EMS physicians and providers arriving on scene is to make sure the ignition is off, remove the key, and disconnect the battery. This shuts down the power source for all electronic control units and avoids any chance of injuries from the electrical components of the vehicle.

Airbags

Emergency medical services physicians and providers need to be especially careful about undeployed airbags. There have been cases where EMS personnel have been injured when an airbag deployed as they were packaging the patient. There are several reasons why an airbag restraint system (ARS) may not have deployed during the crash. For instance, frontal airbags are designed to not deploy in rollover, rear, or side impacts. Side airbags are not designed to deploy in frontal or rear impacts. If the right front passenger seat is not occupied, the firing of those airbags may have been suppressed by design. In some cases, the collision may not have been severe enough to set the airbag off, or there could be a system malfunction that prevented the bags from deploying.

There are clues that an ARS may be present. Sometimes there is a label on the visor, instrument panel, or window. A small, low glove box can indicate a large dash-mounted airbag. Tags or letters may be embossed on the areas containing an ARS, such as the seats, pillars, roof rails, or instrument panel. Some tags to be alert for include: SIR, ARS, SRS, Airbag, SIPS, HPS, ACRS, ITS, and KAS.

Rescue workers should treat undeployed airbag restraint systems as explosive devices.
- Disconnect the battery.
- Disconnect any ARS connectors found.
- Do not place any objects against the module.

- Do not cut into the module.
- Do not strike a sensor, module, or diagnostic module.

Emerging technology

Advanced Automatic Crash Notification

Vehicles in the fleet have a large number of sensors. Some of them monitor the presence of an occupant. Others monitor for data suggesting that a crash may be occurring. These data are constantly analyzed by the computer systems within the vehicle and in the event of a crash, the computers will trigger the deployment of the safety systems in the optimal configuration for the type and severity of the crash being detected. In many vehicles, some of these data will be sent via cellular networks to alert emergency responders and provide useful information that can improve postcrash care for the occupants. The ability to send this information is called Advanced Automatic Crash Notification (AACN) [11]. Currently, crashes sensed as severe enough to be associated with a 20% or greater risk of ISS 15 injury to the occupants are identified by telemetry providers notifying EMS.

Available education

The International Center for Automotive Medicine at the University of Michigan has created a website dedicated to training law enforcement, EMS, and medical personnel. This website is located at www.crashedu.org and contains various educational modules for first responders. Continuing medical education credits are also available.

References

1 Hoyert DL, Xu J. *Deaths: Preliminary Data for 2011*. Hyattsville, MD: National Center for Health Statistics, 2012, p.52.
2 American Automobile Association. *Crashes vs. Congestion: What's the Cost to Society?* Washington, DC: AAA Public Affairs, 2011, p.58.
3 National Highway Traffic Safety Administration. *Traffic Safety Facts: 2011 Data Overview*. Washington, DC: US Department of Transportation, National Highway Traffic Safety Administration, 2013.
4 Peterson TD, Tilman Jolly B, Runge J, Hunt R. Motor vehicle safety: current concepts and challenges for emergency physicians. *Ann Emerg Med* 1999;34(3):384–93.
5 National Highway Traffic Safety Administration. *Traffic Safety Facts: 2011 Data Passenger Vehicles*. Washington, DC: US Department of Transportation, National Highway Traffic Safety Administration, 2013.
6 National Highway Traffic Safety Administration. *Traffic Safety Facts 2011 Data: Pedestrians*, Washington, DC: US Department of Transportation, National Highway Traffic Safety Administration, 2013.

7 International Center for Automotive Medicine. *CrashEdu: Crash Response Training*. Available at: www.crashedu.org/

8 Mackersie RC. History of trauma field triage development and the American College of Surgeons criteria. *Prehosp Emerg Care* 2006:10(3):287–94.

9 American College of Surgeons. Resources for optimal care of the injured patient: an update. Task Force of the Committee on Trauma, American College of Surgeons. *Bull Am Coll Surg* 1990;75(9):20–9.

10 Morris B. *Holmatro's Vehicle Extrication Techniques*. Glen Burnie, MD: Icone Graphic, 2006, p.95.

11 International Center for Automotive Medicine. *AACN Telemetry: What Is It and How Do I Use It?* Available at: www.crashedu.org/ems/mod15/

CHAPTER 29

Penetrating trauma

Michelle Welsford and Alim Pardhan

Introduction

Trauma is the leading cause of death for North Americans aged 1–34 years, only surpassed by cancer and cardiovascular disease in older adults. Penetrating trauma has significant morbidity and mortality and is a common cause for activation of EMS. Injuries due to firearms are particularly lethal and require rapid assessment and decision making in the field to mitigate injury. In 2009, approximately 700 deaths in Canada were associated with firearms, 75% of which were intentional self-harm [1]. In 2010 there were approximately 31,000 firearm-related deaths in the United States, of which approximately 61% were suicides [2].

Other potential causes of penetrating trauma include knives, arrows, nails, glass, wood, and wire. Penetrating trauma can also occur with shrapnel from explosions as well as with foreign objects flying in motor vehicle collisions. The types of weapons/projectiles, the way in which the object imparts its energy, as well as the location of impact, dictate the type and severity of injury.

Physics and mechanics of penetrating trauma

Two physical concepts explain injury associated with penetrating trauma. The energy associated with a moving object is defined by: kinetic energy = ½ mass × velocity². Kinetic injury explains why a small and light projectile (e.g. a bullet) can result in devastating injury. Because the projectile energy is related to the velocity squared, doubling the velocity results in a four-fold increase in kinetic energy; if velocity increases by a factor of 4, kinetic energy increases by a factor of 16. In penetrating trauma, the projectile imparts kinetic energy to the victim's body, resulting in injury.

The second concept is the Law of Conservation of Energy: *Energy cannot be created or destroyed but only transferred from one form to another.* When a projectile enters the body and remains there, it can be inferred that all the projectile's kinetic energy has been transferred to the body. Where the projectile travels through the body and exits, the energy transferred to the body is equal to the kinetic energy of the object before entering minus its energy on leaving the body.

Weapons can usually be classified based on the amount of energy carried by the projectile.

- Low energy: knives, hand-launched missiles
- Medium energy: handguns, smaller bullets, lower velocities (200–400 m/s)
- High energy: military or hunting rifles, larger bullets, higher velocities (600–1000 m/s) [3]

Ballistics

Ballistics, the study of projectiles as they move and hit their target, includes trajectory (the path that that an object follows after launch) and terminal ballistics, a more clinically relevant measure which reports how the projectile acts when it hits its target. Several factors affect terminal ballistics, including missile size, velocity, missile shape, deformity, and stability.

Size

As a general rule, the larger the missile, the more damage caused by direct contact between the missile and tissue. Larger missiles generally have a greater surface area and impart more energy faster. Bullet size is measured by the inside diameter of the gun barrel either in millimeters (e.g. 9 mm) or hundredths of an inch (e.g. 44 caliber). Magnum rounds refer to those with more gunpowder than a normal round, which increases the muzzle velocity and thus the bullet energy by 20–60% [3,4] (Figure 29.1).

Velocity

Missiles traveling through air encounter resistance or drag. Drag increases exponentially with velocity and is inversely proportional to mass. Clinically, this implies that the damage caused by a missile at short range will be greater than one fired at longer range and that heavier missiles are able to maintain

Emergency Medical Services: Clinical Practice and Systems Oversight, Second Edition. Volume 1: Clinical Aspects of EMS.
Edited by David C. Cone, Jane H. Brice, Theodore R. Delbridge, and J. Brent Myers.
© 2015 NAEMSP. Published 2015 by John Wiley & Sons, Inc. Companion Website: www.wiley.com\go\cone\naemsp

their velocity better than light ones. For practical purposes, the impact velocity of bullets will be the same as the muzzle velocity at 45 meters for low-energy firearms, such as handguns, and 90 meters for higher velocity weapons, such as rifles [4].

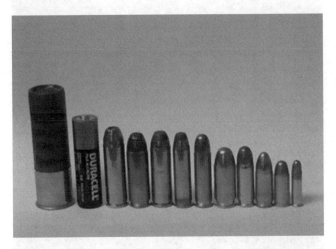

Figure 29.1 Bullets of various lengths and diameters, compared with an AA battery. Source: Reproduced with permission of Robert R. Bass.

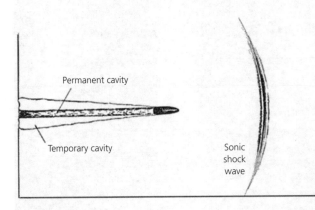

Figure 29.2 Sonic wave and cavitation produced by a high-velocity bullet in tissue. Source: Reproduced with permission of Robert R. Bass.

Slower-moving missiles such as knives or arrows have less kinetic energy and cause injury only where in contact with tissue. Higher energy missiles, such as rifle bullets, create a shockwave and a cavity in the body tissues. This process is known as cavitation (Figure 29.2).

Shape and deformation

The energy imparted by a missile is related to its shape. Missiles that are blunt (i.e. have a higher cross-sectional area) experience more resistance and impart energy to tissues quickly, whereas sharper missiles cut through tissues more effectively and release energy over a longer period of time and distance.

Projectiles may deform on impact, increasing the bullet's cross-sectional area. This mushrooming effect raises the resistance between the missile and tissues, thus increasing the energy transfer rate. Some missiles may fragment on impact, increasing the rate of energy exchange because the total surface area of the fragments is greater than that of the original missile (Figure 29.3).

Stability

Contrary to popular belief, bullets often do not travel in a direct line and may tumble or wobble (yaw) in their course, often decreasing the velocity and accuracy of the missile. If it tumbles or yaws after hitting tissue, the bullet's surface area with respect to tissue is increased, thereby increasing the amount and rate of energy transfer [4] and thus the extent of injury (Figure 29.4).

Types of weapons

Knives and arrows

Knives and arrows are considered to be low-energy weapons. Although the projectile's weight may be significantly higher, the velocity is generally much lower. Tissue damage is typically restricted to direct contact between the projectile and tissue. The extent of tissue damage can be extremely difficult to estimate because the projectile's trajectory cannot be determined based on external injury appearance. The entrance wound will not predict whether the object moved around within the body or what organs it came into contact with. It is, however,

Figure 29.3 Examples of bullet shapes and deformity designed to inflict tissue damage. Source: Reproduced with permission of Robert R. Bass.

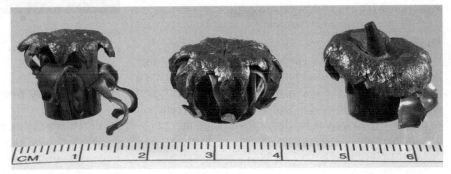

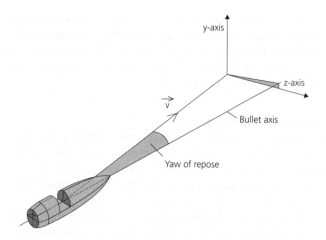
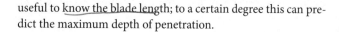

Figure 29.4 Effect of yaw in creating a larger surface area of effect. Source: Reproduced with permission of Robert R. Bass.

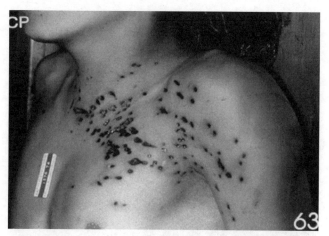

Figure 29.5 Shotgun injuries to chest. Source: Reproduced with permission of Robert R. Bass.

useful to know the blade length; to a certain degree this can predict the maximum depth of penetration.

Handguns

Handguns are typically short-barreled, medium-energy weapons with small bullets. As a medium-energy weapon, a handgun's damage-causing potential is more limited than that of higher energy firearms. Handgun bullets tend to have a blunter shape, causing early release of energy. Despite their shape and composition of softer metal (lead), handgun bullets tend not to deform due to their lower energy. As such, the bulk of the injury is caused in tissues damaged by the bullet's passage.

Rifles

Rifles are named for the rifling in the barrel, which causes the bullet to spin. The spin of the bullet improves accuracy and range due to the conservation of angular momentum. Rifle bullets are larger, retain more kinetic energy, and travel much further with greater accuracy than do handgun projectiles. They are able to transfer significant energy with damage extending outside the bullet's immediate track. Hunting ammunition is designed to expand dramatically (up to three times) on impact [4], increasing the speed of energy delivery and the wound pathway. Military ammunition is fully jacketed so it does not deform, which decreases the energy delivery rate [4].

Shotguns

While shotguns can fire single bullets (slugs), in general they fire a collection of spherical pellets, called shot, which radiate from the muzzle of the gun in a conical distribution. Typical muzzle velocity is 360 m/s [3]. Shot have a high drag coefficient so they lose velocity quite rapidly. At short range, they can be devastating but at longer range they lose much of their destructive potential (Figures 29.5, 29.6).

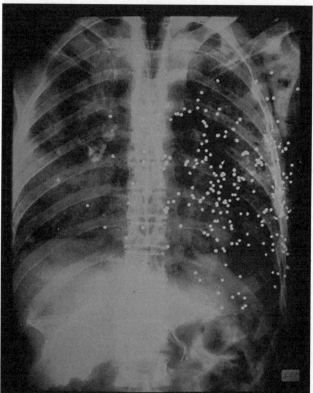

Figure 29.6 X-ray of shotgun injuries to chest. Source: Reproduced with permission of Robert R. Bass.

High-velocity projectile injury

While low-velocity projectiles inflict injury by direct cutting or tearing of tissues, higher velocity projectiles inflict injury in three ways: direct, pressure wave, and cavitation.

Direct injury

Direct injury is caused by a projectile's impact including crushing and lacerating tissues. Direct injury is based on the projectile size, although this may be modified by any deformation and bullet instability as it travels through the body. Crushing and laceration cause serious injury only if the bullet strikes organs or blood vessels [4].

Body armor protects the wearer by spreading the energy of impact over a larger area. Although this means that the projectile is prevented from hitting the body, the kinetic energy strikes a larger area, which can cause significant injury, such as fractured ribs and cardiac contusions.

Pressure wave

When a high-velocity projectile (greater than 750 m/s) hits human tissue, a high-pressure wave moves outward from the missile track in all directions. Caused by the compression ahead of the bullet, the pressure wave moves faster than the bullet itself. The faster and blunter the projectile, the greater the effect. Pressure from higher velocity bullets can exceed 1,000 pounds per square inch. Pressure waves travel better through fluids, higher density tissues, and organs, causing tearing and crushing of tissues. Blood vessels and solid organs (e.g. liver or spleen) can be injured or in some cases fractured. Hollow organs (e.g. large bowel) can rupture, and bones can be broken by the pressure wave (see Figure 29.2) [4].

Cavitation

High-velocity projectiles create a temporary cavity behind the missile path as tissues move away from the track. Cavity size is dependent on energy transferred during the bullet's journey and may be 30–40 times the diameter of the bullet [4]. The cavity will have a lower pressure than the air outside the body, causing air and potentially debris to be pulled in through the entrance and exit wounds. After the bullet has passed, the elasticity of the surrounding tissues tends to collapse the temporary cavity (see Figure 29.2).

Entry and exit wounds

Bullets often have both entry and exit wounds. In general, the exit wound is the same size or larger than the entrance wound but this is not always the case. Although bullets typically follow the path of least resistance, they may not travel in a straight line. Projectiles may have an unpredictable path within body tissues, including rotation or ricochet and deflection off bony structures. Two injury sites do not always represent an entry and an exit wound as they may represent two different entry wounds.

Entrance wounds can be deceptively small. A very small entrance wound can hide a devastating injury, and EMS providers should not be lulled into a false sense of security by a small entrance wound.

Resuscitation and initial assessment

Although the standard approach to patient assessment is described elsewhere, there are several unique considerations in the patient who has suffered a penetrating injury.

Scene safety

Although a thorough assessment of scene safety is always a priority, it takes on particular importance when dealing with penetrating trauma. Almost all potential causes of penetrating trauma harbor risks to the unwary EMS provider, and these must be considered before scene entry.

When penetrating trauma is a result of assault, the prehospital provider must ensure the perpetrator is no longer in the immediate area or has been apprehended or restrained by police. On other scenes where penetrating trauma is a possibility, such as explosions or motor vehicle collisions, the EMS personnel must examine the scene before entry to ensure there is no undue risk. When the scene is unsafe, the provider should withdraw to a safe distance and summon the appropriate assistance, such as police or fire services.

Spine immobilization

Assessment for possible spinal cord injury is important. Numerous case series have challenged the need for spinal immobilization in penetrating trauma patients [5–7]. It is well accepted that cervical spine (c-spine) immobilization is not required for penetrating firearm injuries to the head [8]. Similarly, immobilization for penetrating injuries to the neck and torso is likely only required when there is a high suspicion in an obtunded patient or obvious neurological compromise [9–11].

Extremity bleeding

Most bleeding from extremities, including arterial bleeding and amputations, can be controlled with direct pressure and elevation of the wound. When extremity bleeding persists despite these maneuvers, it may be necessary to apply a tourniquet [12]. Persistent bleeding when constant direct pressure cannot be maintained, such as military-casualty incidents or tactical environments, may also necessitate a tourniquet. Military use of tourniquets has undoubtedly saved lives in combat situations. Similarly, tourniquet use during the Boston Marathon bombing in 2013 allowed over 200 injured patients to be promptly treated and transported to area hospitals [13]. This is discussed more fully in Volume 1, Chapter 35. The letters TK and the time the tourniquet was applied should be written on the patient's limb or forehead.

Permissive hypotensive resuscitation

In managing penetrating trauma patients, IV fluid therapy is controversial. Permissive hypotensive resuscitation advocates that only patients without radial pulses or with a systolic

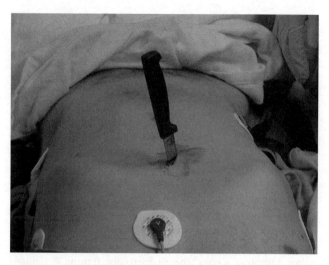

Figure 29.7 Knife left *in situ* in the wound for removal in the operating room. Source: Reproduced with permission of Robert R. Bass.

blood pressure (SBP) of <70 mmHg receive fluid resuscitation in the field [14]. IV access should rarely be obtained on scene and should be reserved for en route in the upper extremities if possible. IV or IO access in the lower limbs is relatively contraindicated because abdominal vascular injuries may lead to direct extravasation rather than reaching the central circulation.

Impaled objects

In general, impaled objects are not removed in the field as the object may be providing tamponade to bleeding soft tissues and blood vessels, and removal could cause exsanguination. Because movement of the object may cause further injury, the object should be well stabilized with bulky dressings and tape. Occasionally this will require cutting the object to a shorter length on scene if it impedes extrication and transportation. Care should be taken to ensure minimal movement of the object during this process. The exceptions are removal of an object that impedes CPR in a pulseless patient or impedes airway management where airway control is required (Figure 29.7).

Transport issues

"Scoop and run" versus "stay and play"

An optimized and efficient trauma system is required to deliver a patient from injury location to definitive care through a coordinated system of public access (9-1-1), EMS care, trauma triage, and trauma center. The corollary to the "golden hour" for the trauma system may be called the "platinum 10 minutes" for EMS, where the goal is to begin transport of the patient within 10 minutes of arrival on scene, barring extrication or other logistical issues that prevent prompt transport.

The platinum 10 minutes, or "scoop and run," is important in penetrating trauma patients who meet trauma triage criteria in which surgical management is likely. The term refers to the strategy of rapid assessment and transport. Interventions such as IV cannulation should be initiated en route to the hospital except in extenuating circumstances, such as a prolonged extrication. Conversely, the term "stay and play" refers to on-scene stabilization and initial management, which is rarely indicated in penetrating trauma.

For the penetrating trauma patient in cardiac arrest, emergency department thoracotomy may be useful if performed within 15 minutes of loss of circulation [15–17]. EMS providers should focus on maintaining the airway, good CPR, and correcting reversible causes of arrest, specifically hypoxia, tension pneumothorax, and hypovolemia, while transporting the patient to the hospital. Communication with the receiving ED or trauma center to notify them of the incoming patient, relevant injuries, and an estimated time of arrival is essential.

Penetrating chest trauma

The consequences of penetrating trauma depend on the mechanism and location of injury, the path of the projectile, and the underlying health of the patient. All patients with penetrating intrathoracic injury are at risk for intraabdominal or neck injury, depending on the entry point and path of the projectile. It is also true that a penetrating traumatic injury to the neck or abdomen can have associated chest injuries. When patients have been stabbed, it is useful to know the approximate length of the blade to understand what structures may have been injured. In the setting of a gunshot wound, any entry wound that does not have an exit wound should be considered to have retained bullet fragments.

Lungs and bronchial tree

Penetrating injury to lungs or bronchial tree can lead to escape of air or blood into the thoracic cavity, resulting in simple pneumothorax, tension pneumothorax, or hemothorax. Treatment for simple pneumothorax is supportive, for tension pneumothorax chest decompression may be required, and hemothorax should be treated with fluids, oxygen, and transport.

Heart and great vessels

Penetrating injury to the "cardiac box" increases the likelihood of myocardial and great vessel injury. The cardiac box is a rectangular shaped area of the anterior chest bounded superiorly by the clavicles, laterally by the midclavicular lines, and inferiorly by the costal margins [18]. It should be noted that the cardiac box includes the epigastric area.

Pericardial tamponade is a potentially rapidly life-threatening condition resulting from accumulation of fluid in the pericardial sac. It occurs more frequently in stab than gunshot wounds:

60–80% of stab wounds involving the heart develop tamponade [19]. Only a small amount of blood (50–100 mL) is necessary for pericardial tamponade to develop. Signs and symptoms of pericardial tamponade are hypotension, tachycardia, muffled heart sounds (Beck triad), dyspnea, cyanosis, and distended jugular veins. These signs may be followed by cardiac arrest with pulseless electrical activity. The treatment for pericardial tamponade is pericardiocentesis (potentially performed by the EMS physician in the field, particularly if ultrasound guidance is available) as a temporizing measure, followed by surgical repair.

Any penetrating thoracic or abdominal trauma can cause a diaphragmatic injury. Because diaphragmatic injuries can result in significant respiratory compromise, respiratory distress associated with injuries to the chest or abdomen should prompt EMS personnel to consider the possibility of a diaphragmatic injury.

Penetrating abdominal trauma

Gunshot wounds to the abdomen most commonly injure the small and large bowel because of the large space they occupy. A projectile passing through a gas-filled bowel will often cause compression of that gas, which may limit the pressure wave and injury. However, a projectile passing through a solid organ, such as the liver and spleen, causes cavitation and more widespread injury. Penetrating abdominal trauma may cause devastating injury to the large vessels (i.e. aorta, inferior vena cava, iliac vessels), leading to immediate exsanguination and death.

Due to the relative lack of skeletal protection and highly vascular structures, penetrating abdominal trauma has a high mortality. As opposed to blunt trauma in which force is more diffuse, transmitted across the abdomen, and leads to primarily solid organ injury, penetrating trauma is often a locally applied force affecting the hollow organs and mesentery. Solid organ injuries are less common with penetrating than blunt trauma, but they can occur, especially in stab wounds, with devastating consequences.

Penetrating wounds should be covered to decrease infection and observed for ongoing bleeding. Any intraabdominal organs visible (evisceration) should simply be covered with sterile saline-soaked dressings and in turn covered with an occlusive dry or plastic dressing.

Penetrating neck trauma

Penetrating neck wounds can be immediately fatal, and seemingly "innocuous" wounds can suddenly become life-threatening. Even the seemingly "benign" penetrating injury to the neck should be treated with careful and expectant management.

Injury to the major blood vessels of the neck may rapidly lead to exsanguination or delayed hemorrhage. Because of the thin overlying muscles and subcutaneous tissue, airway injuries to the larynx or trachea are common and may be devastating. Although somewhat protected by other structures, deeper injury can lead to pharyngeal and esophageal injuries. Lastly, neurological injury can occur to the spinal cord posteriorly, the cranial nerves superiorly, or the brachial plexus inferiorly.

Common carotid injuries occur in approximately 10% of all penetrating neck trauma. Significant carotid artery injuries are usually rapidly fatal, but may occasionally tamponade briefly to allow transport and assessment. History of significant blood loss either at the scene or ongoing is evidence of a major vascular injury. Similarly, expanding hematomas may initially be subtle, but are signs of vascular injury and may lead to airway compromise from direct compression. Hematomas are often visible when the patient's head is in a neutral position and the patient is examined from the feet.

Jugular vein injuries may also be fatal, but they may be successfully managed with direct pressure in the field to allow transport to an operative setting. Venous injuries may be complicated by entrainment of air leading to air emboli, a potentially fatal complication.

Neurological deficits should be carefully documented and relayed to the receiving facility. Unilateral stroke symptoms may be related to carotid artery injury and subsequent brain ischemia. Additionally, unilateral cranial nerve and brachial plexus injuries may also be apparent as facial or arm weakness respectively. Spinal cord injury may result in unilateral or bilateral motor deficits of the arms and legs.

Penetrating neck trauma can lead to airway anatomy distortion due to either a primary direct airway injury or secondarily via compressing hematomas and bleeding. Signs of an expanding hematoma, hoarse voice, stridor, airway compromise, or blood in the airway are warning signs of impending airway compromise and require quick action. Airway compromise should be anticipated, intubation should occur early rather than late, and in most cases, rapid transport should be initiated to a trauma center with basic airway maneuvers if airway intervention is not immediately required.

Although prehospital providers are accustomed to considering a potential spinal injury and providing immobilization to the majority of blunt trauma patients, this is not always required in penetrating injury. Based on case reviews, many have advocated against immobilizing patients with penetrating neck injuries unless neurological signs or symptoms are apparent [6,7]. Isolated stab wounds to the neck are unlikely to cause unstable cervical spine injuries. Although gunshots can lead to cervical spine injury, most spinal cord injuries are complete and obvious on initial evaluation, prompting immobilization. The provider should follow local directions regarding spinal immobilization with the understanding that if no spinal involvement is likely, the patient may be better managed without immobilization.

Penetrating neck injuries should be covered with an occlusive dressing if possible, to reduce the chances of an air embolism if bleeding is minimal. If ongoing bleeding is present, direct manual pressure can be used on one side of the neck. Obvious brisk bleeding from the neck may be best controlled with direct pressure above and below the bleeding site with the provider's two thumbs. Gauze under each thumb may assist with traction on the skin. If this is required to control significant bleeding, care should be taken not to change providers or stop the pressure to inspect the wound until arrival at the trauma center. Bilateral compression and circumferential dressings should be avoided because these may lead to cerebral hypoxia and infarction from bilateral carotid artery compression.

Lastly, IV cannulation, if performed, is preferentially performed on the upper limb opposite the side of neck injury. Because the subclavian vessels may be involved, it is best to avoid infusing fluid that will travel through an injured vessel leading to clot disruption, greater exsanguination, and local hematoma formation.

Penetrating head and facial trauma

The prehospital approach and management of penetrating head trauma is similar to that for head injuries in general and is discussed in Volume 1, Chapter 30. However, the airway management of facial trauma deserves special consideration.

Facial wounds that are otherwise survivable may lead to death due to airway compromise. Penetrating wounds or impaled objects may lead to significantly distorted airway anatomy and blood and foreign bodies in the airway. Any patient with penetrating facial injuries should be carefully considered for airway control. In addition to oral airway and oral endotracheal intubation, surgical airways, such as cricothyrotomy, may be required. Nasal airways should be avoided in patients with significant facial trauma.

Penetrating extremity trauma

Penetrating injury to the extremity can disrupt blood vessels, bones, nerves, muscles, and other soft tissues. This section will focus primarily on vascular and bony injuries.

Vascular injuries are either higher pressure arterial injuries or low-pressure venous injuries, both of which can bleed profusely. Arterial injuries tend to be more serious and should be identified and acted on promptly to prevent further morbidity or mortality. Arterial bleeding is often a brighter red and spurts with each heartbeat. Venous bleeding tends to be darker and tends to flow as opposed to spurt. The majority of active bleeds, including arterial bleeding, can be managed with direct pressure. When these strategies fail, the application of a tourniquet can be considered. Details on indication and use of tourniquets and other modalities may be found in Volume 1, Chapter 35.

Penetrating trauma can also cause bony injuries such as fractures or dislocations. These injuries should be considered open injuries because the penetrating object pathway will have exposed the injury to the outside. They should be treated as other fractures or dislocations by immobilization in the position found and dressing open wounds.

Prevention and public health issues

There are approximately 7.2 million registered firearms in Canada [20], and 223 million registered firearms in the United States [21]. US statistics indicate that approximately 40% of households have access to firearms. EMS personnel face a high probability of responding to locations where firearms may be readily accessible to the occupants. This presents both a challenge and an opportunity. The challenge is that EMS providers must be aware of their surroundings and ensure that the scene is safe to enter before beginning patient care.

Emergency medical services providers also have an opportunity to recognize safety concerns in the home that are not seen by traditional hospital-based health care providers. An example of this would be a home where children are present and a firearm is seen within easy reach of the children. Although it may or may not be appropriate to educate the parents about the dangers of this circumstance at the time, it is an observation that can be relayed to hospital personnel or to the relevant child protection agency. Where children are felt to be at imminent risk, EMS providers may have a legal obligation to report this to the child protection agency (as do other health care providers).

Medicolegal issues

Most jurisdictions require reporting of certain types of injuries. Many require hospitals to notify the police of all patients who present to the ED with gunshot wounds. The role of EMS will vary between jurisdictions. Providers should be familiar with the specific legislation in their jurisdiction and what (if any) requirements exist for reporting gunshot or stab wounds.

Emergency medical services providers should carefully document historical or physical findings. Patient care records are legal documents and can be used as evidence in a court of law. Unless a criminal act is witnessed, EMS providers should document what is seen and heard as opposed to what they are told or what they perceive may have happened. Examples of this include: "The patient states he was shot by his father" rather than "The patient was shot by his father." EMS providers should not make suppositions about which wound is the entrance versus exit, but simply document the locations and descriptions of the two penetrating wounds.

Forensic issues

Emergency medical services often responds to crime scenes or to patients who are the victims or perpetrators of crime. As such, providers need some understanding of forensics and evidence preservation. Wherever possible, the provider should ensure that neither the scene nor evidence is disturbed.

- When a crime is suspected, notify the police immediately. When the police are already on scene, follow the instructions of the officer in charge, especially with respect to scene security and safety. When there is disagreement between law enforcement and EMS, the EMS provider should notify the appropriate supervisor and document all discussions.
- When arriving on scene, ambulances should be parked to allow safe and rapid access to the patient, where possible without being on the immediate crime scene.
- Gloves should be worn at all times.
- Use the minimum number of providers needed.
- Use the same route to get to and from the patient; avoid walking through fluids and other debris.
- Try not to disturb physical evidence
- Do not move or touch anything unless necessary to do so for patient care.
- When it is necessary to move something, document it and notify law enforcement officials.
- Do not cut through or near holes in patient clothing; they may be bullet or knife holes.
- Any removed clothing and any personal articles should be left in the possession of law enforcement.

Prehospital termination of resuscitation in penetrating trauma

Up to one-third of all traumatic deaths occur before arrival at hospital, and prehospital traumatic cardiopulmonary arrest is associated with very poor survival (0–5%). Of patients who sustain traumatic cardiopulmonary arrest, isolated penetrating trauma (stab wound) to the thorax is the most salvageable subset of patients and any signs of life at the time of EMS arrival may reflect a potential survivor if transport time to a trauma center capable of ED thoracotomy is less than 15 minutes. In these very specific circumstances, ED thoracotomy may have up to a 25% survival rate [22]. The higher survival is seen in those patients who did not arrest until after arrival in the ED, but there have been a few survivors where the arrest occurred up to 15 minutes before arrival. Thus, this group of patients requires the most rapid transport with no delay on-scene for additional procedures.

"Futility" of prehospital medical resuscitation has been defined as less than a 1% chance of survival to hospital discharge and this is used to determine guidelines for ceasing resuscitation for non-traumatic cardiac arrest [23]. Using the literature, and a similar definition for "futility," NAEMSP and ACS-COT prepared a joint guideline for termination of resuscitation in prehospital traumatic cardiopulmonary arrest [24].

Conclusion

Trauma is the leading cause of death between the ages of 1 and 34 years in North America. Those penetrating trauma patients who are alive on arrival of EMS providers have a better chance of survival if they are transported rapidly to a designated trauma center. EMS providers should not be fooled by seemingly innocuous penetrating injuries. They can use their knowledge of anatomy and physiology to anticipate potential injuries and intervene before cardiovascular collapse or airway compromise ensues.

References

1 Statistics Canada. Mortality. Summary list of causes, 2009. Available at: www.statcan.gc.ca

2 Murphy SL, Xu J, Kochankek KD. Deaths: Final Data for 2010. *Natl Vital Stat Rep* 2013;61:1–118.

3 American College of Surgeons Committee on Trauma. *Advanced Trauma Life Support For Doctors*, 6th edn. Chicago: American College of Surgeons, 1997.

4 Ordog G, Wasserberger J, Balasubramanium S. Wound ballistics: theory and practice. *Ann Emerg Med* 1984;13:1113–22.

5 Connell R, Graham C, Munro P. Is spinal immobilisation necessary for all patients sustaining isolated penetrating trauma? *Injury* 2003;34:912–14.

6 Arishita GI, Vayer JS, Bellamy RF. Cervical spine immobilization of penetrating neck wounds in a hostile environment. *J Trauma* 1989;29:332–7.

7 Barkana Y, Stein M, Scope A, et al. Prehospital stabilization of the cervical spine for penetrating injuries of the neck – is it necessary? *Injury* 2000;31:305–9.

8 Kaups KL, Davis JW. Patients with gunshot wounds to the head do not require cervical spine immobilization and evaluation. *J Trauma* 1998;44:865–7.

9 Rhee P, Kuncir EJ, Johnson L, et al. Cervical spine injury is highly dependent on the mechanism of injury following blunt and penetrating assault. *J Trauma* 2006;61:1166–70.

10 Cornwell EE 3rd, Chang DC, Bonar JP, et al. Thoracolumbar immobilization for trauma patients with torso gunshot wounds: is it necessary? *Arch Surg* 2001;136:324–7.

11 Hauswald M. A reconceptualisation of acute spinal care. *Emerg Med J* 2013;30:720–3.

12 Lee C, Porter K, Hodgetts T. Tourniquet use in the civilian prehospital setting. *J Emerg Med* 2007;24:584–7.

13 Walls RM, Zinner MJ. The Boston marathon response: why did it work so well? *JAMA* 2013;309(23):2441–2.

14 Bickell W, Wall M, Pepe P, et al. Immediate versus delayed fluid resuscitation for hypotensive patients with penetrating torso injuries. *N Engl J Med* 1994;331:1105–9.

15 Seamon M, Fisher C, Gaughan J. Prehospital procedures before emergency department thoracotomy: "scoop and run" saves lives. *J Trauma* 2007;63:113–20.

16 Powell D, Moore E, Cothren C, et al. Is emergency department resuscitative thoracotomy futile care for the critically injured patient requiring prehospital cardiopulmonary resuscitation? *J Am Coll Surg* 2004;199:211–15.

17 Vanden Hoek TL, Morrison LJ, Shuster M, et al. Cardiac arrest in special situations: 2010 American Heart Association guidelines for cardiopulmonary resuscitation and emergency cardiovascular care. *Circulation* 2010;122:S829–61.

18 Nagy K, Lohmann C, Kim D, Barrett J. Role of echocardiography in the diagnosis of occult penetrating cardiac injury. *J Trauma* 1995; 38:859–62.

19 Asensio JA, Arroyo H, Veloz W, et al. Penetrating thoracoabdominal injuries: ongoing dilemma – which cavity and when? World J Surg 2002;26:539–43.

20 Canadian Firearms Centre. Quick facts about the Canadian Firearms Program: firearms licenses and registration of firearms. Available at: www.cfc-cafc.gc.ca

21 U.S. Department of Justice. Guns used in crime: firearms, crime and criminal justice. Available at: www.ojp.usdoj.gov/

22 Velmahos G, Degiannis E, Souter I, Allwood A, Saadia R. Outcome of a strict policy on emergency department thoracotomies. *Arch Surg* 1995;130(7):774–7.

23 Morrison L, Visentin L, Kiss A, et al. Validation of a rule for termination of resuscitation in out-of-hospital cardiac arrest. *N Engl J Med* 2006;355:478–87.

24 Hopson L, Hirsh E, Delgado J, et al. Guidelines for withholding or termination of resuscitation in prehospital traumatic cardiopulmonary arrest: Joint position statement of the National Association of EMS Physicians and the American College of Surgeons Committee on Trauma. *J Am Coll Surg* 2003;196:106–12.

CHAPTER 30

Traumatic brain injury

Kraigher O'Keefe

Introduction

An estimated 1.7 million people sustain traumatic brain injuries (TBI) annually in the United States, with total costs estimated at $60 billion per year [1,2]. Overall, TBI-related deaths account for one-third of all trauma-related deaths, or 53,000 deaths annually in the United States [2]. Traumatic brain injuries result primarily from falls (35%), motor vehicle collisions (17%), and direct blows to the head (16%) [2]. Men are more likely to sustain TBI than women for virtually all age groups. Children aged 0–14 account for approximately one-third of the cases of TBI [3]. Children (up to age 18) and adults over 75 years old are more likely to present to the ED, and are more likely to die from head injuries [2].

The initial brain insult occurs from direct impact, acceleration/deceleration injury, or penetrating wound resulting in bleeding, contusion, and ultimately cell death. Prevention measures include use of helmets, seat belts, car seats for children, and efforts to reduce falls in the elderly [4]. Once the primary brain injury has occurred, reversal of the insult is impossible. Prevention of secondary brain injury is the goal of therapeutic intervention. Treatment must start with initial management on scene, and continue until the eventual resolution of the patient's injuries. Aggressive treatment of severe head injury patients has been shown to be cost-effective, with an increase in quality-adjusted life-years when all costs are considered [5].

A review of a few physiological concepts is necessary for health care providers to understand how to prevent secondary brain injury. Cerebral perfusion pressure (CPP) is equal to the mean arterial pressure (MAP) minus the intracranial pressure (ICP). Measuring an accurate MAP in the prehospital setting may be difficult, making the systolic blood pressure (SBP) a surrogate that has been used in published guidelines and research. Rapid rises in ICP cause compression of the brain within an enclosed space (skull). As the pressure increases, the brain can be pushed downward, herniating in several possible directions. This herniation can cause compression of cranial nerves, posturing, changes in respiration, paralysis, and sudden death.

Management of severe traumatic brain injury is focused on transport to a trauma center while preventing secondary brain injury. Secondary brain injury occurs through a complex biological cascade, which can continue for hours to days. Both hypotension and hypoxia are independently associated with increased mortality and poorer neurological outcomes [6]. When hypotension and hypoxia occur together, a 75% mortality rate has been reported [7].

Primary assessment

The initial management of all injured patients should begin with airway, breathing, and circulation. Adequate oxygenation must be considered a critical priority in brain-injured patients. Hypoxemia occurs more frequently in brain-injured patients than is clinically suspected or recognized. Even a single episode of hypoxemia (SaO_2 <90%) can add to the overall morbidity, and has been associated with a 150% increase in mortality [8,9]. Supplemental oxygen should be administered to all potential TBI patients with continuous monitoring of the oxygen saturation using pulse oximetry. Adequate circulation is also important in the head-injured patient. Just a single episode of hypotension, defined as a systolic blood pressure less than 90 mmHg, is associated with increased morbidity, and with a 150% increase in mortality [9]. Intravenous fluids should be administered to maintain a systolic blood pressure of at least 90 mmHg [10]. The optimal fluid choice for volume restoration and maintenance of blood pressure has been intensely debated [11,12]. Isotonic crystalloid is recommended in both adults and children. Alterations in mental status due to hypoglycemia can easily be mistaken for those related to a traumatic brain injury. Patients with altered mental status should have a fingerstick glucose checked in the prehospital setting.

Emergency Medical Services: Clinical Practice and Systems Oversight, Second Edition. Volume 1: Clinical Aspects of EMS.
Edited by David C. Cone, Jane H. Brice, Theodore R. Delbridge, and J. Brent Myers.
© 2015 NAEMSP. Published 2015 by John Wiley & Sons, Inc. Companion Website: www.wiley.com\go\cone\naemsp

Secondary assessment

Performing an efficient neurological assessment is essential in the triage and management of brain-injured patients. Providers will need to repeat and reassess a patient's neurological status as it frequently changes rapidly (Table 30.1).

The Glasgow Coma Scale (GCS) was first introduced in 1974 by Teasdale and Jennett as a way to quickly evaluate the neurological status of brain-injured patients [13]. The GCS has been widely adopted as a way to categorize head injury severity (Table 30.2). The GCS should not be used as a static number and prehospital providers must frequently reevaluate neurological status, assessing for improvement or deterioration. A decrease of two or more points suggests increased ICP related to a potentially enlarging mass lesion (hematoma) [14]. A recent National Trauma Data Bank study of 250,000 head-injured patients found that 9% experienced prehospital neurological deterioration, defined as a decrease in two or more points in GCS from EMS to the emergency department measurement. This patient subgroup had higher in-hospital mortality even after adjusting for type of injury and presence of intracranial hemorrhage. Patients with measurable decline in mental status are high risk, and their initial care and evaluation should reflect the seriousness of this clinical finding [15].

The GCS has been criticized for insufficient interrater reliability, especially in the outpatient setting [16]. Recent studies have demonstrated that use of a Simplified Motor Scale (SMS) can be as predictive in outcome when compared to the traditional GCS in head-injured patients in both inpatient and out-of-hospital settings [17]. The SMS scale gives only one score: 2 = obeys commands, 1 = localizes to pain, 0 = withdraws to pain or worse. The SMS has not been widely adopted but data are promising that SMS represents an alternative to traditional GCS, especially in the out-of-hospital setting. Current Brain Trauma Foundation guidelines are to continue using the GCS in the prehospital setting for now [10].

Table 30.1 Glasgow Coma Scale

Eye opening	Verbal response	Motor response
		6–obeys commands
	5–oriented	5–localizes pain
4–spontaneous	4–confused	4–withdraws to pain
3–to speech	3–inappropriate	3–flexor posturing
2–to pain	2–incomprehensible	2–extensor posturing
1–none	1–none	1–none

Table 30.2 Severity of head injury based on GCS

Head injury severity	Glasgow Coma Scale
Mild	14–15
Moderate	9–13
Severe	3–8

The pupils must be evaluated for equality and reactivity to light. Asymmetry is defined as greater than 1 mm difference in diameter, and a fixed pupil is defined as less than 1 mm response to bright light. Unilateral pupillary dilation with decreased reactivity is a sign of increased ICP with uncal herniation causing compression of the ipsilateral third cranial nerve. The eye and orbit should be assessed for signs of direct trauma as unilateral pupillary dilation may be a normal variant. Bilateral pupillary dilation is more likely to be due to a metabolic or toxic cause and, if it is due to trauma, is a poor predictor with mortality reported at 60% [18].

Other assessment considerations

Alcohol use results in higher rates of traumatic injury, including head injuries. Intoxicated patients may be agitated or excessively sedated, making initial evaluation difficult. Blood alcohol concentrations above 80 mg/dL have been shown to have a linear effect on GCS [19]. Safety precautions may prompt the use of sedatives such as benzodiazepines, opioids, and antipsychotics. It is preferable to overtriage potentially intoxicated patients to higher levels of care and assume that their changes in consciousness are related to brain injury and not intoxicants alone. Only with time and serial examinations can alterations in mentation be ascribed solely to alcohol or drugs.

Anticoagulant and antiplatelet therapies are commonly used for a variety of medical conditions. Medications that affect platelet function (aspirin), platelet aggregation (clopidogrel), coagulation (warfarin), and thrombin (dabigatran) increase the risk of intracranial hemorrhage after trauma. EMS providers should inquire about the use of "blood thinners" and these patients should be treated with a high degree of concern for intracranial bleeding even in cases of mild head injury.

Penetrating head injuries can be from missiles or impaled objects. Impaled objects should be left in place during transport as these objects will likely need to be removed in a surgical setting. Firearms are the leading cause of TBI death (40%) in the US, with an estimated 68% self-inflicted [20]. The prognosis for penetrating head injuries is quite variable. Approximately two-thirds of patients die prior to hospital arrival. Poor prognostic indicators for the one-third who arrive alive to the hospital include a GCS of 3–5 on arrival, hypotension, bilateral hemisphere involvement, and bilaterally non-reactive pupils [21].

Prehospital intubation

Endotracheal intubation helps prevent both hypoxia and aspiration in severely head-injured patients. The controversy regards when the intubation should occur and by whom.

A randomized trial of bag-valve-mask ventilation versus intubation in all children requiring prehospital airway management in Los Angeles County showed no difference in survival or neurological outcomes. When looking specifically at head-injured children, there again was no difference in outcome [22]. This remains the best clinical study to date; however, it was performed in children in an urban EMS system, making generalizability to adult or non-urban settings questionable. Investigators in San Diego have published multiple studies on intubation in head-injured patients, showing consistently poor outcomes attributed at least partially to the adverse effects of inadvertent hyperventilation [23]. They also question whether paramedic inexperience may lead to poor outcomes as they report an average of 0.5 intubations per paramedic annually [24,25]. A randomized trial from Australia restricting intubation with end-tidal carbon dioxide monitoring to highly trained prehospital specialists when transport times were over 10 minutes reported a 97% intubation success rate, with no differences in the primary study outcome of extended Glasgow Outcome Scale at 6 months, but improved neurological outcomes at 6 months and no increase in mortality [26].

Previously, hyperventilation was recommended for severely head-injured patients after intubation to decrease intracranial pressure. While hyperventilation does decrease intracranial pressure, it also decreases cerebral blood flow due to cerebral vasoconstriction, leading to decreased oxygenation of the brain. Currently, mild hyperventilation is indicated for brief periods to treat suspected cerebral herniation. Signs of cerebral herniation include dilated and unreactive pupils, asymmetric pupils, a motor exam that identifies either extensor posturing or no response, or decrease in GCS score by 2 points or more [10]. Hyperventilation goal should be end-tidal CO_2 of 30–35 mmHg, monitored with capnography and used only as a *temporizing* measure [10].

An end-tidal carbon dioxide of 35–40 mmHg is recommended for intubated head-injured patients [10]. Unfortunately, inadvertent hyperventilation occurs in as many as 70% of cases, perhaps due to unintentional provider actions or confusion over prior hyperventilation recommendations [27]. Continuous end-tidal capnography is recommended and has been shown to reduce hyperventilation [28].

A Cochrane review article from 2008 suggests that there is no evidence for prehospital intubation in urban, ground transport systems [29]. The Brain Trauma Foundation recommends that EMS systems develop specific protocols that include monitoring of oxygen saturation, blood pressure, and when possible end-tidal carbon dioxide prior to EMS intubations [10]. Prehospital intubation use must be clarified at a local level in the context of transportation distance and time along with local infrastructure and geographical factors.

Additional treatments

Mannitol is widely used in the hospital setting to reduce intracranial pressure, which may reduce relative risk of death. There is currently insufficient evidence to recommend the use of mannitol in the prehospital setting [10,30].

In a recent randomized study, prehospital use of hypertonic saline following severe TBI showed no improved outcomes at 6 months, nor change in survival in patients who were not in shock [31]. Normal saline for volume resuscitation to maintain adequate blood pressure, defined as SBP of greater than 90, is currently recommended. The most recent Brain Trauma Foundation guidelines recommend hypertonic fluid resuscitation as an "option" for patients with GCS <8 [10].

The administration of albumin has been shown to worsen outcome in patients with TBI, therefore its use is not recommended [32]. Steroids have been shown to increase the risk of death and are no longer recommended in head-injured patients and are no longer widely used [33]. Seizures resulting from brain injury place excessive metabolic strain on an already injured brain and should be treated quickly to prevent further hypoxic insult. The risk of post-head injury seizures is noted to be higher in children. There is no evidence to treat head-injured patients prophylactically for seizures in the prehospital setting.

The adoption of therapeutic hypothermia in the context of post-cardiac arrest care has led to research into the use of therapeutic hypothermia in severely brain-injured patients [34]. To date, the effectiveness of therapeutic hypothermia for head injury has largely been inconclusive [35–37]. Some have argued that hypothermia treatment has not been initiated early enough in prior trials, and that a difference in outcome may be noticeable if cooling is started closer in time to the injury [38]. Currently there are no randomized controlled studies to support the use of prehospital therapeutic hypothermia in brain-injured patients.

Sports-related head injuries

Sports-related head injuries occur frequently, estimated at 3.8 million sports-related concussions annually in the US, with the most common sports being football, hockey, rugby, soccer, and basketball [39]. EMS personnel often provide care at youth athletic events and are the first to evaluate these athletes after injury. All athletes with suspected head injuries should be removed from activities and be evaluated by a medical professional. Athletes who sustain head injuries should not return to play that day. Patients with symptoms such as altered mental status, continued vomiting, retrograde amnesia, and loss of consciousness should be transferred to an emergency department.

Pediatrics (Table 30.3)

Prehospital concepts for pediatric traumatic brain injury are similar to those in adults; however, there are some important physiological differences. Children are more susceptible to TBI because of their large heads, thinner bones, and developing brains. Pediatric patients are more prone to brain edema, with more diffuse axonal injuries than primary bleeding or brain contusions. The classic Cushing reflex (hypertension, bradycardia, and respiratory irregularity) is more commonly seen in children. Skull fractures have a significantly higher rate

Table 30.3 Pediatric Glasgow Coma Scale

Eye opening	Verbal response	Motor response
		6–normal spontaneous movement
	5–coos, babbles	5–withdraws from touch
4–spontaneous	4–irritable crying	4–withdraws to pain
3–to speech	3–cries to pain	3–abnormal flexion
2–to pain	2–moans to pain	2–abnormal extension
1–none	1–none	1–none

of having intracranial pathology compared to adults, along with a much higher rate of seizures.

Non-accidental trauma must also be considered in pediatric head injuries, especially with injury patterns that do not match the history given by caregivers, or if there are other concerning injuries such as multiple bruises or old, unexplained fractures are found on exam or imaging.

Therapeutic cooling trials have had some positive studies to date in children; however, currently there is not enough evidence to recommend that cooling be initiated in the prehospital setting in children [40].

Prevention

The frequency and severity of TBI can be reduced through preventive efforts. Prehospital personnel can identify potential hazards or risk-taking behaviors as they are usually the only health care providers who actually enter a patient's living environment or witness the scene of a traumatic event. This allows the provider to either directly educate the patient and family or relate appropriate observations to ED staff when the patient is transported to the hospital.

Examples of preventive environmental modifications to reduce the potential for head injury include window guards and safety gates at staircases to prevent children from falling [41]. Falls in the elderly can be reduced by removing loose rugs and encouraging exercise program participation to maintain or improve muscle strength. Firearms in the home should be kept unloaded in a secure, locked container or cabinet with ammunition stored in a different location. Appropriate protective equipment including a helmet should be worn whenever riding any wheeled device or when engaging in contact sports such as hockey, football, boxing, baseball or softball, riding a horse, skiing, or snowboarding. Seat belts should always be used by adults and appropriately sized child safety and booster seats should always be used by children riding in vehicles.

Transportation and destination decisions

Destination decision making can significantly alter the outcome of a patient with TBI. When an organized trauma system is in place and patients are taken directly to an appropriate

facility, survival from TBI improves [42]. Patients in the moderate or severe TBI group (GCS 13 or less) should be directly transported to a trauma center that is fully equipped and staffed to manage acute neurosurgical emergencies [43]. Patients classified as mild TBI (GCS 14 or 15) can generally be transported to other facilities based on established destination protocols, assuming the patient's other injuries do not require care at a trauma center [44]. A retrospective evaluation of trauma databases suggested that transporting elderly TBI patients (>70 years) with a GCS of 14 directly to a trauma center may reduce this group's higher morbidity and mortality [45]. Transport mode (air versus ground) should consider local factors including but not limited to traffic, weather, available transport vehicles, and provider availability to minimize overall prehospital time [10].

Conclusion

Traumatic brain injury remains a common cause of disability and death. Injury prevention through public health initiatives such as the use of seat belts and helmets is the mainstay of primary brain injury prevention, with the major goal of treatment being to prevent secondary brain injury.

Secondary brain injury is caused by hypoxia and hypotension. Preventing hypotension and hypoxia are the goals of prehospital care. Prehospital intubations, when performed, should be undertaken by experienced providers with the use of continuous end-tidal monitoring, especially in cases of severe injury with long transfer times. Once intubated, providers should avoid hyperventilation. The mental status of head-injured patients should be continually reassessed as those who have a precipitous deterioration in mental status have increased morbidity and mortality. There is not enough consensus to recommend prehospital cooling, hypertonic saline, or prehospital administration of mannitol in severe head injury patients.

References

1 Finkelstein E, Corso PS, Miller TR. *The Incidence and Economic Burden of Injuries in the United States*. New York: Oxford University Press, 2006.
2 Coronado VG, Xu L, Basavaraju SV, et al. Surveillance for traumatic brain injury-related deaths. United States, 1997-2007. CDC. *Surveillance Summaries* 2011;60(SS05):1–32
3 Langlois LA, Rutland-Brown W, Thomas KE. *Traumatic Brain Injury in the United States. Emergency Department Visits, Hospitalizations, and Deaths*. Atlanta, GA: Centers for Disease Control and Prevention, National Center for Injury Prevention and Control, 2006.
4 American Association of Neurological Surgeons. *Head Injury Prevention Tips* Rolling Meadows, IL. American Association of Neurological Surgeons 2008

5 Whitmore RG, Thawani JP, Grady MS, Levine JM, Sanborn MR, Stein SC. Is aggressive treatment of traumatic brain injury cost-effective? *J Neurosurg* 2012;116:1106–13.

6 Yeh DD, Velmahos GC. Prehospital intubation for traumatic brain injury: do it correctly or not at all. *ANZ J Surg* 2012;82:484–5.

7 Findlay G, Martin IC, Smith M, et al. Trauma: who cares? National Confidential Enquiry into Patient Outcome And Death, 2007. Available at: www.ncepod.org.uk

8 Chi JH, Knudson MM, Vassar MJ, et al. Prehospital hypoxia affects outcome in patients with traumatic brain injury: a prospective multicenter study. *J Trauma* 2006;61:1134–41.

9 Cobas MA, de la Peña MA, Manning R, Candiotti K, Varon AJ. Prehospital intubations and mortality: a level 1 trauma center perspective. *Anesth Analg* 2009;109:489–93.

10 Badjatia N, Carney N, Crocco T, et al. Guidelines for the prehospital management of traumatic brain injury, 2nd edn. *Prehosp Emerg Care* 2008;2(s1):S1–52.

11 Cooper DJ, Myles PS, McDermott FT, et al. Prehospital hypertonic saline resuscitation of patients with hypotension and severe traumatic brain injury. *JAMA* 2004;291:1350–7.

12 Tyagi R, Donaldson K, Loftus CM, Jallo J. Hypertonic saline: a clinical review. *Neurosurg Rev* 2007;30:277–89.

13 Teasdale G, Jennet B. Assessment of coma and impaired consciousness. A practical scale. *Lancet* 1974;2:81–4.

14 Servadei F, Nasi MT, Cremonini AM, Giuliani G, Cenni P, Nanni A. Importance of a reliable admission Glasgow Coma Scale score for determining the need for evacuation of post-traumatic subdural hematomas: a prospective study of 65 patients. *J Trauma* 1998;44(5):868–73.

15 Majidi S, Siddiq F, Qureshi AI. Prehospital neurologic deterioration is independent predictor of outcome in traumatic brain injury: analysis from National Trauma Data Bank. *Am J Emerg Med* 2013;21:1215–19.

16 Holdgate A, Ching N, Angonese L. Variability in agreement between physicians and nurses when measuring the Glasgow Coma Scale in the emergency department limits its clinical usefulness. *Emerg Med Australas* 2006;18:379–84.

17 Thompson DO, Hurtado TR, Liao MM, Byyny RL, Gravitz C, Haukoos JS. Validation of the Simplified Motor Score in the out-of-hospital setting for the prediction of outcomes after traumatic brain injury. *Ann Emerg Med* 2011;58:417–25.

18 Signorini DF, Andrews PJ, Jones PA, Wardlaw JM, Miller JD. Predicting survival using simple clinical variables: a case study in traumatic brain injury. *J Neuro Neurosurg Pyschiatry* 1999;66:20–5.

19 Shahin H, Gopinath SP, Robertson CS. Influence of alcohol on early Glasgow Coma Scale in head-injured patients. *J Trauma* 2010;69:1176–81.

20 Adekoya N, Thurman DJ, White DD, Webb KW. Surveillance for traumatic brain injury deaths –United States, 1989–1998. *MMWR* 2002;51(SS10):1–16.

21 Blissitt PA. Care of the critically ill patient with penetrating head injury. *Crit Care Nurse Clin North Am* 2006;18:321–32.

22 Gausche M, Lewis RJ, Stratton SJ, et al. Effect of out-of-hospital pediatric endotracheal intubation on survival and neurological outcome: a controlled clinical trial. *JAMA* 2000;283:783–90.

23 Davis DP, Stern J, Sise MJ, Hoyt DB. A follow-up analysis of factors associated with head-injury mortality after paramedic rapid sequence intubation. *J Trauma* 2003;54:444–53.

24 Davis DP, Peay J, Sise MJ, et al. The impact of prehospital endotracheal intubation on outcome in moderate to severe traumatic brain injury. *J Trauma* 2005;58:933–9.

25 Davis DP, Hoyt DB, Ochs M, et al. The effects of paramedic rapid sequence intubation on outcome in patients with severe traumatic brain injury. *J Trauma* 2003;54:444–53.

26 Bernard SA, Nguyen V, Cameron P, et al. Prehospital rapid sequence intubation improves functional outcome for patients with severe traumatic brain injury: a randomized controlled trial. *Ann Surg* 2010;252:959–65.

27 Thomas SH, Orf J, Wedel SK, Conn AK. Hyperventilation in traumatic brain injury patients: inconsistency between consensus guidelines and clinical practice. *J Trauma* 2002;52:47–52.

28 Davis DP, Dunford JV, Ochs M, Park K, Hoyt DB. The use of quantitative end-tidal capnometry to avoid inadvertent severe hyperventilation in patients with head injury after paramedic rapid sequence intubation. *J Trauma* 2004;56:808–14.

29 Lecky F, Bryden D, Little R, et al. Emergency intubation for acutely ill and injured patients. *Cochrane Database Syst Rev* 2008;16:CD001429.

30 Wakai A, McCabe A, Roberts I, Schierhour G. Mannitol for acute traumatic brain injury. *Cochrane Database Syst Rev* 2013;8:CD001049.

31 Bulger EM, May S, Brasel KJ, et al. Out-of-hospital hypertonic resuscitation following severe traumatic brain injury: a randomized controlled trial. *JAMA* 2010;304:1455–64.

32 SAFE Investigators, Australian and New Zealand Intensive Care Society Clinical Trials Group, Australian Red Cross Blood Service, et al. Saline or albumin for fluid resuscitation in patients with traumatic brain injury. *N Engl J Med* 2007;357:874–84.

33 Roberts I, Yates D, Sandercock P, et al. CRASH trial collaborators. Effect of intravenous corticosteroids on death within 14 days in 10008 adults with clinically significant head injury (MRC CRASH trial): randomized placebo-controlled trial. *Lancet* 2004;364:1321–8.

34 Sagayln E, Band RA, Gaieski DF, Abella BS. Therapeutic hypothermia after cardiac arrest in clinical practice: review and compilation of recent experiences. *Crit Care Med* 2009;37:S223–6.

35 Fox JL, Vu EN, Doyle-Waters M, Brubacher JR, Abu-Laban R, Hu Z. Prophylactic hypothermia for traumatic brain injury: a quantitative systematic review. *CJEM* 2010;12:355–64.

36 Sadaka F, Veremakis C. Therapeutic hypothermia for the management of intracranial hypertension in severe traumatic brain injury: a systematic review. *Brain Inj* 2012;26:899–908.

37 Farag E, Manno EM, Kurz A. Use of hypothermia for traumatic brain injury: point of view. *Minerva Anestesiol* 2011;77:366–70.

38 Boer C, Franschman G, Loer SA. Prehospital management of severe traumatic brain injury: concepts and ongoing controversies. *Curr Opin Anaesthesiol* 2012;25:556–62.

39 Harmon KG, Drezner JA, Gammons M, et al. American Medical Society for Sports Medicine position statement: concussion in sport. *Br J Sports Med* 2013;47:15–26.

40 Sookplung P, Vavilala MS. What is new in pediatric traumatic brain injury? *Curr Opin Anaesthesiol* 2009;22:572–8.

41 Centers for Disease Control and Prevention. Injury prevention and control: traumatic brain injury. Atlanta, GA: Centers for Disease

Control, 2013. Available at: www.cdc.gov/traumaticbraininjury/prevention.html

42 Härtl R, Gerber LM, Iacono L, Ni Q, Lyons K, Ghajar J. Direct transport within an organized state trauma system reduces mortality in patients with severe traumatic brain injury. *J Trauma* 2006;60: 1250–6.

43 Ghajar J. Traumatic brain injury. *Lancet* 2000;356:923–9.

44 Sasser SM, Hunt RC, Faul M, et al. Guidelines for field triage of injured patients: recommendations of the National Expert Panel on Field Triage, 2011. *MMWR Recomm Rep* 2012;61 (RR-1):1–20.

45 Caterino JM, Raubenolt A, Cudnik MT. Modification of Glasgow Coma Scale criteria for injured elders. *Acad Emerg Med* 2011;18: 1014–21.

CHAPTER 31

Electrical injuries

Jeffrey Lubin

Introduction

Although severe electrical injuries are relatively uncommon, the true incidence remains unknown. Many electrocution victims fall from heights, present with dysrhythmias, or are simply found dead; the significance, and even the occurrence, of an electric shock may be unknown.

Electrical injuries tend to follow a bimodal age distribution. The first peak occurs in toddlers, who generally sustain electrical injuries from household electrical outlets and cords. The second peak occurs in adults who work with or around electricity for a living, such as miners, construction workers, and electrical utility workers [1].

The National Electronic Injury Surveillance System from the Consumer Product Safety Commission estimates that emergency departments treated 5,500–6,500 patients annually for product-related electrical shocks from 1992 to 2012 [2]. The majority of these incidents were minor, resulting in emergency department evaluation and subsequent discharge.

Most estimates place the annual death rate from electrical injury at 1,000–1,500 per year, with more than 60% occurring in adults 15–40 years of age. Electrocutions at home account for more than 200 deaths per year and are mostly associated with malfunctioning or misused consumer products [3]. As far as occupational exposure is concerned, according to the Electrical Safety Foundation International, there was an average of approximately 280 fatal electrical injuries per year in all industries from 1992 to 2008; one in 10,000 electrical utility workers in the United States dies from electrical injuries [4,5].

Basic concepts and pathophysiology

Electricity, a flow of electrons across a potential gradient from higher to lower concentration, requires both a complete path, called a circuit, to create continuous flow and a potential difference, measured in volts (V), to drive the electrons through the circuit. The volume of electrons flowing along this gradient is the current, measured in amperes (A). Resistance is the impedance to flow of the electrons and is measured in ohms (Ω).

In direct current (DC), electrons flow constantly in one direction across the voltage potential. Batteries are a common source of DC current, and high-voltage DC current is commonly used as a means for the bulk transmission of electrical power over long distances. Alternating current (AC) results when the direction of electron flow changes rapidly in a cyclic fashion. In the United States, standard household current is AC flowing at 60 cycles per second (Hz) and 110 V. In much of the rest of the world the standard household current is 220–240 V flowing at 50 Hz. Low voltage has been arbitrarily defined as less than 1,000 volts. As a general rule, high voltage is associated with greater morbidity and mortality, although fatal injury can occur with low voltage as well.

Six factors determine the outcome of human contact with electrical current: voltage, type of current, amount of current, resistance, pathway of the current, and duration of contact [6]. In many cases, the magnitude of only a few of these factors is known.

At the same voltage, AC exposure is considered to be about three times more dangerous than DC exposure. The differences in the two types of current have practical significance only at low voltages; at high voltages both currents have similar effects. AC current is more likely to produce explosive exit wounds, while DC current tends to produce discreet exit wounds. AC current is also more likely to cause muscular tetany than DC current. However, high-voltage contacts to both AC and DC current can produce a single violent skeletal muscle contraction, leading to the person appearing to be "thrown" from a voltage source.

The physical effects of different amounts of current vary. A narrow range exists between the threshold of current perception (0.2–0.4 mA) and the "let-go current" (6–9 mA) [7]. The let-go current is the level above which muscular tetany prevents release of subject's grip on the current source. When AC current flows through the arm, even at the standard household frequency of

Emergency Medical Services: Clinical Practice and Systems Oversight, Second Edition. Volume 1: Clinical Aspects of EMS.
Edited by David C. Cone, Jane H. Brice, Theodore R. Delbridge, and J. Brent Myers.
© 2015 NAEMSP. Published 2015 by John Wiley & Sons, Inc. Companion Website: www.wiley.com\go\cone\naemsp

50–60 Hz, flexor tetany of the fingers and forearm can over-power the extensors. If the hand and fingers are properly positioned, the hand will grasp the conductor more tightly, leading to extended contact with the power source [8]. However, current flow through the trunk and legs may cause opisthotonic postures and leg movements if the person has not grasped the contact tightly. Thoracic tetany is also possible and can occur at levels just above the let-go current, usually at 20–50 mA, resulting in respiratory arrest. Ventricular fibrillation (VF) usually occurs at 50–100 mA.

Electrocution causes injury in several ways. As electrical current is conducted through a material, resistance to that flow results in dissipation of both energy and heat, leading to tissue damage from direct heating. The amount of heat produced during the flow of current can be predicted using Joule's First Law, $Q = I^2Rt$, where Q is the amount of heat generated, I is the current flowing through a conductor, R is the amount of electrical resistance, and t is the time of exposure. Using Ohm's Law, $I = V/R$, the relationship between voltage and heat generation can be derived as $Q = V^2t/R$. Therefore, if resistance and other factors remain constant, the heat from current flow through tissue increases proportionately to the duration of current flow, the *square* of the current intensity, and the *square* of the voltage differential. This conversion of electrical energy to thermal energy can result in massive external and internal burns.

In addition, electroporation, defined as the creation of pores in cell membranes by means of electrical current, can be caused by electrical charges insufficient to produce thermal damage but strong enough to cause protein configuration changes that threaten cell wall integrity and cellular function [9,10]. Finally, muscle contractions or falling can result in blunt mechanical injury from exposure to high voltage.

Because electricity requires a complete circuit for continuous flow, the path of electricity flow determines the tissues at risk, the type of injury, and the degree of conversion of electrical energy to heat. For example, current passing through the thorax might cause arrhythmias, direct myocardial damage, or respiratory arrest whereas cerebral current could cause seizures or motor paralysis. Nerves, blood vessels, mucous membranes, and muscles tend to have the least resistance because of their high concentration of electrolytes [11]. The tissues that have the highest resistance to electricity tend to increase in temperature and coagulate. In particular, bone, which has a very high resistance to electrical current, tends to generate a significant amount of heat and often causes damage to nearby muscles. Skin can have a wide range of resistance to electricity, with dry skin having a higher resistance than moist skin. As a result, a patient with dry skin may have extensive superficial tissue damage but more limited conduction of potentially harmful current to deeper structures. On the contrary, wet skin (e.g. electrocution of a person in a bathtub or swimming pool) offers almost no resistance at all, thus generating the maximal intensity of current that the voltage can generate [12].

Evaluation and treatment

Scene safety

Scene safety is of critical importance at the site of an electrical injury. High-voltage power lines are almost never insulated but may *appear* insulated from atmospheric contaminants deposited on the lines over time. A rescuer standing on the ground touching any part of a vehicle that is in contact with a live power line is likely to be killed or seriously injured. In fact, electrocution can occur from ground current simply by walking too close to a downed power line. A common error is establishing a safety perimeter that is too small [13]. The recommended isolation distance is one full span between the adjacent utility poles or towers in all directions from a break in the wire or from the point of contact with the ground. At a minimum, personnel should stay at least 3–9 m (10–30 ft) from downed power lines until the utility company unequivocally confirms that power to the lines is off [14].

Electrical shock is *not* prevented by the rescuer wearing rubber gloves and boots unless they are specifically designed for the voltage present. The equipment must also have been recently tested for insulation integrity. A microscopic hole in a glove can result in an explosive injury to the hand because thousands of volts from the circuit concentrate at the hole to enter the glove [15].

Ideally, it is best to turn off the source of electricity before contact with the victim. Some sources suggest using a non-conductive material, such as a broom handle, to attempt to remove a victim from electrical contact. This should be done only with extreme caution because when voltages are above approximately 600 V, even dry wood may conduct significant amounts of electric current, presenting danger to the rescuer.

The EMS physician must be aware of other hazards at scenes of downed power lines. When voltage is reapplied to downed lines as circuit breakers reset, the lines may physically "jump" forcefully. In addition, although the metal cables that support telephone and power poles are normally grounded, they may become energized if they break or disconnect from an attachment and make contact with a nearby power line.

Management

Cardiac arrhythmia and cardiac arrest are the most common causes of death in electrocution. There are several established and theoretical mechanisms for this:

- accommodation of the ventricular effective refractory period
- asystole from direct current
- direct induction of VF
- induction of an intermediate ventricular tachycardia
- induction of VF from long-term, high-rate cardiac capture
- lowering the VF threshold through ischemia
- respiratory arrest with secondary cardiac arrest
- shock on cardiac T-wave.

It is classically taught that AC current is more likely to cause VF, whereas DC current is more likely to cause asystole. Evidence for this is lacking [16].

Cardiac monitoring is essential in patients who have suffered significant electrical injuries. Almost 50% of these patients exhibit electrocardiographic changes or rhythm disturbances. The most common electrocardiographic alterations are sinus tachycardia and non-specific ST-T-wave changes, which usually correct with time. In fact, if the patient's overall clinical condition is good and he or she has a normal ECG at the time of admission to the ED, the probability of observing any delayed serious dysrhythmia is unlikely [17]. Because most dysrhythmias are transient, therapeutic interventions are rarely needed. Sometimes an injury pattern mimicking infarction may be seen on the ECG; such patterns are generally due to direct myocardial injury and not coronary thrombosis [18]. The difficulty is identifying the existence of new myocardial damage and determining its physiological significance [19].

Cardiopulmonary resuscitation should be initiated as soon as safely possible for victims of electric shock-induced arrest. For line workers, coworkers are trained to begin rescue breathing while still on utility power poles. As soon as the victim is lowered to the ground, chest compressions can be started if the patient is in cardiac as well as respiratory arrest.

Because many victims are young and have no prior cardiovascular disease, resuscitation efforts should be aggressive. It is often not possible to predict the outcome of attempted resuscitation based on age and initial rhythm in electric shock-induced cardiac arrest [20]. Normal BLS or ALS resuscitation protocols should be used, keeping in mind any necessary adjustments for rescuer safety and patient access.

Once cardiac dysrhythmias and respiratory arrest are addressed, patients with electrical injury should be evaluated as trauma patients, treating any blunt injuries and caring for burns. Rescuers should assume that victims of electrical trauma have multiple traumatic injuries. Falls, being thrown from the electrical source by an intense muscular contraction, or blast effect from explosive forces that may occur with electric flashes can cause significant secondary blunt trauma. In addition, fractures and joint dislocations can be caused directly by forceful muscle contractions from an electric current [21]. Therefore, in addition to cardiac monitoring and measurement of oxygen saturation, intravenous access and evaluation of the need for in-line immobilization of the spine should be implemented after the primary survey is completed.

The primary electrical injury is the burn. There are two general patterns: surface burns and internal current flow. Appropriate burn care should be instituted for external burns. Constricting rings and other jewelry should be removed from all extremities whether or not injury is visualized. Patients with burns from high-voltage electricity should be taken to a trauma center. Because visible cutaneous damage generally underestimates internal damage, fluid requirements may exceed prediction using standard thermal burn injury formulas such as the Parkland formula. Most sources advise that an initial fluid volume of 20–40 mL/kg over the first hour is appropriate for a typical patient with a significant electrical injury [14]. Further fluid administration will be guided by continued clinical and hemodynamic assessment.

Lightning injury

Lightning is a unidirectional cloud-to-ground current resulting from static charges that develop when a cold high pressure front moves over a warm moist low pressure area [22–24]. It is neither a direct nor an alternating form of current [24,25]. Although lightning can release greater than 1,000,000 V of energy, generate currents greater than 200,000 A, and reach temperatures as high as 50,000 °F, the actual amount of energy delivered may be less than that typical of high-voltage injuries because its duration is as short as a few milliseconds [12,22,26]. A comparison between lightning, high-voltage, and low-voltage electrical injuries is shown in Table 31.1.

In the United States, lightning kills approximately 80–90 people per year, although 70% of lightning strikes are not fatal [27–30]. Because people tend to seek shelter from lightning storms together, 30% of lightning strikes involve more than one patient [23].

Lightning strikes tend to result in five basic mechanisms of injury [24,25,29].

1 **Direct strike**. A direct strike is more likely to hit a person who is in the open and unable to find shelter. This type of lightning strike is usually fatal [29].

2 **Splash injury**. This occurs when lightning strikes an object, such as a tree or building, or another person, and the current "splashes" to a victim standing nearby. Current can also splash to a victim indoors via plumbing or telephone wires [24].

3 **Contact injury**. This occurs when the victim is in physical contact with an object or a person directly struck or splashed by lightning.

4 **Step voltage/ground current injury**. When lightning hits the ground, the current spreads outward in a radial pattern. Because the human body offers less resistance to electrical current than does the ground, the current will preferentially travel through the body (e.g. up one leg and down the other) between the body's two points of ground contact.

5 **Blunt trauma**. Victims of lightning strike may be thrown by the concussive forces of the shockwave created by the lightning. A lightning strike can also cause significant opisthotonic muscle contractions, which may lead to fractures or other trauma.

The first priority in responding to a lightning strike is scene safety. Contrary to popular myth, lightning can, and often does, strike the same place twice.

Although lightning strikes may cause multisystem injuries, the most common cause of death is immediate cardiorespiratory arrest [24,25,29,31,32]. Unlike the typical trauma patient, however, lightning victims have significant resuscitation potential, which gives rise to the EMS lightning triage mantra, "resuscitate the dead." The cardiac effects of lightning injury can include anything from non-fatal arrhythmias, including bradycardia, tachycardia, premature ventricular contractions, ventricular tachycardia, and atrial fibrillation, to myocardial

Table 31.1 Comparison between lightning, high-voltage, and low-voltage electrical injuries

	Lightning	High voltage	Low voltage
Voltage, V	>30,000,000	>1,000	<600 (<240)
Current, A	200,000	1,000	240
Duration	Instantaneous	Brief	Prolonged
Type of current	Similar to DC	DC or AC	Mostly AC
Cardiac arrest (cause)	Asystole	Ventricular fibrillation	Ventricular fibrillation
Respiratory arrest (cause)	Direct CNS injury	Indirect trauma or tetanic contractions of respiratory muscles	Tetanic contractions of respiratory muscles
Muscle contraction	Single	DC: single AC: tetanic	Tetanic
Burns	Rare, superficial	Common, deep	Usually superficial
Rhabdomyolysis	Uncommon	Very common	Common
Blunt injury (cause)	Blast effect, shock wave	Muscle contraction, fall	Fall (uncommon)
Mortality (acute)	Very high	Moderate	Low

AC, alternating current; CNS, central nervous system; DC, direct current.
Source: Koumbourlis AC. *Crit Care Med* 2002;30:S424–30. Reproduced with permission of Wolters Kluwer Health.

depolarization and asystole [24,30–32]. Lightning may also cause paralysis of the medullary respiratory center, leading to prolonged respiratory arrest. With early and sustained respiratory support by EMS providers, many patients have excellent prognoses [29].

Although lightning produces significant heat and voltage, severe burns are uncommon because of the short duration of exposure [24,25,29,33]. Compared with high-voltage electrical injuries, burn care and aggressive volume resuscitation for deep tissue injury are less important considerations. Full-thickness entry and exit burns are occasionally present, but deep burns and tissue damage are less common than in typical high-voltage electrical injury [25,29]. In many victims struck during rain, the low resistance of wet skin results in a "flashover" effect, decreasing the current transit through the body and thus decreasing the risk of severe internal injury [24,25]. Flashover occurs when the lightning strikes a victim, and the current flashes over the outside of the body along the wet skin surface, vaporizing the moisture and causing superficial burns – and often blasting shoes and clothing off the victim's body [25]. Linear and punctate burns may be seen along the paths of sweat or rainwater accumulation. Full-thickness burns may occur at sites of contact with metal objects, such as jewelry [25]. Lichtenberg figures, or feathering burns, are pathognomonic of lightning injury, but are not true burns [24,26]. They are thought to be the result of electron showers that cause extravasation of red blood cells into the superficial skin layers along the current lines of the flashover [24,25,29,32].

Potential neurological effects of lightning injury include loss of consciousness, confusion, memory loss, seizures, persistent headaches, paralysis, mood disorders, chronic pain syndromes, cerebellar dysfunction, and peripheral neuropathies [23,24,29]. Hearing loss may result from sensorineural damage or from direct otological injury to the tympanic membrane or middle ear [25]. Keraunoparalysis, or "lightning paraplegia," is an immediate effect of lightning injury and consists of paralysis of the limbs with pallor, cool temperature, and absent pulses [34]. It is not actually a neurological phenomenon, but rather the result of severe arterial vasospasm from catecholamine release. It usually resolves within hours, but it can create a difficult and misleading initial patient assessment.

Other considerations in the lightning victim include blunt trauma, either from being thrown or from significant muscle contractions. The lightning victim may also have been struck by falling tree limbs or building debris. The appropriate precautions, including proper spinal immobilization, must be observed. Because deep tissue damage is less common in lightning strike victims than in victims of high-voltage electrical injury, myoglobinuria and acute renal failure are seen less frequently. However, acute renal failure has been reported in 3–15% of victims of major lightning strikes, so appropriate fluid resuscitation should be initiated in the prehospital setting [25].

Rescuers should care for lightning strike victims using standard BLS and ALS principles but should amend multicasualty triage priorities, providing initial care to the apparently dead victims first. Victims who do not suffer immediate cardiac or respiratory arrest are unlikely to die from their injuries [24]. Bystander CPR should be strongly encouraged. Dilated or nonreactive pupils do *not* indicate brain death in the lightning strike victim and therefore should not be used to determine prognosis [29]. Patients should receive cardiac and pulse oximetry monitoring during transport, and trauma precautions, including spinal immobilization, must be observed. Because the extent of injury may not be readily apparent based on external signs, all lightning strike patients require transport for hospital evaluation. Any lightning strike victim with obvious injuries such as long bone fractures, external burns, respiratory compromise, cardiac arrhythmias, hypotension, or altered mental status should be transported to a trauma or burn center for evaluation.

Conclusion

All responders, including the EMS physician, must be familiar with the potential hazards that may be present at an electrical injury scene. The outcome of human contact with electrical current is largely determined by voltage, type, and amount of current, pathway of the current, resistance, and duration of contact. Immediate mortality is generally related to cardiac or respiratory system dysfunction. Because of this, triage schema may need to be altered at the scene of a mass casualty electrical incident. Later sequelae are typically related to burns or other traumatic injuries and often require trauma center or burn center care.

Understanding the nature of electricity can help the EMS physician stay safe, predict injury patterns, and more effectively care for patients.

References

1 John BA, Bena JF, Stayner LT, Halperin WE, Park RM. External cause specific summaries of occupational fatal injuries. Part I: an analysis of rates. *Am J Ind Med* 2003;43:237–50.

2 Consumer Product Safety Commission. *National Electronic Injury Surveillance System (NEISS).* 2013. Available at: www.cpsc.gov/library/neiss.html

3 Hiser S. 1998 Electrocutions Associated with Consumer Products: *Report.* Washington, DC: US Consumer Product Safety Commission, Division of Hazard Analysis, Directorate for Epidemiology, 2001.

4 Electrical Safety Foundation International (ESFI). *ESFI White Paper – Occupational Electrical Accidents in the US, 2003–2009.* Available at: http://esfi.org/index.cfm/pid/10272/cdid/11510

5 Ore T, Casini V. Electrical fatalities among US construction workers. *J Occup Environ Med* 1996;38:587–92.

6 Kouwenhoven WB. Effects of electricity on the human body. *Ind Med Surg* 1949;18(7):269.

7 Cooper MA. Emergent care of lightning and electrical injuries. *Semin Neurol* 1995;15:268–78.

8 Jain S, Bandi V. Electrical and lightning injuries. *Crit Care Clin* 1999;15:319–31.

9 Lee RC, Gaylor DC, Bhatt D, Israel DA. Role of cell membrane rupture in the pathogenesis of electrical trauma. *J Surg Res* 1988;44:709–19.

10 Block TA, Aarsvold JN, Matthews KL 2nd, et al. The 1995 Lindberg Award. Nonthermally mediated muscle injury and necrosis in electrical trauma. *J Burn Care Rehabil* 1995;16:581–8.

11 Jaffe RH. Electropathology: a review of pathologic changes produced by electric currents. *Arch Pathol Lab Med* 1928;5:837–70.

12 Koumbourlis AC. Electrical injuries. *Crit Care Med* 2002;30:S424–30.

13 International Fire Service Training Association. *Fireground Support Operations.* Stillwater, OK: Oklahoma State University, 2002.

14 Fish RM. Electrical injuries. In: Tintinalli JE (ed) *Emergency Medicine: A Comprehensive Study Guide,* 6th edn. New York: McGraw-Hill, 2004.

15 Price T, Cooper MA. Electrical and lightning injuries. In: Marx JA (ed) *Rosen's Emergency Medicine, Concepts and Clinical Practices,* 6th edn. Philadelphia: Mosby Elsevier, 2006.

16 Kroll MW, Fish RM, Lakkireddy D, Luceri RM, Panescu D. Essentials of low-power electrocution: established and speculated mechanisms. *Conf Proc IEEE Eng Med Biol Soc* 2012;2012:5734–40.

17 Akkaş M, Hocagil H, Ay D, Erbil B, Kunt MM, Ozmen MM. Cardiac monitoring in patients with electrocution injury. *Ulus Travma Acil Cerrahi Derg* 2012;18:301–5.

18 Carleton SC. Cardiac problems associated with electrical injury. *Cardiol Clin* 1995;13:263–77.

19 Robinson NM, Chamberlain DA. Electrical injury to the heart may cause long-term damage to conducting tissue: a hypothesis and review of the literature. *Int J Cardiol* 1996;53:273–7.

20 European Resuscitation Council. Part 8: Advanced challenges in resuscitation. Section 3: Special challenges in ECC. 3G: Electric shock and lightning strikes. *Resuscitation* 2000;46:297–9.

21 Fish RM. Electric injury: Part II. Specific injuries. *J Emerg Med* 2000;18:27–34.

22 Rivera J, Romero K, González-Chon O, Uruchurtu E, Márquez MF, Guevara M. Severe stunned myocardium after lightning strike. *Crit Care Med* 2007;35:280–5.

23 Whitcomb D, Martinez JA, Daberkow D. Lightning injuries. *South Med J* 2002;95:1331–4.

24 Gatewood M, Zane R. Lightning injuries. *Emerg Med Clin N Am* 2004;22:369–403.

25 Okafor U. Lightning injuries and acute renal failure: a review. *Ren Fail* 2005;27:129–34.

26 Spies C, Trohman R. Narrative review: electrocution and life-threatening electrical injuries. *Ann Intern Med* 2006;145:531–7.

27 Kisner S, Casini V. Epidemiology of electrocution fatalities: 1998. In: *Worker Deaths by Electrocution: A Summary of NIOSH Surveillance and Investigative Findings.* Publication No. 98–131. Washington, DC: Department of Health and Human Services (NIOSH), 1998.

28 Lopez RE, Holle RL. Demographics of lightning casualties. *Semin Neurol* 1995;15:286–95.

29 Zafren K, Durrer B, Herry J, Brugger H. Lightning injuries: prevention and on-site treatment in mountains and remote areas. Official guidelines of the International Commission for Mountain Emergency Medicine and the Medical Commission of the International Mountaineering and Climbing Federation (ICAR and UIAA MEDCOM). *Resuscitation* 2005;65:369–72.

30 Adekoya N, Nolte K. Struck-by-lightning deaths in the United States. *J Environ Health* 2005;67:45–50.

31 Celik A, Ergun O, Ozok G. Pediatric electrical injuries: a review of 38 consecutive patients. *J Pediatr Surg* 2004:39:1233–7.

32 Jost W, Schönrock L, Cherington M. Autonomic nervous system dysfunction in lightning and electrical injuries. *NeuroRehabilitation* 2005;20:19–23.

33 Zehender M. Images in clinical medicine: struck by lightning. *N Engl J Med* 1994;330:1492.

34 Kleinschmidt-DeMasters BK. Neuropathology of lightning strike injuries. *Semin Neurol* 1995;15:323–8.

CHAPTER 32

Blast injury

John McManus and Richard B. Schwartz

Introduction

A contemporary understanding of explosive injuries is essential for all out-of-hospital health care providers. Although most explosive injuries were previously encountered in austere and/or military environments, civilian attacks with explosive devices have now become more frequent due to the inexpensive nature and ease of access of explosive materials. In fact, the average number of bombings is five per day within the United States, with a total of 36,110 bombing incidents causing almost 700 deaths from 1983 through 2002 [1]. In the most recent explosive events on US soil in Boston, there were over 200 casualties [2]. Newer explosive devices used in recent attacks have resulted in casualties with severe combined penetrating, blunt, and burn trauma. In addition to terrorist bombings, accidental industrial explosions are also common. Although arson has not typically been included in the terrorist's agenda, some explosive agents and materials used in attacks have flammable injury potential because terrorists typically aim their attacks at human beings directly. These explosive and burn types of injuries are not typically different from non-explosive burns; however, the severity and complexity of injury and/or number of burn patients are potentially greater in the former than in the latter. Burn injury and management will be discussed in Volume 1, Chapter 33.

The medical provider treating explosive trauma in the out-of-hospital environment is faced with many unique challenges. Some of these challenges include the possibility of multiple casualties, unsafe environment, lack of medical supplies, prolonged evacuation time and distance, and lack of sophisticated care that is the standard for trauma management in the urban environment. This chapter will cover the evaluation and treatment of explosive injuries in the out-of-hospital environment.

Explosive devices

Because of the current increased terrorist threat and occurrences in many countries, many types of explosive devices can now be purposefully or accidentally encountered by out-of-hospital personnel in the civilian environment. Multiple types of improvised and manufactured explosive devices exist and only a few will be discussed. Most accidental explosive injuries occur from handling or encountering mines, improvised explosive devices (IEDs), or unexploded ordnance (UXO), such as grenades and ammunition. In Afghanistan alone, the combined death and injury rate was 150–300 per month from accidental UXO even before the US conflict [3]. The most common, purposeful explosive injuries currently in combat operations are from IEDs, home-made devices that cause injury or death by using explosives alone or in combination with toxic chemicals, biological toxins, or radiological material. IEDs can use commercial or military explosives, homemade explosives, or military ordnance and can be found in varying sizes and containers, and with various functioning and delivery methods.

Blast injury

An explosion is caused by the rapid chemical conversion of a liquid or solid material into a gas with a resultant energy release. Low explosives (gunpowder) release energy slowly, by a process called deflagration. In contrast, high explosives release energy rapidly through a process called detonation, which involves the almost instantaneous transformation of the physical space occupied by original solid or liquid material into gases, filling the same volume within a few microseconds, thereby expanding under extremely high pressure. The highly pressurized gases compress the surrounding environment, generating a pressure pulse that is

Emergency Medical Services: Clinical Practice and Systems Oversight, Second Edition. Volume 1: Clinical Aspects of EMS.
Edited by David C. Cone, Jane H. Brice, Theodore R. Delbridge, and J. Brent Myers.
© 2015 US Government. Published 2015 by John Wiley & Sons, Inc. Companion Website: www.wiley.com\go\cone\naemsp

Table 32.1 Categories of explosive injuries

Category	Mechanism	Injury type
Primary	A form of barotrauma, unique to explosions, which causes damage to air-filled organs	• Blast lung • Tympanic membrane rupture and middle ear damage • Abdominal hemorrhage and perforation • Globe (eye) rupture • Concussion
Secondary	Trauma caused by the acceleration of shrapnel and other debris by the blast	• Penetrating ballistic (fragmentation) • Blunt injuries (rapid deceleration) • Eye penetration
Tertiary	Casualty becomes a missile and is propelled through the air, with typical patterns of blunt trauma	• Fracture and traumatic amputation • Blunt chest and abdominal trauma • Impalement • Closed and open brain injury
Quaternary	All other explosion-related injuries, illnesses, or diseases which are not due to primary, secondary, or tertiary mechanisms	• Burns (flash, partial, and full thickness) • Crush injuries • Exacerbation of underlying conditions (asthma, angina, etc.) • Inhalation injury
Quinary	The intentional addition of agents that may result in injury	• Radiation • Chemical • Biological (including suicide bombers with hepatitis or HIV)

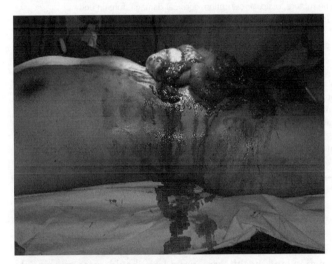

Figure 32.1 Example of an abdominal blast injury.
Source: Reproduced with permission of John McManus.

propagated as a blast wave. As a blast wave passes through the body, it causes damage by several different mechanisms. Patients injured from explosions usually suffer from a combination of blast, blunt, penetrating, and burn injuries. Injuries from explosives are divided up into categories (Table 32.1).

Primary blast injury

As the blast wave passes through tissues of different density, disruption occurs and small particles of tissue and liquids are thrown into the air space. This phenomenon is called *spall*. Not surprisingly, the injuries from this pressure wave tend to occur at sites of a gas/tissue interface (e.g. sinus, lung, middle ear, or bowel) (Figure 32.1). Traumatic brain injury can also occur without other signs of head injury.

Secondary blast injury

Injury from projectiles or secondary blast injury represents the most common cause of trauma from explosive events and causes the most significant mortality and morbidity when the victim(s) survives the primary injury. Most improvised explosive devices have projectiles packed around them (e.g. nails, ball bearings) to increase the injury potential from secondary blast injury.

Tertiary blast injury

Tertiary blast injury results when victims are displaced by the blast wave and they become projectiles themselves. The resulting injuries may be severe and include a mix of blunt and penetrating trauma. In addition, structural collapse may contribute to the injuries under tertiary blast injury.

Quaternary blast injury

These are related to the thermal effect of the blast and exacerbation of existing medical conditions. Many primary, secondary, and tertiary blast injuries will be complicated by quaternary injury. Extensive burns, as well as exacerbation of medical conditions, may be related to explosions. The most common medical conditions affected are respiratory diseases such as asthma or chronic obstructive pulmonary disease; however, many other medical conditions may be exacerbated by explosive events. (It should be noted that some authors use the term "quaternary blast injury" to refer to injuries from a resulting structural collapse, included in this chapter as part of tertiary blast injury.)

Quinary blast injury

Quinary injury is related to the intentional addition of radiological, chemical, or biological compounds to the explosive device with the intent of exposing victims to the additional hazard. This has included the use of suicide bombers who are infected with infectious diseases such as human immunodeficiency virus

Table 32.2 Recommended postexposure management by risk category and specific pathogen

Risk category	HBV[1]	HCV[2]	HIV[3]	Tetanus
Category 1: Penetrating injuries or non-intact skin exposures[4]	Intervene	Consider testing	Generally no action	Intervene
Category 2: Mucous membrane exposures[5]	Intervene		Generally no action	No action
Category 3: Superficial exposure of intact skin[6]	No action	No action	No action	No action

[1]Hepatitis B virus.
[2]Hepatitis C virus.
[3]Human immunodeficiency virus.
[4]Penetration of skin by a sharp object that was in contact with blood, tissue, or other potential infectious fluid (i.e. semen, vaginal fluid, cerebrospinal fluid, synovial fluid, pleural fluid, peritoneal fluid, pericardial fluid, amniotic fluid, or any other visibly bloody body fluid or tissue) before penetration. Non-intact skin exposure is defined as contact of non-intact skin with any of these potentially infectious tissues or fluids.
[5]Contact of mucous membranes (i.e. eyes, nose, mouth, or inner surfaces of the gut or genital areas) with blood, tissue, or other potential infectious fluid (i.e. semen, vaginal fluid, cerebrospinal fluid, synovial fluid, pleural fluid, peritoneal fluid, pericardial fluid, amniotic fluid, or any other visibly bloody body fluid or tissue).
[6]Superficial exposure of intact skin (but not of mucous membranes) with blood, tissue, or other potential infectious fluid (i.e. semen, vaginal fluid, cerebrospinal fluid, synovial fluid, pleural fluid, peritoneal fluid, pericardial fluid, amniotic fluid, or any other visibly bloody body fluid or tissue).

Table 32.3 Overview of explosive-related injuries

System	Injury or condition
Auditory	Tympanic membrane rupture, ossicular disruption, cochlear damage, foreign body
Eye, orbit, or face	Perforated globe, foreign body, air embolism, fractures
Respiratory	Blast lung, hemothorax, pneumothorax, pulmonary contusion and hemorrhage, arteriovenous fistulas (source of air embolism), airway epithelial damage, aspiration pneumonitis, sepsis
Digestive	Bowel perforation, hemorrhage, ruptured liver or spleen, sepsis, mesenteric ischemia from air embolism
Circulatory	Cardiac contusion, myocardial infarction from air embolism, shock, vasovagal hypotension, peripheral vascular injury, air embolism-induced injury
Central nervous system injury	Concussion, closed and open brain injury, stroke, spinal cord injury, air embolism-induced injury
Renal injury	Renal contusion, laceration, acute renal failure due to rhabdomyolysis, hypotension, and hypovolemia
Extremity	Traumatic amputation, fractures, crush injuries, compartment syndrome, burns, cuts, lacerations, acute arterial occlusion, air embolism-induced injury

(HIV) or hepatitis [4,5]. The possibility of biological contamination creates issues regarding postexposure prophylaxis (PEP). Recommendations for PEP by the Centers for Disease Control are summarized in Table 32.2. To determine appropriate actions in response to evaluation of casualties of bombings or other mass casualty events, health care providers should:

1 assess individual exposure risk by categorizing the patient into one of three exposure risk categories that are numbered sequentially:
   • Category 1: penetrating injuries or non-intact skin exposures
   • Category 2: mucous membrane exposures
   • Category 3: superficial intact skin exposures without mucous membrane
2 identify the appropriate risk category and pathogen-specific management recommendation(s)
3 determine the appropriate action to take in response to management recommendations.

Radiological contamination from "dirty bombs" has received a great deal of press attention. Screening for radiation should be considered for all potential terrorist bombings. If there is radiological contamination, although care of injuries takes precedence, patients should undergo appropriate decontamination and health care providers should wear appropriate personal protective equipment to avoid cross-contamination to themselves or others (see Volume 2, Chapter 37). These precautions also apply to potential chemical contamination. An overview of explosive-related injuries is listed in Table 32.3.

Prehospital resuscitation and treatment

Specific recommendations for tactical, military, and mass casualty scenarios will be discussed in other chapters of this text. However, some of these treatment principles do overlap. In explosive environments, there is a significant increase in the number of penetrating traumatic injuries (e.g. gunshot, fragmentary, and blast propellant wounds) [6–8]. Because of the increased complexity and number of casualties and the possibility that civilian providers may be exposed to such, additional training and knowledge of the Tactical Combat

Casualty Care (TCCC) guidelines are important for prehospital personnel. Although advanced trauma life support may be applicable to the emergency department management of trauma patients in both civilian and military hospitals, it was not created for out-of-hospital medicine. The three goals of TCCC are to treat the casualty, to prevent additional casualties, and to complete the mission, while maintaining provider safety [6,9].

Patients exposed to indoor blast are at risk of overpressure primary pulmonary blast injury. Patients with primary pulmonary blast lung are also at risk for arterial gas embolism (AGE). Gas from the damaged alveolus can pass directly into the pulmonary veins and enter the systemic circulation, leading to neurological or pulmonary compromise. Patients with potential pulmonary blast injury who rapidly decompensate after intubation should be considered to have developed AGE. Additionally, in patients with primary pulmonary blast injury, the pulmonary injury may be worsened by overaggressive fluid resuscitation. This must be balanced against the fluid needs for trauma and burn management.

Cervical spine (c-spine) injury must be considered in patients in explosive events. Tertiary injury and structural collapse are common mechanisms for injury. For rescuers, the risk of structural collapse and potential for secondary devices or other threats such as sniper fire must be weighed against the benefits of c-spine control. For patients with only penetrating injury, numerous studies have shown that high-velocity penetrating wounds do not result in occult spinal injury. If there is no clinical sign of spinal injury at the time of the initial insult, c-spine precautions do not need to be maintained in alert and awake patients [10]. For patients with blunt injury mechanisms, c-spine control should be performed when safe for the rescuer and patient.

In a mass casualty incident with blast and burn injuries, CPR should be withheld unless the injuries are the result of an electrical incident. An effort to identify and treat reversible causes (airway obstruction, tension pneumothorax, or hemorrhage) should be undertaken, after which the patient, if pulseless, may be declared dead based on local EMS protocol.

Medical oversight
Training
Practicing effective medical care in an environment involved with explosives (i.e. tactical environment) requires prehospital personnel to be well educated, trained, and equipped. Integrated "team" training allows the medical support members to understand their roles and to learn all aspects of tactical law enforcement operations and fundamentals on how to approach the tactical medical arena. Tactical competency-based guidelines have recently been published to guide the development of Tactical Emergency Medicine Support (TEMS) training curricula [11]. A project has been initiated by the Centers for Disease Control and Prevention to develop a nationally standardized curriculum for tactical medicine training.

This project, using an expert panel and review of the scientific literature, refined the previously published outcome competencies and developed terminal and enabling training objectives to the competencies [11]. In addition, training curricula have been established, such as the National Tactical Officers Association's Specialized Tactics for Operational Rescue and Medicine (STORM) for medics, operators, medical directors, and team commanders. These courses are based on the national TEMS curriculum and use the trainer methodology.

Hazardous materials
Incidents involving clandestine drug laboratories and weapons of mass destruction are also considerations in an explosive environment. Rapid decontamination must be taught and practiced by EMS teams because adequate decontamination is usually not available in the inner perimeter [12].

Forensic science
Basic knowledge of forensic science is important for recognition and preservation of evidentiary items. Documentation of wound and blood patterns should be done. All evidence should be collected appropriately and the chain of custody maintained [13].

Medical threat assessment
Medical threat assessment (MTA) is an important part of medical planning and should be integrated into operations involving response to explosive events. The MTA considers the potential medical threats that may confront the responders during EMS operations and develops the plan to mitigate and respond to the threats. Once the MTA is complete, a plan is then developed on the basis of the medical intelligence to address each possible situation, with the realization that the plan may change as the mission evolves.

Preventive medicine and force health protection
The maintenance of the EMS team's health is an important aspect of an explosive response program. Poor health has been shown to directly correlate with poor job performance and mission failure.

Liability
Because special operations lend themselves to high litigation and possible disability, EMS providers need to ensure that they have proper malpractice and disability coverage for special events.

Conclusion

Explosive injuries present a significant challenge for the medical provider. Explosives are inexpensive and easy to make and use. EMS and hospital providers need to be prepared to confront these events if they occur. Basic ATLS principles should be modified for the possibility of prolonged evacuation times to definitive medical care, as well as the limited availability of medical supplies. The basics, however, remain unchanged with airway control, restoration of effective breathing, and hemorrhage control being the highest priorities. Once the secondary survey is completed, care can be undertaken with minimal wound debridement, copious irrigation, prevention of hypothermia, and early administration of antibiotics and pain medications to decrease morbidity and mortality.

References

1 Kapur BG, Hutson HR, Davis MA, Rice PL. The United States twenty-year experience with bombing incidents: implications for terrorism preparedness and medical response. *J Trauma* 2005;59:1436–44.

2 The Boston Marathon bombings: a post-event review of the robust emergency response. *ED Manag* 2013;25:73–8.

3 Butler FK, Holcomb JB, Giebner SD, et al. Tactical combat casualty care 2007: evolving concepts and battlefield experience. *Mil Med* 2007;172: 1–19.

4 Braverman I, Wexler D, Oren M. A novel mode of infection with hepatitis B: penetrating bone fragments due to the explosion of a suicide bomber. *Isr Med Assoc J* 2002;4:525–9.

5 Recommendations for Postexposure Interventions to Prevent Infection with Hepatitis B Virus, Hepatitis C Virus, or Human Immunodeficiency Virus, and Tetanus in Persons Wounded During Bombings and Similar Mass-Casualty Events – United States, 2008. Available at: http://emergency.cdc.gov/masscasualties/blastinjury-postexposure.asp

6 Mabry R, McManus JG. Prehospital advances in the management of severe penetrating trauma. *Crit Care Med* 2008;36:S258–66.

7 Eastridge B, Mabry R, Seguin P, et al. Death on the battlefield (2001–2011): implications for the future of combat casualty care. *J Trauma Acute Care Surg* 2012;73:S431–7.

8 Jaffe DH, Peleg K, Israel Trauma Group. Terror explosive injuries: a comparison of children, adolescents, and adults. *Ann Surg* 2010;251:138–43.

9 National Association of Emergency Medical Technicians. *PHTLS: Prehospital Trauma Life Support*, 7th edn. St Louis, MO: Mosby, 2011.

10 Ramasamy A. Learning the lessons from conflict: pre-hospital cervical spine stabilisation following ballistic neck trauma. *Injury* 2009;40:1342–5.

11 Schwartz RB, McManus JG Jr, Croushorn J, et al. Tactical medicine – competency-based guidelines. *Prehosp Emerg Care* 2011;15:67–82.

12 Born CT, Briggs SM, Ciraulo DL, et al. Disasters and mass casualties: II. explosive, biologic, chemical, and nuclear agents. *J Am Acad Orthop Surg* 2007;15:461–73.

13 Carmona RH, Rasumoff D. Forensic aspects of tactical emergency medical support. *Tactical Edge* 1992;10:54.

CHAPTER 33

Thermal and chemical burns

John McManus, Richard B. Schwartz, and Sabina A. Braithwaite

Introduction

A contemporary understanding of burn injuries is essential for all out-of-hospital providers. Burn injuries carry high morbidity and mortality, resulting in severe pain, scarring, and permanent disability. Additionally, specialized resources such as burn centers are required for care and recovery.

Deaths from fires and burns are the third leading cause of fatal home injury. The US burn mortality rate ranks eighth among the 25 developed countries [1]. According to the American Burn Association National Burn Repository 2012 statistics, over 450,000 victims received medical treatment for burns in the US in the last decade [1]. The majority of these burns result from fire and/or flame injuries and contact with hot objects. Chemical burns account for approximately 3% of burns and 7% of burn admissions annually. Approximately 3,400 deaths occurred (most from smoke inhalation), including 2,550 deaths from residential fires (most from cooking), 300 from vehicle crash fires, and 550 from other sources (approximately 150 deaths from flame burns or smoke inhalation in non-residential fires, 400 from contact with electricity, scalding liquids, or hot objects). Although the number of fatalities and injuries from residential fires has declined gradually, many residential fire-related deaths remain preventable and pose a significant public health problem. Over 60% of US acute burn hospitalizations were admitted to 127 burn centers [1]. Such centers each average over 200 annual admissions for burn injury and skin disorders requiring similar treatment. The other 4,500 US acute care hospitals average fewer than three burn admissions each per year [1–4]. Fire and burn injuries represent 1% of the incidence of injuries and 2% of the total costs of injuries, or $7.5 billion each year [5]. Risk factors for burn injuries include extreme age groups (<4 years and >65 years), poverty, African and Native American descent, and rural area dwellers.

Pathophysiology

Most adults have sustained burns during their lives. The skin is the largest organ in the body and serves as a barrier to outside insults and injuries. The skin protects against water loss, entrance of undesirable substances (microorganisms, toxins), mechanical shock and forces, extreme environmental temperatures, and ultraviolet light damage to keratin and melanin. Furthermore, the skin is involved in sensory perception, temperature regulation, and biochemical activities (e.g. vitamin D synthesis).

The skin is made up of three basic layers. The outer layer, the epidermis, is the thin outer layer of the skin which consists of the stratum corneum containing fully mature keratinocytes which produce fibrous proteins (keratins) that are continuously shed (prevents the entry of most foreign substances as well as the loss of fluid from the body), the keratinocyte layer containing living keratinocytes (squamous cells), and the basal layer, the deepest layer of the epidermis, containing basal cells (continually dividing and forming new keratinocytes). The middle layer of the skin, the dermis, contains blood vessels, lymph vessels, hair follicles, sweat glands, fibroblasts, and nerves. The dermis is held together by collagen, made by fibroblasts, and gives skin flexibility and strength. The dermis also contains pain and touch receptors. The subcutis is the deepest layer of skin and consists of a network of collagen and fat cells that aid in conserving the body's heat and protect the body from injury by acting as a "shock absorber."

Severity

Accurate assessment of the burn patient and appropriate institution of early care are critical to optimal outcomes. Although burn size and depth are obvious factors in determining burn severity, the location (body part) of the burn, age of the patient,

Emergency Medical Services: Clinical Practice and Systems Oversight, Second Edition. Volume 1: Clinical Aspects of EMS.
Edited by David C. Cone, Jane H. Brice, Theodore R. Delbridge, and J. Brent Myers.
© 2015 US Government. Published 2015 by John Wiley & Sons, Inc. Companion Website: www.wiley.com\go\cone\naemsp

preexisting disease, and presence of trauma, including inhalation injury, may complicate treatment. Specific anatomical locations of burns often result in significant morbidity and mortality disproportionate to burn size (i.e. head, neck, hands, feet, perineum, and genitalia).

Furthermore, patients <2 years or >50 years old are at higher risk of complications and death than the remaining population [1]. In infants, thin skin, limited reserves, and high surface area-to-mass ratios contribute to this risk, whereas thinning skin and medical problems commonly associated with aging are major factors in older individuals. Young children are also at risk for burns caused by abuse. These injuries are most often scald burns from tap water, are deeper than those seen in the general pediatric burn population, and commonly involve the lower extremities, buttocks, and genitalia. Pediatric and elderly burns may often be an initial presentation of abuse and should be considered in the differential diagnosis.

There are several ways to classify burns (depth, severity, and surface area).

Depth

Burn depth is a product of temperature, duration of exposure, and skin thickness, with depth being described in its relationship to total skin thickness. Most burns have areas that are of mixed depth, with deeper burns often occurring in areas of thinner skin. The older classification of describing "degrees" of burn is not often used any more. Rather, the American Burn Association now uses the total body surface area and the severity (partial verses full thickness) of injury as a modern descriptor (Tables 33.1, 33.2). The old descriptive terms are paired with the newer classification system in order to understand the changes.

First-degree (superficial) burn injuries involve only the epidermis or topmost layer of skin and are recognized by their erythematous appearance and lack of blisters or skin separation.

The classic first-degree injury is the sunburn or superficial scald burn from spills. These burns usually have morbidity restricted only to pain, and are therefore not classified into burn size.

Second-degree (superficial or deep partial thickness) burn injuries involve the epidermis and part way through the dermis. Epithelial elements remain in the undestroyed dermal appendages and spontaneous healing usually occurs in 7–28 days. Second-degree burns are very painful and are usually blistered.

Third-degree (full-thickness) burn injuries are those that extend through the dermis, destroying all epidermal and dermal elements. They may initially have blisters containing hemorrhagic fluid and/or dead tissue (eschar). The presence or absence of pain is an unreliable indicator of depth and severity.

Burn size

Accurate initial assessment of burn size is essential for optimal patient care. Burn size is expressed as total body surface area (TBSA) or body surface area (BSA), where approximately 1% of a patient's surface area is equal to the palmar surface of the patient's hand with the fingers closed. This measurement is most useful for small (<5% TBSA) or spotty burns. For larger areas, the rule of nines (Figure 33.1) for adults provides a simple and rapid estimation of burn size in the adult.

When calculating burn size using any method, first-degree burns are not counted and only the proportion of area with at least a partial-thickness burn is calculated. Thus, for an upper extremity to be considered 9% TBSA, the entire extremity from the shoulder to the finger tips must be burned at least to the blistering level. If only the posterior half of the upper extremity is burned, then burn size is considered to be 4.5% TBSA.

Calculating pediatric burns is often challenging and can be inaccurate if the provider is not appropriately trained. The rule of nines (see Figure 33.1) has also been used for pediatric

Table 33.1 Classification of burns based on depth

Classification	Cause	Appearance	Sensation	Healing time	Scarring
Superficial burn	Ultraviolet light, very short flash (flame exposure)	Dry and red; blanches with pressure	Painful	3–6 days	None
Superficial partial-thickness burn	Scald (spill or splash), short flash	Blisters; moist, red and weeping; blanches with pressure	Painful to air and temperature	7–20 days	Unusual; potential pigmentary changes
Deep partial-thickness burn	Scald (spill), flame, oil, grease	Blisters (easily unroofed); wet or waxy dry; variable color (patchy to cheesy white to red); does not blanch with pressure	Perceptive of pressure only	More than 21 days	Severe (hypertrophic) risk of contracture
Full-thickness burn	Scald (immersion), flame, steam, oil, grease, chemical, high-voltage electricity	Waxy white to leathery gray to charred and black; dry and inelastic; does not blanch with pressure	Deep pressure only	Never (if the burn affects more than 2% of the total surface area of the body)	Very severe risk of contracture

Source: Data from US Army Institute of Surgical Research.

Table 33.2 American Burn Association classification of burns by total body surface area (TBSA)

Type of burn	Minor	Moderate	Major
Criteria	<10% TBSA burn in adult <5% TBSA burn in young or old <2% full-thickness burn	10–20% TBSA burn in adult 5–10% TBSA burn in young or old 2–5% full-thickness burn High-voltage injury Suspected inhalation injury Circumferential burn Concomitant medical problem predisposing the patient to infection (e.g. diabetes, sickle cell disease)	>20% TBSA burn in adult >10% TBSA burn in young or old >5% full-thickness burn High-voltage burn Known inhalation injury Any significant burn to face, eyes, ears, genitalia or joints Significant associated injuries (e.g. fracture, other major trauma)
Disposition	Outpatient management	Hospital admission	Referral to burn center

Source: Data from US Army Institute of Surgical Research and American Burn Association.

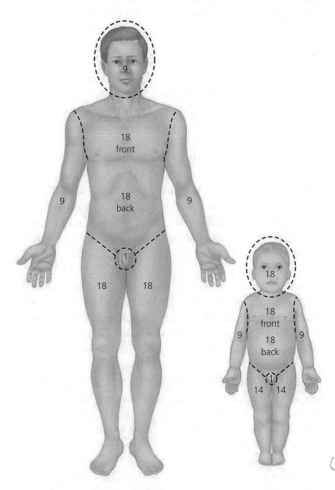

Figure 33.1 Rule of nines. Source: *Dorland's Illustrated Medical Dictionary*, 32nd edn. Philadelphia: Elsevier Saunders, 2011. Reproduced with permission of Elsevier.

patients. However, the Lund and Browder classification can also be used to more precisely calculate the percentage of BSA burned by mapping the injured areas of the body on charts detailing age-appropriate measurements. This method identifies the different body proportions according to the age of the patient (with children having larger heads and smaller lower extremities than adults) and through dividing the body into smaller units, such as dividing the upper extremity into the upper arm, lower arm, and hand. Computer programs are now being used to estimate surface area calculations.

Inhalation injury

Inhalation injury is a complex set of pathophysiological reactions that occur from exposure to smoke and/or chemical products. Systemic and respiratory damage can result in significant morbidity and mortality as well as permanent dysfunction [6,7]. When combined with thermal injury, inhalation injury increases pulmonary compliance and fluid requirements, and doubles mortality. Technically, injury is a misnomer, and inhalation injury is really the result of fluid shifts caused by external burns. These conditions do not necessarily imply pulmonary injury, because they also occur with scald and chemical burns. Edema formation in the posterior pharynx and glottic and subglottic areas associated with deep burns of the upper chest, neck, and lower face has the potential to occlude the upper airway. Tachypnea and stridor are often late signs and when absent are unreliable in ruling out airway injury.

Airway injury is diagnosed by fiberoptic bronchoscopy [8]. Early grading of inhalation injury severity is often inaccurate. The injury is basically a chemical burn from which resulting edema of the small airways creates distal microatelectasis and a clinical picture identical to acute respiratory distress syndrome. Lower airway or "smoke inhalation" injury is caused by the patient inhaling the products of combustion, often as a result of being in a confined space. Specific injuries resulting from specific toxins, cyanide and carbon monoxide, are discussed elsewhere in this text.

Chemical burn

A caustic or corrosive agent is a chemical capable of causing tissue and mucous membrane injury upon contact. These agents are generally made up of extreme pH values (<3 or >11). The

American Burn Association National Burn Repository reported in 2012 that over a 10-year period, chemicals represented 3.3% of all burns in the US [1]. The majority of these burns resulted from accidental exposure at work. Chemical burns have higher complication rates in the very young and old populations with the most common complications being cellulitis, pneumonia, and respiratory failure. Common household and industrial products that result in burns include hydrochloric acid, potassium hydroxide, sodium hydroxide, sulfuric and phosphoric acids, and many others. Hydrofluoric acid (HF) is a weak acid and requires special consideration and specific antidotes that are addressed in Volume 1, Chapter 46. Although the most commonly affected body areas are the face, eyes, and extremities, almost all fatalities are as a result of ingestion [9].

Specific training requirements

The central concepts for prehospital providers and EMS physicians caring for burn patients include the following.

1 Thorough training on a consistent, organized patient assessment algorithm that can be applied to all burn patients, regardless of injury severity, is foundational. It should provide hierarchical management that focuses on life threats, yet incorporates full, sequenced evaluation and integrated management options for actual and potential injuries. Frequent reassessments and ability to integrate information and recognize trends that require urgent intervention are essential.

2 Efficient, appropriate use of local resources (air evacuation, hazardous materials teams, specialized rescue units), and knowledge of hospital capabilities and destination policies (e.g. specialty burn care center) can improve patient outcomes in patients with significant injuries where time is of the essence. EMS systems should have policies and procedures to identify such patients and promote primary transport to the appropriate facility when available. This concept, pioneered by trauma systems, is now being extended effectively to non-trauma disease processes (see Volume 1, Chapter 26 and 39).

3 Proper use of spinal motion restriction, splinting, fluid resuscitation, and pain management to limit additional morbidity. Knowing how and when to properly use infrequent invasive procedures such as cricothyrotomy, needle thoracostomy, and escharotomy is essential for patient safety and care.

4 Recognition of a chemical exposure and proper use of protective equipment is essential in limiting exposure to bystander and health care personnel.

Burn-specific patient assessment and care

The mechanism of injury, while not entirely predictive of actual injury sustained, often alerts the astute clinician to potential injuries that may be encountered during the assessment and management of burn patients. The importance of integration of local EMS and hospital resources, and tailoring guidelines to optimize patient care within these parameters, cannot be overemphasized. Newer telemedicine applications that allow concurrent assessment by EMS and receiving emergency physicians may facilitate triage and continuity of and expedited care at the receiving facility for a number of time-sensitive medical complaints, certainly including burn injuries.

Burn management differs significantly from routine trauma care. Traumatic injuries occur in 5–15% of admitted burn patients [1]. Evaluation and treatment of traumatic injuries take precedence over treatment of the burn, with the caveat that maintenance of body temperature, airway protection, and appropriate burn fluid resuscitation must be achieved.

Distance to the destination burn or trauma center should influence the plan for airway management. If transport time is short (e.g. <10 minutes) and if able to achieve adequate oxygenation and ventilation with basic measures such as a face mask or bag-valve-mask ventilation, time should generally not be taken at the scene for endotracheal intubation (ETI), including pharmacologically assisted intubation. However, in patients with suspected inhalation injury or impending obstruction, prehospital personnel should consider immediate ETI. ETI can be particularly challenging in the burn victim due to altered mental status and/or combativeness, airway secretions or debris, and potential swelling and distortion of anatomy.

The EMS provider must decide if the delay in transport due to placing an advanced airway in a specific patient and situation is clinically beneficial, specifically if it outweighs the potential risk to the patient from either deterioration due to the injuries or due to secondary complications that could occur if the airway cannot be secured in a timely manner [10]. While orotracheal intubation is the preferred route, edema and debris in a burn patient's airway may require a cricothyrotomy to be performed as a last resort. Training EMS personnel in alternative airway techniques may be extremely useful for complicated airway management [11].

Secure the tube with cotton umbilical ribbon. Do not use adhesive tape on the endotracheal tube or any other important device or tube in the burn patient. The patient will become very edematous, the skin will fall off, and the endotracheal tube will fall out if secured only with tape. If this happens, it is very difficult to reestablish the airway due to extensive airway edema. If the patient is not intubated, closely observe for early indicators of impending airway obstruction such as facial or tongue swelling or hoarseness, and intubate the patient if these signs appear.

Careful monitoring of respiratory parameters including pulse oximetry, end-tidal carbon dioxide, ventilatory compliance, and circulation will provide trending that can alert the provider to developing complications in a critical patient [10]. High-flow oxygen should be used in all patients who show signs of respiratory distress and/or hypoxia. Beta-agonists have been used in cases of inhalation injury resulting in increased oxygen delivery and decreased bronchospasm [7]. Outcome prediction metrics based on currently available high-level non-invasive monitoring may help refine destination choices and in-hospital trauma management. Burn eschar on the chest may interfere with ventilation and if this is the case, chest escharotomy should be performed during this assessment.

Those with burn injuries have higher fluid requirements than other trauma patients [7,8,12]. However, prehospital personnel must avoid excessive fluid resuscitation that could paradoxically lead to worsening hemorrhage and/or pulmonary function. Fluid resuscitation is the cornerstone of early burn care. The microvascular structures beneath a burn wound develop increased permeability immediately after injury, resulting in capillary leakage. Capillary leak is roughly proportional to burn size and becomes hemodynamically significant in burns larger than 20% TBSA (10% TBSA in young children or elderly patients). The objective of resuscitation is to replace lost intravascular fluid with the minimal amount of fluid required to maintain normal bodily function [12].

Guidelines in the current literature instruct providers to calculate predicted 24-hour fluid requirements and initial fluid rate based on formulas (Box 33.1) [12]. Although there are multiple formulas for predicting the first 24 hours of fluid required in burn patients, two of the most advocated formulas are as follows.

- **Modified Brooke**. Initial 24 hours: no colloids. Ringer's lactated (RL) solution 2 mL/kg/% burn in adults and 3 mL/kg/% burn in children.
- **Parkland Formula**. Initial 24 hours: RL solution 4 mL/kg/% burn for adults and 3 mL/kg/% burn for children. RL solution is added for maintenance for children:
  ○ 4 mL/kg/hour for children weighing 0–10 kg
  ○ 40 mL/hour + 2 mL/hour for children weighing 10–20 kg
  ○ 60 mL/hour + 1 mL/kg/hour for children weighing 20 kg or higher.

A randomized study of adult, military burn patients comparing these two formulas demonstrated that the modified Brooke formula was successful in lowering fluid requirements without increased mortality [12]. Another burn formula to simplify fluid delivery was also advocated in prehospital patients, labeled "the rule of 10 [13]."

> **Box 33.1** Basic fluid guidelines for burn injuries
>
> - Fluid guidelines should be used in all adults and children with burns >20% total body surface area (TBSA)
> - Common formulas used to initiate resuscitation estimate a crystalloid need for 2–4 mL/kg body weight/% TBSA during the first 24 hours
> - Fluid resuscitation, regardless of solution type or estimated need, should be titrated to maintain a urine output of approximately 0.5–1.0 mL/kg/hour in adults and 1.0–1.5 mL/kg/hour in children
> - Maintenance fluids should be administered to children in addition to their calculated fluid requirements caused by injury
> - Increased volume requirements can be anticipated in patients with full-thickness injuries, inhalation injury, and a delay in resuscitation
>
> Source: Data from US Army Institute of Surgical Research.

- Estimate burn size (using the rule of nines) to the nearest 10% TBSA.
- Multiply that by 10 to calculate the initial fluid rate for patients weighing 40–80 kg.
- Increase fluid rate by 100 cc/hour for every 10 kg of body weight above 80 kg.

Underresuscitation may result in renal failure, hypotension, and multiple organ dysfunction, whereas overresuscitation results in pulmonary and cardiac overload and excessive edema formation [7,9]. The extremes of age are especially sensitive to misestimation of fluid needs. Resuscitation requires an accurate estimation of the time of burn, burn size, and measurement of patient weight. Factors that increase fluid requirements include inhalation injury, late initiation of resuscitation, deep burns, acute intoxication, and preexisting malnutrition [1].

All burn formulas are only starting points in resuscitation. Individual changes to fluid administration rates must be made hourly (or half-hourly in infants and small children) based on urine output and vital signs. The best formula is the one used by the burn center to which the patient is being transferred [13].

Regardless of the type and volume of fluid used in resuscitation of burn patients, awareness and prevention of hypothermia are essential in maintaining circulation. Hypothermia increases burn mortality. Administration of significant volumes of IV fluids at or below room temperature can exacerbate the problem. Preventing heat loss and providing warm fluids to a patient in need of volume resuscitation or rewarming can diminish this potential effect [14–16]. Several commercially available fluid warmers have been studied [17].

All wounds should be exposed for evaluation. In patients with extensive burns, overlying clothes and jewelry should be removed. These items may have melted onto the skin. If this is the case, the burn team may need to excise these items along with the burned skin. Jewelry may have to be cut off with wire cutters or similar devices. Decontamination from toxins and chemicals should also begin during this phase of assessment. Saturated clothing should be removed, powdered chemicals should be brushed off the skin, and the contaminated area(s) irrigated with copious amounts of water until the patient experiences a decrease in pain in the wound. The use of neutralizing solutions in treatment of chemical burns is not routinely recommended except for burns involving hydrogen fluoride. However, control of amount of strong neutralizing solution is the key difficulty. Chemical injuries to the eye are treated by forcing the eyelid open and flushing the eye with water or saline.

Special considerations

Compartment syndrome

Formation of edema beneath full-thickness (usually circumferential) burn eschar has the potential to occlude arterial inflow to the extremity or restrict chest motion and hence ventilation,

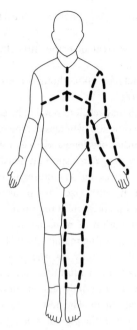

Figure 33.2 Location of escharotomy incisions. Source: US Army Institute of Surgical Research. Reproduced with permission.

resulting in respiratory failure [18]. If available, Doppler signals should be followed; if not, check pulses, skin temperature, and capillary refill at regular intervals. Diminution of the signal or a change in its character may suggest compartment syndrome. Patients receiving massive amounts of fluid may also develop compartment syndrome. This results from an increase in the tissue pressure of an inexpansible compartment of the body. If compartment syndrome is suspected, decompression of the involved compartments with appropriate escharotomy and fasciotomy is indicated as soon as possible [18]. Treatment with escharotomy may be performed in the prehospital setting with either local anesthesia or conscious sedation. Incisions are placed midaxially on the medial and lateral portions of affected extremities and on the midaxillary lines of the trunk connected by an inverted "V" (chevron) incision along the costal margins (Figure 33.2). Escharotomies of the fingers are seldom, if ever, required.

Pain management

The prehospital environment exacerbates the typical challenges found in treatment of acute pain and has the additional obstacles of a lack of supplies and equipment, delayed or prolonged evacuation times and distances, devastating injuries, provider inexperience, and dangerous tactical situations [19,20]. Studies have shown an increase in the incidence of chronic pain and posttraumatic stress disorder (PTSD) with failure to recognize and treat acute pain appropriately, as well as a reduction in PTSD incidence when pain is adequately managed, particularly with early use of ketamine [21,22].

Hydrofluoric acid burn

Hydrofluoric acid is an aqueous solution of the inorganic acid of elemental fluorine and will dissolve anything that has glass or silica content. HF and related products may cause dermal, ocular, pulmonary, gastrointestinal, and systemic injury [1]. When in contact with skin, HF dissociates into hydrogen ions and free fluoride ions. There may be a latent period before a clinically evident burn is apparent, dependent on the concentration of the acid and the length of time it is in contact with the skin. Fluoride ions penetrate tissues deeply, causing tissue damage and the potential for systemic toxicity depending on the HF concentration. In general, exposure to HF solutions of greater than 50% concentration results in immediate pain and tissue destruction. The skin appears blanched, and within 1–2 hours the dermal lines are obliterated by edema. Dermal contact with concentrations of 20–50% HF usually results in burns that develop within a few hours [8,23].

Concentrations greater than 20% HF have a potential for serious toxicity regardless of the degree of surface area involved [23]. Contact with solutions of less than 20% HF concentration results in dermal injury that usually develops within about 24 hours [24]. The clinical presentation of exposure to strong HF solutions of greater than 20% begins with pain at the site that is characteristically intense [24] and often described by patients as "burning," "deep," "throbbing," or "exquisite." Local erythema and edema may or may not be present initially, but later a pale, blanched appearance of the skin is apparent in more severe burns from concentrated HF (e.g. >50%) [8,23,24]. Extensive bullae and maceration of tissue may be seen. Gray areas may develop and progress to frank necrosis and deep ulceration within 6–24 hours.

Guidelines for out-of-hospital management

Guidelines for management of the burn patient should be focused on providing necessary interventions, together with rapid transport to the closest appropriate facility Triage guidelines should also address burn/trauma patients who need different types of specialty care by identifying regional facilities with special capabilities such as pediatric trauma, burn care, hyperbaric therapy, and extremity replantation. Scene time should not be delayed while the provider waits for direct medical oversight. Patient outcomes are significantly better at burn centers than non-burn centers [25]. Burn centers have teams of professionals dedicated to optimal burn care. The American Burn Association has established criteria for transfer of a patient to one of these centers (Box 33.2).

Requirements for transfer

Patients with major burns (>20% TBSA) require IV access, preferably two large-bore peripheral lines. Catheters may be placed through the burned tissue. Central venous access should

---

Box 33.2 American Burn Association burn center referral criteria

1 Partial thickness burns >10% total body surface area
2 Burns that involve the face, hands, feet, genitalia, perineum, or major joints
3 Third-degree burns in any age group
4 Electrical burns, including lightning injury
5 Chemical burns
6 Inhalation injury
7 Burn injury in patients with preexisting medical disorders that could complicate management, prolong recovery, or affect mortality
8 Any patients with burns and concomitant trauma, in which the burn injury poses the greatest risk of morbidity or mortality. In such cases, if the trauma poses the greater immediate risk, the patient may be initially stabilized in a trauma center before being transferred to a burn unit
9 Burned children in hospitals without qualified personnel or equipment for the care of children
10 Burn injury in patients who will require special social, emotional, or long-term rehabilitative intervention

Source: Adapted from *Guidelines for the Operation of Burn Centers. Resources for Optimal Care of the Injured Patient.* Chicago: Committee on Trauma, American College of Surgeons, 2006, pp.79–86.

Box 33.3 Burn injury prevention

Flame burn prevention	Test smoke detectors regularly
	Create an escape plan for the home, and practice it
	Safety device around fireplace and stoves
	Keep matches, lighters away from children
Scald prevention	Use splash guards on stove
	Lower hot water heater maximum temperature to <54°C
	Use thermometer for bath water

Source: Data from US Army Institute of Surgical Research.

---

be avoided because of its high complication rate in the early postburn period when vasospasm, low flow, and a hypercoagulable state contribute to complications. A urinary catheter and a nasogastric tube are recommended for long or delayed transport. Use of ice on a burn wound is absolutely contraindicated because of the risk of a cold injury superposed on the burn. Continual efforts must be made to keep the patient warm. No burn debridement is required before transfer, and the burns should be wrapped in dry sterile or clean sheets or burn-specific water-based gel dressings, and further covered with warm blankets.

Prevention

The prehospital environment offers a unique "teachable moment" for clinicians to educate patients and their families about preventing burns in the future. Prevention programs and safety legislation have made substantial contributions to decreasing the incidence and severity of burn injury, especially for parents and school-age children.

In addition, several initiatives are targeting vulnerable segments of the population for prevention efforts. Mothers with less than high school education who are younger than 20 years and have more than two children are at a much higher risk for fatal fire events [1]. Although prevention initiatives are reaching increasing numbers of people, there is still the need for further education of the public and in particular those subsegments of the population at high risk for burn injury. Specific preventive recommendations are listed in Box 33.3.

References

1 American Burn Association. 2012 National Burn Repository Report of Data from 2002–2011. Available at: www.ameriburn.org/2012NBRAnnualReport.pdf

2 Ahrens M. *Home Structure Fires*. Quincy, MA: National Fire Protection Association, 2011.

3 Karter MJ. *Fire Loss in the United States During 2010*. Quincy, MA: National Fire Protection Association, Fire Analysis and Research Division, 2011.

4 Centers for Disease Control. *Fire Deaths and Injuries Fact Sheet*. Available at: www.cdc.gov/homeandrecreationalsafety/fire-prevention/fires-factsheet.html

5 Corso P, Finkelstein E, Miller T, Fiebelkorn I, Zaloshnja E. Incidence and lifetime costs of injuries in the United States. *Inj Prev* 2006;12(4):212–18.

6 Palmieri TL. Inhalation injury: research progress and needs. *J Burn Care Res* 2007;28:549–54.

7 Colohan SM. Predicting prognosis in thermal burns with associated inhalational injury: a systematic review of prognostic factors in adult burn victims. *J Burn Care Res* 2010;31:529–39.

8 Shirani KZ, Pruitt BA Jr, Mason AD Jr. The influence of inhalation injury and pneumonia on burn mortality. *Ann Surg* 1987;205:82–7.

9 Stuke LE, Arnoldo BD, Hunt JL, Purdue GF. Hydrofluoric acid burns: a 15-year experience. *J Burn Care Res* 2008;29:893–6.

10 Wang HE, Kupas DF, Hostler D, Cooney R, Yealy DM, Lave JR. Procedural experience with out-of-hospital endotracheal intubation. *Crit Care Med* 2005;33:1718–21.

11 Kurola JO, Turunen MJ, Laakso J, et al. A comparison of the laryngeal tube and bag-valve mask ventilation by emergency medical technicians: a feasibility study in anesthetized patients. *Anesth Analg* 2005;101:1477–81.

12 Chung KK, Wolf SE, Cancio LC, et al. Resuscitation of severely burned military casualties: fluid begets more fluid. *J Trauma* 2009;67:231–7.

13 Chung KK, Salinas J, Renz EM, et al. Simple derivation of the initial fluid rate for the resuscitation of severely burned adult combat casualties: in silico validation of the rule of 10. *J Trauma* 2010;69:S49–54.

14 Hildebrand F, Giannoudis PV, van Griensven M, Chawda M, Pape HC. Pathophysiologic changes and effects of hypothermia on outcome in elective surgery and trauma patients. *Am J Surg* 2004;187:363–71.

15 Mizushima Y, Wang P, Cioffi WG, Bland KI, Chaudry IH. Should normothermia be restored and maintained during resuscitation after trauma and hemorrhage? *J Trauma* 2000;48:58–65.

16 Segers MJ, Diephuis JC, van Kesteren RG, van der Werken C. Hypothermia in trauma patients. *Unfallchirurg* 1998;101(10):742–9.

17 Dubick MA, Brooks DE, Macaitis JM, Bice TG, Moreau AR, Holcomb JB. Evaluation of commercially available fluid-warming devices for use in forward surgical and combat areas. *Mil Med* 2005;170:76–82.

18 Kupas DF, Miller DD. Out-of-hospital chest escharotomy: a case series and procedure review. *Prehosp Emerg Care* 2010;14:349–54.

19 Black I, McManus JG. Pain management in current combat operations. *Prehosp Emerg Care* 2009;13:223–7.

20 Wedmore IS, Johnson T, Czarnik J, Hendrix S. Pain management in the wilderness and operational setting. *Emerg Med Clin North Am* 2005;23:585–601.

21 Otis JD, Keane TM, Kerns RD. An examination of the relationship between chronic pain and post-traumatic stress disorder. *J Rehabil Res Dev* 2003;40:397–405.

22 McGhee LL, Maani CV, Garza TH, Gaylord KM, Black IH. The correlation between ketamine and posttraumatic stress disorder in burned service members. *J Trauma* 2008;64:S195–8.

23 Seyb ST, Noordhoek L, Botens S, Mani MM. A study to determine the efficacy of treatments for hydrofluoric acid burns. *J Burn Care Rehabil* 1995;16:253–7.

24 Centers for Disease Control and Prevention. *Hydrogen Fluoride Systemic Agent*. Available at: www.cdc.gov/niosh/ershdb/Emergency ResponseCard_29750030.html

25 Holmes JH 4th, Carter JE, Neff LP, et al. The effectiveness of regionalized burn care: an analysis of 6,873 burn admissions in North Carolina from 2000 to 2007. *J Am Coll Surg* 2011;212:487–93.

CHAPTER 34

Crush injury

Ken Miller

Definition and concepts

Crush injury is the anatomical injury associated with direct trauma due to a compressive force. Extended entrapment with compression may cause crush syndrome, traumatic rhabdomyolysis, or compartment syndrome. *Crush syndrome* is the systemic manifestation of skeletal muscle injury from extended compression. Crush injury-induced traumatic rhabdomyolysis is one form of rhabdomyolysis; however, prolonged immobilization of an individual against a surface (e.g. due to altered level of consciousness) and agitated delirium can cause rhabdomyolysis without external trauma. *Compartment syndrome* is the increase in pressure within a fascial compartment eventually compromising venous outflow then arteriolar inflow with progressive capillary leak and edema leading to skeletal muscle injury that can progress to rhabdomyolysis. All three of these clinical entities may be encountered by EMS physicians, potentially in the same patient.

Pathophysiology of crush injuries

The systemic manifestations of crush syndrome are due to ischemia/reperfusion injury of skeletal muscle and the intense local and systemic inflammatory response due to the physiological, biochemical, and immunological changes that accompany the ischemic and reperfusion periods [1]. Ischemia/reperfusion injury is encountered in EMS practice in acute stroke, head injury, myocardial infarction, and crush injury with crush syndrome. Reactive oxygen species and activated neutrophils are the main contributors to local and systemic effects of ischemia reperfusion. Oxygen is the substrate initiating this response and is provided upon reperfusion. All tissue is sensitive to ischemia reperfusion but skeletal muscle injury can cause major systemic complications.

From the EMS perspective, the critical factors placing a patient at risk of crush syndrome are mass of muscle injured and ischemia time. The critical muscle mass necessary to put an entrapped patient at risk for crush syndrome is poorly defined, but qualitatively requires more than that of a hand or foot. Critical ischemia time is better defined but variable. At body temperature, critical ischemia time (the maximum time a tissue can tolerate ischemia and remain viable) of skeletal muscle is 4 hours [2]. However, critical ischemia time can be shorter when direct trauma is the cause of ischemia rather than just vascular occlusion.

The compression-stretch myopathy and ischemia of crush injury with muscle compression result in sarcolemma membrane leak and the release of myoglobin, urate, potassium, and phosphate out of muscle cells. Water, calcium, and sodium leak into muscle cells. Fluid and electrolyte shifts, myoglobinuria, and hyperkalemia then contribute to the systemic manifestations of crush syndrome after muscle compression is relieved and perfusion is reestablished. Large volumes of intravascular fluid shift into the injured muscle, leading to hypovolemia and hypotension. Hyperkalemia and metabolic acids cause brady-dysrhythmias and reduced cardiac output while uric acid from muscle purines and myoglobin cause acute renal injury. From a clinical management perspective, the early consequences of crush syndrome are hypovolemia, hyperkalemia, and metabolic acidosis and the late consequence is acute renal failure due to myoglobinia and uricosuria.

Clinical setting

Because the compression-stretch myopathy and reperfusion injury of crush injury that goes on to become crush syndrome requires muscle compression of the order of hours rather than minutes, the clinical setting of EMS patients in which crush syndrome is to be suspected will be somewhat unique. Mostly these patients will be entrapped in some way, requiring disentanglement and extrication involving technical rescue, or may require a search operation before extrication is possible. In single-patient or small multicasualty incidents this may involve traffic collisions, industrial, construction or machinery incidents,

Emergency Medical Services: Clinical Practice and Systems Oversight, Second Edition. Volume 1: Clinical Aspects of EMS.
Edited by David C. Cone, Jane H. Brice, Theodore R. Delbridge, and J. Brent Myers.
© 2015 NAEMSP. Published 2015 by John Wiley & Sons, Inc. Companion Website: www.wiley.com\go\cone\naemsp

explosions, structural collapse, debris flows, and below-grade or confined space entrapments.

Although the critical mass of skeletal muscle necessary to cause the systemic effects of crush syndrome is uncertain, the clinical setting would likely involve entrapment of an extremity, possibly as far as the shoulder, hip, or gluteus. Torso compression associated with traumatic asphyxia would be rapidly fatal.

In the large multicasualty or mass casualty/disaster setting, crush syndrome is associated with structural collapse due to earthquakes, floods, tornadoes, hurricane/tropical cyclones, or events of war. Because substantial time might pass before survivors are found in search operations following a disaster, crush syndrome can be a major contributor to delayed morbidity and mortality. Crush syndrome that leads to acute renal failure has been reported to be the second most frequent cause of mortality following disasters, after direct trauma [3–5].

Management of crush injury

The field management of crush injury will depend upon the immediacy of disentanglement and extrication, extent of the anatomical injury, access to and availability of definitive health care infrastructure, transport time, number of casualties, scope of practice of field EMS providers, and availability of advanced field EMS response resources.

Fundamentally, treatment begins with control of external hemorrhage and stabilization of orthopedic and soft tissue injuries following stabilization of the airway, assisted ventilation, and decompression of a tension pneumothorax as needed. Early and effective hemorrhage control can be life-saving.

Following external hemorrhage control, stabilization of the soft tissue and orthopedic injuries through dressings and splinting will contribute to reducing any further injury during patient movement and to pain control. These interventions should not, however, independently delay transport to definitive trauma care, especially when the crush injury is part of other multisystem trauma.

Pain management is both therapeutic and humanitarian during EMS operations. The operational use of analgesics in EMS is defined by two principal considerations: the analgesics available within the scope of practice of the EMS provider, and the spectrum of adverse effects as they relate to the patient and to the rescue environment. Opiates are a common and effective analgesic widely available within EMS practice. In the rescue environment one important consideration is respiratory depression. Access to and management of the airway may be limited during disentanglement and extrication of an entrapped patient, so escalating doses of opiates and their associated effect of respiratory depression must be considered. When scope of practice or availability of advanced EMS responders allows, adjunctive ketamine can be useful during EMS rescue operations. Ketamine in subanesthetic doses (0.1–0.2 mg/kg intravenous or intraosseous) as an adjunct to opiates can reduce the dose of opiates

needed to achieve the degree of analgesia required to improve patient comfort and tolerance of movement necessary during the rescue evolution.

During mass casualty/disaster operations, patient evacuation to definitive care can be delayed by hours or days. If there are open soft tissue injuries or open fractures, empirical antimicrobial therapy can be given. Literature on infection prevention, morbidity, and mortality following crush injury in disasters is lacking but pending clinical evidence, it is reasonable to administer intravenous or intramuscular antistaphylococcal antibiotics, and tetanus toxoid or tetanus immune globulin if those resources are available. Of note, soft tissue injuries with heavy soil contamination (e.g. injuries from tornado debris) have resulted in fungal infections and soft tissue injuries following improvised explosive devices with cross-contamination from bone and tissue of other persons will require HIV, HBV, and HCV prophylaxis and postinjury surveillance.

During the field care of a rescued entrapped survivor, an extremity crush injury may begin to show signs of compartment syndrome. Compartment pressure measurement may not be practical, and the classic signs of pulselessness, pallor, paresthesia, paralysis, and pain out of proportion to injury are all late signs. If compartment syndrome is clinically suspected in association with crush injury in the mass casualty/disaster setting based upon mechanism of injury and pain on passive movement of a distal digit, the therapeutic decision is between adequate and monitored fluid resuscitation and field fasciotomy. Given the absence of outcome data on field fasciotomy and the risk of infection, nerve and other iatrogenic injury, it is likely better to address fluid resuscitation requirements and keep the affected extremity at heart level than to perform a field fasciotomy.

Management of crush injury with suspected crush syndrome

When extremity entrapment has been of the order of hours or longer, treatment extends to the prevention of morbidity and mortality from two additional mechanisms: sudden hypotension and cardiovascular collapse upon extrication, and late renal failure. In the individual patient or multicasualty setting, the duration of entrapment that puts the patient at risk for sudden hypotension and cardiopulmonary arrest has not been well established but traumatic rhabdomyolysis has been reported to occur in less than 1 hour [6]. Myoglobinuric acute renal failure following rhabdomyolysis has been reported to occur in up to 33% of cases and to account for up to 50% of fatalities [7], and was prevalent following the earthquakes in Armenia, China, and Turkey [8]. Morbidity and mortality from immediate postextrication hypovolemia and hyperkalemia as well as late myoglobinuric acute renal failure can be reduced through field interventions.

When crush syndrome is clinically suspected during the management of crush injury, based upon time of entrapment and mass of skeletal muscle compressed, the principal intervention is intravascular fluid resuscitation [7]. Substantial fluid shifts from the intravascular compartment to the interstitial and intracellular compartments during entrapment can result in a precipitous drop in blood pressure following disentanglement and release of the compressing force. A reduction in cardiac output can result from hypovolemia as well as dysrhythmias from hyperkalemia and metabolic acidosis when the injured extremity is reperfused. In single-patient or multicasualty incidents involving crush injury, access to the vascular space will be intravenous or intraosseous. Intraosseous vascular access will have to be in an ipsilateral or contralateral largely uninjured extremity. Proximal and distal long bone as well as manubrium access sites may be limited by local scopes of practice. If advanced practice EMS providers or EMS physicians are available, as well as during mass casualty/disaster events, then central venous access as well as hypodermoclysis (with or without hyaluronidase) may become options for intravascular volume resuscitation.

From a medical logistics perspective, intravenous and intraosseous fluid resuscitation in the rescue environment is probably best done using intermittent bolus infusions. Depending upon the patient's physical position and confinement during entrapment, it may not be practical to hang intravenous solutions to be delivered by gravity, and intravenous infusion pumps may not be available. Pressure infusion bags are a consideration but are difficult to control. Additionally, there may be technical rescue operations going on in close proximity to the patient and intravenous lines, monitoring cables, and oxygen tubing are prone to cutting and dislodgment. Medical and rescue personnel will need to coordinate operations to keep the rescue effort moving. Well-coordinated drug and intravenous fluid bolus therapy along with interval patient assessment will help to optimize patient care as well as rescue operations.

When intravenous or intraosseous vascular access is impossible and central venous access and hypodermoclysis are unavailable, then applying an arterial tourniquet close to the time of disentanglement and release of the compressing force may prevent sudden fluid and electrolyte shifts. Literature on the safety and efficacy of arterial tourniquets for this purpose is lacking, but they should be applied at any point when hemorrhage uncontrolled by other means is part of the problem.

The endpoint of intravascular resuscitation is more difficult to define. Conceptually the goal is to maintain cerebral, coronary, and renal blood flow during the compartmental fluid shifts and/or hemorrhage associated with crush injury, crush syndrome, and extremity reperfusion. The difficulty is defining field-expedient measurable endpoints that reflect those goals. Currently heart rate and heart rate trends, target systolic blood pressure, and presence of pulse oximetry waveforms and measurements of waveform quality from digital capillary beds are practical measureable endpoints in EMS practice. Patient access may be limited if entrapment includes confined space operations. It is also conceivable to monitor urine output, or at least obtain a colorimetric measurement of urine specific gravity if that equipment is available.

Further confounding decision making regarding intravenous fluid resuscitation of a crush injury patient is the concomitant occurrence of head injury, blunt and/or penetrating multisystem trauma, or underlying illness such as chronic heart failure or renal disease. The goal of maintaining end-organ perfusion is favorable when head injury and crush syndrome occur together. However, the strategy of permissive hypotension in penetrating trauma, and perhaps in blunt trauma as well, is in direct conflict with the strategy of intravascular fluid resuscitation for crush syndrome. Evidence-based composite endpoints for systolic blood pressure or other vital signs and fluid resuscitation in the comorbidities of head injury with penetrating or blunt trauma associated with crush syndrome have not been established.

The other intra- and postrescue short-term risk in crush syndrome is hyperkalemia. Whether hyperkalemia evolves during the extrication or is a consequence of limb reperfusion following disentanglement and removal of the compressing force, it can result in bradydysrhythmias and, along with postextrication hypovolemia, contribute to sudden death. Therapeutic options for hyperkalemia will depend upon scopes of practice and availability of medical resources during the rescue.

Maintaining perfusion with intravenous volume resuscitation is the essential therapy. A second generally available strategy is empirical treatment of metabolic acidosis or blood alkalinization using intravenous or intraosseous sodium bicarbonate (e.g. 1 mEq/kg intermittent bolus therapy every few hours). Although field-expedient point-of-care blood analyzers are available, measurement of acid-base parameters is usually limited to specialized medical resources that may not be part of the initial response. Another strategy would be to add 50–100 mEq of sodium bicarbonate to 1 liter of 0.45% sodium chloride, making it approximately isotonic, and use that solution for intravenous fluid replacement. Better goal-directed therapy would be possible if a point-of-care blood analyzer were available, or with continuous or intermittent ECG precordial lead V1 and V2 monitoring for T-wave shape and amplitude; however ECG monitoring for hyperkalemia lacks sensitivity and specificity [9]. Hypotension in spite of intravenous volume resuscitation accompanied by atrioventricular block, tachycardia or bradycardia, or wide QRS complex ('sine wave' ECG appearance) would usually require intravenous or intraosseous administration of calcium chloride or calcium gluconate; however, in the setting of skeletal muscle crush syndrome, calcium is taken up by the injured muscle, making it difficult to raise blood calcium levels, and can aggravate the calcium-dependent apoptosis of myocytes [7].

Another generally available treatment for hyperkalemia is inhaled beta$_2$-agonists like albuterol (e.g. 5 mg every few hours). Atmospheric monitoring and ventilation are important considerations if the rescue involves confined space operations and oxygen is used to drive a nebulizer. Compressed air (breathing air quality) is an alternative to oxygen if hypoxia by pulse oximetry is not present, and is more likely to be a renewable resource in the mass casualty/disaster setting. When available, a very effective treatment of hyperkalemia is intravenous or intraosseous glucose and regular insulin. This therapy requires frequent monitoring of blood glucose.

Late morbidity and mortality from crush injury and crush syndrome can have many causes including sepsis, brain injury, and organ system failure from multisystem trauma. However, myoglobinuric acute renal failure can be prevented or can be reversed by renal replacement therapy (peritoneal dialysis, hemofiltration, or hemodialysis) when fluid resuscitation is begun prior to disentanglement and extrication [7]. Early intravenous or intraosseous fluid resuscitation is the mainstay of treatment, along with empirical sodium bicarbonate to alkalinize the urine to protect the kidneys from the nephrotoxic effects of myoglobin and uric acid. When used early, mannitol, as both an osmotic agent and a polyalcohol free radical scavenger, can be nephroprotective by reducing interstitial fluid volume and muscle compartment pressure, thereby reducing release of myoglobin and purines, and by maintaining renal perfusion [10]. Mannitol can be given alone (e.g. 0.5 g/kg of a 20% solution) or 20–30 g of mannitol and 50–100 mEq of sodium bicarbonate added to 1 L of 0.45% sodium chloride to be given as an infusion or intermittent boluses.

Transport destination considerations

Even in the absence of multisystem trauma, the potential for complex soft tissue, orthopedic, nerve, and vascular injuries resulting from crush injuries makes a designated trauma center the preferred acute care destination. Designated trauma centers will have access to the specialties of plastic and reconstructive surgery, microvascular surgery, and orthopedic surgery as well as critical care, nephrology, and infectious disease consultants. Depending on local standards of care, isolated extremity injury involving crush injury, compartment syndrome, or crush syndrome could be definitively managed at non-trauma-designated hospitals with access to specialty surgical and medical services, or could be stabilized and transferred to a referral hospital. Other than multisystem trauma and head injury, time-sensitive injuries associated with crush injury include uncontrollable external hemorrhage, vascular disruption or occlusion requiring surgical or interventional radiology vascular repair, and compartment syndrome requiring fasciotomy. Hyperbaric oxygen therapy has been used as part of the management of microvascular surgical repair of muscle flaps, partial traumatic amputations, vascular and ischemic muscle injury but its efficacy has only been demonstrated in skin grafts and flaps and chronic ischemic ulcers in patients with diabetes [11]. Hospital destination determination should be based on the availability of surgical and critical care resources rather than the availability of hyperbaric oxygen therapy.

References

1 Gillani S, Cao J, Suzuki T, Hak DJ. The effects of ischemia reperfusion injury on skeletal muscle. *Injury* 2012;43:670–5.

2 Chafin B, Belmont MJ, Quraishi H, et al. Effects of clamp versus anastomotic-induced ischemia on critical ischemic time and survival of rat epigastric fasciocutaneous flap. *Head Neck* 1999;21:198–203.

3 Sever MS, Lameire N, Vanholder R. Renal disaster relief: from theory to practice. *Nephrol Dial Transplant* 2009;24:730–5.

4 Van der Tol A, Hussain A, Sever MS, et al. Impact of local circumstances on outcome of renal casualties in major disasters. *Nephrol Dial Transplant* 2009;24:907–12.

5 Vanholder R, van der Tol A, de Smet M, et al. Earthquakes and crush syndrome casualties: lessons learned from the Kashmir disaster. *Kidney Int* 2007;71:17–23.

6 Agu O, Ackroyd J. Crush syndrome after isolated abdominal crush injury in flood water. *J Trauma* 2002;53:378–9.

7 Better OS, Abassi ZA. Early fluid resuscitation in patients with rhabdomyolysis. *Nat Rev Nephrol* 2011;7:416–22.

8 Portilla D, Shaffer RN, Okusa MD, et al. Lessons from Haiti on disaster relief. *Clin J Am Soc Nephrol* 2010;5:2122–9.

9 Montague BT, Ouellette JR, Buller GK. Retrospective review of the frequency of ECG changes in hyperkalemia. *Clin J Am Soc Nephrol* 2008;3:324–30.

10 Better OS, Rubinstein I, Reis DN. Muscle crush compartment syndrome: fulminant local edema with threatening systemic effects. *Kidney Int* 2003;63:1155–7.

11 Rowe K. Hyperbaric oxygen therapy: what is the case for its use? *J Wound Care* 2001;10:117.

CHAPTER 35

Hemorrhage control

Neil B. Davids and Robert L. Mabry

Introduction

Uncontrolled hemorrhage is the second leading cause of death in the civilian trauma setting [1] and the leading cause of preventable death during armed conflict [2,3]. Traditional methods of hemorrhage control in the prehospital setting were simple dressings, direct pressure, proximal arterial pressure points, elevation of bleeding extremities, and, as a last resort, a tourniquet. These measures are essentially the same as those used in antiquity [4]. Recent military and civilian experiences, as well as technological advances, have made new hemorrhage control tools available to both civilian and military out-of-hospital personnel.

Advances in civilian trauma care have often occurred secondary to military conflict. Because hemorrhage is the leading cause of potentially survivable death on the battlefield, researchers and physicians have focused intensely on prehospital management of severe hemorrhage. Within the past 10 years, significant advances have included several hemostatic dressings, ready-to-use tourniquets, and improved training in their use [5]. Some of these experiences have directly translated into saved lives in the civilian setting as well [6].

Death from compressible hemorrhage is rare in civilian settings [7], being, in most instances, entirely preventable with simple first aid measures [8]. Most civilian patients with severe hemorrhage can be rapidly transported to urban or suburban trauma centers while direct pressure is applied by a prehospital provider to an isolated injury. Hemorrhage control techniques commonly used by the military on the battlefield, such as tourniquets and advanced hemostatic agents, may have a role in EMS systems likely to encounter delayed patient transport, such as the rural and wilderness setting, prolonged extraction from a collapsed structure, enclosed space, or wrecked vehicle, and mass casualty incidents (MCI). This is particularly important in a scenario of mass shootings or deliberate bombings, where penetrating injury is the most common pattern and approximates battlefield situations.

Assessment

Traumatic hemorrhage is the acute loss of circulating blood volume as a result of injury [9]. Hemorrhage severity is largely predicated on the volume of blood lost before hemostatic control can be achieved. This volume will vary as a function of vessel defect, vessel size, type, and location. Large defects result in not only greater bleeding but also greater consumption of clotting factors and platelets, increasing the likelihood of coagulopathy. Brisk, pulsatile bleeding and the bright red hue of oxygenated blood identify arterial hemorrhage. Arterial bleeding control will require the application of pressure sufficient to overcome the systolic blood pressure and compress the muscular wall of the vessel. Constant pressure for 20 or more minutes may be required to stop arterial bleeding. Venous bleeding is non-pulsatile, may be brisk if the vessel is large, and may appear darker until exposed to oxygen. Venous bleeding will occlude at much lower pressures, will require less time to control, and is more amenable to the use of hemostatic agents than arterial bleeding. Capillary bleeding is usually much less brisk than arterial or venous bleeding due to the smaller size of the involved vessels but may be difficult to control if the patient has platelet dysfunction or clotting factor deficiency.

Diagnosis of hemorrhagic shock

Hemorrhagic shock is a failure of the cardiovascular system to deliver oxygen and nutrients to tissues due to blood loss and hypovolemia. Hemorrhagic shock recognition has often depended on abnormalities of vital signs, appearance of the

Emergency Medical Services: Clinical Practice and Systems Oversight, Second Edition. Volume 1: Clinical Aspects of EMS.
Edited by David C. Cone, Jane H. Brice, Theodore R. Delbridge, and J. Brent Myers.
© 2015 US Government. Published 2015 by John Wiley & Sons, Inc. Companion Website: www.wiley.com\go\cone\naemsp

skin, urine output, and mental status [10]. Although providing the basis of shock recognition and assessment, these metrics are limited by a number of important factors. Physiological response in patients on antihypertensives and other pharmacological agents is often blunted. Healthy patients in good physical condition may have sufficient physiological reserves to delay alterations in heart rate, blood pressure, and respiratory rate even with significant blood loss [11]. Urine output can rarely be assessed in the prehospital environment and mental status, while sensitive to hypotension due to blood loss, can be clouded by concomitant head trauma, intoxication, hypoglycemia, pain medications, or mental illness.

Alternative predictors of the severity of shock include the pulse pressure or shock index, both of which can be calculated from traditional vital signs. Pulse pressure is the difference between systolic and diastolic blood pressures. Use of pulse pressure in trauma is based on the principle that hemorrhage will increase the systemic vascular resistance, thus increasing diastolic pressure. At the same time, decreased preload will subsequently produce a reduction in systolic pressure. Narrowing of pulse pressure occurs before significant decreases in systolic blood pressure. Dynamic changes in pulse pressure have been used as a marker for cardiac output and volume status [12,13]. Shock index is calculated by dividing the heart rate by the systolic blood pressure and has been shown to be more sensitive than either of the vital signs alone. Shock index predicts shock states in multiple trauma patients and is predictive of complications once patients are admitted to the hospital [14]. It can also be adjusted to compensate for age-related differences in physiology, especially in the elderly [15].

Serum lactate measurements may identify hypoperfusion; however, this is a late finding and may not be useful in a prehospital setting [16,17]. Point-of-care testing of serum lactate, however, may be useful during long transports.

A novel method for measuring and diagnosing shock is tissue oxygen saturation (which can be measured peripherally); however, it is still undergoing evaluation. Early laboratory studies show it to be an earlier marker than standard vital signs [18,19]. Heart rate variability measurements are able to predict mortality but do not perform better than other common indices, and may not be the best for evaluation of hemorrhagic shock [20]. Sublingual capnography theoretically recognizes local tissue hypoxia and microcirculatory injury, but recent studies suggest it is not present earlier than standard vital signs [21].

Treatment modalities

Pressure

Applying direct pressure to stop bleeding from a wound is one of the most ancient principles of first aid. Steady, firm pressure using gauze or a large dressing (such as an abdominal pad) directly onto the bleeding site remains the method of choice to control hemorrhage in the civilian prehospital setting. The

dressing must be of sufficient thickness so as not to diffuse or reduce the pressure applied to the site of hemorrhage. Once applied, pressure should be continued until the patient arrives at definitive care and is transferred to hospital personnel. The wound should not be periodically examined to see if the bleeding is stopped while en route, as this will result in disruption of the clot and rebleeding. Application of direct pressure requires the full attention of one provider.

If there are multiple casualties or the provider is unable to apply continuous pressure, a pressure dressing may be applied. Pressure dressings are effective and reliable for controlling hemorrhage. They can be fabricated with materials at hand, such as elastic bandages and cravats, or with ready-made commercial dressings [22]. When applying a pressure dressing, the principles are essentially the same as when applying direct pressure. A large pledget of gauze should be applied directly to the wound and compressed with an elastic bandage or cravat. Pressure, not the dressing material itself, is the most important part of attaining hemostasis.

Tourniquets

If pressure fails to control hemorrhage from an extremity injury, a tourniquet should be applied (Figure 35.1). Initially used to curtail bleeding during amputation, the tourniquet was brought to the battlefield in 1674 [4]. Controversy and debate about the appropriateness and circumstances of tourniquet use began soon after and have continued through the current US conflicts in Iraq and Afghanistan [23].

During the Vietnam conflict, Rich described only one case of limb loss secondary to tourniquet use among thousands of casualties with vascular injuries, and Hutton reported that fasciotomies were sometimes needed when tourniquet times were in excess of 2 hours [24].

Over the course of the last decade, the controversy over tourniquet safety and effectiveness has subsided, with almost universal acceptance in severe extremity bleeding or amputation. Every US soldier and Marine carries a tourniquet, and it is used frequently on the battlefield. The most recent review of

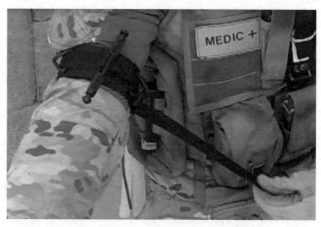

Figure 35.1 The SOF-T tourniquet. Source: www.health.mil/tccc

military use has shown that tourniquets are safe, effective, and have contributed to a significant reduction in deaths from extremity hemorrhage [25,26]. See Video Clip 35.1 for application of a tourniquet.

Civilian prehospital studies evaluating tourniquet safety and effectiveness are lacking. Severe peripheral vascular injures are relatively rare in the civilian setting and transport times to medical facilities are usually rapid. In most instances, civilian EMS providers can maintain continuous direct pressure on a bleeding injury until the patient arrives at the hospital. If direct pressure fails, a tourniquet should be applied. Tourniquets may be useful in MCIs related to explosive blasts, terrorism, or criminal violence. In these cases, there will often be more casualties than skilled providers, and evacuation from the scene may be delayed due to tactical concerns or because of collapsed and unstable structures. This was borne out during the Boston Marathon bombing in 2013. Based on bomb placement, a significant number of lower extremity injuries occurred. Early anecdotal reports conclude that the use of tourniquets (mostly field expedient) saved lives [6]. The American College of Surgeons and the FBI consensus statement (the "Hartford Consensus") recommended tourniquets for life-threatening bleeding from extremity wounds during mass shooting scenarios [27]. The Active Shooter Law Enforcement Rapid Response Training (ALERRT) Center, recognized by the FBI as the national training standard for active shooter response, also recommends the use of tourniquets for extremity hemorrhage.

As tourniquet use became the norm in a combat environment and extremity hemorrhage decreased as a cause of death, control of junctional hemorrhage (hemorrhage in potentially compressible areas not amenable to a standard tourniquet) could be initiated in the prehospital environment [28]. Preliminary research into junctional tourniquets (initially, the Combat Ready Clamp in 2010; Figure 35.2) demonstrated their effectiveness [29,30] and ongoing studies into other potential junctional tourniquet devices continue. See Video Clip 35.2 for application of the Combat Ready Clamp.

The abdominal aortic tourniquet, a device inflated over the abdomen with enough pressure to compress the abdominal aorta, is under investigation. A preliminary study demonstrated effectiveness in human volunteers where an abdominal tourniquet was used to reduce common femoral artery flow; however, it was extremely uncomfortable for the volunteers [31]. Anecdotal evidence in the lay press suggests it may be useful and trials of this device are being conducted with selected groups of military personnel in Afghanistan [32].

Rapid wound closure

Suturing and surgical stapling are common methods for hemorrhage control, but usually require time and clean fields. A novel device, recently introduced in the literature, the IT Clamp (Innovative Trauma Care, San Antonio, TX) looks like a hair clip and uses the teeth of the clip to grasp each side of the wound

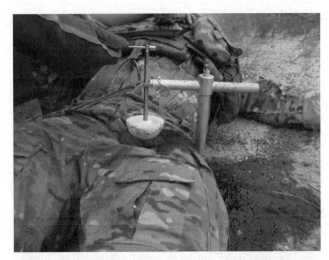

Figure 35.2 The Combat Ready Clamp. Source: www.health.mil/tccc

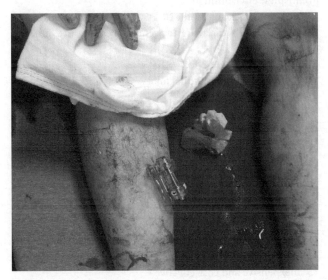

Figure 35.3 The IT Clamp. Source: Dr. John Holcomb

while the clamp portion closes over the wound, approximating the edges and allowing a hematoma to form to serve as a pressure dressing (Figure 35.3). An early study shows that it provides hemostasis in a swine groin injury model compared to standard gauze [33].

Elevation and arterial pressure points are no longer recommended as hemorrhage control methods because of insufficient evidence supporting their use [34].

Internal occlusion

Another potential method for controlling hemorrhage that is being evaluated is the concept of reverse endovascular balloon occlusion of the aorta (REBOA). A balloon catheter is placed through the femoral artery into the aorta and inflated, occluding distal flow and stopping any bleeding distally, which could be extremely important in non-compressible bleeding, such as pelvic fractures. This technique, which effectively becomes an "endovascular thoracotomy," has proven effective in a surgical and hospital setting, and in swine studies provides up to 90 minutes of occlusion without complications [35,36]. Recently, researchers have demonstrated that the catheter can be placed in a prehospital setting [37], providing a potential opportunity to use this method for uncompressible hemorrhage not amenable to other techniques in a prehospital environment [38].

Advanced hemostatic agents

Advanced hemostatic products to control bleeding have been developed for the prehospital environment. Ideally, a hemostatic agent would have the following properties for a prehospital environment.

1 Approved or cleared by the US Food and Drug Administration
2 Stops severe arterial and/or venous bleeding in 2 minutes or less
3 No toxicity or side-effect
4 Causes no pain or thermal injury
5 Poses no risk to medics
6 Ready to use with little or no training
7 Durable and lightweight
8 Flexible enough to fit complex wounds and easily removed without leaving residues
9 Stable and functional at extreme temperatures (-10°C to +40°C) for at least 2 weeks
10 Practical and easy to use under austere conditions (low visibility, rain, wind, etc.)
11 Effective on junctional wounds not amendable to tourniquet
12 Long shelf-life (>2 years)
13 Inexpensive and cost-effective
14 Biodegradable and bioabsorbable [39]

Numerous hemostatic agents have emerged into the marketplace in the last decade and this overview of hemostatic agents is not all-inclusive. Medical directors and EMS purchasing agents should become thoroughly familiar with the vast, confusing, and often contradictory literature regarding hemostatic agents before deciding to add them to their systems.

First generation
Zeolite

QuikClot (QC; Z-Medica, Wallingford, CT) is a granular zeolite powder that is FDA approved for external application in hemorrhage. QuikClot concentrates platelets, red blood cells, and clotting factors at the wound site through rapid adsorption of water. The reaction generates a significant amount of heat ranging from 68°C to 140°C [40]. Initial studies demonstrated effectiveness in a large animal model with lethal groin injury; however, the injuries in these studies were different from those in follow-on studies and when

compared against the more severe model (6 mm femoral arteriotomy), Quikclot failed to provide hemostasis [39]. QC was initially fielded as a granular powder, but difficulty with application and the potential to be washed away by bleeding prompted a repackaging in gauze bags [41]. Concerns with heat generation have led to a newer product called QuikClot ACS+ that uses synthetic zeolite beads in a cotton bag that produce minimal exothermic reaction [42].

Second generation
Celox

Celox (Medtrade Biopolymers, Crewe, UK) is a chitosan-based agent based on a proprietary granular mixture of different chitosan forms. Celox's primary mechanism is similar to that of chitosan in that it is mediated by a mixture of chemical and mechanical (adherence) linkages to red blood cells and tissues which form a physical barrier around the severed vessels [39]. According to the manufacturer, this mechanism is not dependent on the coagulation factors of the patient. Celox is placed on top of a wound in a powder form, leading to the potential to be washed away if not secured to the wound. Attempts to place Celox in a gauze-like bag have been unsuccessful [43]. In a comparison with other agents, it was shown to be inferior to Combat Gauze [44].

Combat Gauze

Created by Z-Medica, Combat Gauze is an FDA-approved hemostatic agent consisting of ordinary cotton rolled gauze impregnated with kaolin, a fine clay-like material used in some antidiarrheal preparations. Kaolin appears to be a potent activator of the intrinsic clotting pathway, inducing the patient's own clotting factors to produce a clot. In a comparison between several other hemostatic dressings, including HemeCon and Celox-D, Combat Gauze proved to be the most effective and safest agent [43]. This lead to Combat Gauze being recommended by the Tactical Combat Casualty Care Committee (the US military's lead agency in guidelines for treatment of wounded service members) as the solitary hemostatic agent in 2009. Combat Gauze also has other factors that make it desirable as a hemostatic agent, including low cost, ease of use, and strong safety profile. See Video Clip 35.3 for application of Combat Gauze to a wound.

Third generation
Celox-XG

Celox-XG Gauze (XG, SAM Medical Products, Wilsonville, OR) is also a chitosan-based product; however, instead of a powder, Celox-XG is a rolled fabric made with non-woven chitosan-derived hemostatic fibers. It works on the same principle as Celox but is much easier to apply than the powder form. It is the standard hemostatic agent for the United Kingdom military in Afghanistan.

In one study, although outcomes were similar, Celox-XG did have shorter clot time than CG or standard gauze [45]. In a more recent study, a comparison of CG, XG, and standard gauze showed less secondary blood loss and faster packing times for XG, but no differences in outcomes [46]. The benefits of Celox-XG are comparable to Combat Gauze, including ease of use and strong safety profile.

Adjunctive therapy

Permissive hypotension
Many studies suggest that limiting prehospital resuscitation protocols to achieve mean arterial pressures in the 60s may improve outcome over standard therapy designed to maintain systolic blood pressures of 100 [47,48]. This "permissive hypotension" is thought to be sufficient to provide adequate perfusion to vital organs without exacerbating bleeding through clot dislodgment or dilution of clotting factors. Multiple studies have shown that permissive hypotension is also beneficial by limiting exposure to crystalloids and fractionated blood products. Crystalloid fluids have been demonstrated to dilute clotting factors and induce inflammatory cascades, which may result in increased hemorrhage and decreased survival [49]. Current Tactical Combat Casualty Care guidelines for the US military also reflect this concept of giving colloid fluids only if there is a weak or absent peripheral pulse or altered mental status.

Prevention of hypothermia
Moderate and severe hypothermia (body temperature of less than 32 °C) inhibit coagulation and contribute to ongoing hemorrhage. Hypothermia reduces the enzymatic activity of coagulation proteins and inhibits the activation of platelets. Dysfunction of the coagulation system is evident below temperatures of 35 °C, and temperatures below 30 °C result in a 50% reduction in platelet function [50]. As part of the "lethal triad" of trauma (acidosis, hypothermia, coagulopathy), it can be avoided by using warmed fluids if possible and using blankets to keep patients warm, especially for longer transports. There are several commercially available hypothermia prevention kits.

Transfusion
Treatment with blood products in the prehospital environment is currently limited to specialized teams and air medical providers [51]. There are trials of using blood product transfusion (plasma and packed red cells) from point of injury care for the US military in Afghanistan, and thus far there have been no known transfusion reactions [52]. Most prehospital providers resuscitate with uncross-matched packed red blood cells, which lack platelets and clotting factors, which may support hemorrhage control. Recent studies of patients requiring massive transfusions have demonstrated that transfusion of platelets and plasma in conjunction with packed cells leads to better hemostatic control, decreased transfusion volumes, and greater survival. Military providers use whole blood before definitive hemorrhage control for similar reasons. Patients with life-threatening hemorrhage should be transfused before or during transport when blood products are available. Although cross-matched blood products are preferable, uncross-matched blood is often all that is available in emergency circumstances.

Freeze-dried plasma (commonly referred to as lyophilized plasma) was originally developed in the United States during World War II. Falling out of favor in the US, it continued to be used successfully by the French military (with some interruption due to HIV transmission concerns) [53]. Use of lyophilized plasma in a prehospital setting would be advantageous in several scenarios, such as MCIs, long transports, or remote locations where access to other blood products might be difficult.

Medications
Recombinant factor VIIA (Novoseven)
Factor VIIa is part of the extrinsic pathway in the coagulation cascade and initiates thrombin generation (activated factor Xa). It is licensed for the treatment of hemophilia patients with antibodies to factor VIII but is also used for the treatment of trauma victims with life-threatening hemorrhage [54]. Boffard demonstrated that administration of factor VIIa reduced the need for packed red blood cell (PRBC) transfusion and massive transfusion in severely bleeding blunt trauma patients [55]. Factor VIIa has not been demonstrated to reduce mortality or critical complications. Furthermore, it has been linked to complications including increased incidence of adult respiratory distress syndrome and is exceptionally expensive. In a more recent Cochrane review, the recommendation was that factor VIIa be used only in its FDA-approved indications unless under a study protocol [56].

Tranexamic acid (TXA)
Intravenous administration of TXA was approved by the FDA in 1986 for prevention or reduction of bleeding in hemophilia patients undergoing dental procedures. Its mechanism of action is an antifibrinolytic that inhibits both plasminogen activation and plasmin activity, thus preventing clot breakdown rather than promoting new clot formation. In the CRASH-2 study, trauma patients were given TXA or placebo with a small but significant reduction in all-cause and bleeding mortality, with the highest improvements in those given TXA in the first 3 hours and in the most severely injured subgroups, as well as a very low incidence of harm [57]. Studies in a combat environment showed similar benefits [58]. Given its low cost, low incidence of adverse events, and importance of early administration, TXA administration may become a useful prehospital intervention.

Conclusion

Uncontrolled hemorrhage is a leading cause of preventable death. Direct pressure remains the primary treatment for hemorrhage and is sufficient for most wounds. Patients who fail management with direct pressure require immediate hemorrhage control. Extremity wounds can be controlled with tourniquets, while advanced hemostatic agents can treat wounds of the trunk and neck, and those in cavities. These agents are now capable of stopping even brisk arterial bleeding and have been shown to improve patient survival. In situations of prolonged transport time or austere environments, consideration should be given to adjunctive therapies such as hypotensive resuscitation, maintenance of euthermia, and transfusion of blood and blood products to address coagulopathy. As has been proven in recent mass casualty incidents such as the Boston Marathon bombing, EMS providers must be prepared to deal with exsanguinating hemorrhage on multiple patients that can parallel battlefield scenarios.

References

1 Sauaia A, Moore FA, Moore EE, et al. Epidemiology of trauma deaths: a reassessment. *J Trauma* 1995;38:185–93.

2 Eastridge BJ, Mabry RL, Seguin P, et al. Death on the battlefield (2001-2011): implications for the future of combat casualty care. *J Trauma Acute Care Surg* 2012;73:S431–7.

3 Bellamy RF. The cause of death in conventional land warfare: implications for combat casualty care research. *Mil Med* 1984; 149:55–62.

4 Schwartz AM. The historical development of methods of hemostasis. *Surgery* 1958;44:604–10.

5 Butler FK Jr, Blackbourne LH. Battlefield trauma care then and now: a decade of Tactical Combat Casualty Care. *J Trauma Acute Care Surg* 2012;73:S395-402.

6 Caterson EJ, Carty MJ, Weaver MJ, Holt EF. Boston bombings: a surgical view of lessons learned from combat casualty care and the applicability to Boston's terrorist attack. *J Craniofac Surg* 2013;24:1061–7.

7 Dorlac WC, DeBakey ME, Holcomb JB, et al. Mortality from isolated civilian penetrating extremity injury. *J Trauma* 2005;59:217–22.

8 Rocko M, Tischler C, Swan KG. Exsanguination in public – a preventable death. *J Trauma* 1982;22:635.

9 American College of Surgeons Committee on Trauma. *Advanced Trauma Life Support Student Course Manual*, 7th edn. Chicago, IL: American College of Surgeons, 2004, p.73.

10 American College of Surgeons Committee on Trauma. *Advanced Trauma Life Support Student Course Manual*, 7th edn. Chicago, IL: American College of Surgeons, 2004, p.74.

11 Zarzaur BL, Croce MA, Fischer PE, Magnotti LJ, Fabian TC. New vitals after injury: shock index for the young and age x shock index for the old. *J Surg Res* 2008;147:229–36.

12 Victorino G, Battistella FD, Wisner DH. Does tachycardia correlate with hypotension after trauma? *J Amer Coll Surg* 2003;196:679–84.

13 Convertino VA, Ryan KL, Rickards CA, et al. Physiological and medical monitoring for en route care of combat casualties. *J Trauma* 2008;64:S342–53.

14 Cannon CM, Braxton CC, Kling-Smith M, Mahnken JD, Carlton E, Moncure M. Utility of the shock index in predicting mortality in traumatically injured patients. *J Trauma* 2009;67:1426–30.

15 Zarzaur BL, Croce MA, Fischer PE, Magnotti LJ, Fabian TC. New vitals after injury: shock index for the young and age x shock index for the old. *J Surg Res* 2008;147:229–36.

16 Cerovic O, Golubovic V, Spec-Marn A, Kremzar B, Vidmar G. Relationship between injury severity and lactate levels in severely injured patients. *Intensive Care Med* 2003;29:1300–5.

17 Pestel GJ, Fukui K, Kimberger O, Hager H, Kurz A, Hiltebrand LB. Hemodynamic parameters change earlier than tissue oxygen tension in hemorrhage. *J Surg Res* 2010;160:288–93.

18 Jones N, Terblanche M. Tissue saturation measurement – exciting prospects, but standardisation and reference data still needed. *Crit Care* 2010;14:169.

19 Soller BR, Zou F, Ryan KL, Rickards CA, Wark K, Convertino VA. Lightweight noninvasive trauma monitor for early indication of central hypovolemia and tissue acidosis: a review. *J Trauma Acute Care Surg* 2012;73:S106–11.

20 Ryan KL, Rickards CA, Ludwig DA, Convertino VA. Tracking central hypovolemia with ECG in humans: cautions for the use of heart period variability in patient monitoring. *Shock* 2010;33:583–9.

21 Chung KK, Ryan KL, Rickards CA, et al. Progressive reduction in central blood volume is not detected by sublingual capnography. *Shock* 2012;37:586–91.

22 Naimer DS, Tanami M, Malichi A, Moryosef D. Control of traumatic wound bleeding by compression with a compact elastic adhesive dressing. *Mil Med* 2006;171:644–7.

23 Mabry RL. Tourniquet use on the battlefield. *Mil Med* 2006;171:352–6.

24 Welling DR, Burris DG, Hutton JE, Minken SL, Rich NM. A balanced approach to tourniquet use: lessons learned and relearned. *J Am Coll Surg* 2006;203:106–15.

25 Kragh JF Jr, Littrel ML, Jones JA, et al. Battle casualty survival with emergency tourniquet use to stop limb bleeding. *J Emerg Med* 2011;41(6):590–7.

26 Kragh JF Jr, O'Neill ML, Walters TJ, et al. Minor morbidity with emergency tourniquet use to stop bleeding in severe limb trauma: research, history, and reconciling advocates and abolitionists. *Mil Med* 2011;176:817–23.

27 Jacobs LM, McSwain NE Jr, Rotondo M, et al. Improving survival from active shooter events: the Hartford Consensus. *J Trauma Acute Care Surg* 2013;74:1399–400.

28 Eastridge BJ, Hardin M, Cantrell J, et al. Died of wounds on the battlefield: causation and implications for improving combat casualty care. *J Trauma* 2011;71:S4–8.

29 Kragh JF Jr, Murphy C, Dubick MA, Baer DG, Johnson J, Blackbourne LH. New tourniquet device concepts for battlefield hemorrhage control. *US Army Med Dep J* 2011;Apr-Jun:38–48.

30 Kragh JF Jr, Murphy C, Steinbaugh J, et al. Prehospital emergency inguinal clamp controls hemorrhage in cadaver model. *Mil Med* 2013;178:799–805.

31 Lyon M, Shiver SA, Greenfield EM, et al. Use of a novel abdominal aortic tourniquet to reduce or eliminate flow in the common femoral artery in human subjects. *J Trauma Acute Care Surg* 2012;73:S103–5.

32 McCloskey M. 'Game changer:' Tourniquet for abdominal wounds is already saving lives. *Stars and Stripes*. Available at: www.stripes.com/news/game-changer-tourniquet-for-abdominal-wounds-is-already-saving-lives-1.235791

33 Filips D, Logsetty S, Tan J, Atkinson I, Mottet K. The iTClamp controls junctional bleeding in a lethal swine exsanguination model. *Prehosp Emerg Care* 2013;17:526–32.

34 Markenson D, Ferguson JD, Chameides L, et al. Part 17: first aid: 2010 American Heart Association and American Red Cross guidelines for first aid. *Circulation* 2010;122:S934–46.

35 Gupta BK, Khaneja SC, Flores L, Eastlick L, Longmore W, Shaftan GW. The role of intra-aortic balloon occlusion in penetrating abdominal trauma. *J Trauma* 1989;29:861–5.

36 Stannard A, Eliason JL, Rasmussen TE. Resuscitative endovascular balloon occlusion of the aorta (REBOA) as an adjunct for hemorrhagic shock. *J Trauma* 2011;71:1869–72.

37 Manning JE. Feasibility of blind aortic catheter placement in the prehospital environment to guide resuscitation in cardiac arrest. *J Trauma Acute Care Surg* 2013;75:S173–7.

38 True NA, Siler S, Manning JE. Endovascular resuscitation techniques for severe hemorrhagic shock and traumatic arrest in the presurgical setting. *J Spec Oper Med* 2013;13:33–7.

39 Kheirabadi, B. Evaluation of topical hemostatic agents for combat wound treatment. *US Army Med Dep J* 2011;Apr-Jun:25–37.

40 Pusateri AE, Delgado AV, Dick EJ Jr, Martinez RS, Holcomb JB, Ryan KL. Application of a granular mineral-based hemo-static agent (QuikClot) to reduce blood loss after grade V liver injury in swine. *J Trauma* 2004;57:555–62.

41 Arnaud F, Tomori T, Saito R, McKeague A, Prusaczyk WK, McCarron RM. Comparative efficacy of granular and bagged formulations of the hemostatic agent QuickClot. *J Trauma* 2007;63:775–83.

42 Arnaud F, Tomori T, Carr W, et al. Exothermic reaction in zeolite hemostatic dressings: QuikClot and ACS+. *Ann Biomed Eng* 2008;36:1708–13.

43 Kheirabadi BS, Scherer MR, Estep JS, Dubik MA, Holcomb JB. Determination of efficacy of new hemostatic dressings in a model of extremity arterial hemorrhage in swine. *J Trauma* 2009;67:450–9.

44 Gerlach T, Grayson JK, Pichakron KO, et al. Preliminary study of the effects of smectite granules (WoundStat) on vascular repair and wound healing in a swine survival model. *J Trauma* 2010;69:1203–9.

45 Watters JM, Van PY, Hamilton GJ, Sambasivan C, Differding JA, Schreiber MA. Advanced hemostatic dressings are not superior to gauze for care under fire scenarios. *J Trauma* 2011;70:1413–19.

46 Kunio NR, Riha GM, Watson KM, Differding JA, Schreiber MA, Watters JM. Chitosan based advanced hemostatic dressing is associated with decreased blood loss in a swine uncontrolled hemorrhage model. *Am J Surg* 2013;205:505–10.

47 Duke MD, Guidry C, Guice J, et al. Restrictive fluid resuscitation in combination with damage control resuscitation: time for adaptation. *J Trauma Acute Care Surg* 2012;73:674–8.

48 Bickell WH, Wall MJ Jr, Pepe PE, et al. Immediate versus delayed fluid resuscitation for hypotensive patients with penetrating torso injuries. *N Engl J Med* 1994;331;1105–9.

49 Hussmann B, Lefering R, Taeger G, Waydhas C, Ruchholtz S, Sven Lendemans and the DGU Trauma Registry. Influence of prehospital fluid resuscitation on patients with multiple injuries in hemorrhagic shock in patients from the DGU trauma registry. *J Emerg Trauma Shock* 2011;4:465–71.

50 DeLoughery T. Coagulation defects in trauma patients: etiology, recognition, and therapy. *Crit Care Clin* 2004;20:13–24.

51 Barkana Y, Stein M, Maor R, Lynn M, Eldad A. Prehospital blood transfusion in prolonged evacuation. *J Trauma* 1999;46:176–80.

52 Malsby RF 3rd, Quesada J, Powell-Dunford N, et al. Prehospital blood product transfusion by U.S. Army MEDEVAC during combat operations in Afghanistan: a process improvement initiative. *Mil Med* 2013;178:785–91.

53 Sailliol A, Martinaud C, Cap AP, et al. The evolving role of lyophi-lized plasma in remote damage control resuscitation in the French Armed Forces Health Service. *Transfusion* 2013;53:65S–71S.

54 Barletta JF, Ahrens CL, Tyburski JG, Wilson RF. A review of recombinant factor VII for refractory bleeding in nonhemophilic trauma patients. *J Trauma* 2005;58:646–51.

55 Boffard KD, Riou B, Warren B, et al. Recombinant factor VIIa as adjunctive therapy for bleeding control in severely injured trauma patients: two parallel randomized, placebo-controlled, double-blind clinical trials. *J Trauma* 2005;59:8–18.

56 Stanworth SJ, Birchall J, Doree CJ, Hyde C. Recombinant factor VIIa for the prevention and treatment of bleeding in patients without haemophilia. *Cochrane Database Syst Rev* 2007;2:CD005011.

57 CRASH-2 Collaborators. Effects of tranexamic acid on death, vascular occlusive events, and blood transfusion in trauma patients with significant haemorrhage (CRASH-2): a randomised, placebo-controlled trial. *Lancet* 2010;376:23–32.

58 Morrison JJ, Dubose JJ, Rasmussen TE, Midwinter, MJ. Military application of tranexamic acid in trauma emergency resuscitation (MATTERs) study. *Arch Surg* 2012;147:113–19.

CHAPTER 36

Orthopedic injuries

Sean Kivlehan, Benjamin T. Friedman, and Mary P. Mercer

Introduction

Epidemiology

Trauma is the leading cause of death worldwide and in the United States for people under the age of 44 [1]. Blunt trauma from motor vehicle accidents, falls, or other mechanisms can result in a range of orthopedic injuries. Recognition and management of orthopedic injuries is an essential component of any EMS system.

General approach to management

The prehospital management of a suspected orthopedic injury begins with assessment of potential life threats. Obtaining a history that includes the mechanism of injury is important to develop an index of suspicion for associated injuries. Prehospital providers should first assess and address the airway, breathing, circulation, and disability of any injured patient. Once the primary survey is complete, an orthopedic evaluation is part of a comprehensive secondary survey. Open fractures and injuries with neurovascular compromise require special attention. Acute hemorrhage control is the first priority for the open fracture in the field and can generally be accomplished with direct pressure. Any exposed bone should be dressed with a sterile saline moistened dressing. The decision to reduce a fracture or dislocation in the field is situation dependent, and should be based on presence of neurovascular compromise, anticipated extrication and transport duration, and provider training and experience [2]. Pain management is an important component of the prehospital care for any orthopedic injury and should ideally be addressed prior to moving the patient to the ambulance. Pain management modalities include immobilization of the affected limb and intravenous opiates [3,4].

Anatomy, fractures, and dislocations

Upper extremity

Upper extremity neurovascular exam

For all upper extremity injuries, both nerve function and vascular patency must be assessed early and repeated frequently,

particularly after any manipulation, splinting, or patient movement. The radial, ulnar, and median nerves should be assessed for both motor and sensory function in all injuries. The axillary and musculocutaneous nerves should be assessed in more proximal injuries (Table 36.1). The vascular exam consists of palpating both the radial and ulnar pulses as well as the brachial artery in more proximal injuries. For injuries distal to the wrist, nailbed capillary refill should be assessed.

Clavicle

Clavicular fractures are generally uncomplicated and can be managed in the field with sling and swathe placement (Table 36.2). Assessment should include a complete neurovascular exam of the limb on the affected side as there is a risk of damage to the underlying subclavian vessels and brachial plexus as well as possibility of pneumothorax.

The clavicular articulations to the sternum (sternoclavicular [SC] joint) and acromion (acromioclavicular [AC] joint) should be assessed as well. AC joint injury can be diagnosed clinically and should be managed with a sling and swathe in the field. SC joint injuries most commonly occur as a result of vehicle accidents or sports injuries and are divided into less serious anterior dislocations and more serious posterior dislocations. While field treatment for both is immobilization, prehospital providers should have a heightened index of suspicion for serious intrathoracic injury with a posterior dislocation, in particular pneumothorax, great vessel injury, and tracheal injury [5].

Scapula

A patient with a scapular fracture will generally present protecting the arm on the affected side and with local tenderness. Management consists of sling and swathe placement and analgesia. Up to 75% of patients with scapular fractures will have additional injuries due to the significant mechanism of injury. Providers should carefully examine the patient for rib fractures, pneumothorax, or upper arm injuries [6].

Emergency Medical Services: Clinical Practice and Systems Oversight, Second Edition. Volume 1: Clinical Aspects of EMS.
Edited by David C. Cone, Jane H. Brice, Theodore R. Delbridge, and J. Brent Myers.
© 2015 NAEMSP. Published 2015 by John Wiley & Sons, Inc. Companion Website: www.wiley.com\go\cone\naemsp

Table 36.1 Upper extremity neurological examination

Nerve	Motor	Sensory
Radial	Wrist or finger extension	First dorsal web space
Ulnar	Index finger abduction	Pinky finger
Median	Thumb and index finger opposition	Index finger
Axillary	Deltoid	Lateral shoulder
Musculocutaneous	Elbow flexion	Lateral forearm

Table 36.2 Upper extremity immobilization approach

Bone	Approach
Clavicle, scapula, shoulder	Sling and swathe
Humerus	Sling and swathe, short board
Elbow	Short board A-splint (bent) or straight with short boards
Forearm	Short board with sling
Wrist, hand	Short board or pillow in position of function with sling
Finger	Malleable metal splint or tongue depressor with buddy splinting

Short or long board splints are generally interchangeable with air or vacuum splints.

Shoulder

Glenohumeral joint dislocations are the most common major joint dislocation encountered, and are generally the result of an indirect blow with the arm in abduction, extension, and external rotation [7]. Anterior dislocations are the most common and can be identified clinically in the field with some reliability. In general, the patient will present guarding the affected arm with mild abduction and external rotation. Posterior dislocations are rare, usually the result of a mechanism of injury such as a seizure, electrical shock, or direct anterior blow to the shoulder, and while carrying a similar associated fracture rate they are less likely to have neurovascular injury. Inferior and superior dislocations are even less common.

When examining a suspected shoulder dislocation, close attention should be paid to the axillary nerve. Vascular injuries are rare but when they do occur, will generally involve the axillary artery [8]. Associated fractures occur in 15–35% of shoulder dislocations and can include the humeral head (Hill–Sachs lesion), anterior glenoid lip, and greater tuberosity. Although these fractures generally do not change management, prereduction x-rays are recommended, and field reduction should typically not be attempted [9]. There are exceptions to this rule, in particular for patients with known recurrent dislocations and athletes on the field with appropriately trained staff [10,11]. Providers should splint the extremity in the position found with a sling and swathe. A short board splint can be placed along the medial upper arm for extra stability, particularly in the presence of a suspected humeral head fracture [9]. In the event of a spontaneous reduction, providers should still splint and transport, as radiographs and follow-up will be needed.

Rotator cuff injuries may be associated with shoulder dislocations or may present independently. Complete evaluation of the rotator cuff could become more commonplace prehospital practice, particularly within a community paramedicine setting. However, no validated rules currently exist to exclude fracture or dislocation, and a patient with an acute shoulder injury would likely benefit from transport to the hospital [9].

Humerus

Fractures of the humerus can be divided into three categories: proximal, midshaft, and distal. Axillary nerve and artery injuries have been recognized in up to 50% of displaced humeral fractures. Humeral shaft injuries are most common in active young men and elderly osteoporotic patients and can be associated with radial nerve injuries or vascular injuries to the brachial artery or vein [7]. Field management is the same as for other shoulder injuries.

Elbow

The elbow joint is composed of the articulations of the distal humerus, proximal radius, and ulna. The brachial artery and the nerves of the forearm and hand travel in close proximity. It is the third most commonly dislocated joint after the shoulder and knee. Supracondylar fractures are among the most common fractures in children [12]. The primary fracture patterns in adults include flexion and extension, the latter being more common. The majority of elbow dislocations (90%) are posterolateral, with the mechanism of injury being fall on an outstretched hand. Commonly associated neurovascular injuries include entrapment of the ulnar nerve and the brachial artery [13].

It is difficult to differentiate an elbow fracture from a dislocation in the field without x-rays, and as such, it is recommended that EMS providers splint all suspected fractures or dislocations in the position found. However, gentle reduction is recommended in a severely angulated fracture or one with significant neurovascular compromise. If reduction is attempted, the elbow then should be splinted at 90° with the forearm in supination with a posterior moldable splint and a sling and swathe placed.

Forearm

While the unique fracture and dislocation patterns of the forearm are of interest to the emergency physician in determining definitive management, they are less important to the prehospital provider. Field management involves splinting with a posterior mold or short boards in the position found. Indications for attempted field reduction are similar to other fractures, although neurovascular compromise in these fractures is less common than in injuries of the humerus or elbow. Fractures to the proximal ulnar, olecranon, and radius are treated similarly to other fractures and dislocations about the elbow.

Wrist

Fractures of the distal radius and ulna are the most common wrist fractures, followed by the carpal bones, notably the scaphoid and triquetrum [14]. Distal forearm fractures should be immobilized in the position of function, if tolerated, or the position found. Carpal fractures can be immobilized in either a short board or commercial wrist splint. Once splinted, the extremity may be placed in a sling and swathe to further reduce movement. Distal neurovascular assessment should be documented. EMS providers may be trained to assess for snuff box tenderness to assist in identifying potential scaphoid fractures [15]. Carpal ligamentous injury frequently occurs in conjunction with bony injury and should be splinted similarly based on physical exam findings of tenderness.

Hand/fingers

Hand and finger injuries are rarely life threatening but can be emotionally disturbing to the patient and provider. Once attention is appropriately turned to the hand injury, function of the median, radial, and ulnar nerves should be assessed as previously outlined. Vascular status can be assessed through capillary refill, which should be less than 2 seconds. Flexor and extensor tendon function should be tested in each finger and compared between hands.

Fractures and dislocations of the phalanx should be splinted as found, and buddy taping can be used to stabilize the finger itself prior to placing the affected hand in a wrist or short board splint. Field reduction may be appropriate in some situations. However, ideally the patient should be transported to the emergency department for a peripheral nerve block prior to reduction. Case reports do exist of successful paramedic performance of a digital block and subsequent reduction, and this is a potential future expansion of practice [16]. While metacarpal fracture management and follow-up vary depending on radiographic findings and patient activity, field management is unchanged and involves splinting. One hand injury that deserves special mention is the high-pressure injection injury, which always requires transport to the ED for evaluation and possible surgical intervention [17].

Pelvis

Although pelvic fractures are relatively rare among orthopedic injuries, they are associated with high mortality (10–15%) due to both the presence of concurrent severe traumatic injuries and the pathophysiology of unstable pelvic fractures [18]. The most common mechanisms associated with pelvic fractures involve the transmission of significant amounts of force such as through high-speed motor vehicle collisions, pedestrians hit by automobiles, or significant falls [19].

Anterior-posterior compressive forces are often associated with the highest degree of hemodynamic instability and mortality [19]. Such fractures cause significant disruption to the pelvic ring, resulting in widening of the pelvis, tearing of the iliac ligaments and shear force injuries of the iliac vessels.

The predominantly venous hemorrhage spills into the retroperitoneum and expanded pelvic cylinder. If left uncontrolled, this hemorrhage can be fatal due to the large potential space of the unstable pelvic vault.

Pelvic injury should be suspected in any patient with significant traumatic injuries of the head, spine, thorax, abdomen, or multiple extremities. Signs of shock should raise suspicion of an unstable pelvic fracture in patients without outward signs of fracture. Other signs and symptoms of pelvic fractures may include perineal or flank hematoma, or blood at the penile meatus or vaginal introitus. Obvious bony instability of the pelvis with light palpation is a clear finding of pelvic fracture. However, the absence of external findings does not exclude the presence of an unstable pelvic fracture [20]. The examiner may gently compress the pelvis to test for stability, but caution is advised, as this may exacerbate an unstable fracture or concomitant bleeding.

Clinical management of the suspected pelvic fracture, as with other major trauma, includes immobilization and rapid transport to a trauma center. Given the risk of vascular and hemodynamic compromise, vital signs and distal neurovascular status should be monitored closely during transport. In addition to general immobilization techniques, use of a pelvic binder may be indicated. Whether it is a commercial product or an improvised sheet, the principle behind the use of a pelvic binder is to reduce the potential space of the pelvis and to tamponade the associated venous bleeding. Epidemiological and biometric data suggest that the application of a pelvic binder reduces mortality [21]. Although routinely used in prehospital care in the past, there is a theoretical concern for worsening of vascular injury and hemorrhage due to vessel laceration by bony fragments. Therefore, care should be taken when applying a binder.

Lower extremity
Lower extremity neurovascular exam

Similar to the upper extremity, a thorough lower extremity neurovascular exam should be completed and documented before and after any intervention or patient movement. The tibial, sural, superficial peroneal, and deep peroneal nerves should be assessed for both motor and sensory function. The femoral and obturator nerves should be assessed when there is concern for pelvic and hip fractures (Table 36.3). The vascular exam involves palpation of the popliteal, dorsal pedal, and posterior tibial pulses.

Hip

Hip fractures are common, accounting for more than 300,000 hospitalizations per year in the United States [22]. Age and sex are major risk factors: 80% of hip fractures occur in patients aged 75 or over, and nearly three out of every four patients are female [23]. More than 90% of hip fractures are due to elderly falls but may also result from high-energy trauma (such as from a motor vehicle collision) [24]. Classically, patients present with pain, and shortening and external rotation of the affected limb [25]. However, these findings can be inconsistent depending on the anatomical location of the fracture.

Table 36.3 Lower extremity neurological examination

Nerve	Motor	Sensory
Tibial	Toe flexion	Plantar foot surface
Sural	N/A	Posterolateral calf and foot
Superficial peroneal	Ankle eversion	Dorsal foot surface
Deep peroneal	Ankle dorsiflexion	First dorsal web space
Femoral	Knee extension	Anterior thigh and knee
Obturator	Hip adduction	Medial thigh

Table 36.4 Lower extremity immobilization approach

Bone	Approach
Hip	Backboard or long board splints, pillows
Femur	Traction splint
Knee	Short board A-splint (bent) or long board splints (straight)
Tibia, fibula	Long board splints
Ankle, foot	Pillow splint
Toe	Buddy taping

Short or long board splints are generally interchangeable with air or vacuum splints.

Prehospital providers should rely on their standard trauma assessments to assess injuries to the hip. As a large amount of force is needed to fracture a hip in younger patients, concomitant injuries are found in 40–75% of cases [26]. Among the elderly, providers should evaluate for precipitating factors, other fall-related injuries, and conditions related to delays in accessing care. Depending on patient condition, further prehospital management could include general orthopedic trauma care, appropriate splinting (Table 36.4), and aggressive analgesia as tolerated. While it is possible to provide skin traction using a commercial device for hip fractures, a 2011 Cochrane review found no benefit from preoperative traction of any sort [27].

Hip joints are inherently stable. Dislocations are generally caused by high-energy trauma, most often motor vehicle crashes. The force required to dislocate a hip is so great that 95% of these patients will have other major injuries as well [28]. Ninety percent of hip dislocations are posterior dislocations of the femoral head, while the remaining 10% are either anterior or medial (associated with acetabular fractures) [29]. Patients will most commonly complain of severe hip pain and limb deformity in the setting of a significant mechanism of injury.

Due to the high rate of concomitant injuries, prehospital providers should generally approach those with suspected hip dislocations as major trauma patients. The focus of care should be on prompt packaging and transport, as these patients have significantly increased rates of serious neurovascular complications if the dislocation is not reduced within 6 hours [30]. However, appropriate splinting and analgesia should not be ignored.

Femur

As with hip dislocations, femoral shaft fractures are often seen in younger patients as a result of major trauma [29]. Of note, large volume hemorrhage can occur in the thigh, with potential development of distal limb ischemia or clinically significant hypovolemia [31]. Owing to the large size of the thigh, compartment syndrome is rare [32].

These fractures can be readily diagnosed in the field, as the thigh is generally painful, swollen, and deformed, while the affected limb appears shortened. Although there are limited data pertaining to their application in the prehospital setting, commercial traction splints have long been the standard of care used by EMS personnel in the management of isolated femoral shaft fractures [25,33,34]. Their use is discussed later in this chapter.

Knee

Knee injuries include fractures, dislocations, and damage to the supporting structures of the joint, including all ligaments and menisci. When splinting knee injuries, it is often best to immobilize the limb in the position found or in the position of comfort [33]. Care should be taken not to splint the leg fully extended, as this may compress the neurovascular bundle against the posterior tibia [35].

Although relatively uncommon, knee dislocations require additional care in the prehospital setting. Tibiofemoral dislocations can result from motor vehicle collision, sports injuries, and even falls [36]. These injuries have the potential to cause severe vascular damage at the site of the popliteal artery, leading to distal ischemia [35]. Prompt treatment and transport are crucial to prevent long-term damage to the affected limb. In extreme cases (such as severely delayed transport or other extenuating conditions significantly delaying definitive care), properly trained and authorized prehospital providers may consider attempting reduction in the field, if necessary to restore distal circulation. Of note, up to 50% of knee dislocations spontaneously reduce prior to ED presentation [37].

Fractures of the tibial plateau can occur from both low- and high-energy trauma and are seen in both young adults and the elderly [38]. Those occurring at the medial plateau have the potential to damage the peroneal nerve and/or the popliteal artery, leading to distal neurovascular impairment [35]. Further complications can include the development of compartment syndrome, although this generally occurs 24–48 hours after the time of injury [39].

Leg injuries

The tibia is the most commonly fractured of all long bones [40]. Eighty percent of the time there is an associated fibular fracture, due to their adjacent positioning and attachment via the syndesmotic ligament [41]. This ligament can transmit energy between the bones such that they may be fractured at non-adjacent sites [35].

The lower leg can be immobilized with a variety of devices, including cardboard, padded wood, and vacuum splints [33]. Similar to the knee, it is best to immobilize the leg with a slight amount of flexion [35]. Care should be taken to also immobilize the ipsilateral knee and ankle, as the long bones of the leg play an important role in stabilizing the adjacent joints [42]. Compartment syndrome is once again a concern, occurring in 8.1% of tibial shaft fractures [43].

Ankle and foot injuries

When splinting ankle or foot injuries, consider pillow splints, air splints, or any other method that avoids pressure on the bony prominences [33]. As with knee dislocations, if patient transport is to be significantly prolonged, properly trained and authorized prehospital personnel may consider reducing dislocated ankle joints that show signs of distal neurovascular compromise.

Many foot and ankle injuries can be subtle and difficult to identify solely on clinical exam, but may be at risk for long-term complications if not evaluated early [44]. To aid in triage of these patients, criteria such as the Ottawa decision rules have been developed to help ED providers determine the need for radiographs [45,46]. However, such methods have not been validated in the prehospital setting. Without a validated method to rule out severe injury in the field, every effort should be made to transport these patients for further evaluation.

Spine

Injuries of the bony spine and spinal column are of concern in patients with multiple system trauma. The cervical spine is the most commonly injured area of the spine, followed by the thoracolumbar spine, lumbar, and thoracic spine, respectively [47]. The incidence of cervical spine fractures in trauma has been estimated to be approximately 4% [48]. However, the incidence of cervical spine injuries is higher (5–10%) in patients with head trauma or trauma above the clavicles [49]. While the overall incidence of concomitant spinal cord injuries in all blunt trauma has been estimated to be less than 2%, it is the possibility of severe neurological impairment, including paralysis, lasting disability, or death that raises the level of concern and caution in the prehospital and acute care environment [48].

Patients with vertebral spine or spinal cord injury can present with a variety of symptoms, from obvious paralysis to subtle neurological deficits or simply neck or back pain. The primary trauma survey may reveal clues to high cervical spine trauma. For example, patients with high cervical injuries may have impairment of the phrenic nerve, presenting with abnormal breathing or respiratory failure that can rapidly progress to death. Neurogenic shock due to impairment of the autonomic pathways presents with hypotension refractory to fluids and is often accompanied by bradycardia.

Assessment of neurological disability may further raise suspicion of severe vertebral column injury. Patients with diminished sensorium have higher potential for harboring occult spinal cord trauma. A careful secondary survey should include a more thorough assessment of neurological status including motor and sensory testing. Further, prehospital providers should be alert for neurological symptoms indicative of central cord, anterior

cord, and Brown-Séquard syndromes. The most common of these, central cord syndrome, occurs frequently in the elderly and classically presents with bilateral weakness, most severe in the distal upper extremities.

Spinal injury should be suspected in any patient with any of the following findings.
- Evidence of multiple traumatic injuries
- Focal neurological symptoms such as weakness or numbness
- Neck pain, back pain, or midline spine tenderness
- Head injuries with significant mechanism AND altered mental status or evidence of significant intoxication
- Distracting painful injuries in the setting of a suspicious mechanism

Maintenance of neutral immobilization of the spine is the standard of care for any patient with suspected spinal injury. Two large, multicenter studies were conducted to explore predictors for safely clearing patients from spinal immobilization without radiographic imaging [50,51]. However, it is important to note that these studies were not conducted in the prehospital setting. Additionally, each study asked the question whether or not to image the spine prior to clearing spinal immobilization, not whether to immobilize the spine during initial assessment.

The most common technique for spinal immobilization includes placing the patient in a hard cervical collar and on a backboard. Once immobilization is initiated, the average amount of time patients spend on a backboard has been estimated to be over 1 hour [52]. Prolonged use of a rigid backboard is associated with several complications such as pain and pressure ulcers as well as respiratory compromise and aspiration events. Additionally, there are several special circumstances of prehospital care, such as wilderness or search and rescue settings, in which total spinal immobilization carries substantial risks of injury to the first responders and is therefore used more judiciously than in standard practice. Given the range of significant complications associated with full spinal immobilization, there is growing interest in the prehospital and trauma literature regarding the utility of limited use of both full spine and cervical spine immobilization [53]. There is increasing utilization of selective spinal immobilization policies among EMS systems (see Volume 1, Chapter 40) Some systems have examined the outcomes associated with these policies, with promising results indicating that such policies could be implemented safely in the prehospital setting [54–56]. More research should be conducted to validate these preliminary studies and to create standardized guidelines for selective immobilization policies.

Splinting

Indications and basic technique

Splinting is the mainstay of emergency immobilization of an injured extremity. Whether the injury is a fracture, dislocation, or sprain, immobilization in the position of comfort will help to reduce pain and chance of further injury. Other indications for splinting include reduction of hemorrhage and maintenance of alignment after reduction of a fracture or dislocation [33,57].

The basic technique for splinting an injured extremity includes protecting the skin and soft tissue, applying a rigid material to immobilize the painful extremity, and securing the rigid material with a flexible material. While immobilization is essential, a splint should also not be applied tightly or circumferentially to the limb, in order to avoid neurovascular compression and compromise. The general rule of thumb is to leave at least one surface of a limb exposed to allow for continued swelling and to prevent complications [33].

Splinting materials

There are many commercial materials made of fiberglass or other durable components. These are primarily used in the ED or wilderness settings for longer term splinting. In the prehospital setting, where transport time is limited to generally less than 1 hour, and patient function and mobility are also limited, temporary materials such as cardboard secured by tape will provide sufficient immobilization and pain control. In austere settings, such as the wilderness or during a disaster response, non-traditional items can easily be repurposed to create a variety of splints or slings. For example, a large sheet or piece of clothing can be tied tightly as a pelvic binder. Hiking backpacks with a hard frame can serve as a partial backboard. Any large stick can be fastened to an extremity with tape or clothing for immobilization [58]. Even prefabricated extremity splints (e.g. fiberglass) can be fashioned into effective, temporary cervical collars [59]. Additionally, larger water bottles or jugs, when filled with water and fastened with rope, can provide the weighted component for a makeshift traction splint [58].

Traction splints

Prehospital use of traction devices for orthopedic trauma has been considered standard treatment of femoral shaft fractures [25,33,34]. Commercial traction splints are considered required ambulance equipment by the American College of Surgeons, the American College of Emergency Physicians, the National Association of EMS Physicians, the Emergency Medical Services for Children Program, and the American Academy of Pediatrics [60]. These recommendations posit that traction reduces pain and limits further blood loss, neurovascular damage, or soft tissue injury.

However, there are downsides to prehospital traction splinting. Proper splint application takes two trained providers approximately 5–6 minutes to perform, contributing to EMS on-scene delays [61]. Case studies have identified episodes of transient peroneal nerve palsies, compartment syndrome, urethral injury, pressure ulcers, and distal ischemia as a result of prolonged use of EMS traction devices [62]. Further research has demonstrated suboptimal rates of proper splint application, much of which is attributed to the infrequency of its usage [63,64]. Additionally, a Cochrane review found no benefit or significant

analgesia related to preoperative hip traction [27]. Further research is needed to better guide prehospital usage of these devices.

Reductions with (and without) medications

Field reduction versus definitive care

The decision to allow field reductions of extremity fractures and dislocations is specific to the individual EMS system and each clinical scenario. There are widely accepted indications for one attempt at gentle reduction, which include distal neurovascular deficit or severe angulation [65]. However, even these should generally be deferred if anticipated transport time is minimal (e.g. less than 10 minutes).

System-specific variations in protocol should be considered for regions with large rural areas and extended transport times. Further, programs that regularly staff large sporting events may provide additional training to their providers that could allow for more aggressive field reduction techniques. When considering implementation of such protocols, availability of both on-scene supervisory personnel (e.g. EMS physician or sports medicine physician) and analgesia should be considered [11].

There are good reasons not to allow field reductions except for the most critical circumstances (e.g. pulse deficit), which include converting a dislocation to a fracture-dislocation, causing further neurovascular compromise, or converting a closed fracture to an open one. Without prereduction films, there is no proof that a fracture preceded a reduction attempt. If a reduction is performed, the extremity should be splinted immediately after in the position of function, distal neurovascular status reassessed, and the patient should always be transported to the emergency department.

Special considerations: partial or complete amputations and neurovascular injuries

Emergency medical services providers are often the first medical personnel to encounter a patient suffering from a traumatic amputation and must be prepared to care for the amputated part as well as the patient. Once priorities such as bleeding control are addressed through either direct pressure or a tourniquet, attention should be turned to recovering and preserving the amputated part in addition to obtaining a thorough history that includes time of amputation, mechanism of injury, and the patient's handedness and occupation. EMS providers should not prognosticate likelihood of replantation.

The stump can be gently cleaned of debris and gross contamination with sterile saline and then covered with saline moistened sterile gauze. The blood vessels of the stump should not be clamped, nor should the stump be manually debrided. An underlying fracture should be assumed, and the extremity should be splinted as such; this is particularly important in the setting of a partial amputation. Efforts should be made by the EMS crew on scene to locate the amputated part, and if the patient is not stable enough to await locating it, then another responder should be instructed to locate, store, and transport it to the hospital urgently.

The amputated part should be wrapped in a saline moistened gauze pad and placed in a plastic bag, which then should be placed in a container of ice. The goal temperature is 4 °C and care should be taken to not freeze the part. The part should not be placed directly on ice or be immersed in saline [66]. The patient should be transferred urgently to a replantation-capable hospital, if available. If the patient meets major trauma criteria and the trauma center is not a replantation center, the patient should preferentially go to the trauma center [66].

Conclusion

Orthopedic injuries commonly present in the prehospital setting. EMS physicians, providers, and systems must be prepared to evaluate and treat these injuries appropriately. EMS physicians can provide a benefit to their systems by understanding the current evidence and best practices.

References

1 Schopper D, Lormand JD, Waxweiler R (eds). *Developing Policies to Prevent Injuries and Violence: Guidelines for Policy Makers and Planners.* Geneva: World Health Organization, 2006.

2 Melamed E, Blumenfeld A, Kalmovich B, Kosashvili Y, Lin G, IDF Medical Corps Consensus Group on Prehospital Care of Orthopedic Injuries. Prehospital care of orthopedic injuries. *Prehosp Disaster Med* 2007;22:22–5.

3 McManus JG, Sallee DR. Pain management in the prehospital environment. *Emerg Med Clin North Am* 2005;23:415–31.

4 Soriya GC, McVaney KE, Liao MM, et al. Safety of prehospital intravenous fentanyl for adult trauma patients. *J Trauma Acute Care Surg* 2012;72:755–9.

5 Groh GI, Wirth MA. Management of traumatic sternoclavicular joint injuries. *J Am Acad Orthop Surg* 2011;19:1–7.

6 Baldwin KD, Ohman-Strickland P, Mehta S, Hume E. Scapula fractures: a marker for concomitant injury? A retrospective review of data in the National Trauma Database. *J Trauma* 2008;65:430–5.

7 Rudzinski JP, Pittman LM, Uehara DT. Shoulder and humerus injuries. In: Tintinalli JE, Stapczynski JS, Ma OJ, Cline DM, Cydulka RK, Meckler GD (eds) *Tintinalli's Emergency Medicine: A Comprehensive Study Guide,* 7th edn. New York: McGraw-Hill, 2011.

8 Beason MS. Complications of a shoulder dislocation. *Am J Emerg Med* 1999;17:288–95.

9 Horn AE, Ufberg JW. Management of common dislocations. In: Roberts JR, Custalow CB, Thomsen TW, et al. (eds) *Roberts & Hedges' Clinical Procedures in Emergency Medicine,* 6th edn. Philadelphia: Saunders Elsevier, 2014.

10 Dudkiewicz I, Arzi H, Salai M, Heim M, Pritsch M. Patients education of a self-reduction technique for anterior glenohumeral dislocation of shoulder. *J Trauma* 2010;68:620–3.

11 Norte GE, West A, Gnacinski M, van der Meijden OA, Millett PJ. On-field management of the acute anterior glenohumeral dislocation. *Phys Sportsmed* 2011;39:151–62.

12 Abzug JM, Herman MJ. Management of supracondylar humerus fractures in children: current concepts. *J Am Acad Orthop Surg* 2012;20:69–77.

13 Bredenkamp JH, Jokhy BP, Uehara DT. Injuries to the elbow and forearm. In: Tintinalli JE, Stapczynski JS, Ma OJ, Cline DM, Cydulka RK, Meckler GD (eds) *Tintinalli's Emergency Medicine: A Comprehensive Study Guide,* 7th edn. New York: McGraw-Hill, 2011.

14 Escarza R, Loeffel MF, Uehara DT. Wrist injuries. In: Tintinalli JE, Stapczynski JS, Ma OJ, Cline DM, Cydulka RK, Meckler GD (eds) *Tintinalli's Emergency Medicine: A Comprehensive Study Guide,* 7th edn. New York: McGraw-Hill, 2011.

15 Shehab R, Mirabelli MH. Evaluation and diagnosis of wrist pain: a case-based approach. *Am Fam Physician* 2013;87:568–73.

16 Simpson PM, McCabe B, Bendall JC, Cone DC, Middleton PM. Paramedic-performed digital nerve block to facilitate field reduction of a dislocated finger. *Prehosp Emerg Care* 2012;16:415–17.

17 Pappou IP, Deal DN. High-pressure injection injuries. *J Hand Surg Am* 2012;37:2404–7.

18 Patterson LA. Pelvic fractures. In: Adams JG (ed) *Emergency Medicine.* Philadelphia: Saunders Elsevier, 2008.

19 Dalal SA, Burgess AR, Siegel JH, et al. Pelvic fracture in multiple trauma: classification by mechanism is key to pattern of organ injury, resuscitative requirements, and outcome. *J Trauma* 1989; 29(7):981–1000.

20 Gonzalez RP, Fried PQ, Bukhalo M. The utility of clinical examination in screening for pelvic fractures in blunt trauma. *J Am Coll Surg* 2002;194:121–5.

21 Krieg JC, Mohr M, Ellis TJ, Simpson TS, Madey SM, Bottlang M. Emergent stabilization of pelvic ring injuries by controlled circumferential compression: a clinical trial. *J Trauma* 2005;59:659–64.

22 Buie VC, Owings MF, DeFrances CJ, Golosinskiy A. *National Hospital Discharge Survey: 2006 Summary, Vital Health Stat 13(168).* Atlanta, GA: National Center for Health Statistics, 2010.

23 Brauer CA, Coca-Perraillon M, Cutler DM, Rosen AB. Incidence and mortality of hip fractures in the United States. *JAMA* 2009; 302:1573–9.

24 Cummings SR, Kelsey JL, Nevitt MC, O'Dowd KJ. Epidemiology of osteoporosis and osteoporotic fractures. *Epidemiol Rev* 1985; 7:178–208.

25 Murray BL. Femur and hip. In: Marx JA, Hockberger RS, Walls RM (eds) *Rosen's Emergency Medicine: Concepts and Clinical Practice,* 8th edn. Philadelphia: Saunders Elsevier, 2014.

26 Sahin V, Karakas ES, Aksu S, Atlihan D, Turk CY, Halici M. Traumatic dislocation and fracture-dislocation of the hip: a long term follow-up study. *J Trauma* 2003;54:520–9.

27 Handoll HH, Queally JM, Parker MJ. Pre-operative traction for hip fractures in adults. *Cochrane Database Syst Rev* 2011;12:CD000168.

28 Hak DJ, Goutlet JA. Severity of injuries associated with traumatic hip dislocation as a result of motor vehicle collisions. *J Trauma* 1999;47:60–3.

29 Anwar R, Tuson K, Khan SA. *Classification and Diagnosis in Orthopaedic Trauma.* New York: Cambridge University Press, 2008.

30 Clegg TE, Roberts CS, Greene JW, Prather BA. Hip dislocations – epidemiology, treatment, and outcomes. *Injury* 2010;41:329–34.

31 Smith RM, Giannoudis PV. Femoral shaft fractures. In: Browner BD, Jupiter JB, Levine AM, Trafton P, Krettek C (eds) *Skeletal Trauma: Basic Science, Management and Reconstruction*, 4th edn. Philadelphia: Saunders Elsevier, 2009.

32 Mithöfer K, Lhowe DW, Vrahas MS, Altman DT, Altman GT. Clinical spectrum of acute compartment syndrome of the thigh and its relation to associated injuries. *Clin Orthop Relat Res* 2004;425:223–9.

33 Klimke A, Furin M. Prehospital immobilization. In: Roberts JR, Custalow CB, Thomsen TW, et al. (eds) *Roberts & Hedges' Clinical Procedures in Emergency Medicine*, 6th edn. Philadelphia: Saunders Elsevier, 2014.

34 National Association of Emergency Medical Technicians and American College of Surgeons Committee on Trauma. *Prehospital Trauma Life Support*, 7th edn. Burlington, MA: Jones and Bartlett Learning, 2011.

35 Pallin DJ. Knee and lower leg. In: Marx JA, Hockberger RS, Walls RM (eds) *Rosen's Emergency Medicine: Concepts and Clinical Practice*, 8th edn. Philadelphia: Saunders Elsevier, 2014.

36 Robertson A, Nutton RW, Keating JF. Dislocation of the knee. *J Bone Joint Surg Br* 2006;88:706–11.

37 Wascher DC, Dvirnak PC, DeCoster TA. Knee dislocation: initial assessment and implications for treatment. *J Orthop Trauma* 1997; 11:525–9.

38 Cole P, Levy B, Schatzker J, Watson JT. Tibial plateau fractures. In: Browner BD, Jupiter JB, Levine AM, Trafton P, Krettek C (eds) *Skeletal Trauma: Basic Science, Management and Reconstruction*, 4th edn. Philadelphia: Saunders Elsevier, 2009.

39 Chang YH, Tu YK, Yeh WL, Hsu RW. Tibial plateau fracture with compartment syndrome: a complication of higher incidence in Taiwan. *Chang Gung Med J* 2000;23:149–55.

40 Russell TA. Fractures of the tibial diaphysis. In: Levine AM (ed) *Orthopedic Knowledge Update: Trauma*. Rosemont, IL: American Academy of Orthopedic Surgeons, 1996, pp.171–9.

41 Court-Brown CM, McBirnie J. The epidemiology of tibial fractures. *J Bone Joint Surg Br* 1995;77:417–21.

42 Trafton PG. Tibial shaft fractures. In: Browner BD, Jupiter JB, Levine AM, Trafton P, Krettek C (eds) *Skeletal Trauma: Basic Science, Management and Reconstruction*, 4th edn. Philadelphia: Saunders Elsevier, 2009.

43 Park S, Ahn J, Gee AO, Kuntz AF, Esterhai JL. Compartment syndrome in tibial fractures. *J Orthop Trauma* 2009;23:514–18.

44 Abu-Laban RB, Rose NG. Ankle and foot. In: Marx JA, Hockberger RS, Walls RM (eds) *Rosen's Emergency Medicine: Concepts and Clinical Practice*, 8th edn. Philadelphia: Saunders Elsevier, 2014.

45 Bachmann LM, Kolb E, Koller MT, Steurer J, ter Riet G. Accuracy of Ottawa ankle rules to exclude fractures of the ankle and mid-foot: systemic review. *BMJ* 2003;326:417.

46 Dowling S, Spooner CH, Liang Y, et al. Accuracy of Ottawa Ankle Rules to exclude fractures of the ankle and midfoot in children: a meta-analysis. *Acad Emerg Med* 2009;16:277–87.

47 Lin M, Mahadevan SV. Spine trauma and spinal cord injury. In: Adams JG (ed) *Emergency Medicine*. Philadelphia: Saunders Elsevier, 2008.

48 Grossman MD, Reilly PM, Gillett T, Gillett D. National survey of the incidence of cervical spine injury and approach to cervical spine clearance in U.S. trauma centers. *J Trauma* 1999;47:684–90.

49 Marion DW. Head and spinal cord injury. *Neurol Clin* 1998;16:485–502.

50 Hoffman JR, Mower WR, Wolfson AB, Todd KH, Zucker MI. Validity of a set of clinical criteria to rule out injury to the cervical spine in patients with blunt trauma. National Emergency X-Radiography Utilization Study Group. *N Engl J Med* 2000; 343:94–9.

51 Stiell IG, Clement CM, McKnight RD, et al. The Canadian C-spine rule versus the NEXUS low-risk criteria in patients with trauma. *N Engl J Med* 2003;349:2510–18.

52 Cooney DR, Wallus H, Asaly M, Wojcik S. Backboard time for patients receiving spinal immobilization by emergency medical services. *Int J Emerg Med* 2013;20:17.

53 National Association of Emergency Medical Services Physicians. EMS spinal precautions and the use of the long backboard. *Prehosp Emerg Care* 2013;17:392–3.

54 Domeier RM, Frederiksen SM, Welch K. Prospective performance assessment of an out-of-hospital protocol for selective spine immobilization using clinical spine clearance criteria. *Ann Emerg Med* 2005;46:123–31.

55 Stroh G, Braude D. Can an out-of-hospital cervical spine clearance protocol identify all patients with injuries? An argument for selective immobilization. *Ann Emerg Med* 2001;37:609–15.

56 Burton JH, Dunn MG, Harmon NR, Hermanson TA, Bradshaw JR. A statewide, prehospital emergency medical service selective patient spine immobilization protocol. *J Trauma* 2006;61:161–7.

57 Fitch MT, Nicks BA, Pariyadath M, McGinnis HD, Manthey DE. Videos in clinical medicine: basic splinting techniques. *N Engl J Med* 2008;359:e32.

58 Kassel MR, Gianotti A. Splints and slings. In: Auerbach PS (ed) *Wilderness Medicine*, 6th edn. Philadelphia: Elsevier Mosby, 2012.

59 McGrath T, Murphy C. Comparison of a SAM splint-molded cervical collar with a Philadelphia cervical collar. *Wilderness Environ Med* 2009;20:166–8.

60 American College of Surgeons Committee on Trauma, American College of Emergency Physicians, National Association of EMS Physicians, Pediatric Equipment Guideline Committee–Emergency Medical Services for Children Partnership for Children Stakeholder Group, American Academy of Pediatrics. Equipment for ambulances. *Prehosp Emerg Care* 2009;13:364–9.

61 Hedges JR, Feero S, Moore B, Shultz B, Haver DW. Factors contributing to paramedic onscene time during evaluation and management of blunt trauma. *Am J Emerg Med* 1988;6:443–8.

62 Agrawal Y, Karwa J, Shah N, Clayson A. Traction splint: to use or not to use. *J Perioper Pract* 2009;19:295–8.

63 Abarbanell NR. Prehospital midthigh trauma and traction splint use: recommendations for treatment protocols. *Am J Emerg Med* 2001;19:137–40.

64 Daugherty MC, Mehlman CT, Moody S, LeMaster T, Falcone RA Jr. Significant rate of misuse of the hare traction splint for children with femoral shaft fractures. *J Emerg Nurs* 2013;39:97–103.

65 Limmer DJ, O'Keefe MF, Grant HT, et al. (eds) *Emergency Care*, 12th edn. Upper Saddle River, NJ: Prentice Hall, 2011.

66 Moorell D. Management of amputations. In: Roberts JR, Custalow CB, Thomsen TW, et al. (eds) *Roberts & Hedges' Clinical Procedures in Emergency Medicine*, 6th edn. Philadelphia: Saunders Elsevier, 2014.

CHAPTER 37

Ocular trauma

Eric Hawkins and Michael D. Mills

Introduction

Traumatic eye injuries are extremely common in the prehospital setting, and may occur as isolated injuries or as part of more extensive maxillofacial or multisystem trauma. These injuries may range from the minor to the sight threatening, and EMS physicians must be prepared to rapidly identify serious problems that could result in permanent blindness or further complications. Once significant eye injuries are recognized, it is important that the patient is stabilized, appropriately treated, and evaluated by a hospital or physician with adequate access to full ophthalmological services to provide definitive care.

Epidemiology

Ocular trauma is common; in the United States an estimated 2–3 million people seek medical attention for eye injuries each year [1,2]. Among many risk factors, the most significant seem to be male sex and age under 30 [3]. Most injuries are not significant, and many never need treatment for minor eye problems [2]. Of those with more serious injuries, 16% have ocular or orbital damage and over 50% of patients with significant facial trauma have associated sight-threatening eye injuries [4]. Trauma is the second most common cause of monocular blindness, trailing only cataracts [5]. Each year, eye injuries are the number 1 cause of ophthalmological hospital admissions in the United States [5].

Evaluation: history and physical exam

Initial assessment and treatment should focus on the ABCs of trauma resuscitation, and any life-threatening injuries should be addressed first, as with any trauma patient [6,7]. Eye injuries can be distracting, and it is important not to divert attention from other sources of serious injury early in the trauma survey process. It is also critical to recognize that associated facial trauma

and swelling may affect airway patency, and this should be secured before further examination of the orbit if needed.

After initial stabilization and primary survey, attention can be focused on the ocular injury and a thorough evaluation should be performed. In the case of known or suspected chemical contact to the face and eye, immediate irrigation with normal saline or clean water should be performed during this evaluation process

The key components in the evaluation of traumatic eye injuries are a thorough history and careful eye examination. The history focuses on key points surrounding the event and should note the type of injury, the time of onset, and any specific symptoms reported by the patient [6]. Mechanism of injury is also recorded and may include blunt or penetrating trauma and thermal or chemical burns to the eye or periorbital areas of the face. Other important points include the patient's visual acuity before the injury, if known, the presence or absence of contact lenses, any past medical history of eye disorders, and any history of ophthalmological surgical or medical treatment [7].

The physical examination of the eye begins with evaluation of visual acuity, establishing a baseline level of function and providing functional assessment of possible damage to the eye [7,8]. In the field, this can be performed using a hand-held Snellen chart to document the smallest objects or letters identifiable at a specific distance from the eye. Visual acuity is recorded for each eye individually and then using both eyes simultaneously [7]. If no chart is available, a newspaper or other source of small print is useful to estimate visual acuity. Patients who normally wear prescription glasses for reading should perform this with those same glasses if available, but those who use contact lenses should not have those replaced for this examination. If the patient's glasses are unavailable, it is possible to use a piece of paper with a small pin-sized hole through which the patient can view the chart and complete the examination [6,7]. This "pin-hole test" corrects for the refractive error of the patient's eyes and should allow completion of the examination. For those who cannot read the Snellen chart due to injury or underlying ocular disease, other options include assessing the

Emergency Medical Services: Clinical Practice and Systems Oversight, Second Edition. Volume 1: Clinical Aspects of EMS.
Edited by David C. Cone, Jane H. Brice, Theodore R. Delbridge, and J. Brent Myers.
© 2015 NAEMSP. Published 2015 by John Wiley & Sons, Inc. Companion Website: www.wiley.com\go\cone\naemsp

patient's ability to count fingers, detect hand motions, or perceive the presence or movement of light [6]. The method of testing and patient performance should be documented for each eye.

After rapid evaluation of visual acuity, attention shifts to the external assessment of the eye and surrounding structures. Each globe is examined for protrusion or proptosis and for external signs of penetration or damage from a foreign body (Figures 37.1–37.3). Ocular movement in the cardinal directions of gaze (vertical up-down, horizontal right-to-left, and diagonal left-to-right and right-to-left) is also tested and any deficit or entrapment recorded. The pupil and iris are then inspected for size, shape, and reaction to light and results compared between eyes. The presence or absence of a hyphema (blood in the anterior chamber that may obscure the iris or pupil) is especially important to assess (Figure 37.4). Finally, the conjunctivae are inspected for erythema, subconjunctival hemorrhage, chemosis, conjunctival swelling, or subconjunctival emphysema. If the

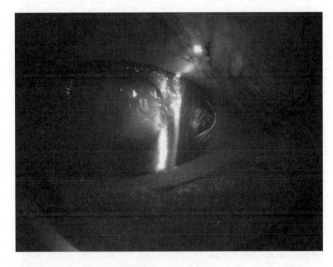

Figure 37.3 Intraocular foreign body on slit lamp. Source: Michael Mills. Reproduced with permission of Michael Mills.

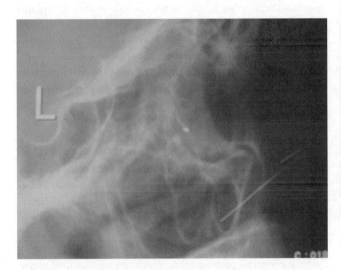

Figure 37.1 Intraocular foreign body x-ray (lateral view). Source: Michael Mills. Reproduced with permission of Michael Mills.

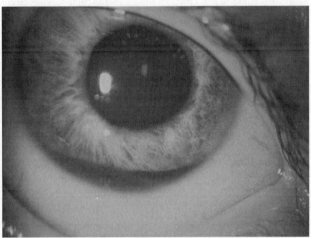

Figure 37.4 Hyphema from air bag injury. Source: Michael Mills. Reproduced with permission of Michael Mills.

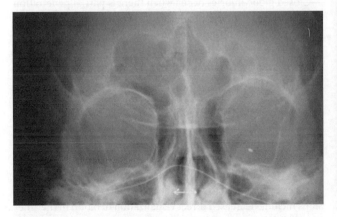

Figure 37.2 Intraocular foreign body x-ray (anterior-posterior view). Source: Michael Mills. Reproduced with permission of Michael Mills.

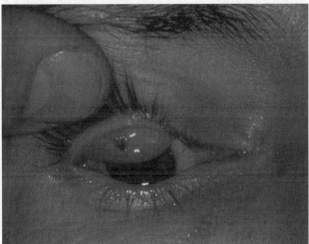

Figure 37.5 Foreign body in eyelid. Source: Michael Mills. Reproduced with permission of Michael Mills.

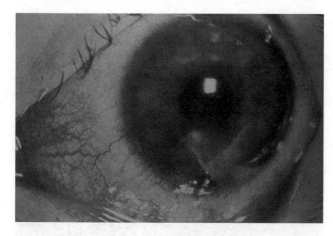

Figure 37.6 Ruptured globe. Source: Michael Mills. Reproduced with permission of Michael Mills.

patient reports a foreign body sensation in the eyelid (Figure 37.5) or if there is any concern for an intraocular foreign body or a punctured globe (Figure 37.6), it is best to end the examination at this point. The affected eye should then be covered with an eye shield or improvised protective device to protect the globe from external pressure before transport for more definitive evaluation and care [7]. The EMS physician should not remove a protruding foreign body (such as a nail) lodged in the globe. A cup or shield may be used to cover the eye with the foreign body in place.

Finally, examination of the surrounding structures of the eye focuses on associated maxillofacial trauma or related complications. The eyelids and periorbital soft tissues are inspected for lacerations, ecchymosis, edema, foreign bodies, and cutaneous evidence of thermal or chemical burns. The orbital rims are similarly inspected and palpated for signs of crepitus or obvious bony deformities. If injuries are unilateral, comparisons are made between the eyes because normal foramina of the surrounding eye rim may be mistaken for fractures. If the patient has obvious periorbital trauma, an orbital blowout fracture is concerning, especially if there is associated diplopia (double vision) or inability to move the eye superiorly. Finally, the patient should have a sensory examination of the skin around the eye. Any numbness or paresthesias could indicate damage to the infraorbital nerve.

Specific eye injuries

Ocular burns
Ocular chemical burns are true ophthalmic emergencies and are best treated in the field with copious irrigation with water. Delays in irrigation have been associated with increased risks to visual acuity and higher rates of subsequent complications when compared with immediate irrigation of the eye [9]. Tap water and normal saline work equally well initially, with the keys being the volume of the fluid and duration of irrigation rather than the type of fluid [10]. Irrigation should continue during

transport for a minimum of 30 minutes for significant exposures. Important historical information to obtain includes the duration of exposure, type of chemical, and the pH of the substance if known. If the chemical is an industrial source, a Material Safety Data Sheet (MSDS) is particularly helpful to identify and categorize the substance in question [10]. Injuries from acid exposures tend to be less serious than alkali substances [11] but this varies by the particular type of chemical involved. In addition to irrigation, proper prehospital management includes pain control and transport to an appropriate center for immediate ophthalmological consultation and evaluation.

Ocular trauma
Direct trauma to the eye can be divided into open or closed globe injuries. Open globe injuries have full-thickness defects in the ocular wall and include lacerations, intraocular foreign bodies, and rupture of the globe from blunt trauma [12]. These signify high-energy mechanisms of injury and are frequently associated with other ocular or periorbital injuries. Symptoms include decreased visual acuity, difficulty with ocular motility, and abnormal or absent pupillary reflexes. On examination, open globe injuries may be evident on gross inspection, as with a visible foreign body, a large scleral laceration with clear penetration, or an obvious deformity of the eye or pupil. However, penetrating injuries may cause negligible external damage to the sclera or globe and a small intraocular foreign body may cause minimal pain after the initial event [13]. The key point for the prehospital physician is to consider an open globe, especially if there is associated significant head injury, periorbital damage, or hyphema. Once an open globe is suspected, all further evaluation of the eye should be postponed until definitive care is available [7]. The eye should be protected with a hard eye shield and the patient should be transported for further emergency evaluation and potential surgical repair by an ophthalmologist. Other appropriate prehospital care includes pain control, elevation of the head of the bed to 30–45°, and antiemetic medication to reduce potential increased intraocular pressure during vomiting.

Closed globe injuries occur when there is partial penetration of the eye and include hyphema, damage to the retina, superficial abrasions and lacerations, and non-penetrating foreign bodies. These can cause significant eye pain, loss of visual acuity, and decreased ocular function, but they vary by the type and location of injury.

Traumatic hyphema
A traumatic hyphema is a collection of blood in the anterior chamber of the eye caused by blunt or penetrating injury. The highly vascular ciliary body or iris is usually the source of bleeding for a hyphema and is often associated with head trauma or other eye injuries to the cornea, iris, lens, or globe [14–16]. Signs include decreased direct visualization of blood in the anterior chamber, poor visual acuity, and decreased pupil reactivity. Hyphema severity is graded on a scale of 1–4 based on the

amount of blood that collects in the anterior chamber when the patient is in a upright position, ranging from a minimal layering (grade 1) to a complete filling of the anterior chamber with blood (grade 4) [14,16]. This classification is important because higher-grade hyphemas have an increased risk of complications and are a threat to permanent damage or loss of visual acuity [17]. Complications include rebleeding into the hyphema, corneal blood staining, and damage of the optic nerve or retina from increased intraocular pressure [15–17]. Prehospital care focuses on pain management, elevation of the head of the bed from 30–45° if possible, covering of the eye with a protective shield, and prompt transport to a medical facility for further ophthalmological evaluation and management [15,16].

Corneal injuries

Corneal injuries are extremely common and may present with ocular pain, sensations of a foreign body in the eye, blepharospasm, or tearing [18]. Decreased visual acuity, blurred vision, and photophobia are also common initial symptoms. Corneal abrasions often result from a direct blow to the eye or a foreign body under the eyelid that irritates the corneal surface. These may be visible on gross exam, but often the lesion can only be seen on slit-lamp examination after staining with fluorescein dye. Similarly, corneal foreign bodies may be seen on visual inspection of the eye and should be suspected in any patient with eye pain associated with high-risk activities like use of power tools, grinding, hammering, or sanding objects with or without use of protective eyewear [11]. If an object is visualized in the eye it should be flushed with saline or removed by a skilled practitioner unless there is concern that it has penetrated the globe, in which case the eye should be covered or patched and the object left in place until appropriate evaluation by a physician.

Prehospital care of corneal injuries focuses on a thorough history, pain management, and transport to a center with appropriate specialty care. Most superficial corneal injuries heal within 24–72 hours, but the prognosis and potential for further complications depend on the depth and overall size of the lesion [18].

Retinal injuries

Trauma of the retina and posterior segments of the eye is less common than injuries to anterior eye structures, but carries a higher risk of blindness and irreversible loss of vision [19]. Common presentations include decreased visual acuity or a sensation of "flashing lights" or "floaters" in the visual field of the affected eye [20]. Retinal injuries require a complete fundus examination for definitive diagnosis, and these techniques are beyond the scope of this review. For the EMS physician, it is important to remember the signs of retinal and posterior segment injury and to obtain a focused eye history and examination, including visual acuity, before transporting the patient for ophthalmological evaluation and treatment.

References

1 McGwin G Jr, Hall TA, Xie A, Owsley C. Trends in eye injury in the United States, 1992–2001. *Invest Ophthalmol Vis Sci* 2006;47:521–7.
2 McGwin G Jr, Xie A, Owsley C. Rate of eye injury in the United States. *Arch Ophthalmol* 2005;123:970–6.
3 Kuhn F, Morris R, Mester V, et al. Epidemiology and socioeconomics. *Ophthalmol Clin North Am* 2002;15:145–51.
4 Poon A, McCluskey PJ, Hill DA. Eye injuries in patients with major trauma. *J Trauma* 1999;46:494–9.
5 US Eye Injury Registry. Eye Trauma Epidemiology and Prevention. Available at: www.useironline.org/epidemiology
6 Harlan JB Jr, Pieramici DJ. Evaluation of patients with ocular trauma. *Ophthalmol Clin North Am* 2002;15:153–61.
7 Juang PS, Rosen P. Ocular examination techniques for the emergency department. *J Emerg Med* 1997;15:793–810.
8 Khaw PT, Shah P, Elkington AR. Injury to the eye. *BMJ* 2004;328:36–8.
9 Schrage NF, Langefeld S, Zschocke J, et al. Eye burns: an emergency and continuing problem. *Burns* 2000;26:689–99.
10 Bhattacharya SK, Hom GG, Fernandez C, Hom LG. Ocular effects of exposure to industrial chemicals: clinical management and proteomic approaches to damage assessment. *Cutan Ocul Toxicol* 2007; 26:203–25.
11 Peate WF. Work-related eye injuries and illnesses. *Am Fam Physician* 2007;75:1017–22.
12 Colby K. Management of open globe injuries. *Int Ophthalmol Clin* 1999;39:59–69.
13 Mester V, Kuhn F. Intraocular foreign bodies. *Ophthalmol Clin North Am* 2002;15:235–42.
14 Sankar PS, Chen TC, Grosskreutz CL, Pasquale LR. Traumatic hyphema. *Ophthalmol Clin* 2002;42:57–68.
15 Walton W, von Hagen S, Grigorian R, Zarbin M. Management of traumatic hyphema. *Surv Ophthalmol* 2002;47:297–334.
16 Brandt MT, Haug RH. Traumatic hyphema: a comprehensive review. *J Oral Maxillofac Surg* 2001;59:1462–70.
17 Wilson F.M. Traumatic hyphema – pathogenesis and management. *Ophthalmology* 1980;87:910–19.
18 Wilson SA, Last A. Management of corneal abrasions. *Am Fam Physician* 2004;70:123–8.
19 Pieramici DJ. Vitreoretinal trauma. *Ophthalmol Clin North Am* 2002;15:225–34.
20 Pokhrel PK, Loftus SA. Ocular emergencies. *Am Fam Physician* 2007;76:829–36.

CHAPTER 38

Bites, stings, and envenomations

Adam Frisch, Andrew King, and Stephanie Outterson

Introduction

Animal bites are estimated to account for 1 million physician visits each year and for 1% of emergency department (ED) visits [1]. The actual number of animal-related injuries is impossible to calculate because many injuries go unreported [1,2]. The infrequent nature of animal-related calls, coupled with the excitement and emotion often found on scene, can lead to poor provider judgment or errors in proper care. This chapter focuses on prehospital management of animal bites, stings, and envenomations and reviews injuries likely to be encountered, with specific prehospital treatments and interventions where appropriate.

Animal bites

Scene safety and preplanning

As with any EMS response, scene safety is a primary concern. When responding to a call involving animals, all personnel should prevent interaction with the offending animal. Prehospital providers and medical directors should be aware of animal control resources available in their coverage areas. Protocols for responding to animal-related calls should include these resources when appropriate. The primary responsibility of EMS personnel is for their own safety and the safety of the patient. Providers should not be primarily responsible for dealing with the animals. While identification of the offending animal may be helpful for treatment, attempting to catch or quarantine the animal exposes the EMS provider to undue risk [3]. For related reasons, transportation of animals, dead or alive, to the hospital for identification is not advised.

Refusal concerns

As many animal-related injuries initially appear benign, both patients and providers often underestimate their potential seriousness, resulting in inappropriate refusal of treatment or transport. Agencies should consider mandatory medical oversight contact for refusal of care in animal encounter situations, as serious risks exist.

Animal-specific concerns

Mammals

Domesticated animals account for the vast majority of mammalian bite wounds, with dogs and cats representing 93–96% of mammalian bites [2]. Bites by both types of animals occur most frequently to the upper extremity, followed by the lower extremity, and finally the face and neck [1]. Acutely lethal wounds tend to occur in young children [1]. Children are often familiar with the offending animal and are more prone to attacks to the face and neck [1,4]. In both cats and dogs, unique oral flora contributes to considerable infection risk. While most wounds do not become infected, those that do often require in-hospital therapy and potential operative management. Two-thirds of hand bites in one study required hospitalization for IV antibiotics, and one-third required at least one surgical procedure [5]. Systemic complications including endocarditis, meningitis, brain abscess, and sepsis must also be considered by providers and medical directors when determining protocols and transport decisions [6].

Human bites carry risks of complications similar to those of other mammalian bites. Hand wounds involving the metacarpal-phalangeal joint and overlying extensor tendons are often "fight bites" (injuries to the hand from striking teeth during an altercation) and are especially prone to infection. More than 30% of fight bites become infected, resulting in decreased functional capacity. Fight bites often coincide with intoxication and/or criminal activity that may act as a barrier to prehospital care through reluctance to disclose the true mechanism, patient refusal, or law enforcement custody.

Very few poisonous mammals exist in North America. Only the short-tailed shrew, found in central and eastern sections of North America, poses a toxic threat. Several non-indigenous mammals have poisonous reputations. The shrew-like solenodon, found in Central America, induces toxins in its saliva

Emergency Medical Services: Clinical Practice and Systems Oversight, Second Edition. Volume 1: Clinical Aspects of EMS.
Edited by David C. Cone, Jane H. Brice, Theodore R. Delbridge, and J. Brent Myers.

through grooved incisors. The platypus, found in Australia, has venomous glands introduced by spurs at the base of its hind feet. In all of these animals, the toxins serve to kill prey and defend from predators [7]. Bites to humans result in unusually painful wounds with local edema, but typically lack serious or systemic effects.

Accounting for less than 10% of animal bites [2], attacks by wild or undomesticated mammalians are rare and usually require only supportive care and basic wound management in the prehospital setting. In general, most bite victims should be transported to the emergency department for wound evaluation, tetanus shots, and possibly antibiotics.

Rabies

Mammalian bites carry the unique risk of rabies virus transmission which is almost universally fatal [8,9]. Current Centers for Disease Control and Prevention (CDC) guidelines recommend postexposure prophylaxis (PEP) including immunoglobulin administration and vaccination series for high-risk bites in vaccine-naive individuals, and a modified vaccination series for those previously vaccinated [10]. Bites from skunks, foxes, raccoons, bats, and some other carnivorous animals are considered at risk and should receive PEP promptly. For domestic animals that appear healthy and can be quarantined for 10 days, PEP can be withheld pending development of symptoms. Patients with bites from other animals should be transported to the hospital so that the need for PEP can be determined [10].

Bats require special consideration because rabies transmission has occurred outside of recognized bites. Although data are conflicting and perhaps viewed as controversial [10], PEP "can be considered for persons who were in the same room as the bat and who might be unaware that a bite or direct contact had occurred (e.g. a sleeping person awakens to find a bat in the room or an adult witnesses a bat in the room with a previously unattended child, mentally disabled person, or intoxicated person) and rabies cannot be ruled out by testing the bat [10]." Thus, EMS providers should have a very low threshold to transport potential victims to the ED for evaluation whether an obvious bite exists or not [10].

Reptiles

Venomous snakes

Of the estimated 45,000 annual snake bites in the United States, roughly 8,000 are reportedly from venomous snakes. There are 25 venomous species of snakes in the United States. The majority of these are in the subfamily of Crotalids (rattlesnakes, cottonmouths, and copperheads), and the remainder in the Elapid subfamily (coral snake) [11]. This division also represents a difference in their respective toxins and clinical manifestations of envenomation.

Crotalid venom is a primarily a hemotoxin (with some cytotoxic and neurotoxic properties) and produces symptoms ranging from local swelling and ecchymosis to systemic coagulopathy, altered consciousness, and shock. The constellation of effects begins within minutes and steadily progresses to its maximal extent over a number of hours (up to 24 hours with leg bites).

Elapid envenomations can remain relatively asymptomatic for up to 12 hours and then manifest neurotoxicity ranging in severity from paresthesia to complete paralysis requiring ventilatory support.

In either case, it is important to avoid underestimating bite severity based on initial patient assessment at the scene. Although "dry bites" occur with relative frequency, the lack of clinical swelling should not lead the provider to assume that no envenomation has occurred. A period of observation of varying lengths depending on the bite site is recommended by toxicologists and should prompt any and all patients with suspected bites to be transported to the emergency department for evaluation.

Much of EMS provider education about snake bites should focus on dispelling common myths. Providers may encounter well-meaning citizens attempting to render "first aid" to snake bite victims. Cold therapy, arterial tourniquets, electricity (from TASERs or car batteries), incision of the wound, and suction (via commercially available device or oral) are popular lay therapies for snake bite that are without scientific backing and may lead to more local tissue damage [3,11–14].

While some of the literature has suggested treatments such as compression immobilization [12–14], all of the major toxicological societies of North America advocate against this technique for US crotalid envenomations [15]. Keeping the patient calm and immobilizing the affected extremity in a neutral position is the best course of action in the prehospital setting.

Insufficient evidence exists for compression immobilization in hemodynamically unstable patients. Effectiveness of pressure immobilization has been suggested in the setting of Australian elapid snake bites and thus, as a corollary, compression immobilization for confirmed North American elapid envenomation may be considered for those with anticipated long transport times [16,17]. Furthermore, if longer transport times are anticipated after elapid envenomation, EMS should be prepared to intervene on the airway and assist with ventilation. Routine use of antivenin therapy is not generally recommended in the prehospital setting, as it requires a significant amount of time and resources to prepare and administer [3].

Adequate analgesia is a significant concern after crotalid envenomation. In the acute phase, toxicologists recommend the use of intravenous fentanyl as opposed to other opioids so as not to confuse the crotalid envenomation symptoms with morphine-induced histamine release, both of which can cause anaphylaxis, hypotension, and local swelling [16].

Nonvenomous snakes

The majority of snake bites in the US are from non-venomous species. Most of these snakes are in the Colubrid family and include the garter snake, hognose snake, banded water snake, rat snake, and parrot snake. Morbidity from these snakes is extremely rare. Transport to a hospital for observation and wound evaluation is recommended. Bites should be considered contaminated since they may contain broken teeth. Antibiotics are generally not necessary with the exception of retained teeth or significant soft tissue injury. Constrictors and pythons are commonly kept as pets and can have very forceful bites. Their teeth are brittle and prone to fracture with attempted extrication. X-rays to assess for retained teeth and tetanus prophylaxis should be considered and thus EMS should recommend transport to the ED for radiographic evaluation of these bites [18].

Other reptiles

Gila monsters and bearded lizards have venom in their saliva injected through grooved teeth and a strong and tenacious bite. Envenomation, however, is usually not lethal and most often causes only local inflammation and pain. Although rare, there have been reports of anaphylactic reactions as well as angioedema, hypotension, myocardial infarction, and coagulopathy [19–21]. Other reptiles have been involved in fatal bite attacks and appropriate trauma care should be used for these wounds. Transport should be advised as these bites are prone to infection with uncommon forms of bacteria.

Marine animals

Marine animals that sting can cause serious pain and tissue damage. North American venomous marine vertebrates (i.e. stonefish, scorpionfish, lionfish, catfish, stingrays) carry heat-labile toxins that generally respond to heat therapy for toxin neutralization and pain reduction [3,14,22–24]. Invertebrate marine animals (i.e. jellyfish) use tentacles or nematocysts to deploy their toxins. Previous recommendations include flooding the area with acetic acid (vinegar) and then scraping off the tentacles [14,23,24]. More recent literature suggests that hot water and topical lidocaine may be more effective for symptom control and acetic acid may be more efficacious for bluebottle jellyfish stings [25]. Gloves or forceps should be used to manually remove visible tentacle remnants. Other therapies are sourced in folklore, including the use of urine, sand, or meat tenderizer, all of which are inappropriate. Often, reimmersion in salt water improves pain. Prehospital personnel should not routinely remove impaled foreign bodies, such as sea urchin spines or stingray barbs, as the spines easily fracture and may require surgical debridement.

Insect bites and stings
Butterflies, moths, and caterpillars

The order Lepidoptera encompasses the families of butterflies, moths, and their larvae, caterpillars. In the United States, the puss caterpillar, flannel moth caterpillar, Io moth, and saddleback caterpillar can have toxic effects. The venom is transmitted via hollow spines, and clinical manifestations may include local pain, burning, swelling, vesicle formation, and, less commonly nausea, vomiting, seizures, and regional adenopathy [26,27]. Treatment is symptomatic and supportive with antiemetics for nausea and vomiting and benzodiazepines for seizures.

Hymenoptera

Hymenoptera account for the majority of severe allergic responses and anaphylaxis in comparison with other insects. There are three families of Hymenoptera: Apidae (honeybees and bumblebees), Vespidae (yellowjackets, hornets, and wasps), and Formicidae (fire ants). About 1% of children and 3% of adults report severe systemic allergic reactions to Hymenoptera venom, and anaphylaxis does not require a previous exposure (or sting) [28,29]. Furthermore, if a person is allergic to one type of Hymenoptera, he or she is likely to be allergic to the others as well [30]. Clinical manifestations of Hymenoptera envenomation range from local reaction to hypersensitivity reactions (including anaphylaxis), fever, rhabdomyolysis, acute renal failure, and death[31,32]. *Apis mellifera scutellata* or "killer bees" are an aggressive hybrid of the honeybee and have the same venom, but are prone to mass attack, thus increasing the risk of a severe reaction [33,34].

Fire ants are named after the burning pain and necrosis victims experience after exposure. Grabbing the skin with its mandibles, the fire ant injects venom from a stinger on its abdomen in a circular pattern an average of seven or eight times. Large areas of swelling develop that later turn into sterile pustules. Anaphylaxis is relatively common and occurs in up to 6% of those envenomated [35].

Allergic reactions should be treated with antihistamines, albuterol, and/or intramuscular epinephrine, depending on the severity. Angioedema, stridor, and signs of upper airway obstruction are of particular concern and should be monitored closely. Cool compresses may help with local pain. Emesis and abdominal pain can be additional symptoms of anaphylaxis and EMS should have a low threshold to transport any of these patients to the hospital [36].

Spiders

There are three clinically significant species of spiders found in North America: the black widow, the brown recluse, and the hobo spider.

Black widow spider bites are often quick and painless, but may be experienced as a pinprick sensation that quickly resolves. Calcium channel-mediated neurotransmitter release of acetylcholine and other excitatory neurotransmitters can result in extremely painful muscle spasm, hypertension, and diaphoresis in the hours following envenomation. Fatalities are rare and therapy should be supportive. Opioids for pain and benzodiazepines to aid in muscle relaxation and minimize hypertension may be considered in the field [3,36]. Some controversy exists among experts about the use of black widow antivenin. EMS should transfer all suspected cases of widow bites to the ED for possible antivenin administration.

Brown recluse and other recluse species are found in the Mississippi River valley and the surrounding states, south east, and south west. The bite has been associated with an evolving necrotic lesion; however, more severe systemic manifestations have been reported, termed "systemic loxoscelism." Signs and symptoms of loxoscelism include fever, vomiting, rhabdomyolysis, hemolysis, disseminated intravascular coagulation, renal failure, and death [37]. Appropriate clinical skepticism should be exercised given the frequency of misdiagnosis and conflicting reports of loxoscelism in areas where recluses are not endemic and the attribution of more common skin lesions, including folliculitis and abscess formation, to a "spider bite [38]." Regardless, transport to the ED for wound evaluation is recommended and intravenous fluids and antiemetics should be administered.

The hobo spider, a European native, is found in the northwestern United States. It is reported to cause dermonecrotic lesions as well. These lesions can be associated with headache, visual impairment, nausea, vomiting, weakness, and lethargy [39,40]. Regardless, as with the brown recluse, treatment is supportive and there are no specific prehospital therapies recommended.

Fifty-four species of tarantula are known to habit the desert south west. Despite their size, their toxicity is relatively minor. New World tarantulas are equipped with urticating hairs they release in self-defense. Depending on the species and type of hairs, clinical manifestations range from local inflammation to severe respiratory inflammation and significant eye injury. Prehospital management includes removal of hairs with cellophane tape and irrigation of the eyes. Antihistamines and corticosteroids may be considered. Any patient with ocular complaints requires transport to the hospital for ophthalmological evaluation.

Scorpions

The only scorpion of toxicological importance endemic to the United States is *Centruroides exilicauda* (the bark scorpion). Scorpions envenomate by stinging with their tails and can cause significant morbidity, especially in children. The venom is a neurotoxin that opens sodium channels, causing catecholamine and acetylcholine release. A scorpion antivenom exists and is used for those with systemic neurotoxic symptoms. Prehospital treatment may consist of symptomatic treatment with opioids and benzodiazepines [41].

Ticks

Ticks are eight-legged arthropods that live off the blood of various animals. Accordingly, they are vectors for viral, bacterial, and parasitic diseases, including Rocky Mountain spotted fever, typhus, tularemia, Lyme disease, babesiosis, ehrlichiosis, Colorado tick fever, and tick-borne encephalitis.42 Certain North American species, namely the Lone Star tick, the American dog tick, and the Rocky Mountain wood tick, secrete venom capable of causing paralysis in a manner similar to botulinum toxin. Discussion of each of the various tick-borne illnesses is outside the scope of this chapter; however, prehospital providers should be aware that prophylactic therapy may be offered to patients with known tick bites and the curative therapy for tick paralysis is removal of the tick. Supportive therapy including close attention to airway and breathing is paramount in any patient with ascending motor paralysis from possible tick-related disease [42,43].

Non-indigenous animals

This chapter has focused on species found in North America. EMS physicians and providers should take the time to learn about non-indigenous animals in their area. There is not enough room to cover all harmful animals in this chapter and providers should look to other toxicological texts for more in-depth information. It is also important to recognize that exposure to non-indigenous animals can occur not only in zoos or known refuges, but in private collections or simply as pets. In the case of private collectors, the owner often is aware of the species as well as its clinical effects, but may be resistant to seeking medical care for fear of legal persecution or confiscation of his or her collection. Poison centers and zoos are the best resources to help find appropriate antivenins. High-quality supportive care should be the standard, with local public health and poison control authorities guiding specific therapy.

Transport

Emergency medical services providers should encourage transport to the hospital. Transport preference should be a facility with a toxicology service or access to a toxicology consultant. If this is not possible within a reasonable time frame, patients should be transported to a local tertiary care facility that has emergency, trauma, and surgical specialties readily available. Prehospital protocols should specify when to contact medical oversight about the use of aircraft for transport of patients to an appropriate facility.

Conclusion

Our environment presents unpredictable encounters with animal bites, stings, and envenomations. Education on animals found locally may help EMS providers feel more comfortable during a response. Providers and medical directors should remember that most care is supportive and symptomatic. Transport to an appropriate facility will give the patient the best chance of a good outcome.

References

1 Ball V, Younggren BN. Emergency management of difficult wounds: part I. *Emerg Med Clin North Am* 2007;25:101–21.

2 Freer L. North American wild mammalian injuries. *Emerg Med Clin North Am* 2004;22:445–73.

3 Singletary EM, Rochman AS, Bodmer JC, Holstege CP. Envenomations. *Med Clin North Am* 2005;89:1195–224.

4 Hon KL, Fu CC, Chor CM, et al. Issues associated with dog bite injuries in children and adolescents assessed at the emergency department. *Pediatr Emerg Care.* 2007;23:445–9.

5 Benson LS, Edwards SL, Schiff AP, et al. Dog and cat bites to the hand: treatment and cost assessment. *J Hand Surg* 2006;31:468–73.

6 Brook I. Management of human and animal bite wounds: an overview. *Adv Skin Wound Care* 2005;18:197–203.

7 Fox RC, Scott CS. First evidence of a venom delivery apparatus in extinct mammals. *Nature* 2005;435:1091–3.

8 Jackson AC. Recovery from rabies. *N Engl J Med* 2005;352:2549–50.

9 Willoughby RE Jr, Tieves KS, Hoffman GM, et al. Survival after treatment of rabies with induction of coma. *N Engl J Med* 2005;352:2508–14.

10 Advisory Committee on Immunization Practices. Human rabies prevention – United States, 1999. Recommendations of the Advisory Committee on Immunization Practices (ACIP). *MMWR Recomm Rep* 1999;48:1–21.

11 Gold BS, Barish RA, Dart RC. North American snake envenomation: diagnosis, treatment, and management. *Emerg Med Clin North Am* 2004;22:423–43.

12 McKinney PE. Out-of-hospital and interhospital management of crotaline snakebite. *Ann Emerg Med* 2001;37:168–74.

13 Pizon AF. Snakebites: prehospital assessment & treatment of envenomations. *J EMS* 2007;32:76–81, 83, 88.

14 Powers DW. Stings and bites: what to do about envenomation injuries. *Emerg Med Serv* 2005;34:67, 69–75.

15 American College of Medical Toxicology, American Academy of Clinical Toxicology, American Association of Poison Control Centers, European Association of Poison Control Centres, International Society of Toxinology, Asia Pacific Association of Medical Toxicology. Position statement: pressure immobilization after North American crotalinae snake envenomation. *J Med Toxicol* 2011;7:322–3.

16 American Pain Society. *Principles of Analgesic Use in the Treatment of Acute Pain and Cancer Pain*, 5th edn. Glenview, IL: American Pain Society, 2003.

17 Sutherland SK, Coulter AR, Harris RD. Rationalisation of first-aid measures for elapid snakebite. *Lancet* 1979;1:183–5.

18 Nelson L, Lewin N, Howland MA, Hoffman RS, Goldfrank LR, Flomenbaum ME. *Goldfrank's Toxicologic Emergencies*, 9th edn. New York: McGraw-Hill Medical, 2011, pp.1601–10.

19 Piacentine J, Curry SC, Ryan PJ. Life-threatening anaphylaxis following gila monster bite. *Ann Emerg Med* 1986;15:959–61.

20 Preston CA. Hypotension, myocardial infarction, and coagulopathy following gila monster bite. *J Emerg Med* 1989;7:37–40.

21 Bou-Abboud CF, Kardassakis DG. Acute myocardial infarction following a gila monster (Heloderma suspectum cinctum) bite. *West J Med* 1988;148:577–9.

22 Atkinson PR, Boyle A, Hartin D, McAuley D. Is hot water immersion an effective treatment for marine envenomation? *Emerg Med J* 2006;23:503–8.

23 Hertelendy A. Aquatic emergencies: pathophysiology of and treatment for underwater stings. *J EMS* 2004;29:86–92, 94, 96, 98, 100.

24 Perkins RA, Morgan SS. Poisoning, envenomation, and trauma from marine creatures. *Am Fam Physician* 2004;69:885–90.

25 Ward NT, Darracq MA, Tomaszewski C, Clark RF. Evidence-based treatment of jellyfish stings in North America and Hawaii. *Ann Emerg Med* 2012;60:399–414.

26 Norris R. Caterpillar envenomations, 2013. Available at: http://emedicine.medscape.com/article/769448-overview

27 Norris R. Millipede envenomations, 2012. Available at: http://emedicine.medscape.com/article/772881-overview

28 Klotz JH, Klotz SA, Pinnas JL. Animal bites and stings with anaphylactic potential. *J Emerg Med* 2009;36:148–56.

29 Yates AB, Moffitt JE, deShazo RD. Anaphylaxis to arthropod bites and stings. *Immunol Allergy Clin North Am* 2001;21:635–51.

30 Graft DF. Insect sting allergy. *Med Clin North Am* 2006;90:211–32.

31 Betten DP, Richardson WH, Tong TC, Clark RF. Massive honey bee envenomation-induced rhabdomyolysis in an adolescent. *Pediatrics* 2006;117:231–5.

32 França FO, Benvenuti LA, Fan HW, et al. Severe and fatal mass attacks by 'killer' bees (Africanized honey bees – Apis mellifera scutellata) in Brazil: clinicopathological studies with measurement of serum venom concentrations. *Q J Med* 1994;87(5):269–82.

33 Lovecchio F, Cannon RD, Algier J, et al. Bee swarmings in children. *Am J Emerg Med* 2007;25:931–3.

34 Bresolin NL, Carvalho LC, Goes EC, Fernandes R, Barotto AM. Acute renal failure following massive attack by Africanized bee stings. *Pediatr Nephrol* 2002;17:625–7.

35 DeSchazo RD, Butcher BT, Banks WA. Reactions to the stings of the imported fire ant. *N Engl J Med* 1990;323:462–6.

36 Nelson L, Lewin N, Howland MA, Hoffman RS, Goldfrank LR, Flomenbaum ME. *Goldfrank's Toxicologic Emergencies*, 9th edn. New York: McGraw-Hill, 2011, pp.1561–81.

37 Saucier JR. Arachnid envenomation. *Emerg Med Clin North Am* 2004;22:405–22.

38 Vetter RS. The distribution of brown recluse spiders in the southeastern quadrant of the United States in relation to loxoscelism diagnoses. *South Med J* 2009;102:518–22.

39 Centers for Disease Control. Necrotic arachnidism – Pacific Northwest, 1988–1996. *MMWR* 1996;45:433–6.

40 Vest DK. Necrotic arachnidism in the northwest United States and its probable relationship to Tegenaria agrestis (Walckenaer) spiders. *Toxicon* 1987;25:175–84.

41 Skolnik AB, Ewald MB. Pediatric scorpion envenomation in the United States: morbidity, mortality, and therapeutic innovations. *Pediatr Emerg Care* 2013;29:98–103.

42 Aurebach PS. *Wilderness Medicine*, 6th edn. Philadelphia: Mosby, 2012, pp.954–74.

43 Diaz JH. A 60-year meta-analysis of tick paralysis in the United States: a predictable, preventable, and often misdiagnosed poisoning. *J Med Toxicol* 2010;6:15–21.

CHAPTER 39

Field trauma triage

Hiren Patel and Scott M. Sasser

Disclaimer

This chapter summarizes the *National Panel Guidelines for Field Triage of Injured Patients Recommendations of the National Expert Panel on Field Triage, 2011*, which has been published previously in *Morbidity, Mortality and Weekly Report (MMWR)*; available at: www.cdc.gov/mmwr/pdf/rr/rr6101.pdf. The text is excerpted from the original publication of current recommendations. In addition, some background materials from an earlier iteration have been included for context; available at: www.cdc.gov/mmwr/PDF/rr/rr5801.pdf. In general, all original *MMWR* text has been excerpted verbatim with a few exceptions (e.g. edits for transition or conciseness that do not affect meaning or interpretation of the recommendations or existing literature). To subscribe to MMWR, visit www.cdc.gov/MMWR.

Introduction

In the United States, unintentional injury is the leading cause of death for persons aged 1–44 years [1]. In 2008, injuries accounted for approximately 181,226 deaths in the United States [2]. In 2008, approximately 30 million injuries were serious enough to require the injured persons to visit a hospital emergency department (ED); 5.4 million (18%) of these injured patients were transported by EMS [3].

Ensuring that severely injured trauma patients are treated at trauma centers has a profound effect on their survival [4]. Ideally, all persons with severe, life-threatening injuries would be transported to Level I or Level II trauma centers, and all persons with less serious injuries would be transported to lower-level trauma centers or community EDs. However, patient differences, occult injuries, and the complexities of patient assessment in the field can affect triage decisions.

The National Study on the Costs and Outcomes of Trauma (NSCOT) identified a 25% reduction in mortality for severely injured adult patients who received care at Level I trauma centers rather than at non-trauma centers [4]. Similarly, a retrospective cohort study of 11,398 severely injured adult patients who survived to hospital admission in Ontario, Canada, indicated that mortality was significantly higher in patients initially undertriaged to non-trauma centers (odds ratio (OR) 1.24; 95% confidence interval (CI) 1.10–1.40) [5].

History of the field triage decision schemes

In 1976, the American College of Surgeons Committee on Trauma (ACS-COT) began publishing resource documents to provide guidance for designation of facilities as trauma centers and appropriate care of acutely injured patients [6–11]. Before this guidance appeared, the typical trauma victim was transported to the nearest hospital, regardless of the capabilities of that hospital, and often with little prehospital intervention [6].

The ACS-COT regularly revised the resource document, which included a decision scheme to provide guidance for the field triage of injured patients. During each revision, the decision scheme was evaluated by a subcommittee of ACS-COT, which analyzed the available literature, considered expert opinion, and developed recommendations regarding additions and deletions to the decision scheme. Final approval of the recommendations rested with the ACS-COT Executive Committee. Following its initial publication in 1986, the decision scheme was updated and revised four times: in 1990, 1993, and 1999 [6].

In 2005, the Centers for Disease Control and Prevention (CDC), with financial support from the National Highway Traffic Safety Administration (NHTSA), collaborated with ACS-COT to convene the initial meetings of the National Expert Panel on Field Triage. The panel comprises persons with expertise in acute injury care, including EMS providers and medical

Emergency Medical Services: Clinical Practice and Systems Oversight, Second Edition. Volume 1: Clinical Aspects of EMS.
Edited by David C. Cone, Jane H. Brice, Theodore R. Delbridge, and J. Brent Myers.
© 2015 US Government. Published 2015 by John Wiley & Sons, Inc. Companion Website: www.wiley.com/go/cone/naemsp

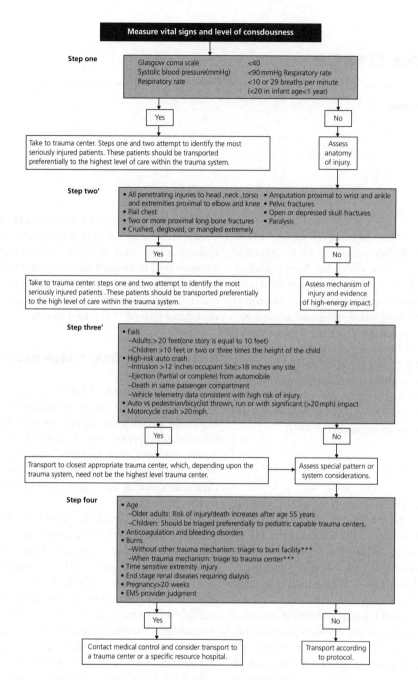

Measure vital signs and level of consdousness

Step one

Glasgow coma scale	<40
Systolic blood pressure(mmHg)	<90 mmHg Respiratory rate
Respiratory rate	<10 or 29 breaths per minute
	(<20 in infant age<1 year)

Yes

Take to trauma center. Steps one and two attempt to identify the most seriously injured patients. These patients should be transported preferentially to the highest level of care within the trauma system.

No

Assess anatomy of injury.

Step two'

- All penetrating injuries to head ,neck ,torso and extremities proximal to elbow and knee
- Flail chest
- Two or more proximal long bone fractures
- Crushed, degloved, or mangled extremely
- Amputation proximal to wrist and ankle
- Pelvic fractures
- Open or depressed skull fractures
- Paralysis

Yes

Take to trauma center. steps one and two attempt to identify the most seriously injured patients .These patients should be transported preferentially to the high level of care within the trauma system.

No

Assess mechanism of injury and evidence of high-energy impact.

Step three'

- Fails
  - Adults:> 20 feet(one story is equal to 10 feet)
  - Children >10 feet or two or three times the height of the child
- High-risk auto crash
  - Intrusion >12 inches occupant Site;>18 inches any site.
  - Ejection (Partial or complete) from automobile
  - Death in same passenger compartment
  - Vehicle telemetry data consistent with high risk of injury.
- Auto vs pedestrian/bicyclist thrown, run or with significant (>20 mph) impact
- Motorcycle crash >20 mph.

Yes

Transport to closest appropriate trauma center, which, depending upon the trauma system, need not be the highest level trauma center.

No

Assess special pattern or system considerations.

Step four

- Age
  - Older adults: Risk of injury/death increases after age 55 years
  - Children: Should be triaged preferentially to pediatric capable trauma centers.
- Anticoagulation and bleeding disorders
- Burns
  - Without other trauma mechanism: triage to burn facility***
  - When trauma mechanism: triage to trauma center***
- Time sensitive extremity injury
- End stage renal diseases requiring dialysis
- Pregnancy>20 weeks
- EMS provider judgment

Yes

Contact medical control and consider transport to a trauma center or a specific resource hospital.

No

Transport according to protocol.

When in doubt, transport to a trauma center

Source: Adopted from American College of Surgeons, Resources from optimal care of the injured patients, Chicago , IL: American College of Surgeons ;2006. Footnotes have been added to enhance understanding of field triage by persons outside the acute injury care field.

* The upper limit of respiratory rate in infants is > 29 breaths per minute to maintain a higher level of over triage for infants.
† Trauma centers are designated Level I-IV, with level I responding the highest level of trauma care available.
§ Any injury noted in steps two and three triggers a "Yes" response.
¶ Age < 15 years.
** Intrusion refers to interior compartment intrusion, as opposed to deformation which refers to exterior damage.
†† Includes pedestrians or bicyclists thrown or run over by a motor vehicle or those with estimated impact >20mph with a motor vehicle.
§§ Local or regional protocol should be used to determine the most appropriate level of trauma center, appropriate center need not be Level I.
¶¶ Age > 55 years.
*** Patients with both burns and concomitant trauma for whom the burn injury poses the greatest risk for morbidity and mortality should be transferred to a burn center. If the non-burn trauma presents a greater immediate risk, the patient may be stabilized in a trauma center and then transferred to a burn center.
††† Injuries such as open fractures or fracture with neurovascular compromise .
§§§ Emergency medical services.
¶¶¶ Patient who do not meet any of the triage criteria in steps 1- 4 should be transported to most appropriate medical facility as outlined in local EMS Protocols.

Figure 39.1 Field triage decision scheme – United States, 2006. Source: Adapted from American College of Surgeons. *Resources for Optimal Care of the Injured Patient*. Chicago, IL: American College of Surgeons; 2006. Reproduced with permission of the American College of Surgeons. Footnotes have been added to enhance understanding of field tirage by persons ouside the acute injury care field.

directors, state EMS directors, hospital administrators, adult and pediatric emergency physicians, nurses, adult and pediatric trauma surgeons, persons in the automotive industry, public health personnel, and representatives of federal agencies.

During 2005 and 2006, the panel met to revise the decision scheme, and the end-product of that comprehensive revision process (Figure 39.1) was published by ACS-COT in 2006 [11]. In 2009, CDC published a comprehensive review of the revision process and the detailed rationale for the triage criteria underlying the 2006 version of the decisions scheme as the "Guidelines for field triage of injured patients: recommendations of the National Expert Panel On Field Triage" (the guidelines) [12].

In 2011, the panel reconvened to review the guidelines in the context of recently published literature as well as the experience of states and local communities working to implement the guidelines and to make recommendations regarding any changes or modifications to the guidelines. A major outcome of the panel's meetings was the revision of the guidelines (Figure 39.2). In 2012, CDC published an update to the guidelines, including the rationale for modifications [13]; this update was endorsed by multiple national organizations.

Accuracy of field triage

The accuracy of field triage can be thought of as the degree of match between the severity of injury and the level of care. Sensitivity and specificity of screening tests are useful indicators of accuracy (Figure 39.3). Maximally sensitive triage would mean that all patients with injuries appropriate for Level I or Level II trauma centers would be sent to such centers. Maximally specific triage would mean that no patients who could be treated at Level III or Level IV centers or community EDs would be transported to Level I or Level II centers. Triage that succeeded in transporting only patients with high injury severity to Level I or Level II centers would maximize the positive predictive value (PPV) of the process, and triage that succeeded in transporting only patients with low injury severity to Level III, IV, or community EDs would maximize the negative predictive value (NPV).

In reality, patient differences, occult injuries, and the complexities of patient assessment in the field preclude perfect accuracy in triage decisions. Inaccurate triage that results in a patient who requires higher-level care not being transported to a Level I or Level II trauma center is termed undertriage. The result of undertriage is that a patient does not receive the specialized trauma care required. Overtriage occurs when a patient who does not require care in a higher-level trauma center nevertheless is transported to such a center, thereby unnecessarily consuming scarce resources. In the triage research literature, all of these measures (sensitivity, specificity, PPV, NPV, undertriage, and overtriage; see Figure 39.3) are used together with measures of association (e.g. odds ratios) to assess the effectiveness of field triage.

As with sensitivity and specificity applied to screening tests, reductions in undertriage usually are accompanied by increases in overtriage, and reductions in overtriage are accompanied by increases in undertriage. Because the potential harm associated with undertriage (i.e. causing a patient in need of trauma center care not to receive appropriate care) is high and could result in death or substantial morbidity and disability, trauma systems frequently err on the side of minimizing undertriage rather than minimizing overtriage. Target levels for undertriage rates within a trauma system range from 0% to 5% of patients requiring Level I or Level II trauma center care, depending on the criteria used to determine the undertriage rate (e.g. death and Injury Severity Score (ISS)) [11]. Target levels of overtriage vary (approximate range: 25–50%) [11]. As field triage continues to evolve on the basis of new research findings, overtriage rates might be reduced while maintaining low undertriage rates.

Field triage decision scheme recommendations

Step one: physiological criteria

Step one of the decision scheme seeks to guide EMS personnel in identifying critically injured patients rapidly through measuring their vital signs and assessing their level of consciousness. The instruction "measure vital signs and level of consciousness" has been included since the 1986 version of the ACS Field Triage Decision Protocol [7]. The sensitivity of physiological criteria to identify severely injured patients has been reported to range from 55.6% to 64.8%, with PPV of 41.8% and specificity of 85.7% [13,14]. A study of 333 patients transported by helicopter to a Level I trauma center during 1993 and 1994 indicated that physiological criteria alone were specific (0.9) but not sensitive (0.6) for identifying ISS >15 [13]. An evaluation of data in the South Carolina EMS registry, conducted to determine undertriage and overtriage rates when EMS personnel used the 1990 version of the ACS field triage guidelines, determined that physiological criteria alone had a sensitivity of 0.65 and PPV of 42% for severe injury (ISS >15) for 753 trauma patients transported to a Level I trauma center in Charleston [14]. Adults meeting such physiological criteria treated at Level I trauma centers had reduced odds of mortality compared with patients treated at lower level trauma centers and non-trauma center hospitals (OR 0.7; 95% CI 0.6–0.9). Multiple peer-reviewed articles published since 2006 continue to support the use of physiological criteria [15–19].

Transport is recommended to a facility that provides the highest level of care within the defined trauma system if any of the following are identified:

- Glasgow Coma Scale ≤13, or
- SBP <90 mmHg, or
- respiratory rate <10 or >29 breaths per minute (<20 in infant aged <1 year), or need for ventilatory support.

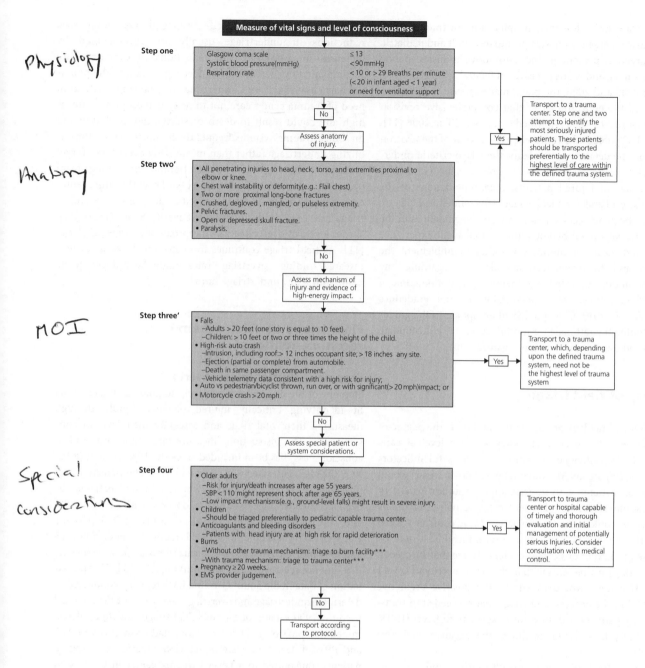

Physiology (handwritten) — *Anatomy* (handwritten) — *MOI* (handwritten) — *Special considerations* (handwritten)

Measure of vital signs and level of consciousness

Step one

Glasgow coma scale	≤ 13
Systolic blood pressure(mmHg)	< 90 mmHg
Respiratory rate	< 10 or > 29 Breaths per minute (< 20 in infant aged < 1 year) or need for ventilator support

No

Assess anatomy of injury.

Yes → Transport to a trauma center. Step one and two attempt to identify the most seriously injured patients. These patients should be transported preferentially to the highest level of care within the defined trauma system.

Step two'

• All penetrating injuries to head, neck, torso, and extremities proximal to elbow or knee.
• Chest wall instability or deformity(e.g.: Flail chest)
• Two or more proximal long-bone fractures
• Crushed, degloved , mangled, or pulseless extremity.
• Pelvic fractures.
• Open or depressed skull fracture.
• Paralysis.

No

Assess mechanism of injury and evidence of high-energy impact.

Step three'

• Falls
  –Adults > 20 feet (one story is equal to 10 feet).
  –Children: > 10 feet or two or three times the height of the child.
• High-risk auto crash
  –Intrusion, including roof:> 12 inches occupant site; > 18 inches any site.
  –Ejection (partial or complete) from automobile.
  –Death in same passenger compartment.
  –Vehicle telemetry data consistent with a high risk for injury;
• Auto vs pedestrian/bicyclist thrown, run over, or with significant(> 20 mph)impact; or
• Motorcycle crash > 20 mph.

Yes → Transport to a trauma center, which, depending upon the defined trauma system, need not be the highest level of trauma system

No

Assess special patient or system considerations.

Step four

• Older adults
  –Risk for injury/death increases after age 55 years.
  –SBP < 110 might represent shock after age 65 years.
  –Low impact mechanisms(e.g., ground-level falls) might result in severe injury.
• Children
  –Should be triaged preferentially to pediatric capable trauma center.
• Anticoagulants and bleeding disorders
  –Patients with head injury are at high risk for rapid deterioration
• Burns
  –Without other trauma mechanism: triage to burn facility***
  –With trauma mechanism: triage to trauma center***
• Pregnancy ≥ 20 weeks.
• EMS provider judgement.

Yes → Transport to trauma center or hospital capable of timely and thorough evaluation and initial management of potentially serious Injuries. Consider consultation with medical control.

No

Transport according to protocol.

Abbreviations: EMS-emergency medical services.
* The upper age limit of respiratory rate in infants is >>29 breaths per minute to maintain a higher level of overtriage for infants.
† Trauma centers are designated level I –IV. A level I center has the greatest amount of resources and personnel for care of the Injured patient and provides regional leadership in education, research and prevention programs. A level II facility offer similar resources to a level I facility, possibly differing only in continuous availability of certain subspecialties or sufficient prevention, education, and research activities for level I designations; level II facilities are not required to be resident or fellow education centers. A level III center is capable of assessment, resuscitation, and emergency surgery, with severely injured patients being transferred to a level I or II facility. A level IV trauma center is capable of providing 24-hour physician coverage, resuscitation, and stabilization to injured patients before transfer to a facility that provides a higher level of trauma care.
§ Any injury noted in step two or mechanism identified in step three triggers a"yes" response.
¶ Age < 15 years
** Intrusion refers to interior compartment intrusion, as opposed to deformation which refers to exterior damage.
†† Includes pedestrians or bicyclist thrown or run over by a motor vehicle or those with estimated impact > 20 mph with a motor vehicle.
§§ Local or regional protocols should be used to determine the most appropriate level of trauma center within the defined trauma system; need not be the highest level trauma center.
¶¶ Age> 55 years
*** Patients with both burns and concomitant trauma for whom the burn injury poses the greatest risk for morbidity and mortality should be transferred to a burn center. If the nonburn trauma presents a greater immediate risk, the patient may be stabilized in a trauma center and then transferred to a burn center.
††† Patients who do not meet any of the triage criteria in steps One through four should be transported to the most appropriate medical facility as outlined in local EMS protocols.

Figure 39.2 Guidelines for field triage of injured patients – United States, 2011. Source: Sasser SM. *MMWR Recomm Rep* 2012;61:1–20.

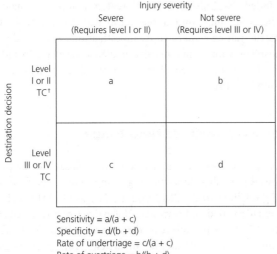

Injury severity

| | Severe (Requires level I or II) | Not severe (Requires level III or IV) |

Level I or II TC†: a, b

Level III or IV TC: c, d

Destination decision

Sensitivity = a/(a + c)
Specificity = d/(b + d)
Rate of undertriage = c/(a + c)
Rate of overtriage = b/(b + d)
Positive predictive value = a/(a + b)
Negative predictive value = d/(c + d)

* In this figure, "a", "b", "c", and "d" represent injured patients, categorized by severity of injury and destination.
†Trauma center.

Figure 39.3 Measures of field triage accuracy. Source: Sasser SM. *MMWR Recomm Rep* 2009;58:1–35.

Step two: anatomical criteria

Step two of the guidelines recognizes that certain patients, on initial presentation to EMS providers, have normal physiology but have anatomical injuries that might require the highest level of care within the defined trauma system. In these cases, reliance on physiological criteria alone might lead to undertriage. In the South Carolina study noted above, the physiological criteria alone had a sensitivity of 0.7 and PPV of 42% for severe injury [14]. Anatomical criteria alone had a sensitivity of 0.5 and PPV of 21.6%. Combining anatomical and physiological criteria to identify severely injured trauma patients produced a sensitivity of 0.8 and PPV of 26.9%. A prospective study of 5,728 patients treated by EMS providers in Washington state included patients who were injured and met at least one of the ACS triage criteria; patients were tracked from EMS contact through hospital discharge [20]. Triage criteria were examined individually and in combination for their ability to identify a major trauma victim (MTV) with ISS of >15 or mortality. Anatomical criteria had a 20–30% yield for identifying major trauma victims and were associated with a hospital admission rate of 86% and a mortality rate slightly below that of the entire study population.

Transport is recommended to a facility that provides the highest level of care within the defined trauma system if any of the following are identified:
- all penetrating injuries to head, neck, torso, and extremities proximal to elbow or knee
- chest wall instability or deformity (e.g. flail chest)
- two or more proximal long bone fractures

- crushed, degloved, mangled, or pulseless extremity
- amputation proximal to wrist or ankle
- pelvic fractures
- open or depressed skull fractures
- paralysis.

Step three: mechanism of injury criteria

An injured patient who does not meet step one or step two criteria should be evaluated in terms of mechanism of injury (MOI) to determine if there might be a severe but occult injury. Evaluation of MOI will help to determine if the patient should be transported to a trauma center. Although different outcomes have been used, recent studies have demonstrated the usefulness of MOI for field triage decisions. A retrospective study of approximately 1 million trauma patients indicated that using physiological and anatomical criteria alone for triage of patients resulted in undertriage, implying that using MOI for determining trauma center need helped reduce the problem of undertriage [21]. Another study of approximately half a million patients determined that MOI was an independent predictor of mortality and functional impairment of blunt trauma patients [22]. Among 89,441 injured patients evaluated by EMS providers at six sites, physiological and anatomical criteria identified only 2,600 (45.5%) of 5,720 patients with ISS >15, whereas MOI criteria identified an additional 1,449 (25.3%) seriously injured patients with a modest (10%) incremental increase in overtriage (from 14.0% to 25.3%) [23].

Transport is recommended to a trauma center if any of the following are identified:
- falls:
  - adults: >20 feet (one story = 10 feet)
  - children: >10 feet or 2–3 times the height of the child
- high-risk auto crash:
  - intrusion, including roof: >12 inches occupant site; >18 inches any site
  - ejection (partial or complete) from automobile
  - death in same passenger compartment
  - vehicle telemetry data consistent with a high risk for injury
- automobile versus pedestrian/bicyclist thrown, run over, or with significant (>20 mph) impact
- motorcycle crash >20 mph.

Step four: special considerations

In step four, EMS personnel must determine whether persons who have not met physiological, anatomical, or mechanism criteria have underlying conditions or comorbid factors that place them at higher risk of injury or that aid in identifying the seriously injured patient. Persons who meet step four criteria might require trauma center care. A retrospective study of approximately 1 million trauma patients indicated that using physiological and anatomical criteria alone for triage of patients resulted in a high degree of undertriage, implying that using special considerations for determining trauma center need helped reduce the problem of undertriage [21]. Among 89,441 injured patients evaluated by EMS providers at six sites, physiological, anatomical, and mechanism of injury criteria identified 4,049 (70.8%) patients with ISS >15; step four identified another 956 (16.7%) seriously injured patients, with an increase in overtriage from 25.3% to 37.3% [23].

Transport to a trauma center or hospital capable of timely and thorough evaluation and initial management of potentially serious injuries is recommended for patients who meet the following criteria:

- older adults:
  - risk for injury/death increases after age 55 years
  - SBP <110 might represent shock after age 65 years; low-impact mechanisms (e.g. ground-level falls) might result in severe injury
- children: should be triaged preferentially to pediatric-capable trauma centers
- anticoagulants and bleeding disorders: patients with head injury are at high risk for rapid deterioration
- burns:
  - without other trauma mechanism: triage to burn facility
  - with trauma mechanism: triage to trauma center
- pregnancy >20 weeks
- EMS provider judgment.

Pediatric concerns

No published data suggest that injured children, in the absence of physiological, anatomical, or MOI triage criteria, are at risk for negative outcomes solely on the basis of their age. The criteria in steps one, two, and three of the 2006 decision scheme are expected to identify nearly all seriously injured children. Therefore, the panel identified no specific age below which all injured children should be transported to a trauma center.

However, children meeting the revised field triage criteria for transport to trauma centers in steps one through three of the decision scheme should be transported preferentially to pediatric-capable trauma centers. Recent studies indicate that organized systems for trauma care contribute to improved outcomes for children [24] and that seriously injured children fare better in pediatric-capable trauma centers. Multiple reports document improved survival in pediatric-capable trauma centers [25–29], including data from the Pennsylvania Trauma Outcome Study registry that demonstrate absolute reductions in injury mortality ranging from 3.8% to 9.7% [30] and improved functional outcomes (e.g. feeding and locomotion) [31] when children aged <16 years with ISS of >15 are treated at pediatric trauma centers or at adult trauma centers that have acquired additional qualifications to treat children. What appears to matter most is the availability of pediatric-specific resources, particularly the availability of a pediatric intensive care unit (ICU), not the designation as a pediatric trauma center *per se* [32,33]. Although some earlier studies

concluded that injured children treated in adult trauma centers had outcomes comparable to those of children treated in pediatric trauma centers, those investigations were conducted in hospitals with comprehensive pediatric services, including pediatric emergency medicine, critical care medicine, and nursing [34–40]

Future research for field triage

In its 2011 analysis, the panel noted an increase in the peer-reviewed published literature regarding field triage from the 2006 guidelines to the 2012 update. The 2011–2012 revision process identified and reviewed 289 articles published during 2006–2011 (~48 articles/year) directly relevant to field triage, 24 times the annual number of articles during 1966–2005 (~2/year) cited in the 2006 guidelines [12]. Despite this increase in the number of articles, the panel concluded that ensuring that the guidelines are based on the best clinical evidence requires expanded surveillance, focused research using robust study designs, and consistent outcome measures.

The preponderance of existing triage studies reviewed by the panel used retrospective data, trauma registry samples, single EMS agencies, and single trauma centers, all of which can result in biased estimates and reduced generalizability. Prospective triage research is needed that includes multiple sites, multiple EMS agencies, trauma and non-trauma hospitals, and population-based study designs that reduce selection bias and increase the generalizability of study findings. In addition, relatively little triage literature exists that evaluates the guidelines in their entirety (as opposed to an individual criterion or component steps of the decision scheme) and the contribution of each step to the full guidelines. Prospective studies evaluating the full guidelines among the broad injury population served by EMS are needed to assess the accuracy of the guidelines appropriately and to better identify targets for improvement. Further, the process of field triage in rural settings, including the effect of geography on triage, issues regarding proximity to trauma centers, use of air medical services, integration of local hospitals for initial stabilization, and secondary triage at non-trauma hospitals, is poorly understood. As a substantial portion of the US population lives >60 minutes from the closest major trauma center, and 28% of US residents are only able to access specialized trauma care within this time window by helicopter [41], field triage in non-urban environments needs to be understood better.

Current peer-reviewed triage literature has described multiple outcome measures, including injury severity, clinical outcomes, need for trauma center resources (with or without a measure of timeliness), or a combination of these metrics. The most common clinical outcome measure is ISS >15, although the Abbreviated Injury Scale (AIS) ≥3 has also been used. Trauma center need has been measured by use of blood products, interventional radiology, major non-orthopedic surgery, or ICU stay. This variability in outcome measures limits comparability among studies and is not always consistent with literature identifying the subgroup of patients most likely to benefit from trauma center care. Future research should address these issues and attempt to match triage evaluation to patients most likely to benefit from trauma center care and clearly define the standard of measure.

The issue of undertriage in older adults was viewed by the panel as a major priority for future research. There is a need to understand the basis for undertriage in this age group and how the guidelines might be modified to reduce this problem. Related topics include the role of age in predicting serious injury, different physiological responses to injury among older adults, different injury-producing mechanisms in older adults, attitudes and behaviors of emergency and trauma care providers regarding triage in older adults, older adults' health care preferences for injury care, end-of-life issues and their relevance to triage, new criteria to identify serious injury in older adults, the role of trauma centers in caring for older injured adults, and other aspects of better matching patient need with hospital capability for this population. How systems respond to patient and/or family preferences regarding hospital destinations that differ from the recommendations in these guidelines should be explored in the context of patients' rights and the moral imperative to provide the optimal chance for improved outcomes from trauma.

Finally, the cost of trauma care, the implications of field triage on cost, and the cost-efficiency of different approaches to field triage require more research. Even after accounting for injury severity and important confounders, the cost of care is notably higher in trauma centers [42,43]. Though the cost-effectiveness of trauma center care has been demonstrated among seriously injured patients (AIS ≥4) [43], it is possible that modest shifts in overtriage might have substantial financial consequences. For example, a recent study that compared the 2006 and 1999 guidelines identified a potential $568 million cost saving at an assumed overtriage rate of 40% [44]. However, further studies are needed to discover new ways to maximize the efficiency and cost-effectiveness of trauma systems and ensure that patients are receiving optimal injury care while considering the importance of the research, education, and outreach mission of trauma centers.

Ongoing collaboration among local, state, and regional EMS agencies with governmental, non-governmental, academic, and public health agencies and institutions will allow the continuing analysis and evaluation of the 2011 guidelines and their effect on the care of acutely injured patients. State-wide EMS and trauma databases provide opportunities for state-wide quality improvement of field triage, research, and adaptation of the guidelines to meet state-specific circumstances. Large, nationally representative databases (e.g. the National EMS Information Systems database, the National Trauma Data Bank–National Sample Program, the Healthcare Cost and Utilization Project–National Inpatient Sample, the National Hospital Ambulatory Medical Care Survey, and NASS-CDS) could be used for future

triage research if advances are made to link these data files across phases of care (e.g. prehospital to in-hospital). Finally, uniform definitions of prehospital variables (including triage criteria) with a standardized data dictionary and data standards (e.g. HL7 messaging) could provide comparable data across study sites and assist with linking data files from the prehospital to the hospital setting.

Conclusion

The current field trauma triage guidelines are based on current medical literature, the experience of multiple states and communities working to improve field triage, and the expert opinions of the panel members. This guidance is intended to assist EMS and trauma systems, medical directors, and EMS physicians and providers with the information necessary to make critical decisions that have been demonstrated to increase the likelihood of improved outcomes in severely injured trauma patients [8].

Improved field triage of injured patients can have a profound effect on the structure, organization, and use of EMS and trauma systems, the costs associated with trauma care, and, most importantly, on the lives of the millions of persons injured every year in the United States. As noted throughout this chapter, improved research is needed to assess the effect of field triage on resource allocation, health care financing and funding, and, most importantly, patient outcomes.

References

1 Holder Y, Peden M, Krug E, Lund J, Gururaj G, Kobusingye O (eds). *Injury Surveillance Guidelines*. Geneva: World Health Organization, 2001. Available at: http://libdoc.who.int/hq/2001/WHO_NMH_VIP_01.02.pdf

2 Butchart A, Harvey AP, Krug E, Meddings D, Peden M, Sminkey L (eds). *Preventing Injuries and Violence: a guide for ministries of health*. Geneva: World Health Organization, 2007.

3 Hofman K, Primack A, Keusch G, Hrynkow S. Addressing the growing burden of trauma and injury in low- and middle-income countries. *Am J Pub Health* 2005;95:13–17.

4 Sasser S, Varghese M, Kellermann A, Lormand JD (eds). *Prehospital Trauma Care Systems*. Geneva, Switzerland: World Health Organization, 2005.

5 Ahmed N, Andersson R. Differences in cause-specific patterns of unintentional injury mortality among 15–44-year-olds in income-based country groups. *Accid Anal Prev* 2002;34:541–51.

6 Mackersie RC. History of trauma field triage development and the American College of Surgeons criteria. *Prehosp Emerg Care* 2006;10:287–94.

7 American College of Surgeons. *Hospital and Prehospital Resources for the Optimal Care of the Injured Patient: Appendices A through J*. Chicago, IL: American College of Surgeons, 1986.

8 American College of Surgeons. *Resources for the Optimal Care of the Injured Patient*: 1999. Chicago, IL: American College of Surgeons, 1999.

9 American College of Surgeons. *Resources for the Optimal Care of the Injured Patient*: 1990. Chicago, IL: American College of Surgeons, 1990.

10 American College of Surgeons. *Resources for the Optimal Care of the Injured Patient*: 1993. Chicago, IL: American College of Surgeons, 1993.

11 American College of Surgeons. *Resources for the Optimal Care of the Injured Patient*: 2006. Chicago, IL: American College of Surgeons, 2006.

12 Sasser SM, Hunt RC, Sullivent EE, et al. Guidelines for field triage of injured patients: recommendations of the National Expert Panel on Field Triage. *MMWR Recomm Rep* 2009;58:1–35.

13 Sasser SM, Hunt RC, Faul M, et al. Guidelines for field triage of injured patients: recommendations of the National Expert Panel on Field Triage, 2011. *MMWR Recomm Rep* 2012;61:1–20.

14 Wuerz R, Taylor J, Smith JS. Accuracy of trauma triage in patients transported by helicopter. *Air Med J* 1996;15:168–70.

15 Norcross ED, Ford DW, Cooper ME, Zone-Smith L, Byrne TK, Yarbrough DR. Application of American College of Surgeons' field triage guidelines by pre-hospital personnel. *J Am Coll Surg* 1995;181:539–44.

16 Cherry RA, King TS, Carney DE, Bryant P, Cooney RN. Trauma team activation and the impact on mortality. *J Trauma* 2007;63:326–30.

17 Edelman DA, White MT, Tyburski JG, Wilson RF. Post-traumatic hypotension: should systolic blood pressure of 90–109 mmHg be included? *Shock* 2007;27:134–8.

18 Codner P, Obaid A, Porral D, Lush S, Cinat M. Is field hypotension a reliable indicator of significant injury in trauma patients who are normotensive on arrival to the emergency department? *Am Surg* 2005;71:768–71.

19 Lipsky AM, Gausche-Hill M, Henneman PL, et al. Prehospital hypotension is a predictor of the need for an emergent, therapeutic operation in trauma patients with normal systolic blood pressure in the emergency department. *J Trauma* 2006;61:1228–33.

20 Esposito TJ, Offner PJ, Jurkovich GJ, Griffith J, Maier RV. Do prehospital trauma center triage criteria identify major trauma victims? *Arch Surg* 1995;130:171–6.

21 Brown JB, Stassen NA, Bankey PE, Sangosanya AT, Cheng JD, Gestring ML. Mechanism of injury and special consideration criteria still matter: an evaluation of the National Trauma Triage Protocol. *J Trauma* 2011;70:38–45.

22 Haider AH, Chang DC, Haut ER, Cornwell EE, Efron DT. Mechanism of injury predicts patient mortality and impairment after blunt trauma. *J Surg Res* 2009;153:138–42.

23 Newgard C, Zive D, Holmes JF, et al. A multi-site assessment and validation of the ACSCOT field triage decision scheme for identifying seriously injured children and adults. *J Am Coll Surg* 2011;213(6):709–21.

24 Hulka F, Mullins RJ, Mann NC, et al. Influence of a statewide trauma system on pediatric hospitalization and outcome. *J Trauma* 1997;42(3):514–19.

25 Pollack MM, Alexander SR, Clarke N, Ruttiman UE, Tesselaar HM, Bachulis AC. Improved outcomes from tertiary center pediatric

intensive care: a statewide comparison of tertiary and nontertiary care facilities. *Crit Care Med* 1991;19(2):150–9.

26 Nakayama DK, Copes WS, Sacco WJ. Differences in pediatric trauma care among pediatric and nonpediatric centers. *J Pediatr Surg* 1992;27:427–31.

27 Hall JR, Reyes, HM, Meller JL, Stein RJ. Traumatic death in urban children, revisited. *Am J Dis Child* 1993;147:102–7.

28 Cooper A, Barlow B, DiScala C, String D, Ray K, Mottley L. Efficacy of pediatric trauma care: results of a population-based study. *J Pediatr Surg* 1993;28:299–305.

29 Hall JR, Reyes HM, Meller JT, Loeff DS, Dembek R. Outcome for blunt trauma is best at a pediatric trauma center. *J Pediatr Surg* 1996;31:72–7.

30 Potoka DA, Schall LC, Gardner MJ, Stafford PW, Peitzman AB, Ford HR. Impact of pediatric trauma centers on mortality in a statewide system. *J Trauma* 2000;49:237–45.

31 Potoka DA, Schall LC, Ford HR. Improved functional outcome for severely injured children treated at pediatric trauma centers. *J Trauma* 2001;51:824–34.

32 Osler TM, Vane DW, Tepas JJ, Rogers FB, Shackford SR, Badger GJ. Do pediatric trauma centers have better survival rates than adult trauma centers? An examination of the National Pediatric Trauma Registry. *J Trauma* 2001;50:96–101.

33 Farrell LS, Hannan EL, Cooper A. Severity of injury and mortality associated with pediatric blunt injuries: hospitals with pediatric intensive care units vs. other hospitals. *Pediatr Crit Care Med* 2004;5:5–9.

34 Knudson MM, Shagoury C, Lewis FR. Can adult trauma surgeons care for injured children? *J Trauma* 1992;32:729–39.

35 Fortune JM, Sanchez J, Graca L, et al. A pediatric trauma center without a pediatric surgeon: a four-year outcome analysis. *J Trauma* 1992;33:130–9.

36 Rhodes M, Smith S, Boorse D. Pediatric trauma patients in an "adult" trauma center. *J Trauma* 1993;35:384–93.

37 Bensard DD, McIntyre RC, Moore EE, Moore FA. A critical analysis of acutely injured children managed in an adult level I trauma center. *J Pediatr Surg* 1994;29:11–18.

38 Partrick DA, Moore EE, Bensard DD, Karrer FM. Operative management of injured children at an adult level I trauma center. *J Trauma* 2000;48:894–901.

39 Sherman HF, Landry VL, Jones LM. Should level I trauma centers be rated NC-17? *J Trauma* 2001;50:784–91.

40 D'Amelio LF, Hammond JS, Thomasseau J, et al. "Adult" trauma surgeons with pediatric commitment: a logical solution to the pediatric trauma manpower problem. *Am Surg* 1995;61:968–74.

41 Branas CC, MacKenzie EJ, Williams JC, et al. Access to trauma centers in the United States. *JAMA* 2005;293:2626–33.

42 Goldfarb MG, Bazzoli GJ, Coffey RM. Trauma systems and the costs of trauma care. *Health Serv Res* 1996;31:71–95.

43 MacKenzie EJ, Weir S, Rivara FP, et al. The value of trauma center care. *J Trauma* 2010;69:1–10.

44 Faul M, Wald MM, Sullivent EE, et al. Large cost savings realized from the 2006 Field Triage Guidelines: reduction in overtriage to US trauma centers. *Prehosp Emerg Care* 2012;16:222–9.

CHAPTER 40

Trauma-stabilizing procedures

Derek R. Cooney and David P. Thomson

Introduction

Physicians providing EMS medical oversight and those providing direct patient care in the prehospital environment must possess a significant level of expertise in the use of non-invasive and invasive procedures for the prehospital stabilization of trauma patients. The nature of the care and the procedures that are appropriate for different levels of providers is based on the education, training, and legal scope of practice of the providers in the EMS system. An EMS physician must be skilled in these procedures and maintain active educational programs and continuous quality improvement activities to insure these procedures are being performed correctly, and under the correct circumstances. In some cases, it may be appropriate that only an EMS physician perform a procedure, either due to special circumstances or due to the provider's ability and/or scope. Appropriate hands-on and didactic training, as well as verification of procedural proficiency, should occur prior to implementing any procedural skill.

Needle thoracostomy

The placement of a needle to relieve tension pneumothorax is often used in ground EMS systems. Some air medical (and critical care) services have also authorized the placement of a formal tube thoracostomy by their crews. The placement of a needle into the pleural space can produce dramatic results in a patient suffering from a tension pneumothorax.

Indication

This procedure should be considered in any patient who suffers from rapid cardiopulmonary decompensation in an appropriate clinical setting. Although tracheal deviation and decreased breath sounds are commonly accepted as signs of a tension pneumothorax, they may not always be present and may not be appreciated in some prehospital environments [1]. Providers should be encouraged to perform this procedure in any blunt chest trauma patient who has a precipitously decreasing course, especially if there is a history of chronic obstructive pulmonary disease or asthma. Trauma patients with obvious subcutaneous emphysema can benefit from the early application of this technique. Eckstein and Suyehara reviewed their experience in a series of over 6,000 trauma patients [2]. Their conclusion, based on the 108 patients in this series who received needle decompression, was that this was a potentially life-saving intervention, with a low complication rate.

If the catheter is placed into the lung parenchyma, the puncture will be small and should heal rapidly. The resultant pneumothorax is an open one, and therefore the patient should suffer little further compromise. If the patient is intubated, the thoracostomy catheter may be placed and left open to the air. If the patient is spontaneously breathing, a one-way valve must be created to prevent reentry of air during inspiration. One-way valves, such as the Heimlich valve, are available with tubing that will connect with a standard venous catheter. Condoms may be used by puncturing the condom with the catheter and then unrolling it after the catheter has been placed in the patient. Surgical gloves have been used, but when compared with condoms, they may produce unacceptable air leakage. Some services will use an aquarium air pump check valve, but despite anecdotal success, there do not appear to be any available scientific data evaluating their use for this purpose. Other devices, such as the McSwain Dart, have also been used for chest decompression, but they confer no demonstrated advantage over a venous catheter.

For most EMS systems, needle thoracostomy is the safest, most rapid, and most effective way of providing pleural decompression.

Technique

Locate the second intercostal space, in the midclavicular line on the anterior chest wall of the affected side. An alternative site is the midaxillary line at the level of the nipple, similar to the usual chest tube site. Apply best possible sterile skin preparation with sterile prep. Load the pneumothorax catheter onto the tip of the

Emergency Medical Services: Clinical Practice and Systems Oversight, Second Edition. Volume 1: Clinical Aspects of EMS.
Edited by David C. Cone, Jane H. Brice, Theodore R. Delbridge, and J. Brent Myers.
© 2015 NAEMSP. Published 2015 by John Wiley & Sons, Inc. Companion Website: www.wiley.com\go\cone\naemsp

10 mL syringe. Direct the catheter perpendicular to the skin, keeping in mind that ideal placement is over the top of the rib and not into the inferior portion of the superior rib which risks damaging the neurovascular bundle. Enter the skin and, while gently withdrawing on the plunger, advance the catheter until air moves freely into the syringe (with or without blood return). The plastic catheter should then be advanced off the needle and into the chest. The syringe (frequently a larger syringe) may be used in conjunction with a stopcock to aspirate the air from the pneumothorax until resistance is noted on the plunger. A one-way valve may then be connected to the end of the catheter. A definitive thoracostomy tube will need to be placed after acute decompression with needle thoracostomy (typically in the hospital setting or in critical care transport situations).

Complications

The rate of significant complications is thought to be low. It is possible to puncture the subclavian vein and/or artery if the second interspace technique is done improperly and the needle is placed too high on the chest. If the lateral approach is used, abdominal organ injury may result from a needle placed too caudad. Laceration of the internal mammary artery and the risk of infection are two other complications to consider. Care is needed to avoid these complications by providing the best available level of preprocedural cleaning and utilization of landmarks when placing the needle.

Tube thoracostomy

This common surgical procedure, mostly limited in the field to air medical services or military situations, is used to evacuate air or blood from the pleural space. It is particularly useful when transport times are sufficiently long. Once the tube has been secured, one must decide what to do with the free end of the tube. If the patient is intubated the tube may be left open, creating an open pneumothorax. For a patient who is not intubated, a one-way valve must be created to prevent entry of air into the thorax during inspiration. The Heimlich valve, essentially a rubber flapper valve in a tube, is the most practical device for the paramedic. It may be connected to suction if required, and if there is a large amount of drainage, a urinary catheter bag may be attached to collect the drainage.

Indication

The ability to rapidly evacuate a large amount of blood from the trauma patient's pleural space, converting a tension hemothorax into an open hemothorax, is this technique's primary advantage. In some cases this may be life-saving but in others, the patient can exsanguinate from the tube, depending on the source of the bleeding. Placement of the formal thoracostomy tube may also be indicated if a large pneumothorax is present and a long transport time is expected. Potential advantages are the lower likelihood of kinking, clotting, and dislodgment of the tube in comparison to the needle technique.

Technique

Abduct and externally rotate the arm on the affected side so that it is up and out of the way. Locate the fifth intercostal space, in the midaxillary line on the chest wall of the affected side. Apply best possible sterile skin preparation with sterile prep. Locally inject the site with anesthetic. Using the #10 blade scalpel, make a 3–4 cm transverse incision onto the fifth rib at the midaxillary line. With a large Kelly clamp, bluntly dissect over the top of the fifth rib into the fourth intercostal space. Some force may be required to enter the pleural space and the operator should feel a definitive pop upon entering the pleural cavity. At this point there may be a rush of air and/or blood. Spread the tips of the Kelly clamp in the pleural cavity to widen access, then turn the clamp 90° and spread again. Insert a gloved finger into the pleural space to verify proper position and to hold the track while guiding the chest tube into place. The Kelly clamp may then be removed at the provider's discretion. The tube may be inserted directly or facilitated by the use of a Kelly clamp to grasp the tip, through the eye, to help guide the tube. The tube should be inserted along the tract and into the pleural cavity, while directing it posteriorly and superiorly. The tube should slide smoothly without significant resistance and all of the fenestrations must be inside the chest wall to allow for suction.

If the tube will not advance, the operator may attempt to turn the tube; however, if the tube is drawn out of the chest, a new tube should be used on the next attempt to place through the same tract.

Once the tube is in position, secure the chest tube to the chest wall with a silk suture. Petroleum gauze with a single cut halfway across the middle of the gauze can then be placed around the tube. Dry gauze, with the same cut, is then placed over the petroleum gauze and the elastic adhesive tape is used to hold the dry gauze in position. The tube is then bolstered and taped to the chest wall. The end of the tube should then be connected to the chest tube drainage apparatus, or a Heimlich (one-way flutter) valve should be placed on the end.

Complications

The tube should be placed under sterile conditions. However, this may be difficult or impossible based on the potential prehospital environments in which this may be performed. This may lead to empyema, should the patient survive. Placement in the wrong interspace can result in injury to the abdominal organs, the heart, or great vessels, and the use of trocars or Kelly clamps to place the tube may cause injury to the lung parenchyma or other thoracic structures.

Pericardiocentesis

Pericardiocentesis is classically taught as the procedure of choice for treating cardiac tamponade. Its use in the prehospital setting has not been fully investigated. In the patient suffering from pulseless electrical activity (PEA) due to cardiac tamponade, pericardiocentesis may theoretically restore a perfusing rhythm. Medical directors may wish to include pericardiocentesis in a traumatic PEA protocol; however, its use should typically be reserved for patients in whom fluid challenge and needle thoracostomy have not resulted in palpable pulses.

Indication

The indication for this intervention is the presence of life-threatening physiological changes with signs of traumatic cardiac tamponade. The Beck triad (muffled heart sounds, jugular venous distension (JVD), and hypotension) and Kussmaul signs (pulsus paradoxus, a drop of >10 mmHg during inspiration, and paradoxical increase in JVD, as a sign of increased jugulovenous pressure) are indications of cardiac tamponade. Cardiac tamponade is present in up to 90% of penetrating injuries to the heart [3].

Pericardiocentesis is also indicated for resuscitation of a patient with PEA when other causes have been ruled out and the patient remains pulseless. Pericardiocentesis has been reported successful even in cases of cardiac tamponade from blunt trauma [4].

Technique without ECG or ultrasound guidance

Expose the subxiphoid region and prep the area with sterile antiseptic solution. Position an 18 G (either 3.5 or 6 inch) spinal needle so that it will enter the skin directly below or adjacent to the xiphoid process. The needle should be held at a 45° angle to the skin, aiming at the left shoulder (assuming normal anatomy). This technique minimizes the likelihood of injuring other important structures. The needle is advanced, maintaining angle and direction, while withdrawing on the plunger. The operator stops advancing when blood returns. After removal of up to 50 mL of blood, vital signs are reassessed. In cases of acute tamponade, removal of as little as 25–30 mL can lead to immediate improvement [4]. If hemodynamic status does not improve, perform additional aspiration of blood in 25 mL increments until condition improves. The stopcock may be place on the Luer-Lok end of the spinal needle and may be used for subsequent drainage (either through tubing into a bag or into a syringe with aspiration). If the needle is left in place it must be stabilized. If removed, the operator should consider drainage of pericardial blood until little to no blood returns, and then check for reaccumulation prior to removal. A sterile dressing should be placed over the site.

At this point, if equipped, the operator may choose to utilize the Seldinger guidewire technique and place a flexible plastic catheter instead of leaving the metal spinal needle.

Technique with ECG guidance

Prior to initiating the procedure described above, the operator uses an alligator clip jumper cable to bridge from the ECG lead (V1 in the case of 12-leads, lead II for 3-lead) to the proximal metal portion of the spinal needle. The same procedure may be used, and advancement of the needle is now additionally guided by blood returned and the change on the ECG lead to ST elevation on the monitor. The rest of the procedure is the same as above.

Technique with ultrasound guidance

If prehospital ultrasound is available, it may be employed to guide placement of the needle into the pericardium. The operator will identify the point of maximal effusion in order to guide site selection. The site should represent a superficial access to the effusion and will not likely be the subxiphoid site, due to the ability of the ultrasound to visualize both the effusion and the needle during the procedure. Angle and depth will be guided by the ultrasound. The operator should use the probe before (to identify the site) and during the procedure (in order to guide the needle to the effusion), and after initial drainage (to check for reaccumulation). The rest of the procedure is the same as the blind technique above.

Complications

Classically, the use of this technique has been discouraged in the patient with a traumatic tamponade as it may delay the implementation of thoracotomy. Thoracostomy is not usually available in the prehospital setting unless a properly trained and equipped EMS physician is present [5]. Theoretically, the needle could also cause injury to the myocardium or puncture or lacerate a coronary vessel.

Spinal immobilization

The most critical aspects of patient packaging are those interventions designed to protect the spinal cord from further injury. Before the appearance of organized EMS services and paramedic training, motor vehicle crash victims were often extricated and transported without the use of any form of spinal immobilization. These patients were simply pulled from their vehicles or placed on stretchers without any consideration of splinting or spinal stabilization. It was reported that patients presented to the hospital with completed spinal cord injuries [6]. Immobilization has since become one of the most fundamental interventions provided by prehospital providers. Although this process has been accepted for decades, no formal studies have assessed its validity or effectiveness, and it is not without its problems. Changes in automotive design since the institution of spinal immobilization in the 1960s have led some to question the need for universal spinal immobilization of motor vehicle crash victims. Like so many prehospital interventions, this is a difficult procedure to study given the current medicolegal climate.

In light of recent studies exposing the lack of evidence of the effectiveness of cervical collars and long spine boards in the maintenance of spinal alignment, coupled with the detrimental effects of routine immobilization, it is important to carefully consider protocol design and quality assurance processes in order to limit the adverse effects of this now ubiquitous but not evidence-based practice [7–20].

Indications

Spinal immobilization has been considered important for a wide variety of mechanisms including motor vehicle crashes, falls, and athletic injuries. Even falls from the standing position, especially in the elderly, may result in spinal injuries. Despite the routine use of spinal immobilization in trauma victims, indications for use in prehospital care remain an active area of research. Although occult spinal injuries may be difficult to detect reliably in the field, studies have noted the discomfort caused by the use of backboards and collars and have questioned whether immobilization should be performed in the absence of signs and symptoms [7].

Recent studies have reported a lack of effectiveness in spinal immobilization using a long spine board [7–9]. Multiple authors have questioned the utility of backboard use due to a lack of data to support their effectiveness in preventing secondary injury, and the documented potential harm associated with backboard use including iatrogenic pain, skin ulceration, increased use of radiographs, aspiration, and respiratory compromise [7,9–19]. The National Association of EMS Physicians (NAEMSP) and the American College of Surgeons Committee on Trauma (ACS-COT) joint position paper on the topic notes the risks associated with the use of long spine boards and cites the need to remove the patient from them as soon as possible [20]. A 2013 paper suggests the mean backboard time for patients might be nearly an hour [21]. Based on available evidence, limiting the use of long spine boards to extrication, and removing the patient from the board while maintaining spinal precautions, may be preferable.

Penetrating trauma

In some geographical areas, gunshot wounds are the leading cause of spinal cord injuries, whereas nationwide they are the third most common source of spinal injury [22]. Although well accepted for blunt trauma, the tactical EMS community, citing data from the WDMET study of Vietnam War casualties, has actively discouraged the use of spinal immobilization for gunshot wounds[23]. These studies suggest that the injuries to the spinal cord from bullets are either complete at the time of wounding or are stable and do not require immobilization [24–28]. Heck et al. also point out that cervical collars may preclude good observation in patients with neck wounds [23]. A review of the Israeli experience with penetrating neck trauma concurs with this view [29]. Jallo agrees that spinal instability is rare with these types of penetrating injuries, but cautions that "optimal management has not been determined" [30]. Other authors have advocated for a middle ground, suggesting that if the cervical collar interferes with patient care then it can safely be removed, but that otherwise it should be left in place [31]. However, the 2013 NAEMSP and ACS-COT joint position statement on use of long spine boards states that patients with penetrating injury and no signs of spinal injury should not be immobilized on long spine boards [21].

Blunt trauma

Immobilization for blunt trauma and falls has been studied in much better detail. Domeier et al. retrospectively reviewed a large group of patients with spinal fractures in Michigan [32]. They concluded that patients with altered mental status, neurological deficit, spinal pain, evidence of intoxication, or suspected extremity fracture were more likely to have significant spinal injuries. In a further study, Domeier et al. prospectively reviewed the above set of spinal immobilization criteria and found that these criteria would have been 95% sensitive and 35% specific, and had a negative predictive value of 99.5% for spinal injury [33]. Domeier suggested that if applied clinically, these criteria might have reduced spinal immobilization by as much as 35%. He pursued this concept by applying the criteria in a prospective clinical study, finding a 39% reduction in spinal immobilization [34]. In this study, the criteria were found to be 92% sensitive and 40% specific. Of the 8% (n = 33) of patients with spinal column injuries that were missed, none had documented spinal cord injuries. Of these 33 patients, 18 had immobilization techniques applied at the hospital. Seventeen of the 33 missed patients were over the age of 70. During retrospective chart review, the authors reported some difficulties with algorithm non-compliance and incorrect assessments by prehospital personnel.

In a similar study, Muhr's group attempted to reduce spinal immobilization use in trauma patients who did not meet trauma system activation criteria. They prospectively applied an eight-point immobilization algorithm. Before algorithm application in their system, 98% of these patients were spinally immobilized. The authors demonstrated a 33% decrease in immobilization [35]. Interestingly, spinal immobilization for blunt trauma is not practiced throughout the world. In a unique comparative study, Hauswald et al. compared neurological outcomes between immobilized and unimmobilized blunt trauma victims in New Mexico and Malaysia [36]. In the Malaysian system, none of the patients received any form of prehospital spinal immobilization, while in the New Mexican system, all studied patients were immobilized. Their results indicated that there was less neurological injury in the Malaysian population than in the New Mexican group. This study has significant limitations, which are described in an accompanying editorial by Orledge and Pepe [37], but the findings are intriguing nonetheless.

Hankins et al. describe another set of clinical criteria that may be used to indicate which patients might be eligible for clinical spinal clearance: no extremes of age (<12 or >65 years old), no altered mental status or language barriers, no neurological deficits, no distracting injuries, and no midline or paraspinal pain or tenderness [38]. Again, it is important to note that NAEMSP/ACS-COT position statement also includes the concept that maintenance of spinal precautions does not require use of a long spine board [20,21].

Application of cervical collar

The first step in spinal immobilization is typically manual stabilization of the head, followed by placement of a rigid cervical collar. Numerous collars are available on the market, ranging from cloth-covered foam rubber to stiff plastics of various designs. The soft collar provides no immobilization and has no place in prehospital care [39].

Indication

Immobilization of the cervical spine is performed to avoid secondary injury in patients who have the potential for unstable fractures. In a 1986 study, McCabe and Nolan compared cervical spine motion on radiographs with volunteers immobilized in Philadelphia, hard extrication, and two versions of the Stifneck collar [40]. The Stifneck collars were better than either the Philadelphia or hard extrication collars in immobilizing the patient in all directions except extension. Dick and Land, in a review of all spinal immobilization devices, found that the Stifneck collar provided the best immobilization among all collars tested [41]. A number of similar plastic collars are currently available, but limited data are available regarding the effectiveness of specific devices. Regardless of the brand utilized, the collar should be made of rigid plastic and sized properly for the patient's neck. Due to the controversy surrounding the utility of the cervical collar and complications it may cause, some authors have advocated very limited use or for spinal precautions only [42,43].

Technique

To ensure the best potential patient outcome, the cervical collar must be properly sized prior to placement. The operator holds out his or her hand and extends all of the fingers. The hand is placed on the side of the neck with the pinky almost touching the shoulder. An imaginary line from the inferior chin is considered and matched up to one of the fingers on the measuring hand. The hand can then be matched up to the cervical collar and the collar adjusted to the correct height based on the distance between the sizing mark/line on the collar and the bottom of the plastic portion of the collar. The chin section of the collar is placed into position first, with the rest of the collar then wrapped around the neck. Allowing for a snug (not tight) fit, close the collar with the hook-and-loop fasteners. The collar should be snug enough to keep your patient from flexing and extending the head, but not so tight as to stop the patient from being able to open the mouth. Immobilization with the cervical collar may be enhanced when used in conjunction with head blocks and the long spine board.

Complications

Application of an improperly sized collar is very uncomfortable for the patient and may be counterproductive to the goal of spinal immobilization. In patients for whom no collar seems to fit properly, padding with towels and securing the head and torso directly to a spine board or extrication device may be preferable, though data are limited. Respiratory compromise and vascular occlusion can occur when not properly fitted.

Application of a long spine board (backboard)

Since the late 1960s the long spine board has been considered an important component of prehospital trauma care in the United States. If immobilization is thought to be clinically useful for a given patient, then proper application and technique should be observed.

Indication

NAEMSP/ACS-COT position paper on use of spinal precautions and long spine boards states that spinal precautions may be appropriate in patients with blunt trauma and altered level of consciousness, spinal pain or tenderness, a neurological complaint (numbness or motor weakness), anatomical deformity of the spine, or a high-energy mechanism of injury and any of the following: drug or alcohol intoxication, inability to communicate, or distracting injury [21].

Equipment

Several immobilization devices are available, each with a slightly different application technique. Devices commonly in use include long spine board, scoop stretcher, vacuum mattress, and the Kendrick Extrication Device (KED).

Long spine board technique

Throughout the procedure, manual inline cervical spine alignment must be maintained until the cervical collar is placed correctly. One team member will maintain manual inline cervical stabilization during all movements. Team members should respond to the leader's commands and count to ensure synchronicity of movement in order to maximize spinal immobility. The team may use the logroll technique or the lift and slide technique to place the patient onto the long spine board. The patient is then strapped to the board. The chest strap is usually secured first, followed by the waist and then the thighs and lower legs. All voids between the board and the patient should be padded. The head is always immobilized last. Head blocks are placed on either side of the head. In some cases, occipital padding may be needed. The head may then be secured using tape or commercially available straps.

Scoop stretcher technique

As with the long spine board technique, the cervical spine should be immobilized and the provider at the head should command the operation. The scoop stretcher is opened and placed with the hinged portion at the head with the open portion toward the feet (or it may be taken completely into two halves). The scoop stretcher is then closed under the patient. If the patient is not on a smooth hard surface, pinching may occur at the buttocks and/or the shoulders. In order to decrease pinching, gentle lateral traction on the patient's clothing may help. If the patient is on a sheet, the sheet should be pulled tight during the procedure to limit the potential for pinching. The head (first) and foot (second) hinges are locked. The patient is then strapped to the stretcher (chest, waist, legs, then head).

Vacuum mattress technique

First the vacuum mattress is inspected and laid flat on the ground. If there are any holes or tears, this technique must not be used. The vacuum valve should be facing up and be positioned at the patient's feet. The patient is then placed on the mattress (lift and slide, logroll off a backboard, placed onto the mattress using a scoop stretcher, or logroll onto a sheet on top of the mattress) and positioned onto the middle of the mattress. The mattress is pumped several times to make it slightly firmer. The mattress is then molded to the patient and the straps are placed. The mattress is molded around the head manually and the mattress pump is used to vacuum the air from the mattress until it is firm and in a molded form. The mattress can be moved on a long spine board or in some cases may be carried with straps if it is sufficiently rigid in the vacuumed state and has been designed for this use.

Extrication device technique

Once a stiff cervical collar is placed, a team member must place the extrication device behind the patient in the upright position, aligning it with the patient. The middle torso strap is secured first, followed by the bottom torso strap. The leg straps and top torso strap are then secured, followed by the head strap, with adequate padding to fill voids. The patient is then extricated using the extrication device haul straps and placed on the long spine board. At this point the operator will disconnect the leg straps, allowing the patient's legs to lie flat on the long spine board. The patient is then secured to the long spine board while still in the extrication device.

Complications

Complications associated with spine board use include discomfort, increased use of x-ray in immobilized patients, potential for decubitus ulcer formation, and risk for respiratory compromise [15,29,44–46]. Medical directors of EMS systems should actively investigate ways to ensure that only those patients who need this intervention receive it, and that those who are immobilized to long spine boards are removed from the boards into less harmful spinal precautions as early as possible.

Pregnant patients who are >20 weeks gestation may experience compression of the abdominal great vessels and should be positioned with the board wedged toward a left lateral slant while maintaining immobilization. Patients with respiratory distress or cardiac decompensation may need to be positioned in the semi-upright to upright position. In this case, use of a short board or extrication device alone may be necessary. If this

is also impractical due to body habitus, the cervical collar may need to be used alone while attempting patient positioning that maintains as much spinal immobilization as possible while avoiding life-threatening cardiopulmonary complications.

Padding

Due to the significant discomfort associated with spinal immobilization, alternative methods of immobilization have been proposed. Additional concern for elderly or bedridden patients is also appropriate considering the associated unequal areas of tissue interface pressures that may lead to tissue damage and breakdown. Hauswald et al. compared four spinal immobilization techniques with healthy volunteers: traditional backboard, blanketed backboard, backboard with gurney mattress, and backboard with gurney mattress and foam pad [47]. Not surprisingly, they found these techniques were rated in the same order, from least to most comfortable. A study by Lerner et al. revealed that occipital padding to produce neutral positioning in spinal immobilization subjects does not reduce pain [7]. Walton et al. described a significant reduction in discomfort, without reduction in the effect of immobilization, when the long board is padded with closed-cell foam [48]. Another alternative to the standard long board is the vacuum mattress device. Multiple studies have shown marked advantages in comfort and some advantages in immobilization when these devices are employed [49–51]. Another option is a specially designed air mattress. Several brands of approved spine board air mattresses are available.

In a study by Cordell et al., a standard long board was compared to standard long board with air mattress [52]. The two groups reported their discomfort on a 100 mm visual analog scale. At 80 minutes the air mattress group reported a mean 9.7 mm rating, versus a 37.5 mm rating in the standard long board group. They also measured tissue interface pressures and found that the air mattress group had significantly less pressure at the occiput, sacrum, and heel. The time of spinal immobilization should be limited and consideration paid to measures to decrease the ill effects, especially in high-risk patients.

Children

Several commercial devices are available for immobilization of children. For smaller children, a short board, well padded under the torso, can be used. Markenson et al. described using the KED for pediatric immobilization [53]. Because of its versatility with both adult and pediatric patients, they suggest that this is "an ideal device" for pediatric immobilization. Although immobilization is meant to protect the spine from further injury, it may compromise ventilation. Even in the majority of children, who would be unlikely to suffer from chronic lung disease, spinal immobilization can produce a significant decrease in forced vital capacity [54]. Providers must be ready to assist with ventilation, should immobilization result in respiratory compromise. Infants and neonates who are found adequately restrained in undamaged car seats, who do not require other assessment and/or interventions, may be best transported immobilized in the car seats.

Selective spine immobilization

Selective spinal immobilization was originally studied in the emergency department and its use has been extrapolated to the prehospital environment.

Indication

It is reasonable to employ protocols that limit spinal immobilization to patients in whom there may be some benefit. A number of studies suggest the validity of this concept and potential for successful implementation [35,55–58].

Technique

The selective spinal immobilization algorithms most commonly used in the emergency department for determining appropriateness of clinical clearance of the cervical spine are the NEXUS and Canadian C-Spine rules. Nexus asks the EMS provider to determine the absence of focal neurological deficit, midline spinal tenderness, altered level of consciousness, intoxication, and distracting injury before electing to omit application of spinal immobilization [59]. The Canadian C-Spine Rule asks three questions.

1 Is there any high-risk factor present that mandates radiography (i.e. age ≥65 years, dangerous mechanism, or paresthesias in extremities)?
2 Is there any low-risk factor present that allows safe assessment of range of motion (i.e. simple rear-end motor vehicle collision, sitting position in ED, ambulatory at any time since injury, delayed onset of neck pain, or absence of midline cervical spine tenderness)?
3 Is the patient able to actively rotate the neck 45° to the left and right? [60]

Both of these rules were developed to more appropriately guide the use of radiography in the emergency department and not to guide paramedics using selective spinal immobilization in the field. However, both rules have been studied in the prehospital environment and found to function effectively [34,61].

Conclusion

Emergency medical services physicians must provide effective and knowledgeable medical oversight for the application of trauma-stabilizing procedures in the prehospital environment. An EMS physician must be skilled in these procedures and maintain active educational programs and continuous quality improvement activities to insure these procedures are being performed correctly, and under the correct circumstances. Appropriate hands-on and didactic training, as well as verification of procedural proficiency, should occur prior to implementing any procedural skill.

References

1 Ross DS. Thoracentesis. In: Roberts JR, Hedges JR (eds) *Clinical Procedures in Emergency Medicine*. Philadelphia: W.B. Saunders, 1985, p.85.
2 Eckstein M, Suyehara D. Needle thoracostomy in the prehospital setting. *Prehosp Emerg Care* 1998;2:132–5.
3 Thourani VH, Feliciano DV, Rozycki G, et al. Penetrating cardiac trauma at an urban trauma center: a 22-year perspective. *Am Surg* 1999;65:811–18.
4 Lu LH, Choi WM, Wu HR, Liu HC, Chiu WC, Tsai SH. Blunt cardiac rupture with prehospital pulseless electrical activity: a rare successful experience. *J Trauma* 2005;59:1489–91.
5 Callaham M. Pericardiocentesis. In: Roberts JR, Hedges JR (eds) *Clinical Procedures in Emergency Medicine*. Philadelphia: W.B. Saunders, 1985, pp.208–25.
6 Green BA, Eismont FJ, O'Heir JT. Pre-hospital management of spinal cord injuries. *Paraplegia* 1987;25:229–38.
7 Lerner EB, Billittier AJ 4th, Moscati RM. The effects of neutral positioning with and without padding on spinal immobilization of healthy subjects. *Prehosp Emerg Care* 1998;2:112–16.
8 Holla M. Value of a rigid collar in addition to head blocks: a proof of principle study. *Emerg Med J* 2012;29:104–7.
9 Kwan I, Bunn F, Roberts I. Spinal immobilisation for trauma patients. *Cochrane Database Syst Rev* 2001;2:CD002803.
10 Ay D, Aktaş C, Yeşilyurt S, Sarikaya S, Cetin A, Ozdogan ES. Effects of spinal immobilization devices on pulmonary function in healthy volunteer individuals. *Ulus Travma Acil Cerrahi Derg* 2011;17: 103–7.
11 Bauer D, Kowalski R. Effect of spinal immobilization devices on pulmonary function in the healthy, nonsmoking man. *Ann Emerg Med* 1988;17:915–18.
12 Hunt K, Hallworth S, Smith M. The effects of rigid collar placement on intracranial and cerebral perfusion pressures. *Anaesthesia* 2001;56:511–3.
13 Johnson DR, Hauswald M, Stockhoff C. Comparison of a vacuum splint device to a rigid backboard for spinal immobilization. *Am J Emerg Med* 1996;14:369–72.
14 March JA, Ausband SC, Brown LH. Changes in physical examination caused by use of spinal immobilization. *Prehosp Emerg Care* 2002;6:421–4.
15 Schafermeyer RW, Ribbeck BM, Gaskins J, Thomason S, Harlan M, Attkisson A. Respiratory effects of spinal immobilization in children. *Ann Emerg Med* 1991;20:1017–19.
16 Thumbikat P, Hariharan RP, Ravichandran G, McClelland MR, Mathew KM. Spinal cord injury in patients with ankylosing spondylitis: a 10-year review. *Spine* 2007;32:2989–95.
17 Vickery D. The use of the spinal board after the pre-hospital phase of trauma management. *Emerg Med J* 2001;18:51–4.
18 Clarke A, James S, Ahuja S. Ankylosing spondylitis: inadvertent application of a rigid collar after cervical fracture, leading to neurological complications and death. *Acta Orthop Belg* 2010;76:413–15.
19 Theodore N, Hadley MN, Aarabi B, et al. Prehospital cervical spinal immobilization after trauma. *Neurosurgery* 2013;72:S22–34.
20 NAEMSP, ACS-COT. EMS spinal precautions and the use of the long backboard. *Prehosp Emerg Care* 2013;17:392–3.
21 Cooney DR, Wallus H, Asaly M, Wojcik S. Backboard time for patients receiving spinal immobilization by emergency medical services. *Int J Emerg Med* 2013;6:17.

22 Kihtir T, Ivatury RR, Simon R, Stahl WM. Management of trans-peritoneal gunshot wounds of the spine. *J Trauma* 1991;31: 1579–83.

23 Heck J, Kepp JJ, Walos G, Vayer J (eds) *Emergency Medical Technician – Tactical Provider*, 16th edn. Bethesda, MD: Casualty Care Research Center, 2001.

24 Shafer JS, Naunheim RS. Cervical spine motion during extrication: a pilot study. *West J Emerg Med* 2009;10:74–8.

25 DuBose J, Teixeira PGR, Hadjizacharia P, et al. The role of routine spinal imaging and immobilisation in asymptomatic patients after gunshot wounds. *Injury* 2009;40:860–3.

26 Stuke LE, Pons PT, Guy JS, Chapleau WP, Butler FK, McSwain NE. Prehospital spine immobilization for penetrating trauma – review and recommendations from the Prehospital Life Support Executive Committee. *J Trauma* 2011;71:763–9.

27 Lustenberger T, Talving P, Lam L, et al. Unstable cervical spine fracture after penetrating neck injury: a rare entity in an analysis of 1,069 patients. *J Trauma* 2011;70:870–2.

28 Ahn H, Singh J, Nathens A, et al. Pre-hospital care management of a potential spinal cord injured patient: a systematic review of the liter-ature and evidence-based guidelines. *J Neurotrauma* 2011;28:1341–61.

29 Barkana Y, Stein M, Scope A, et al. Prehospital stabilization of the cervical spine for penetrating injuries of the neck –is it necessary? *Injury* 2000;31:305–9.

30 Jallo GI. Neurosurgical management of penetrating spinal injury. *Surg Neurol* 1997;47:328–30.

31 Medzon R, Rothenhaus T, Bono CM, Grindlinger G, Rathlev NK. Stability of cervical spine fractures after gunshot wounds to the head and neck. *Spine* 2005;30:2274–9.

32 Domeier RM, Evans RW, Swor RA, Rivera-Rivera EJ, Frederiksen SM. Prehospital clinical findings associated with spinal injury. *Prehosp Emerg Care* 1997;1:11–15.

33 Domeier RM, Swor RA, Evans RW, et al. Multicenter prospective validation of prehospital clinical spinal clearance criteria. *J Trauma* 2002;53:744–50.

34 Domeier RM, Frederiksen SM, Welch K. Prospective performance assessment of an out-of-hospital protocol for selective spine immo-bilization using clinical spine clearance criteria. *Ann Emerg Med* 2005;46:123–31.

35 Muhr MD, Seabrook DL, Wittwer LK. Paramedic use of a spinal injury clearance algorithm reduces spinal immobilization in the out-of-hospital setting. *Prehosp Emerg Care* 1999;3:1–6.

36 Hauswald M, Ong G, Tandberg D, Omar Z. Out of hospital spinal immobilization: its effect on neurologic injury. *Acad Emerg Med* 1998;5:214–19.

37 Orledge JD, Pepe PE. Out-of-hospital spinal immobilization: is it really necessary? *Acad Emerg Med* 1998;5:203–4.

38 Hankins DG, Rivera-Rivera EJ, Ornato JP, et al. Spinal immobiliza-tion in the field: clinical clearance criteria and implementation. *Prehosp Emerg Care* 2001;5:88–93.

39 Podolsky S, Baraff LJ, Simon RR, Hoffman JR, Larmon B, Ablon W. Efficacy of cervical spine immobilization methods. *J Trauma* 1983;23:461–5.

40 McCabe JB, Nolan DJ. Comparison of the effectiveness of differ-ent cervical immobilization collars. *Ann Emerg Med* 1986;15: 50–3.

41 Dick T, Land R. Spinal immobilization devices. Part 1: cervical extrication collars. *J Emerg Med Serv* 1982;7:26–32.

42 Plumb JO, Morris CG. Cervical collars: probably useless; definitely cause harm! *J Emerg Med* 2013;44:e143.

43 Schouten R, Albert T, Kwon BK. The spine-injured patient: initial assessment and emergency treatment. *J Am Acad Orthop Surg* 2012; 20:336–46.

44 Vickery D. The use of the spinal board after the pre-hospital phase of trauma management. *Emerg Med J* 2001;18:51–4.

45 Haut ER, Kalish BT, Efron DT, et al. Spine immobilization in pene-trating trauma: more harm than good? *J Trauma* 2010;68:115–20.

46 Johnson DR, Hauswald M, Stockhoff C. Comparison of a vacuum splint device to a rigid backboard for spinal immobilization. *Am J Emerg Med* 1996;14:369–72.

47 Hauswald M, Hsu M, Stockoff C. Maximizing comfort and minimizing ischemia: a comparison of four methods of spinal immobilization. *Prehosp Emerg Care* 2000;4:250–2.

48 Walton R, DeSalvo JF, Ernst AA, Shahane A. Padded vs. unpadded spine board for cervical spine immobilization. *Acad Emerg Med* 1995;2:725–8.

49 Cross DA, Baskerville J. Comparison of perceived pain with differ-ent immobilization techniques. *Prehosp Emerg Care* 2001;5:270–4.

50 Johnson DR, Hauswald M, Stockhoff C. Comparison of a vacuum splint device to a rigid backboard for spinal immobilization. *Am J Emerg Med* 1996;14:369–72.

51 Luscombe MD, Williams JL. Comparison of a long spinal board and vacuum mattress for spinal immobilisation. *Emerg Med J* 2003;20:476–8.

52 Cordell WH, Hollingsworth JC, Olinger ML, Stroman SJ, Nelson DR. Pain and tissue-interface pressures during spine-board immo-bilization. *Ann Emerg Med* 1995;26:31–6.

53 Markenson D, Foltin G, Tunik M, et al. The Kendrick Extrication Device used for pediatric spinal immobilization. *Prehosp Emerg Care* 1999;3:66–9.

54 Schafermeyer RW, Ribbeck BM, Gaskins J, Thomason S, Harlan M, Attkisson A. Respiratory effects of spinal immobilization in children. *Ann Emerg Med* 1991;20:1017–19.

55 Burton JH, Dunn MG, Harmon NR, Hermanson TA, Bradshaw JR. A statewide, prehospital emergency medical service selective patient spine immobilization protocol. *J Trauma* 2006;61:161–7.

56 Hankins DG, Rivera-Rivera EJ, Ornato JP, et al. Spinal immobiliza-tion in the field: clinical clearance criteria and implementation. *Prehosp Emerg Care* 2001;5:88–93.

57 Dunn TM, Dalton A, Dorfman T, Dunn WW. Are emergency med-ical technician-basics able to use a selective immobilization of the cervical spine protocol?: a preliminary report. *Prehosp Emerg Care* 2004;8:207–11.

58 Stroh G, Braude D. Can an out-of-hospital cervical spine clearance protocol identify all patients with injuries? An argument for selective immobilization. *Ann Emerg Med* 2001;37:609–15.

59 Hoffman JR, Mower WR, Wolfson AB, Todd KH, Zucker MI. Validity of a set of clinical criteria to rule out injury to the cervical spine in patients with blunt trauma. National Emergency X-Radiography Utilization Study Group. *N Engl J Med* 2000;343:94–9.

60 Stiell IG, Wells GA, Vandemheen KL, et al. The Canadian C-spine rule for radiography in alert and stable trauma patients. *JAMA* 2001;286:1841–8.

61 Vaillancourt C, Stiell IG, Beaudoin T, et al. The out-of-hospital val-idation of the Canadian C-Spine Rule by paramedics. *Ann Emerg Med* 2009;54:663–71.

Obstetrics and Gynecological Problems

CHAPTER 41

Physiology of pregnancy: EMS implications

David J. Hirsch

Introduction

Evaluation and treatment of the pregnant patient represent a challenge for all levels of medical providers, from first responder through EMS physician. Thankfully, major complications and acute life-threatening illnesses are rare. However, when they occur, many special considerations must be taken into account in order to provide the best medical care. This chapter will provide an overview of physiological changes in pregnancy and their implications for prehospital care. Although many of the conditions require further diagnostic testing and treatment beyond the current capabilities of EMS, familiarization by EMS providers and EMS medical directors is critical. This will enable EMS providers to consider life-threatening conditions that require immediate intervention, formulate a preliminary differential diagnosis, initiate treatment, and make the best determination for transport destination.

General considerations

Anatomical

The anatomical changes that a woman undergoes during pregnancy are not confined to the reproductive organs. One of the most apparent changes is weight gain. By full term, a woman of average weight should be expected to gain between 25–35 pounds (11.5–16 kg) [1]. Most of this weight is made up of the fetus and uterus, but contributions are also made by the breasts and additional fluid in the form of blood volume and extracellular fluid. This additional weight, particularly its distribution, provides distinct challenges for EMS providers in certain circumstances such as airway management and traumatic injury, which will be discussed in detail later.

Physiological

Innumerable physiological changes occur during pregnancy. Discussion will be limited to those with the most direct prehospital effects. The increase in blood volume, on average 48% above that of a non-pregnant patient, is one of the most dramatic changes. This is an absolute increase of about 1500 mL [2]. This increased volume improves blood flow and provides nutrients to the growing uterus and fetus, protects the fetus from impaired venous return from maternal supine position, and protects the mother from the effects of blood loss during delivery [3]. Other notable changes include increased baseline heart rate, increased cardiac output, and normal to low blood pressure (Box 41.1).

Critical care and trauma

The core of any EMS provider's training is based on initial evaluation and stabilization of the most critically ill or injured patient. This is best accomplished by using a systematic method such as the ABCs (airway, breathing, circulation). The pregnant patient should be approached in a similar manner, with specific additional considerations. Any resuscitation during pregnancy places at least two lives at stake, considering the mother and one or more fetuses.

Airway

Airway management is among the most critical skills for the EMS provider to master. Without proper airway maintenance, a patient has a small chance of even arriving at the hospital alive. Several anatomical changes to the airway during pregnancy can complicate airway management in the prehospital setting [4]. Edema, caused by increased extracellular fluid volume, can lead to more profound airway obstruction in states of decreased responsiveness, complicating basic airway maneuvers such as bag-valve-mask ventilation. Edema may also lead to swelling of the glottic structures, causing a decreased glottic opening and complicating advanced airway interventions. Additional important considerations are listed in Box 41.2.

Emergency medical services providers must anticipate these issues, and pay close attention to basic airway techniques, with more liberal use of airway adjuncts such as oral or nasal airways as appropriate. Suctioning devices must be ready and available at all

Emergency Medical Services: Clinical Practice and Systems Oversight, Second Edition. Volume 1: Clinical Aspects of EMS.
Edited by David C. Cone, Jane H. Brice, Theodore R. Delbridge, and J. Brent Myers.
© 2015 NAEMSP. Published 2015 by John Wiley & Sons, Inc. Companion Website: www.wiley.com\go\cone\naemsp

Box 41.1 Physiological changes in pregnancy

Blood volume increased by 50%
Baseline heart rate increased 10–15%
Respirations increased 10–15%
Cardiac output increased
Blood pressure decreased or normal

Box 41.2 Airway and breathing considerations

Increased airway edema
Increased risk of regurgitation and aspiration
Increased risk of bleeding due to capillary engorgement
Decreased functional residual capacity (20%)
Increased oxygen consumption (30–60%)

Source: Lewin et al. 2000 [4]. Reproduced with permission of Elsevier.

times to address vomiting. For advanced airway interventions, ALS providers should perform an airway assessment using standardized scoring systems such as Mallampati to help predict the presence of a difficult airway. A smaller sized endotracheal tube than anticipated should be kept on hand in case of difficulty passing the tube through the glottic opening. Standard monitoring such as oxygen saturation and waveform capnography is critical.

Breathing

The gravid uterus causes significant upward displacement of the diaphragm, restricting lung function. Functional residual capacity is decreased by approximately 20% in pregnancy [4]. This, in combination with increased oxygen consumption of 30–60% and decreased venous return due to inferior vena cava compression, can lead to rapid desaturation with any medical or traumatic insult. The patient with respiratory distress or who is requiring ventilation should be placed as upright as feasible to decrease abdominal pressure on the thorax. Oxygen should be used more liberally to ensure the fetus is receiving adequate oxygenation.

Circulation

As described earlier, pregnancy is accompanied by increased blood volume which may allow initial compensation for even major blood loss, followed by rapid deterioration. Given this, patients should be treated aggressively with fluid resuscitation for potential hypovolemic states. The shift toward a permissive hypotension approach to trauma patients should likely not be applied to pregnant patients, though data on this are lacking. Given the relative anemia of pregnancy, blood transfusion may be necessary earlier in resuscitative efforts than in a non-pregnant patient. Vasopressors may be used if necessary to correct shock.

Complications such as pulmonary edema and third spacing with crystalloid infusions due to lower oncotic pressure should be anticipated. Patients with hypotension and/or those who are

supine should always be placed tilted to the left 15–30° using sandbags or pillows. This allows the gravid uterus to be moved off the inferior vena cava, improving venous return to the heart.

Disease states by system

In the preceding section, the evaluation and management of the pregnant patient *in extremis* were discussed. In the following sections, a general overview of disease states by system will be presented. Particular attention will be paid to pathophysiology seen in the pregnant patient compared to standard pathophysiology.

Cardiovascular

Aside from the gynecological system, the cardiovascular system undergoes the most dramatic changes during pregnancy. The heart of the pregnant woman actually remodels, increasing contractile force [5], and when combined with the increased blood volume, increased heart rate, and decreased vascular resistance, a 50% increase in cardiac output results.

When evaluating the pregnant patient, the ALS provider must be aware of ECG changes that occur normally in pregnancy. Due to elevation of the diaphragm and pressure on the heart, ECG changes including left axis deviation, ST-wave flattening, and T-wave inversions are seen particularly near full term. The ST- and T-wave changes seem to appear primarily in the inferior and precordial leads [6]. While most of the cardiovascular changes are beneficial, pathophysiological states can occur. Arrhythmias during pregnancy are fairly common, including supraventricular tachycardia (SVT), paroxysmal atrial fibrillation or flutter, or, more rarely, ventricular tachycardia [7].

Because safety data on many of the antiarrhythmic medications for treatment of the tachyarrhythmias are limited, pharmacological therapy is best avoided when possible during pregnancy [8]. That being said, patients who enter the EMS system often require emergency treatment and medications will be necessary. In cases of SVT, vagal maneuvers should be attempted first. Adenosine is considered a relatively safe intervention if vagal maneuvers fail. Calcium channel blockers such as verapamil and diltiazem are not felt to be as safe, but may be considered [8].

In patients who present in ventricular tachycardia with a pulse, lidocaine is indicated, with procainamide considered a second-line treatment. Amiodarone should be avoided unless absolutely necessary due to reports of fetal bradycardia and other serious adverse effects on the fetus [9]. Electrical cardioversion is considered safe if the patient is unstable or presents with pulseless ventricular tachycardia or ventricular fibrillation.

One of the feared cardiovascular complications of pregnancy is idiopathic cardiomyopathy. Patients present with findings consistent with standard congestive heart failure but may be otherwise young and healthy without the standard cardiovascular risk factors. Symptoms include shortness of breath, dyspnea on exertion, orthopnea, and increased peripheral edema. Prehospital management is similar to that of non-pregnant patients, with supplemental oxygen, positive pressure ventilation, and nitrates in the acute setting. For volume overload and chronic treatment, diuretics are used. After the pregnancy is completed, some patients have return of normal cardiac function, and some do not. Subsequent pregnancies carry a significant risk of recurrence of cardiomyopathy.

Pulmonary

Several changes occur during pregnancy that affect the pulmonary system. Because of the deviation of the diaphragm upward into the thorax, respiratory mechanics are affected. The functional residual capacity, vital capacity, residual volume, and inspiratory capacity all decrease [10]. Patient position greatly affects the patient's mechanics, and EMS providers should place the patient in as much inclination as feasible.

Patients with underlying chronic pulmonary disorders, most commonly asthma, are at risk for worsening status during pregnancy due to the restricted respiratory mechanics. Fortunately, standard prehospital treatments for asthma exacerbations are considered safe in pregnancy. Standard therapy with supplemental oxygen, bronchodilators, and corticosteroids is indicated. Continuous monitoring with pulse oximetry and waveform capnography is critical. Positive pressure ventilation should be used as needed to help avoid the need for endotracheal intubation.

Toxicological

While many medications have different and largely unknown effects in pregnant patients, one of the most relevant toxicological exposures for EMS providers to be aware of is carbon monoxide (CO). This exposure deserves particular attention because it is fairly unique in that the fetus is at higher risk of adverse effects than the mother [11]. Pregnant patients have higher susceptibility to CO due to increased minute ventilation, in addition to increased endogenous production from the fetus [12]. Fetal hemoglobin has a higher affinity for CO than maternal hemoglobin, and the fetus is at risk for life-threatening exposure even if the mother appears relatively well.

Treatment includes removing the patient from the source of exposure, initiating high-flow oxygen, and considering hyperbaric oxygen (HBO). EMS providers should consider transport to a specialty center that can provide HBO if indicated (see Box 41.3) according to local protocols.

Neurological

One of the most serious neurological complications associated with pregnancy is seizures of eclampsia. Preeclampsia can affect almost every organ system in the body, and is typically diagnosed based on the combination of hypertension and proteinuria. Other associated symptoms include headaches, epigastric

---

Box 41.3 Indications for hyperbaric oxygen therapy in the pregnant patient

Carboxyhemoglobin level ≥20%
Mental status depression
Seizures
Metabolic acidosis
Fetal distress
Cardiotoxicity
Any neurological findings in the mother

Source: Shannon 2007 [11]. Reproduced with permission of Elsevier.

---

pain, and visual changes. If the syndrome progresses, the patient may develop eclampsia, with generalized seizure activity and significantly elevated blood pressure (see Volume 1, Chapter 42).

Thromboembolic conditions

Venous thromboembolism is an important cause of maternal morbidity and mortality that EMS providers should be aware of. The most important of these conditions includes deep venous thrombosis (DVT) and pulmonary embolism (PE). Pregnant women are 4–5 times more likely to develop venous thromboembolism than non-pregnant women [13] due to the hypercoagulable state that is associated with pregnancy. Some studies have quoted rates of 1.72 per 1000 deliveries with 1.1 deaths per 100,000 [14].

The major concern regarding DVT is the possibility of dislodgment of the thrombus and travel to the lungs. Pulmonary embolism is a serious life-threatening condition, and prompt diagnosis and treatment are imperative. Diagnosis of DVT is best performed by duplex ultrasonography. PE can be diagnosed by computed tomography angiogram. Treatment includes anticoagulation with heparin or low molecular weight heparin. In cases of massive PE with persistent shock or cardiac arrest, thrombolytics can be considered.

Genitourinary

Due to anatomical changes, pregnant women are at higher risk for urinary tract infections (UTI) than non-pregnant women [15]. UTI can progress to pyelonephritis, or kidney infection, which is the most common cause of serious bacterial infection in pregnant women [16]. Serious bacterial infections in the mother can put the pregnancy at risk, and so early treatment is important.

Gastrointestinal

Most women in pregnancy have some degree of nausea and vomiting. This is most common in the first trimester and then typically improves. In some patients, this condition is severe and is referred to as hyperemesis gravidarum, defined as vomiting that is severe enough to produce weight loss, dehydration, and electrolyte abnormalities, particularly hypokalemia [3]. For patients with hyperemesis gravidarum, treatment is centered around antiemetics, IV fluid replacement, and correction of electrolytes.

Two surgical emergencies, appendicitis and cholecystitis, deserve specific attention. The evaluation, diagnosis, and treatment are more difficult than in the non-pregnant patient, and missed diagnosis can have adverse outcomes for the mother and fetus.

Appendicitis is the most common non-obstetric surgical diagnosis in pregnancy [17]. Diagnosis is more difficult than in the non-pregnant patient due to a variety of factors. Typical presenting signs and symptoms of appendicitis commonly occur under normal conditions during pregnancy. These include nausea and vomiting, decreased appetite, and abdominal pain. In addition, the anatomical location of the appendix has been described as having the tendency to shift superiorly and posteriorly due to displacement by the uterus [18]. Due to these confounding variables, pregnant patients have a higher rate of missed early diagnosis and perforation of the appendix. This puts the fetus at risk, and there is a risk of premature labor and miscarriage.

Emergency medical services providers should consider this diagnosis in patients presenting with right-sided abdominal pain. The location may not be necessarily limited to the right lower quadrant, and may be located in the right upper quadrant or right flank area.

A second common cause of right-sided abdominal pain in pregnancy is biliary disease. Patients may suffer from recurrent postprandial pain due to biliary colic, or develop acute inflammation and pain in the gallbladder from cholecystitis. Acute cholecystitis is the second most common general surgical condition during pregnancy [19] and can, like appendicitis, put the mother and fetus at risk. Symptoms of cholecystitis include right-sided abdominal pain as described above, as well as nausea, vomiting, and fever. Management may be conservative initially and surgical intervention may be delayed until after delivery if possible.

Endocrine

While there are many endocrine changes that occur in the pregnant patient, the most commonly encountered and most relevant to the EMS provider is gestational diabetes. Although many patients are diagnosed through routine prenatal screening with glucose tolerance tests, some patients may not be aware of the condition. In cases of hyperglycemia, patients may have typical symptoms of diabetes including polydipsia and polyuria. Rarely, patients may present with hyperglycemic hyperosmolar non-ketotic syndrome or diabetic ketoacidosis (DKA). EMS providers should treat with IV fluids for dehydration, and perform an ECG to evaluate and treat for life-threatening hyperkalemia states which can be associated with DKA. The mainstay of treatment for these conditions in the hospital is insulin therapy and electrolyte management.

Complications which may occur due to diabetes for the fetus include macrosomia (increased fetal size) which can lead to difficulties with delivery. In addition, neonates may have episodes of profound hypoglycemia in the minutes after delivery due to high compensatory circulating levels of insulin. EMS providers should anticipate this if necessary and be prepared to give dextrose to the neonate according to local protocol.

Conclusion

There are many anatomical and physiological changes in pregnancy which require specific awareness and knowledge by EMS providers. With the appropriate training, continuous quality improvement, and medical oversight, providers can have confidence in initiating the best emergency medical care and transporting safely to the appropriate receiving facility.

References

1 Rasmussen KM, Committee to Reexamine IOM Pregnancy Weight Guidelines, Food and Nutrition Board, Board on Children, Youth and Families, Institute of Medicine, Division of Behavioral and Social Sciences and Education, National Research Council. *Weight Gain during Pregnancy: Reexamining the Guidelines*. Atlanta, GA: National Academies Press, 2009.

2 Prichard JA. Changes in blood volume during pregnancy and delivery. *Anesthesiology* 1965;26:393–9.

3 Cunningham FG, Leveno KJ, Bloom SL, et al. *Williams Obstetrics*, 23rd edn. New York: McGraw-Hill; 2010.

4 Lewin SB, Cheek TJ, Deutschman CS. Airway management in the obstetric patient. *Crit Care Clin* 2000;16:505–13.

5 Thornburga KL, Jacobsona SL, Girauda GD, Morton MJ. Hemodynamic changes in pregnancy. *Semin Perinatol* 2000; 24:11–14.

6 Perrotta E, Carillo C, Celli P. Electrocardiographic changes during at term labor. *G Ital Cardiol* 1999;29:48–53.

7 Silversides CK, Harris L, Haberer K, et al. Recurrence rates of arrhythmias during pregnancy in women with previous tachyarrhythmia and impact on fetal and neonatal outcomes. *Am J Cardiol* 2006;97:1206–12.

8 Page RL. Treatment of arrhythmias during pregnancy. *Am Heart J* 1995;130:871–6.

9 Cox JL, Gardner MJ. Treatment of cardiac arrhythmias during pregnancy. *Prog Cardiovasc Dis* 1993;36:137–78.

10 Prowse C, Gaensler EA. Respiratory and acid-base changes during pregnancy. *Anesthesiology* 1965;26:381–92.

11 Shannon MW, Borron SW, Burns MJ. *Haddad and Winchester's Clinical Management of Poisoning and Drug Overdose*, 4th edn. Philadelphia: Saunders Elsevier, 2007.

12 Longo LD. The biological effects of carbon monoxide on the pregnant women, fetus, and newborn infant. *Am J Obstet Gynecol* 1977;129:69–103.

13 Heit JA. Trends in the incidence of venous thromboembolism during pregnancy or postpartum: a 30-year population-based study. *Ann Intern Med* 2005;143:697–706.

14 James AH, Jamison MG, Brancazio LR, Myers ER. Venous thromboembolism during pregnancy and the postpartum period: incidence, risk factors, and mortality. *Am J Obstet Gynecol* 2006;194:1311–15.

15 Foxman B. Epidemiology of urinary tract infections: incidence, morbidity, and economic costs. *Am J Med* 2002;113:5–13.

16 Cunningham FG, Lucas MJ. Urinary tract infections complicating pregnancy. *Baillières Clin Obstet Gynaecol* 1994;8:353–73.

17 Tracey M, Fletcher HS. Appendicitis in pregnancy. *Am Surg* 2000;66:555–9.

18 Baer JL, Reis RA, Arens RA. Appendicitis in pregnancy with changes in position and axis of the normal appendix in pregnancy. *JAMA* 1932;98:1359–64.

19 Indar AA, Beckingham IJ. Acute cholecystitis. *BMJ* 2002;325: 639–43.

CHAPTER 42

Emergencies of pregnancy

W. Scott Gilmore

Introduction

Human pregnancy is generally divided into three 13-week trimesters. While this terminology is useful, it is easier to divide the pregnancy into two halves, each lasting about 20 weeks. The first half is commonly referred to as early pregnancy and the latter as late pregnancy. Each half of pregnancy has its own unique emergencies that the EMS physician should keep in mind.

The most common disorder of early pregnancy is miscarriage. Only 20% of miscarriages occur after the first trimester. Ectopic pregnancy is the most life-threatening emergency of early pregnancy. High suspicion for ectopic pregnancy should always be maintained for females of child-bearing age, and prompt diagnosis and therapy should be reflexive. The most common emergencies of late pregnancy include placenta previa and placental abruption.

Evaluation of the pregnant patient

An EMS physician should rapidly ascertain pertinent information from any pregnant patient. This includes estimated due date or weeks of gestation, last menstrual period, number of previous pregnancies, number and type of deliveries, contraction intervals, membrane rupture, bleeding, and complications with previous pregnancies such as gestational diabetes, preeclampsia, or preterm labor. The EMS physician's challenge is to identify life threats and initiate treatment in spite of the fact that pregnancy status is often unknown by the patient.

Miscarriage

Miscarriage is the most common complication of early pregnancy. Approximately 15–20% of clinically evident pregnancies are miscarried [1]. Eighty percent of all miscarriages occur before the 12th week of gestation [2]. In most cases, the primary focus for the EMS physician is to provide psychological support to the patient and her family. If the patient has passed tissue it should be transported with the patient to the receiving facility. If the patient is showing signs or having symptoms of hemorrhagic shock, a large-bore intravenous catheter should be inserted for access and the patient appropriately resuscitated with boluses of normal saline.

Ectopic pregnancy

Ectopic pregnancy is the implantation of a fertilized ovum outside the endometrial cavity. It occurs in approximately 1.5–2.0% of pregnancies [3], with some studies reporting the incidence of ectopic pregnancy as high as 2.6% of all pregnancies [4–7]. The reported rise in incidence of ectopic pregnancy is strongly associated with an increased incidence of pelvic inflammatory disease [8].

The clinical use of sensitive pregnancy testing, transvaginal sonography, and diagnostic laparoscopy has had a major effect on the diagnosis of ectopic pregnancy before rupture. Nevertheless, ruptured ectopic pregnancies continue to occur, often because the clinician or the patient did not recognize the early signs and symptoms of the condition, and such pregnancies account for 6% of all maternal deaths and remain the leading cause of first-trimester pregnancy-related death [3]. The most frequent causes of death for women with ectopic pregnancies in the United States are hemorrhage, infection, and anesthetic complications.

The etiology of ectopic pregnancy is multifactorial and as many as 50% of women with ectopic pregnancies have no identifiable risks [9]. Factors that are strongly associated with an increased risk of ectopic pregnancy include damage to the ovarian tubes from pelvic inflammatory disease, previous tubal surgery, or a previous ectopic pregnancy. A history of cigarette smoking, age over 35 years, and many lifetime partners have been identified as minor factors (Table 42.1).

The risk of recurrence of ectopic pregnancy is approximately 10% among women with one previous ectopic pregnancy and at

Emergency Medical Services: Clinical Practice and Systems Oversight, Second Edition. Volume 1: Clinical Aspects of EMS.
Edited by David C. Cone, Jane H. Brice, Theodore R. Delbridge, and J. Brent Myers.
© 2015 NAEMSP. Published 2015 by John Wiley & Sons, Inc. Companion Website: www.wiley.com\go\cone\naemsp

Table 42.1 Relative risk factors for ectopic pregnancy

High	Moderate	Low
Prior ectopic	Chlamydia	Age <18
Tubular sterilization	Infertility	Age >35
Use of intrauterine contraceptive device (IUD)	Partners >1	
Pelvic inflammatory disease	Smoking	

least 25% among women with two or more previous ectopic pregnancies [10]. Women in whom the affected fallopian tube has been removed are at increased risk for ectopic pregnancy in the remaining tube.

Ectopic pregnancies that involve implantation outside the fallopian tube account for less than 10% of all ectopic pregnancies. These unusual pregnancies are difficult to diagnose and are associated with high mortality [11]. Abdominal pregnancies occur in 10.9 per 100,000 pregnancies and in 9.2 per 1,000 ectopic pregnancies. The maternal mortality rate has been reported to be 7.7 times higher than that observed in tubal ectopic pregnancies, and 90 times higher than in an intrauterine pregnancy [12].

Heterotopic pregnancy, the co-occurrence of an ectopic pregnancy and intrauterine pregnancy, has increased in incidence and occurs in 0.3–0.8% of the general population and 1–3% of women pregnant as a result of assisted reproduction [13,14].

The patient history (including an assessment for risk factors) and physical examination are the principal tools used to evaluate a patient with possible ectopic pregnancy. In the out-of-hospital setting, any woman of reproductive age with abdominal pain or vaginal bleeding should be considered to have an ectopic pregnancy until proven otherwise.

Patient history

The location, nature, and severity of pain with ectopic pregnancy are highly variable. Colicky pain presents mainly in the hypogastric or iliac regions and is most likely due to small-volume intraperitoneal hemorrhage. Localized abdominal or pelvic pain is caused by acute distension of the fallopian tube at the site of implantation. Tubal rupture is typically associated with a longer-lasting, more generalized pain due to hemoperitoneum, but rupture may also be associated with a decrease in or resolution of pain altogether. Pain referred to the shoulder, indicating irritation of the diaphragm from intraperitoneal blood (Kehr's sign), is a late sign. Vaginal bleeding may be small in volume (spotting) or equivalent to a menstrual period. The passage of tissue does not distinguish failing intrauterine from ectopic pregnancy and may simply represent a cast of endometrial tissue.

Classic signs and symptoms of tubal ectopic pregnancy include abdominal pain, vaginal bleeding, and delay of an expected menses with classic presentation around 6 to 8 weeks

of gestation [9]. However, fewer than half of women with ectopic pregnancy have the classically described symptoms of abdominal pain and vaginal bleeding. In fact, these symptoms are more likely to indicate miscarriage [15].

Physical examination

Women with ectopic pregnancy may have pelvic or adnexal tenderness and vaginal bleeding. Hypovolemia, tachycardia, hypotension, diaphoresis, and shock are late signs that may indicate ruptured ectopic pregnancy with intraperitoneal hemorrhage. Although it is less common for women to present with these signs, due to improved diagnostic methods, a woman with hemodynamic instability or peritoneal signs and a positive pregnancy test result or a delay of an expected menses potentially has a ruptured ectopic pregnancy, and should have prompt evaluation by an obstetrician.

Management

For the EMS physician, the key to treating a pregnant patient with early obstetrical complaints is maintaining a high index of suspicion for a possible ectopic pregnancy and recognizing hemodynamic instability secondary to hemorrhagic shock. If the patient is in shock, large-bore intravenous access should be obtained and the patient resuscitated appropriately with crystalloids. In a woman of child-bearing age with abdominal pain and hypotension, the finding of free abdominal fluid on prehospital ultrasound should increase the suspicion of ruptured ectopic pregnancy.

Placental abruption

Placental abruption, defined as the premature separation of the placenta from the uterine wall, complicates approximately 1% of births [16]. Abruption is believed to account for approximately 30% of episodes of bleeding during the second half of pregnancy. It is associated with significant perinatal mortality and morbidity.

Abruption may be "revealed," in which case blood tracks between the placenta and the endometrium, and escapes through the cervix into the vagina. The less common "concealed" abruption occurs when blood accumulates behind the placenta, with no obvious external bleeding. Finally, abruption may also be classified as total, involving the entire placenta, in which case it typically leads to fetal death, or partial, with only a portion of the placenta detached from the uterine wall.

Placental abruption has a wide spectrum of clinical significance, varying from minor bleeding with few or no consequences to massive abruption with fetal death and severe maternal morbidity. Maternal risks include massive bleeding, disseminated intravascular coagulopathy, and death. The risk to the fetus depends on both the severity of the abruption and the age at which the abruption occurs, whereas the danger to the mother is posed primarily by the severity of the abruption.

Table 42.2 Risk factors for placental abruption

High	Moderate	Low
Cocaine and drug use	Cigarette smoking	Maternal age and parity
Chronic hypertension with preeclampsia	Multiple gestations	Oligohydramnios
	Chronic hypertension	Dietary and nutritional deficiencies
	Preeclampsia	Carrying a male fetus
	Premature rupture of membranes	
	Chorioamnionitis	

prior abruption (handwritten)

Source: Oyelese 2006 [18]. Reproduced with permission of Lippincott Williams & Wilkins Inc.

The incidence of placental abruption is reported to be between 1% and 3.8% of deliveries [17–22]. The incidence of abruption peaks at 24–26 weeks gestation and drops precipitously with advancing gestation [18,19]. Other risk factors include trauma, thrombophilias, dysfibrinogenemia, hydramnios, advanced maternal age, and intrauterine infections (Table 42.2) [23].

Bleeding in early pregnancy carries an increased risk of abruption in later pregnancy [24,25]. Placental abruption is usually the result of shearing forces, may occur without direct abdominal trauma, and is independent of placental location. Approximately 6% of all trauma cases [26] and 20–25% of major trauma cases are associated with placental abruption [27] but placental abruption is difficult to predict based on the severity of trauma [26]. Placental abruption usually manifests within 6–48 hours after trauma but can occur up to 5 days later [26,28,29]. Perhaps the greatest determination of abruption risk, however, is an abruption in a prior pregnancy [30]. When examined, the risk increased 15–20-fold in subsequent pregnancies when an earlier pregnancy was complicated by abruption [31].

The diagnosis of abruption is a clinical one and the condition should be suspected in women who present with vaginal bleeding or abdominal pain or both, a history of trauma, and those who present in otherwise preterm labor. The differential diagnosis includes all causes of abdominal pain and bleeding in pregnancy, such as placenta previa, appendicitis, urinary tract infection, preterm labor, ovarian pathology, and muscular pain.

Patient history

The clinical presentation of abruption varies widely. Classically, placental abruption presents with vaginal bleeding and abdominal pain. It is important to realize, however, that severe abruption may occur with neither or just one of these signs. Vaginal bleeding occurs in 80% of cases. The amount of vaginal bleeding correlates poorly with the degree of abruption [32]. The severity of symptoms depends on the location of the abruption, whether it is revealed or concealed, and the degree of abruption. Backache may be the only symptom, especially when the placental location is posterior [33]. Finally, abruption may present as idiopathic preterm labor.

In addition to the standard obstetric history, a history should be obtained that focuses on cocaine and drug use, hypertension, preeclampsia, and other predisposing factors.

Physical examination

Upon physical examination, typically there is uterine hypotonus with associated high-frequency, low-amplitude uterine contractions. The uterus is frequently tender and may feel hard on palpation. In cases of severe abruption, typically, the uterus is contracting vigorously and labor rapidly progresses. The remainder of the physical examination should be performed looking for signs of trauma, preeclampsia, or other predisposing factors.

The ultrasonographic appearance of abruption depends to a large extent on the size and location of the bleed, as well as the duration between the abruption and the time the ultrasonographic examination was performed. In cases of acute revealed abruption, the examiner may detect no abnormal ultrasonographic findings. The ultrasonographic appearance of abruption in the acute phase is hyperechoic to isoechoic when compared with the placenta [34]. The sensitivity, specificity, and positive and negative predictive values of ultrasonography for placental abruption are 24%, 96%, 88%, and 53% respectively [35]. Thus ultrasound will fail to detect at least one half of cases of abruption.

Management

A patient with signs or symptoms of placental abruption should have a large-bore IV catheter inserted for access and transport expeditiously to a facility with obstetrical capabilities. The patient should be monitored closely during transport, observing for the development of signs of shock.

Bleeding caused by placental abruption can lead to maternal hypovolemic shock. Blood loss may be underestimated because of a concealed abruption. If the patient exhibits signs or symptoms of shock, she should be resuscitated with boluses of normal saline.

In the case of trauma, transport expeditiously to a trauma center where the patient can be evaluated by both a trauma surgeon and an obstetrician and undergo fetal monitoring.

Placenta previa

Placenta previa is another cause of bleeding episodes during the second half of pregnancy. Placenta previa refers to a placenta that overlies or is proximate to the internal os of the cervix. Normally, the placenta implants in the upper uterine segment. In placenta previa, the placenta is either totally or partially within the lower uterine segment.

> **Box 42.1** Risk factors for placenta previa
>
> Prior cesarean section
> Termination of pregnancy or uterine surgery
> Smoking
> Increasing age
> Multiparity
> Cocaine use
> Multiple pregnancies

Morbidities associated with placenta previa include antepartum bleeding, need for hysterectomy, morbid adherence of the placenta, intrapartum hemorrhage, postpartum hemorrhage, blood transfusion, septicemia, and thrombophlebitis [36]. Placenta previa is also associated with an increase in preterm birth. In the United States, maternal mortality occurs in 0.03% of cases with placenta previa [37]. Placenta previa complicates approximately 0.3–0.5% of pregnancies [37]. The annual incidence in the United States is reported to be 4.8 per 1,000 deliveries [37].

The likelihood of placenta previa increases in a dose–response fashion with a greater number of prior cesarean sections and with greater parity, with a relative risk of placenta previa rising from 4.5 (95% confidence interval (CI) 3.6–5.5) in women with one prior cesarean section to 44.9 (95% CI 13.5–149.5) in women with four prior cesarean sections (Box 42.1) [38].

Patient history

The classic presentation is painless bleeding in the late second trimester or early third trimester. However, some patients with placenta previa will experience painful bleeding, possibly due to uterine contractions or placental separation, whereas others will experience no bleeding at all before labor [39].

Physical examination

Women who present with bleeding in the second half of pregnancy should have a sonographic examination for placental location. Digital vaginal examination with a placenta previa may provoke catastrophic hemorrhage and should not be performed, either in the field or in the emergency department.

Management

A large-bore intravenous cannula should be inserted and the patient transported expeditiously to a hospital. She should be closely monitored during transport. If at any time she shows signs of shock, fluid resuscitation with normal saline should be performed.

Hypertension during pregnancy

Hypertension is observed in approximately 6–8% of pregnancies and is generally divided into several categories [40]. Gestational hypertension occurs during pregnancy, resolves during the postpartum period, and is recognized by a new blood pressure reading of 140/90 mmHg or higher. Preeclampsia is gestational hypertension with proteinuria, and eclampsia is the occurrence of seizures in the patient with signs of preeclampsia. Progression of preeclampsia to eclampsia is unpredictable and can occur rapidly [40].

Approximately 2–7% of pregnancies are complicated by pregnancy-induced hypertension. Hypertensive emergencies during pregnancy are the second leading cause of maternal deaths in the United States, with a 15% occurrence [41,42]. The incidence of eclampsia has progressively declined, but it is still one of the major causes of maternal mortality.

Preeclampsia

Preeclampsia is a multisystem disorder characterized by the presence of hypertension and proteinuria after 20 weeks of gestation [42]. It affects 12% of pregnancies and is responsible for nearly 20% of maternal deaths in the United States [44]. Urinary protein excretion greater than 300 mg daily is required for diagnosis [45]. This amount of proteinuria usually corresponds to a positive reaction (+1) on a urine dipstick via random urine sample [46–51]. Severe preeclampsia is defined by blood pressure readings higher than 160/110 mmHg and more than 5 g of urinary protein excretion daily.

Preeclampsia may also be associated with many other signs and symptoms, such as edema, visual disturbance, headache, and epigastric pain. Features of severe preeclampsia include hypertensive emergency, acute renal failure, cerebral and visual disturbances, and pulmonary edema or cyanosis. Common risk factors for the development of preeclampsia include primiparity, multiple gestations, previous preeclampsia, obesity, diabetes mellitus, and connective tissue disorders [52].

Management

The use of magnesium sulfate in all patients with preeclampsia for the prevention of eclampsia is controversial. The large "Magpie" prospective trial suggested that the prophylactic use of magnesium sulfate in preeclampsia decreased the overall risk of eclampsia and may reduce maternal death [53]. Prehospital treatment should be centered around supportive care and transport to an appropriate receiving facility.

Eclampsia

Eclampsia is defined as the presence of new-onset grand mal seizures in a woman with preeclampsia [51]. Eclampsia is rare and occurs in less than 1% of preeclamptic patients and may occur in the absence of preeclampsia [43,51]. In 10–15% of patients with eclampsia, hypertension is absent or modest and/or proteinuria is not detected [54]. The incidence of eclampsia is about 1 in 3,250 pregnancies in the United States [55–57]. More than 90% of eclamptic seizures present after gestational week 28, but reports exist of eclampsia presenting as early as gestational week 16 [58] and as late as 23 days postpartum [59,60].

Eclampsia is associated with increased rates of abruptio placentae, microangiopathic hemolytic anemia, pulmonary edema, acute renal failure, and preterm delivery [61].

Eclamptic seizures can occur at any time during pregnancy and infrequently 48 hours to 1 month post partum. One-third or more of patients having eclamptic seizures in the postpartum period present without ever having manifested signs and symptoms of preeclampsia [62].

The rate of preeclampsia in subsequent pregnancies following a pregnancy complicated by eclampsia is as high as 25% [63].

Seizures from eclampsia are usually grand mal. Other clinical features of eclampsia include nausea, vomiting, hyperreflexia, severe headaches, and altered mental status. However, many of these features are also seen in preeclampsia. Rarely cortical blindness occurs with severe preeclampsia/eclampsia. Focal neurological signs are unusual, but have been reported [63].

Management

Several large randomized controlled trials have demonstrated that parenteral magnesium sulfate is superior to both phenytoin and diazepam in preventing the initial and recurrent seizures and lowering maternal mortality. In the Collaborative Eclampsia Trial, magnesium sulfate reduced the risk of recurrent seizures in eclamptic women by 52% when compared to diazepam and by 67% when compared to phenytoin [64].

The American College of Obstetricians and Gynecologists recommends a 4–6 g loading dose given intravenously over 15–20 minutes, followed by a continuous infusion rate of 2 g/hour [51]. There is concern for magnesium toxicity while administering such high doses. Toxicity is manifested by loss of tendon reflexes, respiratory depression, muscular paralysis, respiratory arrest, and maternal cardiac arrest. Tendon reflexes disappear considerably before serious toxicity such as cardiac arrhythmias and respiratory arrest occur.

Conclusion

The most important action that an EMS physician can undertake in any emergency of pregnancy is to maintain a high index of suspicion and protect the life of mother and child.

References

1 Wilcox AJ, Weinberg CR, O'Connor JF, et al. Incidence of early loss of pregnancy. *N Engl J Med* 1988;319:189–94.
2 Coppola PT, Coppola M. Vaginal bleeding in the first 20 weeks of pregnancy. *Emerg Med Clin North Am* 2003;21:667–77.
3 Chang J, Elam-Evans LD, Berg CJ, et al. Pregnancy related mortality surveillance – United States, 1991–1999. *MMWR Surveill Summ* 2003;52:1–8.
4 Hoover KW, Tao G, Kent CK. Trends in the diagnosis and treatment of ectopic pregnancy in the United States. *Obstet Gynecol* 2010;115:495–502.
5 Trabert B, Holt VL, Yu O, van den Eeden SK, Scholes D. Population-based ectopic pregnancy trends, 1993–2007. *Am J Prev Med* 2011;40:556–60.
6 Van den Eeden SK, Shan J, Bruce C, Glasser M. Ectopic pregnancy rate and treatment utilization in a large managed care organization. *Obstet Gynecol* 2005;105:1052–7.
7 Zane SB, Keike BA Jr, Kendrick JS, Bruce C. Surveillance in a time of changing health care practices; estimating ectopic pregnancy incidence in the United States. *Matern Child Health J* 2002;6:227–36.
8 Kamwendo F, Forslin L, Bodin L, Danielsson D. Epidemiology of ectopic pregnancy during a 28-year period and the role of pelvic inflammatory disease. *Sex Transm Infect* 2000;76:28–32.
9 Marion LL, Meeks GR. Ectopic pregnancy: history, incidence, epidemiology, and risk factors. *Clin Obstet Gynecol* 2012;55:376–86.
10 Seeber BE, Barnhart KT. Suspected ectopic pregnancy. *Obstet Gynecol* 2006;107:399–413.
11 Barnhart KT. Clinical practice. Ectopic pregnancy. *N Engl J Med* 2009;361:379–87.
12 Atrash HK, Friede A, Hogue CJ. Abdominal pregnancy in the United States: frequency and maternal mortality. *Obstet Gynecol* 1987;69:333–7.
13 Kirk E, Bourne T. Diagnosis of ectopic pregnancy with ultrasound. *Best Pract Res Clin Obstet Gynaecol* 2009;23:501–8.
14 Rojansky N, Schenker JG. Heterotopic pregnancy and assisted reproduction – an update. *J Assist Reprod Genet* 1996;13:594–601.
15 Ramakrishnan K, Scheid DC. Ectopic pregnancy: forget the "classic presentation" if you want to catch it sooner. *J Fam Pract* 2006;55:388–95.
16 Ananth CV, Berkowitz GS, Savitz DA, Lapinski RH. Placental abruption and adverse perinatal outcomes. *JAMA* 1999;282:1646–51.
17 Ananth CV, Wilcox AJ. Placental abruption and perinatal mortality in the United States. *Am J Epidemiol* 2001;153:332–7.
18 Oyelese Y, Ananth CV. Placental abruption. *Obstet Gynecol* 2006;108:1005–16.
19 Rasmussen S, Irgens LM, Bergsjo P, Dalaker K. The occurrence of placental abruption in Norway 1967–1991. *Acta Obstet Gynecol Scand* 1996;75:222–8.
20 Sheiner E, Shoham-Vardi I, Hallak M, et al. Placental abruption in term pregnancies: clinical significance and obstetric risk factors. *J Matern Fetal Neonatal Med* 2003;13:45–9.
21 Salihu HM, Bekan B, Aliyu MH, Rouse DJ, Kirby RS, Alexander GR. Perinatal mortality associated with abruptio placenta in singletons and multiples. *Am J Obstet Gynecol* 2005;193:198–203.
22 Ananth CV, Oyelese Y, Yeo L, Pradhan A, Vintzileos AM. Placental abruption in the United States, 1979 through 2001: temporal trends and potential determinants. *Am J Obstet Gynecol* 2005;192:191–8.
23 Hasegawa J, Nakamura M, Hamada S, et al. Capable of identifying risk factors for placental abruption. *J Matern Fetal Neonat Med* 2014;27:52–6.
24 Ananth CV, Oyelese Y, Prasad V, Getahun D, Smulian JC. Evidence of placental abruption as a chronic process: associations with vaginal bleeding early in pregnancy and placental lesions. *Eur J Obstet Gynecol Reprod Biol* 2006;128:15–21.
25 Weiss JL, Malone FD, Vidaver J, et al. Threatened abortion: a risk factor for poor pregnancy outcome, a population-based screening study. *Am J Obstet Gynecol* 2004;190:745–50.
26 Pearlman MD, Tintinallli JE, Lorenz RP. A prospective controlled study of outcome after trauma during pregnancy. *Am J Obstet Gynecol* 1990;162:1502–7.
27 Vaizey CJ, Jacobson MJ, Cross FW. Trauma in pregnancy. *Br J Surg* 1994;81:1406–15.

28 Higgins SD, Garite TJ. Late abruptio placentae in trauma patients: implications for monitoring. *Obstet Gynecol* 1984;63:S10–12.

29 Curet MJ, Schermer CR, Demarest GB, Bleneik EJ 3rd, Curet LB. Predictors of outcome in trauma during pregnancy: identification of patients who can be monitored for less than 6 hours. *J Trauma* 2000;49:18–24.

30 Toivonen S, Heinonen S, Anttila M, Kosma VM, Saarikoski S. Obstetric prognosis after placental abruption. *Fetal Diagn Ther* 2004;19:336–41.

31 Ananth CV, Savitz DA, Williams MA. Placental abruption and its association with hypertension and prolonged rupture of membranes: a methodologic review and meta-analysis. *Obstet Gynecol* 1996;88:309–18.

32 Tikkanen M. Etiology, clinical manifestations, and prediction of placental abruption. *Acta Obstet Gynecol Scand* 2010;89:732–40.

33 Oyelese Y, Ananth CV. Placental abruption. *Obstet Gynecol* 2006;108:1005–16.

34 Nyberg DA, Cyr DR, Mack LA, Wilson DA, Shuman WP. Sonographic spectrum of placental abruption. *Am J Roentgenol* 1987;148:161–4.

35 Glantz C, Purnell L. Clinical utility of sonography in the diagnosis and treatment of placental abruption. *J Ultrasound Med* 2002;21:837–40.

36 Crane JM, van den Hof MC, Dodds L, Armson BA, Liston et al. Maternal complications with placenta previa. *Am J Perinatol* 2000;17:101–5.

37 Iyasu S, Saftlas AK, Rowley DL, Koonin LM, Lawson HW, Atrash HK. The epidemiology of placenta previa in the United States, 1979 through 1987. *Am J Obstet Gynecol* 1993;168:1424–9.

38 Ananth CV, Wilcox AJ, Savitz DA, Bowes WA Jr, Luther ER. Effect of maternal age and parity on the risk of uteroplacental bleeding disorders in pregnancy. *Obstet Gynecol* 1996;88:511–16.

39 Oyelese Y, Smulian JC. Placenta previa, placenta accreta, and vasa previa. *Obstet Gynecol* 2006;107:927–41.

40 Sibai BM. Diagnosis and management of gestational hypertension and preeclampsia. *Obstet Gynecol* 2003;102:181–92.

41 ACOG Committee on Practice Bulletins. ACOG practice bulletin. Chronic hypertension in pregnancy. *Obstet Gynecol* 2001;90:177–85.

42 ACOG Committee on Practice Bulletins. ACOG practice bulletin. Clinical management guidelines for obstetrician-gynecologists. *Obstet Gynecol* 2003;102:203–13.

43 Wagner LK. Diagnosis and management of preeclampsia. *Am Fam Physician* 2004;70:2317–24.

44 Koonin LM, MacKay AP, Berg CJ, Atrash HK, Smith JC. Pregnancy-related mortality surveillance – United States, 1987–1990. *MMWR CDC Surveill Summ* 1997;46:17–36.

45 Vidaeff AC, Carroll MA, Ramin SM. Acute hypertensive emergencies in pregnancy. *Crit Care Med* 2005;33:S307–12.

46 Waugh JJ, Clark TJ, Divakaran TG, Khan KS, Kilby MD. Accuracy of urinalysis dipstick techniques in predicting significant proteinuria in pregnancy. *Obstet Gynecol* 2004;103:769–77.

47 Waugh J, Bell SC, Kilby MD, Lambert P, Shennan A, Halligan A. Urine protein estimation in hypertensive pregnancy: which thresholds and laboratory assay best predict clinical outcome? *Hypertens Pregnancy* 2005;24:291–302.

48 Meyer NL, Mercer BM, Friedman SA, Sibai BM. Urinary dipstick protein: a poor predictor of absent or severe proteinuria. *Am J Obstet Gynecol* 1994;170:137–41.

49 Gribble RK, Fee SC, Berg RL. The value of routine urine dipstick screening for protein at each prenatal visit. *Am J Obstet Gynecol* 1995;173:214–17.

50 Higby K, Suiter CR, Phelps JY, Siler-Khodr T, Langer O. Normal values of urinary albumin and total protein excretion during pregnancy. *Am J Obstet Gynecol* 1994;171:984–9.

51 ACOG Committee on Practice Bulletins – Obstetrics. ACOG practice bulletin 33. Diagnosis and management of pre-eclampsia and eclampsia. *Obstet Gynecol* 2002;99:159–67.

52 McCoy S, Baldwin K. Pharmacotherapeutic options for the treatment of preeclampsia. *Am J Health Syst Pharm* 2009;66:337–44.

53 Altman D, Carroli G, Duley L, et al. Do women with pre-eclampsia, and their babies, benefit from magnesium sulphate? The Magpie Trial: a randomised placebo-controlled trial. *Lancet* 2002;359:1877–90.

54 Vollard ES, Zeeman G, Alexander JM. Delta eclampsia: a hypertensive encephalopathy of normotensive women [abstract]. *Am J Obstet Gynecol* 2008;197:S140.

55 Sibai BM. Diagnosis, prevention, and management of eclampsia. *Obstet Gynecol* 2005;105:402–10.

56 Douglas KA, Redman CW. Eclampsia in the United Kingdom. *BMJ* 1994;309:1395–400.

57 Wallis AB, Saftlas AF, Hsia J, Atrash HK. Secular trends in the rates of pre-eclampsia, eclampsia, and gestational hypertension, United States, 1987–2004. *Am J Hypertens* 2008;21:521–6.

58 Sibai BM, Abdella TH, Taylor HA. Eclampsia in the first half of pregnancy. A report of three cases and review of the literature. *J Reprod Med* 1982;27:706–8.

59 Lubarsky SL, Barton JR, Friedman SA, Nasreddine S, Ramadan MK, Sibai BM. Late postpartum eclampsia revisited. *Obstet Gynecol* 1994;83:502–5.

60 Chames MC, Livingston JC, Ivester TS, Barton JR, Sibai BM. Late postpartum eclampsia: a preventable disease? *Am J Obstet Gynecol* 2002;186:1174–7.

61 Mattar F, Sibai BM. Eclampsia. VIII. Risk factors for maternal morbidity. *Am J Obstet Gynecol* 2000;182:307–12.

62 Hirshfeld-Cytron J, Lam C, Karumanchi SA, Lindheimer M. Late postpartum eclampsia: examples and review. *Obstet Gynecol Surv* 2006;61:471–80.

63 Karumanchi SA, Lindheimer MD. Advances in the understanding of eclampsia. *Curr Hypertens Rep* 2008;10:305–12.

64 [No authors listed] Which anticonvulsant for women with eclampsia? Evidence from the Collaborative Eclampsia Trial. *Lancet* 1995;345:1455–63.

CHAPTER 43
Normal childbirth

Stephanie A. Crapo

Introduction

Pregnancy is commonly encountered in the prehospital setting, and its management typically requires little more than a focused history and physical examination along with safe and timely transport to an appropriate hospital. There are notable exceptions, such as imminent delivery, that have the potential to be catastrophic. These are stressful, time-sensitive emergencies.

Pregnancy

Definitions

Gravidity is the number of times a woman has been pregnant and parity is the number of times a woman has given birth to a fetus of 20 weeks or more, regardless of whether the fetus was alive or stillborn. Neither gravidity nor parity is increased for twin pregnancies. For example, a woman who has one twin pregnancy with successful delivery of both infants is denoted G_1P_1.

Gestational age

Ovulation occurs around day 14 of the menstrual cycle. The egg is fertilized usually in the oviduct and migrates through the fallopian tubes into the uterus. The egg implants in the uterus around day 6 following fertilization. The heartbeat is first detected by ultrasound in weeks 8–12. The first fetal movements are felt in weeks 18–20 for a primigravid patient and 2 weeks earlier in the multiparous patient [1]. A full pregnancy lasts approximately 40 weeks. It is divided into trimesters and usually measured by weeks. The first trimester is weeks 0–13, the second trimester is weeks 14–27, and the third trimester is weeks 28–42. A pregnancy is considered viable between 22 and 26 weeks [2]. Term pregnancy is carried to at least 37 weeks.

Gestational age can be estimated by both last menstrual period and fundal height. Nine months and 7 days are added to the first day of the last menstrual period (Nagele rule) to obtain the estimated due date. Calculation from the last menstrual period usually overestimates gestational age. Fundal height is a rapid clinical tool to estimate gestational age. It is measured in centimeters from the pubic symphysis to the top of the fundus. Centimeters = weeks of gestation +/- 2 weeks. Using this estimation, a 20-week pregnancy reaches the umbilicus.

Physiological changes of pregnancy

Many physiological changes occur in pregnancy induced both by hormones and/or by the enlarging uterus (Box 43.1) [1].

Evaluation of the pregnant patient

All levels of EMS providers, from first responders to physicians, should be capable of rapidly ascertaining pertinent information from the ill or injured pregnant patient. In addition to questions relating to the chief complaint, an obstetrical and gynecological history is important to elicit, including last menstrual period, contraceptive use, gravidity, and parity. Providers should be expected to expand that history and determine if the patient has had complications associated with the current pregnancy such as gestational diabetes, preeclampsia, or preterm labor or if the patient has had complications with prior pregnancies. If delivery is imminent, history should include frequency and strength of contractions, and fluid/water leakage. As soon as it is determined that the patient is not going to deliver imminently, vital signs should be obtained and viewed in context of the normal physiological changes of pregnancy.

Examination includes thorough evaluation of the mother as well as the fetal status. If the patient has signs of active labor such as contractions, urge to defecate or push, rupture of membranes, or any other concerning signs, a visual examination of the perineum should be performed. Medical directors should carefully craft protocols that specify when visual inspection of the perineum is appropriate. Failure to have a written document

Emergency Medical Services: Clinical Practice and Systems Oversight, Second Edition. Volume 1: Clinical Aspects of EMS.
Edited by David C. Cone, Jane H. Brice, Theodore R. Delbridge, and J. Brent Myers.
© 2015 NAEMSP. Published 2015 by John Wiley & Sons, Inc. Companion Website: www.wiley.com\go\cone\naemsp

---

Box 43.1 Physiological changes in pregnancy

Blood volume increased by greater than 50%
Baseline heart rate increased by 10–15%
Cardiac output increased
Blood pressure decreased or normal
Respirations increased 10–15%
Delayed gastric emptying
Increased kidney size and renal blood flow

Box 43.2 Stages of active labor

Stage 1	Begins with uterine contractions causing progressive dilation of the cervix and ends with full dilation of the cervix (10 cm)
Stage 2	Begins with full cervical dilation and ends when the fetus is delivered
Stage 3	Begins when the neonate is separated from mother and ends with placenta delivery

---

for the EMS provider to follow opens the provider, medical director, and system to potential liability.

Ultrasound in pregnancy

Many prehospital providers are including ultrasound in the evaluation of patients (see Volume 1, Chapter 69). Ultrasound is especially useful in the evaluation of pregnant patients to confirm intrauterine pregnancy as well as to evaluate fetal well-being with heartbeat and fetal movement.

The earliest definitive sonographic finding in pregnancy is the gestational sac, detected at 6–8 weeks on transabdominal ultrasound [1,3]. Later in pregnancy, fetal viability can be assessed by observing fetal movement and fetal heart tones. Fetal heart tones should be 120–160 beats per minute after 12 weeks' gestation. They are first detected on ultrasound around 8 weeks' gestation but it may be up to 12 weeks before heart tones are seen, depending on the habitus of the patient and quality of ultrasound used [3].

A major concern in pregnant patients with abdominal pain is ectopic pregnancy. While it is not expected to be diagnosed in the field, ultrasound can assist in the recognition of ectopic pregnancy. An intrauterine pregnancy visible on ultrasound essentially excludes ectopic pregnancy. Some ultrasound findings suspicious for ectopic pregnancy include pelvic free fluid and adnexal mass other than simple cyst. A gestational sac, yolk sac, or fetal pole with heartbeat outside the uterus confirms the diagnosis of ectopic pregnancy [3].

Labor and delivery

Active labor

Labor is "the presence of uterine contractions of sufficient frequency, duration, and intensity to cause demonstrable effacement and dilation of the cervix [4]." Active labor is divided into three stages [5] (Box 43.2). A nulliparous woman has a longer labor phase (slower cervical dilation) than does a multiparous woman.

Imminent delivery

All women who are in active labor should receive supplemental oxygen and IV access. If a delivery is deemed imminent, crews should ensure they have appropriate personnel to provide resuscitative care for the mother and baby. Obstetric and neonatal

resuscitation equipment should be readied. Direct medical oversight should be notified of an impending delivery, in case emergency assistance and advice are required, though deliveries in most cases progress with little intervention.

Delivery of the neonate

If the fetus' head is visible in the vaginal outlet, the EMS providers should be prepared for imminent delivery. The patient should be placed in the lithotomy position. Using both hands on the anterior and posterior aspects of the head, constant pressure should be placed to maintain control of the delivery. Head delivery should be slow to decrease damage done to the perineum. The occiput should pass below the symphysis pubis and the face should be pointed toward the anus. Once the head is delivered, the nares then mouth should be suctioned out with a bulb syringe. The provider should use one finger at this point to evaluate for a nuchal cord (described in Volume 1, Chapter 44). The baby then rotates, and shoulders begin to appear at the vulva. Both hands of the provider should be placed on either side of the infant's head, maintaining control and applying downward pressure until the anterior shoulder passes under the symphysis pubis. An upward movement will then deliver the posterior shoulder followed by completion of the anterior shoulder. The rest of the body is typically delivered without difficulty, but some traction may be applied. The umbilical cord should be double-clamped and cut. Separation of the infant from the mother ends stage 2 of labor and marks the beginning of stage 3. The neonate should be immediately dried and evaluated [5,6].

Post delivery

Care of the neonate

Once the umbilical cord is clamped and cut, the neonate should be placed in a supine, head-down position with the head turned to the side. Normally, the newborn begins to breathe and cry almost immediately after birth. If respirations do not occur or are infrequent, suctioning of the mouth and pharynx should be performed. Stimulating the feet or back may also initiate breathing. The neonate should be dried and kept warm. If the neonate is stable, the infant can be held close to the mother's chest to decrease heat loss and should be encouraged to nurse. This will aid in delivery of the placenta due to release of oxytocin in the mother.

Table 43.1 APGAR scoring system

Sign	0	1	2
Heart rate	Absent	Below 100	Over 100
Respiratory effort	Absent	Slow, irregular	Good, crying
Muscle tone	Flaccid	Some flexion of extremities	Active motion
Reflex irritability	No response	Grimace	Vigorous cry
Color	Blue, pale	Body pink, extremities blue	Pink

A standardized method to evaluate the newborn's condition is the 1- and 5-minute APGAR scores (Table 43.1). Scores between 4 and 6 at 1 minute may indicate a mildly to moderately depressed infant, whereas scores below 3 represent a severely depressed infant [7]. If warming and stimulating the neonate do not initiate the infant's respirations, the prehospital provider will need to begin resuscitating the infant according to standard Pediatric Advanced Life Support (PALS) algorithms.

Intravenous access is not necessary in the prehospital setting unless the neonate requires ongoing and active resuscitation. Even then, it should only be performed if adequate resources exist to accomplish all other first-line resuscitative efforts. Consider umbilical vein cannulation or intraosseous access if required. If the baby is in distress, transport should be immediately initiated to the closest appropriate facility.

Delivery of the placenta

Stage 3 of labor is the delivery of the placenta, which usually occurs spontaneously about 10–30 minutes after delivery of the fetus [6]. The prehospital care provider should not delay transport for delivery of the placenta. Physical signs that the placenta is about to be delivered include the uterus becoming globular in shape, the umbilical cord lengthening, and a potential gush of blood just prior to the delivery. The gush of blood marks the separation of the placenta from the uterus. The uterus should be externally massaged at the fundus to assist with contractions. Avoid strong traction on the umbilical cord due to possible complications such as separation of the umbilical cord or uterus inversion [5]. Loss of approximately 500 mL blood is expected throughout the delivery.

Challenges of prehospital deliveries

Complicated in-hospital deliveries are often attended by multiple providers including obstetricians, labor nurses, and a neonatal resuscitation team composed of neonatologists and neonatal intensive care unit (NICU) nurses. In contrast, unplanned out-of-hospital deliveries have limited equipment and personnel resources and unpredictable environments. They are often managed by two or three EMS providers who likely have limited experience in labor and delivery. Successful delivery of the neonate also doubles the patient load for the EMS providers.

Deliveries encountered in the prehospital setting are frequently from known high-risk pregnancies and can be significantly premature. One study found that four factors contribute to unplanned out-of-hospital deliveries: multiparity, lack of or poor prenatal care, extended travel time to the hospital, and unemployment [8]. These factors lend to the increased maternal and infant morbidity and mortality found in the prehospital setting [9].

The role of the EMS medical director is to ensure that crews are properly trained and equipped. This includes adequate high-quality educational offerings for the field crews on this broad range of topics and aggressively reviewing patient care reports to ensure that appropriate, compassionate, and evidence-based care is being consistently delivered. Clear protocols and guidelines must be in place to protect and guide the EMS provider.

Special considerations

Pregnant trauma patient

The pregnant trauma patient represents an especially difficult challenge in the prehospital setting. Basic trauma life support should be carried out according to local trauma management protocols. Airway and hemorrhage control, high-flow oxygen, immobilization, and rapid transport to an appropriate facility remain top priorities. Severity of injury can be difficult to determine in the pregnant trauma patient. Although normal physiological vital sign changes seen with pregnancy can mimic shock (see Box 43.1), the pregnant patient's elevated blood volume can allow for massive blood loss before decompensation. Respiratory reserve becomes increasingly limited as the pregnancy advances. EMS protocols should reflect that seemingly minor trauma (e.g. ground-level falls, low-speed motor vehicle collisions) can cause placental abruption and require transport to an appropriate facility.

All supine pregnant trauma patients in the second and third trimester should be transported tilted roughly 15° to the left. (The right side of a long backboard can be lifted approximately 15° with blankets.) This positioning allows the uterus to be moved off the inferior vena cava, facilitates blood return to the heart, and maintains uterine perfusion [10–13].

Pregnant patient in cardiac arrest

Cardiac arrest resuscitation strategy for the pregnant patient who is more than 20 weeks differs fundamentally from the non-pregnant patient in that scene interventions should be minimal and immediate transport is the highest priority. Similar to the scene evaluation of a trauma patient, EMS providers are directed to "load and go" and perform all interventions and resuscitation measures en route to the hospital. The primary directive during transport is to maximize maternal resuscitative measures. EMS providers must focus on external chest compressions in an attempt to maintain some degree of perfusion to the fetus. The success of perimortem cesarean section in the ED correlates directly with the length of time the patient has been in cardiac arrest (see Volume 1, Chapter 45). There are reported cases of good neurological outcome of the neonate if the cesarean section is done within the first 5 minutes of the arrest [14–16].

References

1 Bardsley CH. Normal pregnancy. In: Tintinalli JE, Kelen GD, Stapczynski JS, Ma OJ, Cline DM (eds) *Tintinalli's Emergency Medicine: A Comprehensive Study Guide*, 7th edn. New York: McGraw-Hill, 2011.

2 Kaempf JW, Tomlinson M, Arduza C, et al. Medical staff guidelines for periviability pregnancy counseling and medical treatment of extremely premature infants. *Pediatrics* 2006;177:22–9.

3 Broder J. Imaging the genitourinary tract. In: *Diagnostic Imaging for the Emergency Physician*. Philadelphia: Saunders, 2011.

4 ACOG Practice Bulletin Number 49. Dystocia and augmentation of labor. *Obstet Gynecol* 2003;102:1445–54.

5 Mercado J, Brea I, Mendez B, et al. Critical obstetric and gynecologic procedures in the emergency department. *Emerg Med Clin North Am* 2013;31:207–36.

6 Drage JS, Berendes H. APGAR scores and outcome of the newborn. *Pediatr Clin North Am* 1966;13:637–43.

7 VanRooyen MJ, Scott JA. Emergency delivery. In: Tintinalli JE, Kelen GD, Stapczynski JS, Ma OJ, Cline DM (eds) *Tintinalli's Emergency Medicine: A Comprehensive Study Guide*, 7th edn. New York: McGraw-Hill, 2011.

8 Renesme L, Garlantezec R, Anouilh F, et al. Accidental out-of-hospital deliveries: a case-control study. *Acta Paediatr* 2013;102:e174–7.

9 Verdile VP, Tutsock G, Paris PM, Kennedy R. Out-of-hospital deliveries: a five-year experience. *Prehosp Disaster Med* 1995;10: 10–13.

10 Cruikshank DP. Anatomic and physiologic alterations of pregnancy that modify the response to trauma. In: Buchsbaum HJ (ed) *Trauma in Pregnancy*. Philadelphia: WB Saunders, 1979.

11 Pearlman MD, Tintinalli JE. Evaluation and treatment of the gravida and fetus following trauma during pregnancy. *Obstet Gynecol Clin North Am* 1991;18:371–81.

12 Lavery JP, Staten-McCormick M. Management of moderate to severe trauma in pregnancy. *Obstet Gynecol Clin North Am* 1995;22: 69–90.

13 Neufield JD, Moore EE, Marx JA, Rosen P. Trauma in pregnancy. *Emerg Med Clin North Am* 1987;5:623–40.

14 Weber CE. Postmortem caesarean section: review of the literature and case reports. *Am J Obstet Gynecol* 1971;110:158–65.

15 Katz VL, Dotters DJ, Droegemueller W. Perimortem caesarean delivery. *Obstet Gynecol* 1986;68:571–6.

16 Lopez-Zeno JA, Carlo WA, O'Grady JP, et al. Infant survival following delayed postmortem ceasarean delivery. *Obstet Gynecol* 1990;76: 991–2.

CHAPTER 44

Childbirth emergencies

Angus M. Jameson and Micha Campbell

General considerations and resource management

Out-of-hospital deliveries not attended by physicians or midwives are a rare occurrence, comprising less than 2% of all births in the US [1]. The majority of out-of-hospital deliveries encountered by EMS personnel are uncomplicated vertex presentations and require only routine supportive care of both mother and neonate [1–3]. Maternal risk factors for unattended out-of-hospital delivery include younger maternal age, multiparity, and poor prenatal care [3]. These same risk factors are associated with not only prematurity but higher incidence of fetal morbidity and mortality [3]. Literature over the last two decades shows a trend towards increasing numbers of unattended out-of-hospital deliveries and an increasing medicolegal burden of such cases [1]. It is imperative that medical directors provide robust training, protocol, and direct medical oversight support to crews managing out-of-hospital births.

Due to the low frequency and high-risk nature of unattended out-of-hospital births, along with the significant emotional component of these situations for both patient and provider, catastrophic outcomes are possible and do occur. It is important for EMS personnel to realize that the same risk factors that contribute to unattended out-of-hospital birth also contribute to prematurity (often extreme) and neonatal morbidity. Some complications are not amenable to successful resolution within the scope of practice of prehospital providers and will necessitate temporizing measures and rapid transport. The most practical approach is to focus training on the methodical application of interventions within the scope of care and whenever possible to expedite transport to an appropriate receiving facility.

Resource management at the scene of an unattended out-of-hospital childbirth also presents challenges as there will be at minimum two patients for the prehospital personnel to manage. As the proportion of overall pregnancies involving multiple gestations continues to rise, it is reasonable to expect EMS personnel to encounter increasing numbers of multiple birth situations, further complicating resource management. The request for additional resources, if available, should be made as soon as a multiple gestation birth, an abnormal presentation, or other childbirth emergency is identified. In some systems mother and neonate may also require transport to separate receiving facilities. Finally, given the emotionally charged nature of an out-of-hospital childbirth, attention must be paid to caring for other family members or loved ones on scene to ensure not only their support but also that they do not interfere with the provision of appropriate care.

Management of abnormal presentations

Umbilical cord prolapse

Umbilical cord prolapse is a rare complication characterized by an umbilical cord descending through the cervix prior to the presenting fetal part, and may lead to fetal distress if the fetus compresses the cord as it subsequently traverses the birth canal. Incidence of prolapsed unbiblical cord has been variously reported but is generally felt to occur in approximately 0.5–1% of all deliveries [4–6]. Although no specific data have been offered on the incidence of prolapsed umbilical cords encountered in the prehospital environment, it is reasonable to expect a rate generally similar to overall incidence.

Risk factors for prolapsed cord include abnormal presentation of the fetus (particularly breech), lack of prenatal care, twinning (particularly the second-born twin), and gestational diabetes/macrosomia [4,5]. The presence of a prolapsed cord is associated with lower Apgar scores and increased perinatal mortality, and it is imperative that the prehospital provider assesses for this potentially disastrous condition by visualizing the perineum. For crews with advanced fetal monitoring capability, unexplained fetal distress should prompt sterile vaginal exam to assess for the presence of this complication [5,7,8].

Emergency treatment of umbilical cord prolapse centers on the temporizing decompression of cord by elevation of the presenting fetal part followed by rapid delivery to remove the neonatal dependence on umbilical cord blood flow for oxygenation.

Emergency Medical Services: Clinical Practice and Systems Oversight, Second Edition. Volume 1: Clinical Aspects of EMS.
Edited by David C. Cone, Jane H. Brice, Theodore R. Delbridge, and J. Brent Myers.
© 2015 NAEMSP. Published 2015 by John Wiley & Sons, Inc. Companion Website: www.wiley.com/go/cone\naemsp

Using a gloved hand, the provider gently elevates the presenting part. The exposed cord may be covered in a moist sterile towel. If Doppler is not available to assess cord blood flow, an attempt may be made detect pulsation in the cord; however, this may be faint and care must be taken to avoid further manual compression of the cord during palpation [7,8]. Because prolapsed cord is associated with abnormal presentations, rapid completion of delivery, particularly in the prehospital setting, may be less likely. Providers should expedite transport if at all possible in these situations while attempting to preserve cord blood flow via manual elevation of the presenting part as described above and positioning of the mother in the knee-to-chest position or steep Trendelenburg to aid in reducing pressure on the cord [8]. Most often, cesarean section is undertaken to expedite delivery once at the hospital [4,5,8].

Breech

Breech presentations are encountered in 3–4% of deliveries overall [9]. In the prehospital environment, one series showed a breech incidence of 2.5% (2/81). Both were feet-first breeches and neither was completely delivered in the field [2]. Breech presentations may be of three types: complete, with flexion at both hips and knees; incomplete or footling, where one or both hips are not flexed, resulting in a foot as the presenting part; and frank, where both hips are flexed and both knees are extended so that the legs lie along the abdomen of the fetus.

Complications during breech presentation are related to incomplete dilation of the cervix by a small presenting part, entrapment of the after-coming head, prolapsed cord (particularly with footling presentation), and injury due to excessive traction by the attendant [8,9]. There is general agreement that once a breech presentation is recognized, every effort should be made to obtain obstetric expertise and rapid availability of c-section. EMS clinicians should therefore initiate transport as soon as possible. If delivery is already in progress, the presenting body part should be wrapped in a towel and supported but not elevated. Providers should be alert for a prolapsed cord as this is a known complication of breech presentation. Traction should be avoided. If only an after-coming head remains undelivered, crews may be instructed to place fingers on the maxilla to gently flex the neck to facilitate passage of the head.

Shoulder dystocia

Shoulder dystocia is defined as failure of the fetal shoulders to deliver following delivery of the fetal head and occurs in between 0.2–3% of deliveries [7–11]. Some authors have proposed a more concrete definition based on a time interval of >60 seconds between delivery of the fetal head and shoulders and the necessity for maneuvers beyond simple gentle downward traction to facilitate delivery of the anterior shoulder, but there is not consensus [8,10]. Physiologically, shoulder dystocia results from the impaction of the fetal shoulders against the maternal pelvic inlet. Most commonly, the anterior fetal shoulder is impacted against the pubic symphysis, but the posterior fetal shoulder may also

impact against the sacral promontory. The most common cause is fetal macrosomia. Dystocia may also be precipitated by very rapid delivery of the fetal head without time for the shoulders to appropriately rotate and possibly by overzealous external rotation of the fetal head by an inexperienced attendant [8]. There are no reliable prediction criteria for dystocia.

Shoulder dystocia is classically heralded by the "turtle sign" which involves the retrograde movement of the fetal head back into the introitus following its initial delivery. Shoulder dystocia should be suspected whenever delivery does not complete with gentle downward movement of the fetal head. It constitutes a true emergency and is associated with significant fetal morbidity and mortality resulting from mechanical injury to the brachial plexus and neck of the neonate and frank suffocation [7,8]. Fortunately, if the dystocia is relieved within a few minutes, the incidence of permanent injury and perinatal death is very low, having been reported to be between 0–1.6% and 0–2.9% respectively [10].

Disagreement exists over the optimal combination and sequence of maneuvers designed to relieve shoulder dystocia [11]. Interventions in the prehospital environment will likely be limited by the scope of practice of personnel unless an EMS physician is on scene. The primary focus should be on positioning and gentle suprapubic pressure to attempt to reduce the anterior shoulder impaction and facilitate completion of delivery.

The most commonly applied maneuver is McRoberts, which consists of hyperflexion of the maternal hips which results in increased sacral–pubic distance. This maneuver is easy to perform and is in fact used routinely by many obstetricians to prevent development of dystocia. McRoberts should be accompanied by application of suprapubic — not fundal — pressure. Application of the McRoberts maneuver alone has been reported to relieve approximately 40% of dystocias, and when suprapubic pressure was added, success climbed to nearly 60% [10]. If the combination of McRoberts and suprapubic pressure fails to relive the dystocia, a trial of rolling the patient to the "all fours" position (Gaskin maneuver) should be undertaken [11,12]. If the dystocia cannot be relieved with this sequence of maneuvers, focus should shift to immediate emergency transport for more invasive maneuvers.

Emergency medical services physicians may elect to attempt fetal rotation maneuvers (Woods corkscrew and Rubin) to complete delivery, or direct their crews to perform these maneuvers via on-line consult; however, providing adequate and effective guidance via radio or cell phone in these situations will likely be difficult [11,13–15]. If on scene, an EMS physician may also attempt replacement of the fetus into the uterus (Zavenelli maneuver) as a temporizing measure until cesarean section can be completed [14,15]. While episiotomy may be useful in facilitating such maneuvers, it is unlikely itself to relieve the bone-on-bone impaction of a shoulder dystocia [10]. Deliberate fracture of the fetal clavicle has also widely been described, but is not universally accepted as an appropriate practice [10].

Vaginal hemorrhage

Postpartum hemorrhage is the leading cause of maternal death worldwide and may be classified into primary and secondary hemorrhage. Primary occurs in the first 24 hours following delivery, and secondary occurs after 24 hours until weeks following delivery. Primary postpartum hemorrhage complicates 4–6% of pregnancies, although the incidence has recently been shown to be on the rise [16,17]. Most (80%) primary hemorrhage is due to uterine atony. Other causes include inherited coagulopathies (i.e. von Willebrand), retained placenta, placenta accreta, uterine inversion, and pelvic/vaginal trauma [16]. Secondary postpartum hemorrhage is most often due to retained products of conception with or without infection, and coagulopathies both inherited and acquired [16].

Prehospital management of postpartum hemorrhage centers on treatment of uterine atony, as this represents the majority of cases encountered. Fundal massage using a circular motion over the uterine fundus should be the first maneuver attempted by clinicians of all levels. Specialty or critical care transport units may also have the capacity to administer pharmacological agents to assist with uterine contraction such as oxytocin, misoprostol (Cytotec), methylergonovine (Methergine), and prostoglandins (Hemabate and Dinoprostone) [8,9,16]. Crews should establish large-bore IV access if not already done, and initiate fluid resuscitation per protocol for hemorrhagic shock.

Prehospital efforts to complete delivery of the placenta if it does not spontaneously deliver (i.e. traction on the umbilical cord) have the potential to exacerbate hemorrhage and may precipitate uterine inversion. They should be attempted under the direction of medical oversight, if at all. Bleeding from lacerations to the perineum and vagina should be controlled using standard hemorrhage control techniques, including direct pressure and vaginal packing if necessary [16]. If an inverted uterus is identified, direct medical oversight may consider having crews attempt manual reduction to facilitate hemorrhage control in remote locations with prolonged transport times.

References

1 McLelland GE, Morgans AE, McKenna LG. Involvement of emergency medical services at unplanned births before arrival to hospital: a structured review. *Emerg Med J* 2014;31:345–50.

2 Verdile VP, Tutsock G, Paris PM, Kennedy RA. Out-of-hospital deliveries: a five-year experience. *Prehosp Disaster Med* 1995; 10:10–13.

3 Moscovitz HC, Magriples U, Keissling M, Shriver JA. Care and outcome of out-of-hospital deliveries. *Acad Emerg Med* 2000;7:757–61.

4 Qureshi NS, Taylor DJ, Tomlinson AJ. Umbilical cord prolapse. *Int J Gynecol Obstet* 2004;86:29–30.

5 Kahana B, Sheiner E, Levy A, et al. Umbilical cord prolapse and perinatal outcomes. *Int J Gynecol Obstet* 2004;84:127–32.

6 Katz Z, Shoham Z, Lancet M, et al. Management of labor with umbilical cord prolapse: a 5-year Study. *Obstet Gynecol* 1988;72:278–81.

7 Burg MD, Biesbroeck D. Emergency delivery. In: Wolfson AB (ed) *Harwood-Nuss' Clinical Practice of Emergency Medicine*, 5th edn. Philadelphia: Lippincott Williams and Wilkins, 2010, pp.695–700.

8 Delke I. Delivery in the emergency department. In: Benrubi GI (ed) *Handbook of Obstetric and Gynecologic Emergencies*, 4th edn. Philadelphia: Lippincott Williams and Wilkins, 2010, pp.160–74.

9 Gabbe SG, Niebyl JR, Galan HL, Jauniaux ERM. *Obstetrics: Normal and Problem Pregnancies*, 6th edn. Philadelphia: Saunders, 2012, pp.396–444.

10 Gherman RB, Chauhan S, Ouzounian JG, et al. Shoulder dystocia: the unpreventable obstetric emergency with empiric management guidelines. Am J Obstet Gynecol 2006;195:657–72.

11 American College of Obstetricians and Gynecologists. ACOG Practice Bulletin Number 40. Clinical management guidelines for obstetrician-gynecologists: shoulder dystocia. *Obstet Gynecol* 2002;100:1045–50.

12 Bruner JP, Drummond SB, Meenan AL, Gaskin IM. All-fours maneuver for reducing shoulder dystocia during labor. *J Reprod Med* 1998;43:439–43.

13 Woods CE. A principle of physics as applicable to shoulder dystocia. *Am J Obstet Gynecol* 1943;45:796–804.

14 Ramsey PS, Ramin KD, Field CS. Shoulder dystocias: rotational maneuvers revisited. *J Reprod Med* 2000;45:85–8.

15 Gherman RB. Shoulder dystocia: an evidence-based evaluation of the obstetric nightmare. *Clin Obstet Gynecol* 2002;45: 345–62.

16 American College of Obstetricians and Gynecologists. ACOG Practice Bulletin Number 76. Clinical management guidelines for obstetrician-gynecologists: postpartum hemorrhage. *Obstet Gynecol* 2006;108:1039–47.

17 Mehrabadi A, Hutcheon JA, Lee L, et al. Trends in postpartum hemorrhage from 2000 to 2009: a population-based study. *BMC Pregnancy Childbirth* 2012;12:108.

CHAPTER 45

Perimortem cesarean section

Christian Martin-Gill

Introduction

While the origin of the perimortem cesarean section is debated, the procedure is reported to have been performed in all cultures dating back to ancient times [1]. The term "cesarean section" is said to come from the performance of the postmortem section, dating back to 715 BC when Roman king Numus Pompilius decreed that no child should be buried within its mother [1,2]. This was first known as Lex Regis (the law of the king) and later translated into Lex Cesare (the law of Caesar), leading to the term cesarean section. This procedure was described widely through the Middle Ages to aid with baptism, and multiple royal and religious decrees reinforced the performance of postmortem sections. While initially performed to aid in burial, the procedure was later performed in an attempt to save the infant and mother [3]. Literature from the 1800s demonstrates a debate over the pros and cons of the procedure, and medical reports of infants surviving surface at that time [2]. Because of the high frequency of maternal mortality, as well as high rates of sepsis, dehydration, and hemorrhagic shock as the causes of maternal death, infants often died before the mother and survival following postmortem sections remained low for centuries [2,4].

Over time, the leading causes of maternal mortality in pregnancy have changed to trauma, cardiac disease, and embolism [4–6]. In these cases, the mother and infant are generally in good health until an insult results in maternal cardiac arrest. Thus, performance of a postmortem c-section could be more likely to result in birth of a live infant than described historically. The term perimortem cesarean section (PMCS) began to be used widely following a landmark literature review of postmortem cesarean section cases by Katz et al. [5] Of 269 cases reported from 1879 to 1985, 188 infants (70%) survived, a higher infant survival rate than previously considered. The majority of surviving infants (with timing records) were delivered within 5 minutes from death of the mother. All but one neurologically intact infant was delivered within 15 minutes. Katz et al. recommended performance of PMCS within 4 minutes of maternal arrest, with delivery by 5 minutes, in any case with fetal viability. This became known as the "4-minute rule" and remains widely referenced today [7]. A follow-up review of 38 cases between 1985 and 2004 supported this recommendation [4].

Potential benefits of perimortem cesarean section

The reasons for performing PMCS have changed over time. While first primarily performed for burial and religious reasons and later to attempt survival of the fetus who would otherwise meet certain death, cases of maternal survival after PMCS reveal the additional potential benefit of the procedure as part of maternal resuscitation. In a pregnant woman at term, the great vessels are compressed by the uterus, which leads to a reduction in cardiac output by two-thirds [1,2,4,7–9]. Considering that cardiopulmonary resuscitation (CPR) already produces a cardiac output that is only one-third of normal, chest compressions in a supine pregnant mother under the best circumstances produce a cardiac output that is 10% of normal. Emptying the uterus through PMCS alleviates compression of the inferior vena cava, improves venous return, and allows redistribution of uterine blood to other organs, which under normal conditions at term contributes up to 25% of cardiac output. Emptying the uterus also increases the functional residual capacity of the mother's lungs, allowing for better oxygenation [1,10]. In combination, this may improve the effectiveness of CPR and lead to successful resuscitation of the mother after delivery of the infant.

In the landmark review by Katz et al., 12 cases were identified where there was sudden and often profound improvement in the mother's condition once the uterus was emptied [5]. There have been multiple additional reports of maternal survival after PMCS, including 13 of 38 mothers discharged in good condition in Katz et al.'s follow-up review of PMCS cases [4]. Dijkman et al. reviewed all cases of maternal cardiac

Emergency Medical Services: Clinical Practice and Systems Oversight, Second Edition. Volume 1: Clinical Aspects of EMS.
Edited by David C. Cone, Jane H. Brice, Theodore R. Delbridge, and J. Brent Myers.
© 2015 NAEMSP. Published 2015 by John Wiley & Sons, Inc. Companion Website: www.wiley.com\go\cone\naemsp

arrest in The Netherlands from 1993 to 2008 and found eight of 12 mothers who regained cardiac output after PMCS, though only two ultimately survived [11]. In none of these cases was PMCS performed within 5 minutes, and timing may have contributed to the ultimate outcomes. In another review of 94 PMCS cases, the authors determined that PMCS was beneficial to the mothers in 31.7% of cases, without demonstration of harm in any case [12]. Because of this potential effect on maternal resuscitation, it has been suggested that physicians should perform PMCS regardless of the gestational age or fetal viability, without delays to assess the status of the infant [11].

Performance of perimortem cesarean section in the field

Only a few cases of PMCS performed in the field have been reported in the modern medical literature. In all of these cases, PMCS was performed by a physician working as part of an EMS team. Kupas et al. reported the performance of a PMCS on a 39-year-old woman at 39 weeks gestation who suffered a myocardial infarction [13]. PMCS was performed by an emergency medicine resident functioning as a flight physician, along with a physician neighbor. Neither mother nor infant survived. Bowers and Wagner similarly described a 31-year-old woman at 37 weeks gestation who was involved in a motor vehicle crash into a building [14]. PMCS was performed by an emergency medicine resident as part of a physician/nurse flight team. Neither mother nor infant survived. Kue et al. reported the performance of a PMCS on a 21-year-old woman at unknown gestation involved in a motor vehicle collision [15]. PMCS was also performed by a flight physician, who first performed an ultrasound and determined there was no maternal cardiac activity, but there was fetal cardiac activity. CPR had been ongoing for over 25 minutes prior to PMCS and both mother and infant ultimately died. In each of these cases, cardiac arrest likely ensued for at least 25 minutes prior to PMCS, which may have contributed to the ultimate outcomes.

The performance of PMCS in the out-of-hospital setting involves a number of challenges not encountered in the hospital. PMCS is not commonly part of a nurse or paramedic scope of practice and the absence of a physician as part of an EMS team will severely limit the ability to perform this procedure, regardless of maternal or fetal outcome [14]. Therefore, even when medical oversight is contacted, performance of PMCS is almost certainly outside the nursing or paramedic scope of practice. At least one case of PMCS performed by paramedics has been reported in the lay press, and the appropriateness of the providers in performing the procedure was brought into question [16]. It is important for EMS medical directors and EMS providers to review regulations from medical control boards and state licensing bodies in order to develop policies and procedures for how to manage this rare field presentation.

On the rare occasion that a physician is present, resources in the prehospital setting may still be limited. Following PMCS, lack of sufficient personnel to resuscitate two patients may result in the need to cease resuscitation efforts on the mother in order to focus on resuscitation of the newly delivered infant. Furthermore, due to the rare in-field presentation of a pregnant woman in cardiac arrest, an EMS physician may not have adequate experience or training in performance of a PMCS. In these cases, if transport can be completed within 5 minutes of maternal arrest, one may consider delaying the procedure in order to transport the patient to a facility with the appropriate obstetrical and neonatal resources to manage this emergency. Similarly, transport teams without practitioners who are licensed to perform this procedure should be dissuaded from performing PMCS in the prehospital setting, focusing on rapid transport with ongoing resuscitation of the mother.

Indications for perimortem cesarean section

Performance of PMCS within 4–5 minutes of maternal arrest beyond 20–24 weeks gestation is widely supported for the potential survival of both the infant and the mother [1–5,7,10,13,17]. The fundus can be identified 2 cm or 1 fingerbreadth above the umbilicus for every 2 weeks past 20 weeks and many experts recommend PMCS for any gestation that is 2 fingerbreadths above the umbilicus (24 weeks gestation). Other experts recommend that maternal resuscitation incorporate a determination of the likelihood of fetal viability by Doppler, audible fetal heart tones, or ultrasonography prior to the performance of PMCS [15,18–23]. However, the value of performing these assessments versus potential delays to the time-dependent PMCS has been debated. There have been cases reported in the literature with good fetal outcomes in spite of no fetal heart tones being audible [10]. Also, both ultrasonography and Doppler may be difficult to perform concurrently with CPR, and the fetus may be experiencing a period of bradycardia during resuscitation that complicates assessment of fetal heart rate. Therefore, authors have argued that time should not be spent looking for fetal viability, as it only wastes time to performance of the procedure, decreasing the likelihood that it will be successful in saving the mother or baby [2,3,10,13]. Furthermore, the American Heart Association recommends that PMCS be considered after the 20th week of gestation, or for any obviously gravid uterus that is deemed clinically to be sufficiently large to cause aortocaval compression [24].

The "4-minute rule" may be challenging to apply in the out-of-hospital setting, as the patient is likely to be in cardiac arrest for longer than 5 minutes at the time that appropriate resources and providers arrive on scene. PMCS should still be considered in these situations, as many neurologically intact infants have survived after more than 25 minutes of maternal death [1,6,25–27]. In these or other cases where the mother is determined to not be viable, in-field ultrasound may have its optimal role when considering PMCS solely for the infant [15].

Education

Considering that most EMS physicians will never have the opportunity to perform a PMCS in the field, the hesitancy to perform this potentially life-saving intervention could be partly overcome by special training and education. Special courses have been developed to train physicians in maternal resuscitation in cardiac arrest, including the performance of PMCS. These include the Advanced Life Support in Obstetrics (ALSO), Managing Obstetric Emergencies and Trauma (MOET), and Advances in Labour and Risk Management (ALARM) courses [7,11]. In a study of the management of cardiac arrest in pregnant women over a 15-year period in The Netherlands, there was an increase from 0.36 to 1.6 PMCS procedures per year following the introduction of the MOET course [1,11]. It is intuitive that without adequate training, physicians would lack the capability and willingness to perform this procedure, especially in the resource-limited prehospital setting. Performance of PMCS should therefore be incorporated in the training of all EMS physicians who may encounter the need to perform this procedure in the field.

Procedure

As soon as maternal cardiac arrest is identified, resuscitation should begin immediately. While tilting of the mother to the left during CPR has been described, manual leftward displacement of the uterus may be more effective in relieving aortocaval compression [28]. This necessitates one provider focusing on displacement of the uterus, a resource that may not be available in the limited environment of the field setting. Two EMS providers may alternate providing chest compressions with providing manual displacement of the uterus. Defibrillation should be performed for the appropriate rhythms at the same dosages as other adults (Class I, Level C evidence) [24].

The PMCS is a relatively simple procedure, which can be performed with limited equipment [3,10,17,23,29–31]. Once a decision has been made to perform a PMCS, the operator should proceed without delay. A suggested list of equipment to be used in the out-of-hospital setting is provided in Box 45.1. During the procedure, CPR of the mother should continue to increase chances of survival for both the mother and baby.

A generous vertical midline incision of the abdomen has been described most commonly as the preferred method to gain rapid access to the peritoneal cavity [3,10,13,17,21]. In the gravid woman, the linea nigra runs in the midline of the abdomen and serves as a guide for the incision. The incision should run from pubis to umbilicus and should be carried down through the fascial layers. If needed for access, the incision may be extended to the xiphoid. Alternately, a Pfannenstiel incision, which runs horizontally just above the pubic symphysis, could be performed [14,21,31]. The operator should select the incision he or she is most familiar with to facilitate a rapid intervention. Once in the

Box 45.1 Recommended equipment for an out-of-hospital perimortem cesarean section

Essential equipment

Scalpel with No. 10 blade
Toothed forceps
Bandage scissors
Bulb syringe
2 umbilical clamps
Towels
Suction device with suction catheter
Packing gauze

Optional equipment

Antiseptic solution
2 medium-sized Richardson retractors
Bladder retractor
Foley catheter
Needle driver
No. 0 or No. 1 delayed-absorbable (e.g. chromic) suture on a large needle

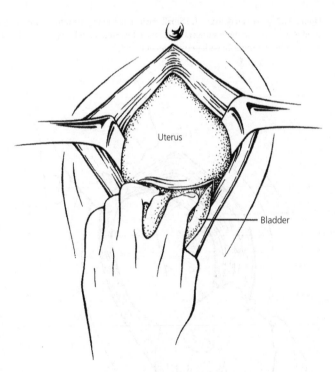

Figure 45.1 Cesarean delivery. Retraction of abdominal wall and displacement of bladder. Source: Roberts JR and Hedges JR. Emergency childbirth. In: *Clinical Procedures in Emergency Medicine*, 4th edn, p.1139. Reproduced with permission of Elsevier.

peritoneal cavity, two Richardson retractors may be used to provide access to the uterus and the bladder should be displaced caudally, either manually or with a bladder retractor (Figure 45.1). A distended bladder may be quickly drained with a Foley catheter. If time does not permit, a stab incision of the bladder can be made, which can be easily repaired if the mother is successfully resuscitated.

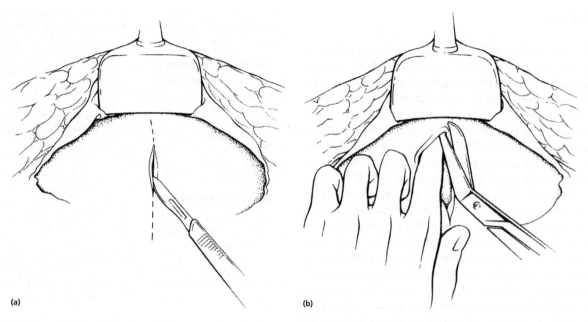

(a) (b)

Figure 45.2 Cesarean delivery. (a) Small vertical incision made into the lower uterine segment. (b) Bandage scissors are used to extend the incision toward the fundus while the operator's fingers shield the fetus. Source: Roberts JR and Hedges JR. Emergency childbirth. In: *Clinical Procedures in Emergency Medicine*, 4th edn, p.1139. Reproduced with permission of Elsevier.

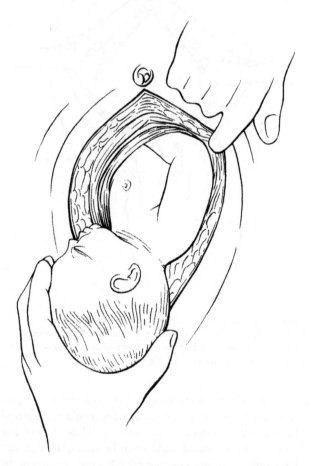

Figure 45.3 Cesarean delivery. Delivery of the infant from a vertex position. Source: Roberts JR and Hedges JR. Emergency childbirth. In: *Clinical Procedures in Emergency Medicine*, 4th edn, p.1139. Reproduced with permission of Elsevier.

Once the bladder has been retracted, a short vertical incision should be performed in the lower uterine segment, just cephalad to the bladder (Figure 45.2a). This incision is then extended cephalad using bandage scissors. The fingers of the operator's free hand should be placed inside the uterus to lift the uterine wall and protect the infant as the incision is extended (Figure 45.2b). The incision should be long enough to allow rapid delivery of the infant. If the placenta is embedded in the anterior wall of the uterus, it should be transected while entering the uterus. Though this may result in a significant amount of blood loss, it will facilitate the rapid delivery of the infant.

When the uterine incision is complete, all retractors should be removed to avoid injury to the baby. If the fetus is in a vertex position, the operator's hands should be inserted into the uterine cavity between the fetal head and the pubic symphysis, and the head and shoulders should be elevated out of the incision (Figure 45.3). If the fetus is in a breech or transverse presentation or if the uterine incision is too high to adequately access the head, a feet-first delivery may be easiest.

Once the infant is delivered, the mouth and nose should be suctioned with a bulb syringe and the cord clamped and cut while the infant is held at the level of the mother's abdomen. The child should be assessed, cleaned, and warmed immediately. Resuscitation should ensue as appropriate. The uterus should be palpated to evaluate for the possibility of twins and the placenta may be removed if resources and time allow. Packing or suturing the uterus closed will decrease bleeding if maternal circulation is restored. The uterus may be sutured with No. 0 or No. 1 delayed-absorbable sutures using a continuous locking one-layer closure. Direct pressure may also be applied to the mother's aorta, minimizing bleeding from the pelvic vessels and limiting the functional volume of the patient.

Ethical and legal considerations

The decision to perform a PMCS may invoke ethical and legal concerns. On one hand, there may be concern that the provider could be charged with battery for performing PMCS if consent is not obtained. On the other hand, failing to perform PMCS would result in near-certain death for the infant and mother. Since PMCS was described in 1986, no physician in the United States has been held liable for performing a PMCS, even when this was against the wishes of the mother's family [2,10,29]. However, at least two cases have been identified where a lawsuit was brought against physicians and hospital staff for failure to perform a PMCS [2]. Even if PMCS is successful, a concern may be that the provider may deliver an infant who will have persistent neurological deficits. However, a case review of PMCS over 25 years identified no reported cases where an infant surviving beyond the early neonatal period had neurological disability [9], and multiple neurologically intact infants have survived following PMCS after even prolonged maternal resuscitation [1,6,25–27]. In addition to considering the potential benefits to the infant, one must also consider the risks to the mother. In this case, there is no maternal risk, as withdrawal of support will certainly result in death of both mother and fetus [1].

Ultimately, peer-reviewed resuscitation guidelines may provide the simplest recourse for the EMS physician in deciding whether to perform a PMCS. The American Heart Association recommendation is for the performance of PMCS in any case of maternal cardiac arrest when the gestational age is ≥20 weeks, regardless of fetal viability [24]. This is recommended to be performed within 4 minutes of the onset of maternal cardiac arrest if there is no return of spontaneous circulation (Class IIb, Level C evidence), but may be considered sooner in cases of obvious non-survivable injury, when the maternal prognosis is grave, and the resuscitative efforts deemed futile [24].

The emotional impact of performing PMCS in the field must be considered, both for the provider who performs the procedure and the rest of the EMS team who contribute to the resuscitation of mother and infant. The effect on any family or friends on scene must also be considered. Procedures should be in place to provide critical incident stress management to EMS personnel within 24 hours, with individual follow-up care determined on an individual basis [14]. Community resources may be sought to assist family members as well.

Conclusion

The out-of-hospital management of cardiac arrest in a pregnant patient is a rare and challenging event. Performance of perimortem cesarean section within 4 minutes and delivery within 5 minutes in pregnant patients beyond 20–24 weeks gestation are recommended to provide the highest likelihood of survival for both baby and mother. EMS physicians should be trained in performance of this procedure as they are most likely to be capable to perform it in the field. EMS systems should have established policies and procedures for this challenging situation and take into account state and local scope of practice for prehospital providers.

References

1 Fadel HE. Postmortem and perimortem cesarean section: historical, religious and ethical considerations. *J IMA* 2011;43:194–200.

2 Katz VL. Perimortem cesarean delivery: its role in maternal mortality. *Semin Perinatol* 2012;36:68–72.

3 Lanoix R, Akkapeddi V, Goldfeder B. Perimortem cesarean section: case reports and recommendations. *Acad Emerg Med* 1995;2:1063–7.

4 Katz V, Balderston K, DeFreest M. Perimortem cesarean delivery: were our assumptions correct? *Am J Obstet Gynecol* 2005;192:1916–20.

5 Katz VL, Dotters DJ, Droegemueller W. Perimortem cesarean delivery. *Obstet Gynecol* 1986;68:571–6.

6 Guven S, Yazar A, Yakut K, Aydogan H, Erguven M, Avci E. Postmortem cesarean: report of our successful neonatal outcomes after severe trauma during pregnancy and review of the literature. *J Matern Fetal Neonat Med* 2012;25:1102–4.

7 Engels PT, Caddy SC, Jiwa G, Douglas Matheson J. Cardiac arrest in pregnancy and perimortem cesarean delivery: case report and discussion. *CJEM* 2011;13:399–403.

8 Cardosi RJ, Porter KB. Cesarean delivery of twins during maternal cardiopulmonary arrest. *Obstet Gynecol* 1998;92:695–7.

9 Whitten M, Irvine LM. Postmortem and perimortem caesarean section: what are the indications? *J R Soc Med* 2000;93:6–9.

10 Page-Rodriguez A, Gonzalez-Sanchez JA. Perimortem cesarean section of twin pregnancy: case report and review of the literature. *Acad Emerg Med* 1999;6:1072–4.

11 Dijkman A, Huisman CM, Smit M, et al. Cardiac arrest in pregnancy: increasing use of perimortem caesarean section due to emergency skills training? *BJOG* 2010;117:282–7.

12 Einav S, Kaufman N, Sela HY. Maternal cardiac arrest and perimortem caesarean delivery: evidence or expert-based? *Resuscitation* 2012;83:1191–200.

13 Kupas DF, Harter SC, Vosk A. Out-of-hospital perimortem cesarean section. *Prehosp Emerg Care* 1998;2:206–8.

14 Bowers W, Wagner C. Field perimortem cesarean section. *Air Med J* 2001;20:10–1.

15 Kue R, Coyle C, Vaughan E, Restuccia M. Perimortem Cesarean section in the helicopter EMS setting: a case report. *Air Med J* 2008;27:46–7.

16 Chen DW. 2 Paramedics Face Inquiry Over Surgery in Emergency. *New York Times*, 1997. Available at: www.nytimes.com/1997/09/27/nyregion/2-paramedics-face-inquiry-over-surgery-in-emergency.html

17 Hauswald M, Kerr NL. Perimortem cesarean section. *Acad Emerg Med* 2000;7:726.

18 Brun PM, Chenaitia H, Dejesus I, Bessereau J, Bonello L, Pierre B. Ultrasound to perimortem caesarean delivery in prehospital settings. *Injury* 2013;44:151–2.

19 Gunevsel O, Yesil O, Ozturk TC, Cevik SE. Perimortem caesarean section following maternal gunshot wounds. *J Res Med Sci* 2011;16:1089–91.

20 Knobloch K. Re: Perimortem Cesarean section in the helicopter EMS setting. *Air Med J* 2008;27:152–3.

21 McDonnell NJ. Cardiopulmonary arrest in pregnancy: two case reports of successful outcomes in association with perimortem Caesarean delivery. *Br J Anaesth* 2009;103:406–9.

22 Morris JA Jr, Rosenbower TJ, Jurkovich GJ, et al. Infant survival after cesarean section for trauma. *Ann Surg* 1996;223:481–8.

23 Phelan HA, Roller J, Minei JP. Perimortem cesarean section after utilization of surgeon-performed trauma ultrasound. *J Trauma* 2008;64:E12–14.

24 Vanden Hoek TL, Morrison LJ, Shuster M, et al. Part 12: cardiac arrest in special situations: 2010 American Heart Association Guidelines for Cardiopulmonary Resuscitation and Emergency Cardiovascular Care. *Circulation* 2010;122:S829–61.

25 Awwad JT, Azar GB, Aouad AT, Raad J, Karam KS. Postmortem cesarean section following maternal blast injury: case report. *J Trauma* 1994;36:260–1.

26 Capobianco G, Balata A, Mannazzu MC, et al. Perimortem cesarean delivery 30 minutes after a laboring patient jumped from a fourth-floor window: baby survives and is normal at age 4 years. *Am J Obstet Gynecol* 2008;198:e15–16.

27 Lopez-Zeno JA, Carlo WA, O'Grady JP, Fanaroff AA. Infant survival following delayed postmortem cesarean delivery. *Obstet Gynecol* 1990;76:991–2.

28 Jeejeebhoy FM, Zelop CM, Windrim R, Carvalho JC, Dorian P, Morrison LJ. Management of cardiac arrest in pregnancy: a systematic review. *Resuscitation* 2011;82:801–9.

29 Strong TH Jr, Lowe RA. Perimortem cesarean section. *Am J Emerg Med* 1989;7:489–94.

30 Doan-Wiggins L. Emergency childbirth. In: Roberts JR, Hedges JR (eds) *Clinical Procedures in Emergency Medicine*, 4thedn.Philadelphia: W.B. Saunders, 2004, pp.1117–43.

31 Cunningham FG, Leveno KJ, Bloom SL, Spong CY, Dashe JS. Cesarean delivery and peripartum hysterectomy. In: Cunningham FG, Leveno KJ, Bloom SL, Spong CY, Dashe JS (eds) *Williams Obstetrics*, 23rd edn. New York: McGraw-Hill Medical, 2010, pp.549–55.

Toxicological Problems

CHAPTER 46
Principles of toxicology

Christine M. Murphy

Introduction

Emergency personnel commonly encounter toxicological emergencies from accidental exposures (e.g. workplace incidents or drug interactions) or intentional exposures (e.g. drug abuse or suicide attempts). In 2011, over 2.3 million human toxin exposures were reported to the American Association of Poison Control Centers [1]. More than 93% of exposures were reported from residences, with routes of exposure by ingestion (83%), through the skin (7%), inhalation (6%), and through the eye (4%). Eighty percent of exposures were unintentional and 62% involved patients under the age of 20 years.

The outcome following a poisoning depends on numerous factors, including dose taken, time to first medical contact, and the patient's preexisting health status. Poisonings recognized early and treated quickly often do well. The case fatality rate for self-poisonings in the modern health care setting is approximately 0.5%; however, in the developing world it is 10–20% [2]. Therefore, it is imperative that EMS personnel understand the basic management of the poisoned patient.

Evaluation

When evaluating a patient with a potential toxicological emergency, it is important to maintain a broad differential diagnosis [3]. A comatose patient who smells of alcohol may be harboring an intracranial hemorrhage; an agitated patient who appears anticholinergic may actually be encephalopathic from an infectious etiology. Patients must be thoroughly assessed and appropriately stabilized. There is often no specific antidote or treatment for a poisoned patient and supportive care is the most important intervention.

History

Emergency medical services personnel should gather as much information as possible about the type of toxin(s) to which the patient was exposed. Poisoned patients are commonly unreliable historians, particularly if suicidal or presenting with altered mental status [4]. If information cannot be obtained from the patient, it is beneficial to obtain information from others at the scene, such as family and friends. Bottles of possibly ingested substance or pills, even if not in the original containers, can assist hospital personnel and poison centers. Other helpful information includes the time of exposure (acute versus chronic), amount taken, route of exposure (e.g. ingestion, IV, inhalation, or dermal), reason for the exposure (e.g. accidental, suicide attempt, or abuse), other medicines routinely taken by the patient (including prescription, over the counter, vitamins, alternative medical preparations), and suicide note, if available. With any unknown exposure, a list of all medications in the home should be obtained, including those of current visitors to the home. This is especially important in an unknown pediatric exposure.

Physical examination

In the emergency setting, patient stabilization takes precedence over a meticulous physical examination. However, a rapid directed examination can yield important diagnostic clues. Once the patient is stable, a more comprehensive physical examination can reveal additional signs suggesting a specific poison/exposure. Additionally, a dynamic change in clinical appearance over time may be a more important clue than findings on the initial examination. Taking note of odors emanating from the patient or the environment can provide valuable information. Some poisons produce odors characteristic enough to suggest the diagnosis upon first encounter (Table 46.1). A complete set of vital signs can further assist the provider in narrowing the differential diagnosis [5]. The skin should be carefully examined by removing patient clothes and assessing for color, temperature, and the presence of dryness or diaphoresis. Absence of diaphoresis is an important clinical distinction between anticholinergic and sympathomimetic poisoning. The presence of bites or similar marks may suggest spider or snake envenomations. The presence of erythema or bullae over pressure points may suggest rhabdomyolysis in the comatose patient, while

Emergency Medical Services: Clinical Practice and Systems Oversight, Second Edition. Volume 1: Clinical Aspects of EMS.
Edited by David C. Cone, Jane H. Brice, Theodore R. Delbridge, and J. Brent Myers.
© 2015 NAEMSP. Published 2015 by John Wiley & Sons, Inc. Companion Website: www.wiley.com\go\cone\naemsp

Table 46.1 Odors that suggest a toxicological exposure

Odor	Possible source
Bitter almonds	Cyanide
Fruity	Isopropanol, acetone
Garlic	Organophosphates
Gasoline	Petroleum distillates
Mothballs	Naphthalene, camphor
Pears	Chloral hydrate
Minty	Methylsalicylate
Rotten eggs	Hydrogen sulfide
Freshly mowed hay	Phosgene

Table 46.2 Examples of diverse classes of agents that can potentially cause seizures

Category	Examples of specific agents
Analgesics	Meperidine, propoxyphene, tramadol
Antihistamines	Diphenhydramine
Antimicrobials	Isoniazid, penicillin
Botanicals	False morel mushrooms, tobacco, water hemlock
Drugs of abuse	Amphetamines, cocaine, phencyclidine
Inhalants	Carbon monoxide, chlorinated hydrocarbons
Methylxanthines	Caffeine, theophylline
Psychiatric medications	Bupropion, cyclic antidepressants, venlafaxine
Pesticides	Lindane, organophosphates
Withdrawal	Antiepileptic medications, ethanol, sedative hypnotics

Table 46.3 Examples of potential toxins associated with miosis or mydriasis

Miosis	Mydriasis
Antipsychotic agents	Anticholinergics
Carbamates	Sympathomimetics
Clonidine	Selective serotonin reuptake inhibitors
Opiates	Withdrawal syndromes
Organophosphates	
Sedative-hypnotics	

track marks suggest IV or subcutaneous drug abuse. Finally, a systematic neurological evaluation is important, particularly with patients exhibiting altered mental status. While the Glasgow Coma Scale (GCS) is useful for evaluating trauma victims, it has little role in predicting the prognosis of the poisoned patient [6].

Seizures are a common presentation of an unknown overdose, and the list of toxins that can induce a convulsion is lengthy (Table 46.2). Ocular findings helpful in narrowing the differential diagnosis include miosis and mydriasis (Table 46.3). Other useful general neurological signs include fasciculations (from organophosphate poisoning), rigidity (tetanus and strychnine), tremors (lithium and theophylline), and dystonic posturing (neuroleptic agents).

Toxidromes

A toxidrome is a toxic syndrome or constellation of signs and symptoms associated with a certain class of poisons. Rapid recognition of a toxidrome can determine the class or, in some cases, the specific poison responsible for a patient's condition. Table 46.4 lists characteristics of selected toxidromes. It is important to note that patients may not present with every component of a toxidrome and that toxidromes are difficult to identify in mixed ingestions.

Certain aspects of a toxidrome can have great significance. For example, noting dry axilla may differentiate an anticholinergic patient from a sympathomimetic patient, and miosis may distinguish opioid toxicity from a benzodiazepine overdose. There are notable exceptions to the recognized toxidromes. For example, several opioid agents (meperidine, propoxyphene, and tramadol) are not always associated with miosis. In most cases, a toxidrome will not indicate a specific poison but rather a class of poisons. Several poisons have unique presentations that make their presence virtually diagnostic. For example, clonidine is associated with sedation, miosis, bradycardia, shallow respirations, and hypotension, yet the patient will become alert with stimulation and then drift rapidly back to sedation with no stimulation.

Cardiac monitor and electrocardiogram

Electrocardiogram interpretation of in the poisoned patient can be challenging. Numerous drugs can cause ECG changes. The incidence of ECG changes in the poisoned patient is unclear, and the significance of various changes may be difficult to define [7]. Despite the fact that drugs have widely varying indications for therapeutic use, many unrelated drugs share common electrocardiographic effects if taken in overdose. Toxins can be placed into broad classes based on their cardiac effects. Agents that block the cardiac fast sodium channels and agents that block cardiac potassium efflux channels cause characteristic ECG changes, QRS prolongation, and QT prolongation, respectively. The recognition of specific ECG changes associated with other clinical data (toxidromes) can be potentially life saving [8].

The ability of drugs to induce cardiac sodium channel blockade prolonging the QRS complex has been well described in the literature [9]. Cardiac voltage-gated sodium channels reside in the cell membrane and open in conjunction with cell depolarization. Sodium channel blockers bind to the transmembrane sodium channels, decreasing the number available for depolarization. This creates a delay of sodium entry into the cardiac myocyte during phase 0 of depolarization. As a result, the upslope of depolarization is slowed and the QRS complex widens [10]. In some cases, the QRS complex may take the pattern of recognized bundle branch blocks [11,12]. With tricyclic antidepressant poisoning, rightward axis deviation of the terminal 40 msec of the QRS axis can be present, in addition to QRS widening [13,14]. In the most severe cases, QRS

Table 46.4 Toxidromes

Toxidrome	Signs and symptoms	Potential agent example
Opioid	Sedation, miosis, decreased bowel sounds, decreased respirations	Codeine, fentanyl, heroin, hydrocodone, methadone, morphine, oxycodone
Anticholinergic	Mydriasis, dry skin, dry mucous membranes, decreased bowel sounds, sedation, altered mental status, hallucinations, urinary retention	Atropine, antihistamines, cyclic antidepressants, cyclobenzaprine, phenothiazines, scopolamine
Sedative hypnotic	Sedation, decreased respirations, normal pupils, normal vital signs	Benzodiazepines, barbiturates, zolpidem
Sympathomimetic	Agitation, mydriasis, tachycardia, hypertension, hyperthermia, diaphoresis	Amphetamines, cocaine, ephedrine, phencyclidine, pseudoephedrine
Cholinergic	Miosis, lacrimation, diaphoresis, bronchospasm, bronchorrhea, vomiting, diarrhea, bradycardia	Organophosphates, carbamates, nerve agents
Serotonin toxicity	Altered mental status, tachycardia, hypertension, hyperreflexia, clonus, hyperthermia	Overdose of serotonergic agents alone or in combination (i.e. selective serotonin reuptake inhibitors, dextromethorphan, meperidine)

prolongation becomes so profound that it is difficult to distinguish between ventricular and supraventricular rhythms [15,16]. Continued QRS prolongation may result in a *sine wave* pattern and eventual asystole. It has been theorized that the sodium channel blockers cause slowed intraventricular conduction, unidirectional block, the development of a reentrant circuit, and a resulting ventricular tachycardia [17]. This can then degenerate into ventricular fibrillation. Differentiating a QRS prolongation due to sodium channel blockade in the poisoned patient versus other non-toxic etiologies can be difficult.

Drugs blocking myocardial sodium channels comprise a diverse group of pharmaceutical agents (Box 46.1). Patients poisoned with these agents have varied clinical presentations. For example, sodium channel-blocking medications such as diphenhydramine, propoxyphene, and cocaine may also develop anticholinergic, opioid, and sympathomimetic syndromes, respectively [18–20]. In addition, specific drugs may affect not only the myocardial sodium channels but also calcium influx and potassium efflux channels, resulting in ECG changes and rhythm disturbances not related entirely to the drug's sodium channel-blocking activity [21,22]. All the agents listed in Box 46.1 induce myocardial sodium channel blockade and may respond to therapy with sodium bicarbonate or hypertonic saline. Displacement of the sodium channel-blocking agents by hypertonic saline or sodium bicarbonate can improve inotropy and prevent arrhythmias.[9] It is therefore reasonable to treat poisoned patients with prolonged QRS intervals, particularly those with hemodynamic instability, empirically with 1–2 mEq/kg of sodium bicarbonate (the gold standard for treatment of sodium channel blockade). Shortening of the QRS can confirm the presence of a sodium channel-blocking agent.

Approximately 3% of all non-cardiac prescriptions are associated with the potential for QT prolongation [23]. Myocardial repolarization is driven predominantly by outward movement of potassium ions [24]. Blockade of the outward potassium currents prolongs the action potential [25]. This subsequently results in QT interval prolongation and the potential emergence

---

Box 46.1 Sodium channel-blocking drugs

Amantadine	Diphenhydramine
Carbemazepine	Hydroxychloroquine
Chloroquine	Loxapine
Class IA antiarrhythmics	Orphenadrine
Disopyramide	Phenothiazines
Quinidine	Propranolol
Procainamide	Propoxyphene
Class IC antiarrhythmics	Quinine
Flecainide	Verapamil
Propafenone	
Citalopram	
Cocaine	
Cyclic antidepressants	

---

of T- or U-wave abnormalities on the ECG [26]. The prolongation of repolarization causes the myocardial cell to have less charge difference across its membrane, which may result in the activation of the inward depolarization current (early afterdepolarization) and promote triggered activity. These changes may lead to reentry and subsequent polymorphic ventricular tachycardia (VT), most often as the torsades de pointes variant of polymorphic VT [27]. QT prolongation is considered to occur when the QTc interval is greater than 440 msec in men and 460 msec in women, with arrhythmias most commonly associated with values greater than 500 msec. However, the potential for an arrhythmia for a given QT interval will vary from drug to drug and patient to patient [24]. Drugs associated with QT prolongation are listed in Box 46.2 [28]. Management of QT prolongation includes infusion of magnesium and possibly calcium to prevent the development of polymorphic VT.

There are many agents that can induce human cardiotoxicity, and the resultant ECG changes range from bradycardia (e.g. calcium channel blocker and beta-blocker toxicity) to tachycardia (e.g. sympathomimetics and anticholinergics). EMS personnel managing patients who have taken medication overdoses should be aware of the various ECG changes that can potentially occur.

QT pwlong.

Box 46.2	Drugs that block efflux from potassium channels

Antihistamines	Class III antiarrhythmics
Diphenhydramine	Amiodarone
Loratadine	Dofetilide
Antipsychotics	Ibutilide
Chlorpromazine	Sotalol
Droperidol	Cyclic antidepressants
Haloperidol	Erythromycin
Pimozide	Fluoroquinolones
Quetiapine	Hydroxychloroquine
Risperidone	Methadone
Thioridazine	Pentamidine
Ziprasidone	Quinine
Arsenic trioxide	Tacrolimus
Chloroquine	Venlafaxine
Cisapride	
Citalopram	
Clarithromycin	
Class IA antiarrhythmics	
Disopyramide	
Quinidine	
Procainamide	

Treatment

All patients presenting with potential toxic exposures should be aggressively managed, as the majority of outcomes are good. Airway patency and adequate ventilation should be ensured. If necessary, endotracheal intubation should be performed. Too often, EMS personnel are lulled into a false sense of security by adequate oxygen saturations on high-flow oxygen. A poor gag reflex or inadequate ventilation may increase risk for subsequent aspiration or carbon dioxide retention with worsening acidosis. Intravenous access is generally recommended for poisoned patients, and hypotension should initially be treated with IV fluids. The patient's pulmonary status should be closely monitored for the development of pulmonary edema as fluids are infused. Continuous cardiac monitoring, pulse oximetry, and frequent neurological checks should be documented, noting any changes over time. Glucose should be checked in all patients with altered mental status. EMS personnel must have a low threshold for suspecting carbon monoxide exposure in altered mental status patients. Carbon monoxide is a relatively common, potentially deadly, and easily missed poisoning. Carbon monoxide levels should be measured as early as feasible because these levels can diminish greatly during transport, especially when supplemental oxygen is administered.

Many toxins can also cause seizures. In general, toxin-induced seizures are treated similarly to epileptic seizures. EMS personnel should ensure a patent airway and measure blood glucose. Most toxin-induced seizures are self-limited. However, for seizures requiring treatment, the first-line agent should be parenteral benzodiazepines for all poisonings. The use of long-acting paralytic agents should be avoided in intubated poisoned patients because these agents may mask seizures.

After initial evaluation and stabilization, toxin-specific therapies should be initiated, and decontamination should be considered. Several poisons have specific antidotes which can be of great benefit if used in a timely and appropriate manner (see Volume 1, Chapter 47).

Decontaminating the poisoned patient

External decontamination may be necessary for poisoning by dermal or ocular exposure. Additionally, 83% of poisonings occur by ingestion, which has prompted studies examining the use of gastrointestinal decontamination, which may be required, in the prehospital setting [1].

Dermal decontamination

Patients with dermal contamination pose a potential risk of secondary exposure to health care personnel. Decontamination should occur before EMS transport. Personnel conducting dermal decontamination should don personal protective equipment (PPE) appropriate for the contaminating agent. Gas or vapor exposure does not require decontamination (the exception being a need for ocular decontamination in some cases); removal from the site should be sufficient. Potential off-gassing can be avoided by removing and sealing contaminated clothing in a plastic bag [29]. Exposure to liquids or solids requires dermal decontamination [29]. Proceeding from head to toe, brush all solids off the patient's skin and clothing, irrigate the exposed skin and hair for 10–15 minutes with water or saline, and scrub with a soft surgical sponge, being careful not to abrade the skin. Patient privacy should be respected if possible, and warm water should be used to avoid hypothermia [29]. Irrigate all wounds for an additional 5–10 minutes. Stiff brushes and abrasives should be avoided because they enhance dermal absorption of the toxin and can produce skin lesions that may be mistaken for chemical injuries. Sponges and disposable towels are effective alternatives.

Ocular decontamination

When required, ocular decontamination should be performed immediately by gentle irrigation of the affected eye(s) and contiguous skin [30]. Ocular irrigation with sterile normal saline or lactated Ringer's solution should continue for at least 15–30 minutes [31]. Tap water is acceptable if that is the only solution available. However, due to its hypotonicity relative to the stroma, tap water may facilitate penetration of corrosive substances into the cornea and potentially worsen outcome [30,32]. Lactated Ringer's solution may be a preferable irrigant due to its buffering capacity and neutral pH [30,32]. Irrigation should be directed away from the medial canthus to avoid forcing contaminants into the lacrimal duct. Longer irrigation times may be needed with specific substances and the endpoint of irrigation should be normalization of the eye's pH. Because pH paper is not typically carried by EMS units (although it may be available on hazardous materials units), continuing irrigation during transport is frequently required.

Gastrointestinal decontamination

Significant controversy exists concerning the need for routine gastric decontamination in the poisoned patient, and gastric lavage is no longer recommended. Gastric decontamination may be considered in select cases and specific scenarios, but in general, the prehospital care provider should focus on rapid transportation of the poisoned patient to the hospital. Before performing any gastrointestinal decontamination techniques, including the oral administration of activated charcoal, EMS personnel must clearly understand the hazards of these procedures. Personnel must carefully weigh the risks and benefits prior to making any decisions about the use of gastrointestinal decontamination. Contacting the local poison center (i.e. US poison centers at 1-800-222-1222) can guide decisions to pursue gastric decontamination.

Syrup of ipecac, previously a mainstay of poisoning management, is no longer recommended in the management of poisoning [33–35]. Emesis, either by mechanical stimulation (i.e. placing a finger down the throat) or by use of syrup of ipecac, should be avoided. The prehospital use of activated charcoal is currently controversial, and it is premature to recommend the administration of activated charcoal by EMS personnel without poison center guidance [34]. Activated charcoal is given orally to prevent gastrointestinal absorption of an ingested substance. The administration of charcoal is contraindicated in any person who demonstrates compromised airway protective reflexes unless he or she is intubated [36]. Intubation will reduce the risk of charcoal aspiration but will not totally eliminate its occurrence [37]. Charcoal is also contraindicated in persons who have ingested corrosive substances (acids or alkalis). Charcoal not only provides no benefit in corrosive ingestions, but its administration could precipitate vomiting, obscure endoscopic visualization, or lead to complications if a perforation develops and charcoal enters the mediastinum, peritoneum, or pleural space. Charcoal should be avoided in cases of pure aliphatic petroleum distillate ingestion. Hydrocarbons are not well adsorbed by activated charcoal, and its administration could lead to further aspiration risk. Other commonly encountered substances that do not readily bind to charcoal include lithium, solvents, most metals (iron, lead), potassium chloride, sodium chloride, fluoride, cyanide, and alcohols (to include ethylene glycol, methanol, diethylene glycol).

Antidotes

The number of pharmacological antagonists or antidotes that EMS personnel may have access to in prehospital management is quite limited. There are few agents that will rapidly reverse toxic effects and restore a patient to a previously healthy baseline state. Administering some pharmacological antagonists actually may worsen patient outcome compared with simply optimizing basic supportive care. As a result,

Table 46.5 Antidotes

Agent or clinical finding	Antidote
Acetaminophen	N-acetylcysteine
Benzodiazepines	Flumazenil*
Beta-blockers	Glucagon
Cardiac glycosides	Digoxin immune Fab
Crotalid envenomation	Crotalidae polyvalent immune Fab
Cyanide	Sodium thiosulfate*
	Sodium nitrite
	Hydroxycobalamin*
Ethylene glycol	Fomepizole
Iron	Deferoxamine
Isoniazid	Pyridoxine
Methanol	Fomepizole
Methemoglobinemia	Methylene blue
Opioids	Naloxone*
Organophosphates	Atropine*
	Pralidoxime*
Sulfonylureas	Glucose*
	Octreotide

*Antidotes that may be available to EMS personnel.

antidotes should be used cautiously and with clearly understood indications and contraindications. Table 46.5 gives a list of potential antidotes available to EMS providers. Many antidotes are covered in Chapter 47 but two specific antidotes will be discussed here.

Flumazenil

Benzodiazepines are involved in many intentional overdoses. Although these overdoses are rarely fatal when a benzodiazepine is the sole ingestant, they often complicate overdoses with other central nervous system depressants (e.g. ethanol, opioids, and other sedatives) due to their synergistic activity. Flumazenil should *not* be administered as a non-specific coma reversal drug and should be used with extreme caution after intentional benzodiazepine overdose because it has the potential to precipitate withdrawal in benzodiazepine-dependent individuals and/or induce seizures in those at risk [38,39]. The initial flumazenil dose is 0.2 mg administered intravenously over 30 seconds. If no response occurs after an additional 30 seconds, a second dose is recommended. Additional incremental doses of 0.5 mg may be administered at 1-minute intervals until the desired response is noted or until a total of 3 mg has been administered. At present, flumazenil is very rarely used in the out-of-hospital setting.

Naloxone

Opioid poisoning from the abuse of morphine derivatives or synthetic narcotic agents may be reversed with the opioid antagonist naloxone [40]. Naloxone is commonly used in comatose patients as a therapeutic and diagnostic agent. The standard dosage regimen is to administer from 0.4 to 2 mg slowly, preferably intravenously. The IV dose should be readministered at 5-minute intervals until the desired endpoint is achieved – restoration of respiratory function, ability to protect airway, and an improved level of consciousness [41]. If the IV route of administration is not viable, alternative routes include intramuscular injection, intraosseous, intranasal, or via nebulization [41]. Intramuscular administration is an accepted alternative route but if the patient is hypotensive, naloxone may not be absorbed rapidly from the intramuscular injection site. Intransal and intramuscular naloxone have been distributed to bystanders for use in heroin and opioid overdose situations [42–44]. The onset of action is longer with the intranasal form than the IV form (8–12 minutes versus 6–8 minutes), but similar to that of intramuscular naloxone [45,46]. One study suggests intranasal naloxone may induce a gentler reversal with less agitation compared to IV naloxone [45]. Early reports suggest an increased need for redosing with intranasal delivery but it is not clear if this is truly needed or a provider response to the longer onset of action [46]. There are no published data on the optimal dose of intranasal naloxone, but in studies investigating intranasal naloxone delivery a 2 mg dose is frequently used and 1 mg is delivered in each nostril [42,47,48]. The cost of the mucosal atomization device that allows for intranasal drug delivery is prohibitive in many areas of the US and worldwide [42,49]. There is ongoing research on both intramuscular and intranasal naloxone in the prehospital setting for both bystanders and EMS providers.

A patient may not respond to naloxone administration for a variety of reasons: insufficient dose of naloxone, the absence of an opioid exposure, a mixed overdose with other central nervous and respiratory system depressants, or medical or traumatic reasons. When it does reverse opioid intoxication, naloxone can precipitate profound withdrawal symptoms in opioid-dependent patients. Symptoms of withdrawal include agitation, vomiting, diarrhea, piloerection, diaphoresis, and yawning [41]. There are reports of patients developing noncardiogenic pulmonary edema in response to naloxone and as an effect of opioid intoxication itself without a clear understanding of the mechanisms behind this. Providers should use care in administering this agent, and only give the amount that is necessary to restore adequate respiration and airway protection.

Special considerations: caustic exposures

Acids and bases are routinely grouped into a more general category called caustics. In most cases, the concentration of the product, duration of exposure/contact time, and route of exposure (ingestion, inhalation, dermal, ocular) determine the extent of injury suffered by an exposed patient.

Traditionally, acids and bases have been associated with different injury patterns. *Liquefactive necrosis* is a term often used to describe the type of tissue damage encountered with caustics that are characterized as "bases" [50,51]. Bases can deeply penetrate the tissue, causing fat saponification, protein disso-

lution, and emulsification of cell membranes. *Coagulation necrosis* is the type of injury associated with caustics characterized as "acids." With coagulation necrosis, tissues become erythematous and ulcerated, mucous membranes slough, and eschars can form which theoretically prevent deeper penetration of the acid [50,51]. While these injury patterns apply to most caustics classified as acids or bases, there are exceptions to the rule.

One of these frequently encountered exceptions is hydrofluoric acid. Found in wheel cleaners and glass etching creams, hydrofluoric acid is considered an acid but rarely causes visible tissue damage. Instead, it penetrates the tissues and binds to intracellular calcium and magnesium, leaching them out of the cells, depleting the cells of these ions, and causing significant pain [52,53]. Patients exposed to this compound develop hyperkalemia, hypocalcemia, and hypomagnesemia, which can result in cardiac dysrhythmias and death. Thorough decontamination of the skin and eyes is necessary for any possible exposures. Antacids containing calcium and magnesium can be given orally in an effort to bind the fluoride molecule of the ingested hydrofluoric acid early, but this should not be done without poison center involvement, especially if multiple agents are ingested [54]. Additionally, treatment consists of aggressive IV electrolyte repletion and cardiac monitoring.

Once the patient has been removed from any caustic exposure source, stabilization of the airway, breathing, and circulation remains the initial priority. Stridor or drooling may indicate airway involvement/impending airway compromise, and EMS providers should pay close attention to these patients. The presence or absence of oral lesions does not provide an accurate indication of whether or not significant ingestion has occurred [55]. Decontamination at the scene is preferred if possible to prevent continued injury. The type of decontamination will depend on the route of exposure. The same principles of decontamination previously discussed can be used – for example, if the patient has been exposed to sodium hydroxide crystals, brushing the solid crystals off prior to removing clothing and washing the skin is necessary. For exposures involving inhalation and vapor exposure, removing the patient from the source and flushing the eyes is important. There are a few instances where dilutional therapy with milk or water may be recommended by the poison center [56–60]. This may be recommended prior to EMS arrival and has better results when performed within minutes of ingestion, but should not be attempted without poison center recommendation. Basic wound care dressings can be applied to injured skin after the wound has been decontaminated with water or normal saline.

Protocols

The development of specific protocols for treating each individual type of poisoning is unrealistic due to the vast number of potential toxins. It is also impractical to have one protocol that could easily pertain to all cases of poisoning. It may be necessary to construct protocols for the different problems that require different treatments in the field (e.g. suspected opioid intoxication, carbon monoxide toxicity, and chemical dermal contamination). Integral to these protocols is an outline of the relevant history and physical findings that guide the provider to appropriate generalized management of the intoxicated patient. In addition, each protocol should contain the toll-free national poison center number (1-800-222-1222) where the EMS provider can obtain guidance 24/7 from experts in the field of medical toxicology.

Conclusion

Emergency medical services providers are often required to care for poisoned patients. Many of these patients do well with standard medical management and never develop significant toxicity. However, for patients who present with serious toxic effects or after potentially fatal exposures, prompt action must be taken. As many poisons have no true antidote and the poison involved may initially be unknown, the first step is good supportive care. Attention to supportive care, vital signs, and prevention of complications are the most important steps. Taking care of these issues will often be all that is necessary to ensure recovery.

Acknowledgment

Christopher P. Holstege and David Lawrence contributed to this chapter in the previous edition.

References

1 Bronstein AC, Spyker DA, Cantilena LR Jr, Rumack BH, Dart RC. 2011 Annual Report of the American Association of Poison Control Centers' National Poison Data System (NPDS). *Clin Toxicol* 2012;50: 911–1164.

2 Eddleston M, Haggalla S, Reginald K, et al. The hazards of gastric lavage for intentional self-poisoning in a resource poor location. *Clin Toxicol* 2007;45:136–43.

3 Lawrence DT, Bechtel L, Walsh JP, Holstege CD. The evaluation and management of acute poisoning emergencies. *Minerva Med* 2007;98:543–68.

4 Taylor RL, Cohan SL, White JD. Comprehensive toxicology screening in the emergency department: an aid to clinical diagnosis. *Am J Emerg Med* 1985;3:507 11

5 Erickson TB, Thompson TM, Lu JJ. The approach to the patient with an unknown overdose. *Emerg Med Clin North Am* 2007;25:249–81.

6 Merigian KS, Hedges JR, Roberts JR, Childress RA, Niehaus MA, Franklin N. Use of abbreviated mental status examination in the initial assessment of overdose patients. *Arch Emerg Med* 1988;5: 139–45.

7 Delk C, Holstege CP, Brady WJ. Electrocardiographic abnormalities associated with poisoning. *Am J Emerg Med* 2007;25:672–87.

8 Holstege C, Baer A, Brady WJ. The electrocardiographic toxidrome: the ECG presentation of hydrofluoric acid ingestion. *Am J Emerg Med* 2005;23:171–6.

9 Kolecki PF, Curry SC. Poisoning by sodium channel blocking agents. *Crit Care Clin* 1997;13:829–48.

10 Harrigan RA, Brady WJ. ECG abnormalities in tricyclic antidepressant ingestion. *Am J Emerg Med* 1999;17:387–93.

11 Heaney RM. Left bundle branch block associated with propoxyphene hydrochloride poisoning. *Ann Emerg Med* 1983;12: 780–2.

12 Fernandez-Quero L, Riesgo MJ, Agusti S, Cidoncha B. Left anterior hemiblock, complete right bundle branch block and sinus tachycardia in maprotiline poisoning. *Intensive Care Med* 1985;11:220–2.

13 Wolfe TR, Caravati EM, Rollins DE. Terminal 40-ms frontal plane QRS axis as a marker for tricyclic antidepressant overdose. *Ann Emerg Med* 1989;18:348–51.

14 Berkovitch M, Matsui D, Fogelman R, Komar L, Hamilton R, Johnson D. Assessment of the terminal 40-millisecond QRS vector in children with a history of tricyclic antidepressant ingestion. *Pediatr Emerg Care* 1995;11:75–7.

15 Brady WJ, Skiles J. Wide QRS complex tachycardia: ECG differential diagnosis. *Am J Emerg Med* 1999;17:376–81.

16 Clark RF, Vance MV. Massive diphenhydramine poisoning resulting in a wide-complex tachycardia: successful treatment with sodium bicarbonate. *Ann Emerg Med* 1992;21:318–21.

17 Joshi AK, Sljapic T, Borghei H, Kowey PR. Case of polymorphic ventricular tachycardia in diphenhydramine poisoning. *J Cardiovasc Electrophysiol* 2004;15:591–3.

18 Zareba W, Moss AJ, Rosero SZ, Haij-Ali R, Konecki J, Andrews M. Electrocardiographic findings in patients with diphenhydramine overdose. *Am J Cardiol* 1997;80:1168–73.

19 Stork CM, Redd JT, Fine K, Hoffman RS. Propoxyphene-induced wide QRS complex dysrhythmia responsive to sodium bicarbonate – a case report. *J Toxicol Clin Toxicol* 1995;33:179–83.

20 Kerns W 2nd, Garvey L, Owens J. Cocaine-induced wide complex dysrhythmia. *J Emerg Med* 1997;15:321–9.

21 Bania TC, Blaufeux B, Hughes S, Almond GL, Homel P. Calcium and digoxin vs. calcium alone for severe verapamil toxicity. *Acad Emerg Med* 2000;7:1089–96.

22 Dorsey ST, Biblo LA. Prolonged QT interval and torsades de pointes caused by the combination of fluconazole and amitriptyline. *Am J Emerg Med* 2000;18:227–9.

23 De Ponti F, Poluzzi E, Montanaro N. QT-interval prolongation by non-cardiac drugs: lessons to be learned from recent experience. *Eur J Clin Pharmacol* 2000;56:1–18.

24 Yap YG, Camm AJ. Drug induced QT prolongation and torsades de pointes. *Heart* 2003;89:1363–72.

25 Anderson ME, Al-Khatib SM, Roden DM, Califf RM. Cardiac repolarization: current knowledge, critical gaps, and new approaches to drug development and patient management. *Am Heart J* 2002;144:769–81.

26 Sides GD. QT interval prolongation as a biomarker for torsades de pointes and sudden death in drug development. *Dis Markers* 2002;18:57–62.

27 Nelson LS. Toxicologic myocardial sensitization. *J Toxicol Clin Toxicol* 2002;40:867–79.

28 De Ponti F, Poluzzi E, Cavalli A, Recanatini M, Montanaro N. Safety of non-antiarrhythmic drugs that prolong the QT interval or induce torsade de pointes: an overview. *Drug Saf* 2002;25:263–86.

29 Houston M, Hendrickson RG. Decontamination. *Crit Care Clin* 2005;21:653–72.

30 Kuckelkorn R, Schrage N, Keller G, Redbrake C. Emergency treatment of chemical and thermal eye burns. *Acta Ophthalmol Scand* 2002;80:4–10.

31 Wagoner MD. Chemical injuries of the eye: current concepts in pathophysiology and therapy. *Surv Ophthalmol* 1997;41:275–313.

32 Saidinejad M, Burns M. Ocular irrigant alternatives in pediatric emergency medicine. *Pediatr Emerg Care* 2005;21:23–6.

33 Krenzelok EP, McGuigan M, Lheur P. Position statement: ipecac syrup. American Academy of Clinical Toxicology; European Association of Poisons Centres and Clinical Toxicologists. *J Toxicol Clin Toxicol* 1997;35:699–709.

34 American Academy of Pediatrics Committee on Injury, Violence, and Poison Prevention. Poison treatment in the home. *Pediatrics* 2003;112:1182–5.

35 Bond GR. Home syrup of ipecac use does not reduce emergency department use or improve outcome. *Pediatrics* 2003;112:1061–4.

36 Chyka PA, Seger D. Position statement: single-dose activated charcoal. American Academy of Clinical Toxicology; European Association of Poisons Centres and Clinical Toxicologists. *J Toxicol Clin Toxicol* 1997;35:721–41.

37 Moll J, Kerns W 2nd, Tomaszewski C, Rose R. Incidence of aspiration pneumonia in intubated patients receiving activated charcoal. *J Emerg Med* 1999;17:279–83.

38 Seger DL. Flumazenil – treatment or toxin? *J Toxicol Clin Toxicol* 2004;42:209–16.

39 Bledsoe BE. No more coma cocktails. Using science to dispel myths and improve patient care. *J EMS* 2002;27:54–60.

40 Chamberlain JM, Klein BL. A comprehensive review of naloxone for the emergency physician. *Am J Emerg Med* 1994;12:650–60.

41 Clarke SFJ, Dargan PI, Jones AL. Naloxone in opioid poisoning: walking the tightrope. *Emerg Med J* 2005; 22:612–16.

42 Doe-Simkins M, Walley A, Epstein A, Moyer P. Saved by the nose: bystander-administered intranasal naloxone hydrochloride for opioid overdose. *Am J Public Health* 2009;99:788–791.

43 Kerr D, Kelly A, Dietze P, Jolley D, Barger B. Randomized controlled trial comparing the effectiveness and safety of intranasal and intramuscular naloxone for the treatment of suspected heroin overdose. *Addiction* 2009;104:2067–74.

44 Wheeler E, Davidson P, Jones S, Irwin K. Community-based overdose prevention programs providing naloxone – United States 2010. *MMWR Morb Mortal Wkly Rep* 2012;61:101–5.

45 Kelly A, Kerr D, Dietz P, Patrick I, Walker T, Koutsogiannis Z. Randomized trial of intranasal versus intramuscular naloxone in prehospital treatment for suspected opioid overdose. *Med J Aust* 2005;182: 24–7.

46 Robertson T, Hendey G, Stroh G, Shalit M. Intranasal naloxone is a viable alternative to intravenous naloxone for prehospital narcotic overdose. *Prehosp Emerg Care* 2009; 13:512–15.

47 Barton E, Ramos J, Colwell C, Benson J, Baily J, Dunn W. Intranasal administration of naloxone by parmedics. *Prehosp Emerg Care* 2002;6:54–8.

48 Barton E, Colwell C, Wolff T, et al. Efficacy of intranasal naloxone as a needleless alternative for treatment of opioid overdose in the prehospital setting. *J Emerg Med* 2005; 29:265–71.

49 Dasgupta N, Brason II F, Albert S, Sanford K. Project Lazarus: overdose prevention and responsible pain management. *N Carolina Med Board Forum* 2008;1:8–12.

50 Weigert A. Caustic ingestion in children. *Contin Educ Anaesth Crit Care Pain* 2005;5:5–8.

51 Schaffer SB, Hebert AF. Caustic ingestion. *J La State Med Soc* 2000;152:590–6.

52 Boink AB, Wemer J, Meulenbelt J, Vaessen HA, de Wildt DJ. The mechanism of fluoride-induced hypocalcemia. *Hum Exp Toxicol* 1994;13:149–55.

53 Lepke S, Paasow H. Effects of fluoride on potassium and sodium permeability of the erythrocyte membrane. *J Gen Physiol* 1968;51:S365–72.

54 Kao WF, Deng JF, Chiang SC, et al. A simple, safe and efficient way to treat severe fluoride poisoning – oral calcium or magnesium. *J Toxicol Clin Toxicol* 2004;42:33–40.

55 Crain EF, Gershel JC, Mezey AP. Caustic ingestions: symptoms as predictors of esophageal injury. *Am J Dis Child* 1984;138:863–5.

56 Rumack BH, Burrington JD. Caustic ingestions: a rational look at diluents. *Clin Toxicol* 1977;11:27–34.

57 Homan CS, Maitra SR, Lane BP, Thode HC Jr, Davidson L. Histopathologic evaluation of the therapeutic efficacy of water and milk dilution for esophageal acid injury. *Acad Emerg Med* 1995;2:587–91.

58 Homan CS, Maitra SR, Lane BP, Thode HC, Sable M. Therapeutic effects of water and milk for acute alkali injury of the esophagus. *Ann Emerg Med* 1994;24:14–19.

59 Homan CS, Maitra SR, Lane BP, Geller ER. Effective treatment of acute alkali injury of the rat esophagus with early saline dilution therapy. *Ann Emerg Med* 1993;22:178–82.

60 Homan CS, Singer AJ, Henry MC, Thode HC. Thermal effects of neturalization therapy and water dilution for acute alkali exposure in canines. *Acad Emerg Med* 1997;4:27–32.

CHAPTER 47

Treatment and evaluation of specific toxins

Michael C. Beuhler

Introduction

This chapter discusses several chemicals often inhaled, but ingestion and dermal exposures are encountered for a few. EMS physicians and personnel must have appropriate training, personal protective equipment (PPE), and medical protocols to deal with a variety of potential toxic exposures. The offending agent is often unidentified or misidentified during early phases of the response (see Volume 2, Chapter 46); extreme caution should be exercised until the situation has been fully defined.

The toxic effects of most chemicals can be classified into a general range of syndromes, and appropriate triage, decontamination, treatment, and transport often will be based on signs and symptoms. Responders may use patterns of vital signs, mental status, pupil size, mucous membrane irritation, lung examination, and skin examination (for burns or discoloration) to identify suspected toxidromes. Irritant gas exposure, such as chlorine or ammonia, results in irritation of upper airways and mucous membranes. Acetylcholinesterase inhibitors such as organophosphate and carbamate pesticides and nerve agents result in cholinergic symptoms including wheezing, salivation, lacrimation, vomiting, sweating, diarrhea, and sometimes seizures or coma. Solvent exposure may cause lightheadedness, nausea, confusion, and loss of consciousness. On contact with skin or mucous membranes, most solvents cause skin irritation or injury. Metabolic poisons such as cyanide (CN), carbon monoxide (CO), or hydrogen sulfide (H_2S) can result in rapid loss of consciousness and cardiorespiratory collapse. Finally, fear of potential exposure may cause persons to present with symptoms such as chest pain, palpitations, shortness of breath, and syncope, attributable to generalized autonomic arousal.

Recognition of potential clinical syndromes will guide prehospital care and notification of authorities and receiving facilities. Poison centers are a resource that should be considered for additional clinical information regarding antidotal therapy, local trends or uncommon clinical presentations; this resource is available to any health care provider.

Some of the agents discussed in this chapter injure the skin and mucous membranes on contact by chemical reaction. Decontamination must be approached in a knowledgeable and focused manner. It is impractical and dangerous to conduct unnecessary decontamination when there is no need; precious minutes will be lost donning excessive protective gear and establishing decontamination stations when not necessary – minutes that may result in greater casualties. Overall, victims exposed to gas or vapors only, without skin or eye irritation and with no grossly apparent deposition of toxins on their person, have very low risk of secondary contamination and may be evacuated immediately; eye irritation alone may be addressed with gentle irrigation during transport.

Organophosphates and nerve agents

Organophosphates have widespread civilian use as agricultural pesticides and have been used in military campaigns and terrorist attacks as highly lethal nerve agents. Although organophosphate pesticides are less potent than the military versions, both have the capability to cause significant morbidity or death. In Japan, the Aum Shinrikyo cult used sarin (a nerve agent) in two terrorist events resulting in 19 deaths, 1,000 hospitalizations, and 5,000 people seeking medical attention [1].

Pathophysiology and clinical presentation

Toxicity from organophosphate compounds can occur via almost any route of exposure, including dermal, ocular, inhalation, ingestion, or injection. The onset, severity, and duration of effects depend on the potency of the agent; the route, concentration, and duration of exposure; and the use of antidotal therapy. Patients with vapor exposure experience a rapid onset of effects, whereas dermal exposure will often have a delayed onset of toxicity.

Organophosphates bind to the enzyme responsible for acetylcholine hydrolysis, acetylcholinesterase, resulting in an elevated

Emergency Medical Services: Clinical Practice and Systems Oversight, Second Edition. Volume 1: Clinical Aspects of EMS.
Edited by David C. Cone, Jane H. Brice, Theodore R. Delbridge, and J. Brent Myers.
© 2015 NAEMSP. Published 2015 by John Wiley & Sons, Inc. Companion Website: www.wiley.com\go\cone\naemsp

synaptic concentration of acetylcholine at both nicotinic and muscarinic receptors. Initially the binding is reversible; water may enter the enzyme active site and hydrolyze the organophosphate moiety off. However, after a time, depending upon the organophosphate, the moiety bound to the enzyme undergoes a chemical change and is no longer able to undergo hydrolysis. This is called aging and results in permanent inhibition of the acetylcholinesterase enzyme. The carbamate pesticides are very similar clinically and pharmacologically to the organophosphosphate compounds, the main difference being that they will not age and pralidoxime is not necessary for therapy.

Acetylcholinesterase inhibition results in prolongation and potentiation of acetylcholine action at cholinergic synapses. In the central nervous system, this causes confusion, agitation, and seizures. In the autonomic nervous system, increased cholinergic transmission results in diaphoresis, bradycardia (tachycardia is seen for other reasons), miosis (not always present), lacrimation, salivation, vomiting, defecation, and urination due to overstimulation of muscarinic receptors. The latter constellation of symptoms is represented by the cholinergic toxidrome mnemonic DUMBBELS (diarrhea, urination, miosis, bronchorrhea/bronchospasm/bradycardia, emesis, lacrimation, and salivation). Increased cholinergic activity at neuromuscular junctions results in muscle fasciculations and motor weakness.

Late effects of organophosphate poisoning include "intermediate syndrome," a return of weakness and neuromuscular symptoms 1–4 days after initial clinical improvement. Patients may require additional supportive therapy or reintubation. Late neurological sequelae include peripheral neuropathies, persistent miosis, and neuropsychiatric sequelae (nightmares, headache, anxiety); this effect is likely to compound the psychological effect of a nerve agent attack.

Decontamination and personal protective equipment

The risk of provider poisoning by an organophosphate depends upon the class of the agent. With the highly lethal war nerve agents (GA, GB, VX, etc.), most are volatile (except VX) and very small doses will potentially be lethal. For protection, a level A fully encapsulated garment is required. Personnel responding to war nerve agent attacks are at significant risk of becoming secondarily exposed and suffering from adverse effects from insufficiently decontaminated victims. In the Tokyo sarin attack, first responders and nurses suffered adverse effects from the vapors of insufficiently decontaminated patients in poorly ventilated areas, but injuries were mild with improvement once they ventilated the vehicles during transport [2].

Exposures to organophosphate pesticides are more common and less lethal to humans. These agents have much lower volatility than the war agents; the smell reported is partially due to the solvent hydrocarbon. Unless the patient is completely drenched in concentrated organophosphate pesticide, standard universal precautions with double nitrile gloves should be sufficient to prevent any significant exposure. The vomitus from patients ingesting concentrated organophosphate pesticide should be handled with caution. Although there is a report about secondary ED staff contamination by "pesticide vapors," there are uncertainties about the exact etiology of this event [3].

Decontamination includes removal of all clothing and jewelry, physical removal of visible residue, and irrigation with water or soap and water; for the organophosphate pesticides, significant scrubbing with soap and water will be required. Items of leather and cloth are difficult to clean and should not be returned to the patient. There is no consensus regarding gastric decontamination of pesticide organophosphates. In many cases, the patient will already have vomited and so the utility of lavage is questionable. Activated charcoal could be of benefit, but this should only be considered when the airway is secure (i.e. intubation) to prevent possible aspiration.

Detection and diagnosis

First responders should be vigilant for potential organophosphate exposures in instances in which there are multiple casualties presenting with similar symptoms. In the 1995 sarin attacks in Tokyo, the most common physical sign was miosis, with presenting symptoms ranging from eye pain, headache, and bronchorrhea to apnea and death [1]. The miosis was a very useful sign to separate those suffering from toxicity from those who were "worried well." Note that miosis is not useful in organophosphate toxicity with other routes of exposure (such as ingestion). Rapid development of the cholinergic toxidrome in a number of casualties should prompt immediate consideration of an organophosphate. Activity of red blood cell cholinesterase and plasma cholinesterase may assist diagnosis in hospital.

Treatment and disposition

After decontamination, supportive care includes airway maintenance and support of ventilation, as respiratory failure is the primary reason for death with organophosphates. Aggressive suctioning may be required because of copious airway secretions and vomiting; aspiration is not uncommon with organophosphate pesticide ingestion. If intubation is required, succinylcholine should be avoided because it may lead to prolonged neuromuscular blockade due to the organophosphate inhibition of butyrylcholinesterase. The mainstay of treatment in nerve agent and organophosphate poisoning consists of antidotal therapy with atropine, pralidoxime, and diazepam.

Atropine competitively antagonizes excess acetylcholine effects at central and peripheral muscarinic receptors but has no effect at nicotinic receptors. Atropine can effectively reverse bronchorrhea, bradycardia, and gastrointestinal symptoms and treat seizures, but has no effect on nicotinic symptoms such as fasciculations, weakness, or paralysis [4]. Side-effects may include delirium, tachycardia, and agitation. The initial dose of atropine is 2 mg in adults (0.05 mg/kg in children, minimum

0.1 mg) administered intravenously or intramuscularly. Although it can be administered via the endotracheal route, this has disadvantages because of the excessive secretions and ventilation difficulties. The dose is titrated to effect and may be repeated every 1–5 minutes; although tachycardia may develop, atropine is given until the patient is well ventilated as demonstrated by reduced secretions and resolution of bronchoconstriction and/or is no longer bradycardic. Atropine will also potentially decrease vomiting, diarrhea, and bradydysrhythmia. The required dose of atropine can be very large for oral pesticide poisoning, with some patients requiring hundreds of milligrams of atropine; much less is required to treat war nerve agent poisoning. Unless symptoms resolve with a single dose of atropine, patients who require administration of atropine following organophosphate exposure should also receive pralidoxime.

Pralidoxime chloride is an oxime that reactivates acetylcholinesterase by reacting with the phosphorus moiety, resulting in an oxime-phosphate compound that leaves the regenerated enzyme. Oxime therapy must be administered before the aging of that bond is complete, a process that can begin within minutes of exposure and depends upon the organophosphate. The initial dose is 1–2 g for adults (25–50 mg/kg for children), and repeated dosing may be required; continuous infusions of 8–10 mg/kg/hour have been recommended. Slow administration over 15–30 minutes has been advocated to minimize side-effects which include hypertension, headache, blurred vision, weakness, epigastric discomfort, nausea, and vomiting. Rapid administration can result in laryngospasm, muscle rigidity, and transient impairment of respiration.

Benzodiazepines are used for the treatment and prevention of seizures. Diazepam 5–10 mg intravenously may be used, but repeated dosing may potentiate organophosphate-induced respiratory depression.

All three of these agents are available as autoinjectors; the commercially available MARK I autoinjector contains both 2 mg of atropine and 600 mg of pralidoxime and requires two injections. A new autoinjector, the Antidote Treatment Nerve Agent Auto-Injector (ATNAA or DuoDote®), allows for both atropine (2.1 mg) and pralidoxime (600 mg) to be injected simultaneously; one disadvantage to this device is the inability to give more atropine without also giving more pralidoxime [5].

Gases (irritants and hydrocarbons)

Irritant gases include a number of chemicals found or produced throughout our modern society; this section will be limited to chlorine, phosgene, anhydrous ammonia, and hydrofluoric acid (HF). Irritant gases, such as chlorine and phosgene, have had extensive military use as chemical warfare agents. In addition to military use, these agents, as well as anhydrous ammonia, are used in industrial processes and are sometimes transported in massive quantities. Phosgene is rarely transported in bulk; however, it can be formed in small quantities by the heating of

chlorinated hydrocarbons. Compounds like hydrogen fluoride and hydrogen chloride are commonly used as aqueous solutions as hydrofluoric acid and hydrochloric acid, although there are some industrial processes that use the gas form. See Volume 1, Chapter 46 for discussions on caustic exposures, noting that HF also has systemic toxicity from large and/or concentrated exposures.

The solubility of a gas in water allows prediction of its warning properties and clinical presentation. Chlorine (good water solubility), HF (excellent water solubility), and ammonia (excellent water solubility) have pungent odors and cause rapid onset of irritant symptoms, a warning property that may prompt victims to escape and limit their exposure. These gases dissolve rapidly on contact with the water in the eyes and upper airway mucosa, where they cause eye irritation, lacrimation, corneal burns, rhinorrhea, and sneezing. With longer duration or higher concentrations of exposure, lower respiratory effects also manifest with alveolar damage and pulmonary edema. However, phosgene (low water solubility) has a subtle odor reported to be similar to newly mown hay that may not be perceptible to all individuals. Phosgene has poor warning properties; it does not cause immediate symptoms and it results in a lower respiratory injury as the lack of water solubility allows for penetration deep into the distal airways, potentially resulting in a more severe exposure.

Injury is caused through production of reactive chemical species in the aqueous environment (i.e. pulmonary tract, mucous membranes). Chlorine reacts with water to release hydrochloric acid, hypochlorous acid, and free radicals. Anhydrous ammonia combines with water to form the caustic ammonium hydroxide. Phosgene combines with water to release hydrochloric acid; it also reacts directly with cellular macromolecules. The alveolar damage from phosgene causes delayed-onset non-cardiogenic pulmonary edema and sometimes hypovolemic shock. HF gas is a "weak" acid, meaning it does not completely dissociate in an aqueous environment (but weak ≠ benign). Being undissociated, the fluoride ion is readily absorbed systemically where it binds with calcium to form insoluble calcium fluoride. Fatal hypocalcemia and hyperkalemia occur with significant fluoride exposures.

Because these agents are gases at ambient temperatures and pressure, there is little need for decontamination with the gaseous form of these compounds once patients are evacuated to a safe environment. Removal of clothing and gentle eye irrigation for those with ocular irritation are all that is usually required; note that patients with eye exposure to anhydrous ammonia gas may suffer significant corneal injury. There are no specific antidotes for respiratory irritants, although the use of nebulized sodium bicarbonate has been reported to potentially neutralize the acidic compounds formed by chlorine exposure.

More severe upper airway exposures can result in development of upper airway edema and laryngospasm. Respiratory distress or stridor mandates intubation to prevent airway compromise. Other supportive measures include supplemental oxygen, suctioning, beta-agonists, anticholinergic agents for broncho-spasm, and fluid resuscitation for hypovolemic shock. Steroids (inhaled, oral) have been used following exposure to irritant gas exposure; they may be beneficial but there is not strong clinical evidence to routinely recommend their use. Patients with mild exposures to water soluble agents who remain asymptomatic 6 hours after exposure are unlikely to worsen, whereas delayed pulmonary edema is common with exposure to poor water sol-ubility compounds such as phosgene thus requiring prolonged observation.

For hydrogen fluoride exposures, field administration of IV calcium gluconate to individuals with significant inhalation exposure should be considered prophylactically as the onset of fatal arrhythmias often occurs without warning and the calcium may be normal when first checked; large amounts of IV calcium may be required.

Hydrocarbon gases such as methane and propane have minimal physiological effect. At high levels, some can be narco-tizing but the primary mechanism for causing human illness is oxygen displacement and resulting hypoxia. Individuals exposed to high levels of volatile hydrocarbons should be removed from the source and provided with 100% oxygen. The initial responder should consider the flammable and explosive nature of the hydrocarbon gas in their initial management; also, care should be taken not to enter a potentially hypoxic environment resulting when hydrocarbon gas levels are extremely high.

Hydrocarbon abuse where the individual deliberately inhales the hydrocarbon for euphoric reasons is called huffing (from a rag), sniffing (from a container), or bagging (from a bag). The greatest initial concerns are the cardiac sensitization that occurs with many of the chlorinated or fluorinated hydrocarbons. This is manifested by "sudden cardiac death" when a surge of epi-nephrine triggers a fatal ventricular arrhythmia. For the first responder, awareness of this phenomenon and restraint from using epinephrine are important. The bio-accumulation of the desired hydrocarbon, its metabolite, or other hydrocarbons in the product may also have consequences. Individuals who huff methanol-containing products may develop acidosis and visual disturbances. Huffing metallic spray paints for the toluene results in an acidosis and severe hypokalemia, sometimes to the point of paralysis. Solvents containing methylene chloride will be metabolized to carbon monoxide in the body, necessitating treatment as discussed below.

Carbon monoxide

Carbon monoxide is an odorless, colorless gas responsible for thousands of ED visits annually. Unintentional CO poisonings occur with the use of malfunctioning equipment that utilizes combustion, generators and portable heaters in poorly venti-lated areas during power outages or with people riding behind mechanized vehicles such as boats or farm machinery. Carbon monoxide may be produced chemically; this has rarely been used as a suicide method [6]. The manifestations of CO poisoning form a spectrum ranging from mild, non-specific symptoms to severe illness with hemodynamic instability and central nervous system toxicity.

Carbon monoxide binds to hemoglobin 240 times more avidly than oxygen and causes a leftward shift in the oxygen hemoglobin dissociation curve that further decreases oxygen delivery to tissues. CO also binds directly to heme-containing cellular proteins, including cytochromes, myoglobin, and guanylate cyclase. Binding to cardiac myoglobin may cause myocardial depression, hypotension, and cardiac arrhythmias. CO may increase nitric oxide levels, creating free radicals and leading to further systemic hypotension and cellular injury.

Acute CO poisoning initially causes non-specific symptoms such as headache, nausea, and dizziness progressing to altered mental status, confusion, syncope, seizures, and coma. Cardiovascular effects include hypotension, cardiac ischemia, infarction, and arrhythmias. Patients with underlying cardio-vascular disease are prone to exacerbation of their underlying disease. Other organs may be affected, producing a range of clinical effects including rhabdomyolysis, renal failure, skin bullae, and non-cardiogenic pulmonary edema. Delayed effects of CO poisoning after initial recovery may manifest as long as 40 days after the initial exposure. Memory loss, ataxia, seizures, emotional lability, psychosis, and motor disturbances have been described.

Chronic low-level CO poisoning has caused headaches, light-headedness, cerebellar dysfunction, and cognitive and mood changes. It is often difficult to identify and quantify as the symp-toms may not be recognized as manifestations of CO poisoning. Symptoms are often alleviated by removal of the patient from the environment.

In pregnancy, severe CO toxicity is associated with poor fetal outcomes. Maternal levels do not correlate with fetal exposure, and poor fetal outcomes have been noted with maternal levels that are not extremely elevated. Fetal hypoxia likely contributes to this; the injury is not due to an increased innate fetal hemoglobin affinity for CO over maternal hemoglobin, as was previously believed [7].

Prehospital workers must rely on clinical suspicion and clinical syndromes to recognize CO poisoning. Fire and haz-ardous material units usually carry CO gas detection equipment, permitting measurement of environmental CO levels. These levels can be useful in making treatment decisions and should be communicated to ED caregivers. The gold standard for diag-nosing CO poisoning is CO-oximeter measurement of venous carboxyhemoglobin levels. However, the severity of exposure depends on both the concentration and duration of exposure; therefore blood levels serve to guide, not dictate therapy.

A new commercially available non-invasive CO-oximeter is available for clinical use. The CO-oximeter uses eight wave-lengths of light instead of the usual two used by traditional pulse oximeters and has a reported error of ±3% (1 SD) absolute car-boxyhemoglobin level. However, one study demonstrated a false-positive rate of 9% and a false-negative rate of 18% so when clinical suspicion is high, formal CO-oximetry should be used to confirm the level [8,9]. The role of prehospital CO-oximetry remains undefined.

Rescuers should initiate field treatment based on clinical symptoms, history, and possibly environmental levels. Prehospital treatment of CO poisoning begins with evacuation of victims from the exposure, initiating high-flow supplemental oxygen by non-rebreather mask, and supporting cardiovascular and respiratory function. The half-life of carboxyhemoglobin decreases from a range of 240–320 minutes in ambient oxygen to a range of 50–100 minutes with inhalation of 100% oxygen at atmospheric pressure [10].

Although the primary treatment for CO poisoning is supplemental oxygen, hyperbaric oxygen therapy (HBO) is likely beneficial for selected patients with severe poisoning and neurological symptoms. HBO rapidly corrects the relative anemia from the carboxyhemoglobin by decreasing the half-life of carboxyhemoglobin to approximately 20 minutes and increasing dissolved oxygen in the blood, augmenting oxygen delivery. HBO also reduces CO binding to other heme-containing cellular proteins. Benefit from HBO may exist even for the patient with a normal carboxyhemoglobin level as HBO may reduce tissue and free radical-mediated cellular injury by reducing endothelial neutrophil adhesion and lipid peroxidation.

Potential complications of HBO include barotrauma, claustrophobia, and oxygen toxicity and unless it is a multiplace chamber, there is no capacity to access the patient when the chamber is pressurized. The Undersea and Hyperbaric Medical Society maintains a directory of hyperbaric facilities (www. uhms.org). EMS agencies should have preestablished protocols for medical oversight consultation. Depending upon the region and resources, an EMS system may preferentially take stable CO-poisoned patients to an ED within a system that can also offer HBO. This could potentially decrease the time delay for the patient to receive HBO therapy.

Despite years of study, the exact indication for HBO for CO-poisoned patients is not clear. A clinical policy paper by ACEP [11] determined that there was the lowest level of evidence for recommending HBO therapy for CO-poisoned patients and such therapy cannot be mandated. However, considering extensive animal and reasonable human evidence, it is common practice for many to recommend HBO therapy for CO-poisoned patients with loss of consciousness (transient or persistent) and/ or neurological symptoms (especially cerebellar) and also for the pregnant patient with evidence of fetal distress. There are no studies in pregnant patients with HBO for CO toxicity, but there is good clinical evidence that HBO therapy will not be harmful to the fetus. Adult patients who have been resuscitated from cardiac arrest from CO poisoning have nearly universally fatal outcomes; only pediatric patients or those with witnessed cardiac arrest should be considered for HBO [12].

Some physicians use cardiovascular manifestations as an indication to perform HBO; others feel that a telemetry admission and cardiac work-up are more beneficial. Some have proposed absolute carboxyhemoglobin levels as indications for HBO therapy; levels proposed include greater than 25% or greater than 15% in pregnant patients. These levels are not evidenced based; it is known that carboxyhemoglobin levels do not correlate with toxicity, and fetal injury can occur with low maternal levels.

If a patient will receive benefit from HBO therapy, it should be provided as soon as possible (ideally within 6 hours) and no later than 24 hours after the exposure. One well-designed clinical trial randomizing patients with elevated carboxyhemoglobin levels or neurological or cardiac symptoms showed statistically significant improvements in symptoms and in neuropsychiatric sequelae with HBO [13].

Cyanide

Cyanide (CN⁻) is widely used in industries such as mining, metallurgy, electroplating, and plastic polymer production. Cyanide is encountered as a salt such as sodium cyanide or as the gas hydrogen cyanide (HCN), but there are naturally trace amounts found in certain foods. HCN gas is produced when a cyanide salt is mixed with acid. Cyanide has been used in warfare without great success; however, CN⁻ is a potential agent for terrorism, as evidenced by interest in the mubtakar, an improvised cyanide delivery device [14]. HCN is commonly generated during pyrolysis of natural and synthetic substances such as paper, silk, wool, and plastics. Although smoke inhalation usually results in CO poisoning, toxicity may also result from concurrent HCN exposure and this represents one of the most the most common source in society today.

The cyanide ion binds to the ferric ion of cytochrome c oxidase, halting mitochondrial electron transport and stopping aerobic generation of adenosine triphosphate, so tissues switch to anaerobic respiration. Cyanide first affects tissues with high levels of oxygen consumption such as cardiac myocytes and central nervous system neurons. Inhibition of cellular enzymes leads to increased susceptibility to oxidative stress and lipid peroxidation, and neuronal damage ensues. Increased brain glutamate levels may result in excitatory neurotoxicity, whereas decreased gamma-aminobutyric acid levels may lead to seizures.

Clinical effects from cyanide exposure depend on the dose, route, and duration of exposure. Low-level exposures to cyanide produce non-specific symptoms such as dyspnea, headache, nausea, anxiety, and altered mental status. Higher levels may result in hyperpnea within seconds, and loss of conscious, apnea, and death within minutes. Cyanide-containing hydrocarbons such as acetonitrile require metabolism to free the cyanide and so symptoms may not develop for several hours after exposure, which is quite different from any other cyanide exposure.

Combined with an appropriate history of exposure, the finding of a lactic acidosis and hemodynamic or respiratory compromise that does not respond to supplemental oxygen should prompt consideration for cyanide. Some experts propose lactate levels greater than 10 mmol/L as suggestive of CN poisoning [15]. Other clinical clues to the nature of the exposure may include a bitter almond odor from hydrogen cyanide gas emitted from the patient's lungs, as well as a cherry red color to the skin or bright red venous blood resulting from the inability to use oxygen. These signs are unreliable as many people cannot recognize the bitter almond odor and the cherry red skin color may not be present. Victims exposed to only HCN gas will not require any decontamination beyond disrobing; cases of secondary cyanide poisoning have resulted from dermal contamination or ingestions of cyanide salts with vomiting or when the stomach is opened during autopsy.

Currently, there are three antidotal therapies approved for use in the United States: sodium nitrite, sodium thiosulfate, and hydroxocobalamin. Sodium nitrite and sodium thiosulfate are sold as part of one antidotal kit but are available separately as well. Amyl nitrite is no longer part of the FDA-approved cyanide antidotal kit and has very limited use in the USA.

Sodium nitrite produces methemoglobin by oxidizing the hemoglobin iron from 2+ to 3+ with the standard dose resulting in a methemoglobin level of around 12%. Cyanide has a higher chemical affinity for methemoglobin (Fe^{3+}) than for the cytochrome c oxidase, which results in displacing cyanide from mitochondria and binding to the methemoglobin. The toxicity from sodium nitrite includes hypotension and excessive methemoglobinemia. When administered inappropriately, fatalities have occurred. Additionally, oxygen delivery in patients with concomitant carbon monoxide toxicity from smoke inhalation may be reduced due to methemoglobinemia. However, the peak of methemoglobinemia after IV sodium nitrite occurs in about 15 minutes, and the probable decline in carbon monoxide level on 100% oxygen closely matches the increase in methemoglobinemia. The sodium nitrite dose in adults is 300 mg over 2–3 minutes; the pediatric dose is based on weight as well as serum hemoglobin.

Sodium thiosulfate is a sulfur donor which enables the endogenous conversion of cyanide to thiocyanate, a relatively non-toxic compound, which is excreted by the kidneys. Sodium thiosulfate is cheap, is packaged in a liquid form ready for injection, and has an extremely safe profile with minimal side-effects reported. Sodium thiosulfate takes time ($\approx$15 minutes) for an effect to be noted. The dose is 12.5 g in adults and in pediatrics it is 0.42 g/kg up to the adult dose; the dose may be repeated once, at half initial dose, if necessary.

The newest approved antidote for cyanide is hydroxocobalamin, a derivative of vitamin B_{12}. A reddish-colored, light-sensitive powder requiring reconstitution before its use, hydroxocobalamin's mechanism of action is similar to sodium nitrite but instead of turning the hemoglobin into a cyanide scavenger, the hydroxocobalamin is the scavenger. Cyanide has an extremely high affinity for hydroxocobalamin; it binds to the cobalt metal center and forms vitamin B_{12} (cyanocobalamin), which is excreted by the kidneys. Hydroxocobalamin has a favorable safety profile and causes only minor adverse effects: self-limited reddish skin, urine and serum discoloration, pustular skin rashes, allergic reactions, and elevations in blood pressure [16]. The latter is potentially advantageous because it may reverse the hypotension from cyanide toxicity. However, the discoloration of serum is known to interfere with colorimetric serum assays and has caused problems when attempting hemodialysis [17,18]. The adult dose of hydroxocobalamin is 5 g, with a pediatric dose of 70 mg/kg up to 5 g; it may be repeated in cases of massive cyanide poisoning. It is recommended to be administered over 15 minutes. It is incompatible in the same IV line with many other medications, including sodium thiosulfate.

When considering which antidotal therapy to use, sodium thiosulfate is cheap, safe, and may be administered immediately when IV access is achieved. Hydroxocobalamin is expensive, has some side-effects, has storage stability issues, requires reconstitution before administration, and has a 15-minute infusion time, a time delay not addressed in most comparative studies. For prehospital care, with a weak clinical suspicion of cyanide toxicity, sodium thiosulfate may be administered empirically, immediately with almost no risk. The combination of thiosulfate and hydroxocobalamin (not given simultaneously through the same IV line) has been proposed as an advantage, as suggested by some animal studies. Sodium nitrite is not as safe and will decrease oxygen-carrying capacity, so if there is a choice, hydroxocobalamin should be administered in smoke inhalation victims.

Hydrogen sulfide

Hydrogen sulfide is a toxin similar to cyanide in that it causes inhibition of cellular aerobic respiration, but the inhibition of the cytochrome c oxidase is not as profound as with cyanide. It is more irritating than hydrogen cyanide and has a strong odor, but individuals experience odor fatigue and thus may mistakenly believe that the gas has dissipated when the odor disappears. Hydrogen sulfide is produced by decaying organic materials and can collect in enclosed spaces. Most tragedies involving hydrogen sulfide occur when the initial victim enters an area and is overcome, followed by one or more rescuers who are also poisoned. There are only a few substances that can cause rapid loss of consciousness like this (CO, hypoxic environments, and nerve agents, to name the most common). It has also been used in suicide events where an individual mixes calcium polysulfide and acid together, evolving hydrogen sulfide gas. Often this is performed in a closed car; the first responder should be aware of this potential etiology and the danger of this gas. Treatment is supportive, with removal from exposure and 100% oxygen being most important. The standard cyanide antidotal therapies are usually not required as the hydrogen sulfide will spontaneously unbind from the cytochrome c oxidase; for those who are critically ill, there is some limited evidence to support the use of sodium nitrite.

Vesicants

Sulfur mustard and lewisite are vesicants – potent alkylating agents that interact with cellular macromolecules and DNA to cause cell death via necrosis or apoptosis. Sulfur mustard has been used since WWI and still occasionally resurfaces to cause illness in fishermen when old munitions are brought up in their nets. The nitrogen mustards (HN1, HN2, HN3) are a group that uses nitrogen rather than sulfur; now these have new life as chemotherapeutic agents: cyclophosphamide, chlorambucil, ifosfamide, and melphalan. Sulfur mustard melts at 57.0 °F (14.4 °C), meaning that if the environment is above this temperature, there will be possible vapor injury.

The injury caused by vesicants is proportional to the concentration times the duration of exposure, considering the tissue susceptibility, with delicate tissues (cornea) having high sensitivity to injury. With sulfur mustard, there is a delay of several hours between exposure and development of the initial lesions. Skin and mucous membrane exposure results in desquamation and formation of painful blisters. These blisters are filled with straw-colored liquid on an erythematous base; they become confluent as the injury progresses. Severe corneal damage and eye pain occur with eye exposure; gentle early eye irrigation is recommended along with ophthalmological consultation but permanent blindness from vapor exposure is rare. Inhalation of vesicants results in irritation and necrosis of upper airways and possibly pulmonary edema. Bronchoscopy may be necessary to clean out necrotic upper airway tissue to allow for ventilation. Secondary pulmonary infections often ensue. With significant exposures to sulfur mustard, bone marrow suppression occurs, potentially complicating infections. Sulfur mustard is carcinogenic and theoretically increases risk for neoplasias, although the risk from a single exposure is probably low. Lewisite (an arsenic-containing vesicant) is very similar to sulfur mustard, except the onset of symptoms is much faster (immediate ocular irritation, faster skin changes) rather than hours with sulfur mustard.

Vesicants pose a significant risk of secondary contamination of rescuers. Sulfur mustard penetrates most materials and it has no warning properties. Typically, level A PPE is required for operations in the hot zone and during initial decontamination; cases of secondary caregiver injury exist where decontamination was not adequate. All visible chemical agent and victims' clothing, jewelry, and personal items must be removed, followed by copious soap and water. The sulfur mustard reacts rapidly with tissues and after about 15 minutes it has all been internalized or locally reacted; however, sulfur mustard on objects has very long persistence. The bullae fluid does not have any sulfur mustard in it, so universal precautions as protection are sufficient.

Conclusion

Priorities for treatment of toxic exposures include recognizing a potential chemical source, adopting appropriate PPE if necessary, removing victims from the exposure, and appropriate decontamination of victims if necessary. Therapeutic priorities for toxic exposures include supportive care, including stabilization of airway and cardiorespiratory status. Specific measures such as hyperbaric oxygen and antidotal therapy may be appropriate in selected instances of CO, organophosphate, or

CN poisoning. Poison centers remain a resource for the first responder that should be considered for additional clinical information regarding local trends or uncommon clinical presentations.

References

1 Okumura T, Nobukatsu T, Shinichi I, et al. Report on 640 victims of the Tokyo subway sarin attack. *Ann Emerg Med* 1996;28:129–35.

2 Okumura T, Suzuki K, Fukuda A, et al. The Tokyo subway sarin attack: disaster management, part 1: community emergency response. *Acad Emerg Med* 1998;5:613–28.

3 Geller RJ, Singleton KL, Tarantino ML. Nosocomial poisoning associated with emergency department treatment of organophosphate toxicity – Georgia 2000. *MMWR* 2001;49:1156–8.

4 Shih T-M, Rowland TC, McDonough JH. Anticonvulsants for nerve agent-induced seizures: the influence of the therapeutic dose of atropine. *J Pharmacol Exp Ther* 2007;320:154–61.

5 Package Insert, ATNAA (Antidote Treatment- Nerve Agent, Auto-Injector) Atropine Injection, Pralidoxime Chloride Injection. Meridian Medical Technologies.

6 Prahlow JA, Doyle BW. A suicide using a home carbon monoxide "death machine". *Am J Forensic Med Pathol* 2005;26:177–80.

7 Westphal M, Weber TP, Meyer J, et al. Affinity of carbon monoxide to hemoglobin increases at low oxygen fractions. *Biochem Biophys Res Commun* 2002;295:975–7.

8 Barker SJ, Curry J, Redford D, Morgan S. Measurement of carboxyhemoglobin and methemoglobin by pulse oximetry. *Anesthesiology* 2006;105:892–7.

9 Weaver LK, Churchill SK, Deru K, et al. False positive rate of carbon monoxide saturation by pulse oximetry of emergency department patients. *Respir Care* 2013;58:232–40.

10 Weaver LK, Howe S, Hopkins R, et al. Carboxyhemoglobin half-life in carbon monoxide-poisoned patients treated with 100% oxygen at atmospheric pressure. *Chest* 2000;117:801–8.

11 Wolf SJ, Lavonas EJ, Sloan EP, Jagoda AS. Clinical policy: critical issues in the management of adult patients presenting to the emergency department with acute carbon monoxide poisoning. *Ann Emerg Med* 2008;51:138–52.

12 Hampson NB, Zmaeff JL. Outcome of patients experiencing cardiac arrest with carbon monoxide poisoning treated with hyperbaric oxygen. *Ann Emerg Med* 2001;38:36–41.

13 Weaver LK, Hopkins RO, Chan KJ, et al. Hyperbaric oxygen for acute carbon monoxide poisoning. *N Engl J Med* 2002;347:1057–67.

14 http://publicintelligence.net/ufouo-dhs-mubtakar-improvised-cyanide-gas-device-warning/

15 Baud FJ, Barriot P, Toffis V, et al. Elevated blood cyanide concentration in victims of smoke inhalation. *N Engl J Med* 1991;325:1761–6.

16 Uhl W, Nolting A, Golor G, et al. Safety of hydroxocobalamin in healthy volunteers in a randomized, placebo-controlled study. *Clin Toxicol (Phila)* 2006;44:17–28.

17 Sutter M, Tereshchenko N, Rafii R, et al. Hemodialysis complications of hydroxocobalamin: a case report. *J Med Toxicol* 2010;6:65–7.

18 Curry SC, Conner DA, Raschke RA. Effect of the cyanide antidote hydroxocobalamin on commonly ordered serum chemistry studies. *Ann Emerg Med* 1994;24:65–7.

Environmental Problems

CHAPTER 48

Cold exposure illness and injury

Jonnathan Busko

Introduction

Humans live in a wide range of environments. Below 82 °F, a healthy naked human being can no longer produce enough heat to maintain body temperature [1] and requires protection from the cold. Cold illness and injuries are common and EMS physicians must be familiar with their epidemiology, presentation, and treatment to improve patient outcomes. Common cold injuries include hypothermia, non-freezing tissue injuries, freezing tissue injuries, and cold water immersion. These four processes account for the majority of cold-related EMS care.

Hypothermia

Definition

Hypothermia is a core body temperature below 95 °F (35 °C). Stages include mild hypothermia (90–95 °F/32–35 °C), moderate hypothermia (82–90 °F/28–32 °C), and severe hypothermia (below 82 °F/28 °C). Measuring a "true" core body temperature can be a challenge in the hospital, let alone in the prehospital environment, and individual physiological responses to cold can vary widely. From a practical perspective, hypothermia is best defined from a physiological standpoint: cold stress exceeding the body's ability to produce sufficient heat to maintain body temperature [2]. The stages can then be based on clinical presentation and a patient's ability to self-rewarm if the cold stress is eliminated (Table 48.1). In this approach, the core temperature is adjunctive but the clinical picture guides the provider's actions.

Types

From 1999 to 2011, there were on average 1301 deaths annually in the United States attributed to hypothermia [3]. While the classic image of hypothermia is the lost hiker huddled in the snow, EMS providers are more likely to encounter urban hypothermia, a multifactorial hypothermia resulting from cold exposure and some combination of medical conditions, medications, changes in temperature perception, substance abuse, inadequate nutrition, and inadequate social circumstances [4–7]. Urban hypothermia is a chronic disease and while the clinical presentation of hypothermia may precipitate the call for EMS and may well be the immediate life threat, it is rarely the only active disease process. It is often considered to be secondary hypothermia.

Wilderness or environmental hypothermia, by contrast, is primary hypothermia caused by exposure to cold stress that exceeds the body's heat production capacity. It is either acute, as in immersion, or subacute hypothermia (over days), as seen in the inadequately prepared hiker in a cold (although not necessarily freezing) environment.

Mechanisms of thermoregulation

Humans maintain a core temperature within a narrow range of (95–100.7 °F/35–38 °C) for optimal metabolic functioning. Four mechanisms, radiation, conduction, convection, and evaporation, contribute to heat loss from the body; homeostasis is maintained by balancing these mechanisms against heat production.

Infrared radiation emission accounts for up to 40% of all heat loss. The greater the temperature difference between the individual and the environment, the greater the rate of heat loss [8]. This can occur even when the air temperature is warm if the surrounding environmental features (such as a cave or concrete structure) are colder.

Evaporation via sweating dissipates excess heat, with approximately 575 calories of heat lost for each cubic centimeter of evaporated sweat [8]. Unfortunately, this mechanism is just as effective at removing heat during periods of cold stress. Individuals who become wet will rapidly lose heat via evaporation in a cold environment.

In conduction, direct transfer of heat from one object to another, a colder object becomes an important source of heat loss for the recumbent ill or injured individual. The greater the area of uninsulated contact, the more heat is lost.

Convection, particularly combined with evaporation, also contributes to heat loss. The body heats a small local environment to minimize heat transfer. If this buffer zone is lost, the body is

Emergency Medical Services: Clinical Practice and Systems Oversight, Second Edition. Volume 1: Clinical Aspects of EMS.
Edited by David C. Cone, Jane H. Brice, Theodore R. Delbridge, and J. Brent Myers.
© 2015 NAEMSP. Published 2015 by John Wiley & Sons, Inc. Companion Website: www.wiley.com\go\cone\naemsp

Table 48.1 The stages of hypothermia can be defined based on the clinical presentation, and the ability of the patient to self-rewarm if cold stress is removed

Clinical presentation	Ability to self-rewarm	Likely temperature
Mild hypothermia Shivering, general loss of fine then gross motor function with progressive loss of intellectual function and development of confusion	Good initially but limited as temperature decreases	90–95°F/32–35°C
Moderate hypothermia Loss of shivering, progressive vulnerability of the heart to atrial fibrillation, and progression of confusion to unconsciousness	Poor progressing to none	82–90°F/28–32°C
Severe hypothermia Muscular rigidity, loss of detectable vital signs, progressive cardiac vulnerability to ventricular fibrillation due to rough handling with progression to spontaneous ventricular fibrillation, coma	None	Below 82°F/28°C

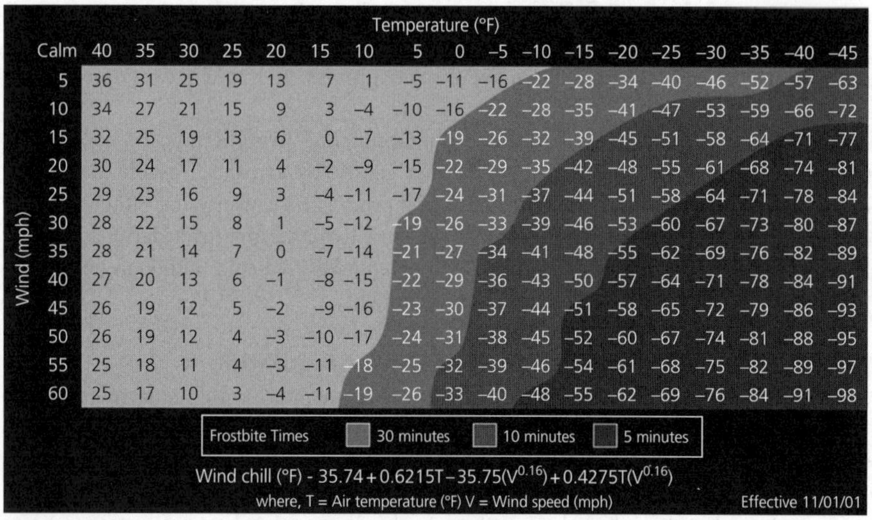

Temperature (°F)

Wind (mph)	40	35	30	25	20	15	10	5	0	−5	−10	−15	−20	−25	−30	−35	−40	−45
5	36	31	25	19	13	7	1	−5	−11	−16	−22	−28	−34	−40	−46	−52	−57	−63
10	34	27	21	15	9	3	−4	−10	−16	−22	−28	−35	−41	−47	−53	−59	−66	−72
15	32	25	19	13	6	0	−7	−13	−19	−26	−32	−39	−45	−51	−58	−64	−71	−77
20	30	24	17	11	4	−2	−9	−15	−22	−29	−35	−42	−48	−55	−61	−68	−74	−81
25	29	23	16	9	3	−4	−11	−17	−24	−31	−37	−44	−51	−58	−64	−71	−78	−84
30	28	22	15	8	1	−5	−12	−19	−26	−33	−39	−46	−53	−60	−67	−73	−80	−87
35	28	21	14	7	0	−7	−14	−21	−27	−34	−41	−48	−55	−62	−69	−76	−82	−89
40	27	20	13	6	−1	−8	−15	−22	−29	−36	−43	−50	−57	−64	−71	−78	−84	−91
45	26	19	12	5	−2	−9	−16	−23	−30	−37	−44	−51	−58	−65	−72	−79	−86	−93
50	26	19	12	4	−3	−10	−17	−24	−31	−38	−45	−52	−60	−67	−74	−81	−88	−95
55	25	18	11	4	−3	−11	−18	−25	−32	−39	−46	−54	−61	−68	−75	−82	−89	−97
60	25	17	10	3	−4	−11	−19	−26	−33	−40	−48	−55	−62	−69	−76	−84	−91	−98

Frostbite Times: 30 minutes, 10 minutes, 5 minutes

$$\text{Wind chill (°F)} - 35.74 + 0.6215T - 35.75(V^{0.16}) + 0.4275T(V^{0.16})$$

where, T = Air temperature (°F) V = Wind speed (mph)   Effective 11/01/01

Figure 48.1 Windchill chart. Source: www.nws.noaa.gov/om/windchill/

constantly reheating new air (or water) and heat losses increase dramatically. Moving air (wind) augments this effect. Heat loss is a function of the square of wind velocity so doubling the wind speed quadruples heat loss [8] up to a maximum speed of 40 mph (64 km/h), after which the air is moving too quickly to absorb heat [9]. This phenomenon is referred to as wind chill (Figure 48.1). Wind chill describes the rate of heat loss from exposed skin. This has implications for how urgently a rescue must be effected. Use of windproof garments or shelters eliminates the wind chill effect.

Two primary defenses guard against heat loss. First, in response to cold stress, there is a behavioral imperative to add additional layers of clothing and to seek sources of warmth [8]. The second defense is heat production. Any muscular activity produces heat. The body can uncouple heat production from useful activity via shivering [3]. While shivering will produce additional heat to counter cold stress, it will not prevent worsening hypothermia if the environmental conditions don't change. Shivering should serve as a signal to take other actions to decrease the environmental cold stress. Performing useful activity that increases the chances of survival also generates heat and is the preferred method of muscular heat production.

Prevention

Preventing wilderness hypothermia requires recognizing cold stress and taking actions to decrease it. Sufficient calorie and water intake is crucial to allow effective metabolism and heat generation. Clothing that maintains a microclimate of trapped air, prevents heat loss though convection, and wicks moisture away through all the layers of the clothing decreases the risk of hypothermia. Avoidance of substances that promote vasodilation (e.g. alcohol) or that impair judgment and temperature perception (e.g. alcohol or illicit drugs) will decrease the risk of primary hypothermia.

Preventing urban hypothermia is a far more complex issue with public health and social welfare implications [10]. Programs such as the Low Income Home Energy Assistance Program likely decrease the incidence of urban hypothermia, as do homeless shelters.

Recognition

While classification based on core body temperatures is useful for research and statistical purposes [1,11–14], an individual's performance at a given core body temperature can vary widely [15] and so the assessment and treatment should be based on clinical presentation (see Table 48.1).

In the early stages of hypothermia, a perception of being cold and a behavioral imperative to change or exit the cold environment will predominate. Unless sufficient heat is being developed from useful activity, the patient will shiver and may be mildly agitated. Loss of fine motor control follows. At this stage, if the patient has sufficient calorie reserves and is removed from the cold stress, he will be able to rewarm himself.

Left untreated, hypothermia will progress and symptoms will include confusion, slurred speech, loss of gross motor coordination, and loss of judgment. This stage is described as the "umbles": the patient stumbles, mumbles, grumbles, fumbles, and tumbles. Eventually as caloric reserves are depleted, shivering stops. At this point, the patient is no longer able to self-rewarm even if cold stress is eliminated.

The patient will progress to a state of unresponsiveness. Cardiac dysrhythmias occur, particularly atrial fibrillation. Metabolic demand decreases and the patient becomes bradycardic. As the myocardium becomes more irritable, the risk of ventricular fibrillation with minimal or no stimulation increases. Respiratory rate decreases and the patient may appear apneic.

Once the patient is comatose, effort must be focused on minimizing physical movements that could trigger ventricular fibrillation, including bumping, dropping, or otherwise physically stimulating the patient.

Treatment

Treatment of hypothermia depends on whether or not the patient is able to self-rewarm if the cold stress is eliminated. Therefore, the most important action is to eliminate the cold stress. This may be as simple as moving the patient to a heated ambulance. If a heated sheltered environment is not readily available, efforts to eliminate further heat loss include insulating the patient from the ground to prevent conduction, removal of wet clothing to minimize evaporation, and sheltering from wind to prevent convection. Although studies have evaluated mechanisms to decrease radiant heat loss [15], to date none have been particularly successful.

Once the cold stress is removed, an assessment must be made of the patient's ability to self-rewarm. For the patient with mild hypothermia who still has adequate caloric and metabolic reserves (that is, still shivering or recently stopped shivering), elimination of cold stress and feeding the patient should be sufficient to restore normothermia [8,13,16].

For patients who are metabolically depleted and unable to self-rewarm, active interventions will be necessary. The historical dogma has been that out-of-hospital interventions are sufficient only to prevent further heat loss and are not adequate to restore normothermia. Such interventions have included heated IV fluids, heated (and preferably humidified) inhaled oxygen, application of heat packs or heated water bottles to the neck, axilla, and inguinal creases, and rescuer/patient skin-to-skin contact [8,17,18]. More invasive procedures such as warm water irrigation of the stomach, bladder, peritoneal, and pleural

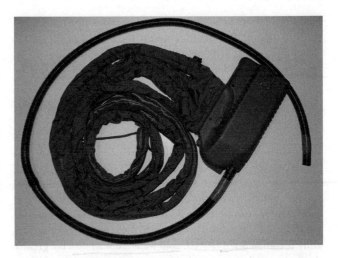

Figure 48.2 Charcoal vest. Charcoal inserts are burned in the body of the device and a small fan blows warm air through the green tubes that are wrapped around the patient's torso. The black tube carries exhaust away. Source: Jonnathan Busko. Reproduced with permission of Jonnathan Busko.

cavity as well as heated dialysis and cardiopulmonary bypass have been reserved for the hospital setting [8,19,20].

Over the last decade, research has demonstrated that effective prehospital interventions exist. These include a 600 W heater with a soft rewarming blankets (a forced warm air full-body blanket) [21,22], 600 or 850 W heater with rigid torso cover [21,23], and charcoal vest forced hot air heaters (Figure 48.2) [21]. Of these devices, the charcoal heater is the only one that does not require electricity beyond a D-cell battery to run the fan, is light enough that a single rescuer could carry two, and is inexpensive. On the other hand, it does use a flame source to generate heat (burning charcoal) and therefore poses a risk when used with oxygen. All of these devices have been demonstrated to attenuate afterdrop (the tendency for the core temperature to drop even after the initiation of rewarming) and to actually rewarm the patient. If EMS agencies and providers function in an environment where hypothermia is prevalent, acquisition of at least one of these types of devices should be considered. Avoid immersion in warm water as this increases mortality [15].

Disposition

Due to concomitant medical and social issues, the patient with urban hypothermia must be transported to an emergency department for further evaluation.

For the patient with primary hypothermia in a wilderness setting, the disposition is less clear. A patient with mild hypothermia who recovers to normothermia may not need evacuation if changes can be made to the patient's clothing system or to the route so recurrent cold stress is minimized. For the patient with moderate hypothermia, evacuation is mandatory with one exception. In the case of an expedition with provisions for active rewarming, the decision to evacuate the moderately hypothermic patient restored to normothermia is made in conjunction with the patient, the expedition leader, and medical support staff in the context of the risks of evacuation.

For the patient with severe hypothermia and signs of life, evacuation is mandatory. The method of evacuation must be such that the patient experiences as little unnecessary movement and as few bumps as possible. Evacuation may not be possible and *in situ* rewarming may be necessary.

The patient without signs of life presents a challenge. While the mantra "no one is dead until warm and dead" is always operative, it is not always practical. Rescuer safety is primary and while successful resuscitation of severely hypothermic patients has been reported, the risk:benefit ratio of the operation must be considered. In addition, there are indeed patients who are cold and dead. These include those with a core temperature less than 50 °F (10 °C), cold water submersion for greater than 1 hour, obvious fatal injuries, and frozen patients (i.e. ice formation in the airway or chest walls that are so rigid compressions cannot be performed [24]. Cardiopulmonary resuscitation (CPR) is difficult in the wilderness environment and effective performance during patient transport is impossible. Some experts recommend performing rewarming in place [8] while others recommend transporting without CPR if definitive care (any provider capable of providing effective active rewarming) is available within 3 hours [24]. Guidelines for defibrillation, CPR techniques, and medication administration vary widely [8,19,24] and the American Heart Association in 2010 noted a lack of research identifying optimal resuscitation techniques [25].

Non-freezing cold injuries

Non-freezing cold injury to the foot (trenchfoot or immersion foot) occurs with subacute exposure in cold but non-freezing conditions. The foot becomes macerated with vasomotor instability and anesthesia. Temperature affects the time to onset; for shipwrecked sailors whose feet are immersed in cold water, onset may take as little as 24 hours [26] while the minimum time to onset on land is 4–5 days [8].

Injury occurs from local maceration due to water exposure, cold-induced vasoconstriction, and circulatory compromise from excessively tight footwear and immobility [8,27]. Prolonged vasoconstriction leads to damage to the blood vessels and results in injury to the tissues they feed [28].

Non-freezing cold injuries progress through three phases. In the pretreatment (prehyperemic) phase, the limbs are blanched and yellowish white. Local edema may be present and the patient may complain of anesthesia, particularly as cold exposure progresses. Pain is rare at this phase [27]. In the urban setting, alcoholism and chronic homelessness may contribute to a complete non-awareness of this condition.

Once treatment is initiated, the patient enters the hyperemic phase lasting hours to weeks [28]. The vasoconstriction reverses and, due to vasomotor instability, the extremities become hot, red, swollen, and painful [29]. Blisters in this phase indicate more serious injury and gangrene may occur in the most severe cases.

The posthyperemic phase may be absent in mild cases or may persist for years after the injury. It is characterized by ongoing symptoms after the resolution of the hyperemic phase, including vasomotor instability, persistent cold sensitivity, and limb coolness. After periods of exertion, blistering, edema, and paresthesias may also reoccur [27]. This phase may last for years.

Clean, dry socks changed at least once and preferably twice a day will markedly decrease the risk of non-freezing cold injury. Avoiding immobility, taking breaks from the cold, wet environment, limiting activity to minimize sweating, and keeping the feet dry for 8 out of every 24 hours are important prevention techniques [27].

Remove the wet garments, keep the feet dry and elevated, and keep bedclothes from pressing on the feet [8]. Tissue rewarming is not necessary, but warming the core temperature (if necessary) while providing cooling with a fan to the injured area will markedly decrease pain, edema, and blistering [29]. Remember that the social and environmental conditions that predispose to trenchfoot also contribute to hypothermia.

Frostbite

Frostbite is a freezing injury to soft tissues. A combination of local (tissue-level) freezing temperatures and an inability of the body to produce or provide sufficient heat allows the tissues to freeze. Frostnip may precede freezing. Frostnip is a condition of superficial ice crystal formation without resulting tissue damage. Cyclic vasoconstriction and vasodilation in the extremities (known as the "hunting response") may be present. This process, which occurs more in cold-acclimatized individuals, protects at-risk tissue from freezing. While it contributes to additional heat loss, cyclic rewarming permits greater dexterity in the hands, improving function in cold environments [30,31].

Environmental conditions that predispose to frostbite are the same conditions that predispose to hypothermia. Peripheral vasoconstriction may cause blood flow to the distal extremities to essentially cease [8]. The cold also induces vascular endothelial damage with plasma leakage.

With continued cooling, freezing occurs and extracellular ice crystals form. This leads to changes in local solute concentrations and intracellular dehydration. Additional injury comes from denaturation of lipid-protein complexes, toxic concentrations of intracellular electrolytes, thermal shock, and, in the event of rapid freezing (seconds to minutes), intracellular ice crystals [32]. However, tissue freezing does not necessarily result in permanent damage. Frozen cells are metabolically inactive and so cell death may not occur when the tissues are frozen. Instead, when rewarming occurs and the tissues become metabolically active, oxygen demand increases. The endothelial damage to the microvascular circulation that occurred during freezing now contributes to local thrombosis and watershed ischemia [8].

Early signs of incipient frostbite include a cold sensation, pain, and pallor. As freezing occurs, pain resolves and anesthesia ensues. The loss of sensation may be accompanied by a sense that the limb is clumsy or that the affected body part is absent. The tissue becomes paler. A noticeable progression of superficial to deep freezing occurs. The skin will begin to feel firm and non-pliable although the underlying tissues will be soft. Ultimately, the entire affected part becomes solid. In severe cases, purplish discoloration may occur.

Several grading systems have evolved. The best grading system is one that allows early and accurate prognostication of treatment resource requirements and prognosis. Unfortunately, the ideal system has not yet been developed [32]. For prehospital providers, a grading system of "degrees" based on findings after freezing and rewarming is commonly used. First-degree injuries are characterized by numbness, erythema, white or yellow plaques in the area of injury, and edema without tissue loss. Second-degree injuries add blisters surrounded by erythema and edema. In a third-degree injury, blisters are more extensive and contain blood. A fourth-degree injury involves the subcuticular tissues. It may be difficult to clinically distinguish fourth-degree from third-degree injuries in the immediate postrewarming period [32].

Prevention of frostbite includes preventing hypothermia so that peripheral circulation is maintained, avoiding constricting garments and boots (including too many layers of socks), and remaining active.

Treatment of frostbite is less about what to do and more about what not to do. The two key principles are to avoid thawing and refreezing the frozen part and preventing burns. Honoring these two principles, any appropriate treatment to rapidly thaw the tissue is acceptable, although controlled rewarming with warm water immersion of affected limbs remains the preferred treatment. While there is no additional benefit to rewarming a frozen part that has completely thawed, there is also no harm. If there is any doubt about whether the part is completely thawed, rewarming should be instituted.

Rewarming is best accomplished by treating the hypothermia to a core temperature of at least 93 °F (34 °C) and then completely immersing the frozen part in a warm water bath (99–108 °F/37–42 °C). All clothing, constricting bands, or items that would decrease peripheral circulation should be removed. The bath should be brought to the appropriate temperature without the part immersed to prevent scalds. Except when rewarming the bath, the part should remain fully immersed until the tissues become pliable and there are no further color changes. The temperature of the bath should be continuously monitored. Rewarming will typically take 30–60 minutes. Avoid massage of the injured part since this may increase local damage [8,32].

Although older guidelines based on the work of Baron Larrey cautioned against rapid rewarming [33], recent work has demonstrated the superiority of a rapid rewarming approach [34].

In a wilderness or uncontrolled environment, thawing of a frozen part should only occur if the following conditions can be met [8].

1 The person will not need to use the frostbitten part for evacuation until healing is complete.
2 The person can be kept warm during thawing and until healing is complete.
3 Thawing can be completed in a controlled, uninterrupted manner with accurate temperature management of the rewarming bath.

If these conditions cannot be met, the extremity should not be thawed [32].

During rewarming, pain can be intense. Adjunctive parenteral narcotics may be necessary to control this pain. Additional therapies include thromboxane inhibitors (ibuprofen 400 mg PO every 12 hours), tetanus immunization as needed, and strict wound care of the injured part [32]. Antibiotics are indicated for any signs of infection [8]. Sterile dressings should be placed between the digits once they are thawed to decrease tissue adhesion. Unless another traumatic condition or an abscess exists, surgery is contraindicated until the extent of the tissue death is clear, often 3–6 months [32].

Cold water immersion

Cold water immersion (head above the water, as opposed to submersion or drowning with the head below the water) is immersion in water less than 77 °F (25 °C) [35,36]. In water below 77 °F (25 °C), no amount of exertion can maintain a normal core body temperature in an unprotected individual [37]. In water temperatures below 68 °F (20 °C), a variety of physical and behavioral responses create hazardous conditions that put the immersion victim at increased risk of death either from drowning or eventually from hypothermia.

In cold shock response, the first phase of cold water immersion, respiratory patterns change with hyperventilation and a gasp response predominating; unacclimatized individuals also lose breath-holding ability [38]. Breathing becomes erratic and the individual cannot entrain coordinated physical activity with the respiratory cycle. While this phase lasts only a few minutes, the victim may hyperventilate to unconsciousness, panic or aspirate water and, if not wearing a personal flotation device (PFD), may drown. A victim wearing a PFD can focus on controlling breathing and successfully survive the initial immersion.

If the victim recovers from the initial cold shock response, a period of approximately 10 minutes remains for useful activity [36] before loss of fine and gross motor function progresses to complete inability to perform any meaningful survival actions [39]. This phase is called cold incapacitation. Core temperatures may increase as significant peripheral vasoconstriction shunts blood centrally. For a victim without a PFD, this phase will typically conclude with drowning as the ability to maintain the head above water is lost. Useful actions that promote recovery or survival should be performed. However, unnecessary physical activity should be avoided as movement promotes heat loss at a rate greater than metabolic heat generation [40]. If the shore is sufficiently close (within 800 m) the victim may consider attempting to swim to shore [36]. While this decision should be made as soon as possible during the cold incapacitation phase, it should not be made lightly as the rate of cooling will increase and, if the swim attempt is unsuccessful, hypothermia will be accelerated [36].

After 30–60 minutes, the victim will begin to face a significant risk of hypothermia. Many factors influence the time to onset of hypothermia (body morphology, sea state, protective garments, exercise, shivering, and behaviors) [36]. Nonetheless, even if the victim becomes unconscious from hypothermia, as long as submersion can be prevented, the victim may not actually die from hypothermia for up to 2 hours [36].

Sudden death in the period immediately preceding rescue as well as in apparently recovered survivors of cold water immersion has been described up to 24 hours after rescue [36,41]. This occurs in approximately 20% of immersion victims [42]. Although no one cause has been identified, a number of factors such as afterdrop and return of cold, acidotic or alkalotic blood to the heart, catecholamine release, decreased hydrostatic pressure upon removal from the water, cold-dulled baroreceptor reflexes, increased blood viscosity, intravascular volume depletion, and decreased work capacity of the heart may explain why this happens [36,42]. Rescuers must make all efforts to keep cold water immersion victims horizontal, prevent unnecessary physical activity (including walking to an aid room or ambulance), and maintain vigilance for this potentially delayed lethal event [42].

Cold water immersion is a threat to rescuers and patients alike. First, and most importantly, anyone at risk for cold water immersion must wear a PFD and preferably protective insulating garments appropriate to the degree of risk. While each circumstance is unique, it is important for anyone immersed in cold water to remember and act based on the 1-10-1 rule [36]. Upon immersion, the victim has 1 minute to control ventilation and prevent panic. This is followed by 10 minutes of useful activity to either signal for rescue or improve the situation to increase the chances of survival and rescue. Finally, it will take approximately 1 hour until unconsciousness occurs due to hypothermia, so any actions taken in the first 10 minutes that result in rescue before 1 hour may well prevent death from hypothermia.

Conclusion

Cold illness and injury are common in the EMS environment. EMS physicians and providers must be familiar with their epidemiology, presentation, and treatment. Hypothermia, non-freezing tissue injuries, freezing tissue injuries, and cold water immersion account for the vast majority of cold-related EMS care. It is important for the EMS provider to understand the pathophysiology and treatment of these disease processes to improve patient outcomes.

References

1 Wilkerson JA , Giesbrecht GG. Baby it's cold outside: basic human cold physiology. In: Giesbrecht GG, Wilkerson JA (eds) *Hypothermia, Frostbite, and other Cold Injuries: Prevention, Survival, Rescue, and the Treatment*. Seattle, WA: Mountaineers Books, 2006, p.11–22.
2 Ulrich AS, Rathlev NK. Hypothermia and localized cold injuries. *Emerg Med Clin North Am* 2004;22:281–98.
3 Xu J. Number of hypothermia-related deaths, by scx – National Vital Statistics System, United States, 1999–2011. *MMWR* 2013;61:1050.
4 White JD. Hypothermia: the Bellevue experience. *Ann Emerg Med* 1982;11:417–24.
5 Shields CP, Sixsmith DM. Treatment of moderate-to-severe hypothermia in an urban setting. *Ann Emerg Med* 1990;19:1093–7.
6 Collins KJ, Exton-Smith AN, Dore C. Urban hypothermia: Preferred temperature and thermal perceptions in old age. *BMJ* 1981;282:175–7.
7 Rango N. The social epidemiology of accidental hypothermia among the aged. *Gerontologist* 1985;25:424–30.
8 Wilkerson JA. Cold Injuries. In: Wilkerson JA, Moore EE, Zafren K (eds) *Medicine for Mountaineering and Other Wilderness Activites*, 6th edn. Seattle,WA: Mountaineers Books, 2010, p.272–89.
9 Wilkerson JA. Don't lose your cool: mechanisms of heat loss. In: Giesbrecht GG, Wilkerson JA (eds) *Hypothermia, Frostbite, and Other Cold Injuries: Prevention, Survival, Rescue, and Treatment*. Seattle: Mountaineers Books, 2006, pp.31–7.
10 Hislop LJ, Wyatt JP, McNaughton GW, et al. Urban hypothermia in the west of Scotland. *BMJ* 1995;311:725.
11 Jolly BT, Ghezzi KT. Accidental hypothermia. *Emerg Med Clin North Am* 1992;10:311–27.
12 Hanania NA, Zimmerman JL. Accidental hypothermia. *Crit Care Clin* 1999;15:235–49.
13 Reuler JB. Hypothermia: pathophysiology, clinical settings, and management. *Ann Intern Med* 1978;89:519–27
14 Hamilton RS, Paton BC. The diagnosis and treatment of hypothermia by mountain rescue teams: a survey. *Wilderness Environ Med* 1996;7:28–37.
15 Giesbrecht GG, Wilkerson JA: Too cool to breathe: evaluation and treatment of hypothermia. In: Giesbrecht GG, Wilkerson JA (eds) *Hypothermia, Frostbite, and Other Cold Injuries: Prevention, Survival, Rescue, and Treatment*. Seattle: Mountaineers Books, 2006, pp.38–56.
16 Shields CP, Sixsmith DM. Treatment of moderate-to-severe hypothermia in an urban setting. *Ann Emerg Med* 1990;19:1093–7.
17 Giesbrecht GG, Bristow GK, Uin A, Ready AE, Jones RA. Effectiveness of three field treatments for induced mild (33.0°C) hypothermia. *J Appl Physiol* 1987;63:2375–9.
18 Giesbrecht GG, Sessler DI, Mekjavic IB, Schroeder M, Bristow GK. Treatment of mild immersion hypothermia by direct body-to-body contact. *J Appl Physiol* 1994;76:2373–9.
19 Danzl DF. Accidental hypothermia. In: Auerbach PS (ed) *Wilderness Medicine*, 6th edn. Philadelphia: Elsevier, 2012, pp.116–42.

20 Sultan N, Theakston KD, Butler R, Suri RS. Treatment of severe accidental hypothermia with intermittent hemodialysis. *CJEM* 2009;11:174–7.

21 Hultzer MV, Xu X, Marrao C, Bristow G, Chochinov A, Giesbrecht GG. Pre-hospital torso warming modalities for severe hypothermia: a comparative study using a human model. *CJEM* 2005;7:378–86.

22 Giesbrecht GG, Schroeder M, Bristow GK. Treatment of mild immersion hypothermia by forced-air warming. *Aviat Space Environ Med* 1994;65:803–8.

23 Giesbrecht GG, Pachu P, Xu X. Design and evaluation of a portable rigid forced-air warming cover for prehospital transport of cold patients. *Aviat Space Environ Med* 1998;69:1200–3.

24 Alaska Department of Health and Social Services, Division of Public Health, Section of Community Health and EMS. *State of Alaska Cold Injuries Guidelines*, 2003 version revised 1/2005.

25 Vanden Hoek TL, Morrison LJ, Shuster M, et al. Part 12: Cardiac arrest in special situations: 2010 American Heart Association guidelines for cardiopulmonary resuscitation and emergency cardiovascular care. *Circulation* 2010;122:S829–61.

26 Ungley CC, Blackwood W. Peripheral vasoneuropathy after chilling. *Lancet* 1942;2:447–51.

27 Imray CHE, Castellani JW. Nonfreezing cold induced injuries. In: Auerbach PS (ed) *Wilderness Medicine*, 6th edn. Philadelphia: Elsevier, 2012, pp.171–80.

28 Thomas JR, Oakley HN. Nonfreezing cold injury. In: Pandolf KB, Burr RE (eds) *Textbook of Military Medicine: Medical Aspects of Harsh Environments*, Vol 1. Washington, DC: Office of the Surgeon General, Borden Institute, 2002, pp.467–90.

29 Webster DR, Woolhouse FM, Johnson JL. Immersion foot. *Am J Bone Joint Surg* 1942;42:785–94.

30 Arvesen A, Rosén L, Eltvik LP, Kroese A, Stranden E. Skin microcirculation in patients with sequelae from local cold injuries. *Int J Microcirc Clin Exp* 1994;14:335–42.

31 Greenfield ADM, Shepard IT, Whelan RF. Cold vasoconstriction and vasodilatation. *Irish J Med Sci* 1951;309:415.

32 Freer L, Imray CHE. Frostbite. In: Auerbach PS (ed) *Wilderness Medicine*, 6th edn. Philadelphia: Elsevier, 2012, pp.181–200.

33 Larrey DJ. *Memoirs of Military Surgery*, Vol 2. Baltimore, MD: Joseph Cushing, 1814.

34 Mills WJ Jr. Summary of the treatment of the cold injured patient. *Alaska Med* 1973;15:56.

35 Marino F, Booth J. Whole body cooling by immersion in water at moderate temperatures. *J Sci Med Sport* 1998;1:73–82.

36 Giesbrecht GG, Steinman AM. Immersion in cold water. In: Auerbach PS (ed) *Wilderness Medicine*, 6th edn. Philadelphia: Elsevier, 2012, pp.143–70.

37 Sagawa S, Hiraki K, Youset MK, Knoda N. Water temperature and intensity of exercise in maintenance of thermal equilibrium. *J Appl Physiol* 1988;65:2413–19.

38 Giesbrecht GG. Keep your head up: cold water immersion. In: Giesbrecht GG, Wilkerson JA (eds) *Hypothermia, Frostbite, and other Cold Injuries: Prevention, Survival, Rescue, and Treatment.* Seattle, WA: Mountaineers Books, 2006, pp.57–67.

39 Ferretti G. Cold and muscle performance. *Int J Sports Med* 1992;13:S185–7.

40 Hayward JS, Eckerson JD, Collis ML. Effects of behavioral variables on cooling rate of man in cold water. *J Appl Physiol* 1975;38:1073–7.

41 Golden FSC. Problems of immersion. *Br J Hosp Med* 1980;23:371–83.

42 Golden F, Tipton M. *Essentials of Sea Survival.* Champaign, IL: Human Kinetics, 2002, pp.243–89.

Further resources

The cold water boot camp is a project to teach the public about the hazards of cold water immersion and to provide survival strategies for cold water immersion.

www.youtube.com/watch?v=J1xohI3B4Uc
www.youtube.com/watch?v=nwETEkmVAeE
www.youtube.com/watch?v=aowQ9bthgBQ

CHAPTER 49

Heat-related illness

Gerald (Wook) Beltran

Introduction

Heat-related illnesses are a spectrum of disorders more commonly seen when the patient is in a warm environment, has underlying comorbidities, is physically active, and/or has attire which does not readily permit easy removal of body heat (such as firefighter "turnout gear"). If not diagnosed and managed appropriately, significant morbidity and mortality may result. This chapter will discuss the physiology of thermoregulation and the various heat-related illnesses, including management strategies.

According to the Centers for Disease Control and Prevention (CDC), an average of 688 people die annually from heat-related illness [1]. Between 1999 and 2003, an estimated 3,442 deaths were attributed to heat injury. Males accounted for 66% of the deaths. Fifty-three percent of those who died were between the ages of 15 and 64 years, while 40% were greater than 64 years of age.

Emergency medical services protocols should reflect the most up-to-date science on the management of patients with heat-related illness. The best management strategies incorporate expected transport times given the acuity of the patient's illness, local geography, weather, hospital proximity, and local traffic patterns.

Physiology of thermoregulation

Normal oral temperature has been demonstrated to be 33.2–38.2 °C [2]. Rectal temperature averages 34.4–37.8 °C, while the normal tympanic temperature is 35.4–37.8 °C.

The human body generates heat through metabolism. Basal metabolic rate is a measure of the number of calories expended at rest while sedentary. The maintenance of body temperature to a narrow window, or thermoregulation, is a complex task controlled by the hypothalamus. The body's extremities have a greater variation in temperature, dependent on environmental factors, including clothing. Generally, the extremities tend to be cooler than the rest of the body, while the core temperature fluctuates very little.

While metabolism of the various body tissues generates heat, the majority of body heat comes from skeletal muscle activity. Endocrine function can also affect metabolic rate and increase temperature. For example, epinephrine and norepinephrine can increase basal metabolic rate and subsequent heat generation. Similarly, thyroid hormones can produce an elevation of metabolic rate as well as an increase in body temperature.

Body temperature homeostasis occurs with heat generation in balance with heat dissipation. The narrow homeostatic range prevents enzymatic and cellular dysfunction or injury. Several reflexes or semi-reflexes help to maintain temperature. The reflexes or semi-reflexes activated by cold include shivering, hunger, increased voluntary activity, curling up, decreased heat loss, cutaneous vasoconstriction, epinephrine and norepinephrine release, and erection of the short body airs (i.e. "goose bumps"). The reflexes or semi-reflexes activated by heat include cutaneous vasodilation, sweating, decreased voluntary movement, anorexia, decreased heat production, and increased respiration. The posterior hypothalamus controls the reflexes activated by cold, while those for warmth are located in the anterior hypothalamus. Sweating and cutaneous vasodilation occur with activation of the anterior hypothalamus [3]. Sensors in the spinal cord, skin, deep tissues, hypothalamus, and extrahypothalamic regions of the brain provide feedback to the hypothalamus on body temperature [3]. The hypothalamus is activated by core temperature increases of less than 1 °C [4]. Lesions of the anterior area of the hypothalamus cause hyperthermia.

Heat is dispersed from the body by several different mechanisms including conduction, convection, evaporation, and radiation. Heat loss by conduction occurs through direct contact with an object or environment that is cooler. Skin temperature greatly affects the amount of body heat lost or gained through conduction. The amount of heat dispersed from the body's core to the skin is reliant on cutaneous blood flow. When the cutaneous vessels dilate, more blood flows to the skin, allowing for greater heat transfer from the deeper tissues (tissue conductance). Horripilation is the erection of

Emergency Medical Services: Clinical Practice and Systems Oversight, Second Edition. Volume 1: Clinical Aspects of EMS.
Edited by David C. Cone, Jane H. Brice, Theodore R. Delbridge, and J. Brent Myers.
© 2015 NAEMSP. Published 2015 by John Wiley & Sons, Inc. Companion Website: www.wiley.com\go\cone\naemsp

the cutaneous hairs which helps to trap air near the skin and inhibit heat transfer from the skin. Clothing also inhibits tissue conductance by limiting transfer of heat from the skin to the environment. Convection refers to the removal of heat as cooler air passes over exposed skin. The more air passes over the skin (e.g. from a fan), the more heat can be dispersed. Evaporation is the heat lost via converting a liquid to a gas. In the human body, about 600 kcal/hour in ideal conditions can be removed through evaporation [5]. Radiation is the transfer of heat by infrared electromagnetic waves. Approximately 250–300 kcal/hour can be transferred to the human body by solar radiation, with clothing acting as a barrier and providing some protection, estimated at 100 kcal/hour [6]. Additionally, the body disperses heat by radiating to cool objects in the vicinity [3].

At an ambient temperature of 21 °C and while at rest, heat loss from the body occurs through radiation and conduction (70%), evaporation (27%), respiration (2%), and urination and defecation (1%) [3]. As the ambient temperature increases, radiation losses decline and heat loss through evaporation increases [3]. At higher ambient temperatures, evaporation plays a more critical role in body heat removal. The removal of heat is reliant upon the gradients of moisture and temperature. As the environmental temperature and humidity increase, the exchange of heat becomes impaired. Therefore, hot humid environments confer the greatest risk to patients for heat-related illness (Figure 49.1).

The body adapts over time to more efficiently manage heat stress, primarily through salt retention and increased fluid secretion from sweat glands to increase the rate of evaporation [6]. Other adaptations include increased circulating plasma volume, improved renal filtration, and increased resistance by the kidney to exertional rhabdomyolysis [7]. Adaptation through production of acute-phase reactants also protects tissues from heat stress [8]. Individual cells produce intracellular heat shock proteins which protect them from

sudden heating [9,10]. The mechanism is believed to occur through the binding of heat shock proteins to cellular proteins which inhibit the cellular proteins from denaturing (or unfolding) in hot environments.

Pathophysiology

Regardless of the etiology, if hyperthermia is not addressed, tissue and cellular swelling and disruption will occur with widespread hemorrhage. Heat injury causes denaturation of proteins, a severe inflammatory response, and disruption of the coagulation cascade. The denaturation of proteins causes direct injury to the cells and cellular function. Pyrexia above 41.6 °C for a few hours can cause cellular damage. Temperatures above 49 °C can cause nearly immediate cell death. Organs most susceptible to apoptosis secondary to hyperthermia include the mucosa of the small intestine, thymus, lymph nodes, and spleen. Injury caused by inflammatory response is due to the release of several inflammatory cytokines including tumor necrosis factor-alpha, interleukin (IL)-1 (beta), and interferon gamma. Several anti-inflammatory cytokines are also released during heat stress, including IL-6, IL-10, and tumor necrosis factor receptors p55 and p75. Animal models with injection of IL-1 and tumor necrosis factor-alpha have demonstrated changes similar to heat stroke [11]. Heat injury causes activation of the coagulation cascade, injury to the vascular endothelium, and increased permeability of the vasculature. This has been demonstrated through surrogate markers of endothelial damage or activation as seen in heat stroke patients. Some of these markers include von Willebrand factor antigen, endothelin, and intracellular adhesion molecule 1 [11–14].

Minute ventilation, heart rate, and cardiac output increase in response to elevated body temperature, while at the same time, perfusion to the viscera decreases. Medications may

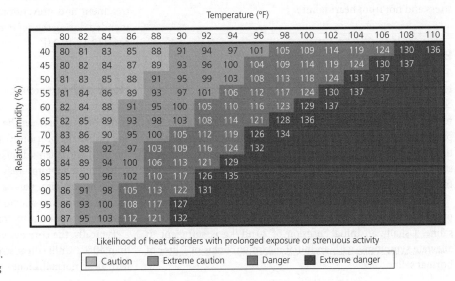

Figure 49.1 NOAA's National Weather Service Heat Index. Source: National Weather Service National Oceanic and Atmospheric Administration: www.nws. noaa.gov/os/heat/images/heatindex.png

Temperature (°F)

Relative humidity (%)	80	82	84	86	88	90	92	94	96	98	100	102	104	106	108	110
40	80	81	83	85	88	91	94	97	101	105	109	114	119	124	130	136
45	80	82	84	87	89	93	96	100	104	109	114	119	124	130	137	
50	81	83	85	88	91	95	99	103	108	113	118	124	131	137		
55	81	84	86	89	93	97	101	106	112	117	124	130	137			
60	82	84	88	91	95	100	105	110	116	123	129	137				
65	82	85	89	93	98	103	108	114	121	128	136					
70	83	86	90	95	100	105	112	119	126	134						
75	84	88	92	97	103	109	116	124	132							
80	84	89	94	100	106	113	121	129								
85	85	90	96	102	110	117	126	135								
90	86	91	98	105	113	122	131									
95	86	93	100	108	117	127										
100	87	95	103	112	121	132										

Likelihood of heat disorders with prolonged exposure or strenuous activity

□ Caution   ■ Extreme caution   ■ Danger   ■ Extreme danger

impede body heat removal. For example, vasoconstrictors and beta-blockers can prevent the body from transferring warm blood from the core to the skin for dissipation [13,15,16].

Underlying chronic medical conditions can also predispose individuals to heat illness. The elderly are at risk as they often have reduced cardiopulmonary reserve. Additionally, they are more often prescribed medications that put them at risk, tend to be less mobile, and are often volume depleted secondary to a decreased thirst mechanism. Age-related decreases in heat shock proteins, lessening their ability to tolerate increased temperatures, also put the elderly at increased risk [14]. Chronic metabolic conditions (e.g. thyrotoxicosis) predispose individuals to heat-related illness. Obesity increases hyperthermic risk, as adipose tissue impedes cooling, and decreases cardiac reserve. Those who are physically active in hot and humid environments are also at risk. For example, those in the military, athletes (e.g. high school athletes have an increased risk of heat illness over other sports by about 10 fold), and outdoor workers are at increased risk for heat-related illness (e.g. 20-fold increased rate of heat-related death compared to individuals in other employment) [1,17–19].

Heat edema

In the continuum of heat-related illness, heat edema is one of the mildest forms. Presenting as edema of the hands and/or feet, heat edema is caused by vasodilation and pooling of interstitial fluid, usually in the dependent extremities [12,17]. Limited to the extremities, the patient's core temperature is unaffected. Heat edema is most commonly observed in the elderly and those unacclimatized to hot environment.

Heat edema is managed symptomatically. Elevation of the affected extremities and compression stockings are the mainstay of treatment, in addition to moving the patient to a cooler environment [20]. Medication interventions are not recommended. Use of diuretics in these patients should be avoided, unless they present with signs of heart failure, as the edema is from heat stress and not from heart failure.

Heat syncope

Heat syncope is constellation of symptoms that can include syncope, dizziness, and orthostatic hypotension. These symptoms are related to venous pooling and peripheral vasodilation [17]. The patients often experience syncope after standing following exertion, or quickly changing their body position during exertion (e.g. standing after completing heavy bench presses). Patients suffering from this ailment usually have an unremarkable core temperature.

The mainstay of treatment for this ailment is to move the patient to a cooler environment and provide intravenous normal saline. Usually an initial infusion of 20 mL/kg is sufficient to alleviate symptoms, with an initial maximum bolus of 1 liter of normal saline.

Heat tetany

Heat tetany refers to spontaneous muscle spasm, such as carpopedal spasm or laryngospasm. Often a Chvostek or Trousseau sign may be elicited. This arises from a respiratory alkalosis from hyperventilation due to heat stress [21]. Patients may also complain of circumoral paresthesias. The tetany appears to be related to the rate of PCO_2 change more than the absolute pCO_2 change [22]. The core temperature in these patients may be either normal or elevated.

Treatment for heat tetany consists of removal from the warm environment. Once the heat stress is removed, the compensatory hyperventilation, subsequent hypocarbia, and associated spasms will resolve. Using a paper bag for rebreathing may also help resolve the symptoms, but does create the risk of hypoxemia [6,23]. Given this risk, the use of a paper bag is generally not recommended. The recommended management strategy to alleviate these symptoms is simply removal from the heat stress.

Heat cramps

The cramping of skeletal muscle during or after exertion in a warm environment is called heat cramps. The muscles most commonly involved include the legs (typically the larger muscle groups of the legs such as the quadriceps), calves, abdomen wall, and least commonly the arms. Heat cramps arise from heavy sweating and repletion with hypotonic fluids, causing a dilutional hyponatremia. Core temperature is either normal or may be elevated, but usually not in excess of 40 °C.

Treatment consists of rehydration with oral electrolyte solutions or intravenous normal saline as well as stretching and massage of the affected muscle and rest. Gradual rehydration is preferred, as an aggressive rehydration strategy might worsen hyponatremia. Oral rehydration with electrolyte solutions may be of benefit in preventing additional cramping of the same or other muscles [17,20]. In the past, salt tablets were used for both treatment and prevention. Currently, their use is not recommended during the acute management stage of this disease process [12,13,15,23].

Heat exhaustion

Some overlap between heat exhaustion and heat stroke occurs and unlike the previously described milder forms of heat-related illness, these patients display systemic symptoms. Heat exhaustion signs and symptoms may include anorexia, dizziness, fatigue, headache, malaise, nausea, sweating, visual changes, weakness, anxiety, confusion, diaphoresis, fever, hypotension, oliguria, skin flushing, tachycardia, or vomiting.

Typically, the core temperature is elevated, but is usually less than 40 °C. Unlike heat stroke, heat exhaustion patients present with near-normal mental status (although in some cases mild confusion is present which resolves after a short course of treatment). Seizures or coma are not part of the heat exhaustion spectrum.

Treatment consists of cooling. Moving the patient out of the hot environment is important (e.g. moving to a shaded or air-conditioned area). Removal of unneeded clothes will facilitate cooling. Cooling by immersing in cool water, running cold water over the patient, or evaporative cooling are all effective cooling methods. Rehydration is also important, with oral rehydration preferred as long as the patient is conscious, able to safely swallow, and does not have vomiting or diarrhea.

Heat stroke

The most serious of the heat-related illnesses is heat stroke. While there is some overlap between this entity and heat exhaustion, these patients are hyperthermic with central nervous dysfunction. In population studies, this diagnosis carries up to a 10% mortality risk [24]. A medical emergency, heat stroke may present with anorexia, dizziness, fatigue, headache, malaise, nausea, visual changes, or weakness. More concerning symptoms include anhydrosis, cardiac dysrhythmias, hepatic failure, hyperthermia, neurological signs (e.g. ataxia, coma, confusion, irritability, seizures), pulmonary edema, renal failure, rhabdomyolysis, shock, tachycardia, and tachypnea [25]. Core temperature is often between 40°C and 44°C. Temperatures may be higher in some cases. Although anhydrosis is described in the classic case of heat stroke, this is not a reliable sign and patients may be diaphoretic and still have this illness.

When severe, heat stroke can lead to multiorgan dysfunction. Factors associated with high case fatality rates include delay in presentation, delay in initiation of treatment, and increased disease severity upon presentation [25].

Heat stroke is classified in two forms: classic and exertional. Classic heat stroke often occurs during heat waves, is more common in the elderly and debilitated, and typically develops over days, not hours or minutes. The inciting etiology is due to external heat stress. Physical activity, or exertion, is usually not a contributing factor to development of classic heat stroke. Patients are often anhydrotic due to the time period over which this condition develops. Exertional heat stroke often occurs in healthy, young adults who are physically active in hot and humid environments without sufficient acclimatization [26]. Developing secondary to internal heat generation (i.e. body metabolism), it is more commonly seen in athletes, firefighters, foundry workers, and military recruits.

Treatment for heat stroke is similar to that for heat exhaustion. Cooling the patient is critical. Moving the patient from the warm environment to a cooler one is important (e.g. moving to a shaded or air-conditioned area). Removal of excess clothing will help facilitate cooling. Cooling by any of the previously mentioned methods will work (e.g. immersing in cool water, running cold water over the patient, or mist sprayer and fans).

Rehydration is also important, with intravenous rehydration preferred given the patient's neurological changes. Seizures should be managed according to protocol, usually with benzodiazepines.

Cooling techniques

One of the key elements in treating patients with heat exhaustion and heat stroke is rapid cooling. Decreased mortality and improved outcomes have been observed with rapid cooling to a temperature of 38.3°C [27–29]. Evaporation combined with convection (e.g. mist spray and a fan) is practical in a clinical setting, commonly employed, and efficient, but does depend on ambient humidity [30]. Ice water immersion is an efficient way of rapidly cooling patients and a metaanalysis supported its use with heat stroke [31]. There are, however, practical challenges when using ice water immersion which include difficulty in monitoring and difficulty in obtaining intravenous access after immersion. There are also several commercial body cooling units available. Ice packs to the groin and axilla may have utility when used in combination with evaporative cooling to lower body temperature [32].

In the prehospital environment, ice water immersion is often impractical due to equipment requirements, difficulty in moving a wet patient, placing defibrillation pads, monitoring the patient, maintaining the airway (i.e. aspiration risk), and obtaining intravenous access. Commercial cooling units are also impractical in the prehospital setting. They require special equipment which does not readily fit into an ambulance, can be cost prohibitive, and adds another piece of equipment with components that have a limited shelf-life.

There are few studies comparing the various methods of rapid cooling. Most have methodological challenges. Given the practical challenges (including expense) with the various cooling methods in the prehospital environment, evaporative cooling with convection may be the best alternative, especially in a patient with altered mental status [31]. In an ambulance, this could entail cool mist spray with air conditioning. Supplementary cooling with ice packs to the groin and axilla may also help expedite cooling. Simply removing the patient from the warm environment to the shaded ambulance will also help reduce the patient's heat stress.

Conclusion

The heat-related illness continuum ranges from minor illness with mild discomfort to life-threatening heat stroke. The human body is able to acclimatize to heat stress but once those adaptive strategies have been overwhelmed, illness ensues. Early recognition by EMS providers, in combination with patient treatment protocols that the medical director creates incorporating state, regional, and local practices, will help to reduce patient discomfort, morbidity, and mortality in the spectrum of disease. Management usually involves removal from the heat stress, cooling, and hydration as appropriate.

References

1 Centers for Disease Control and Prevention. Heat-related deaths – United States, 1999–2003. *MMWR* 2006;55:796–8.

2 Sund-Levander M, Forsberg C, Wahren LK. Normal oral, rectal, tympanic and axillary body temperature in adult men and women: a systematic literature review. *Scand J Caring Sci* 2002;16:122–8.

3 Barrett KE, Barman SM, Boitano S, Brooks HL. Hypothalamic regulation of hormonal functions. In: Barrett KE, Boitano S, Barman SM, Brooks HL (eds) *Ganong's Review of Medical Physiology*, 24th edn. Philadelphia: McGraw-Hill Medical, 2012.

4 Mackowiak P. *Fever: Basic Mechanisms and Management*, 2nd edn. Philadelphia: Lippincott-Raven, 1997, p.5–40.

5 Buono MJ, Sjoholm NT. Effect of physical training on peripheral sweat production. *J Appl Physiol* 1985;65:811–14.

6 Auerbach P. *Wilderness Medicine*, 4th edn. St Louis, MO: Mosby, 2001.

7 Knochel J. Catastrophic medical events with exhaustive exercise: white collar rhabdomyolysis. *Kidney Int* 1990;38:709–19.

8 Gabay C, Kushner I. Acute-phase proteins and other systemic response to inflammation. *N Engl J Med* 1999;340:448–54.

9 Polla BS, Bachelet M, Elia G, Santoro MG. Stress proteins in inflammation. *Ann NY Acad Sci* 1998;851:75–85.

10 Tsan MF, Gao B. Cytokine function of heat shock proteins. *Am J Cell Physiol* 2004;286:C739–44.

11 Bouchama A, Hammami MM, Haq A, Jackson J, al-Sedairy S. Evidence for endothelial cell activation/ injury in heatstroke. *Crit Care Med* 1996;24:1173–8.

12 Lugo-Amador NM, Rothenhaus T, Moyer P. Heat-related illness. *Emerg Med Clin North Am* 2004;22:315–27.

13 Barrow MW, Clark KA. Heat-related illnesses. *Am Fam Physician* 1998;58:749–56, 759.

14 Bouchama A, Knochel JP. Heat stroke. *N Engl J Med* 2002;346:1978–88.

15 Wexler RK. Evaluation and treatment of heat-related illness. *Am Fam Physician* 2002;65:2307–14.

16 Lee-Chiong TL Jr, Stitt JT. Heatstroke and other heat-related illnesses. The maladies of summer. *Postgrad Med* 1995;98:26–28, 31–33, 36.

17 Howe AS, Boden BP. Heat-related illness in athletes. *Am J Sports Med* 2007;35:1384–95.

18 Centers for Disease Control and Prevention. Heat illness among high school athletes – United States 2005–2009. *MMWR* 2010;59:1009–13.

19 Centers for Disease Control and Prevention. Heat-related deaths among crop workers – United States. *MMWR* 2008;57:649–53.

20 DeFranco MJ, Baker CL 3rd, DaSilva JJ, Piasecki DP, Bach BR Jr. Environmental issues for team physicians. *Am J Sports Med* 2008; 36:2226–37.

21 Ishmine P. Hyperthermia. In: Baren JM, Rothrock SG, Brennan J, Brown L (eds) *Pediatric Emergency Medicine*. Philadelphia: Saunders Elsevier, 2008.

22 Iampietro PF, Mager M, Green EB. Some physiological changes accompanying tetany induced by exposure to hot, wet conditions. *J Appl Physiol* 1961;16:409–12.

23 Seto CK, Way D, O'Connor N. Environmental illness in athletes. *Clin Sports Med* 2005;24:695–718.

24 Centers for Disease Control and Prevention. Heat-related illnesses and death – United States, 1994–1995. *MMWR* 1995;44:465–8.

25 Centers for Disease Control and Prevention. Heat-related mortality – Arizona, 1993–2002, and United States 1979–2002. *MMWR* 2005;54:628–30.

26 Yaqub B, Al Deeb S. Heat strokes: aetiopathogenesis, neurological characteristics, treatment and outcome. *J Neurol Sci* 1998;156:144–51.

27 Dematte JE, O'Mara K, Buescher J, et al. Near-fatal heat stroke during the 1995 heat wave in Chicago. *Ann Intern Med* 1998;129:173–81.

28 Vicario SJ, Okabajue R, Haltom T. Rapid cooling in classical heatroke: effect on mortality rates. *Am J Emerg Med* 1986;4:394–8.

29 Inter-Association Task Force on Exertional Heat Illness. Consensus Statement 2002. Available at: www.nata.org/sites/default/files/inter-association-task-force-exertional-heat-illness.pdf

30 Slovis C. Features and outcomes of classical heat stroke. *Ann Intern Med* 1999;130:614–15.

31 Smith J. Cooling methods used in the treatment of exertional heat illness. *Br J Sports Med* 2005;39:503–7.

32 Kielblock AJ, van Rensburg JP, Franz RM. Body cooling as a method for reducing hyperthermia. An evaluation of techniques. *S Afr Med* 1986;69:378–80.

CHAPTER 50

High-altitude illnesses

Hawnwan Philip Moy

Introduction

Altitude illness can be life-threatening if not recognized and adequately treated in a timely manner. Altitudes as low as 1,500 meters (m) cause physiological changes as the body adapts to the unique environment [1]. Rapid physiological adjustments can become pathological and perhaps fatal. More than 40 million tourists annually visit locations in the United States with elevations greater than 2,400 m [1]. Consequently, an increasing number of health professionals encounter high altitude pathologies. Despite research in altitude medicine, significant morbidity and mortality related to high altitude environments persist. This continual and growing public health risk emphasizes the need for education about altitude medicine not only for the lay person, but for all health professionals. In particular, the EMS physician must understand the pathophysiology and treatment for high altitude illness both as a potential responder and as a medical director for responders.

Physiology

High altitude is considered to be heights between 1,500 and 3,500 m (4,921 to 11,483 feet (ft)), very high altitude is between 3,500 and 5,500 m (11,483 to 18,045 ft) and extreme altitude is greater than 5,500 m (18,045 ft) [1]. No matter how high you climb, the percentage of oxygen in the air remains roughly 21%. What changes as you climb is the density of the air molecules. At sea level, the air molecules are densely packed together from the weight of the air above them. As you climb, there is less pressure on the air molecules and so they are more dispersed. This air pressure is called barometric pressure or atmospheric pressure.

Air molecules that are more dispersed translate into fewer molecules taken in with each breath. Thus, a breath at 3,500 m contains about 60% as much oxygen as at sea level. The concentration of the oxygen is still 21%, but there are fewer oxygen molecules available. At 5,000 m (the altitude of Everest Base Camp), each breath has about half the oxygen available at sea level and at 8,848 m (Mount Everest summit), each breath takes in about one-third as much as at sea level. As the level of inhaled oxygen decreases, the body responds with altitude acclimatization.

Many physiological changes occur as the human body is subjected to the stress of high altitude. Erythropoietin is released from the kidneys once hypoxic conditions are sensed. This hormone stimulates bone marrow to increase red blood cell production. Within 2 hours of ascent, erythropoietin can be measured [2]. Within 4–5 days, new red blood cells are in circulation. Over a period of weeks to months, red blood cell mass increases in proportion to the degree of hypoxia, allowing for an improved oxygen uptake and delivery.

The lungs respond by utilizing normally unused portions. As the human body ascends to altitude, breathing is deeper and faster. Sensing a fall in pO_2, the carotid bodies located within the carotid artery signal the central respiratory center in the medulla to increase the rate of pulmonary ventilation. Increased ventilation decreases alveolar and blood concentrations of carbon dioxide, while trying to maintain a normal oxygen concentration. As carbon dioxide continues to fall, pH becomes alkalotic. This alkalosis will reach a maximum threshold in which the central respiratory center limits further increase in ventilation so as to prevent severe alkalosis.

Within 24–48 hours of persistent alkalosis, the kidneys begin to excrete bicarbonate in the urine. Bicarbonate diuresis reverses alkalosis and returns the body's pH to a normal physiological level. This adjusted pH stimulates the cycle to begin again as the ventilatory response again increases, resulting in alkalosis, which prompts the kidneys to excrete bicarbonate. Ventilatory compensation reaches a maximum after 4–7 days at the same altitude [3]. For each increase in altitude, the cycle of pulmonary-renal events recurs.

Other physiological changes at altitude include dehydration, edema, and periodic breathing. The lower humidity and air pressure cause the skin and lungs to lose water through evaporation at a faster rate, resulting in dehydration if meticulous attention is not paid to fluid intake. As water is lost, the body tries to maintain

Emergency Medical Services: Clinical Practice and Systems Oversight, Second Edition. Volume 1: Clinical Aspects of EMS.
Edited by David C. Cone, Jane H. Brice, Theodore R. Delbridge, and J. Brent Myers.

fluid balances by minimizing the excretion of water and sodium. Fluid leaks from capillaries into tissues, causing edema. Most noticeable in the face, hands, and feet, high altitude edema seems to affect women more commonly than men. The edema usually worsens with ascent and resolves with descent. Periodic breathing is common at high altitude. As the body attempts to regulate oxygen and carbon dioxide, breathing may fall into a cycle of decreased breathing, followed by complete apnea for 3–15 seconds. Once the $paCO_2$ has built up again, breathing resumes.

The circulatory system responds to altitude with an increase in sympathetic activity, which causes a mild increase in blood pressure. After 24 hours, bicarbonate diuresis begins to decrease pH as well as stroke volume. Fortunately, this decrease in blood volume rarely causes myocardial strain as echocardiographic studies demonstrate a lack of myocardial stress with a decreased stroke volume [4]. Additionally, with acclimatization, resting heart rate returns to normal, except at extreme altitudes. Paradoxical pulmonary hypoxic vasoconstriction shunts blood away from poorly aerated, injured, or diseased lung alveoli to healthy alveoli so as to maintain adequate oxygenation. When exposed to a high altitude environment, this phenomenon occurs throughout the lungs, leading to complete pulmonary vasoconstriction and mild pulmonary hypertension which is usually managed well by the body. Cerebral blood flow depends on the overall balance of hypoxic vasodilation and hypocapnia-induced vasoconstriction. This balance is rigorously tested in high altitude hypoxic environments. One study demonstrated a cerebral blood flow increase of 24% on abrupt ascent to 3,810 m and subsequent return to normal over 3–5 days [5]. With severe hypoxia at high altitude, this delicate autoregulation of vasodilation and vasoconstriction becomes impaired, leading to several pathophysiological states discussed below.

Acute mountain sickness

Pathophysiology

Acute mountain sickness (AMS) is the most common of the attitude illnesses. AMS has been described in altitudes as low as 2,500–2 700 m [1]. We do not fully understand the exact pathophysiology of AMS but it is thought that genetics may play a role. The pathophysiology of AMS includes minor hypoventilation, interstitial edema, and increased sympathetic drive [6,7].

Several theories regarding the cause of AMS are circulating. One theory suggests that AMS results from mild brain swelling. A study using brain imaging of patients with moderate-to-severe AMS showing white matter edema with an elevated intracranial pressure (ICP) supports this concept [8]. However, those with mild AMS do not have cerebral edema [9–14]. Hence, this hypothesis only partially explains AMS. Other investigators have postulated that an increase in ICP causes AMS. Although some studies demonstrate an increase of ICP in AMS using optic nerve sheath diameter and lumbar puncture pressure, other studies demonstrate no change in

pressure [14–17]. Thus, evidence that ICP is elevated in mild AMS remains limited. A third hypothesis, known as the tight fit hypothesis, theorizes that persons with smaller intracranial and intraspinal cerebral spinal fluid capacity are predisposed to develop AMS, because they cannot tolerate brain swelling compared to those who have more room to accommodate [18].

Symptoms

Most unacclimatized persons traveling to high altitude experience a mild form of AMS. The most common complaint is headache followed by fatigue, anorexia, and dizziness [14,19]. Headache is described as throbbing, bitemporal, and worse at night. Additionally, Valsalva maneuvers or bending over exacerbate the headache. Anorexia and nausea are common. Frequent waking from sleep, periodic breathing, and a feeling of suffocation are exaggerated in patients with AMS. Symptoms are often described as similar to an alcohol hangover [1]. Additionally, persons with AMS may complain of a deep inner chill, vomiting, dyspnea on exertion (although pulmonary symptoms vary widely), and lassitude. Symptoms typically begin within 24–48 hours of reaching altitude and resolve in 3–5 days at the same altitude.

There are no pathognomonic physical exam findings associated with AMS. Pulse may range from bradycardia to tachycardia [7,14,20]. Blood pressure may range from normal to postural hypotension. Rales may be present and oxygen saturation changes correlate poorly in the diagnosis of AMS [21]. Fundoscopic examination may reveal venous dilation as well as retinal hemorrhages, but are not diagnostic. Finally, a decrease in urine output demonstrating poor alkalotic diuresis may also be an early finding of AMS. It is always key to remember that there are *no* neurological deficits associated with AMS [14,22–25].

Treatment

Management depends on the severity of AMS. Mild AMS can be treated by halting further ascent to allow for acclimatization. This may take 3–4 days. Additionally, acetazolamide accelerates acclimatization by increasing bicarbonate diuresis. This may prevent AMS or accelerate treatment if given early enough [26,27]. Acetazolamide is typically given as 250 mg by mouth (PO) twice a day or as a single dose. Symptomatic treatment with analgesics such as ibuprofen (or other non-steroidal antiinflammatories), acetaminophen (650–1,000 mg PO), or aspirin (500–650 mg PO) should be considered [28]. Antiemetics such as ondasetron can be provided. Dexamethasone (4–8 mg PO, intramuscularly (IM) or intravenously (IV)) appears to treat symptoms of AMS by an unknown mechanism. However, it has been shown that symptoms increased when dexamethasone was removed in 24 hours [1]. AMS patients should avoid alcohol and other respiratory depressants to avoid further hypoxemia.

For moderate-to-severe AMS, descent is the treatment. One may descend as far as necessary, but a drop of 500–1,000 m is usually effective. Also, lightweight portable hyperbaric chambers mirror descent and can also effectively treat AMS. These hyperbaric chambers are manually inflated fabric pressure bags. Typically an inflation of 2 psi is roughly equivalent to a drop in altitude of 1,600 m, though the exact equivalent of psi to altitude drop depends on the initial altitude [29,30]. Additionally, oxygen given at 0.5–1 L/min by mask or nasal cannula (NC) is an effective treatment for moderate-to-severe AMS.

High altitude cerebral edema

Pathophysiology
High altitude cerebral edema (HACE) is life threatening. With increasing altitude and decreasing atmospheric pressure, capillaries begin to leak, causing edema. When fluid leaks into the closed space of the brain, HACE occurs. Studies demonstrate cerebrospinal fluid pressures of more than 300 millimeters of water and severe edema on cerebral imaging, and autopsies demonstrate petechial hemorrhages along with severe edema [10,31]. Much like AMS, there is a spectrum of HACE ranging from reversible HACE to severe, end-stage HACE. Reversible HACE demonstrates vasogenic edema whereas end-stage HACE produces gray matter (cytotoxic) edema [32]. As cytotoxic edema progresses, cerebral cells are separated from capillaries, resulting in failure to transport oxygen and nutrients to the cells, leading to brain cell death. Intracranial pressure increases as edema continues on a systemic level [33]. As compression of the brain develops, third and sixth nerve palsies may present, as well as other neurological symptoms [34].

Symptoms
Unlike AMS, HACE has a more dramatic presentation. The classic symptoms are ataxic gait, severe lassitude, and altered consciousness. Altered consciousness can range from confusion to drowsiness to coma. Additionally headache, nausea, and vomiting may occur. Other neurological presentations such as hallucinations, cranial nerve palsies, seizures, and paralysis have been described, but may not be as common [10,14,35–37]. The progression from AMS to HACE can be as quick as 12 hours, but typically develops in 1–3 days.

Treatment
Recognition and treatment of HACE must be swift. At first presentation of ataxia or altered mentation, descent should begin immediately. Treatment with dexamethasone (4–8 mg IV, IM, or PO) followed by 4 mg every 4–6 hours should also be started. Additionally, oxygen therapy via mask or NC at 4 L/min should be initiated and titrated to an oxygen saturation of greater than 90%. If the patient is comatose, rescuers should proceed to advanced airway management. Hyperventilation should be used with caution as hyperventilation in an already alkalotic patient can be catastrophic. Furosemide has been successfully used to reduce fluid overload in the cranial vault [14,38]. It is also reasonable to postulate that hypertonic saline and mannitol can reduce ICP, even without the appropriate studies. Coma for severe HACE can last from an average of 5.6 days to up to 3 weeks, with full recovery in about 2.4 weeks [9]. However, if not recognized and treated appropriately, death will occur.

High altitude pulmonary edema

Pathophysiology
Three physiological factors drive high altitude pulmonary edema (HAPE): excessive pulmonary hypertension, high-protein permeability leak, and persistent hypoxic exposure. Excessive pulmonary hypertension is a direct result of the paradoxic pulmonary hypoxic vasoconstriction. In the case of high altitude environments, the entire lung is hypoxic, resulting in diffuse vasoconstriction of the pulmonary capillaries. The degree of constriction varies among individuals. While pulmonary hypertension is one of the three necessary factors of HAPE, it is not necessarily the cause, as all persons exposed to high altitude environment have some form of pulmonary hypertension. It is hypothesized that uneven hypoxic pulmonary vasoconstriction results in overshunting of blood to relatively non-constricted vessels. This leads to high pressures and eventual capillary leakage, causing lung edema [39–42].

Symptoms
The most common cause of death related to high altitude illness is HAPE. Victims are typically young athletic males with a rapid ascent from sea level who may not have had HAPE on previous high altitude adventures. Typically, HAPE occurs within the first 2–4 days of ascent higher than 2,500 m, and most commonly on the second night [15]. The earliest signs may be decreased exercise performance and increased recovery time. Additionally, fatigue, weakness, and dyspnea on exertion become more obvious. Persistent dry cough develops with other signs of increasing hypoxia, including cyanotic nail beds and lips. AMS occurs in 50% of individuals with HAPE [39]. Symptoms are worse at night and eventually tachycardia and tachypnea develop at rest. More severe forms of HAPE result from increasing respiratory distress.

Treatment
Treatment for HAPE depends on the severity of the illness. The earlier HAPE is recognized, the better the outcome. The best treatment is *early* descent of only 500–1,000 m. After 2–3 days at this altitude, the patient may re-ascend. Supplemental high-flow oxygen (4 L/min or more) for more than 24 hours is also essential. If descent is too slow or delayed, administration of high-flow oxygen is life saving. Climbers should not wait for rescue and should descend immediately. Oftentimes waiting for help has proven fatal.

Other treatments include resistance on expiration (expiratory positive airway pressure) or continuous positive airway pressure, which can act as a temporizing measure [43]. If unavailable, pursed lip breathing can be effective. Additionally, diuretics such as furosemide (80 mg every 12 hours) may be used [14]. Phosphodiesterase-5 inhibitors (e.g. sildenafil) demonstrate potential for prevention for HAPE, but have not been approved for treatment [44–46]. Calcium channel blockers such as nifedipine (30 mg slow release every 12–24 hours) reduce pulmonary vascular resistance while improving arterial oxygenation [47]. However, clinical improvement remains minimal with diuretics and calcium channel blockers when compared to descent and supplemental oxygen.

Once at a more appropriate elevation, recovery is the rule before any re-ascent can be attempted [48]. Typically, bed rest and oxygen sufficient to keep oxygen saturation greater than 90% are key, and medications are rarely necessary. If treated promptly and correctly, intubation is rarely required. Patients should be warned that recovery may take up to 2 weeks and return to normal activity should be gradual.

Considerations for the medical director

Education for altitude illnesses is key for any EMS physician or medical director. Instruction to medics, first responders, rescuers, and potential patients should be emphasized. Education should be focused on recognition of altitude illness, especially early signs of HACE and HAPE. Differentiation of temporizing treatments, including acetazolamide, from definitive life-saving treatments, like descent, must also be stressed.

Climbers themselves should also be made aware. Although direct education for all potential patients is impossible, indirect education through pamphlets, websites, and frequently asked questions can be made readily available. Instruction should also focus on ensuring frequent contact with appropriate parties, such as a base camp or climbing partner, as well as dispelling treatment myths, such as that simple hydration can treat all climbing pathologies. Identification of climbers can be acquired through the National Park Service, which requires registration of individuals who want to climb to high altitudes.

Finally, interagency cooperation and training with multiple services must be considered by the medical director. Frequent communication and training with rescue teams, first responders, EMS agencies, and hospitals can further facilitate a smoother response should such illnesses present. Input from a variety of personnel may aid in the modification or creation of flexible protocols that allow responders to think critically while simultaneously providing definitive end goals. These exercises can also help the system anticipate unforeseen barriers such as weather, resources, and communications. Such interdepartmental options can facilitate the identification and acquisition of pertinent equipment, from supplemental oxygen to portable hyperbaric chambers, needed for response.

Conclusion

Travel to high altitude locations can be fun and incredibly gratifying. However, there remains a real risk to health and potentially life when exposed to such extreme environments. Hypoxia is the main insult the body endures. The delicate balance of physiological compensation for hypoxia aids in the comprehension of pathology that may follow.

Of all pathologies described, AMS is the most benign. However, it must be remembered that mild AMS can evolve into severe life-threatening HACE. Like HACE, HAPE can kill very quickly. HAPE remains the most common cause of death of all high altitude illnesses. Definitive treatment for AMS, HACE, and HAPE is descent of about 500–1,000 m as well as supplemental oxygen. Other medical treatments are available, but only as temporizing measures.

There are many factors that a medical director has to be concerned with, but chiefly the EMS system's knowledge of altitude illnesses in conjunction with cooperation between rescue teams, first responders, and hospitals play an important role in the treatment of these patients. The risk of high altitude illness increases as more people participate in travel and recreational activities in these environments. The challenges of high altitude illness are many, but preparation through education and training can help save lives and keep such adventures fun, entertaining, and safe.

References

1 Auerbach PS, Hackett PH, Roach RC. High-altitude medicine and physiology. In: Auerbach PS, Hackett PH, Roach RC (eds) *Wilderness Medicine*, 6th edn. Philadelphia: Elsevier Mosby, 2012, pp.2–33.

2 Semenza GL. Regulation of erythropoietin production: new insights into molecular mechanisms of oxygen homeostasis. *Hematol Oncol Clin North Am* 1994;8:863–4.

3 Huang SY, Alexander JK, Grover RF, et al. Hypocapnia and sustained hypoxia blunt ventilation on arrival at high altitude. *J Appl Physiol* 1984;56:602–6.

4 Suarez J, Alexander JK, Houston CS. Enhanced left ventricular ventricular systolic performance at high altitude during Operation Everest II. *Am J Cardiol* 1987;60:137–42.

5 Severinghaus JW, Chiodi H, Eger EI 2nd, Brandstater B, Hornbein TF. Cerebral blood flow in man at high altitude: role of cerebrospinal fluid pH in normalization of flow in chronic hypoxia. *Circ Res* 1966;19:274–82.

6 Bärtsch P, Maggiorini M, Schobersberger W, et al. Enhanced exercise-induced rise of aldosterone and vasopressin preceding mountain sickness. *J Appl Physiol* 1991;71:136–43.

7 Bärtsch P, Shaw S, Francioli M, Gnädinger MP, Weidmann P. Atrial natriuretic peptide in acute mountain sickness. *J Appl Physiol* 1988;65:1929–37.

8 Fischer R, Vollmar C, Thiere M, et al. No evidence of cerebral edema in severe acute mountain sickness. *Cephalalgia* 2004;24:66–71.

9 Hackett PH, Yarnell PR, Hill R, Reynard K, Heit J, McCormick J. High-altitude cerebral edema evaluated with magnetic resonance imaging: clinical correlation and pathophysiology. *JAMA* 1998;280:1920–5.

10 Houston CS, Dickinson JG. Cerebral form of high altitude illness. *Lancet* 1975;2:758–61.

11 Kronenberg RS, Safar PA, Wright F, et al. Pulmonary artery pressure and alveolar gas exchange in man during acclimatization to 12, 470 ft. *J Clin Invest* 1971;50:827–37.

12 Levine BD, Yoshimura K, Kobayashi T, Fukushima M, Shibamoto T, Ueda G. Dexamethasone in the treatment of acute mountain sickness. *N Engl J Med* 1989;321:1707–13.

13 Matsuzawa Y, Kobayashi T, Fujimoto K, Shinozaki S, Yoshikawa S. Cerebral edema in acute mountain sickness. In: Ueda G, Reeves JT, Sekiguchi M (eds) *High Altitude Medicine*. Matsumoto, Japan: Shinshu University Press, 1992, pp.300–4.

14 Singh I, Khanna PK, Srivastava MC, Lal M, Roy SB, Subramanyam CS. Acute mountain sickness. *N Engl J Med* 1969;280:175–84.

15 Fagenholz PJ, Gutman JA, Murray AF, Noble VE, Camargo CA Jr, Harris NS. Evidence for increased intracranial pressure in high altitude pulmonary edema. *High Alt Med Biol* 2007;8:331–6.

16 Kallenberg K, Bailey DM, Christ S, et al. Magnetic resonance imaging evidence of cytotoxic edema in acute mountain sickness. *J Cereb Blood Flow Metab* 2007;27:1064–71.

17 Sutherland AI, Morris DS, Owen CG, Bron AJ, Roach RC. Optic nerve sheath diameter, intracranial pressure and acute mountain sickness on Mount Everest: a longitudinal cohort study. *Br J Sports Med* 2008;42:183–8.

18 Shapiro K, Marmarou A, Shulman K. Characterization of clinical CSF dynamics and neural axis compliance using the pressure volume index: I. The normal pressure volume index. *Ann Neurol* 1980;7:508–14.

19 Honigman B, Theis MK, Koziol-McLain J, et al. Acute mountain sickness in a general tourist population at moderate altitudes. *Ann Intern Med* 1993;118:587–92.

20 O'Connor T, Dubowitz G, Bickler PE. Pulse oximetry in the diagnosis of acute mountain sickness. *High Alt Med Biol* 2004;5:341–8.

21 Maggiorini M, Bühler B, Walter M, Oelz O. Prevalence of acute mountain sickness in the Swiss Alps. *BMJ* 1990;301:853–5.

22 Bärtsch P, Shaw S, Wiedmann P, Franciolli M, Maggiorini M, Oelz O. Aldosterone, antidiuretic hormone and atrial natriuretic peptide in acute mountain sickness. In: Sutton JR, Coates G, Houston CS (eds) *Hypoxia and Mountain Medicine*. Burlington, VT: Queen City Press, 1992.

23 Hackett PH, Rennie ID, Hofmeister SE, Grover RF, Grover EB, Reeves JT. Fluid retention and relative hypoventilation in acute mountain sickness. *Respiration* 1982;43:321–9.

24 Roach RC, Riboni K, Maes DP, et al. Fluid redistribution and acute mountain sickness (AMS) (abstract). *FASEB J* 2000;14:A82.

25 Swenson ER. High altitude diuresis: fact or fancy. In: Houston CS, Coates G (eds) *Hypoxia: Women at Altitude*. Burlington, VT: Queen City Publishers, 1997, pp.272–83.

26 Grissom CK, Roach RC, Sarnquist FH, Hackett PH. Acetazolamide in the treatment of acute mountain sickness: clinical efficacy and effect on gas exchange. *Ann Intern Med* 1992;116:461–5.

27 Maggiorini M, Merki B, Pallavicini E, et al. Acetazolamide and almitrine in acute mountain sickness (AMS) treatment (abstract).

In: Sutton JR, Houston CS, Coates G (eds) *Hypoxia and the Brain*. Burlington, VT: Queen City Press, 1995.

28 Broome JR, Stoneham MD, Beeley JM, Milledge JS, Hughes AS. High altitude headache: treatment with ibuprofen. *Aviat Space Environ Med* 1994;65:19–20.

29 Kasic JF, Yaron M, Nicholas RA, Lickteig JA, Roach R. Treatment of acute mountain sickness: hyperbaric versus oxygen therapy. *Ann Emerg Med* 1991;20:1109–12.

30 Roach RC, Hackett PH. Hypobaria and high altitude illness. In: Sutton JR, Coates G, Houston CS (eds) *Hypoxia and Mountain Medicine*. Burlington, VT: Queen City Press, 1992.

31 Wilson R. Acute high altitude illness in mountaineers and problems of rescue. *Ann Intern Med* 1973;78:421–8.

32 Klatzo I. Pathophysiological aspects of brain edema. *Acta Neuropathol (Berl)* 1987;72:236–9.

33 McGillicudy JE: Cerebral protection. Pathophysiology and treatment of increased intracranial pressure. *Chest* 1985;87: 85–93.

34 Ropper AH. Raised intracranial pressure in neurologic diseases. *Semin Neurol* 1984;4:397.

35 Dickinson JG. High altitude cerebral edema: cerebral acute mountain sickness. *Semin Respir Med* 1983;5:151.

36 Hamilton AJ, Cymmerman A, Black PM. High altitude cerebral edema. *Neurosurgery* 1986;19:841–9.

37 Wu T, Ding S, Liu J, et al. Ataxia: an early indicator in high altitude cerebral edema. *High Alt Med Biol* 2006;7:275–80.

38 Dickinson J. *Acute Mountain Sickness*. Oxford: Oxford University Press, 1981.

39 Hultgren HN. High-altitude pulmonary edema: current concepts. *Annu Rev Med* 1996;47:267–84.

40 Hultgren HN, Honigman B, Theis K, Nicholas D. High-altitude pulmonary edema at a ski resort. *West J Med* 1996;164:222–7.

41 Hultgren HN, Lopez CE, Lundberg E, Miller H. Physiologic studies of pulmonary edema at high altitude. *Circulation* 1964; 29:393–408.

42 Hultgren HN, Spickard WB, Hellriegel K, Houston CS. High altitude pulmonary edema. *Medicine* 1961;40:289–313.

43 Schoene RB, Roach RC, Hackett PH, Harrison G, Mills JW Jr. High altitude pulmonary edema and exercise at 4400 meters on Mt. McKinley: effect of expiratory positive airway pressure. *Chest* 1985;87:330–3.

44 Ghofrani HA, Reichenberger F, Kohstall MG, et al. Sildenafil increased exercise capacity during hypoxia at low altitudes and at Mount Everest base camp: a randomized, double-blind, placebo-controlled crossover trial. *Ann Intern Med* 2004;141:169–77.

45 Ricart A, Maristany J, Fort N, Leal C, Pagés T, Viscor G. Effects of sildenafil on the human response to acute hypoxia and exercise. *High Alt Med Biol* 2005;6:43–9.

46 Richalet JP, Gratadour P, Robach P, et al. Sildenafil inhibits altitude-induced hypoxemia and pulmonary hypertension. *Am J Respir Crit Care Med* 2005;171:275–81.

47 Bärtsch P, Maggiorini M, Ritter M, Noti C, Vock P, Oelz O. Prevention of high-altitude pulmonary edema by nifedipine. *N Engl J Med* 1991;325:1284–9.

48 Zimmerman GA, Crapo RO. Adult respiratory distress syndrome secondary to high altitude pulmonary edema. *West J Med* 1980; 133:335–7.

CHAPTER 51

Effects of flight

David P. Thomson

Introduction

For humans to fly, they must adapt to a very dynamic environment. The Wright brothers were successful because they understood that stability was not possible. To stay in the air, the pilot and aircraft had to be able to adjust to the changing conditions [1]. To care for critically ill and injured patients in this setting requires a basic knowledge of both the forces affecting an aircraft and the forces that affect humans within that aircraft. There are the classic forces of aerodynamics: lift, gravity, thrust, and drag. The forces affecting humans also include vibration, barometric pressure, acceleration, spatial disorientation, and thermal stresses, among others.

Aerodynamic forces

In order to understand how the flight environment affects patients and air medical providers, the EMS physician must have a basic understanding of aerodynamic forces and terminology.

For an aircraft to fly, there must be a source of lift. For the fixed wing airplane, that source is the wing. In the helicopter, the rotor blade supplies the lift. In both cases, the wing or rotor passing through the air encounters two phenomena. Bernoulli's principle states that when air is accelerated, it has a lower pressure. A wing with a curved upper surface and a straight lower surface causes air traveling over the upper surface to speed up to catch its counterpart moving beneath the wing. The pressure on the upper surface is reduced compared to that of the lower surface, producing lift.

Helicopters often have essentially symmetrical airfoils for their rotors; thus the speed of the air relative to the rotor is the same for the upper and the lower surface. For these rotors, and for the wings of many aerobatic aircraft, lift depends on the angle of attack. This is the angle that develops between the chord line (the imaginary line formed between the most forward point in the leading edge and the farthest aft point in the trailing edge) and the direction of the air.

Children who put their hands outside the car window and feel the air move their arm up and down take advantage of this phenomenon.

The density of air determines how much lift a given wing or rotor can generate. Hot air does not have as much density as does cold air. Air pressure also decreases with altitude. The combination of the actual altitude above sea level and the effect of the temperature is expressed as the density altitude. Thus an aircraft that might be able to generate enough lift to take off in the winter at JFK airport (at sea level) might not be able to take off in Denver, the Mile High City, in August.

Gravity, or weight, is the force that opposes lift. For aircraft, the weight of the aircraft, its fuel, and its passengers or load determines the effects of gravity. An aircraft that is too heavily loaded cannot overcome the effects of gravity with the effects of lift. Aircraft are tested to determine their useful load, which is the remainder when the weight of the aircraft and its necessary supplies (e.g. fuel, oil) is subtracted from the amount of lift that can be generated.

Thrust is the ability of the engine, or the main rotor, to move the aircraft through the air. A propeller, or a jet engine, provides the thrust for airplanes. For helicopters, the main rotor provides this thrust.

The Wright brothers were among the first to understand that an aircraft propeller is essentially a rapidly spinning wing. The term airscrew has been used to describe how a propeller pulls the aircraft through the air. Just as a screw pulls itself through a piece of wood, the propeller bites into the air and pulls the airplane forward through the air. This pulling allows the wing to pass through the air and generate lift.

Drag is the force that opposes the aircraft's movement through the air. Thin, smooth, gradually curved shapes move through a fluid more easily than boxy shapes. If one has rowed a jon boat, with its squared bow and flat bottom, then paddled a long, slender kayak, it is easy to appreciate the effects of drag. A slender, tapered business jet experiences much less drag than a biplane.

Emergency Medical Services: Clinical Practice and Systems Oversight, Second Edition. Volume 1: Clinical Aspects of EMS.
Edited by David C. Cone, Jane H. Brice, Theodore R. Delbridge, and J. Brent Myers.
© 2015 NAEMSP. Published 2015 by John Wiley & Sons, Inc. Companion Website: www.wiley.com\go\cone\naemsp

Effects on humans

The first recorded ascents of humans into the air occurred in the 1780s, with the French balloonists, Montgolfier, Charles, and de Rosier. Charles, using a hydrogen-filled balloon, was the first to note that when he ascended rapidly he became exceptionally cold and that when he descended he developed ear pain. Others ascended even higher, with Glaisher and Coxwell noting the effects that occurred when they climbed to 9,450 meters, nearly perishing in the attempt. Even before powered flight was achieved, the effects of altitude on the organism had become apparent [2].

Atmospheric effects

The atmosphere has a significant effect on humans in flight. Temperature decreases with altitude at a rate of about 2 °C (3.5 °F) per 1,000 feet – the adiabatic lapse rate [3]. For patients and medical crews this phenomenon can become important, as even in helicopters an ascent to 5,000 feet above ground level is not uncommon, resulting in an uncomfortable temperature change. While the Commission on Accreditation of Medical Transport Systems (CAMTS) standard 02.05.15 requires "climate control [4]," knowing the extent of the changes that may occur during a flight is an important consideration in patient packaging.

Barometric pressure at 18,000 feet/5,500 meters is half of that found at sea level, resulting in a doubling of the gas volume, in accordance with Boyle's law [5]. The most familiar manifestation of this phenomenon is the ear discomfort that many people experience as an airliner descends for landing. Barotitis media and barosinusitis may occur because of these gas volume changes and should be taken seriously as they can incapacitate crew members during critical phases of flight [6]. Although the middle ear and the sinuses are dramatic examples, any gas-filled structure or device can be affected. A pneumothorax or an endotracheal balloon may expand or contract depending on the pressure/altitude change.

While common sense might suggest that any patient transported by air with a pneumothorax should have a thoracostomy, the research is not as clear. A case series from Somalia is illustrative: two patients, treated with needle thoracostomy, survived a trip at 3,000 meters without difficulty. A third patient, who was transported at a lower cabin altitude, also survived his trip but later succumbed to his wounds. The latter patient had extensive adhesions secondary to tuberculosis, making thoracic drainage more difficult [7]. Although they caution the reader against air transport of a pneumothorax, the writers of another case report note that the patient underwent a 2-hour airplane flight without complication, the pneumothorax being discovered incidentally after her arrival at the receiving burn center [8].

Placing a needle or a tube in a patient's chest is not without risk in itself. In an elegant study from the University of Oklahoma, an experimental model of pneumothorax was flown in a helicopter and the volume changes measured at 1,000 and 1,500 feet above ground level (AGL), altitudes commonly encountered in helicopter EMS (HEMS) transport. The authors noted a 1.5% increase in pneumothorax size per 500 ft increment. They also suggest that the use of oxygen may mitigate some of the effects [9]. It appears that prophylactic placement of a tube, even in a known pneumothorax, may not be needed. Pneumocephalus and penetrating eye trauma also produce worries regarding pressure changes, but there is little literature surrounding the effects of flight on these [10].

Concerns have been raised about endotracheal tube cuff pressures exceeding 30 cmH_2O and producing tracheal mucosal injury. A Swiss group adjusted the pressure of the cuff prior to departure, and then measured the pressures during flight, noting that almost all of their patients' cuff pressures exceeded 30 cmH_2O during flight [11]. A group from France notes that it is their practice to fill the cuff with saline when treating intubated patients in a hyperbaric chamber, suggesting that this may be useful for helicopter transfers [12]. However, few follow this practice in air medical transport. On descent, the converse problem can become apparent: the cuff can contract and the patient may develop an air leak [13]. Regular monitoring of cuff pressures with a manometer is recommended.

The pressure decrease associated with altitude also produces hypoxia, with its obvious effects on both the patient and providers (see Volume 1, Chapter 50). Pulse oximetry and routine use of supplemental oxygen can be employed to mitigate these effects, but providers should be particularly cautious in managing patients with cardiovascular compromise or anemia.

Aircraft effects

The type of aircraft can have a significant effect on both patient and crew. A smooth flight in a newer jet aircraft may produce little fatigue for the passengers. A helicopter flight, even through smooth air, subjects the passengers to constant vibrations of several different frequencies [14], which can have a pronounced effect on crew fatigue [15]. Some have postulated that back pain, a common problem among helicopter pilots, is in part due to vibration [16]. Vibration may affect the spinal muscles [17–19], as well as the vertebrae, depending on the frequencies produced by the individual aircraft type [20]. Vibration may also affect monitors, pumps, and other patient care devices. These devices, and the cables and wires associated with them, must be inspected regularly.

In addition to the issue of vibration is the problem of noise. From the perspective of human physiology, these are closely related [21]. Aircraft engines, propellers, transmissions, and rotors generate significant levels of noise in many different frequency bands [22]. In commercial transport airplanes the engines are at a distance from the cabin, and the pressure hull of the fuselage tends to attenuate engine and wind noise. Modern high-bypass jet engines also tend to produce less noise [23]. Most helicopters, however, have little structure to attenuate the noise, and the engines, transmission, and rotor system are located directly above the passenger cabin [24]. Vibration and noise contribute to fatigue and may be part of the accident chain [21]. Helicopter companies have recognized the importance of this problem and have embarked on studies to better address this issue [25]. At the present time, the best solution is the use of headphones or helmets. Helmets are required by CAMTS for helicopter operations [4]. Both the HGU-56/P and the HGU-86/P helmets, worn by the US military and many HEMS programs, provide substantial hearing protection [26]. Testing of other helmets has yielded similar results [27].

Aircraft motion may have significant effects on patients and crew members. Most medical aircraft are not flown in a manner that produces substantial G forces [28]. The one notable exception to this may occur during takeoff and landing in fixed wing aircraft, where the acceleration may cause patients, crew, and, most importantly, equipment to shift. Crews must package patients and secure equipment accordingly. If the patient has a condition that is likely to be affected by the aircraft movement (e.g. fractures), the crew should discuss this with the pilot to see if the takeoff or landing profile can be modified.

Motion sickness is the most commonly reported side-effect of aircraft travel. Unusual head positions, unexpected turbulence, and the need to concentrate on tasks in the aircraft cabin contribute to this phenomenon. Patients, especially those with conditions that preclude their ability to look out a window or who have nauseogenic medications or conditions, may benefit from prophylactic administration of antinausea medications prior to departure. Crew members may occasionally require antiemetics in order to remain functional. Sedating medications such as the phenothiazine-based antiemetics or antihistamines such as dimenhydrinate should be avoided if at all possible by crew members. Ondansetron, especially in its quick-dissolving form, may be useful for crew members. Other motion sickness remedies, such as ginger root or Sea Bands (Sea-Band Ltd, www.sea-band.com) are used by many who seek natural remedies for this malady. Some crew members may be able to overcome motion sickness by looking outside when patient care duties permit.

The conflict between what the instruments say and what the pilot's vestibular system is experiencing produces spatial disorientation, a sensation that is difficult to overcome. Spatial disorientation is a particular problem for pilots. The most profound and deadly manifestation of spatial disorientation occurs during inadvertent or unexpected flight into instrument conditions. Dark night conditions can produce this same problem, in which the pilot cannot distinguish ground from sky. General Jimmy Doolittle, best known for the "Doolittle Raid" on Tokyo in 1942, demonstrated that aircraft could be flown solely with reference to instruments in September 1929 [3]. Since that time thousands of pilots have become "instrument rated." Nevertheless, pilots who crash after unexpectedly encountering instrument flight conditions remain a serious problem [29]. Repetitive practice, either in a simulator or with a safety pilot acting as a lookout for the hooded training pilot, allows a pilot to safely manage spatial disorientation. Pilots must keep "instrument current" by performing a series of instrument procedures every 6 months.

Flicker vertigo is a problem that primarily affects helicopter crews. Most noticeable on a sunny day, the rotors produce a visual flicker as they spin. Helicopter rotor systems often produce flicker within a range that produces vertigo (4–20 Hz) [30]. When motion detected by the eyes is in conflict with that perceived by the vestibular system, nausea, or at least a sopite syndrome, can be induced [31–34]. Flicker vertigo produces nausea and disorientation; in rare cases seizures have been reported. Visors or other headgear that limit the view of the rotor system may be helpful in preventing flicker vertigo. Night vision goggles do not appear to enhance or decrease this problem [30].

Other concerns in the flight environment

Many HEMS services in the United States use night vision goggles (NVGs) when operating after dark, a practice encouraged by the National Transportation Safety Board [35]. NVGs enhance the available light and present what is essentially a black and white picture in front of the crew member's eyes. Although NVGs improve the ability of pilots and crews to see at night, they are not without their problems. They have a markedly reduced field of view, and their visual acuity is equivalent to approximately 20/200 [36]. The ANVIS goggles weigh about 800 grams including their mount [37]. When a counterweight is added to the occiput, the NVG, helmet and counterweight weigh about 3.7 kg [38]. This results in neck pain being a common complaint among helicopter crews [39]. Because of these concerns, it is important that helmets fit the crew member well [40].

The air medical service has been described as one of the most dangerous jobs in the United States [41]. In order to mitigate risks, crews wear helmets, flame-retardant uniforms, and boots. Like many other forms of personal protective garb, this flight equipment can make it difficult for individuals to cool during hot and humid operations. Attention must be paid to fluid intake to prevent heat injuries.

Conversely, cold weather operations can pose a threat as many cold weather garments are made of synthetic materials that melt when exposed to a heat source. Flight crew members should wear natural fiber underwear and socks (i.e. cotton, wool, silk). Boots and outerwear should be made of leather or flame-retardant fabrics, such as Nomex®.

Conclusion

The provision of emergency care in the aerospace environment poses a number of challenges. Providers must be mindful of the unique characteristics of the airplane or helicopter in which they are caring for their patient. Pressure and temperature changes can significantly affect the patient and the crew. Noise, vibration, and other aircraft effects will alter the way in which care can be delivered. Special consideration must be given to protect the patient and the crew from the environment and the emergencies that can arise as the result of flight.

References

1 Culick FEC, Dunmore S. *On Great White Wings: The Wright Brothers and the Race for Flight*. New York: Hyperion, 2001.

2 DeHart RL. The historical perspective. In: *Fundamentals of Aerospace Medicine*, 2nd edn. Baltimore, MD: Williams & Wilkins, 1996, pp.3–22.

3 Sanderson J. *Aviation Fundamentals*. Englewood Cliffs, NJ: Jeppesen Sanderson Inc, 1991.

4 Commission on Accreditation of Medical Transport Systems. *Commission on Accreditation of Medical Transport Systems*, October 2012. Available at: http://camtsshelley.homestead.com/Approved_Stds_9th_Edition_for_website_2-13.pdf

5 Hart KR. The passenger and the patient in flight. In: DeHart RL (ed) *Fundamentals of Aerospace Medicine*, 2nd edn. Baltimore, MD: Williams & Wilkins, 1996, pp.667–83.

6 Rayman RB. Otolaryngology. In: Rayman RB (ed) *Rayman's Clinical Aviation Medicine*, 5th edn. New York: Castle Connolly Graduate Medical Publishing, 2006, pp.297–307.

7 Haid MM, Paladini P, Maccherini M, et al. Air transport and the fate of pneumothorax in pleural adhesions. *Thorax* 1992;47:833–4.

8 Hurren JS, Dunn KW. Spontaneous pneumothorax in association with a major burn. *Burns* 1994;20:178–9.

9 Knotts D, Arthur AO, Holder P, et al. Pneumothorax volume expansion in helicopter emergency medical services transport. *Air Med J* 2013;32:138–43.

10 Milligan JE, Jones CN, Helm DR, Munford BJ. The principles of aeromedical retrieval of the critially ill. *Trends Anaesthes Crit Care* 2011;1:22–6.

11 Bassi M, Zuercher M, Erne JJ, Ummenhofer W. Endotracheal tube intracuff pressure during helicopter transport. *Ann Emerg Med* 2010;56:89–93.

12 Bessereau J, Coulange M, Jacquin L, et al. Endotracheal tube intra-cuff pressure during helicopter transport: letter to the editor. *Ann Emerg Med* 2010;56:583.

13 Miyashiro R, Yamamoto L. Endotracheal tube and laryngeal mask airway cuff pressures can exceed critical values during ascent to higher altitude. *Pediatr Emerg Care* 2011;27:367–70.

14 Pearson JT, Goodall RM, Lyndon I. Active control of helicopter vibration. *Comput Control Engine J* 1994;5:277–84.

15 Bateman RP, White RP Jr. Helicopter crew evaluations on the effects of vibration on performance. *Proceedings of the Human Factors and Ergonomics Society Annual Meeting* 1985;29:550–3.

16 Bongers PM, Hulshof CT, Dijkstra L, et al. Back pain and exposure to whole body vibration in helicopter pilots. *Ergonomics* 1990;33:1007–26.

17 De Oliveira CG, Simpson DM, Nadal J. Lumbar back muscle activity of helicopter pilots and whole-body vibration. *J Biomech* 2001;34:1301–15.

18 De Oliveira CG, Nadal J. Back muscle EMG of helicopter pilots in flight: effects of fatigue, vibration, and posture. *Aviat Space Environ Med* 2004;75:317–22.

19 Bazrgari B, Shirazi-Adl A, Kasra M. Seated whole body vibrations with high-magnitude accelerations – relative roles of inertia and muscle forces. *J Biomech* 2008;41:2639–46.

20 De Oliveira CG, Nadal J. Transmissibility of helicopter vibration in the spines of pilots in flight. *Aviat Space Environ Med* 2005;76:576–80.

21 Von Gierke HE, Nixon CW. Vibration, noise and communication. In: DeHart RL. *Fundamentals of Aerospace Medicine*, 2nd edn. Baltimore, MD: Williams & Wilkins, 1996, pp.261–308.

22 Mucchi E, Vecchio A. Acoustical signature analysis of a helicopter cabin in steady-state and run up operational conditions. *Measurement* 2010;43:283–93.

23 Pike AC. Helicopter noise certification. *Acoustics* 1988;23:213–30.

24 Padfield RR. *Learning to Fly Helicopters*. New York: TAB Books, 1992.

25 Caillet J, Marrot F, Unia Y, Aubourg PA. Comprehensive approach for noise reduction in helicopter cabins. *Aero Sci Technol* 2012;23:17–25.

26 Gordon E, Ahroon WA, Hill ME. *Sound Attenuation of Rotary-Wing Aviation Helmets with Oregon Aero Earcup Replacement Products*. Ft Belvoir, VA: US Army Aeromedical Research Laboratory, 2006.

27 Pääkkönen R, Kuronen P. Noise attenuation of helmets and headsets used by Finnish Air Force pilots. *Appl Acoust* 1996;49:373–82.

28 Holleran RS. *ASTNA Patient Transport Principles and Practice*, 4th edn. St Louis, MO: Elsevier Mosby, 2010.

29 AOPA Air Safety Institute. *22nd Joseph T. Nall Report*. Frederick, MD: AOPA Air Safety Institute, 2010.

30 Rash CE. Awareness of causes and symptoms of flicker vertigo can limit ill effects. *Human Fact Aviat Med* 2004;51:1–6.

31 Bubka A, Bonato F, Urmey S, Mycewicz D. Rotation velocity change and motion sickness in an optokinetic drum. *Aviat Space Environ Med* 2006;77:811–15.

32 Bos JE, Bles W. Motion sickness induced by optokinetic drums. *Aviat Space Environ Med* 2004;75:172–4.

33 Johnson D. *Introduction to and Review of Simulator Sickness Research*. Arlington, VA: US Army Research Institute for the Behaviorial and Social Sciences, Rotary Wing Aviation Research Unit, 2005.

34 Kiniorski ET, Weider SK, Finley JR, et al. Sopite symptoms in the optokinetic drum. *Aviat Space Environ Med* 2004;75:872–5.

35 Sumwalt RL. *National Transportation Safety Board*. Available at: www.ntsb.gov/doclib/speeches/sumwalt/sumwalt050411.pdf

36 Salazar G, Temme L, Antonio JC. Civilian use of night vision goggles. *Aviat Space Environ Med* 2003;74:79–84.

37 Own the Night. Available at: www.ownthenight.com/catalog/i105.html

38 Harrison MF, Neary JP, Albert WJ, et al. Physiological effects of night vision goggle counterweights on neck musculature of military helicopter pilots. *Mil Med* 2007;172:864–70.

39 Parush A, Gauthier MS, Arseneau L, Tang D. The human factors of night vision goggles: perceptual, cognitive, and physical factors. *Rev Human Fact Ergonom* 2011;7:238–79.

40 Van den Oord MH, Steinman Y, Sluiter JK, Frings-Dresen MH. The effects of an optimised helmet fit on neck load and neck pain during military helicopter flights. *Appl Ergonom* 2012;43:958–64.

41 Blumen IJ. National Transportation Safety Board. Available at: www.ntsb.gov/news/events/2009/hems_public_hearing/presentations/NTSB-2009-8a-Blumen-revised-final-version.pdf

CHAPTER 52

Diving injury

Anthony J. Frank Jr

Historical perspective

Water comprises 70% of the surface of our planet. It is only natural that given this large percentage of our home, human beings would be drawn to explore this environment. It is currently estimated that there are 1.2 million active scuba divers worldwide [1] and that approximately 200,000 new divers are certified every year [2]. Although diving is considered to be a relatively safe sport, operating in an environment with unique hazards where life-supportive breathing gases must be carried leaves little margin for error. Comparing the total hours involved, diving is estimated to be 96 times more dangerous than operating a motor vehicle [3].

Introduction

Emergency medical services physicians and medical directors of EMS systems need not be certified scuba divers, but will benefit from developing a fundamental knowledge of dive-related physiology and hazards. There are four main categories of diving injury: injuries on the surface, injuries of descent, injuries at depth, and injuries of ascent. This chapter deals with injuries below the surface.

Due to the high density of water, small changes in depth cause significant changes in the pressure exerted on an object. At the surface, a body is subjected to the weight of the earth's atmosphere, which is equal to 1 atmosphere absolute (ATA). During descent, for every 33 feet of seawater (fsw) or 34 feet of freshwater (ffw) traveled below the surface, pressure increases by 1 atmosphere (atm). Typical units of measure for pressure include: 33 fsw = 34 ffw = 1 atm = 760 mmHg = 760 torr = 14.7 psi. The majority of recreational diving occurs between 33 and 120 fsw (2 to <5 ATA).

The gas laws

To appreciate the physiology of diving injury, EMS physicians must be familiar with Boyle's law, Dalton's law, and Henry's law.

Boyle's law

Governing the physiology of barotrauma and recompression therapy, Boyle's law states that given a constant temperature, the volume and pressure of an ideal gas are inversely related. It also deals with conditions related to changes in pressure in hollow, air-filled organs and structures in the body.

As an example, during descent the pressure is doubled; on a descent from the surface (1 ATA) to a depth of 33 fsw (2 ATA), the volume of a gas is halved (Figure 52.1). The law is typically stated as:

$$P_1 V_1 = P_2 V_2$$

As a diver is descending in the water column, the volume of air in gas-filled organs will decrease. If the volume of air in the lungs at the surface is V then at 33 fsw the volume will be 1/2 V, at 66 fsw 1/3 V, etc.

If using compressed air, as in scuba diving, when a breath is taken at 66 fsw, lung volume returns to V. If ascent occurs at this point without exhalation, as in an unconscious diver, the lung volume will expand to 1.5 V at 33 fsw and 3 V at the surface, with potential for barotrauma.

Liquids and liquid-filled organs are non-compressible. The body tissues are composed primarily of water and thus there is no change in volume with pressure increases and decreases.

Dalton's law

Dalton's law explains the physiology of conditions such as oxygen toxicity and nitrogen narcosis. The law states that total pressure exerted by a mixture of gases is the sum of the partial pressures of the gases in the mix. Thus for fresh air:

$$P_{total} = P_{02} + P_{CO2} + P_{N2}$$

As total pressure is increased, the partial pressures of each gas in the mixture will increase proportionally. Fresh air is composed of 79% nitrogen and 21% oxygen. These ratios remain constant as pressure is increased at depth.

Emergency Medical Services: Clinical Practice and Systems Oversight, Second Edition. Volume 1: Clinical Aspects of EMS.
Edited by David C. Cone, Jane H. Brice, Theodore R. Delbridge, and J. Brent Myers.
© 2015 NAEMSP. Published 2015 by John Wiley & Sons, Inc. Companion Website: www.wiley.com\go\cone\naemsp

Pressure	Depth	Gas bubble volume
1 ATA	Surface	100%
2 ATA	33 fsw	50%
3 ATA	66 fsw	33%
4 ATA	99 fsw	25%
5 ATA	132 fsw	20%

Figure 52.1 Boyle's law.

The partial pressure of nitrogen in air at sea level is approximately 600 mmHg or 0.79 ATA (0.79×760 mmHg), and of oxygen is 160 mmHg or 0.21 ATA (0.21×760 mmHg). At a depth of 66 fsw, the partial pressure of each would be $3 \times 600 = 1800$ mmHg (2.37 ATA) for nitrogen and $3 \times 160 = 480$ mmHg (0.63 ATA) for oxygen.

Henry's law

Henry's law is the foundation for decompression sickness ("the bends"). The law states that at equilibrium, the concentration of a gas dissolved *in* a liquid is directly proportional to the partial pressure of the gas *above* the liquid (Figure 52.2). This is stated as:

$$P = kC$$

where P is the partial pressure of the gas above the liquid, k is a constant, and C is the concentration of the gas in the liquid. The common example is opening a carbonated beverage container. As the pressure is reduced by opening the can, the CO_2 dissolved in solution escapes, forming bubbles as the gas equalizes with the atmospheric partial pressure of the gas.

Injury of descent: barotrauma of descent

Barotrauma is an injury that occurs due to changes in pressure of an air-filled structure during descent or ascent. Barotrauma is the most common medical problem associated with diving and can involve almost any structure that can have entrapment of gases. Barotrauma causes injury by a change in volume of free gas in an air-filled organ resulting in a pressure disequilibrium. Both increasing and decreasing pressure can cause mechanical injury to body structures. Pain is typically the initial complaint.

Middle ear barotrauma

Middle ear barotrauma, also known as barotitis media or "ear squeeze," is the most common complaint and medical problem of scuba divers. It is experienced by 30–40% or novice scuba divers and 10% of experienced divers [4]. As a diver descends in the water column, water pressure against the tympanic membrane (TM) increases. A diver will employ various methods to force air into the middle ear through the eustachian tube to equalize this pressure across the TM. If the diver is unsuccessful at "clearing" his ears, continued attempts may be futile due to the collapsible nature of the medial third of the eustachian tube. Ascent and reattempts at clearing are the only option for resolution. Further descent may cause TM rupture and result in cold water caloric stimulation and vertigo which may precipitate panic, disorientation, rapid ascent with other associated types of barotraumas, or drowning.

Treatment of middle ear barotrauma is usually with decongestants and analgesics and it will typically resolve over 3–7 days [5]. Refraining from diving with a cold or other symptoms

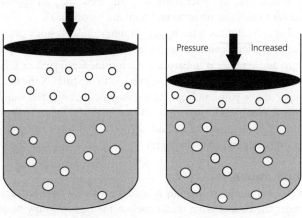

Figure 52.2 Henry's law.

that may cause difficulty with pressure equalization and early recognition of symptoms are common prevention strategies.

Inner ear barotrauma

Inner ear barotrauma is much less common than middle ear barotrauma, but has a higher morbidity. Damage to the cochleovestibular apparatus is the result of a large negative pressure gradient in the middle ear that occurs due to a forceful Valsalva maneuver against an occluded eustachian tube. As a result of the increased pressure during the attempted Valsalva, the pressure differential between the cerebrospinal fluid through the vestibular and cochlear structures and the middle ear may result in several injuries, including round or oval window rupture, middle ear hemorrhage, Reissner's membrane tear, fistualization of the windows, or a combination of these.

A triad of findings are associated with inner ear barotrauma: vertigo, unilateral roaring tinnitus, and hearing loss. In addition, a feeling of ocular fullness, nystagmus, disorientation, ataxia, and nausea and vomiting may be seen. Immediate concerns relate to the occurrence of panic in the underwater environment, uncontrolled ascent, or drowning.

Treatment of inner ear barotrauma includes elevating the head of the bed to 30°, bed rest, avoidance of strenuous physical activity, and symptomatic treatment. Early otolaryngology consultation should be obtained for further treatment recommendations as surgical repair options remain relatively controversial [6].

External ear barotrauma

A less common condition than middle ear barotrauma, external squeeze may occur with a tight-fitting wetsuit hood creating a relative negative pressure in the external canal. The TM is pulled outward due to trapped air in the canal. Cerumen, earplugs, and structural abnormalities may also contribute to this condition.

Sinus barotrauma

The sinus cavities are susceptible to pressure-volume changes according to Boyle's law. The ethmoid, maxillary, and frontal sinuses require patent nasal passages for equalization of pressure. Any mechanical abnormalities such as deviated septum, polyps, or physical conditions such as bacterial and viral infection, or upper respiratory infections may predispose a diver to sinus barotrauma and resultant barosinusitis.

The frontal sinus is the most commonly affected sinus cavity due to the long connection to the nasal passage [4]. Common signs and symptoms in barosinusitis include facial pain or fullness during descent or ascent, numbness to the front of the face, upper tooth pain, and epistaxis. Systemic decongestants and topical nasal vasoconstrictors are the mainstay of treatment. Some authors advocate a short corticosteroid burst to hasten recovery and return to diving [5].

Mask squeeze

A face mask must seal tightly around the face and forehead, and under the nose. Diving masks enclose the nose to allow nasal exhalation when equalizing the pressure between the mask and the outside environment. Equalization failure may result in capillary rupture with facial petechiae, ecchymosis, and scleral/conjunctival hemorrhage.

Suit barotrauma

Suit squeeze develops where folds in wet or dry suit material become compressed during descent, causing a partial vacuum and resulting in an impressive area of ecchymosis post dive. Despite the dramatic appearance, the condition is benign and will resolve in days to weeks.

Dental barotrauma

Tooth squeeze or barodontalgia is an infrequent but dramatic type of barotrauma. Air trapped below decayed teeth or in other dental structures may cause pain during ascent or descent as air bubbles expand, causing a negative or positive pressure related to ambient pressure. This condition is mostly benign and self-limited, although may be quite painful.

Injury at depth

Nitrogen narcosis

Nitrogen is an inert gas and does not interact biochemically in the body. Nitrogen narcosis, also known as inert gas narcosis or "rapture of the deep," develops typically at depths greater than 100–120 fsw. Nitrogen begins to have anesthetic properties at 3.2 ATA. The symptoms result from the intoxicating effects of increased nitrogen tissue concentrations. Divers may become euphoric, have a false sense of well-being, inappropriate laughter, and develop numbness and tingling in the face, lips, or legs. Decreased decision making and judgment combined with loss of fine motor skills and delayed reaction times may result in drowning or contribute to a dive emergency. As in most physiological states, the effects are variable and there are no absolutes as to who is likely to develop this condition and at what depth. The diving "martini rule" describes that every 1 ATA (33 fsw) descended greater than 100 fsw equates to the consumption of one martini.

The condition improves rapidly with ascent, assuming that it is recognized in time. Divers may be unaware that they were affected by the condition. Cold temperature, workload, alcohol, hangovers, and fatigue may contribute to the onset and severity. It is generally recommended that recreational divers not dive with compressed air to depths greater than 120 fsw. Commercial divers use other inert gases, such as helium, neon, and argon, in their compressed gas mix to offset the effects of narcosis. Oxygen itself may become narcotic if left unmetabolized in tissues [7].

Oxygen toxicity

Despite the necessity for oxygen to sustain life, increased pressures and lengthy durations of exposure can be damaging to living organisms. The damaging effects are a result of increased partial pressures of oxygen and not necessarily the inspired oxygen percentage in the gas mixture. Although all organs may suffer oxygen's toxic effects, brain, lung, and eye function are often the first to be disrupted. Oxygen free radicals are believed to be responsible for the deleterious effects of high partial pressures of oxygen. Intermediates such as superoxide anions, hydroxyl radicals, and hydrogen peroxide are potentially toxic to cell membranes [8].

Two types of oxygen toxicity relevant to diving are central nervous system (CNS) and pulmonary ("whole body"). CNS toxicity has a more rapid onset even after short exposures (A). Whole-body toxicities usually follow prolonged exposures to oxygen at lower partial pressures (B).

A. Oxygen is generally considered to become toxic to the CNS when the partial pressure exceeds 1.6 ATA. Partial pressures less than 1.4 are unlikely to produce toxicity. These partial pressures are highly variable among individuals and make planning for dives riskier as high pressures are used for aggressive dive profiles.

   The toxicity experienced may range from visual changes to the extreme of convulsive activity. The convulsion experienced is not damaging in itself, but obviously in an aquatic environment can lead to life-threatening sequelae. The mnemonic VENTIDC [4] may be used to recall the range of toxicity.

   V: Visual changes (tunnel or blurry vision)

   E: Ear ringing/tinnitus

   N: Nausea

   T: Tingling, twitching, or muscle spasms (usually facial muscles or lips)

   I: Irritability, anxiety, agitation, confusion

   D: Dyspnea, dizziness, fatigue, problems with coordination

   C: Convulsions

   Any diver experiencing any of these symptoms should ascend from depth at the earliest opportunity to prevent the potential catastrophic consequences of unconsciousness or convulsions.

B. In pulmonary or whole-body toxicities, the lung is the primary organ affected, but many other parts of the body can be affected as well. The term whole-body toxicity is used to include any organ systems other than the CNS. Pulmonary irritation due to prolonged exposure of oxygen at lower partial pressures is an example of whole-body toxicity. Other symptoms that may be experienced in the whole-body category are itching, skin numbness, nausea, dizziness, and headache.

Immersion pulmonary edema

Cases of immersion pulmonary edema (IPE) have become widely recognized since 1989 [9]. IPE, typically occurring in divers with no underlying medical diseases, presents as a rapid onset of dyspnea at the bottom and continued dyspnea on the surface associated with cough and blood-tinged, frothy sputum. Because the fluid builds up in the air-containing spaces of the lungs and interrupts gas exchange, IPE resembles drowning. The important difference is that the obstructing fluid comes from within the body rather than from inhalation of surrounding water.

The cause of IPE has yet to be determined. Aggressive hydration prior to diving may be a contributing factor. It has been seen in triathletes and Navy SEALs doing high-intensity surface swims. Divers get IPE when swimming on the bottom without clear evidence of stress. In some cases, the diver mentions a tight-breathing regulator, and in others no evident stress or equipment problems are noted.

Immersion pulmonary edema is not a manifestation of decompression sickness and does not require recompression. The treatment is oxygen and diuretics to remove water from the lungs.

Injury of ascent: barotrauma of ascent

During ascent, the volume of all gases in air-containing structures will increase as the pressure decreases (Boyle's law). This type of barotrauma is the result of expansion of gases as pressure is decreased during ascent.

Reverse sinus or ear barotrauma (reverse squeeze)

Reverse sinus or ear barotrauma is less common than its counterparts during descent. The process of equalization on ascending is normally easier. As the ambient pressure is reduced, the pressure in the middle ear passively diffuses through the eustachian tube or through the sinus cavities. Initial descent problems may lead to inflammation and subsequent swelling of the passages, disrupting the ability to easily equate these pressures in these structures. Complications can range from blood from the ear or nose to tympanic membrane rupture, sinus fracture, or pneumocephalus.

Alternobaric vertigo

Alternobaric vertigo may occur during ascent as the middle ear pressures become unequal. Onset is sudden and usually preceded by a full feeling in the ears. The difference in pressures causing asymmetric stimulation of the vestibular system may result in significant vertigo. Nausea and vomiting may accompany the vertigo. Typically a self-limited condition, the real danger of alternobaric vertigo is a possibility of diver panic with rapid ascent and resultant pulmonary barotrauma or arterial gas embolism. Near drowning may also occur. Descent of a few feet should result in improvement of symptoms.

Gastrointestinal (GI) barotrauma

Aerogastralgia is a rare type of ascent barotrauma in divers, usually novice divers. Expansion of bowel gas during ascent may cause GI discomfort and abdominal pain. Causes include eating large meals or gas-producing foods (legumes) prior to a dive or drinking carbonated beverages. Swallowing air or

Valsalva maneuver with the head down may also contribute to the condition. The standard cure is evacuation of gas through the two anatomical venting orifices with the resultant decrease in pressure.

Pulmonary barotrauma

Pulmonary barotrauma (PBT) is the most serious type of barotrauma. Overexpansion of gas trapped in the lungs can result in pulmonary overpressurization. Sudden rapid and uncontrolled ascent in sport divers breathing compressed air at depth is the most common cause for PBT. Situations involving panic such as breath-holding out-of-air scenarios, buoyancy compensator malfunctions, loss of regulator, or accidental loss of weight belt can all contribute to these events.

During ascent without exhaling, the volume of gas in the lungs will double from a depth of 33 fsw to the surface. The greatest risk for pulmonary barotrauma occurs in less than 10 feet of water [4]. A pressure differential of 80 mmHg (alveolar air) above ambient water pressure on the chest wall, equivalent to 3–4 feet of seawater depth, is all that is necessary to force air bubbles across the alveolar–capillary membrane [10]. Conditions that may result from this physiology are alveolar hemorrhage, pneumothorax, pneumomediastinum, subcutaneous emphysema, and the most feared complication – arterial gas embolism (AGE).

Arterial gas embolism

The most striking and dramatic condition associated with PBT is AGE. The second most common cause of mortality, among sport divers, following drowning, AGE accounts for roughly 30% of diving-related deaths [4]. Victims of AGE manifest symptoms during ascent or within 10 minutes of reaching the surface.

Patients suffering AGE can be classified into three groups. The first group is composed of those patients who suffer immediate loss of consciousness, apnea, and cardiac arrest on reaching the surface. This group represents 4% of AGE patients and in these cases, recompression, cardiopulmonary resuscitation, and advanced life support are unlikely to be successful [10]. These patients are suspected to have suffered a large bolus of air to the central vascular bed, particularly the pulmonary arteries and right ventricle. The resulting vascular obstruction leads to pulseless electrical activity and death.

A second group of patients accounts for an additional 5% of deaths; these patients reach the hospital and will die as a result of the AGE or severe near-drowning accompanying AGE. Fifty percent of the remaining patients will have a complete functional recovery [10].

Victims suffering from AGE present with a variety of systemic and neurological findings. The severity and location of AGE depend on the amount and distribution of the air embolus. The most common initial findings are neurological in nature and include loss of consciousness, confusion, or stupor. AGE may

Table 52.1 Presenting signs and symptoms of patients with arterial gas embolism

Neurological	Pulmonary	Visual	Other
Loss of consciousness	Chest pain	Blindness	Nausea
Focal paralysis	Hemoptysis	Nystagmus	Vomiting
Confusion	Crepitance	Gaze preference	Cardiac arrest
Coma	Dyspnea		
Convulsions			
Vertigo			
Ataxia			
Unilateral motor/ sensory deficit			
Bilateral motor/ sensory deficit			
Dizziness			
Headache			
Memory difficulty			

involve multiple organ systems and the presentation is variable (Table 52.1).

Decompression sickness: "the bends"

Decompression sickness (DCS) occurs after a reduction in ambient pressure usually due to decompression back to ambient pressure from either a dive or hyperbaric chamber exposure. The pathophysiology of DCS results from the inflammatory and obstructive effects of inert gas bubbles in the vascular system and tissues. DCS represents a spectrum of clinical illnesses previously classified as DCS types I, II, III and now more commonly referred to by the affected organ system (Table 52.2). The incidence of DCS is 2.8 cases per 10,000 dives [5].

Risk of DCS is increased by the length and depth of a dive, and DCS may result despite strict adherence to appropriate dive tables. Contributing factors include age, obesity, dehydration, exercise prior to diving, fever, cold ambient temperatures post dive, exertion, and flying after diving. Men are 2.6 times more likely to experience DCS than women, perhaps due to variable risk-taking behaviors. A patent foramen ovale may also increase risk of DCS, having been found in 65% of divers with serious DCS [5].

The clinical diagnosis of DCS is suspected based on a history of exposure to increased atmospheric pressure and development of characteristic signs and symptoms. Most patients are symptomatic within 1 hour of reaching the surface. The remainder of patients will develop symptoms within 3 hours. Cases have been reported days following a dive although this amounts to less than 2% of cases [5].

Shallow water blackout

Shallow water blackout is a loss of consciousness caused by cerebral hypoxia towards the end of a breath-hold dive, when the alveolar PCO_2 is lowered to 20–30 mmHg without a significant increase in PO_2. During the dive or swim, exercise-induced hypoxia sufficient to cause loss of consciousness may occur before CO_2 reaccumulates to provide stimulation to

Table 52.2 Organ systems affected by decompression sickness (DCS)

DCS type	Location	Symptoms	Other names/cautions	Incidence
Musculoskeletal – "the bends"	Major joints	Pain – boring, deep ache, may be sharp or throbbing	Pain only bends, joint or limb bends	Most common 70% of patients
Skin or cutaneous	Skin	Rash, pruritus, formication	Cutis marmorata, mottling or marbling of skin may indicate more severe decompression sickness	Relatively uncommon, usually benign
Pulmonary or "the chokes"	Substernal on inhalation	Non-productive cough, dyspnea, cyanosis	Represents massive pulmonary gas embolism	Unusual but serious
Neurological	Any level of central nervous system; typically spinal cord (low thoracic/lumbar)	Random and may be diffuse: paresis, paraplegia, paresthesia, dysesthesia, bowel or bladder dysfunction	Decompression sickness of the brain produces symptoms that may be indistinguishable from arterial gas embolism	Found in 50–60% of scuba diving casualties [5]
Inner ear or vestibular, "the staggers"	Inner ear	Vertigo, dizziness, nausea, vomiting, nystagmus	High incidence of residual inner ear damage as opposed to inner ear barotrauma	Usually seen in saturation divers or very deep heliox dives
Vasomotor	Vascular system	Hypotension unresponsive to fluids	Decompression shock	Rare, rapidly life threatening, most do not survive
Dysbaric osteonecrosis	Major joints	Avascular or aseptic necrosis of bone	Long-term sequela to inadequate decompression	<1% to more than 80% based on age and type of diving performed in lifetime
Dysbaric retinopathy	Eye	Variable	Suspected to be related to small bubble microembolization	Uncommon

breathe. Victims are often established practitioners of breath-hold diving (sport free divers), are fit, strong swimmers, and have not experienced problems before.

Transport and destination hospital considerations

Patients suspected of suffering from AGE or DCS should be transported as rapidly as possible to a facility with resources for evaluation by a diving physician and possible hyperbaric oxygen therapy. Early treatment is more efficacious than delayed care, but there are numerous cases reported to have benefited even with delays of greater than 6 hours [10]. Recompression is the essential and primary treatment for these disorders.

Prehospital care should consist of supplemental oxygen at a flow rate of at least 10 L/min by non-rebreather mask, or appropriate airway management in patients suffering near drowning. Maintenance of intravascular volume is also important to support capillary perfusion and assist with elimination of bubbles from the arteriolar-capillary level. Intravenous isotonic fluids should be administered to maintain urine output of 1–2 cc/kg/hour.

Historically, it was recommended to position a patient in Trendelenburg position for transport. Current recommendations are to position AGE and DCS patients throughout their evaluation and treatment in a manner that allows the greatest access to and care of the patient [5,10].

The Divers Alert Network (DAN: 919.684.9111) is a 24 hour a day, 7 day a week international resource for dive-related injury

management and referral. On-call diving physicians, paramedics, and emergency medical technicians are available to provide medical information, referrals, and evacuation assistance as needed.

Conclusion

In general, diving is considered to be a relatively safe sport. Most diving operations will be free from major medical problems provided that divers pay attention to some general rules and have been properly trained.

Barotrauma of the ears and sinuses is the most common dive injury experienced. Pulmonary barotrauma is an infrequent complication but should be suspected when neurological or pulmonary symptoms are present.

The two main dive conditions that may benefit from recompression treatment and hyperbaric oxygen therapy are arterial gas embolism and decompression sickness. Decompression sickness occurs in deep long dives and in about 1% of divers. Arterial gas embolism occurs rapidly upon resurfacing. Rapid diagnosis and appropriate referral to definitive care may prevent additional decline in condition, further injury, and long-term sequelae of dive-related injuries.

Emergency medical services physicians and medical directors should have a fundamental knowledge of dive-related physiology and hazards. An understanding of the basic conditions encountered during a dive, combined with the knowledge of the dive phase at which an injury occurred and chief complaint, will help to diagnose and treat an injured diver.

References

1 Davison B. So how many divers are there, really? *Undercurrent* 2007;22:11.
2 WikiAsk. http://wiki.answers.com/Q/How_many_recreational_scuba_divers_in_the_world
3 Lansche JM. Deaths during skin and scuba diving in California in 1970. *Calif Med* 1972;116:18–22.
4 Byyny RL, Shockley LW. Scuba diving and dysbarism. In: Marx JA, Hockberger RS, Walls RM (eds) *Rosen's Emergency Medicine: Concepts and Clinical Practice*, 7th edn. Philadelphia: Mosby Elsevier, 2010, pp.1903–16.
5 Van Hoesen KB, Bird NH. Diving medicine. In: Auerbach PS (ed) *Wilderness Medicine*, 6th edn. Philadelphia: Mosby Elsevier, 2012, pp.1520–49.
6 Hunter SE, Farmer JC. Ear and sinus problems in diving. In: Bove AA (ed) *Bove and Davis' Diving Medicine*, 4th edn. Philadelphia: Saunders Elsevier, 2004, pp.431–59.
7 NOAA. Diving physiology. In: *NOAA Diving Manual: Diving for Science and Technology*, 4th edn. Flagstaff, AZ: Best Publishing, 2010, pp.3–36.
8 Clark JM, Thom SR. Toxicity of oxygen, carbon dioxide, and carbon monoxide. In: Bove AA (ed) *Bove and Davis' Diving Medicine*, 4th edn. Philadelphia: Saunders Elsevier, 2004, pp.241–59.
9 Bove AA. Cardiovascular disorders and diving. In: Bove AA (ed) *Bove and Davis' Diving Medicine*, 4th edn. Philadelphia: Saunders Elsevier, 2004, pp.485–506.
10 Van Hoesen K, Neuman TS. Gas embolism: venous and arterial gas embolism. In: Neuman TS, Thom SR (eds) *Physiology and Medicine of Hyperbaric Oxygen Therapy*. Philadelphia: Saunders Elsevier, 2008, pp.257–81.

Further reading

Ellerman RL. *Diver Medical Technician: Care of the Injured Diver*. North Charleston: Robert L. Ellerman, 2012.
Ellerman RL. *Diver Medic Field Operations: A Practical Guide*. North Charleston: Robert L. Ellerman, 2012.
Fuller FF. Environmental emergencies. In: Pollak AN (ed) *Nancy Caroline's Emergency Care in the Streets*, 7th edn. Burlington, VA: Jones and Bartlett Learning, 2013, pp.1804–31.
Hart AJ, White SA. Open water scuba diving accidents at Leicester: five years' experience. *J Accid Emerg Med* 1999;16:198–200.
Snyder B, Neuman TS. Dysbarism and complications of diving. In: Tintinalli JE (ed) *Tintinalli's Emergency Medicine: A Comprehensive Study Guide*, 7th edn. New York: McGraw-Hill, 2011, pp.1213–18.
Whitaker AJ, Bodiwala GG. Immediate management of diving emergencies. *Br J Sports Med* 1982;16:102–6.

SECTION IX

Special Populations

CHAPTER 53

The special needs of children

Susan Fuchs

Epidemiology of prehospital pediatric care

Despite the fact that pediatric calls account for only 13% of ambulance runs [1], they provoke a disproportionate degree of concern and anxiety for prehospital care providers and, in turn, medical oversight physicians. A recent study by the Pediatric Emergency Care Applied Research Network (PECARN) from 14 EMS ground agencies across 11 states found that the most common chief complaints were traumatic injury (29%), general illness (10%), respiratory distress (9%), behavioral/psychiatric disorder (8.6%), seizure (7.45%), pain/non-chest/non-abdomen (6.5%), abdominal pain/problems (4.5%), and asthma (3.9%) [2] (Table 53.1) [3].

Prehospital care providers may be uncomfortable with pediatric patients. This can be due to limited knowledge and skills obtained during initial training, infrequent field experience, or a lack of continuing education. It can also be due to weight-based drug doses and equipment size variations in children. In addition, empathy in treating ill and injured children plays a large role. NAEMSP model pediatric protocols were developed so they would not have to be started from scratch in each system [4]. The particular protocol or algorithm chosen should be based on several factors including the structure of the system (e.g. one-tiered versus two-tiered; EMT versus paramedic), scope of practice decisions, transport times, continuing education requirements, skills retention, system quality improvement, and, of course, resources.

Evaluation of children

Evaluation is an area in which children are truly different. An accurate assessment of a pediatric patient is the key to proper field evaluation and treatment and, in turn, appropriate direct medical oversight. Evaluation should be tailored to each child in terms of age, size, and developmental level.

Pediatric Assessment Triangle

A useful learning tool that may be beneficial for providers is the Pediatric Assessment Triangle (PAT), which looks at Appearance, work of Breathing, and Circulation –a variation on the classic ABCs of primary assessment. This tool was developed by the Pediatric Education for Paramedics Task Force [5] and has been incorporated into the Pediatric Education for Prehospital Professionals (PEPP) program [6] and Advanced Pediatric Life Support (APLS) course [7].

The PAT allows the prehospital provider to develop a general impression of the child and determine if life support is needed urgently. The three parts of the triangle are done by watching and listening to the patient and do not require equipment. They can be accomplished from across the room and can be completed in 30–60 seconds.

Appearance

This is the most important component as it determines the severity of injury or illness. It consists of five characteristics, the TICLS mnemonic: Tone, Interactiveness, Consolability, Look/gaze, and Speech/cry. Assessment of tone includes: Is the child moving vigorously or is he limp? Interactiveness reflects how alert the child is: does she react to a voice or an object? Does the child reach for a toy or is he uninterested? Is the child consolable; can she be comforted? Look/gaze: Does the child look at the EMS provider or caregiver, or does the child have a blank expressionless face? Speech/cry: Is the cry or voice strong or weak? [6].

Work of Breathing

This portion of the tool can give the provider a quick indication of oxygenation and ventilation and can be done without a stethoscope. The characteristics to note include:
- abnormal airway sounds such as grunting, wheezing, or muffled phonation
- abnormal positioning such as the tripod position, sniffing position, or refusing to lie down
- presence and location of retractions presence of nasal flaring [6].

Emergency Medical Services: Clinical Practice and Systems Oversight, Second Edition. Volume 1: Clinical Aspects of EMS.
Edited by David C. Cone, Jane H. Brice, Theodore R. Delbridge, and J. Brent Myers.
© 2015 NAEMSP. Published 2015 by John Wiley & Sons, Inc. Companion Website: www.wiley.com\go\cone\naemsp

Table 53.1 Top three chief complaints by age [3]

<1 year	1–5 years	6–12 years	13–18 years
Respiratory distress (27.2%)	Trauma (22.4%)	Trauma (32.8%)	Trauma (31.3%)
General illness (22.4%)	General illness (16.9%)	Behavioral/ psychiatric (10.3%)	Behavioral/ psychiatric (13.9%)
Trauma (9.8%)	Seizure (16.0%)	Seizure (7.3%)	Pain non-chest/ non-abdomen (9.2%)

Source: Lerner EB. (Abstract) *Prehosp Emerg Care* 2012;16:161. Reproduced with permission of NAEMSP.

Table 53.2 Vital signs

Age	Weight (kg)	Respiration (min–max)	Heart rate (min–max)	Systolic blood pressure (min–max)
Premie	1–2	30–60	90–190	50–70
Newborn	3–5	30–60	90–190	50–70
6 month	7	24–40	85–180	65–106
1 year	10	20–40	80–150	72–110
3 year	15	20–30	80–140	78–114
6 year	20	18–25	70–120	80–116
8 year	25	18–25	70–110	84–122
12 year	40	14–20	60–110	94–136
15 year	50	12–20	55–100	100–142
18 year	65	12–18	50–90	104–148

Circulation to the skin

This helps determine the adequacy of perfusion to vital organs, using three characteristics:

- pallor, which reflects inadequate blood flow
- mottling, which is due to vasoconstriction
- cyanosis, which is blue coloration of the skin and mucous membranes [6].

If there is an abnormality in one or more aspects of the triangle, this can help the provider decide how severely ill or injured the child is and the most likely physiological abnormality. For example, abnormal appearance and breathing point to a respiratory problem, whereas abnormal appearance and circulation point to a circulatory disorder. Abnormalities in all three areas point to a critically ill child who requires rapid scene interventions.

The next step in patient assessment is the ABCDEs.

A – Airway: Assessment of the patient's airway should include: Is it patent? Is the child maintaining his or her own airway or is assistance needed in the form of airway positioning: jaw thrust, chin-lift, oral airway, nasal airway, bag-mask, or endotracheal (ET) tube?

B – Breathing: Respiratory rate varies with age and can be very difficult to obtain in a crying child. Children in respiratory distress will usually breathe fast but as they tire, the rate will decrease, which is an ominous sign. When one listens to the chest, are there any adventitious sounds (grunting, stridor, wheezing, rales, rhonchi) or no sounds (no air movement)? Depending on available equipment, the use of a pulse oximeter can help determine oxygen saturation and the need for supplemental oxygen and/or assisted ventilation.

C – Circulation: Determining heart rate and strength of peripheral pulses (radial) can be accomplished together. Heart rate varies with age and can also increase with fever and anxiety, but a heart rate below the normal range is worrisome and can imply hypoxia or pending arrest. If peripheral pulses are weak, central pulses should be checked as a means of assessing circulation. Capillary refill, which should be less than 2 seconds, can be assessed with the evaluation of the temperature and color of the extremity. Cold, blue, pale, or mottled extremities indicate poor circulation and shock. Although obtaining a blood pressure is part of the vital signs, in children it is often inaccurate because of the wrong size cuff or a fighting child. A normal blood pressure in the face of some of the above abnormalities should not make a prehospital care provider comfortable. In fact, hypotension in a child is a late finding of shock.

D – Disability: This is a brief assessment of level of consciousness (mental status). The key is a quick assessment done initially as general appearance, so this is a recheck. It is not necessary to memorize a pediatric Glasgow Coma Scale, as a rapid assessment uses the mnemonic AVPU: Awake, responsive to Voice, responsive to Pain, and Unresponsive.

E – Exposure: Although parts of the ABCDEs require that parts of the body be exposed for a complete assessment, it is necessary to ensure that all of the child's body has been examined to fully evaluate any abnormalities. At the same time, it is also important to prevent heat loss and hypothermia.

Vital signs

One of the most challenging aspects for prehospital care providers in the assessment of infants and children is that their vital signs change with age, so it is difficult to remember what is within a normal range. Having a table with appropriate vital signs for age is an easy way to solve this problem (Table 53.2).

Heart rate

A child's heart rate decreases with age. Counting an infant's very fast heart rate can be difficult by auscultation in a screaming child. It is often easier to feel the pulse as this is not as threatening. In an infant, the brachial pulse can be used while in a child or adolescent, the radial pulse is useful. While counting the pulse, one can also assess pulse quality (strong versus weak). A fast heart rate can be due to fever, pain, anxiety, or fear but can also be due to shock or hypoxia. Watching the trend of the heart rate is also useful once you intervene, to see if the patient is improving. Any heart rate >220 in an infant or >180 in a child deserves prompt action. While this may be due to sinus tachycardia, it is also important to determine if this is supraventricular tachycardia. A slow heart rate (<60) in a symptomatic child (altered mental status, hypoxia, poor pulse quality) should prompt cardiopulmonary resuscitation (CPR) [6].

Respiratory rate

A child's respiratory rate also decreases with age. When counting respirations, especially in infants, it is important to count for 30 seconds, then double the number, as very young infants may have periodic breathing (short periods of apnea of 5 seconds, followed by rapid breathing). Try to count respirations when the child is calm, as crying does not provide an accurate respiratory rate. A child's respiratory rate can be elevated due to fever, pain, fear, or anxiety, as well as respiratory distress. It is important to assess the respiratory rate with additional information provided by the PAT such as signs of increased work of breathing (e.g. retractions, abnormal airway sounds). Beware of a slow respiratory rate, as this can signal respiratory failure [6].

Blood pressure

Blood pressure determination is often difficult in a child due to lack of proper cuff size or agitation of the child caused by the cuff tightening. The proper size cuff has a width two-thirds the length of the upper arm (or thigh). In children under age 3 years, it may be difficult to obtain an accurate blood pressure, so use of other information such as heart rate, pulse quality, and capillary refill time (normally less than 2–3 seconds) can provide needed information about the child's condition. (An infant or young child with a rapid heart rate, weak pulses, and delayed capillary refill is in shock whether the blood pressure is normal or not.) In a child, it is often difficult to obtain both the systolic and diastolic blood pressure due to movement, so obtaining a systolic pressure by palpation (rather than auscultation) is useful. For children older than 1 year of age, the systolic blood pressure should be greater than 70 + (2 × age of child in years). If it is less than this, there is hypotension [6].

Pain

Pain is now considered the fourth vital sign but once again, assessing pain in children is not easy. A crying infant can be in pain, hungry, or just wet. A toddler may not understand the word "pain" but recognize "boo-boo" or "owie." In older children, use of self-reporting scales such as the visual analog scale (VAS) (e.g. 0 no pain to 10 the worse pain in my life) is possible; however, language barriers may prevent understanding. The Wong-Baker FACES scale has been used in hospital settings. There are other scales, including the FLACC observational scale and CHEOPS, which use observations on the infant/child's cry, facial expression, and leg movement to provide a total score. The Oucher and Faces Pain Scale-revised use a 0–10 score that has the child match his or her facial expression, similar to the Wong-Baker FACES scale. No matter which scale is used, once

pain is assessed and treated, it should be reassessed to see if the pain has decreased [6].

Weight measurement

While parents may know their child's weight in pounds, medication dosing in children is by kilograms. While it is possible to mentally divide the weight in pounds by 2.2 to get kilograms, it may be easier and more reliable to use a calculator or phone application. If the parent does not know the child's weight or no parent/caregiver is available, there are a few tools one can use. The easiest is a length-based tape that takes the child's length and provides a weight in kilograms. The Broselow Pediatric Emergency Tape is the one commonly in use. This tape goes from 3 to 36 kg and should be placed with the red portion at the child's head, and the weight is measured at the child's heel. A benefit of this device is that it provides equipment size as well as medication doses in mg, except for resuscitation medications that are in mL. Other formulas for weight include: 1–10 years: (age × 2) + 10 (kg), or for those >10 years: (age × 2) + 20 kg [8], and Luscombe and Owens (3 × age + 7) [9]. The midarm circumference formula (weight (kg) = (mid-arm circumference [cm]-10) × 3) was useful to estimate body weight in Chinese children [10]. Another device called the MERCY Tape is based upon weight estimation using the mid-upper arm circumference and humeral length, and estimates weight more accurately in obese children than the Broselow tape [11,12].

A recent concern is that the Broselow tape underestimates a child's weight due to the obesity epidemic in the US. The length-based tape assumes lean body mass, and the weight given is the 50th percentile for any measured length. Resuscitation drugs (epinephrine) have a small volume of distribution and clearance, which is associated with lean body mass, not the actual body weight. Lean body weight is similar to ideal body weight, so these drugs are best dosed by ideal body weight [13]. Those drugs that are lipid soluble are best dosed by actual body weight, but if a child is overweight, toxicity can occur if the drug has a narrow therapeutic window [13]. In realistic terms, if the calculated drug dose for an obese child is greater than the adult dose, use the adult dose. In addition, length is the best predictor of equipment size needed as well, so adding a few kilograms to the weight estimated by the Broselow tape is *not* recommended!

Specialized equipment needs

As mentioned above, children of different ages and sizes require different sized equipment. The length-based tape or computer or telephone applications can provide this information, but they are all useless unless you have the right equipment in your ambulance. Numerous organizations, including NAEMSP, recently revised the 2009 Policy Statement: Equipment for Ground Ambulances. This new policy includes a list of core equipment for both BLS and ALS ambulances, for adults and children. While states may mandate equipment or allow EMS regions or medical directors to dictate what equipment is carried based on scope of practice and other factors, this consensus document represents the latest guidelines [14].

Developmental approach

Another important consideration in taking care of pediatric patients is the various developmental levels. A 6-month-old crying infant cannot tell you where it hurts while an injured 15 year old can, but may not disclose important information in front of his or her parents or friends. Understanding some of the developmental characteristics of children can assist you in your evaluation of the patient.

Infants

Infants under 2 months have a very limited repertoire. They cannot tell the difference between you and their caregivers by sight, but may turn to their mother's voice. When evaluating them, it is important to keep them warm, allow the parents to hold them if possible, and speak in a soothing voice.

Those from 2 to 6 months can make eye contact and recognize their caregivers. They are also more active, and those older than 3 months can roll over. They may follow objects or light with their eyes, and they bring objects to their mouths, so don't offer anything small! Once again, evaluate them in a parent's lap, and try to get down to their level (squat down or evaluate them when you are on your knees). Those between 6 and 12 months are gaining gross motor skills, which include going from sitting by themselves to crawling, to cruising (walking while holding onto an object), and some can walk by 12 months. Their verbal skills are still limited, saying only a few simple words (mama, dada). A key development during this time is that they experience stranger anxiety. This means that they know you are not their parent/caregiver, and do not like to be separated from them. Once again, during your evaluation keep the child with the parents and, if possible, during transport, keep the parents in eyesight or within voice range.

Other tips for evaluating infants is allowing parents to offer a pacifier, toy, or blanket, and allowing the parents to remove or lift the infant's clothes. Evaluate them based on their activity level: if they are calm, listen to the heart rate and respiratory rate first. If not, save this for later as they become more accustomed to you. Perform the most uncomfortable or distressing part of the exam last [15].

Toddlers

Toddlers are considered ages 1–3, and are gaining verbal and fine and gross motor skills rapidly. They can walk, run, play with toys, and feed themselves. Some say only a few words but others speak in phrases, and definitely say "no." They are very fearful of strangers, curious but not aware of danger, and very opinionated. On the other hand, they are playful and enjoy make-believe. During your evaluation, use the toddler's name and talk to them

in a friendly tone of voice. Use distraction and play to gain their confidence and cooperation. Ask the parent/caregivers to help with the exam. Speak in simple terms and give the patient limited choices. If there is a critical portion of the exam, do that first, then work from toes to head. Despite their small size, they can put up quite a fight during your exam and therefore a combination of patience and parental assistance may be needed [15].

Preschoolers

Preschoolers include those 3–5 years of age. They are very mobile, speak in sentences and have a large vocabulary. They are creative thinkers but also illogical. They have many misconceptions about bodily functions and illness, and fear being left alone. Evaluation tips include distraction (use one of their toys to demonstrate what you will be doing), choosing your words carefully, and allowing the patient to participate in the exam (hold the stethoscope or let them listen to their heart) [15].

School-aged children

School-aged children are those who attend elementary and middle schools. They are independent, talkative, and have a fair understanding of illness and injury. They fear being different from friends and being separated from parents and friends, and do not like loss of control. When ill or injured, this independence is threatened, so the child may be angry and put up resistance to evaluation, especially in front of friends. It is important to establish trust with the patient and explain to them in simple terms what you are going to do, but don't negotiate. It may be beneficial to give the patient privacy by completing the evaluation in the ambulance, and praise them for their cooperation. You can perform the evaluation in a head-to-toe manner [15].

Adolescents and teenagers

Adolescents can be rational and can express themselves well. They often like to take risks, even though they may understand the possible consequences. Friends take a front seat to parents and they like to appear independent of their parents. When evaluating adolescents, use their name and respect their modesty and privacy. They may not provide all past medical information in front of their friends, and may not divulge drug or alcohol use in front of their parents. Speak directly to them, explain what you are going to do, and be honest. If they are uncooperative, friends may be able to provide some assistance [15].

Children with special health care needs

One of the most important aspects of evaluating a child with special health care needs is to ask a parent or caregiver their developmental level and baseline activities. The child may have physical disabilities but be developmentally normal for age, or have severe impairments in speech and mental abilities. This affects not only their baseline vital signs, weight, and size, but their response to illness and injury. Evaluation includes asking the parent/caregiver what is different from normal, asking them the best approach to the child, and enlisting their help. Ask if they have a special emergency information form, which can provide EMS with past medical history, allergies (especially latex allergy), medications, and where they usually receive their medical care. Ask the parent if they have a "go bag" which has all the special equipment they need for transport and hospital visits. In many cases, these children obtain their care at a children's hospital farther than the local hospital, and that is where the parents are most comfortable. EMS personnel may need to contact medical oversight for approval if transport to the preferred hospital is outside their protocols [15].

Consent issues

When taking care of pediatric patients, consent issues may arise. While parents commonly provide consent for treatment, if an injury occurs without them, several legal issues can arise. Obtaining *informed consent* is required by law but children cannot provide informed consent, because they are considered to be *minors* (less than 18 years of age), unless they are *emancipated minors*. Emancipated minor laws vary from state to state but in most states, emancipated minors include those who are married, have a child, are pregnant, are on active military duty, or are not living at home and are self-supporting, no matter what their age [16]. The emancipated minor can consent to treatment as well as refuse treatment by EMS.

There are emergency situations when no parent or legal guardian is available and the child needs medical care and transport. In this case the *emergency exception rule/implied consent* is in effect, but the following four conditions must be met:

- the child's legal guardian is unavailable or unable to provide consent for treatment or transport
- the child is suffering from an emergency condition that places his or her life or health in danger
- treatment or transport cannot be delayed until consent can be obtained
- only treatment for the emergency condition is administered by EMS [16].

In cases where implied consent is used, excellent documentation is required, including that attempts were made to contact the guardian, the nature of the injury and treatment provided, and why it was an emergency. The EMS provider should contact medical oversight if guardians are not available or if unsure about transporting the patient.

Mature minors are those who have been declared adults by the court. The age also varies by state but is usually older than 14 years. A mature minor can refuse treatment and transport for him or herself, as long as he or she is not on a psychiatric hold and is competent to make the decision to refuse [16].

If the guardians refuse transport of a child, a few conditions should be met. They must be alert, mentally competent, and oriented. In these cases, the EMS provider should contact medical oversight to either have a physician control speak to the parent to convince him or her to allow treatment and transport, or get approval for the refusal. If medical oversight feels that emergency treatment and transport are needed, or if the parent is not competent, law enforcement may be needed to take *temporary protective custody* of the child. Each state differs somewhat in who can take temporary protective custody but law enforcement is one of the groups in all states. A key fact is that, if temporary protective custody is taken, this allows EMS to transport the child to a hospital for a medical evaluation but not to treat a non-life-threatening illness or injury [16].

References

1 Shah MN, Cushman JT, Davis CO, et al. The epidemiology of emergency medical services use by children: an analysis of the National Hospital Ambulatory Medical Care Survey. *Prehosp Emerg Care* 2008;12;269–76.
2 Lerner EB, Dayan P, Brown K, et al. Characteristics of the pediatric patients treated by the Pediatric Emergency Care Applied Network's affiliate EMS agencies. *Prehosp Emerg Care* 2014;18:52–9.
3 Lerner EB, Dayan P, Brown K, et al. An analysis of pediatric prehospital patients: can we aggregate data among emergency medical services systems? (Abstract) *Prehosp Emerg Care* 2012;16:161.
4 National Association of EMS Physicians. Model Pediatric Protocols, 2003 Revision. Available at: www.childrensnational.org/EMSC
5 Dieckmann RA, Brownstein D, Gausche-Hill M. The pediatric assessment triangle: a novel approach to pediatric assessment. *Pediatr Emerg Care* 2010;26:312–15.
6 Pediatric assessment. In: Fuchs S, Pante MD (eds) *Pediatric Education for Prehospital Professionals*, 3rd edn. Burlington, MA: Jones and Bartlett Learning, 2014, pp.2–29.
7 Fuchs S, Yamamoto L (eds). *American Academy of Pediatrics/American College of Emergency Physicians. APLS/The Pediatric Emergency Medicine Resource*, 4th rev. edn. Burlington, MA: Jones and Bartlett Learning, 2012.
8 Los Angeles County Department of Health. *Pediatric Surge Pocket Guide*. Los Angeles, CA: Los Angeles Department of Public Health, 2009.
9 Luscombe M, Owens B. Weight estimation in resuscitation: is the correct formula still valid? *Arch Dis Child* 2007;92:412–25.
10 Cattermole GN, Leung PY, Mak PS, et al. Mid-arm circumference to be used to estimate children's weights. *Resuscitation* 2010;81:1105–10.
11 Abdel-Rahman SM, Ahlers N, Holmes A, et al. Validation of an improved pediatric weight estimation strategy. *J Pediatr Pharmacol Ther* 2013;18:112–21.
12 Abdel-Rhaman SM, Paul IM, James LP, et al. Evaluation of the MERCY Tape: performances against the standard for pediatric weight estimation. *Ann Emerg Med* 2013;62:332–9.
13 Luten R, Zaritsky A. The sophistication of simplicity…optimizing emergency dosing. *Acad Emerg Med* 2008;15:461–5.
14 American College of Surgeons, Committee on Trauma. Equipment for ambulances – 2013. *Prehospital Emerg Care* 2014;18:92–97.
15 Using a developmental approach. In: Fuchs S, Pante MD (eds) *Pediatric Education for Prehospital Professionals*, 3rd edn. Burlington, MA: Jones and Bartlett Learning, 2014, pp.274–87.
16 Medicolegal and ethical considerations. In: Fuchs S, Pante MD (eds) *Pediatric Education for Prehospital Professionals*, 3rd edn. Burlington, MA: Jones and Bartlett Learning, 2014, pp.30–47.

CHAPTER 54

Pediatric medical priorities

Toni Gross and Susan Fuchs

Introduction

Approximately half of the EM responses to calls for pediatric patients are for medical complaints [1–3]. Calls for medical complaints outnumber traumatic calls in patients under 5 years. Seizures and respiratory distress are common pediatric medical complaints [2]. Other less common conditions, such as shock, cardiac arrest, and apparent life-threatening events (ALTE), require careful education and training. Controversies exist over management of the pediatric airway, and there is still a need to address the research agendas calling for improved evidence for out-of-hospital pediatric care [4].

Respiratory and airway problems

Cardiopulmonary arrest in the majority of infants and children is respiratory in origin [5]. Appropriate and timely treatment of a child in respiratory distress may prevent respiratory and subsequent cardiac arrest. Many respiratory diseases are unique to children; however, the underlying treatment is the same as for adults: maintenance of the airway and adequate oxygenation and ventilation.

Evaluation of the very young patient with respiratory complaints should take place in the parent's/guardian's arms if possible. The respiratory rate can increase with fear, and an anxious child may resist therapy and become more distressed. Signs of respiratory distress include a child in tripod position or refusing to lie down, nasal flaring or retractions, and grunting or head bobbing in infants. Interventions may be accomplished more easily with the parent's assistance. Moving a child from a position of comfort might worsen the respiratory distress. During transport, a child in respiratory distress should be safely restrained in an upright position, unless specific treatments require the supine position.

All children in respiratory distress require supplemental high-flow oxygen, such as a face mask at 12–15 L/min. The "blow-by O_2" method administers oxygen by holding the face mask 1–2 inches in front of the child's face, and is useful when a face mask increases the child's agitation and work of breathing. If the child is cyanotic, oxygen with assisted bag-valve-mask (BVM) ventilation may be required. The airway should be managed in the least invasive way possible – supraglottic devices and endotracheal intubation (ETI) should be used only if BVM ventilation fails [6,7].

Anatomical differences in infants and children affect airway management. The occiput is proportionally larger and causes neck flexion in the supine position. Placing a towel roll under the shoulders can improve airway alignment. The tongue is large relative to the oral cavity and is a source of upper airway obstruction. Children have larger tonsils and adenoids. Attempts at nasopharyngeal airway placement or intubation may cause bleeding. During endotracheal intubation, the straight blade is preferred to the curved blade due to the weaker hyoepiglottic ligament and relatively large and floppy epiglottis. The trachea is narrow, increasing the effect of even small decreases in the airway size due to secretions, edema, or external compression. The subglottic region and the non-distensible cricoid cartilage are the narrowest portion of the pediatric airway, unlike in adults, where the vocal cords are the narrowest portion [8].

Wheezing is a frequent EMS pediatric encounter. First-line treatment for acute asthma episodes includes bronchodilators, such as the beta-agonist albuterol, and the anticholinergic ipratropium. Other therapy may include corticosteroids, IV magnesium sulfate, and epinephrine (nebulized or IM injection) (Table 54.1). Continuous positive airway pressure (CPAP) should be administered for severe respiratory distress of any cause. Bag-valve-mask ventilation should be utilized in children with respiratory failure [9,10]. It is very difficult to manage ventilation in asthmatic patients who are intubated; therefore, intubation should only occur when high-quality BVM ventilation fails [7,10,11].

Other respiratory processes such as bronchiolitis, pneumonia, and airway foreign bodies can cause wheezing. Bronchiolitis is associated with a large amount of mucus production and airway edema, and neonates are at risk of apnea.

Emergency Medical Services: Clinical Practice and Systems Oversight, Second Edition. Volume 1: Clinical Aspects of EMS.
Edited by David C. Cone, Jane H. Brice, Theodore R. Delbridge, and J. Brent Myers.

Table 54.1 Pediatric medication doses

Drug	Dose
Respiratory	
Albuterol	2.5 mg nebulized or 6 puffs MDI (+/−aerochamber/mask)
Ipratropium	0.5 mg nebulized
Methylprednisolone	2 mg/kg IV, IM, IO (max. 125 mg)
Dexamethasone	0.6 mg/kg IV, IM (max. 10 mg)
Prednisolone	2 mg/kg PO (max. 60 mg)
Magnesium sulfate	40 mg/kg IV (max. 2 g)
Epinephrine	0.01 mg/kg of 1:1,000 IM (max. 0.3 mg) 5 mL of 1:10,000 nebulized
Metabolic	
Dextrose	0.5 g/kg IV (max. 25 g)
Glucagon	0.02 mg/kg IM (max. 1 mg)
Neurological	
Midazolam	0.2 mg/kg buccal, IN, IM (max. 4 mg) 0.1 mg/kg IV (max. 4 mg)
Diazepam	0.1 mg/kg IV (max. 4 mg)
Lorazepam	0.1 mg/kg IV (max. 4 mg)

IM, intramuscular; IV, intravenous; IO, intraosseous; MDI, metered dose inhaler; PO, per os.

The airway should be maintained by suctioning the nose and/or mouth when excessive secretions are present [12]. Bronchodilators may be ineffective in bronchiolitis but albuterol should be administered to all children in respiratory distress with signs of bronchospasm [13–15]. Nebulized epinephrine should be administered if the above treatments fail.

Pneumonia usually presents with fever and cough, associated with dyspnea, tachypnea, chest pain, and/or vomiting. Prehospital interventions include oxygen and ventilatory support by the least invasive means. IV access should be obtained if the patient's status warrants treatment of dehydration with IV fluids. Suspected foreign body airway obstruction is managed according to AHA/ILCOR guidelines.

Laryngotracheobronchitis, or croup, causes a characteristic barking cough and can present with stridor. Nebulized epinephrine should be administered to all children in respiratory distress with signs of stridor and can be repeated with unlimited frequency for ongoing distress [16,17]. Patients who receive nebulized epinephrine should be transported to a receiving facility for continued observation [18].

While key history and physical exam findings can lead the provider to the correct treatment guideline, a key principle should be to treat respiratory distress first, by ensuring an open airway and providing supplemental oxygen, and then consider the differential diagnosis.

Controversies over airway management

The current literature highlights shortcomings associated with prehospital pediatric ETI. Few studies show improved outcomes, and several studies describe worsened outcomes.

ETI and intubation medications may inadvertently interact with other physiological processes key to resuscitation. Adverse events and errors are frequent. Significant system-level barriers limit training and clinical experiences for prehospital providers and students, and ETI is a complex procedure, requiring a significant amount of training to learn and maintain proficiency. Fortunately, few situations necessitate prehospital ETI.

One review documented that ETI was attempted in only 0.7% of all calls for children less than 15 years of age. Paramedics were unable to intubate 18% of these patients [19]. A review from a largely rural state documented that fewer than half of the state's paramedics attempt at least one pediatric intubation per year; only 2% of providers attempted any pediatric intubation during the 5-year study period [20].

A large prospective controlled trial comparing BVM ventilation to ETI in pediatric medical and trauma patients under 13 years of age demonstrated no survival or neurological outcome benefits in the ETI group [10]. The ETI group had longer scene and total prehospital times. In a review of the National Pediatric Trauma Registry, mortality and abnormal functional outcome scores were more likely in children who were intubated in the prehospital setting versus the hospital setting, controlling for injury severity scores. Observed versus expected rate of mortality was higher for patients intubated in the prehospital setting across all injury severities [21].

Supraglottic airway devices have not been studied in pediatric patients in the prehospital setting; however, use by prehospital providers on pediatric high-fidelity simulators has been studied [22–26]. Of the available devices, the laryngeal mask airway is available in a range of sizes that allows its use in all ages, including neonates. The King airway device (Kingsystems, Noblesville, IN) is limited in pediatric use due to available sizes. The smallest size is recommended for patients as small as 3 feet tall or 12 kg, making them unavailable for patients under the age of approximately 2 years.

One key fact remains: proficiency in pediatric BVM ventilation is mandatory for all prehospital providers [27]. The method of airway support used in the system should be based on the skill level of the providers, equipment and medications available, ongoing training and experience, transport times, and medical oversight.

Apparent life-threatening events

Apparent life-threatening events (ALTE) may present as a call to 9-1-1 from a frantic parent stating that his or her child has stopped breathing or turned blue. The child may have already recovered to baseline status. An ALTE is defined as "an episode that is frightening to the observer and that is characterized by some combination of apnea (central or occasionally obstructive), color change (usually cyanotic or pallid but occasionally erythematous or plethoric), marked change in muscle tone (usually marked limpness), choking, or gagging. In some cases, the observer fears that the infant has died [28]."

Apparent life-threatening event is a diagnosis usually reserved for infants up to age 12 months. ALTE has a reported incidence of 1–9 infants per 1,000 live births, but accounts for 7.5% of infant EMS encounters [29], 2% of hospitalized children, and 0.7% of infant ED visits [30]. ALTE is more common in younger infants less than 3 months [31]. The literature reports mortality associated with ALTE as being anywhere between <1% and 6% [28].

Greater than 80% of these patients will recover quickly and be well-appearing at the time of evaluation, with no signs of distress. Nearly all will have normal vital signs [29]. The on-scene evaluation for children with ALTE should include close examination of the patient and surroundings for evidence of occult trauma, and a blood glucose measurement. Despite the patient's well appearance, all those with a chief complaint consistent with ALTE should be transported to the hospital. At least 75% of patients presenting to the ED with ALTE are admitted to hospital [32]. Thirteen percent may need significant intervention during hospitalization [33]. It is prudent to recommend contact with direct medical oversight for caregivers who are refusing medical care and/or transport.

The differential diagnosis of ALTE is broad, encompassing gastrointestinal, respiratory, neurological, cardiac, and metabolic disorders. Serious illness causing an ALTE is difficult to exclude during a brief EMS evaluation. Of the very serious causes of ALTE, child abuse has been found in as many as 11% of cases, metabolic disease in 1.5%, ingestion of drugs or toxins in 1.5%, meningitis in 0.5–1%, and cardiac problems in 0.8% [30,32,34]. One study noted that a call to 9-1-1 for ALTE was associated with an almost five times greater odds of abusive head trauma being diagnosed as the cause of the ALTE [35], clearly emphasizing the high index of suspicion EMS providers must have when responding to these calls.

Long-term prognosis for infants with ALTE is generally very good. Recurrence of ALTE has been reported as being as high as 24% [30]. ALTE has not been shown to be a risk factor for subsequent sudden infant death syndrome (SIDS) [34].

Seizures and seizure mimics

Seizures account for 10% of pediatric calls to 9-1-1 [2]. They often are associated with anxiety on the part of the family and bystanders. The EMS physician should be concerned about the cause of the seizure as well as field treatment; however, providers should not diagnose the cause of the seizure before initiating appropriate therapy and transport [36]. The management of seizure is covered in Volume 1, Chapter 20 and Table 54.1.

For actively seizing patients, a blood glucose level should be measured. A blood glucose of <45 mg/dL in neonates or <60 mg/dL in infants, children, and adolescents should be treated with IV dextrose or IM glucagon (see Table 54.1). Hypoglycemic

Table 54.2 Conditions that mimic seizures

Generalized paroxysms	Apnea
	Pathological startles
	Breath-holding spells
	Vagal syncope
	Cardiac syncope
	Complicated migraine
	Benign paroxysmal vertigo
	Psychological disorders
Abnormal movements and postures	Neonatal jitteriness and clonus
	Benign paroxysmal torticollis of infancy
	Sandifer syndrome (reflux)
	Movement disorders
	Motor tics
	Benign myoclonus of early infancy, shuddering attacks, and chin trembling
	Autonomic storms (diencephalic seizures)
Oculomotor abnormalities	Opsoclonus myoclonus syndrome
	Daydreaming and behavioral staring
Sleep disorders	Benign sleep myoclonus and neonatal sleep myoclonus
	Sleep transition disorders
	Narcolepsy-cataplexy syndrome

Source: Mikati 2011 [56]. Reproduced with permission of Elsevier.

pediatric patients should be transported to the hospital, even if they return to baseline mental status after treatment.

Febrile seizures occur in 5% of the population and are strictly defined as occurring between ages 6 months and 6 years. Simple febrile seizures are generalized seizures lasting less than 15 minutes and not associated with focal neurological findings. Complex febrile seizures, defined as focal, lasting longer than 15 minutes, or recurring within 24 hours, carry a higher association with serious bacterial infection.

Fever associated with seizures can be the result of heat illness or toxin exposure. Patients with epilepsy have a lower seizure threshold during the course of a febrile illness and may have breakthrough seizures at that time. If a high fever is suspected as the cause of seizure, the child can be cooled with wet towels en route, not with ice or cold packs.

A list of conditions that mimic seizures can be found in Table 54.2. Notable pediatric-specific conditions include breath-holding spells, which are common in toddlers and usually associated with a painful or temperamental episode. In the neonatal period, benign myoclonus, sleep myoclonus, and jitteriness or exaggerated Moro reflex can mimic motor seizures. Sandifer syndrome is epistotonic posturing associated with gastroesophageal reflux.

Shock

Many providers equate shock with hypotension, which may be useful for adults but presents problems when caring for children. Normal blood pressure varies with age (Table 54.3) and

Table 54.3 Definition of hypotension by systolic blood pressure and age

Age	Systolic blood pressure (mmHg)
Term neonates (0–28 days)	<60
1 month–12 months	<70
1–10 years	<70 + (2 × age in years)
>10 years	<90

Source:Kleinmann 2010.[39] Reproduced with permission of Lippincott Williams & Wilkins.

Table 54.4 Normal heart rate by age

Age	Heart rate (beats/min)
Newborn	130
3 months	140
6 months	130
1 year	120
2 years	115
3–6 years	100
8 years	90
12 years	85

Source:Arcara 2012 [57]. Reproduced with permission of Elsevier.

obtaining an accurate blood pressure in a child can be difficult. Due to children's unique physiology, when hypotension is present, the body's compensatory mechanisms have failed and providers should recognize that the child is in a critical condition and at significant risk of death. While compensated shock may persist for hours, once the patient is hypotensive, cardiopulmonary failure may occur within only minutes [37].

Heart rate, initially and on repeated assessments, is the key parameter for recognition of compensated shock. Tachycardia without fever, anxiety, or hypoxia requires immediate intervention. Heart rate varies with age and knowledge of the norms is needed (Table 54.4). Assessing pulse quality and comparing peripheral to central pulses is an easy clinical assessment of stroke volume. Delayed capillary refill (>2 seconds) and skin that appears pale, mottled, cool, or diaphoretic are also common signs of shock [37,38].

A change in the level of consciousness demonstrates the effects of shock on the brain. Although this may be subtle, in children as young as 2 months, irritability or failure to recognize the parents is a sign of cerebral hypoperfusion [37]. A decreasing level of consciousness is an ominous sign. Other parameters to assess include muscle tone and pupillary responses.

Shock in children tends to result from *hypovolemia*, which most commonly occurs in gastroenteritis/dehydration and trauma. Other forms of shock include *distributive* (maldistribution of blood as occurs in sepsis, anaphylaxis, or spinal cord injury), *cardiogenic* (resulting from an arrhythmia, congestive heart failure, congenital heart disease, or post arrest), and *obstructive* (impaired cardiac output due to obstruction of blood flow as from a tension pneumothorax or cardiac tamponade).

Restoring adequate intravascular volume by the administration of 20 mL/kg of a crystalloid (normal saline or Ringer's lactate) should be initiated quickly (over 5–20 minutes). This can be accomplished by using a 30–60 mL syringe to push fluids through an IV or IO line [37]. If a child's weight is unknown, a length-based resuscitation tape should be used for fluids, drug dosing, and equipment size [39]. Patients in hypovolemic shock may require up to 60 mL/kg of crystalloid fluid resuscitation. If cardiogenic shock is suspected, smaller fluid boluses of 5–10 mL/kg should be used. In diabetic ketoacidosis with compensated shock, a bolus of 10–20 mL/kg should be administered over 1 hour [37]. If signs of pulmonary edema or worsening tissue perfusion are noted during fluid resuscitation, IV fluids should be stopped. Serum glucose should be measured.

A major difficulty in these situations may be the ability of the provider to establish IV access. It has been demonstrated that it is very difficult and time-consuming to establish IV access in young ill children [40]. In some situations, rather than waste precious moments of transport time, it may be useful to "load and go" and search for access en route [41]. Another method is to limit the number of attempts or time allowed for IV access before IO cannulation is attempted in the appropriate patient [42].

In children with cardiac lesions, where there is mixing of the pulmonary and systemic circulations, careful attention must be directed to the child's clinical response to interventions [43]. While oxygen is considered empiric therapy for patients in shock, supplemental oxygen relaxes pulmonary vascular resistance and can lead to increased left-to-right shunting. This decreases systemic blood flow, worsening metabolic acidosis. Providers must ascertain from caregivers what the patient's baseline oxygen saturations are, and should not provide supplemental oxygen that raises saturations above the patient's baseline.

Cardiac arrest

Out-of-hospital cardiac arrest (OHCA) is a rare occurrence in childhood, with an incidence of 2.6–19.7 annual cases per 100,000 pediatric population [44]. Survival rates for children who suffer OHCA are 6–12%, and overall intact neurological survival is reported to occur in 4% [44–46]. In contrast to adults, cardiac arrest in infants and children is usually the end result of respiratory failure or shock, and not of primary cardiac etiology. It is important to emphasize this principle when considering all pediatric prehospital emergencies and educating providers. Despite recent AHA recommendations to teach "Circulation-Airway-Breathing," when treating children, airway and ventilation skills are critical to preventing the need for cardiopulmonary resuscitation (CPR).

Sudden cardiac arrest (SCA) is much less common in children than in adults. Predisposing conditions for SCA in children include anatomical anomalies, genetic mutations causing channelopathies, and myocarditis, though these may not be diagnosed at the time of SCA. Blunt trauma to the chest and drug intoxication are also associated with SCA. Many cases of SCA in children occur during exercise. SCA in children should be treated as in adults, with immediate high-quality CPR and early defibrillation [39].

The highest incidence of pediatric OHCA occurs in infants, where the majority of cases are unwitnessed [45,46]. Survival to hospital discharge is higher for patients with witnessed arrests: 13% versus 4.6% for unwitnessed arrest [44]. Favorable neurological outcomes are more common in adolescents than in younger children and adults [45]. Return of spontaneous circulation (ROSC) is achieved in 30% of children with OHCA [44]. Survival to hospital discharge after ROSC is 31–38%, with 31–54% of these survivors having good Cerebral Performance Category scores [46–48].

The initial rhythm in pediatric cardiac arrest is asystole in 78–80%, pulseless electrical activity (PEA) in 12–13%, and ventricular fibrillation (VF) or pulseless ventricular tachycardia (VT) in only 4-8% [44–46] The most common first documented rhythm in traumatic cardiac arrest is PEA, and in adolescent arrests is VT/VF. Traumatic cardiac arrest is associated with higher morbidity and mortality than non-traumatic cardiac arrest, although survival to hospital discharge is 5–18%, and neurologically favorable outcomes occur in 1–8% [45,49,50].

Bystander CPR rates for pediatric patients in cardiac arrest vary greatly (8–85%), but average 30% [44,46].A Japanese nationwide prospective study of pediatric cardiac arrest compared patients receiving traditional CPR versus chest compression-only CPR from bystanders. Forty-seven percent of patients received bystander CPR; these patients had significantly higher rates of favorable neurological outcome 1 month after OHCA. Traditional CPR was associated with five times higher odds of a favorable outcome for OHCA from non-cardiac causes and had similar outcomes to chest compression-only CPR for OHCA from cardiac causes [51].

American Heart Association Pediatric Advanced Life Support guidelines recommend early defibrillation for VF and pulseless VT. A dose attenuator is recommended for use with an automated external defibrillator (AED) for children up to 25 kg (approximately 8 years of age). In infants <1 year of age, an AED with a dose attenuator may be used but a manual defibrillator is preferred. If neither is available, a regular AED may be used [52]. There is insufficient evidence to make a recommendation for or against the use of vasopressin for cardiac arrest in children [39].

Therapeutic hypothermia has not been proven to be of benefit in pediatric cardiac arrest. Review of 18 non-randomized studies showed no effect on mortality or good neurological outcome [53]. Ongoing randomized controlled trials may provide definitive evidence in the future. Until there is evidence showing benefit of hypothermia after pediatric cardiac arrest, EMS should not routinely cool children after ROSC. There is evidence that hypothermia improves survival and neurodevelopment

in newborns with moderate-to-severe hypoxic ischemic encephalopathy from intrapartum asphyxia [54].

It has been shown that paramedics are uncomfortable terminating CPR in children [55]. Decisions on if and when to terminate resuscitation in the field should be determined by the medical director, ideally with consultation from local pediatric providers. A model offline protocol for termination of resuscitation in children does not exist, and there are very few resources to help guide the medical oversight of this difficult situation. No reliable predictors of outcome have been identified to guide when to terminate resuscitative efforts. Some variables associated with survival are duration of CPR, number of doses of epinephrine, age, witnessed versus unwitnessed arrest, and the first rhythm [39].

Conclusion

Although pediatric calls account for only a small percent of EMS runs, they cause anxiety for providers. Some factors, such as training and appropriate equipment, can be addressed beforehand; other aspects cannot. The physician's level of comfort when providing direct medical oversight on pediatric calls will be discerned by the prehospital care providers.

Patient assessment skills are the cornerstone of therapy because treatment and triage decisions are based on this information. Providing oxygen is basic but decisions regarding IV access, medications, and airway interventions should be based on the age of the child, transport time, and the information related by the prehospital care providers. Frequent reassessment should be performed en route; in many cases, a child will be stabilized on arrival in the ED due to prehospital care and expertise.

References

1 Joyce SM, Brown DE, Nelson EA. Epidemiology of pediatric EMS practice: a multistate analysis. *Prehosp Disaster Med* 1996;11:180–7.

2 Richard J, Osmond MH, Nesbitt L, Stiell IG. Management and outcomes of pediatric patients transported by emergency medical services in a Canadian prehospital system. *CJEM* 2006;8:6–12.

3 Shah MN, Cushman JT, Davis CO, et al. The epidemiology of emergency medical services use by children: an analysis of the National Hospital Ambulatory Medical Care Survey. *Prehosp Emerg Care* 2008;12:269–76.

4 EMSC National Resource Center, Children's National Medical Center. *Gap Analysis of EMS Related Research. Report to the Federal Interagency Committee on EMS,* 2009. Available at: www.childrensnational.org/emsc

5 Field JM, Hazinski MF, Sayre MR, et al. Part 1: executive summary. 2010 American Heart Association Guidelines for Cardiopulmonary Resuscitation and Emergency Cardiovascular Care. *Circulation* 2010; 122:S640–56.

6 Wang HE, Mann NC, Mears G, et al. Out-of-hospital airway management in the United States. *Resuscitation* 2011;82:378–85.

7 Denver Metro Area Study Group. A prospective multicenter evaluation of prehospital airway management performance in a large metropolitan region. *Prehosp Emerg Care* 2009;13:304–10.

8 Nagler J. Emergency airway management in children: unique pediatric considerations. UpToDate. Available from: www.uptodate.com/contents/emergency-airway-management-in-children-unique-pediatric-considerations

9 Ehrlich PF, Seidman PS, Atallah O, et al. Endotracheal intubations in rural pediatric trauma patients. *J Pediatr Surg* 2004;39:1376–80.

10 Gausche M, Lewis RJ, Stratton SJ, et al. Effect of out-of-hospital pediatric endotracheal intubation on survival and neurological outcome. *JAMA* 2000;283:783–90.

11 Stiell IG, Spaite DW, Field B, et al. Advanced life support for out-of-hospital respiratory distress. *N Engl J Med* 2007;356:2156–64.

12 Mussman GM, Parker MW, Statile A, et al. Suctioning and length of stay in infants hospitalized with bronchiolitis. *JAMA Pediatr* 2013;167:414–21.

13 Mallory MD, Shay DK, Garrett J, Bordley WC. Bronchiolitis management preferences and the influence of pulse oximetry and respiratory rate on the decision to admit. *Pediatrics* 2003; 111:e45–51.

14 Camargo CA, Rachelefsky G, Schatz M. Managing asthma exacerbations in the emergency department: Summary of the National Asthma Education and Prevention Expert Panel Report 3 Guidelines for the Management of Asthma Exacerbations. *J Emerg Med* 2009;37:S6–17.

15 Chavasse RJ, Seddon P, Bara A, McKean MC. Short acting beta2-agonists for recurrent wheeze in children under two years of age. *Cochrane Database Syst Rev* 2002;3:CD002873.

16 Westley CR, Cotton EK, Brooks JG. Nebulized racemic epinephrine by ippb for the treatment of croup: a double-blind study. *Am J Dis Child* 1978;132:484–7.

17 Bjornson C, Russell KF, Vandermeer B, et al. Nebulized epinephrine for croup in children. *Cochrane Database Syst Rev* 2011;2:CD006619.

18 Kunkel NC. Baker MD. Use of racemic epinephrine, dexamethasone, and mist in the outpatient management of croup. *Pediatr Emerg Care* 1996;12:156–9.

19 Vilke GM, Steen PJ, Smith AM, Chan TC. Out-of-hospital pediatric intubation by paramedics: the San Diego experience. *J Emerg Med* 2002;22:71–4.

20 Burton JH, Baumann MR, Maoz T, et al. Endotracheal intubation in a rural EMS state: procedure utilization and impact of skills maintenance guidelines. *Prehosp Emerg Care* 2003;7:352–6.

21 DiRusso SM, Sullivan T, Risucci D, et al. Intubation of pediatric trauma patients in the field: predictor of negative outcome despite risk stratification. *J Trauma* 2005;59:84–91.

22 Ritter SC, Guyette FX. Prehospital pediatric King LT-D use: a pilot study. *Prehosp Emerg Care* 2011;15:401–4.

23 Mitchell MS, White ML, King WD, Wang HE. Paramedic King laryngeal tube airway insertion versus endotracheal intubation in simulated pediatric respiratory arrest. *Prehosp Emerg Care* 2012; 16:284–8.

24 Byars DV, Brodsky RA, Evans D, et al. Comparison of direct laryngoscopy to pediatric King LT-D in simulated airways. *Pediatr Emerg Care* 2012;28:750–2.

25 Guyette FX, Roth KR, LaCovey DC. Feasibility of laryngeal mask airway use by prehospital personnel in simulated pediatric respiratory arrest. *Prehosp Emerg Care* 2007;11:245–9.

26 Chen L, Hsiao AL. Randomized trial of endotracheal tube versus laryngeal mask airway in simulated prehospital pediatric arrest. *Pediatrics* 2008;122:e294–7.

27 American Heart Association. Management of respiratory distress and failure. In: Chameides L, Samson RA, Schexnayder SM, Hazinski MF (eds) *PALS Provider Manual*. Dallas, TX: American Heart Association, 2011.

28 Infantile Apnea and Home Monitoring. NIH Consensus Statement Online, Sep 29–Oct 1 1986. Available at: http://consensus.nih.gov/1986/1986InfantApneaMonitoring058html.htm

29 Stratton SJ, Taves A, Lewis RJ, et al. Apparent life-threatening events in infants: high risk in the out-of-hospital environment. *Ann Emerg Med* 2004;43:711–17.

30 McGovern MC, Smith MB. Causes of apparent life threatening events in infants: a systematic review. *Arch Dis Child* 2004;89:1043–8.

31 Davies F, Gupta R. Apparent life threatening events in infants presenting to an emergency department. *Emerg Med J* 2002;19:11–16.

32 Mittal MK, Sun G, Baren JM. A clinical decision rule to identify infants with apparent life-threatening event who can be safely discharged from the emergency department. *Pediatr Emer Care* 2012;28:599–605.

33 Claudius I, Keens T. Do all infants with apparent life-threatening events need to be admitted? *Pediatrics* 2007;119:679–83. [Erratum in *Pediatrics* 2007;119:1270.]

34 Bonkowsky JL, Guenther E, Filloux FM, Srivastava R. Death, child abuse, and adverse neurological outcome of infants after an apparent life-threatening event. *Pediatrics* 2008;122:125–31.

35 Guenther E, Powers A, Srivastava R, Bonkowsky JL. Abusive head trauma in children presenting with an apparent life-threatening event. *J Pediatr* 2010;157:821–5.

36 Fuchs S. Managing seizures in children. *Emergency* 1990;22̣47̣52̣.

37 American Heart Association. Recognition of shock. In: Chameides L, Samson RA, Schexnayder SM, Hazinski MF (eds) *PALS Provider Manual*. Dallas, TX: American Heart Association, 2011.

38 American Academy of Pediatrics. Cardiovascular emergencies. In: Dieckmann RA (ed) *Pediatric Education for Prehospital Professionals*, 2nd edn. Sudbury, MA: Jones and Bartlett, 2006.

39 Kleinman ME, Chameides L, Schexnayder SM, et al. Part 14: pediatric advanced life support. 2010 American Heart Association Guidelines for Cardiopulmonary Resuscitation and Emergency Cardiovascular Care. *Circulation* 2010;122:S876–908.

40 Rosetti VA, Thompson BM, Aprahamian C, et al. Difficulty and delay in intravascular access in pediatric arrests. *Ann Emerg Med* 1984;13:406.

41 Gausche M, Henderson DB, Brownstein D, et al. Education of out-of-hospital emergency medical personnel in pediatrics: report of a national task force. *Ann Emerg Med* 1998;31:58–64.

42 Carcillo JA, Han K, Lin J, Orr R. Goal-directed management of pediatric shock in the emergency department. *Clin Ped Emerg Med* 2007;8:165–75.

43 Sacchetti A, Wernovsky G, Paston C, Fernandes M. Hypoventilation and hypoxia in reversal of cardiogenic shock in an infant with congenital heart disease. *Emerg Med J* 2004;21:636–8.

44 Donoghue AJ, Nadkarni V, Berg RA, et al. Out-of-hospital pediatric cardiac arrest: an epidemiologic review and assessment of current knowledge. *Ann Emerg Med* 2005;46:512–22.

45 Nitta M, Iwami T, Kitamura T, et al. Age-specific differences in outcomes after out-of-hospital cardiac arrests. *Pediatrics* 2011;128:e812–20.

46 Atkins DL, Everson-Stewart S, Sears GK, et al. Epidemiology and outcomes from out-of-hospital cardiac arrest in children: the ROC epistry-cardiac arrest. *Circulation* 2009;119:1484–91.

47 Moler FW, Donaldson AE, Meert K, et al. Multicenter cohort study of out-of-hospital pediatric cardiac arrest. *Crit Care Med* 2011;39:141–9.

48 Young KD, Gausche-Hill M, McClung CD, Lewis RJ. A prospective, population-based study of the epidemiology and outcome of out-of-hospital pediatric cardiopulmonary arrest. *Pediatrics* 2004;114:157–64.

49 Zwingmann J, Mehlhorn AT, Hammer T, et al. Survival and neurologic outcome after traumatic out-of-hospital cardiopulmonary arrest in a pediatric and adult population: a systematic review. *Crit Care* 2012;16(4):R117.

50 DeMaio VJ, Osmond MH, Stiell IG, et al. Epidemiology of out-of-hospital pediatric cardiac arrest due to trauma. *Prehosp Emerg Care* 2012;16:230–6.

51 Kitamura K, Iwami T, Kawamura T, et al. Conventional and chest-compression-only cardiopulmonary resuscitation by bystanders for children who have out-of-hospital cardiac arrests: a prospective, nationwide, population-based cohort study. *Lancet* 2010;375: 1347–54.

52 Link MS, Atkins DL, Passman RS, et al. Part 6: electrical therapies: automated external defibrillators, defibrillation, cardioversion, and pacing: 2010 American Heart Association Guidelines for Cardiopulmonary Resuscitation and Emergency Cardiovascular Care. *Circulation* 2010;122:S706–19.

53 Scholefield B, Duncan H, Davies P, et al. Hypothermia for neuroprotection in children after cardiopulmonary arrest. *Cochrane Database Syst Rev* 2013;2:CD009442.

54 Tagin MA, Woolcott CG, Vincer MJ, et al. Hypothermia for neonatal hypoxic ischemic encephalopathy. *Arch Pediatr Adolesc Med* 2012;166:558–66.

55 Hall WL II, Myers JH, Pepe PE, et al. The perspective of paramedics about on-scene termination of resuscitation efforts for pediatric patients. *Resuscitation* 2004;60:175–87.

56 Mikati MA, Obeid M. Conditions that mimic seizures. In: Kliegman RM, Stanton BMD, St Geme J, et al (eds) *Nelson Textbook of Pediatrics*, 19th edn. Philadelphia: W.B. Saunders, 2011.

57 Johns Hopkins Hospital, Arcara K, Tschudy M (eds) *The Harriet Lane Handbook: A Manual for Pediatric House Officers*, 19th edn. Philadelphia: Elsevier Mosby, 2012.

CHAPTER 55

Pediatric trauma priorities

Joseph L. Wright

Introduction

Injury is the leading cause of death and disability in children, and adolescents, young adults, and pediatric patients constitute 25% of all injured patients in the United States. While overall mortality is one-third the rate of trauma deaths in adults, case fatality rates for children are higher [1]. In other words, for equivalent trauma severity, children are more likely than adults to die during transport and resuscitation. Although prehospital encounters with pediatric patients represent a small fraction of EMS transports, traumatic injury is the most common chief complaint for EMS response in the pediatric age range [2].

Most injuries in children fall into the category of minor trauma, such as contusions and lacerations, and typically require straightforward application of the basic tenets of wound care, splinting, and immobilization. However, being prepared to manage major multisystem pediatric trauma involves a thorough understanding of the unique anatomical and physiological characteristics of the pediatric patient, as well as a working appreciation of pediatric growth and development [3,4]. The effect that these factors can bring to bear upon injury presentation and patient assessment, and thus the establishment of resuscitation and treatment priorities, is significant.

The following discussion is organized around a system-based inventory of what makes children different and an analysis of how these differences can affect the approach to the pediatric trauma patient. The clinical implications of these unique attributes are highlighted in the context of the trauma survey. Also important is a basic appreciation of injury mechanisms in children, as they differ from those in older patients. The recognition of particular injury patterns can be important clues in the field assessment and management of the pediatric trauma patient.

Anatomical and physiological considerations

There are several key anatomical and physiological characteristics unique to the pediatric patient of which the prehospital professional needs to be aware when evaluating an injured child. These characteristics can affect the presentation of traumatic injuries, especially in young children, and require a heightened index of suspicion during the trauma survey for subtle signs and symptoms of occult injury.

General

Because of a child's smaller body size, traumatic forces can be distributed over a larger area, thus making multisystem trauma the rule rather than the exception with childhood injuries. Children often sustain internal injuries with little or no external evidence of trauma. Thus, as a general rule, internal injury cannot be ruled out in a child merely based on the absence of external signs of trauma. Children also have a large surface area to body mass ratio and are particularly vulnerable to thermoregulatory derangements from prolonged environmental exposure. Particularly in infants, the relatively large head can be a source of significant unrecognized heat loss in a trauma resuscitation situation. The simple placement of a cap on the head of an infant during transport and turning up the heat in the ambulance can help to obviate this problem.

Head

Head injury is the most common cause of serious trauma in children. The disproportionately large head in young children functions like a "lawn dart," causing them to lead head-first during falls or rapid deceleration mechanisms, such as car crashes. More than 80% of multisystem pediatric trauma cases involve the head and nearly one-third of all childhood injury deaths result from head injury [1,4]. Among the highest priority early

Emergency Medical Services: Clinical Practice and Systems Oversight, Second Edition. Volume 1: Clinical Aspects of EMS.
Edited by David C. Cone, Jane H. Brice, Theodore R. Delbridge, and J. Brent Myers.
© 2015 NAEMSP. Published 2015 by John Wiley & Sons, Inc. Companion Website: www.wiley.com\go\cone\naemsp

interventions in the management of multisystem pediatric trauma are those directed at limiting the severity of traumatic brain injury and preserving brain function.

Airway

The pediatric airway has several unique anatomical features with which the prehospital professional must be familiar to ensure successful airway management. These features are usually present until about 8 or 9 years of age when the airway assumes more of an adult configuration. Because of the relatively short neck, particularly in young children, the larynx is more cephalad and far more anterior than what would be visualized on direct laryngoscopy of an adult patient. In fact, the cricoid pressure provided by the Sellick maneuver is not only necessary to occlude the esophagus during endotracheal intubation, but is often required to actually bring the airway into view. The diameter of the pediatric airway is obviously much smaller than the adult airway and is far more vulnerable to compromise from relatively small amounts of obstructive material, blood, or edema. The tongue is a relatively larger structure within the mouth and is actually the most common cause of upper airway obstruction in the young child.

The epiglottis is a floppier, U-shaped structure that generally requires use of the straight Miller blade to control it directly and provide adequate visualization during intubation. The narrowest part of the pediatric airway is the subglottic region, below the vocal cords, as opposed to at the cords themselves. This "physiological cuff" obviates the need for cuff inflation or for cuffed endotracheal tubes altogether before 8 years of age. Children are obligatory abdominal breathers and depend on sufficient diaphragmatic excursions to ventilate properly. Swallowing air, or aerophagia, with subsequent gastric distension is common in the trauma resuscitation setting. Gastric decompression with an orogastric or nasogastric tube is required to prevent disruption of ventilatory mechanics [5,6].

Spinal column

Although vertebral injuries in children are uncommon, the cervical spine has a high injury risk potential due to the large head being supported by relatively weak neck muscles and elastic supporting ligaments. Through the age of 8, anatomically, the pediatric c-spine has a higher fulcrum (C1–C2) compared to adults upon extreme flexion-extension of the neck. Therefore disruption of innervation to the diaphragm (phrenic nerve) and accompanying ventilatory impairment must be a consideration in high-energy mechanisms in which neck injury with vertebral fracture is a possibility [7,8]. Compression fractures to the thoracolumbar vertebral bodies are a possibility in rapid deceleration from a motor vehicle crash when a child hyperflexes over a lap belt which is improperly positioned across the abdomen. This circumstance is typically the result of young children being prematurely advanced to adult restraint systems when they still require the use of belt-positioning booster seats [9].

Cardiovascular

The cardiovascular response to hemodynamic instability from bleeding in young children is one of rapid and accentuated vasoconstriction with limited stroke volume boosting capacity. The ability to increase cardiac output is almost entirely dependent on the capacity to increase heart rate because of the diminished compliance of the immature ventricular myocardium. Tachycardia is the earliest and most sensitive sign of impending hemorrhagic shock in children and must always be explained in the evaluation of any injured child. The prehospital professional must also appreciate that normal ranges for pediatric vital signs are age dependent, and that convenient access to a reference guide is prudent. The total circulating blood volume in a child is 70–80 cc/kg and children will maintain compensatory vasoconstrictive mechanisms in the face of hemorrhage until 25% blood volume loss, after which uncompensated shock rapidly ensues [3,10]. Particularly in young children, relatively small volumes of blood loss can precipitate hemorrhagic shock and it is incumbent upon the prehospital professional to note external evidence of blood loss on the scene and maintain a high index of suspicion for occult blood loss, especially in the face of tachycardia. Even an isolated laceration to the highly vascularized scalp of an infant can produce significant enough blood loss to warrant volume resuscitation.

Musculoskeletal, chest, and abdomen

The pediatric musculoskeletal system is generally more pliable and elastic than an adult's and, therefore, less likely to yield fractures in response to equivalent mechanical force. For example, significant blunt force trauma can be distributed to the intrathoracic cavity without evidence of rib fractures. Therefore, injuries like flail chest are uncommon in children, yet high-energy transfers can exert significant injury directly to the heart and lungs. The mediastinum in a child is hypermobile and can be significantly displaced, for instance, by a tension pneumothorax with concomitant kinking of the great vessels. Loss of pulses or other sudden change of vital signs should raise suspicion for this possibility.

The ribcage itself is more horizontally oriented than in adults, exposing the liver and spleen which themselves are poorly protected by underdeveloped abdominal muscles and by the absence of a fat pad. This same orientation is responsible for excursion of the diaphragm on full exhalation as high as the nipple line with concomitant presentation of underlying abdominal organs high in the thoracoabdominal cavity. The clinical implication is that injuries to abdominal organs can occur after chest trauma alone.

In the developing long bones, the ligamentous structures are actually stronger than the nearby growth plates, explaining why fractures at the epiphyseal-metaphyseal region, the weak cartilaginous areas, are more common in children.

Injury patterns

Children in the United States are far more likely to sustain blunt trauma than are adults; blunt force mechanisms represent nearly 90% of the pediatric injury burden. Motor vehicle occupant injuries remain the leading cause of death in the pediatric age group [1]. Although penetrating injury mechanisms are far more typical of adult patients, firearm injuries among children, especially unintentional, are a growing concern, as are intentional firearm injuries among adolescents for whom gun violence is the most common cause of penetrating trauma [11]. Children are typically injured as a function of their activity or location. Thus, being aware of common patterns of injury based on mechanism as part of the assessment of the pediatric trauma patient is important. Three examples are Waddell's triad, handle bar injuries, and the lap belt complex.

- Waddell's triad refers to the multisystem injury pattern seen when a child pedestrian is struck by a vehicle. This mechanism can produce lower extremity (femur) fractures from direct contact with the bumper, chest and abdominal trauma caused by being thrown onto the hood, and, finally, head injury when the child strikes the pavement, as described above, lawn dart style.
- Bicycle falls produce a range of injuries from minor abrasions and contusions to major head injury in unhelmeted riders. However, contact with the bicycle handle bars during a fall can cause intraabdominal trauma, such as a duodenal hematoma, which, clinically, may be very subtle and notoriously late-presenting. The prehospital professional must have a high index of suspicion for such injury when soliciting a history that reveals this mechanism.
- The lap belt complex refers to a constellation of signs and possibly symptoms associated with hyperflexion over the top of an abdominally positioned lap belt during rapid deceleration in a motor vehicle crash. The presence of an ecchymotic bruise across the abdomen can be an important clue to underlying intraabdominal (especially hollow viscus) injuries, as well as vertebral compression fractures to the thoracolumbar spine. These injuries can also have a delayed clinical presentation, thereby making recognition of the mechanism and associated injury pattern essential [9].

The prehospital professional may encounter traumatic injuries that seem inconsistent with the developmental motor capability of a young child to have sustained as a result of an unintentional mechanism. This circumstance should be a red flag for suspected intentional injury or child abuse. Child abuse is the most important cause of visceral injuries in children under the age of 3 [3,12].

Pain management

Due to the wide range of developmental and communication variability in assessing pain in children and unfounded concern about masking injury, pediatric trauma patients are frequently undertreated with analgesics. Recent national efforts to define an evidence-based approach to pain management in all injured patients strongly support weight-based opioid dosing, with either intravenous morphine sulfate, 0.1 mg/kg, or intranasal or intravenous fentanyl, 0.1 µg/kg. Redosing if pain persists upon 5-minute reassessment is also strongly recommended [13,14].

Resuscitation and management priorities

The approach to the trauma survey is basically the same as in adults. The sequencing of the steps in assessment of the injured child must be primarily attendant to the integrity of the airway and adequacy of ventilation, along with protection and immobilization of the cervical spine as necessary. Controlling bleeding, establishing vascular access, and supporting circulation are also primary management priorities. As the prehospital professional completes the trauma survey and head-to-toe secondary assessment, there are several pitfalls and caveats based on the aforementioned unique characteristics that must be kept in mind [3].

- Failure to recognize the subtle signs of early shock. Tachycardia is the most sensitive measure of compensated traumatic shock, usually hemorrhagic, in an injured child and should never be dismissed [10]. Also crucial is understanding that responsiveness inconsistent with expected developmental stage suggests a derangement in sensorium secondary to early shock and compromise of cerebral perfusion.
- Failure to suspect abdominal injury in multiple trauma. Small size, greater surface to mass ratio, poor protection of viscera by muscle or fat, and compliant musculoskeletal system all contribute to the widespread internal distribution of kinetic energy forces in multisystem trauma. The absence of external signs of injury should never rule out intrathoracic or intraabdominal injuries.
- Acute gastric dilation mimics visceral injury. Swallowed air with gastric distension can not only mimic injury but may interfere with diaphragmatic excursion and thus impair ventilation. Decompression with passage of an orogastric or nasogastric tube will ameliorate this preventable complication.
- Inadequate pain management. Oligoanalgesia, or underdosing of pain medications in the field, may be more common in pediatric patients due to communications challenges in the way that children manifest and express pain and/or in the way that providers may subjectively interpret it. Appropriate weight-based dosing of opioid analgesics (morphine or fentanyl) should always be offered in the management of moderate-to-severe pain associated with traumatic injury [13,14].

Field triage

The Centers for Disease Control and Prevention's 2011 Guidelines for the Field Triage of Injured Patients introduced a modification to the Step 1 criteria that recognizes that patients requiring ventilatory support, independent of respiratory rate, require immediate transport to a trauma center. This revision is particularly appropriate for pediatric patients acknowledging that adults and children in need of ventilatory support, including both bag-mask ventilation and intubation, represent a high-risk group, whether or not their respiratory rate falls outside the specified ranges of <10 or >29 breaths per minute (<20 in infant aged <1 year) [15].

References

1 Tuggle D, Krug SE, American Academy of Pediatrics, Section on Orthopedics, Committee on Pediatric Emergency Medicine, Section on Critical Care, Section on Surgery, Section on Transport Medicine, Committee on Pediatric Emergency Medicine, and Pediatric Orthopedic Society of North America. Management of pediatric trauma. *Pediatrics* 2008;121:849–54.

2 Lerner EB, Dayan PS, Brown K, et al. Characteristics of the pediatric patients treated by the Pediatric Emergency Care Applied Research Network's affiliated EMS agencies. *Prehosp Emerg Care* 2014; 18:52–9.

3 Wright J, Patterson M. Resuscitating the pediatric patient. *Emerg Med Clin North Am* 1996;14:219–31.

4 American Academy of Pediatrics. Trauma. In: Fuchs S, Pante M (eds) *Pediatric Education for Prehospital Professionals*, 3rd edn. Burlington, MA: Jones and Bartlett, 2014.

5 American Academy of Pediatrics, American College of Emergency Physicians, American College of Surgeons Committee on Trauma, Emergency Medical Services for Children, Emergency Nurses Association, National Association of EMS Physicians, National Association of State EMS Officials. Equipment for ground ambulances – Joint Policy Statement. *Prehosp Emerg Care* 2013 Oct 29 (Epub ahead of print).

6 Wright JL, Krug SE. Emergency medical services for children. In: Kliegman R et al. (eds) *Nelson Textbook of Pediatrics*, 19th edn. Philadelphia: Elsevier, 2011.

7 Leonard JC, Kuppermann N, Olsen C, et al. Factors associated with cervical spine injury in children after blunt trauma. *Ann Emerg Med* 2011;58:145–55.

8 Kim EG, Brown KM, Leonard JC, et al., for the C-Spine Study Group of the Pediatric Emergency Care Applied Research Network (PECARN). Variability of prehospital spinal immobilization in children at risk for cervical spine injury. *Pediatr Emerg Care* 2013;29:413–18.

9 Newman KD, Bowman LM, Eichelberger MR, et al. The lap belt complex: intestinal and lumbar spine injury in children. *J Trauma* 1990;30:1133–8.

10 Schwaitzberg SD, Bergman KS, Harris BH. A pediatric trauma model of continuous hemorrhage. *J Pediatr Surg* 1988;23:605–9.

11 Dowd MD, Sege RD, for the American Academy of Pediatrics. Firearm-related injuries affecting the pediatric population. *Pediatrics* 2012;130:e1416–23.

12 American Academy of Pediatrics. Child maltreatment. In: Fuchs S, Pante M (eds) *Pediatric Education for Prehospital Professionals*, 3rd edn. Burlington, MA: Jones and Bartlett, 2014.

13 Brown KM, Hirshon JM, Alcorta RA, Weik TS, Lawner BJ, Ho S, Wright JL. Implementation and evaluation of an evidence-based prehospital pain management protocol developed using the national prehospital model process. *Prehosp Emerg Care* 2014;18:–51.

14 Gaushe-Hill M, Brown KM, Oliver ZJ, et al. An evidence-based guideline for prehospital analgesia in trauma. *Prehosp Emerg Care* 2014;18:25–34.

15 Centers for Disease Control and Prevention. Guidelines for field triage of injured patients. *MMWR* 2012;61:1–21.

CHAPTER 56

Technology-dependent children

Brent D. Kaziny and Manish I. Shah

Introduction

As technology advances, medicine has become better equipped to extend the life expectancy of individuals who have complex medical conditions. Children with conditions such as hearing impairment, seizures, and extreme prematurity are living with technology that can be both life-sustaining and life-enriching. EMS physicians and prehospital personnel must be familiar with this technology in order to better care for the patients they encounter.

According to a recent data query from the Child and Adolescent Health Measurement Initiative, the percentage of children with special needs is on the rise. In 2001, only 12.8% of children in the nation were defined as having "special needs." This number increased to 15% in 2013 [1]. Not only are these children increasing in numbers, they also have significant increases in the number of hospitalizations and percentage of hospital days and charges when compared to children without special health care needs. For example, one study showed that this population had an increase in hospitalizations of over 19% from 2004 to 2009, and accounted for 81.7% of the hospital days for all children admitted at 28 children's hospitals across the country [2].

One study that reviewed hospital discharges from a large pediatric tertiary care center found that 41% of all patients sent home relied on some form of technology. For children included in this retrospective cohort, the most common medical devices were gastrostomy or jejunostomy tubes (10%), central venous catheters (7%), medication nebulizers (7%), ventriculoperitoneal cerebrospinal fluid shunts (2%), and tracheostomies (1%) [3].

As this population has grown, there has also been a growing interest in how best to care for these children in the prehospital setting. While focused training programs specifically designed to deal with these patients have been conducted and studied, it is still unclear whether or not they provide a true benefit to either the prehospital provider or the patient. One study reviewing such training programs noted that even in children with special health care needs, simple Basic Life Support (BLS) procedures were much more common than advanced procedures [4]. Such research points out that despite these children's complex conditions, BLS is likely all that is needed during their prehospital care.

While caring for these children, it is important to recognize that the medical and technological complexity of their conditions may greatly compound the likelihood for medical errors to be made. These potential errors range from simple to complex. Something as simple as forgetting to transport a patient with his or her required equipment could pose great problems, not just during the child's transport but also upon arrival at the health care facility. Of course, more complex errors can be made, such as the failure to distinguish between an obstructed tracheostomy and a ventilator malfunction [5]. Though BLS is what is needed to manage most technology-dependent children in the prehospital setting, familiarity with how to manage common situations in this population is essential for both EMS physicians and field providers.

The caregiver as a resource and the emergency information sheet

A family member and/or home nurse care for the vast majority of children with special health care needs at home. As such, supplies for their routine care are usually present in the home, and caregivers have a great deal of knowledge with regard to both the child's medical issues as well as the maintenance and routine functioning of their medical devices. It is essential to recognize the family member and/or caregiver as a vital resource during the prehospital care and transport of these children. However, at least one study showed that over half of caretakers at a specialty clinic visit were unable to report some of the child's specific diagnoses, and almost 30% could not provide a list of medications. Interestingly, in this same study of 49 caregivers, none of the children wore any medical identification jewelry [6]. While primary caregivers should be considered as the first source for information regarding the child's care and accompanying medical technology, EMS agencies should also engage with their local hospitals to facilitate the exchange of health information for transported patients.

Emergency Medical Services: Clinical Practice and Systems Oversight, Second Edition. Volume 1: Clinical Aspects of EMS.
Edited by David C. Cone, Jane H. Brice, Theodore R. Delbridge, and J. Brent Myers.
© 2015 NAEMSP. Published 2015 by John Wiley & Sons, Inc. Companion Website: www.wiley.com\go\cone\naemsp

As a result of this potential lack of information on the caretakers' part, especially in times of stress or in their absence, both the American Academy of Pediatrics and the American College of Emergency Physicians have endorsed the use of an emergency information form for children with special health care needs. In addition, many states ask parents to place one in the freezer of the child's home, so that they can be located quickly and easily in the event of a medical emergency. Even when parents are home, the prehospital provider should ask about the emergency information form and verify that it is up to date, since the parent may not be the primary caregiver and/or the person with the child may be distracted in the midst of an emergency situation [7,8].

The technology

DOPE mnemonic

When evaluating any device that requires troubleshooting, it is essential to use a systematic approach, such as the DOPE mnemonic. Though this is routinely used with a failing endotracheal intubation, similar concepts can be applied to almost all the devices discussed below. The original DOPE mnemonic reminds us to think about:

D - Dislodgment
O - Obstruction
P - Pneumothorax (for airway) or Peritonitis/Perforation/Pseudocyst (for gastrostomy tubes and ventriculoperitoneal shunts)
E - Equipment malfunction

Tracheostomy tubes

A tracheostomy may become dislodged or obstructed, leading to complications in management of airway and breathing. When tracheostomy tubes are connected to ventilators, pneumothorax and/or equipment malfunction can also lead to respiratory distress or failure.

Tracheostomies serve to maintain the airway in a tracheostomy-dependent patient, but they also preserve stoma integrity. Many reasons exist for needing to replace a tracheotomy tube, the most common being difficulty with breathing or ventilation due to a clogged tube, and the second being decannulation, or accidental removal of the tube. The first priority must be maintained airway and breathing for the patient while decisions are made regarding tracheostomy management. EMS providers should assemble appropriate equipment prior to considering replacing a tracheostomy tube. Key equipment includes suction and suction catheters, replacement tracheostomy tube and cannula, if available (families often have their own equipment), and tracheostomy tape or the patient's preferred method of stabilizing the tracheostomy tube.

If the child is in distress, first attempt to ventilate via bag and mask, either via the tracheostomy or via the mouth with the stoma site covered. Administering several drops of saline in the stoma prior to suctioning may help to clear debris and/or secretions. If the tracheostomy tube is clogged despite suctioning, remove it with the head and neck slightly hyperextended after releasing the securing ties and deflating the balloon, if present. If the tracheostomy tube is to be reused, cleanse secretions and debris and ensure that the balloon is still functional prior to reinserting it. The tube can be stiffened for reinsertion by inserting the obturator or placing it in cold water. If no replacement tube is available and the old tube is not functional, use an endotracheal tube of similar size by removing the connector portion of the tube, trimming the tube to a similar length as the prior tracheostomy tube, and replacing the connector. Gently insert the lubricated tube, holding it by the flange using pressure in a posterior/inferior direction. Gentle traction above and below the stoma may make passage easier. Once in place, remove the obturator. If unable to pass the tube, a repeat attempt may be tried with a smaller size tracheostomy tube, if available, or a smaller endotracheal tube placed in the stoma. After placement and confirmation, secure it with clean tracheostomy ties or clean stabilization device.

Home oxygen

Many technology-dependent children require home oxygen. The patient's home oxygen settings can be assessed by observing the flow and FiO_2 on an oxygen concentrator and/or oxygen tank in the home. The patient should be transferred over to the ambulance oxygen supply for the transport, but any personal tanks should be brought with the child as they may be needed for the return trip home.

Ventilators

Children with tracheostomies may require ventilator support for part of the day, if not 24 hours a day. These ventilators generally have battery packs; however, the ventilator should be placed on the ambulance's power supply for transport. The settings should remain standard per the caregiver's instructions, unless concerns for poor O_2 saturations, or other signs of poor oxygenation and/or ventilation, are present. For example, if the oxygen saturation is lower than what is normal for the patient or breath sounds are unequal, pneumothorax or equipment failure may be present. Also, if the airway pressures are higher than normal on the ventilator, this may be a sign of airway obstruction. With any of these situations, the prehospital provider should consider maintaining oxygenation and ventilation with a bag-valve attached to the tracheostomy rather than the ventilator. Noting chest rise and an age-appropriate respiratory rate is important in these situations.

Gastrostomy/gastrojejunostomy tubes

Many technology-dependent children require a method of obtaining nutrition other than by mouth. Most of these children have surgically created stomas into the stomach (a gastrostomy tube) or both the stomach and jejunum (a gastrojejunostomy tube). These tubes can present with a number of complications, but most commonly present with either displacement or obstruction.

The more quickly the tube is found to be out, the more likely the success of replacing the gastrostomy tube (G-tube). Families often have replacement G-tubes, or previous G-tubes can be cleansed in gentle solution, rinsed well, and reused. Inspect the site to ensure the stoma is open and no tear is present, and cleanse the site of secretions or debris. Check the G-tube, making sure the balloon is intact and functional. If the tube is in place but seems obstructed, attempt to flush it with 5–10 mL of a carbonated beverage (soda, soda water, or sodium bicarbonate solution). If it is dislodged and a replacement tube is unavailable, a Foley catheter can be used in its place. Once the G-tube or Foley catheter is lubricated, gently insert it using light pressure into the stoma. If resistance is met, repeat the attempt with a red rubber catheter. If successful, remove the red rubber catheter and reattempt placement of G-tube or Foley. If still unable to pass, replace the red rubber catheter or use a smaller Foley. Inflate the balloon with 3–5 mL of saline or water and once in, check placement by pulling back with a syringe for gastric contents, followed by instillation of air while auscultating with a stethoscope.

Vagus nerve stimulators

A vagus nerve stimulator (VNS) is a small device that is surgically implanted under the skin. Typically, it is placed near the patient's clavicle and can be felt with palpation. The device has a wire that leads from the device to the vagus nerve. It is then programmed to deliver a weak electrical current, similar to a pacemaker, which travels along the vagus nerve to the brain. These signals help prevent seizures. In addition, an external magnet can be passed over the device if the patient is seizing or if the patient feels he or she is about to seize, in an effort to abort the seizure. The prehospital provider may be required to pass this magnet over the device, in order to stimulate the device to prevent or stop a seizure. However, despite the presence of a VNS, prehospital providers should continue to provide the same level of care and perform the same general interventions they would normally perform for a seizing patient.

Cochlear implants

A cochlear implant is generally located behind and above the external ear and aids individuals with significant auditory impairment. In general, these should be left in place and not adjusted or removed during prehospital care. However, the presence of this hardware means that patients with these implants are at higher risk for meningitis, mastoiditis, and intracranial abscesses. So these complications should be considered in the setting of fever, neck stiffness, headache, vomiting, or severe ear pain.

Ventriculoperitoneal shunts

A ventriculoperitoneal (VP) shunt is placed in children with obstructive hydrocephalus. Obstructive hydrocephalus is common in patients with neural tube defects, such as spina bifida, meningocele, and myelomeningocele. Since the cerebrospinal fluid (CSF) in the ventricles of the brain does not

adequately drain, a VP shunt is placed to prevent ventricular swelling, brain herniation, and death. The VP shunt tubing leads from the ventricle and generally courses behind one ear, down the neck, and into the peritoneal space, where the fluid is deposited and reabsorbed by the body. While other types of shunts exist that lead the CSF into various places (ventriculoatrial, ventriculopleural), the VP shunt is the most common.

Patients with VP shunts can present with various complications including infection or malfunction, due to blockage or a break in the tubing. Infection may be associated with fever, and both infection and malfunction can be associated with headache, nausea, vomiting, altered mental status, or focal neurological deficits. There is almost never a need for the prehospital provider to access this tubing, but being able to identify it on exam may provide great insight into what may be affecting the patient.

Central venous catheters

Central venous catheters can exist in a variety of places with varying levels of permanence. If the child has one of these present and it is currently in use, it can be used emergently to deliver intravenous medications and fluids, if a peripheral IV or intraosseous access cannot be obtained first. Patients with central venous catheters are prone to bacteremia and sepsis, so when these children have fever and tachycardia, the prehospital provider should strongly consider giving rapid IV fluids.

Conclusion

Though children who are technology dependent often only require BLS care, at times it is beneficial to utilize pediatric-specific and specialized transport teams when caring for these children. Regional resources for patient transport should be reviewed and assessed to determine the need to involve a pediatric specific transport service for an individual patient [9,10].

While technology-dependent children are not the most common patients encountered in the prehospital setting, becoming familiar with commonly used devices can increase one's confidence significantly. In addition, EMS agencies should identify patients who are technology dependent in their local area in order to know their individual needs prior to an emergency. Remembering to use the caregiver as a resource and to ask for an emergency information form can provide providers with valuable information regarding the patient's specific medical conditions. Finally, relying on home equipment during transport can ensure an uneventful transport with the necessary supplies for a safe arrival.

References

1 NS-CSHCN 2009/10. Data query from the Child and Adolescent Health Measurement Initiative, Data Resource Center for Child and Adolescent Health. Available at: www.childhealthdata.org

2 Berry J, Hall M, Hall DE, et al. Inpatient growth and resource use in 28 children's hospitals. *JAMA Pediatr* 2013;167:170–7.

3 Feudtner C, Villareale NL, Morray B, et al. Technology-dependency among patients discharged from a children's hospital: a retrospective cohort study. *BMC Pediatrics* 2005;5:8.

4 Spaite DW, Conroy C, Karriker KJ, et al. Improving emergency medical services for children with special health care needs: does training make a difference? *Am J Emerg Med* 2001;19:474–8.

5 Sacchetti A, Sacchetti C, Carraccio C, Gerardi M. The potential for errors in children with special health care needs. *Acad Emerg Med* 2000;7:1330–3.

6 Carraccio CL, Dettmer KS, duPont ML, Sacchetti AD. Family member knowledge of children's medical problems: the need for universal application of an emergency data set. *Pediatrics* 1998;102: 367–70.

7 American College of Emergency Physicians. Emergency information form for children with special health care needs. *Ann Emerg Med* 2010;56:315–16.

8 American Academy of Pediatrics, Committee on Pediatric Emergency Medicine and Council on Clinical Information Technology;, American College of Emergency Physicians, Pediatric Emergency Medicine Committee. Policy statement – emergency information forms and emergency preparedness for children with special health care needs. *Pediatrics* 2010;125:829–37.

9 Lerner CF, Kelly RB, Hamilton LJ, Klitzner TS. Medical transport of children with complex chronic conditions. *Emerg Med Int* 2012. Available at: 10.1155/2012/837020

10 O'Neil J, Yonkman J, Talty J, Bull MJ. Transporting children with special health care needs: comparing recommendations and practice. *Pediatrics* 2009;124:596–603.

CHAPTER 57

Approach to the geriatric patient

Thomas V. Caprio and Manish N. Shah

Introduction

The older adult (age ≥65 years) group is the fastest growing segment of the US population. In 2000, 40 million older adults lived in the United States and comprised 13% of the population. The Census Bureau estimates that this number will double by 2040 to 80 million, and older adults will then comprise 21% of the US population [1].

This large number of older adults and the rapid increase in their numbers will significantly affect prehospital physicians and providers. Assuming that use rates remain constant, EMS must prepare for a significant increase in the number of older adult patients requesting assistance, with approximately half of the EMS call volume being comprised of older patients by 2030. EMS leaders must ensure that the EMS system is prepared for this massive demographic change.

Changes of normal aging

The physiological changes of normal aging are important considerations in the approach to the geriatric patient. Aging itself is not a disease. Age should be viewed as a risk factor, but not sufficient in and of itself to cause disease. Aging produces a diminished physiological capacity; therefore, older adults may not have the same functional reserve in organ systems to recover from injury or illness. Even healthy and active older adults may need prolonged periods to recover from acute illness or trauma due to this reduced physiological capacity.

There are normal and predictable physiological changes that occur with normal aging (Box 57.1). The EMS medical director must consider these changes when developing protocols, and the EMS physician must be aware of these changes when caring for older patients in the field. For instance, as skin becomes thinner and less elastic with a reduction in subcutaneous fat, trauma patients can suffer skin tears, and pressure ulcers can form more easily when patients are on backboards. The EMS

medical director must ensure that EMS providers understand these concepts. Otherwise, the providers may encounter difficulty while caring for their patients. For instance, there is a predictable reduction in pulmonary and cardiac function with older age. When an older adult is physiologically stressed, he or she will have reduced ability to compensate for changes in blood pressure or respiratory illness, leading to significant clinical consequences.

Assessment of the geriatric patient

For EMS professionals caring for the geriatric patient, the initial steps are unchanged. A primary survey should be completed, evaluating the patient's ABCs. Vital signs should be obtained and considered while accounting for existing medical problems and medications. Any immediate interventions necessary should be completed. A full history should be taken, including the symptoms the patient has experienced, allergies, medications (including over-the-counter and herbal medications, and medications that the patient is not taking despite prescription), and past medical history. A full examination should be completed. Although not traditionally considered, an environmental assessment should also be completed because the environment can provide clues as to the extent of the disease or the precipitating factors for disease. Finally, a social history should be obtained because psychosocial issues could either be the primary reason for the request for assistance or could precipitate or exacerbate medical issues.

Communication with older patients is key in performing an effective assessment. A common error is to assume that an older patient is deaf, has dementia, or is otherwise unable to communicate or participate in medical evaluation or care. It is common for medical personnel to rely on family members of older patients to contribute collateral information regarding current illness or medical history. However, this often comes at the cost

Emergency Medical Services: Clinical Practice and Systems Oversight, Second Edition. Volume 1: Clinical Aspects of EMS.
Edited by David C. Cone, Jane H. Brice, Theodore R. Delbridge, and J. Brent Myers.
© 2015 NAEMSP. Published 2015 by John Wiley & Sons, Inc. Companion Website: www.wiley.com\go\cone\naemsp

of speaking exclusively to others and entirely excluding the older patient. The general rule of thumb when caring for older patients is to always speak to the patient first and establish his or her level of understanding and participation. Use a strong, clear voice, but avoid shouting as this tends to distort words and makes it more difficult to understand. If hearing aids or eyeglasses are available and practical for the patient to use in the situation, these can make a dramatic difference in communication.

When obtaining the history, it is important to establish the baseline cognitive and physical functioning of the patient. If EMS is responding to a patient with reported "confusion" or "weakness," does this patient have a history of dementia or physical limitations from a prior stroke or other condition? It is also relevant to consider the social context of the patient. Does he or she reside in an assisted living facility, nursing home, or his or her own home? This may influence the decision to transport a patient to the hospital if there are other caregivers available to be with the patient compared with one who lives alone without support. Family members and caregivers can also provide valuable information about the patient. A report by those present during a fall, episode of syncope, or witnessed seizure becomes a crucial element of the medical history, and it is important to communicate this information to subsequent emergency personnel.

The final area to consider is the presence of advance directives and communicating these treatment preferences and goals of care throughout the health system. Patient decisions regarding resuscitation, hospitalization, and appointment of health care agents (health care poxy or durable power of attorney for medical care) are relevant care directives for EMS personnel to quickly identify, honor, and transfer across care settings. Most states have standardized out-of-hospital "do not resuscitate" forms for patients which should be available for immediate review in a patient's place of residence, whether it is a home or a long-term care facility. For patients with advanced chronic or life-threatening illness, these advance directive papers may be the most important tools in guiding subsequent decision making with regard to emergency care. See Volume 1, Chapter 64 for further information on this topic.

Geriatric medical conditions

Cognitive impairment

Cognitive impairment is a common condition among older adults and has been shown to increase as people age. Estimates show that up to 10% of non-institutionalized older adults, 13% of EMS patients, and approximately a quarter of older adult emergency department (ED) patients suffer from it [2]. Because cognitive impairment has been associated with significant morbidity and mortality, it is important to identify this condition, even in the EMS setting. A validated instrument to assess a patient's cognitive function, particularly suited to EMS, is the Six-Item Screener (Box 57.2). This has been shown to have a sensitivity of 89% and specificity of 88% to identify cognitive impairment in a community sample and can be easily used by EMS professionals [3].

Depression

Depression is a common problem among older adults, with studies reporting that up to 20% of community-dwelling older adults suffer from depressed mood [4]. Depressive symptoms are a risk factor for increased use of medical services and for death and disability [5]. Thus, this could be a precipitating factor for repeated EMS use by a patient or deterioration of a patient's medical condition. Due to this increased risk of morbidity and mortality, identification of depression is critical. However, estimates suggest that fewer than one half of depressed older adults receive the correct diagnosis or treatment [4,6]. A number of screening instruments exist for use in the outpatient setting with reasonable sensitivity and specificity to identify potential depression. The Patient Health Questionnaire-2, or PHQ-2, has been shown to be effective in identifying patients who may be depressed (Box 57.3). This tool can be easily used by EMS because it is short and has a simple scoring scheme and excellent sensitivity and specificity for major depressive disorder [7,8]. Recommendations can then be provided to the ED or primary care physician to ensure that the mood issues are considered.

Box 57.1 Common changes in normal aging

- Skin is thinner and susceptible to trauma
- Greater difficulty in temperature regulation
- Risk of fractures from bone loss
- Reduced spine flexibility and loss of height
- Reduced cardiac and pulmonary reserve
- Reduced renal function and drug clearance
- Decline in hormone levels
- Reduced vision from cataracts
- Hearing loss from noise exposure

Box 57.2 Six-Item Screener for cognitive impairment

Ask the patient to repeat three words after you: apple, table, and penny. If not repeated correctly, the test cannot continue.
1 What year is this?
2 What month is this?
3 What is the day of the week?
What were the three objects I asked you to remember?
4 apple
5 table
6 penny
One point for each question answered correctly.
Three or more errors indicate possible dementia.

Source: Callahan CM. *Medical Care* 2002;40:771–81. Reproduced with permission from Lippincott Williams & Wilkins, Inc.

Falls

Falls are a leading and preventable cause of morbidity, mortality, and loss of quality of life among community-dwelling older adults. Among older adults, 30% fall annually and 50% of them fall repeatedly [9]. Falls result in fear, functional deterioration, and even institutionalization. Up to 25% of those who fall suffer serious physical injuries including fractures, joint injuries, and intracranial injuries, and the remainder may suffer emotional consequences [10].

Medications and drug toxicity

A common problem in geriatric medicine is the phenomenon of "polypharmacy." This problem stems from the fact that many older adults are on numerous medications, either due to their medical needs or because multiple medical providers have prescribed medications without full knowledge of the patient's current medication list. The metabolism, distribution, elimination, and excretion of medications can be altered with aging. As patients take an increasing number of prescribed medications, the potential for adverse drug reactions and drug-to-drug interactions also increases. There are also inappropriate medications, particularly those with cardiovascular or anticholinergic side-effects, that can contribute significantly to cardiac or respiratory compromise, falls, urinary problems, delirium, hospitalizations, and even death. Older patients presenting to EMS and the ED are often taking many of these potentially inappropriate medications [11].

Patients may not report medication lists accurately, so it is important for EMS personnel to observe the environment for medications and to consider prescription, over-the-counter, herbal, and dietary supplement use. It often is helpful to ask the patient and family members or caregivers about other medical providers prescribing medications. For example, an older patient may consider medications prescribed by a cardiologist to be different from those prescribed by the primary care physician.

A patient with cognitive difficulties may find it challenging to remember when and how to take prescribed medications, especially if he or she has multiple prescriptions. This cognitive impairment places older patients at risk for errors in taking medications and increases the chance for unintentional overdose. EMS physicians and personnel should look for pill-taking strategies and reminders in the patient's home, including pill boxes, calendars, and prescription bottles. An empty (or full) prescription bottle may sometimes be the only clue as to the patient's actual medication use at home.

Altered mental status

Altered mental status refers to a disturbance in consciousness and a change in the behavior of a patient. In geriatric medicine, this acute change in mental status is often referred to as "delirium." Delirium usually occurs over a relatively short period of time and is marked by a reduced ability to focus, a change in cognition, and a fluctuation throughout the course of a day. Patients with delirium tend to have poor attention, are often disoriented, and have altered levels of consciousness ranging from alert, or even hypervigilant, to profound lethargy [12]. Older patients may be at risk for developing delirium simply because of their acute illnesses. Patients with dementia, cancer (especially brain tumors), stroke, renal or hepatic disease, and metabolic disturbances are at highest risk for developing delirium. A common condition such as pneumonia or a urinary tract infection is sometimes enough to precipitate an older patient's decline in mental status with the development of acute confusion and altered behavior. Medication side-effects, drug toxicity, and overdosage of medications can also be precipitants of delirium.

A careful history from the patient or family caregivers is important in establishing if newly observed behavioral and cognitive symptoms are a change from a person's baseline function, especially in cases with preexisting cognitive impairment or dementia. A recent history of an unwitnessed fall may raise the clinical suspicion for head trauma and resultant traumatic brain injury or even the development of an intracranial hemorrhage (subdural hematoma) which sometimes can manifest several days after the traumatic event. A focused neurological assessment is critical in establishing the urgency of new symptoms and communicating findings to hospital personnel for further evaluation.

Cardiac arrest

Approximately one half of EMS patients suffering from cardiac arrest are older adults. The overall survival rate for all patients suffering cardiac arrest is poor, with most studies reporting fewer than 10% of patients surviving to discharge home [13]. One challenge for field personnel is determining which patients suffering cardiac arrest should be transported to an ED and which should have interventions terminated in the field. Traditionally, EMS professionals have depended on direct medical oversight communication to terminate resuscitation efforts. However, Morrison et al. have found that for BLS systems, a patient who suffers a cardiac arrest not witnessed by EMS, does not receive a shock from an automated external defibrillator during resuscitation, and fails to have return of spontaneous circulation in the field can have the resuscitation appropriately terminated in the field (positive predictive value 99.5%). Applying these criteria to patients receiving ALS care has been reported to be 100% predictive by the same group [14]. These criteria should be considered but must be weighed against psychosocial issues related to leaving the newly deceased in the home or another setting and related to each family's response to the death. These criteria should also be weighed against local system issues related to handling of the body. Local EMS protocols should address all of these issues.

Trauma

The Guidelines for the Field Triage of Injured Patients, developed by the Centers for Disease Control and Prevention, guide EMS personnel in their trauma triage decisions and determining the receiving hospital to which an injured patient should be transported. The goal of the Guidelines is to minimize undertriage (patients who need the resources of a trauma center but are taken elsewhere) without excessive overtriage. Despite these formal guidelines, numerous studies suggest that older adults are less likely to receive trauma center care than younger adults with similar injury severity [15–17].

This variation in care may occur because the Guidelines are not age specific. No age-specific cut-offs for anatomical or physiological parameters exist, despite older adults having different physiological responses to injury and significantly worse outcomes than younger adults from minor injuries [18,19]. Additionally, the Guidelines poorly consider preexisting medical conditions and the use of multiple medications, both of which can affect response to injury and lead to worse outcomes.

The most recent revision of the Guidelines recognizes this and includes an expanded section on geriatric patients under Step Four, the "Special Considerations" section. Age >55 is a "special consideration," meaning EMS providers should consider transporting those patients to trauma centers. However, age as a "special consideration" is subjective and does not *require* transport to a trauma center. Ultimately, the considerations rely on the ability of EMS personnel to recognize serious injury in older adults with limited testing and time, which studies suggest may be inadequate and result in undertriage [15,17,20].

Since time to definitive care is considered important in trauma care, EMS medical directors must focus their attention on destination decisions for older adults trauma patients to ensure that EMS providers can appropriately transport these patients to the correct destination.

Social emergencies

Social issues can be the primary reason for which EMS was requested or may be an important precipitating issue that led to the need for EMS assistance. EMS physicians and medical directors must be sensitive to these issues. Efforts must be made to recognize and address them when caring for older adults. Gaps in social support, caregiver crisis, or evolving family conflicts could all be major underlying reasons for an older adult's acute decompensation in health status or the reason behind requesting EMS. Addressing social issues may require system changes to truly integrate EMS into the health care system, including collaboration with social service agencies, primary care physicians, and others.

Medication and alcohol abuse

Substance abuse is actually quite common among older adults, with over 17% of adults aged 60 and older misusing alcohol or prescription drugs [21]. This can result in frequent ED visits, as well as an increased risk for falls and hip fractures. Because older adult medication abusers tend to be more socially isolated and less public regarding their addiction and related problems, EMS professionals may be the first to truly identify the problem when they enter the home.

Elder abuse and maltreatment

Unlike child abuse, elder abuse and mistreatment have not received much public attention. They are common, with studies reporting that 1–2 million older adults have been injured, exploited, or mistreated [22]. Elder mistreatment includes financial, psychological, physical, and sexual abuse. EMS professionals need training on the risk factors for mistreatment and ways to identify potential abuse. A number of risk factors for elder abuse have been examined and the literature is somewhat inconsistent. Risk factors that have been validated include social isolation of the older adult, dementia, and a shared living arrangement with the abuser. Characteristics of the abuser that have been identified include mental illness, alcohol abuse, and dependency on the older adult [23]. Each EMS agency should have an established protocol for reporting suspected cases of abuse, particularly if EMS providers are mandated reporters by state law.

Caregiver distress

A third social emergency is sometimes identified by the EMS professionals: caregiver distress and burnout. Family members and friends may provide the majority of care for older adults with medical, psychological, or behavioral problems. Over time, this can be exhausting and lead to significant stress for families without sufficient social supports or opportunities for periods of respite. As such, when a request for assistance for elderly patients is made, EMS professionals should pay attention to the family members as much as the primary patient. If the primary caregiver seems to be stressed, overwhelmed, or unable to manage the patient, then he or she may also be in need of assistance. A caregiver may also feel a personal sense of failure if a loved one becomes ill under his or her care, adding to the perceived burden, and the caregiver may be seeking reassurance and support. The EMS professional can help address caregiver needs by reporting information to the ED providers, calling family or friends to provide further support, and by being a calm and professional presence during the care of the patient.

Special considerations

There are a number of special considerations that EMS leaders must acknowledge and address in their systems. EMS professionals may need special equipment to care for older adults. Padding at the upper back is needed to properly stabilize and transport older adults with kyphosis. Padded backboards are needed to prevent the rapid development of decubitus ulcers. Protocols that minimize the use of backboards should be considered. Proper temperature control mechanisms and blankets are needed to prevent hypothermia or hyperthermia. Electronic medical records, preferably integrated through a regional health information organization, would be of particular benefit because older adults tend to have a number of comorbidities and medications, and having these data readily available can result in improved care.

The medical and social condition of an older adult who refuses transport to a hospital needs to be considered carefully before allowing him or her to "sign off." Research has shown that approximately half of older adults cared for by EMS and transported to the ED are admitted to the hospital, and also that older adults experience a decline in functional status after ED visits [24]. Therefore, older adults are a high-risk group and EMS providers should not merely accept the refusal of care, but should instead work to convince the patient to accept transport so he or she can benefit from care in the ED. Potential options to convince a patient to accept transport may include speaking to a medical oversight physician or the patient's primary care physician, or involving family. If the patient persists in refusing, EMS should consider notifying the patient's primary care physician to ensure that careful follow-up occurs. An EMS physician on scene may be able to convince a patient to accept treatment and transport.

Nursing homes and assisted living facilities

Long-term care facilities encompass a spectrum of services and housing options that are designed to address many of the needs of an older adult population. These facilities may include group homes, senior apartments, assisted living facilities, and nursing homes. Nursing homes remain key providers for the frailest older adults: those with complex care needs, high levels of functional dependence, advanced dementia, and those without sufficient social or financial supports to meet their needs at home.

Emergency medical services are often called to evaluate and transport residents of long-term care facilities to and from the hospital. Most commonly, the resident has experienced an acute illness, sustained traumatic injury following a fall, or exhibited a change in behavior. The transfer of appropriate information between these facilities and the hospital is often inadequate and has been recognized as a vital component in ensuring proper continuity of care for these patients [25]. Assisted living facilities

and other senior housing centers are much more varied in the level of documentation available for their residents. It is of value for each EMS agency to collaborate with long-term care facilities in the community to improve access to information and ensure that copies of relevant documentation are readily available when patients are transported to and from the hospital.

Public health

Although the EMS system was originally developed primarily to care for patients with acute injuries and illnesses [26], it is being increasingly recognized that EMS personnel can fulfill an important public health role, including preventing injuries and illnesses and helping patients maintain physical, social, and emotional function. This public health role is being called "community paramedicine." Surveys of EMS providers have indicated that they believe that prevention is a core mission of EMS systems and should be implemented [27]. Work has shown that EMS personnel can successfully screen older adults and perform other public health roles [28,29]. However, the ideal structure, effectiveness, and cost-effectiveness of the screening programs and associated intervention programs still need to be evaluated.

One obstacle to EMS personnel involvement in public health activities is the fragmentation of the US health care system. This prevents EMS personnel from confirming public health needs and ensuring that interventions are provided. Furthermore, the financial fragmentation prevents EMS organization from realizing financial benefits from community paramedicine programs. EMS system leaders and medical directors are encouraged to work with the local medical and social service community to better integrate public health and medical care activities of the EMS system into the health care system, improve communications, and ensure patients receive the highest quality and safest care possible.

Conclusion

Geriatric patients require a thoughtful and focused approach when they are experiencing acute illness or injury. Their chronic medical conditions, functional impairments, and social settings make the older adult population among the most complex that EMS providers may encounter. At the same time, the data gathered in the home setting, treatment interventions, and transfer of information to other providers can have a profound effect on the quality of health care for the most vulnerable of geriatric patients.

References

1 Howden LM, Meyer JA. *Age and Sex Composition: 2010*. Available at: www.census.gov/prod/cen2010/briefs/c2010br-03.pdf

2 Shah MN, Jones CMC, Richardson TM, et al. Prevalence of depression and cognitive impairment in older adult emergency medical services patients. *Prehosp Emerg Care* 2011;15:4–11.

3 Callahan CM, Unverzagt FW, Hui SL, et al. Six-item screener to identify cognitive impairment among potential subjects for clinical research. *Med Care* 2002;40:771–81.

4 Beekman AT, Copeland JR, Prince MJ. Review of community prevalence of depression in later life. *Br J Psychiatry* 1999;174:307–11.

5 Penninx BW, Guralnik JM, Ferrucci L, et al. Depressive symptoms and physical decline in community-dwelling older persons. *JAMA* 1998;279:1720–6.

6 Claassen CA, Larkin GL. Occult suicidality in an emergency department population. *Br J Psych* 2005;186:352–3.

7 Depression Management Tool Kit, Accessed November 1, 2005. Available at: www.depressionprimarycare.org

8 Kroenke K, Spitzer RL, Williams JBW. The Patient Health Questionnaire – 2. Validity of a two-item depression screener. *Med Care* 2003;41:1284–92.

9 Tinetti ME, Speechley M, Ginter SF. Risk factors for falls among elderly persons living in the community. *N Engl J Med* 1988;319:1701–07.

10 Tinetti ME, Williams CS. Falls, injuries due to falls, and the risk of admission to a nursing home. *N Engl J Med* 1997;337:1279–84.

11 Hustey FM, Wallis N, Miller J. Inappropriate prescribing in an older ED population. *Am J Emerg Med* 2007;25:804–7.

12 Inouye SK. Delirium in older persons. *N Engl J Med* 2006;354:1157–65.

13 Hostler D, Thomas EG, Emerson SS, et al. Increased survival after EMS witnessed cardiac arrest. Observations from the Resuscitation Outcomes Consortium (ROC) epistry-cardiac arrest. *Resuscitation* 2010;81:826–30.

14 Morrison LJ, Verbeek PR, Zhan C, et al. Validation of a universal termination of resuscitation clinical prediction rule for advanced and basic life support providers. *Resuscitation* 2009;80(3):324–28.

15 Lane P, Sorondo B, Kelly JJ. Geriatric trauma patients – are they receiving trauma center care? *Acad Emerg Med* 2003;10:244–50.

16 Chang DC, Bass RR, Cornwell EE, et al. Undertriage of elderly trauma patients to state-designated trauma centers. *Arch Surg* 2008;143:776–82.

17 Ma MH, MacKenzie EJ, Alcorta R, et al. Compliance with prehospital triage protocols for major trauma patients. *J Trauma* 1999;46:168–75.

18 Helling TS, Watkins M, Evans LL, et al. Low falls: an underappreciated mechanism of injury. *J Trauma* 1999;46:453–6.

19 Spaniolas K, Cheng JD, Gestring, ML, et al. Ground level falls are associated with significant mortality in elderly patients. *J Trauma* 2010;69:821–25.

20 Newgard CD, Nelson MJ, Kampp M, et al. Out-of-hospital decision making and factors influencing the regional distribution of injured patients in a trauma system. *J Trauma* 2011;70:1345–53.

21 Substance Abuse and Mental Health Services Administration. Available at: www.oas.samhsa.gov

22 Pillemer K, Finkelhor D. The prevalence of elder abuse: a random sample survey. *Gerontologist* 1988;28:51–7.

23 Lachs MS Berkman L, Fulmer T, et al. A prospective community based pilot study of risk factors for the investigation of elder mistreatment. *J Am Geriatr Soc* 1994;42:169–73.

24 Chin MH, Jin L, Karrison TG, et al. Older patients' health-related quality of life around an episode of emergency illness. *Ann Emerg Med* 1999;34:595–603.

25 Terrell KM, Miller DK. Challenges in transitional care between nursing homes and emergency departments. *J Am Med Dir Assoc* 2006;7:499–505.

26 Shah MN. The formation of the emergency medical services system. *Am J Public Health* 2006;96:414–23.

27 Lerner EB, Shah MN, Fernandez AR. Do EMS providers think they should participate in disease prevention? *Prehosp Emerg Care* 2008;12:108–9.

28 Mosesso VN, Packer CR, McMahon J, et al. Influenza immunizations provided by EMS agencies: the Medivax project. *Prehosp Emerg Care* 2003;7:74–8.

29 Shah MN, Caprio TV, Swanson P, et al. A novel emergency medical services based program to identify and assist older adults in a rural community. *J Am Geriatr Soc* 2010;58:2205–11.

CHAPTER 58

Bariatric patient challenges

Jeremy T. Cushman

Introduction

Obesity is a major health problem in the United States. Body mass index (BMI) is used to quantify obesity and is calculated by dividing the weight in kilograms by the height in meters. More than 69% of the US population is considered overweight, and 36% are obese as determined by BMI (Table 58.1) [1].

Obesity has numerous effects on health, and is a risk factor for many diseases and health conditions such as hypertension, dyslipidemia, type 2 diabetes mellitus, coronary artery disease, stroke, gallbladder disease, osteoarthritis, obstructive sleep apnea, pulmonary hypertension, and some cancers (notably endometrial, breast, and colon) [2]. Obesity does not only contribute to medical conditions, but may also affect one's risk for, and recovery from, trauma. Obese individuals are at increased risk for traumatic injury [3], may have increased risk of chest, pelvis and extremity fractures, and of pulmonary, renal, and thromboembolic posttraumatic complications [4]. Obstructive sleep apnea, being relatively common in the obese, increases seven-fold the risk of motor vehicle accidents [5].

The variety of anatomical and physiological changes that occur with the bariatric patient not only affects their risk for disease, but can dramatically affect their prehospital management. Mask ventilation can be difficult and poor respiratory mechanics can predispose the bariatric patient to rapid desaturation and hypercarbia. Medication administration can be complicated based upon various drug dosing calculations, and high-quality cardiopulmonary resuscitation (CPR) can be hindered by the habitus of the bariatric patient. Increasing numbers of bariatric surgery procedures present the prehospital provider with unique pathologies, while more practically speaking, the bariatric patient can pose significant challenges to patient packaging, lifting, and movement. This chapter reviews the key anatomical and physiological changes and identifies the critical management considerations that the overweight patient poses to our prehospital care systems.

Airway

The bariatric patient can provide significant challenges to airway management as a BMI of greater than 26 kg/m^2 is an independent predictor of difficulty in maintaining oxygen saturation with mask ventilation [6]. Redundant soft tissue about the face and neck can complicate both BLS and ALS airway interventions, and positioning of the bariatric patient is critical for successful management of airway and breathing. Whenever practical, the obese patient should be allowed to sit in a Fowler's or semi-Fowler's position. This will displace redundant soft tissue around the neck inferiorly, allowing for easier airway management, and will improve the patient's respiratory dynamics, which is critical as bariatric patients do not tolerate periods of apnea.

Mask ventilation of the bariatric patient requires two-person techniques to be effective, where one provider is assigned to establish and maintain a mask seal with a two-hand grip, while the other provides ventilations. Often this simple but important intervention is not performed either because of a perception of "adequacy" with one-person techniques, or because in some systems there may not be enough personnel to accomplish this. Additionally, the use of a properly sized mask with oral or nasal airway adjuncts is critical to achieving effective mask ventilation in the obese patient. Ramp positioning, where the patient's external auditory canal is aligned with the sternal notch, has been identified as an important tool to improve laryngoscopic view and also improves mask ventilation and subsequent oxygenation [7]. This positioning can be accomplished by aggressive padding behind the shoulders, neck, and head with towels and blankets. Soft tissue displacement during laryngoscopy may be difficult, thus worsening visualization of the glottic opening, and the ramp placement assists with this.

Interestingly, although increased BMI does predict difficulty with mask ventilation, there is mixed literature to support a similar correlation with tracheal intubation [8]. Regardless, since the obese patient is clearly difficult to effectively mask ventilate,

Emergency Medical Services: Clinical Practice and Systems Oversight, Second Edition. Volume 1: Clinical Aspects of EMS.
Edited by David C. Cone, Jane H. Brice, Theodore R. Delbridge, and J. Brent Myers.
© 2015 NAEMSP. Published 2015 by John Wiley & Sons, Inc. Companion Website: www.wiley.com/go/cone\naemsp

Table 58.1 Body mass index (BMI) classification

BMI (kg/m²)	Classification
<18.5	Underweight
18.5–24.9	Normal
25.0–29.9	Overweight
30.0–39.9	Obese
>40.0	Morbidly obese

and such a technique is the basis for initial and failed airway management attempts, the bariatric patient must be approached as if any airway intervention will be difficult.

Surgical airway placement may be challenging in the bariatric patient, regardless of the open or percutaneous technique used. Due to the additional soft tissue about the neck, surgical landmarks are often obscured and conventional cuffed tracheostomy tubes may not have adequate length to assure tracheal placement. As a result, a cuffed endotracheal tube is recommended when performing a surgical airway on a bariatric patient. Supraglottic airway devices may be effective in the bariatric prehospital patient based on operating room data [5]; however, there is scant prehospital literature on the topic, and no published experience with the commonly used King airway.

The bariatric patient with respiratory distress or airway compromise can create significant clinical management challenges for higher-risk procedures such as rapid sequence intubation. A patient who is inherently unable to tolerate hypoxia, coupled with predictable difficulty in effective mask ventilation, requires a thoughtful and methodological approach to airway management. Preparation is critical, including adequate preoxygenation with continuous positive airway pressure, two-person mask ventilation techniques, and ramp positioning. Having immediate access to surgical airway equipment and supraglottic airways is also required. Most importantly, developing the critical clinical decision-making skills amongst providers who may perform rapid sequence intubation is imperative to balance the risks and benefits of the procedure in the bariatric patient.

Breathing

The effects of obesity can dramatically affect the acutely ill patient's respiratory system. The overweight and obese have poor pulmonary reserves as a result of multiple factors. The obese patient demonstrates a restrictive pulmonary physiology as a result of the additional chest wall mass, as well as an increase in resting intraabdominal pressure [9]. Intraabdominal compartment pressure of greater than 12 cmH$_2$O is often considered a compartment syndrome, and the morbidly obese often have intraabdominal pressures at or exceeding this level [10]. This decreases the effectiveness of the diaphragm for inspiratory effort and decreases venous return. Further, the bariatric patient will have decreased lung volumes, a decrease in functional reserve capacity and expiratory reserve volume,

and reduced lung and chest wall compliance. These features impart poor respiratory mechanics and are coupled with an increased ventilation/perfusion mismatch compared to a non-obese patient [5,6]. Thus the bariatric patient has a smaller oxygen reserve, but because of increased metabolic activity has increased oxygen demand and CO$_2$ production [5]. This constellation of physiological insults results in a rapid onset of hypoxemia in even the "healthy" morbidly obese patient.

To combat this inherently poor baseline physiology, a few important interventions can enhance the oxygenation of the obese patient. Whenever possible, the obese patient should be positioned in either a semi-Fowler's or ramped position, even during preoxygenation for advanced airway procedures. For the immobilized patient, even slight reverse Trendelenburg positioning can displace body mass to decrease pressure on the diaphragm or the upper chest muscles and therefore improve respiratory muscle mechanics. When considering continuous positive airway pressure (CPAP), bilevel positive airway pressure (BiPAP), or mechanical ventilation, obese patients generally require more positive end-expiratory pressure (PEEP) to maintain alveolar ventilation than their lean counterparts and should generally be started at 10 cmH$_2$O [11]. Thus the advantages of PEEP to recruit atelectatic alveoli in the bariatric patient have to be balanced with its negative effects on cardiac output, particularly given the elevated intraabdominal pressures that reduce cardiac preload. Extremely important, however, is remembering that lung volumes are calculated on ideal body weight and not total body weight. This is important for both mask ventilation and when placing the bariatric patient on a ventilator. Exceeding the recommended 6–8 mL/kg tidal volume calculated based on the patient's ideal body weight can increase the risk of acute lung injury and ultimately the morbidity and mortality of the obese patient [12].

The increase in chest wall tissue found in the overweight and obese can also affect the efficacy of needle thoracostomy attempts. The mean chest wall thickness in a Netherlands study was 3.5 cm, and a catheter length of 4.5 cm was found to not penetrate the pleural space in 9.9–35.4% of patients, depending on age and sex [13]. A US study found more concerning results, as the mean chest wall thickness was 4.5 cm, and concluded that the standard 4.4 cm catheter would not be successful in 50% (95% confidence interval (CI) 40.1–59.3%), requiring emergency pleural decompression [14]. Proper equipment selection and rescuer knowledge of conventional needle catheter success are thus paramount for a successful intervention.

Circulation

The bariatric patient has an increased circulatory blood volume, a hyperkinetic circulatory system, and often myocardial hypertrophy and diastolic dysfunction [2]. This may limit the physiological response to an acute pathological insult, putting the patient at increased risk for rapid decompensation. Basic staples of resuscitative care such as blood pressure monitoring may be difficult to obtain accurately because of excess adipose tissue, further challenging objective measurements of perfusion in the morbidly obese. Assuring response personnel are using the appropriate sized blood pressure cuff, and understanding limitations of automatic blood pressure machines compared to manual blood pressures, remain essential, important skills when managing the bariatric patient.

Effective, high-quality CPR may be negatively affected by obesity. In addition to the challenges of airway and breathing found in the bariatric patient, obtaining proper CPR positioning, sufficient compression depth, and good chest recoil may be difficult. Further, many CPR assistive devices may not fit the bariatric patient, placing increased reliance on conventional CPR techniques. Despite these considerations, there is no clear correlation between BMI and outcome for in-hospital cardiac arrest [15], and there is scant literature on its effects in the prehospital setting and what, if any, practical implications obesity has on performing high-quality CPR.

Venous access can be particularly challenging in the bariatric patient. Excess adipose tissue may limit peripheral venous access, and redundant neck tissue may make external jugular approaches nearly impossible. Longer intravenous catheters may be required, if a suitable site can be found at all. Intramuscular approaches may not effectively administer the medication to the muscle body and instead enter the excess adipose tissue, whose absorption of drug is erratic at best. Various peripheral venous access assistive devices have emerged, including ultraviolet vessel detection, ultrasound, and intraosseous devices, all with their inherent benefits and disadvantages. Intraosseous venous access is a common option in the bariatric patient, and manufacturers have created longer needles to address the limitations of traditional shorter length needles in the overweight subject. Even with advances in intraosseous technology, the bariatric patient often remains a vascular access challenge, primarily related to greater difficulty in establishing the proper landmarks for needle insertion as a result of excess adipose tissue.

Once venous access is obtained, there remain unique challenges to drug dosing in the bariatric patient. Drugs are classically dosed based on lean or ideal body weight (IBW), total body weight (TBW), or adjusted body weight. In the bariatric patient, the pharmacokinetic parameters of volume of distribution, clearance, and protein binding can be markedly affected, particularly those medications that are lipophilic [16,17]. This becomes important when managing the bariatric patient since EMS personnel may provide significantly more medication than is required because of a general tendency to calculate the dose based on TBW. Table 58.2 outlines common EMS medications and their recommended initial doses based on pharmacokinetic literature or expert opinion [16–19].

To generalize, lipophilic medications should be dosed according to TBW, while hydrophilic medications should be dosed according to IBW. To add to the confusion, some medica-

Table 58.2 Dose considerations for common prehospital medications

Dosing calculation	Medication
No weight consideration	Adenosine, amiodarone, metoprolol, ondansetron, dobutamine, epinephrine
Ideal body weight	Dopamine, ketamine, lidocaine, morphine, norepinephrine, procainamide, rocuronium, vecuronium
Total body weight	Diltiazem, etomidate, fentanyl, lorazepam, midazolam, propofol, succinylcholine

tions, such as lorazepam and midazolam, should have bolus doses calculated based on TBW and continuous infusions based on IBW. Notably, most vasoactive medications (epinephrine and norepinephrine) are generally titrated to achieve a target goal (mean arterial pressure) and therefore pharmacokinetic data have less effect on the dose regimen. Dopamine is the exception to this and dose is based on IBW in addition to the target goal.

Importantly, drug dosage recommendations are typically made based upon the pharmacokinetic or clinical data from individuals with normal weights, so there may be unique variations in the bariatric patient's pharmacokinetic parameters that are simply not known or appreciated. In short, there is a significant paucity of data in dose recommendations for the obese and morbidly obese, and providers and EMS physicians must be prepared for the possibility of erratic absorption, longer onset, and prolonged duration of medications administered to the obese patient.

Bariatric surgery

As the incidence of morbid obesity has grown, so has the number of patients receiving bariatric surgery. Bariatric surgery is generally reserved for those with a BMI ≥ 40 kg/m^2 (or ≥ 35 kg/m^2 with comorbid conditions) and may be accomplished through a number of surgical techniques [2]. Bariatric surgery has the same short-term complications as other surgical procedures including infection, sepsis, delayed wound healing, deep venous thrombosis, and pulmonary embolism. Additional short-term complications unique to bariatric surgery include anastomotic or staple leak which may occur in up to 3% of Roux-en-Y bypass procedures [20], and approximately 3% of bariatric surgeries will experience postoperative hemorrhage which usually occurs within the first 24 hours after the procedure [21]. Long-term complications found with all procedures can include small bowel obstruction, gastric or small bowel ulcers, and nausea and vomiting. Laparoscopic adjustable gastric banding can be complicated by erosion or slippage of the band, or leakage from the port or band tubing, while Roux-en-Y can be complicated by anastomotic stricture, gastrogastric fistula, and dumping syndrome [22]. Many who undergo bariatric surgery develop gallstones as a result of such rapid weight loss and some surgeons elect to perform prophylactic cholecystectomy because of this frequent postoperative complication.

Patient packaging and movement

Facilitating the movement and maintaining the dignity of the bariatric patient has received increased attention over the last decade. Industry has responded with numerous features designed to enhance patient comfort, promote patient and provider safety, and decrease injury to prehospital personnel. These include specialized lifting devices such as bariatric transfer sheets, reinforced and wider backboards capable of carrying larger loads, lateral transfer aids to facilitate bed to EMS and EMS to hospital transitions, and various improvements to stretchers and stair chairs such as hydraulic lifts, lateral expansion "wings" to accommodate a larger girth patient on the standard stretcher, wider stretchers, and stretchers with enhanced load limits.

Despite this, the bariatric patient poses unique packaging and movement challenges to prehospital personnel. Common disposable cervical collars often do not fit correctly nor provide adequate immobilization because of the additional adipose tissue found around the neck. Personnel must be familiar with other immobilization techniques using towels, blankets, or manual stabilization when caring for an injured victim with high concern for cervical spine injury. Further, because of the excess adipose tissue often found in the upper back, additional padding behind the head may be required to maintain the neck in a neutral position.

Older backboards often have lower weight limits than more modern boards and are therefore at risk for breakage. The standard modern backboard is 16 inches wide and most can safely handle up to 450 lbs, which may not be adequate for moving the bariatric patient. Many manufacturers are now offering wider, reinforced backboards that are capable of supporting up to 1,000 lbs. Other immobilization devices such as the Kendrick Extrication Device and various traction splints may not be able to accommodate larger torsos or proximal thighs, requiring improvisation by the responding personnel to meet the immobilization needs of the bariatric patient.

The standard EMS stretcher is 23 inches wide and is able to support between 550 and 700 lbs. Often, the challenge is with the girth of the patient and not necessarily the weight; most patients in excess of 400 lbs will not fit safely or comfortably on standard stretchers. Bariatric stretchers often have a width of 29 inches, with stretcher adapters that can expand up to 40 inches, and increased load limits of 850–1600 lbs depending on height position. These increased load capacities come at a cost as these stretchers are significantly heavier than the standard stretcher. Critical to the movement of the bariatric patient is to assure that the stretcher is kept in the lowest position possible in order to minimize the risk of tipping. Equally important is to assure that no fewer than four, and ideally six, personnel are used to move the loaded bariatric stretcher.

Once safely secured on the stretcher, the loading of that stretcher into specialized ambulances has become commonplace. The so-called "bariatric" ambulance is generally a Type I or III ambulance that includes a ramp or hydraulic system to completely remove the need for personnel to lift the patient and the stretcher into the ambulance. Ramp systems use a set of ramps and a winch to pull the stretcher into the patient compartment, while hydraulic systems use an elevator lift that brings the stretcher from the ground to the level of the patient compartment, allowing the stretcher to be rolled directly in. Both systems have weight limits that are device specific but generally can accommodate up to 1,300 lbs inclusive of stretcher, patient, equipment, etc. Bariatric ambulances also often carry bariatric stair chairs, transfer devices, and other adjuncts that can facilitate the movement of the bariatric patient while maintaining some dignity and potentially reducing the risk of provider lifting injury. Having policies or procedures in place outlining the safe movement of a bariatric patient is critical, as this outlines the capabilities and resources of a community. For example, specific limitations of regional air medical services should be determined well in advance of a request for service.

The lifting and moving of bariatric patients represent a significant injury hazard to prehospital personnel, who already experience higher injury rates than workers in most other industries [23]. The majority of these injuries are related to strains and sprains of the back, and represent an important area for injury prevention. Given the increased frequency of caring for bariatric patients, EMS agencies should establish programs to assure personnel are using the proper lifting and moving techniques for all patients, along with frequent familiarization with the specialized bariatric lifting and moving equipment that is available. Training mannikins that approach 540 lbs are available and are an important tool to assist EMS personnel in learning how to safely extricate, package, and move the bariatric patient.

Conclusion

The bariatric patient poses unique challenges to prehospital personnel. Airway management can be complicated and poor respiratory mechanics can predispose the bariatric patient to rapid desaturation and hypercarbia; however, basic airway skills, preparation, and patient positioning may reduce this risk. An increased potential for barotrauma can result from improperly calculated tidal volumes while vascular access can be challenging despite modern technologies due to difficulties in identifying anatomical landmarks. Medication administration can be complicated based upon various drug dosing calculations, and familiarity with the unique pharmacokinetics of the bariatric patient is critical. The bariatric patient can also pose significant challenges and hazards to patient packaging, lifting, and movement; however, industry responses to this demand provide EMS personnel with new tools to respond to this challenge.

Proper lifting techniques and adequate numbers of personnel to safely move the bariatric patient are imperative to reduce injury regardless of the assistive devices used.

Whether it is the ABCs or extrication and movement, being familiar with the alterations in physiology along with the pitfalls of management requires familiarization and preparation to improve the care of the bariatric patient.

References

1 National Center for Health Statistics. Health, United States, 2012: With special feature on emergency care. Hyattsville, MD. 2013. Available at: www.cdc.gov/nchs/data/hus/hus12.pdf#063

2 National Heart, Lung, and Blood Institute. Clinical Guidelines on the Identification, Evaluation, and Treatment of Overweight and Obesity in Adults. NIH Publication 98-4083. Bethesda, MD, 1998. Available at: www.nhlbi.nih.gov/guidelines/obesity/ob_gdlns.htm

3 Xiang H, Smith GA, Wilkins JR III, et al. Obesity and risk of nonfatal unintentional injuries. *Am J Prevent Med* 2005;29:41–5.

4 Meroz Y, Gozal Y. Management of the obese trauma patient. *Anesthesiol Clin* 2007;25:91–8.

5 Findley LJ, Unverzagt MF, Suratt PM. Automobile accidents involving patients with obstructive sleep apnea. *Am Rev Respir Dis* 1988; 138:337–40.

6 Langeron O, Masso E, Huraux C, et al. Prediction of difficult mask ventilation. *Anesthesiology* 2000;92:1229–36.

7 Collins JS, Lemmens HJ, Brodsky JB, et al. Laryngoscopy and morbid obesity: a comparison of the "sniff" and "ramp" positions. *Obes Surg* 2004;14(9):1171–5.

8 Dargin J, Medzon R. Emergency department management of the airway in obese adults. *Ann Emerg Med* 2010;56:95–104.

9 Porhomayon J, Papadakos P, Singh A, Nader ND. Alteration in respiratory physiology in obesity for anesthesia critical care physician. *HSR Proc Intensive Care Cardiovasc Anesth* 2011;3(2):109–18.

10 Lambert DM, Marceau S, Forse RA. Intra-abdominal pressure in the morbidly obese. *Obes Surg* 2005;15(9):1225–32.

11 Gander S, Frascarolo P, Suter M, et al. Positive end-expiratory pressure during induction of general anesthesia increases duration of nonhypoxic apnea in morbidly obese patients. *Anesth Analg* 2005;100:580–4.

12 Acute Respiratory Distress Syndrome Network. Ventilation with lower tidal volumes as compared with traditional tidal volumes for acute lung injury and the acute respiratory distress syndrome. *N Engl J Med* 2000;342:1301–8.

13 Zengerink I, Brink PR, Laupland KB, et al. Needle thoracostomy in the treatment of tension pneumothorax in trauma patients: What size needle? *J Trauma* 2008;64(1):111–14.

14 Stevens RL, Rochester AA, Busko J, et al. Needle thoracostomy for tension pneumothorax: failure predicted by chest computed tomography. *Prehosp Emerg Care* 2009;13(1):14–17.

15 Jain R, Nallamothu BK, Chan PS. Body mass index and survival after in-hospital cardiac arrest. *Circulation* 2010;3:490–7.

16 Erstad BL. Dosing of medications in morbidly obese patients in the intensive care unit setting. *Intensive Care Med* 2004;30:18–32.

17 Cheymol G. Effects of morbid obesity on pharmacokinetics: implications for drug therapy. *Clin Pharmacokinet* 2000;39(3):215–31.

18 DeBaedemaeker L, Morier EP, Struys M. Pharmacokinetics in obese patients. *Cont Ed Anes, Crit Care Pain* 2004;4(5):152–5.

19 Ingrande J, Lemmens HJ. Dose adjustment of anaesthetics in the morbidly obese. *Br J Anaesth* 2010;105(S1):i16–i23.

20 Papasavas PK, Caushaj PF, McCormick JT, et al. Laparoscopic management of complications following laparoscopic Roux-en-Y gastric bypass for morbid obesity. *Surg Endosc* 2003;17(4):610–14.

21 Spaw AT, Husted JD. Bleeding after laparoscopic gastric bypass: case report and literature review. *Surg Obes Relat Dis* 2005;1(2):99–103.

22 Karmali S, Stoklossa CJ, Sharma A, et al. Bariatric surgery: a primer. *Can Fam Physician* 2010;56:873–9.

23 Maguire BJ, Hunting KL, Guidotti TL, Smith GS. Occupational injuries among emergency medical services personnel. *Prehosp Emerg Care* 2005;9:405–11.

CHAPTER 59

Behavioral health emergencies

Jay H. Reich and Aaron Stinton

Introduction

A psychiatric or behavioral health emergency can be defined as an acute change in conduct that results in a behavior that is intolerable for the patient, family, or society [1]. These changes range from the inability to cope with a stressful situation to agitated or violent patients who present a danger to themselves or others.

Little has been written directly about behavioral health emergencies in the prehospital setting. The "standard of care" is extrapolated from emergency departments and psychiatric units. EMS professionals receive little training regarding behavioral conditions during their initial and continuing education [2,3].

Evaluation of the problem

The "standard" approach field personnel use may be inadequate for the assessment of behavioral health patients for multiple reasons. Providers may be unsure how to evaluate an uncooperative or dangerous patient without involving law enforcement, whose specialized training can help EMS pursue appropriate treatment options [4]. EMS may elect to contact direct medical oversight for help, but it can be equally difficult for the medical oversight physician to assess the patient remotely. Under these circumstances, it is imperative that patients who might pose a threat to themselves or others are fully evaluated. It may require the patient to be brought into the hospital against his or her will. It is important for the EMS medical director to ensure that the prehospital provider and medical oversight physician have the appropriate training and knowledge to deal with these patients before they are encountered. This may include issuing a hold order for cases where the patient lacks capacity for medical decision making. General management guidelines should be provided by protocol.

Remember, as with all patients encountered by EMS, behavioral patients have legitimate health problems. Unfortunately, they are sometimes mislabeled as "uncooperative" or "difficult," resulting in inappropriate treatment. Education should reinforce that the patient's behavior is a manifestation of disease, and patience and compassion are essential to providing excellent, supportive care to this vulnerable population.

Emergency departments and EMS are common points of entry into the health care system for the psychiatric patient [1]. Medical direction should be familiar with local psychiatric resources as well as common diagnoses including their presentations, complications, and management. These include anxiety disorders, major depression, schizophrenia, and bipolar disorder [5].

Assessment and treatment

Making an accurate psychiatric diagnosis in the field is frequently impossible and generally irrelevant. Treatment protocols should describe assessment and care for clinical symptom patterns, not specific diagnoses. Policies and procedures must also be put in place to ensure safety of patient and provider [6].

The first step when confronted by a patient with a behavioral disorder is to evaluate scene safety. If not safe, EMS should withdraw and await the arrival of law enforcement before intervention is attempted. If safe, providers may carefully approach and attempt a brief medical assessment. They should determine if the behavioral changes are due to an organic etiology and/or if the patient is in imminent danger secondary to a medical emergency.

There are multiple medical conditions, many reversible, which can present with behavioral changes (Box 59.1). Presentation may vary from lethargy and confusion to agitation and violence. Classic examples include the confused patient with acute hypoglycemia, the agitated patient with hypoxia, and the lethargic patient in shock. Initial evaluation must include a thorough history (medical and psychiatric) and physical examination, including measurement of blood sugar level and pulse oximetry. Mental status changes of acute onset without a previous history of psychiatric disorder are highly suggestive of an organic etiology. EMS should inquire about prescribed medications or

Emergency Medical Services: Clinical Practice and Systems Oversight, Second Edition. Volume 1: Clinical Aspects of EMS.
Edited by David C. Cone, Jane H. Brice, Theodore R. Delbridge, and J. Brent Myers.
© 2015 NAEMSP. Published 2015 by John Wiley & Sons, Inc. Companion Website: www.wiley.com\go\cone\naemsp

suspected drug/alcohol abuse. Special attention should be paid during physical examination to eliciting abnormal neurological findings. If vital sign abnormalities are observed, the patient should be considered medically unstable and mental status changes a consequence of an organic problem until proven otherwise. The provider should effect appropriate interventions. Delayed stabilization or failure to transport patients with organic problems is dangerous, especially when dealing with mentally disturbed patients.

Occasionally, the patient may not cooperate with the initial assessment and stabilization. In these situations, EMS personnel should try to gain the patient's confidence by providing reassurance, explaining who they are, and describing every step before it is performed. If the patient remains non-compliant, the presence of an EMS physician, as a figure of authority, may be of assistance in obtaining the patient's cooperation. Unfortunately, this is often not possible. Other appropriate alternatives include the indirect medical oversight physician speaking directly to the patient via radio, phone, or video phone or attempting to reach the patient's psychiatrist or primary care physician. If the patient does not cooperate with the initial assessment, physical and/or chemical restraints may be considered. This should be done in cooperation with law enforcement. Patients with behavioral changes must receive at a minimum an appropriate prehospital assessment or be transported to the hospital.

Once deemed medically stable, the next step is to determine if the patient's mental status represents a danger to himself or herself or to others. Each case needs to be evaluated on an individual basis as not every patient with abnormal behavior will require transport.

If the patient is refusing transport, he or she must meet the following criteria before the non-transport request should be honored.

1 The patient has the capacity to refuse.
2 Organic etiology has been reasonably ruled out by an appropriate medical evaluation.
3 No evidence of suicidal, homicidal, or aggressive behavior is present.
4 There is a known past history of psychiatric disorder with similar behavior.
5 Appropriate social, family, or mental health support is available.

Many EMS systems have adopted policies permitting the use of alternative transport destinations such as psychiatric EDs and detoxification facilities. Selected patients may be more amenable to routing to these facilities rather than EDs. Strict criteria must be established in order to assure success and safety. The National Association of EMS Physicians and the American College of Emergency Physicians jointly issued a policy identifying important elements which must be in place to have a successful alternative transport destination program. Examples include EMS physician medical director oversight, medical director-led program development, implementation and quality improvement, as well as education programs at all levels. These programs

may result in up to 25% of psychiatric patients being directly transported to psychiatric EDs. They have also demonstrated high sensitivity in detecting the need for medical evaluation [7,8].

It is the responsibility of the medical director to make sure that a thorough evaluation is completed before EMS personnel release a patient at the scene. Given that most adult patients presenting to the ED with new acute psychiatric symptoms will have an organic etiology [9] and the evaluation and "medical clearance" of patients in the field can be more challenging than when performed in the ED, protocols should direct providers to err on the side of caution and to transport these patients (see Box 59.1).

The suicidal patient

Suicidal ideation is the existence of thoughts pertaining to ending one's own life. *Passive suicidal ideation* refers to thoughts without a plan. *Active suicidal ideation* refers to thoughts with a

---

Box 59.1 Organic disorders with behavioral manifestations

Neurological

Central nervous system infections (meningitis, encephalitis, brain abscess)
Head trauma
Hypertensive encephalopathy
Stroke
Mass lesion
Seizure disorder
Dementia

Drug intoxication/poisoning

Alcohol
Amphetamines
Anticholinergic syndromes
Bath salts
Cocaine
LSD
Marijuana
Phencyclidine (PCP)

Withdrawal syndromes

Alcohol
Barbiturates
Opiates

Metabolic

Hypoxia
Hypoglycemia
Renal failure (acidosis/electrolytes imbalance)
Hepatic failure

Endocrinological

Hypothyroidism/hyperthyroidism
Addison disease
Cushing disease

Source: Goldberg[10], Larkin[11].

plan, and thus a greater risk. A *suicidal gesture* is self-inflicted harm without a realistic expectation of death, whereas a *suicide attempt* is an act with a clear expectation of death [12].

More people die from suicide than homicide in the United States [13]. In 2010, a total of 38,364 Americans took their own lives, compared with 16,259 homicides, making suicide the 10th leading cause of death [13]. There were 12.4 suicides per 100,000, an increase from 10.7 in 2005 [13,14]. Suicide is a serious problem among young people, being the third leading cause of death for 15–24 year olds [15,16]. The most common methods include firearms, suffocation/asphyxiation, and poisonings. Suicide rates tend to increase with age and are highest among white men aged >65 [17].

Always take a suicide threat seriously. Suicidal statements indicate a crisis the individual feels he or she is unable to handle. Up to two-thirds of those who commit suicide have visited physicians or health care facilities during the preceding month [18]. It is therefore important to recognize the signs and symptoms, not just declaration of intent, with which a suicide-prone patient could present. Intervention by EMS may be the last opportunity to provide help and prevent tragedy. Initial and ongoing training coupled with comprehensive treatment protocols will help to ensure that EMS provide maximum assistance while ensuring their own safety.

After arrival, EMS should perform a complete scene assessment to ensure proper situational awareness, including checking for weapons or potential weapons. Immediately remove any objects that the patient could use to inflict physical harm to him/herself or others. If guns or knives are present, the crew should withdraw to safety and await the police to remove the weapons and secure the scene. Once secured, attempts to initiate communication with the patient should be made as soon as possible. Communication with direct medical oversight, the patient's psychiatrist, or the family physician may be beneficial in understanding the current scenario. During the negotiations, using friends or family members whom the patient trusts and respects can be effective. However, if the patient identifies an individual as being part of the crisis, that individual should be removed. Encourage the patient to discuss the situation. Most patients are relieved to be empowered just to discuss their thoughts [18].

It is important to emphasize during EMS education the need to show sympathy, empathy, and concern, and to avoid potentially frightening or agitating the patient. Providers do not have to agree or disagree with the patient, but should listen to what he or she has to say. Providers should avoid statements such as "Don't do that!" or "You know that is not true!" The suicidal patient may consider these comments to be a challenge or that EMS are being judgmental and not supportive. If the patient perceives a negative attitude, it may worsen their already low self-esteem. The provider should offer reassurance that the crisis can be resolved and that authorities are only there to be of assistance. Promises that EMS providers are unable or unwilling to keep will make the patient more suspicious and should be avoided.

Suspicion by providers of non-verbalized suicidal ideation or the presence of specific risk factors should prompt a further exploration. If the patient admits to any current or past depression, hopelessness, or despair, he should be asked directly whether he has any thoughts about self-harm. There has been no evidence to support the concern that posing such questions could actually induce suicidal thoughts and behaviors; more often, once broached directly, in a non-judgmental and sensitive manner, the patient typically welcomes the opportunity to unburden himself to caregivers.

Often, such patients present with a level of anxiety and agitation that once alleviated will reduce suicidal feelings. Protocols should allow for the use of fast-acting benzodiazepines, such as lorazepam, midazolam, or diazepam, which often prove effective in low doses when titrated as necessary. If there are contraindications to benzodiazepines, such as suspicion of their abuse, another agent such as diphenhydramine or a low dose of a high-potency neuroleptic (e.g. haloperidol) may be employed [12]. Similarly, suicidal patients suffering from severe or chronic pain may become markedly less despondent after adequate analgesia.

As cooperation develops, all actions and activities should be clearly explained, in advance if possible. At this point, pharmacological interventions may be considered or may be found to be unnecessary. Before initiating transport, policies should require the patient be fastened on the stretcher and not permitted to sit next to the exit door or in the front seat of the ambulance. EMS personnel should explain that these are security measures for the patient's safety. The provider who has established the best rapport with the patient should ride along with him or her to the hospital. Additional members of the response team should then sit next to the exits.

If all reasonable efforts have failed to persuade the patient to cooperate, the question of whether to commit the patient to an involuntary transport must be addressed. This is a decision in which direct medical oversight is often involved. There are several factors that correlate with a higher risk for committing suicide (Table 59.1). If it is decided that the patient is in immediate danger of committing suicide, the provider should be directed to proceed with the transport, never leaving the patient unattended. Laws pertaining to involuntary transport and admissions vary from state to state. EMS medical directors must be familiar with the specifics of their state and local statutes. When in doubt, it is always better to direct an involuntary transport and to have the patient evaluated at an ED or psychiatric institution. If, subsequent to the decision for involuntary transport, the patient becomes agitated and/or violent, the use of physical or chemical restraints may be required. This option should be addressed within protocol.

The agitated and violent patient

Encounters with agitated patients total 1.7 million in the US annually [19]. Agitation may be a component of a medical emergency, established psychiatric illness, intoxication, suicidal ideation, or a precursor to potentially violent behavior.

Table 59.1 Factors that correlate with a higher risk for committing suicide

Factors	High risk
Suicide intentions	Affirmation of suicide intention
	Detailed and violent plan with poor probability for rescue and accessible resources (e.g. gun)
	History of previous attempts
Psychiatric diagnosis	Schizophrenia
	Bipolar disorder
	Major depression
	Acute psychosis
Medical problems	Diagnosis of terminal diseases (e.g. cancer, AIDS)
	Diagnosis of chronic illness (e.g. diabetes)
Drug abuse	Alcohol, cocaine, other illicit drugs
Social history	Marital status –widowed or divorced
	Recent significant loss – death of a loved one
	Unemployment
	No family support
Family history	Suicide
	Psychiatric disorders
Sex	Women – attempt suicide more often
	Men – successful attempts more often
Age	Over 45 years old

Historically, there have been varied approaches to the assessment and treatment of agitated patients, at times based on anecdote and tradition. With a push for further research and additional training [19], the Project BETA Workgroup, a consensus group organized by the American Association of Emergency Psychiatrists and comprising emergency psychiatrists, emergency physicians and others, published a series of articles attempting to address agitation and violence in the emergency setting. Many of their findings can be extrapolated to EMS.

The acutely agitated patient must be approached with caution and with a high clinical suspicion. As with the suicidal patient, scene and crew safety is of primary concern. EMS personnel should receive ongoing education on interacting with the agitated and violent patient, as well as assessing and evaluating these patients before they erupt [20]. The patient's level of agitation should be assessed and documented. A patient who is talking in a loud voice, moving around constantly, gesticulating with the arms, or displaying closed fists should be considered potentially violent [3,21,22].

To the extent which the patient will allow, a medical examination should be completed. Organic etiologies must be considered and either ruled out or managed (see Box 59.1). In the prehospital setting, this would include tests such as blood glucose, oxygen saturation, and observation for signs of possible ingestions or intoxication. The patient's history is crucial and should be corroborated by others if possible. Patient history has a 94% sensitivity and physical exam a 51% sensitivity for detecting medical problems in agitated patients. Further clues to suggest an organic etiology include atypical presentations of known psychiatric disorders and new-onset agitation in patients over the age of 45 without a previous psychiatric history [23]. Special consideration should be given to those with a history of psychosis, paranoia, bipolar and antisocial personality disorder, as these diagnoses are indicators of a higher incidence of violent behavior [10].

After an initial evaluation, there should be a better understanding of the patient's condition and risk for violence. Even if assessed as low risk for aggressiveness, EMS personnel should remain vigilant and ready to react if necessary. However, if the patient is considered to be at high risk for violence, the following measures should be taken [1,10].

- Never leave the patient unattended.
- Maintain a safe distance from the patient and protect the exit at all times.
- Do not allow the patient to block the escape route or exits. Providers should remain positioned between the patient and the provider's own route of egress.
- Remove any objects at the scene that could be used by the patient as a weapon.
- When facing a violent individual, the EMS provider should avoid prolonged eye contact as it may be considered a challenge.
- One responder should become the "negotiator." If the patient is medically stable, providers should be prepared to spend a prolonged time talking. If the negotiator seems to be losing patience, someone else should assume that role. It is better to spend the extra minutes for peaceful solutions than to rush into a physical confrontation.
- EMS should attempt to "verbally deescalate" the situation while maintaining a calm and reassuring tone.
- Identify reasons for the crisis and let the patient vent his or her thoughts. EMS providers should be supportive, never argumentative.
- A tacit "show of force," with members of the response team backing the negotiator, is suggestive to the patient of the presence of an overwhelming force and is often enough to calm him or her.

Other situations

As a consequence of the aging of society, an increasing percentage of EMS responses involve geriatric patients. The elderly, especially those with limited familial and financial resources, occasionally disregard their own personal well-being. Frequently these patients will rebuff treatment and/or transport. Faced with a self-neglectful patient found in unkempt surroundings, providers may be hard-pressed to accomplish transport for an otherwise competent patient. The EMS physician or direct medical oversight must be directly involved in determining the patient's final disposition. EMS personnel should carefully describe the patient's medical condition as well as the physical environment. Occasionally, direct communication with the patient by the EMS physician is beneficial. A preestablished "geriatric referral program" may provide some reassurance that needed resources and services are available on an expedited basis.

Patients who present with substance abuse or intoxication are a risk not only to themselves, but to the providers as well. Although many mind-altering substances may generate violent behavior, cocaine and phencyclidine are the two most common; less commonly, marijuana, amphetamines, and hallucinogens may do so as well [24]. Many new synthetic drugs are now available with similar effects. Methylenedioxypyrovalerone (MDPV), often referred to as "bath salts" among other names, has effects similar to amphetamines and cocaine [25]. Patients with a history of recent exposures should be handled in a manner similar to that of the violent patient.

Patient restraint

The major indication for restraining a patient in the prehospital environment occurs when the patient is considered to have lost medical decision-making capacity and his or her behavior precludes a thorough evaluation and/or treatment. NAEMSP, in its position paper "Patient restraint in emergency medical services systems," recognizes that prehospital personnel may find themselves in situations requiring the use of restraints to protect the patient, the public, or themselves from harm [26].

There are three methods of patient restraint: verbal deescalation, physical restraint, and chemical restraint. Treatment protocols should be developed to address the specific clinical scenario encountered, and methods that may be employed individually or in combination; however, the least restrictive method that accomplishes the task while maintaining safety should be employed.

NAEMSP position paper establishes 17 principles that are recommended for incorporation in an EMS system's prehospital patient restraint protocol. Key among these are personnel safety, patient dignity, methods of restraint, indications for restraint, documentation requirements, and, most importantly, medical oversight and quality improvement [26].

Medical oversight must be involved and help decide if the patient should be transported against his or her will. This is a decision with medicolegal implications given the litigious society in which we currently practice. The legal justification for physical or chemical restraint is based on the professional judgment by the EMS physician in charge that the patient lacks capacity to refuse treatment and transport [27]. The EMS medical director must be involved in the decision-making process and should therefore be familiar with the state and local legal statutes. In general, the medicolegal exposure of permitting patients who are at risk of harming themselves or others to remain unevaluated is much higher than the exposure involved in the involuntary transport of that patient for further evaluation.

Documentation is of crucial importance not only for legal protection but also for good patient care. "Documentation of patient assessment, reason for restraint, restraint procedure, frequency of reassessment, and care during transportation should occur for all patients who require restraint"[26]. It is very important to document how the patient represented a threat to him/herself or to others.

Verbal deescalation

The Project BETA Workgroup highly advocates for verbal deescalation as the initial method for controlling the agitated or violent patient. These techniques require initial and continuing education, but mastery requires actual practice. There are ten recommended domains to improve deescalation attempts [28].

- Respect personal space
- Do not be provocative
- Establish verbal contact
- Be concise and simple
- Identify wants and needs
- Listen closely – active listening
- Agree or agree to disagree
- Lay down the law and set limits
- Offer choices and optimism
- Debrief patient and staff

Effective use of these techniques will result in fewer chances for injury to both the patient and provider. Taking sufficient time to deescalate the patient will ultimately save time overall. Patients who can be deescalated by verbal means may also develop more trust in the system and effectively seek help in the future [28].

Physical restraint

Coercive restraint of patients should be limited due to short- and long-term negative effects, especially on the relationship between patient and health care workers. Surveys of patients have shown that even without injury, restraint can be a very stressful situation. Studies have shown an effective decrease of restraint use in the inpatient setting, but this does not necessarily apply to ED or prehospital situations [29]. In the EMS setting there is often insufficient time and possibly dangerous environmental situations which do not allow for all potentially appropriate non-coercive interventions to take place. Before proceeding, EMS personnel should assemble a "restraint team," identifying a team leader and assigning each member specific responsibilities. The ideal number of persons on the team is five: one for each extremity and one for the head and neck. The leader should preferably be the same person who to this point has been the "negotiator."

The patient should be given a last opportunity to cooperate while at the same time explaining that otherwise he will be restrained for his own safety, and to help him maintain self-control.

The following is a commonly recommended procedure for physical restraint, although multiple other techniques are available [1,27].

1 The leader should continue to communicate.
2 Two persons should approach from behind, while two approach from the front. This will make it difficult for the patient to concentrate in one direction or attack from one flank.

3 If the patient attacks to one side, the persons left behind should grasp both arms at the elbows simultaneously. By placing the rescuer's legs in front of the patient's and pushing forward, the patient can be forced to the floor face down.

4 At this point, the other two members of the team will hold the patient's legs by the knees, while the leader restrains the head to prevent injury and to preclude biting and spitting.

5 The patient should be restrained face-up to the stretcher using the four-point restraint technique. Leather restraints are recommended.

6 One hand should be restrained over the patient's head and the other by the patient's side. This will decrease the amount of force generated in any one direction.

7 Providers should continue talking to the patient throughout.

8 The patient should not be left unattended! Providers should maintain constant monitoring of the patient's vital signs and respiratory status, and the neurovascular status of all extremities distal to the restraints.

9 Clothing should be searched for dangerous objects. Ideally, this should be done in the presence of a law enforcement officer.

10 Once applied, the use of restraints should not be negotiated during transport, and not removed until arrival at the receiving facility.

11 If the patient continues to struggle and poses a potential harm to himself or others, the addition of chemical restraints should be considered.

12 At the receiving facility, providers should ensure the ED staff have all necessary equipment and personnel before removing the restraints.

There are multiple risks, to the patient and EMS, involved with the restraint procedure. Patient deaths while in the prone restraint position have been attributed to "positional asphyxia"; however, a combination of other factors such as underlying medical conditions, drug or alcohol intoxication, and patient resistance to restraint may prove to be the true culprit [30]. Nevertheless, patients should never be transported in a prone, "hog-tied", or wrapped position.

Emergency medical services personnel generally have limited education and experience in appropriate restraint techniques and may become physically injured during the procedure. Ideally, law enforcement officers should be involved in the restraint procedure, as well as during transport. EMS and law enforcement personnel should work closely together, but EMS professionals should not allow police officers to influence the evaluation and treatment of the patient [3]. It is desirable to have frequent interagency training sessions. This can improve interagency communication and cooperation in an actual situation.

Chemical restraint

Sometimes physical restraint is not enough. It is impossible to perform an adequate evaluation if the patient is still agitated, and needed care may be obstructed by his or her behavior. The use of chemical restraint is more effective and more humane than physical restraint alone. Rapid tranquilization is the technique of giving a psychotropic drug to control behavioral disturbances [31]. The combination of physical and chemical restraints is the best approach to gain control of the patient and proceed with evaluation and transport. The use of medications in the physically restrained patient may reduce the risk of injury or death in cases of excited delirium. The patient may actually be willing to accept medication prior to physical restraint. The option should be presented and the route discussed. The medical director must develop policies and protocols to assist EMS professional in this decision-making process. Direct medical oversight may be required for difficult scenarios. Pharmaceuticals are indicated only when the provider or physician believes that the patient is not competent, his behavior represents an immediate danger, or his behavior hinders a safe transport. The goal is to control agitation and psychotic symptoms.

When considering medications for use in the prehospital environment, certain characteristics are of vital importance. The medication should:
- be available for oral, intramuscular, intranasal, or intravenous administration. Frequently, the patient may not have nor cooperate with an IV line
- have a rapid onset of action
- have a short half-life to facilitate a complete evaluation at the receiving facility
- cause limited central nervous system or respiratory depression
- have a low incidence of side-effects.

Rapid tranquilization is a fairly common technique used in the ED and psychiatric wards and has been extrapolated for use in the prehospital setting; however, state or regional lists of approved medications may limit the availability of specific medications for EMS usage [32]. Among the several classes of medications used for rapid tranquilization, butyrophenones and benzodiazepines are the two most commonly used by EMS.

Butyrophenones

Probably the most popular neuroleptic used in the out-of-hospital setting today is haloperidol, which is a first-generation antipsychotic of the butyrophenone class. It may be administered by the oral, IM, or IV route [33]. This high-potency neuroleptic has been shown to be effective in controlling agitation [32]. The classic regimen is administration of 5 mg IM or IV (in extremely agitated or large patients a 10 mg initial dose may be used), repeated every 30–60 minutes if needed [34]. One advantage of haloperidol is that the patient remains responsive to commands and is not overly sedated [35]. The onset of effect is 20 minutes via IM and 5–10 minutes via the IV route [36]. If the patient cooperates, a 10 mg oral dose may be used with effects similar to that of the IM injection [37]. Haloperidol has a low incidence of side-effects, the most common being extrapyramidal symptoms (<10%), which are easily reversible with diphenhydramine 50 mg IV or benztropine 2 mg IM.

Extrapyramidal symptoms can occur after a single dose and up to 12–24 hours after administration. Other less common side-effects include akathisia, hypotension, neuroleptic malignant syndrome, and decreased seizure threshold [10,32,36,38].

Another butyrophenone, droperidol, was used for the same indications as haloperidol. "Black box" warnings from the Food and Drug Administration regarding proarrhythmogenic effects and the requirements surrounding its implementation have largely eliminated its usage. There have been several studies which have refuted the FDA's statements. If given in appropriate dosing, 5–10 mg IM, there is a very low rate of complications or clinically significant QT prolongation. A direct comparison with midazolam showed more predictable sedation as well as fewer instances of oversedation and airway compromise with the use of droperidol [32,39,40].

Second-generation antipsychotics such as olanzapine are also available and have a lower incidence of side-effects. While there have not been any studies looking at their use in the prehospital setting, these medications are being used more commonly in the ED and inpatient settings. However, due to concern about excessively decreased oxygen saturation in alcohol-intoxicated patients, first-generation antipsychotics remain the primary agent [32].

Benzodiazepines

The other major group of medications used for prehospital rapid tranquilization are the benzodiazepines. Lorazepam and midazolam both have good IM absorption. Typical regimens are lorazepam 0.05 mg/kg or midazolam 0.1–0.2 mg/kg IM every 30–60 minutes (Table 59.2). The most important indication for benzodiazepine use is in controlling alcohol or sedative withdrawal symptoms, and they are the drug of choice. Side-effects are excessive sedation and respiratory depression [38,41]. Preexisting diminished mental status and respiratory depression represent relative contraindications to their use.

Benzodiazepines and butyrophenones may be used together. Several investigators have reported the use of lorazepam in combination with haloperidol with good results, achieving a synergistic effect while reducing the amount of each drug [10,32,37]. A recommended regimen is 5 mg of haloperidol with 2 mg of lorazepam given intramuscularly.

Controversies and common mistakes

Scenes involving mentally unstable patients may be chaotic. Therefore, it is very easy to commit serious treatment errors. One of the most common is the failure to perform a complete medical evaluation. Failure to perform a physical examination and vital sign assessment may give the false impression that the patient is "just nuts," a critical mistake with possible tragic consequences. Conversely, after determining medical stability, there is also a tendency for EMS to minimize the need for intervention. For a variety of reasons, there tends to be a significant lack of empathy engendered by psychiatric patients. This may lead providers to inappropriately believe the patient is "just faking it" or "wasting our time." This can be disastrous, especially in the situation of a patient with suicidal ideation. Every patient who is suspected of having suicidal thoughts should be transported for additional psychiatric evaluation. It is better to err on the side of treatment and transport.

When faced with an agitated and/or aggressive patient, it is unnecessarily dangerous to simply use force to manage him or her. Not spending sufficient time deescalating the patient and establishing rapport is another common mistake. Providers should convey assurance to the patient and attempt to gain his or trust. Becoming argumentative or trying to reason with a psychotic patient will just cause further agitation.

Emergency medical services safety is of paramount importance. Personnel should be instructed to withdraw immediately if the patient is armed and/or extremely agitated. Law enforcement agencies should be notified and assume control of the scene until it is safe for EMS to return. EMS should not attempt to "fight" or restrain the patient without the appropriate personnel and equipment.

After a physical or chemical restraint has been applied, the patient should never be left unattended. Close monitoring of vital signs and mental status must be maintained. Providers must be ever watchful for unintentional oversedation or side-effects from pharmacotherapy.

Patients and EMS personnel should not be subjected to unnecessary injuries. The medical director should ensure that sufficient policies and protocols are in place to empower providers when treating these types of patients.

Finally, a common pitfall is the lack of interagency coordination and cooperation. The approach to the violent or agitated patient must be well organized and preplanned. Arguments among responders, especially in view of the patient, must be avoided. All providers should clearly understand and accept their roles and responsibility before caring for the patient. Coordinated training should be held with law enforcement and other responsible agencies on a periodic basis.

Table 59.2 Common medications for rapid tranquilization

Medication	Dose	Route	Onset of action	Peak effect
Haloperidol	5–10 mg	PO, IM	10–20 min	30–60 min
		IV (do not use deconate salt IV)	5–10 min	30–60 min
Diazepam	0.1–0.2 mg/kg	IV (over 1 min)	5–10 min	30–60 min
Lorazepam	0.05–0.1 mg/kg	IM, IV	15–20 min	60–90 min
Midazolam	0.05–0.1 mg/kg	IV	5–10 min	30–60 min
	0.01–0.2 mg/kg	IM	15 min	30–60 min
	0.2 mg/kg (max. 10 mg)	IN	6–8 min	15 min

IM, intramuscular; IV, intravenous; PO, by mouth.
Source: Benitez [34], DiPiro [35], PDR Staff [36], Knoester [42].

Conclusion

Psychiatric and behavioral health emergencies represent a unique challenge for the prehospital professional. EMS physicians, paramedics, and EMTs frequently face patients and situations that are difficult to manage regardless of their level of training. Their own safety is even sometimes in jeopardy. Active participation by the EMS medical director and direct medical oversight medical control when needed is important to guarantee that the highest quality of care is provided for the patient as well as to provide reassurance to the EMS provider. Strong treatment protocols and frequent training sessions, including with other public safety agencies, yield the best results.

References

1 Bledsoe BE. Behavioral and Psychiatric Emergencies. In: Bledsoe BE, Porter RS, Shade BR (eds) *Brady Paramedic Emergency Care*, 2nd edn. Upper Saddle River, NJ: Brady, 1994.

2 Tintinalli JE, McCoy M. Violent patient and the out-of-hospital provider. *Ann Emerg Med* 1993;22:1276–9.

3 Verdile VP. Out-of-hospital management of the violent patient. *Out-of-Hospital Care Rep* 1992;2:17–24.

4 Judd RL. Behavioral and psychological crisis in emergency medical services. *Top Emerg Med* 1983;4:1–7.

5 Dorland WA. *Dorland's Illustrated Medical Dictionary*, 27th edn. Philadelphia: W.B. Saunders, 1988.

6 Doyle TJ, Vissers RJ. An EMS approach to psychiatric emergencies. *Emerg Med Serv* 1999;28:87, 90–3.

7 Cheney P, Haddock T. Safety and compliance with an emergency medical service direct psychiatric center transport protocol. *Am J Emerg Med* 2008;26:750–6.

8 National Association of EMS Physicians. Alternate ambulance transportation and destination. National Association of EMS Physicians/ AmericanCollege of Emergency Physicians Joint Position Paper. *Prehosp Emerg Care* 2001;5:289.

9 Henneman PL, Mendoza R, Lewis RJ. Prospective evaluation of emergency department medical clearance. *Ann Emerg Med* 1994; 24:672–7.

10 Goldberg RJ, Dubin WR, Fogel BS. Review: behavioral emergencies, assessment of psychopharmacologic management. *Clin Neuropharm* 1989;12:233–48.

11 Larkin GL, Beautrais AL. Behavioral disorders: emergency assessment. In: Tintinalli JE, Stapczynski JS, Cline DM (eds) *Emergency Medicine: A Comprehensive Study Guide*, 7th edn. New York: McGraw-Hill Medical, 2011.

12 Harwitz D, Ravizza L. Psychiatric emergencies: suicide and depression. *Emerg Med Clin North Am* 2000;18:263–71.

13 Centers for Disease Control and Prevention, Murphy SL, Jiaquan X, Kochanek KD. Deaths: final data for 2010. *National Vital Statistics Reports* 2013;61(4).

14 Centers for Disease Control and Prevention, Kung HC, Hoyert DL. Deaths: Preliminary data for 2005. *Health E-Stats*, Sept 2007. Available at: www.cdc.gov/nchs/data/hestat/prelimdeaths05/ prelimdeaths05.htm

15 National Vital Statistics System, National Center for Health Statistics, Centers for Disease Control and Prevention. 10 Leading Causes of Death by Age Group, United States – 2003. Available at: www.cdc. gov/nchs/data/hestat/leadingdeaths03/leadingdeaths03.htm

16 Centers for Disease Control and Prevention. Suicide trends among youths and young adults aged 10–24 – United States 1990–2004. *MMWR* 2007;56(35):905–8.

17 Centers for Disease Control and Prevention. Suicide and Suicidal Behavior. In: *Fact Book of the Year 2000: Working to Prevent and Control Injury in the United States*. Washington, DC: National Center for Injury Prevention and Control, 2001.

18 Hirschfeld R, Russel J. Assessment and treatment of suicidal patients. *N Engl J Med* 1997;337:910–15.

19 Holloman GH Jr, Zeller SL. Overview of project BETA: best practices in evaluation and treatment of agitation. *West J Emerg Med* 2012;13:1–2.

20 Lehman LS, Padilla M, Clark S, et al. Training personnel in the prevention and management of violent behavior. In: *Management of Violent Behavior*. Washington, DC: Hospital and Community Psychiatry Service, American Psychiatric Association, 1988, p.24–7.

21 Fredrick L. Defending your life: how to manage the violent patients and scenes. *JEMS* 1992;17:64–7.

22 Blummenreich P, Lippman S, Bacani-Oropilla T. Violent patients: are you prepared to deal with them? *Post Grad Med* 1991;90: 201–6.

23 Nordstrom K, Zun LS, Wilson MP, et al. Medical evaluation and triage of the agitated patient: consensus statement of the American Association for Emergency Psychiatry Project BETA Medical Evaluation Workgroup. *West J Emerg Med* 2012;13:3–10.

24 Tueth MJ. Management of behavioral emergencies. *AM J Emerg Med* 1995;13:344–50.

25 3,4-Methylenedioxypyrovalerone (MDPV). Drug Enforcement Administration Drug & Chemical Evaluation Section. www.deadiversion. usdoj.gov/drug_chem_info/mdpv.pdf

26 Kupas DF, Wydro GC. Patient restraint in emergency medical services systems. *Prehosp Emerg Care* 2002;6:340–5.

27 Tardiff K. Management of the violent patient in an emergency situation. *Psychiatr Clin North Am* 1988;11:539–49.

28 Richmond JS, Berlin JS, Fishkind AB, et al. Verbal de-escalation of the agitated patient: consensus statement of the American Association of Emergency Psychiatry Project BETA De-escalation Workgroup. *West J Emerg Med* 2012;13:17–25.

29 Knox DK, Holloman GH. Use and avoidance of seclusion and restraint: consensus statement of the American Association of Emergency Psychiatry Project BETA Seclusion and Restraint Workgroup. *West J Emerg Med* 2012;13:35–40.

30 Chan TC, Vilke GM, Neuman T, Clausen JL. Restraint position and positional asphyxia. *Ann Emerg Med* 1997;30:578–86.

31 Pilowsky LS, Ring H, Shine PJ, et al. Rapid tranquilization: a survey of emergency prescribing in a general psychiatric hospital. *Br J Psychiatry* 1992;160:831–5.

32 Wilson MP, Pepper D, Currier GW, et al. The psychopharmacology of agitation: consensus statement of the American Association of Emergency Psychiatry Project BETA Psychopharmacology Workgroup. *West J Emerg Med* 2012;13:26–34.

33 Larkin GL, Beautrais AL. Behavioral disorders: emergency assessment. In: Tintinalli JE, Stapczynski JS, Cline DM (eds) *Emergency Medicine: A Comprehensive Study Guide*, 7th edn. New York: McGraw-Hill Medical, 2011.

34 Benitez JG. How to control the violent patient. *UPMC Trauma Rounds* 1994;5:6–7.

35 DiPiro JJ, Talbert FL, Yee GC, et al. Pharmacotherapy: A Pathophysiologic Approach, 8th edn. New York: McGraw-Hill Medical, 2011

36 Physicians' Desk Reference Network. *Physicians' Desk Reference*, 67th edn. Montvale, NJ: PDR Network, 2012.

37 Circaulo DA. Psychotropic drug therapy in the emergency department. *Top Emerg Med* 1983;4:17–23.

38 Dubin WR. Rapid tranquilization: antipsychotics or benzodiazepines. *J Clin Psychiatry* 1988;49: 5–12.

39 Isbister GK, Calver LA, Page CB, et al. Randomized controlled trial of intramuscular droperidol versus midazolam for violence and acute behavioral disturbance: the DORM study. *Ann Emerg Med* 2010;56:392–401.

40 Kao LW, Kirk MA, Evers SJ, et al. Droperidol, QT prolongation, and sudden death: what is the evidence? *Ann Emerg Med* 2003;41:546–58.

41 Stewart SM. Droperidol. *Crit Care Nurse* 1987;7:86.

42 Knoester PD, Jonker DM, Van der Hoeven RT, et al. Pharmacokinetics and pharmacodynamics of midazolam administered as a concentrated intranasal spray. A study in healthy volunteers. *Br J Clin Pharmacol* 2002;53:501–7.

Special Considerations

CHAPTER 60

Intimate partner violence

Petra Norris

Introduction

Woman abuse, wife assault, domestic violence, relationship terrorism, and intimate partner violence (IPV) are all terms that have been used to describe the violence that occurs between two people in an intimate relationship. Although domestic violence includes IPV, it also refers to violence against other family members; therefore, for the purpose of this chapter, the term IPV will be defined as the intentional use of tactics to gain and maintain power and control over the thoughts, beliefs, and conduct [1] of an intimate partner. The term partner may be defined as a current or former girlfriend, boyfriend, spouse, or common-law spouse.

Tactics used to gain control in IPV create fear, isolation, and the entrapment of one partner. The majority of non-fatal intimate partner victimizations occur at home [2]. The EMT or EMS physician is in the unique position to attend to the patient in the home and observe the environment in which the violence took place, as well as the behaviors of the victim and abuser along with their interactions with each other. Being aware of these behaviors will allow the EMS provider to identify situations in which abuse may not yet have escalated to physical violence, thereby allowing early intervention.

Scope of the problem

Violence against women is well documented by the World Health Organization (WHO). IPV occurs in all countries, regardless of social, economic, religious, or cultural status [3]. Although it is recognized that violence occurs against men in both opposite and same-sex relationships, the prevalence of women as victims is overwhelmingly greater than men. Therefore, this chapter will focus on male violence against female partners.

About one in four women and one in seven men have experienced severe physical violence [4]. Women are three times more likely to report that they have been beaten, choked, sexually assaulted, or threatened with a gun or knife [5] and therefore more likely to require medical attention. Domestic violence is a leading cause of injury to American women between the ages of 15 and 44 and is estimated to be responsible for 20–25% of emergency department (ED) visits by women [6]. One in five homicides involves killing of an intimate partner [7].

High-risk groups

Part of identifying IPV is awareness of the high-risk groups. Although it already has been established that women are a risk group, there are subgroups that are at even higher risk. Women who are separated or divorced report higher rates than women of other marital status [2]. Aboriginal women are three times more likely to experience spousal violence than non-aboriginal [7]. Visible minorities report a rate of IPV of 5% [8]. Women with disabilities are 1.5–10 times as likely to be abused as non-disabled women, depending on whether they live in the community or in institutions [9]. At least 4–8% of pregnant women report suffering abuse during pregnancy [10], and 39.2% of same-sex cohabiting women, and 23.1% of men, reported being raped, physically assaulted, and/or stalked by a marital or cohabiting partner at some time in their lifetime [11].

Understanding intimate partner violence

Abuse often begins in a close, mutual relationship, which over time becomes exclusive, allowing the abuser to isolate the victim. Violence can appear gradually or suddenly, but generally there is a period of "testing [12]." This may begin with verbal abuse and then progress to sexual and physical abuse (Box 60.1). Shoving and pushing can escalate to punching, kicking, and assault with blunt and penetrating weapons.

Cycle of violence

Many abusive relationships undergo a cycle of violence, which occurs in three stages (Figure 60.1) [12]. In phase one, tension builds and the woman increases her efforts to please the abuser

Emergency Medical Services: Clinical Practice and Systems Oversight, Second Edition. Volume 1: Clinical Aspects of EMS.
Edited by David C. Cone, Jane H. Brice, Theodore R. Delbridge, and J. Brent Myers.
© 2015 NAEMSP. Published 2015 by John Wiley & Sons, Inc. Companion Website: www.wiley.com\go\cone\naemsp

Box 60.1 Forms of abuse found in intimate partner violence

Physical	Use of physical force often resulting in injury (e.g. hitting, slapping, punching)
Verbal	Attacking someone's self-esteem by calling her derogatory names (e.g. stupid, slut)
Emotional/psychological	Emotional trauma experienced by the victim (e.g. making threats, putting her down, blackmail, or continuous blaming)
Sexual	Any form of sexual activity with another person without their consent
Spiritual	Denying the ability to practice or express her religion or spirituality or being forced to practice another religion
Financial/material	Controlling someone through the restriction of financial or necessary material items (e.g. not being able to work or being forced to hand over her paycheck, being denied material things such as food and/or medications)

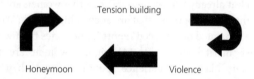

Figure 60.1 Cycle of violence.

in hopes of avoiding violence. The woman may intentionally trigger the abuse at a time when she feels the violence is inevitable to decrease the stress she feels about the impending violence, or to be in control as to where and when the violence will occur. In phase two, violence erupts and may increase in frequency and severity over time. Phase three represents a "honeymoon" phase in which the abuser apologizes for the abuse, may purchase gifts, blames the victim, and offers rationalizations (e.g. "If you only didn't… I wouldn't…."). This phase may become shorter over time.

The cycle of violence can also occur generationally because it is passed through the family. Children witnessing abuse learn that it is tolerated or even appropriate behavior and a way of gaining power and control, and therefore may repeat the behavior in their own relationships.

Intimate partner violence as a health care issue

Studies report that about one in four women seeking care in the ED for any reason is a victim of violence (one in three treated for trauma), and 37% of female patients who are treated in the ED for violent injury have been injured by intimate partners [13].

Health care providers are being encouraged to universally screen for violence in the ED and primary health care settings. This means that all women over the age of 12 are asked about abuse, not only those in whom injuries appear suspicious. The National Violence Against Women survey revealed that 125,000 (17.5%) female victims of assault used ambulance services [14]. Because EMS personnel are often the first responders to situations that involve violence, it is critical to be able to identify, ask about, and respond appropriately to the unique situations that involve IPV. If violence can be identified early then there is an opportunity to intervene, thereby improving the health and lives of women and children and stopping the cycle of abuse.

Health effects of abuse

Many women living with abuse experience more than just physical injuries such as fractures and soft tissue injuries; they may present with psychiatric and medical conditions such as those listed in Box 60.2 [1]. Between 2001 and 2005 the US Department of Justice statistics reported that fewer than one-fifth of victims reporting an injury sought treatment following the injury. Approximately 8% of female and 10% of male victims were treated at the scene of the injury or in the home. Females who experienced an injury were slightly more likely than their male counterparts to seek treatment at a hospital [2]. EMS might be called to a scene at which the patient is experiencing any of the aforementioned conditions. Through noticing the environment, patient injuries, and/or interactions between the patient and her partner at the scene, the EMS provider may be able to identify IPV.

Emergency medical services provider safety

If EMS is activated through a 9-1-1 call for IPV, it is important to have law enforcement secure the scene before EMS access. If EMS personnel arrive at the scene of a non-disclosed IPV situation and feel that they are at risk, law enforcement should

Box 60.2 Health effects of intimate partner violence

Physical effects	Broken bones, burns, bruises, headaches, chronic (often abdominal or pelvic) pain, gastrointestinal problems
Emotional/psychological effects	Anxiety, insomnia, low self-esteem, phobias, flashbacks, memory loss
Psychiatric effects	Self-harm, suicide, eating disorders, depression, dissociation, posttraumatic stress disorder
Sexual effects	Multiple pregnancies close together, unwanted pregnancy, miscarriage, sexually transmitted infections, sexually addictive behaviors

be called. Once the scene is secure, the providers can proceed with assessing safety in the immediate area where the patient is located to provide medical assistance. Patients should be assessed in the appropriate sequence with the primary survey, ABCs, and life-saving interventions undertaken, followed by a secondary survey and further history.

While on the scene, EMS providers should keep the following in mind.

• Avoid confronting the abuser.
• Do not place yourself physically between a couple who are arguing.
• Ensure that an escape route such as the door is available.
• Do not let the abuser get between you and your escape route.

Be aware of your jurisdiction's legal requirements with respect to reporting to law enforcement. Some states require EMTs responding to an injury sustained during a crime to report to police; others will allow or mandate the patient to decide the best action to take. Requirements may be different for physicians.

Assessment and examination

On the initial interaction with the patient, EMS personnel may find there was a delay in seeking help and/or that this patient may have experienced repeated calls and visits to the ED for injuries.

Physical assessment

The physical assessment may reveal injuries such as abrasions, bruises, burns, dislocations, lacerations, bites, fractures, abrasions, or marks on the neck consistent with strangulation, petechial hemorrhage in the eyes, a combination of old and new injuries, and/or patterned injuries to the head, face, neck, throat, chest, breasts, back, abdomen, or genitals. Injuries that suggest a defensive posture, such as those found on the hands or ulnar aspect of the arms, are suspicious. Patients may also experience mouth and dental trauma. It may also be found that the patient's or partner's description of accident is inconsistent with the observed injury. If this is the case, EMS should document both what is reported and objective observations.

Behavioral assessment

Once the patient is medically stable, EMS personnel should observe the environment as well as the behaviors and interactions between the people at the scene. The abusive partner's behavior may include: hovers over her, insists on being present while she is being examined, answers for the woman [15], is overly friendly with the care provider, or appears kind or overly concerned. Conversely, he may also minimize the injury, lack sympathy, make remarks about her, or blame her for the violence/accident. The woman's behavior may be evasive and guarded interactions, including saying nothing in front of her partner, minimizing the seriousness of her injury, avoiding eye contact, and looking to her partner for guidance [1].

Asking about abuse

Once an EMS provider has made a determination that this call or injury could be a result of IPV, as part of the overall patient assessment, he or she should ask about abuse in a confidential environment, and respond appropriately to support the patient. The goal of asking about abuse is to make a supportive connection and convey the message that abuse is a health issue. This may help to lessen the patient's isolation. Options may then be reviewed so that the patient is empowered to make informed choices for herself and her children. If the patient denies abuse, she will at least be left with the awareness that she can access EMS assistance when required, if and when she chooses to disclose.

Separating couples

Asking about abuse must be done in private, away from anyone who may intimidate the victim. Ideally, children should not be present because they may repeat information they hear to others. This could create a dangerous situation if disclosed information were repeated to the abuser. Separating the abuser may require some creativity and is a challenge in the out-of-hospital setting. Two options are to have one EMT take the partner into another room to ask more health history questions or wait until the patient is alone in the back of the ambulance. It is important to make clear to the partner beforehand that the ambulance is for patients only. The EMT should be conscious of what he or she is saying and tone of voice. Do not inadvertently give messages that the patient is to blame or should follow your advice, such as saying, "What did you do to cause this?" or "How can you love this guy?"

Encouraging disclosure

There is no question that will elicit a disclosure if the patient is not ready. Do not force a disclosure. Should the EMS provider suspect abuse based on physical or behavioral observations, use the observation in the question, such as, "I am concerned that this injury may have been caused by someone hurting you. Did someone hurt you?" or "I noticed your partner doesn't like to leave you alone, how do you feel about that?" If the EMS provider is practicing universal asking/screening, then something that contextualizes the question would be more appropriate, such as, "Violence against women has become a health care issue; therefore, I ask all my female patients if they have ever experienced abuse/violence as a child, adolescent, or adult."

If she says "yes", the EMS provider can respond with the following questions.

• "Are you safe now?" (Determine the location of the perpetrator.)
• "Would you like to talk about it?" (If the EMS provider does not have the time, then provide 24-hour IPV hotline/helpline numbers for support.)

- "Have you talked to anyone else about this?" (This helps determine the patient's support systems or just how isolated she may be.)
- "What do you need right now?" (Demonstrates that the EMS provider is focused on her and her needs at this time and can pass the information to ED staff.)

If she says "no", the EMS provider can respond with the following message: "I ask all my patients about violence and want to make sure they are aware of resources that are available to them in case their relationship changes." The patient may deny abuse because she is experiencing barriers to disclosure such as fear the abuser will find out, fear that the police and/or a child protection agency will become involved, or shame and embarrassment. Or she may not have been abused; in any case, most patients appreciate the question. Again, do not force a disclosure.

When people experience IPV their power and self-determination are taken away. EMS care should endeavor to empower the patient. Ways in which this can be done are explaining and asking permission before performing medical procedures, if the patient's condition allows; sitting at or below the patient's eye level; building trust by being direct and compassionate in responding to her questions; and being clear about violence against women being a crime and that this was not her fault.

Even in the out-of-hospital environment, women need a supportive, non-judgmental atmosphere in which to feel safe disclosing abuse. Expressing concern, conveying that you believe her, and providing validation for her experience are effective ways of offering support. If possible, provide options such as a sexual assault/domestic violence care or response center, police involvement, safety planning, and shelter referrals. The EMS provider should respect the decisions the patient makes; it might not be what the provider would have done given the situation, but the patient is the expert of her life and knows what she can deal with at this time.

High-risk indicators and concerns

Factors that have been shown to be related to increased risk of further violence in relationships include increasing frequency and severity of violence, using or threatening to use a weapon or to kill the woman, access to guns, perpetrator using drugs and alcohol excessively, and violence in pregnancy [16].

Women who have been injured through IPV often decline transport to the hospital [17]. Therefore, they will not have the availability of resources such as nurse examiners or social workers to provide them with support or referrals. Hence, the EMS provider's knowledge of safety plans and the resources in the local community may be beneficial.

Culture and domestic violence

North America has become very culturally diverse and continues to attract people with a range of cultural norms, values, attitudes, and beliefs about illness and violence and the treatment

response to a variety of conditions. As each individual responds to stress and violence differently, much of each person's reaction will be influenced or affected by his or her cultural background. During times of physical/emotional stress, verbal understanding may be decreased whether or not the patient is English speaking. It is important to have as accurate an account of the events as possible in order to collect appropriate evidence and medically clear the individual. It is helpful to limit the amount of technical language, professional jargon, and common expressions that may be interpreted literally, such as "tachycardia" or "I am feeling under the weather." Speak slowly, not loudly. Face the person; it may or may not be appropriate to make/sustain eye contact. Use short, simple sentences. Repeat and/or rephrase questions and summarize often to ensure your understanding. Ask open-ended questions. Questions that require only a "yes or no" answer do not tell you if the questions have been correctly understood [18].

If the interpreter is a spouse or other family member, bear in mind that not all facts may be disclosed due to the potential ramifications of reporting a domestic violence call. Abusive men of all cultures use similar power and control tactics. However, when a family has immigrated to North America there may be some additional tactics employed such as those listed in Box 60.3.

It is important to consider the family structure in diverse cultures, particularly what is the hierarchy and who has the power within the family. On an individual level, women may feel fear, shame, and powerlessness, and therefore remain silent. Their view on marriage may be that they are there to provide a sexual service and therefore sexual assault does not exist in a marriage. They may also be struggling with how they will be perceived if they disclose; going against the family and getting a spouse in trouble may be interpreted as a sign of weakness, as may seeking help [18].

When considering the impact on the family/community, the family may deny that sexual/domestic violence exists

Box 60.3 Control tactics relevant to immigrants experiencing intimate partner violence

Isolation	Not allowing her to learn English, isolating her from anyone who speaks her language
Emotional	Failing to file papers to legalize her immigration status or lying about her status, writing her family lies about her, calling her racist names
Intimidation	Withdrawing or threatening to withdraw papers filed for her residency, threatening deportation, hiding/destroying important papers
Economic	Threatening to report her if she works "under the table," not allowing job training or schooling
Children	Threatening to send children to their country of origin or report them to immigration
Sexual	Calling her a prostitute or "mail-order bride," alleging she is a prostitute on legal documents

in the desire to succeed and reestablish oneself. Other considerations are [18]:

- fear of being ostracized for bringing shame upon the family
- fear of retaliatory violence from the perpetrator and his supporters
- fear of being shunned by the community
- uncertainty and mistrust about how the police/system will respond
- fear of deportation.

Cultures differ in their styles and attitudes toward decision making and disclosure. Assume there will be differences between cultures and within cultures. Use your power and privilege to empower others. Create safe spaces for these sensitive conversations and respect others' decisions even if you do not agree.

Safety planning

Women seek strategies aimed at preventing and responding to violence [17]. The EMS provider should ascertain what she has done in the past to keep herself safe, what is working, and what is not working. Because a woman's level of risk may change over time, safety plans need to be flexible. Assess what the patient's major concerns are at this time by asking open-ended questions such as, "What are you worried about most right now?" This aids in building a trusting relationship and views the patient not as a victim but as a strong capable participant in her future. The more she directs the safety planning, the more likely she is to adhere to it. The resources listed at the end of this chapter provide more information about safety planning.

Referrals

There are many options that EMS and other emergency providers may offer to victims of IPV. The EMS physician should make referrals in a way as to empower the patient to make her own decisions. The person in the situation is the best judge of what is safe to do right now. It is important for emergency providers to be aware of crisis lines, along with the appropriate agencies and organizations in their jurisdiction which offer services for victims of IPV. Sexual assault/domestic violence care or response centers can offer crisis intervention and support, documentation of injuries and photographs, safety planning and risk assessments, referrals to shelters, and other advocacy services. There may be mandatory reporting policies in your jurisdiction and all EMS personnel should be familiar with police services and mandatory reporting requirements. Shelters usually have counselors available 24 hours a day and provide a safe place for someone to flee relationship violence. Child protection agencies offer protective and referral services as well. Legal agencies may be available for victims of IPV.

Preserving evidence and documentation

When performing a physical assessment, the EMS provider may note patterns of blunt injury, lacerations, or penetrating wounds. It is therefore important to know these patterns and appropriately document if the injury does not fit the mechanism described. Be careful not to disturb the crime scene or destroy possible evidence, such as by removal of the patient's clothing. If anything needs to be removed to attend the patient, describe the condition of the clothing and place it in a paper bag. Cut around bullet holes or stab wounds, not through them [12]. The manner in which clothing is removed or altered should be noted (e.g. "during resuscitation, patient's shirt torn open, tearing off four buttons"). If any furniture needs to be moved to get to the patient, this should also be documented.

Use the patient's own words when describing how she received the injuries, who assaulted her, and when. A detailed history of all aspects of the assault need not be taken as part of immediate care. The EMS provider should write what is pertinent to the care and treatment of injuries. Documentation should occur at the scene or as soon as possible after attending to the patient. Should a case go to court, the patient care record will be the only documentation the EMS provider will have of this event (Box 60.4). Documentation should be objective, without accusations or value statements, accurate, specific, legible, and complete.

Realistic expectations

It can be difficult to bear witness to abuse. Often health care providers feel powerless in their efforts to make a significant difference in someone's life. It is important to remember that

---

Box 60.4 Key aspects of IPV documentation

- Location of injuries (best done on body diagrams)
- Full description of all injuries (type, color)
- Size of injuries; if no measuring device is available, compare with a well-known item like size of a quarter
- Other injury characteristics (e.g. scabbed, bleeding, or presence of foreign body)
- Mechanism of injury
- Areas of tenderness/pain
- Injury patterns
- Distinguish between her or the partner's reports and your observations
- Excited utterances made by the patient such as, "I really thought I was going to die this time"
- Patient's/perpetrator's behaviors
- Other persons (such as children) present and their behaviors
- Police officers' names and badge numbers
- Any safety planning information or referrals provided
- If drugging is suspected, any body fluids such as emesis or urine should be collected and preserved if possible

Box 60.5 Potential reasons why a victim of IPV may return to an abusive relationship

- Fear of personal safety and/or safety of their children/pets
- Low self-esteem, fear of the unknown
- Economic issues
- Isolation, no friends, no support system
- Cultural/religious beliefs
- Fear of deportation, unsure of legal rights
- Family pressures, blame for failure of the relationship
- Unsure of options
- Abuse may be considered "normal"
- Threat of sexual orientation revealed
- "He's not always abusive"
- Systemic barriers

dealing with abuse is a process and each person has the right to set his or her own agenda and work at his or her own pace. The role of EMS is to provide medical treatment and support and empower patients to make the decisions that are right for them at a time when they feel it is safe. EMS cannot "fix" a victim or the situation. At times, providers may not agree with the decisions patients make, but they are the experts of their lives.

Domestic violence does not always end when women leave the relationship. Statistics show that the most dangerous time is when she has decided to leave or soon after she has left [19]. Women can be trapped in and may return to relationships many times for a variety of reasons before making a final break (Box 60.5).

Understanding why people stay in abusive relationships and how to keep them safe is key when providing care to a victim of IPV. A strong multidisciplinary team approach is essential and will result in the most appropriate and beneficial patient-focused care for people experiencing violence in their lives. Therefore, ensure that all essential information and impressions are communicated to ED staff.

Conclusion

A call to a residence where IPV has taken place can be one of the most difficult calls to which EMS respond. It is vital for the scene to be secure before the EMS personnel enter the premises. On calls where IPV is not initially identified in the call, but is suspected once on the scene, it is the responsibility of EMS personnel to ask and assess the patient's immediate safety. In instances where the patient declines transportation, knowledgeable EMS personnel can provide support and resources and suggest immediate safety planning. If the patient accepts transport to the ED, ensure that all relevant information is reported to the health care provider taking responsibility for the patient.

Complete the call report as soon as possible to ensure that documentation provides an accurate, comprehensive, and timely account of the call. EMS documentation of the events/injuries could be vital if and when the patient chooses to press assault charges. All providers should be aware of and compliant with local legislative requirements.

References

1 Task Force on the Health Effects of Woman Abuse, Middlesex-London Health Unit. *Final Report*. London, ON: Task Force on the Health Effects of Woman Abuse, 2000.

2 Catalano S. Intimate partner violence in the United States. US Department of Justice, Bureau of Justice Statistics. Available at: http://bjs.ojp.usdoj.gov/content/pub/pdf/ipvus.pdf

3 World Health Organization. World report on violence and health. Available at: www.who.int/violence_injury_prevention/violence/world_report/en/summary_en.pdf

4 Black MC, Basile KC, Breiding MJ, et al. *The National Intimate Partner and Sexual Violence Survey (NISVS): 2010 Summary Report*. Atlanta, GA: National Center for Injury Prevention and Control, Centers for Disease Control and Prevention, 2011.

5 Registered Nurses' Association of Ontario. *Woman Abuse: Screening, Identification and Initial Response*. Toronto: Registered Nurses' Association of Ontario, 2005, p.17.

6 Baby Centre Medical Advisory Board. Domestic violence during pregnancy. Available at: www.babycenter.com/0_domestic-violence-during-pregnancy_1356253.bc?page=1

7 Statistics Canada. Measuring violence against women: statistical trends 2006. Ottawa: Ministry of Industry. Available at: www.statcan.gc.ca/pub/85-570-x/85-570-x2006001-eng.pdf

8 Sinha M. Victimization among visible minority and immigrant populations. Canadian Centre for Justice Statistics, Statistics Canada. Available at: www.phac-aspc.gc.ca/ncfv-cnivf/EB/2012/february-fevrier/1-eng.php#anchor1

9 Health Canada, National Clearing House of Family Violence. Woman abuse overview paper. Available at: www.phac-aspc.gc.ca/ncfv-cnivf/publications/femviof-eng.php

10 Centers for Disease Control and Prevention. Intimate partner violence during pregnancy: a guide for clinicians. Available at: www.cdc.gov/reproductivehealth/violence/IntimatePartnerViolence/sld011.htm

11 Tjaden P, Thoennes N. Extent, nature, and consequences of intimate partner violence (No. NCJ 181867). Washington, DC: US Department of Justice, Office of Justice Programs. Available at: www.ncjrs.gov/pdffiles1/nij/181867.pdf

12 Polsky S, Markowitz J. *Color Atlas of Domestic Violence*. St Louis, MO: Mosby, 2004.

13 Eisenstat S, Bancroft L. Domestic violence. *N Engl J Med* 1999;341:886–92.

14 Husni ME, Linden JA, Tibbles C. Domestic violence and out-of-hospital providers. *Acad Emerg Med* 2000;7:243–8.

15 Salvatore SL, Jones P, Bentzien V. *EMS and The Domestic Violence Patient*. New Jersey: Backdraft Publications, 1999.

16 Campbell J. Danger assessment. Available at: www.dangerassessment.org/

17 Davies J, Lyon E, Monti-Catania D. *Safety Planning with Battered Women: Complex Lives, Difficult Choices*. California: Sage Publications, 1998.

18 Srivastava R. *The Healthcare Provider's Guide to Clinical Cultural Competence*. Toronto: Elsevier, 2007.

19 Shipway L. *Domestic Violence: A Handbook for Health Professionals*. New York: Routledge, 2004.

Recommended resources

Peel Committee Against Woman Abuse (safety plans in a variety of languages). Available at: www.pcawa.org

National Centre on Domestic and Sexual Violence (a variety of power and control wheels). Available at: www.ncdsv.org/

CHAPTER 61

Sexual assault

Petra Norris

Introduction

Sexual violence is a critical global issue that affects millions of people worldwide, claiming a victim every 45 seconds according to the American Medical Association [1]. EMS personnel are certain to encounter sexual assault victims, and are often the first to interact with the victim after the assault. It is crucial that EMS physicians and personnel, as well as EMS medical directors, understand the psychosocial, medical, and legal aspects of sexual assault.

Sexual violence has been defined as any form of sexual activity with another person without her or his consent. The assault may include forced kissing, fondling, attempted or completed penetration, forced masturbation by the victim or to the assailant, forced participation in or looking at sexually explicit photos, sexual harassment, exhibitionism, and voyeurism [2]. Both women and men can be victims of sexual assault; however, the majority of assaults are perpetrated by men against women and children [3]. Therefore, for ease of pronoun use, she or her will be used here in any reference to a victim.

The National Intimate Partner and Sexual Violence Survey reports that nearly one in five women (18.3%) and one in 71 men (1.4%) in the United States have been raped at some time in their lives, including completed forced penetration, attempted forced penetration, or alcohol/drug-facilitated completed penetration [4]. It is important to note that sexual assault is one of the most underreported crimes. Fewer than one in ten victims report the crime to the police [5]. Most women will confide in family, friends, co-workers, doctors, and/or nurses [6].

Reasons for not reporting include embarrassment, fear of being blamed or not being believed, and fear of reprisal from the assailant or court proceedings. Sexual assault is often attributed to overwhelming sexual desire. It is anything but. All forms of sexual assault are the misuse of power and control over another person with the intention of abusing and humiliating the victim [7].

Drug-facilitated sexual assault

Drug-facilitated sexual assault (DFSA) is the term used to describe cases of sexual assault in which the victim is unable to consent or resist because she has been rendered incapacitated or unconscious due to the effects of alcohol and/or drugs [8]. DFSA may result when drugs or alcohol are administered without the victim's knowledge, or through the perpetrator taking advantage of a person who is already under the influence of drugs/alcohol. These crimes are less likely to be reported to law enforcement agencies because of the inability of the victim, due to drug-induced amnesia or fear, to describe the events.

Consent issues

Sexual assault occurs when there is no consent on the part of the other person. Consent is an active choice and constitutes a voluntary agreement between two persons of legal age to engage in sexual activity. A spouse can be charged with sexually assaulting the other spouse in cases of intimate partner violence. Previous consent to sexual activity does not mean that consent is not required the next time the other person seeks a sexual encounter.

The following are examples of situations of non-consent and sexual assault [9].

- Someone who is under the influence of medication, drugs, and/or alcohol
- A child
- Someone who expresses in words, gestures, or by his or her conduct a refusal to engage in or continue sexual activity
- Someone who submits to sexual activity because of force or threats against her or others
- Lies are used to obtain consensual sex
- A third person says "yes" for someone else
- The accused is in a position of power/authority over someone
- The accused is a blood relative
- A doctor, nurse, or other health care professional performing an unnecessary internal examination

Emergency Medical Services: Clinical Practice and Systems Oversight, Second Edition. Volume 1: Clinical Aspects of EMS.
Edited by David C. Cone, Jane H. Brice, Theodore R. Delbridge, and J. Brent Myers.
© 2015 NAEMSP. Published 2015 by John Wiley & Sons, Inc. Companion Website: www.wiley.com\go\cone\naemsp

Myths

Myths are used to condone or deny sexual assault. Accepting myths as reality contributes to the way society responds to and may influence the reporting of sexual assault. Some of the widely held myths are:

- the only way a rapist can really force a woman to have intercourse is by using a weapon
- women who do not actually physically fight back have not been raped
- if the attacker is drunk at the time of the assault, then he cannot be accused of rape.

Providers should understand that sexual assault can affect anyone (including males, children, and the elderly) and is not typically accompanied by physical injury or signs of trauma.

Male sexual assault

Use of weapons and brutality are reported more often in male sexual assault. Therefore, males may sustain more physical trauma than females [10]. The most common forms of assault that males experience are receptive anal and/or oral intercourse and forced manual genital stimulation [10]. The male patient may feel guilty about having been assaulted because of a belief that males are supposed to be able to protect themselves. This feeling can be compounded if the male also experienced an erection and/or ejaculation during the assault. Both these responses can occur as involuntary reactions to extreme stress. A male does not have to be sexually aroused to have an erection [10].

Given that most assaults committed against men are perpetrated by other males, a common misunderstanding for assaulted heterosexual males is that he will become homosexual after the assault.

Psychological care of the patient

Many victims of sexual assault do not suffer life-threatening injuries; however, they do experience psychological trauma. Therefore, after assessment for and management of physical injuries, support becomes the EMT's priority. During a sexual assault, power and control are taken away from the person; care should be directed at restoring the person's self-determination through decision making with respect to her care. Sexual assault is the only crime in which the victim is often considered to have some responsibility and have contributed to the assault by the way she dressed, spoke, or acted, or her location at the time of the assault. No one asks or deserves to be sexually assaulted: EMTs should always treat patients with respect. The patient will experience a multitude of emotions, including but not limited to shock, disbelief, confusion, guilt, self-blame, terror, anger, and lack of trust.

These emotions may be evident or the patient may be very composed. The patient may even block out the events if they are too much for her to cope with at the time [10]. The type of response she receives from the first person to whom she discloses can affect how she views her situation and subsequently deals with it.

Some of the most important things an EMT can do in the initial interaction is to connect with the patient through introducing himself or herself, using the patient's name, maintaining eye contact, and using a calm, even tone when speaking. It is important that the EMT proceed on the presumption that an assault has occurred; it is not the EMT's role to decide whether or not an assault occurred. Responses to the patient should be non-judgmental and intended to reassure the patient that she is safe and that the assault was not her fault. Many victims buy into the myths surrounding sexual assault, and it is thus important to be able to help the patient distinguish between myth and reality.

People respond to crisis in a variety of ways, from crying to being calm and cooperative to laughing nervously. All are normal responses and it is important to help the patient understand this if she is concerned about how she is responding. A controlled response from a patient does not mean that the assault did not happen. She may also be concerned that she did not do enough to resist the assault; therefore, she should be reassured that she did what was necessary to prevent any further harm. If she is alone, the EMT should ask her if she would like a support person to be called.

Physical care of the patient

In addition to suffering severe emotional trauma, the patient is at risk of genital or other physical injuries.

Police-reported data show that the victim and accused were known to each other in 82% of sexual assault incidents [5]. Perpetrators can include a family member, friend, neighbor, or work colleague. Tactics used in these cases may focus less on physical force but rely on verbal intimidation, tricks, and administration of drugs or alcohol. Therefore, the absence of injuries is as consistent with sexual assault as their presence. In rape by a stranger, the likelihood of force is increased, either through verbal threats and physical force, or the element of surprise.

People respond differently when confronted with sexual assault. Some may succumb to escape any further injury or death, whereas others may fight to escape. Regardless of how the patient responded to the situation, it is important that the EMT reassure her that she handled the situation appropriately.

After securing the scene and ensuring provider safety, life-saving medical care is the EMT's top priority; therefore the patient's ABCs should always be assessed and assisted as needed.

The EMT should make detailed notes of any physical side-effects and injuries of sexual assault, among which may be:

- loss of consciousness, drowsiness, dizziness, disorientation, difficulty speaking or moving, or hallucinations. Note: it is important in cases in which DFSA is suspected that the EMT document the patient's level of consciousness, affect, and any symptoms or signs of drug effects
- bites on the face/breasts
- suction injuries of the neck
- skeletal muscle tension and general soreness
- complications of strangulation: marks, petechiae in the face and conjunctiva
- evidence of being restrained, such as any patterned injury, rope marks around wrists/ankles, or fingertip bruising on arms or legs
- abrasions, lacerations, and bruises on a variety of areas on the body, head, behind the ears, neck, thighs, knees
- broken teeth, jaw, black eyes
- clumps of hair missing due to hair pulling [10].

Unless there is severe hemorrhage or other evidence of life-threatening genital injury, this area should not be examined. Genital and/or anal injuries sustained in a sexual assault can be difficult to visualize and therefore assessment of these areas should be left to a trained sexual assault examiner in the emergency department. Unnecessary examination may leave the patient feeling revictimized and may disturb vital forensic evidence. Typical injuries include small tears, bruises, abrasions, redness, and swelling. In forced oral penetration the EMT may note similar injuries around the mouth along with petechiae on the palate and uvula and a torn frenulum [8]. Bruising behind the ears may occur from the assailant's use of physical force in an oral assault.

It is the EMT's responsibility to ask appropriate questions, assess, and document observations and findings. Questioning should be kept to a minimum: the EMT should only ask questions that are required to do a physical assessment. Hospital staff and law enforcement will conduct a more thorough examination and investigation.

Depending on the circumstances of the sexual assault, the patient may be at risk of sexually transmitted infections and/or pregnancy. She should be advised that medical treatment for pregnancy and human immunodeficiency virus is time-sensitive and can be obtained from a sexual assault care center or emergency department (ED).

Culture and sexual assault

As each individual responds to stress and violence differently, much of their reaction will be influenced or affected by their cultural background [11]. Some immigrants have a command of the English language and others may require an interpreter to assist them in communication. Remember, during times of physical/emotional stress, understanding may be decreased. In cases of sexual assault it is important to have as accurate an account of the events as possible in order to collect appropriate evidence [11].

- Limit the amount of technical language, professional jargon, and common "expressions" that may be interpreted literally.
- Speak slowly, not loudly.
- Face the patient; it may or may not be culturally appropriate to make/sustain eye contact.
- Use short, simple sentences.
- Repeat or rephrase questions and summarize often to ensure your understanding.
- Ask open-ended questions. Questions that require only a "yes" or "no" do not tell you if the questions have been understood correctly.

Touch is a major part of health care response, used to provide physical care and emotional comfort. While all humans require some degree of touch, cultural norms and context will influence what is appropriate. In cases of sexual assault, a person may not wish to be touched in any way. It is best to ask prior to touching if it is OK, i.e. "May I touch your arm, to look at the injury?" Let the patient know when you are going to touch her. Experiences of touch will vary depending on the patient's age and sex, the body part involved, and her interpretation of touch. The interpretation could be that of a caring gesture or control [11].

In order to respond to a patient with the bigger picture in mind, it is important to understand the role of the individual, the family, and the community with respect to attitudes towards violence, sexuality, and sexual behaviour. There will be gender variations and the value of virginity to be considered. Other effects on decision making will be with respect to "saving face" and the effect this disclosure will have on the family and the community and what social supports they may have. Affecing their decision to report may be their understanding of trust, power, and privilege with respect to the authorities, their immigration and resettlement experience, and the effect of racism and fear of retaliatory violence from the perpetrator and his supporters [11].

Expect that there will be differences between cultures and within cultures when people experience sexual assault. While you may feel the most appropriate plan of care is to take the patient to the hospital and involve police, this may not be the best course of action in the long run. Focus on the patient's strengths and avoid judgment by altering your perspective and seeing it from her point of view.

Legal aspects

In cases of sexual assault, there are two crime scenes where evidence can be collected immediately: the location where the assault occurred, and the victim of the assault herself. There are several aspects that need to be proven for a sexual assault to have occurred.

- Both victim and perpetrator were together at the same location.
- There was a sexual act.
- There was no consent.

Documentation should be prepared on the assumption that the information may eventually be presented in a court of law. It is imperative that the documentation be accurate, comprehensive, objective, legible, and timely, either during or immediately after giving care.

Preservation of evidence

Evidence can be verbal or physical. The EMT should document any information that the patient volunteers, using exactly the same words the patient uses in quotes. This information may be used later in court as an "excited utterance," which is a spontaneous statement that concerns a shocking event while under stress caused by that event. For example, the patient makes a statement such as, "He threatened to kill me if I told anyone." This might influence the sentencing process after the perpetrator is apprehended and convicted.

When considering physical evidence, every effort must be made to preserve that which might link the perpetrator to the victim and the sexual assault. DNA evidence can be collected from blood, hair, saliva, semen, and skin. Therefore any areas on the patient that may have been exposed to any of the aforementioned body fluids or substances must be protected. For example, if the perpetrator kissed, licked, or bit any area of the patient, care should be taken not to disturb this area. If the patient is aware of having scratched the assailant, then the fingernails should be protected by either advising the patient not to scratch or do anything with her hands or by wrapping them in a paper bag or linen of some sort to preserve whatever evidence might be present. Do not use plastic (i.e. plastic gloves) because plastic may cause biological evidence to deteriorate [12].

Do not remove clothing or disturb bodily evidence unless necessary for medical assistance due to injuries [12]. Clothing and other items removed during examination should be placed in separate paper bags. The appearance of the clothing should be carefully documented (e.g. torn, stained). Bullet holes or other defects mechanically inflicted should be cut around and not through because these may be instrumental in determining the angle or distance from which a weapon was used [13].

Characteristics of wounds (e.g. location, type, size, color) should be documented as they appeared before any medical interventions. If a ruler or measuring tape is not available for precise measurement of any wounds, a well-known comparison should be used (e.g. size of a quarter, length of a dollar bill). Any foreign debris or objects embedded in the wound should be noted. Debris removed from a wound should be inserted into a paper bag or clean container. Tubes or drains should not be inserted into wounds. Therapeutic puncture sites should be indicated with circular markings so that these areas can be distinguished from injuries received during the assault.

Should the patient need to urinate, defecate (if she cannot wait), or vomit, this evidence should be preserved. Generally a sterile or clean container will suffice (e.g. urine specimen container). This is especially important if a DFSA is suspected. Any containers the patient believes may have been used in the drugging, such as a water bottle or coffee mug, should also be collected.

Food or drink should not be given to any patient who has been orally assaulted. Patients should avoid brushing teeth or gargling until evidence has been collected. Forensic evidence deteriorates quickly; the highest quality evidence is collected within 72 hours of the sexual assault [10]. If at all possible, it is important to get the patient to a sexual assault care center for evidence collection as soon as possible, should she decide to involve law enforcement. The EMT must be aware of legal obligations and requirements with respect to reporting to law enforcement. Some jurisdictions require EMTs responding to an injury sustained during a crime to report to police; others will let the patient decide the best action to take.

Chain of custody

Evidence collected from the patient becomes part of a chain of custody. This is the method of obtaining, transporting, and storing evidence that demonstrates proof that evidence collected at the crime scene or from the patient is the same as that being presented in court [13]. Paper bags, sterile containers, tamper-resistant tape, and chain of custody forms are rarely carried on ambulances. If these are not available, the EMT should devise a way to preserve evidence in which the item is sealed. The date and time the item was collected and removed, a description of the item, the location from where it was collected, and the EMT's initials should be documented on the item. Items collected should be placed in an area where their integrity can be maintained, allowing the EMT to testify that there has been no opportunity for tampering with the item. Once law enforcement is involved, the item(s) should be signed over to the police. This may include the ambulance stretcher sheet because there may have been a transfer of hair, debris, or other fibers from the patient/perpetrator. This sheet should be carefully folded on itself and provided to the police or ED.

Sexual assault nurse examiners/sexual assault response teams programs

Many states and provinces have sexual assault response teams (SART) or sexual assault care centers (SACC) that have specially trained sexual assault nurse examiners (SANE) available 24 hours a day. These nurses attend to the medicolegal needs of a sexual assault patient. They provide prophylactic treatment for sexually transmitted infections and pregnancy along with a thorough physical assessment and evidence collection. EMS physicians and EMTs should be aware of the treatment centers in their area.

Conclusion

The manner in which the EMS physician and EMT react to a disclosure of sexual assault will affect how the patient will view her situation, respond to treatment, and engage in the recovery process. The life of a person who is sexually assaulted is changed forever. A thoughtful and supportive response along with appropriate evidence preservation by the EMT can be the first step in a patient's journey to recovery and prosecution of the perpetrator. Local sexual assault crisis hotline numbers should be readily available and the patient encouraged to seek counseling or to speak to someone she feels would be supportive.

References

1 Sexual Assault: The Silent, Violent Epidemic. Available at: www.infoplease.com/ipa/A0001537.html

2 Basile KC, Saltzman LE. Sexual Violence Surveillance: Uniform Definitions and Recommended Data Elements Version 1.0. Atlanta, GA: Centers for Disease Control and Prevention, National Center for Injury Prevention and Control, 2002. Available at: www.cdc.gov/violenceprevention/pdf/sv_surveillance_definitionsl-2009-a.pdf

3 Tjaden P, Thoennes N. Extent, Nature and Consequences of Rape Victimization: Findings from the National Violence Against Women Survey. US Department of Justice Publication No. NCJ 210346, 2006. Available at: www.ncjrs.gov/pdffiles1/nij/210346.pdf

4 Black MC, Basile KC, Breiding MJ, et al. The National Intimate Partner and Sexual Violence Survey (NISVS): 2010 Summary Report. Atlanta, GA: National Center for Injury Prevention and Control, Centers for Disease Control and Prevention, 2011. Available at: www.cdc.gov/violenceprevention/pdf/nisvs_executive_summary-a.pdf

5 Brennan S, Taylor-Butts A. Sexual Assault in Canada 2004 and 2007. Ottawa: Canadian Centre for Justice Statistics Profile Series. Available at: www.statcan.gc.ca/pub/85f0033m/85f0033m2008019-eng.pdf

6 Statistics Canada. Impacts of Victimization. Ottawa: Statistic Canada. Available at: www.statcan.gc.ca/pub/85f0033m/2008019/findings-resultats/victim-eng.htm

7 Family Service of the Piedmont Inc. Sexual Assault. Available at: www.familyservice-piedmont.org/sexual-assault

8 LeBeau MA, Mozayani A (eds). *Drug-Facilitated Sexual Assault: A Forensic Handbook*. San Diego, CA: Academic Press, 2001.

9 Kinsey Confidential. Sexual Assault and Consent. Kinsey Institute. Available at: http://kinseyconfidential.org/resources/sexual-assault/

10 Girardin B, Faugno D, Seneski P, et al. *Color Atlas of Sexual Assault*. St Louis, MO: Mosby, 1997.

11 Srivastava R. *The Healthcare Provider's Guide to Clinical Cultural Competence*. Toronto: Elsevier, 2007.

12 Lynch VA. *Forensic Nursing*. St Louis, MO: Mosby, 2006, p.343.

13 Polsky SS, Markowitz J. *Color Atlas of Domestic Violence*. St Louis, MO: Mosby, 2004 p.76.

CHAPTER 62

Child maltreatment

Deborah Flowers and Molly Berkoff

Introduction

Child maltreatment is a serious public health problem. In 2011, an estimated 3.4 million referrals involving approximately 6.2 million children were made to Child Protective Service (CPS) agencies nationally [1]. An estimated 676,569 children were determined to be victims of abuse or neglect [1]. Of these, 78.5% experienced neglect, 17.6% were physically abused, 9.1% were sexually abused, and approximately 9% experienced emotional or psychological abuse [1]. An estimated 1,570 children died of abuse or neglect in 2011, with a rate of 2.10 per 100,000 in the total US population [1]. Although any child may fall victim to child abuse, the most vulnerable groups are infants, preverbal children, and children with chronic diseases and disabilities.

Role of the prehospital provider

Emergency medical services physicians and personnel play an important role in recognizing and reporting child maltreatment. They frequently have the opportunity to assess the scene and home environment as well as the interactions between the child and the caregiver(s). If there are any suspicions for maltreatment, it is vitally important that appropriate interventions are implemented to protect the child as mortality is known to be significantly higher in children who experience repeated episodes of non-accidental trauma [2]. Observations made by prehospital providers can be invaluable to physicians, nurses, other health care providers, child welfare workers, and law enforcement personnel who are charged with evaluating and investigating child maltreatment.

Child maltreatment

Child maltreatment involves acts of commission and omission that result in harm or threat of potential harm to a child [3]. Acts of commission involve physical, psychological, and sexual abuse. Acts of omission (neglect) may involve failure to provide adequate food, shelter, medical and dental care, and education [3]. A caregiver may also fail to provide adequate supervision or may expose a child to a dangerous or injurious environment, which may be considered neglect.

Assessment and general approach

Providing the appropriate level of medical care is the first priority when responding to any illness or injury. This priority does not change when responding to children who are victims of maltreatment. BLS and ALS measures should be implemented as indicated after provider safety is assured. Scene assessment and investigation, although very important in understanding mechanisms of injury and the relationship to real or potential maltreatment, should not impede the delivery of expedient and appropriate medical care. Pediatric ABCs and the primary survey are discussed elsewhere (see Chapters 54 and 55) and will not be specifically addressed in this chapter.

Secondary survey: signs and symptoms suggestive of abuse or neglect

The secondary survey should involve a careful examination of the child, especially the skin surfaces. The most common manifestations of child abuse are cutaneous injuries; therefore, a detailed physical examination is essential in identifying suspicious findings [4]. Bruising, burns, and bite marks are often observed in children who have sustained physical abuse. However, children may have no obvious cutaneous findings and still be victims of physical abuse. For example, the presence of bruising with inflicted rib and extremity fractures has been shown to be uncommon [5].

Bruising

The age and developmental level of the child should be considered when understanding mechanisms and resulting injuries. Bruising is rare in infants before they begin to walk or crawl. When bruising is identified in this age group and a credible

Emergency Medical Services: Clinical Practice and Systems Oversight, Second Edition. Volume 1: Clinical Aspects of EMS.
Edited by David C. Cone, Jane H. Brice, Theodore R. Delbridge, and J. Brent Myers.
© 2015 NAEMSP. Published 2015 by John Wiley & Sons, Inc. Companion Website: www.wiley.com\go\cone\naemsp

history is not obtained from the caregiver, abuse should be considered and the child should receive an appropriate medical evaluation.

For mobile children, accidental bruising is more common to certain areas of the body. Skin overlying bony prominences is more likely to bruise from accidental causes such as play activities or falls. Areas over the knees, anterior tibial area, forehead, hips, lower arms, and spine commonly demonstrate bruising from accidental causes. However, this does not guarantee that bruising over these areas cannot result from inflicted trauma.

Bruising over more protected areas such as the upper arms, medial and posterior thighs, hands, torso, cheeks, ears, neck, genitalia, and buttocks is more frequently associated with inflicted trauma. The observation of bruising over these areas should raise suspicions for maltreatment. However, bruising over these areas can also occur accidentally; therefore, obtaining a careful history regarding the injuries that may have led to the bruising becomes important in assessing whether or not the injuries are compatible with the caregiver's account and the child's developmental abilities.

Observations that increase concerns for inflicted trauma include multiple sites of bruising and bruising that demonstrates a pattern. Research has shown that dating of bruises (e.g. by the progression of colors) is unreliable [6]. A finding of multiple bruises over the body of a child should increase concerns for inflicted trauma.

Burns

Burns are common injuries in children and may occur from both accidental and inflicted causes. Abusive burns represent about 10% of pediatric burns [7]. Most common abusive burns will be scald burns such as immersion burns. Abusive burns may also occur from contact with hot thermal sources, chemicals, electricity, and even microwaves [8].

Obtaining information concerning the history of the burn, to include the mechanism and timing, is important in understanding if an abusive or neglectful injury may have occurred. The history should be correlated not only with the physical presentation of the injury but also with the developmental level of the child if the caregiver is reporting an action on the behalf of the child that led to the burn. Any mismatch with respect to the reported history, a changing history, mechanism, appearance and developmental level of the child should be documented. Delays in seeking care for burns may also represent abuse and neglect, and therefore documenting the reported timing of the burn is important.

Fractures

It is estimated that 11–55% of pediatric fractures are the result of physical abuse [9]. Younger children are particularly at risk for sustaining abusive fractures: 55–70% of all abusive fractures occur in infants less than 1 year of age [9]. With respect to orthopedic injuries, a careful history and secondary survey are

vital when assessing the young child. EMS providers do not have the advantage of radiography in determining if a child has a fracture. Some children may not exhibit signs such as guarding, deformity, swelling, or pain, thus creating difficulty in making safe and accurate assessments.

Transport decisions

Before determining that a child does not require EMS transport, careful consideration should be given to the age of the child, the ability to adequately determine if a fracture or other injury exists, and the history given by the caregivers. Any child with a suspicious or concerning history surrounding the injury should be transported to medical care.

Scene survey

Emergency medical services providers are in an excellent position to provide valuable information about the scene and circumstances of the call. In many instances, they will be able to observe and confirm or refute the details provided by the caregiver and communicate these to the medical providers. This type of information becomes very important when determining the credibility of the history and the injuries sustained by the child.

Obtaining the history

Obtaining a concise and detailed history will obviously depend on the acuity of the child's condition. The ability of the child to respond to questions is contingent on age and developmental level as well as the degree of injury. A verbal child may be able to answer simple questions such as "what happened?" but he or she may not be able to answer questions relating to how, where, or when. The following questions should be asked of the caregiver.

- How did the injury occur?
- Where did the injury occur?
- When did it happen?
- Who witnessed the event?
- What is the child's medical history?
- Who is the child's regular medical provider?

The provider should think about the responses to the questions in terms of a credible explanation for the observed injuries.

- Is the explanation credible? Does the injury pattern fit the manner in which the caretaker describes the incident?
- Does the scene assessment support the alleged mechanism of injury?
- Was there a long delay before seeking medical attention?
- If there are histories from more than one source, are they consistent?
- Was there adequate supervision of the child?
- Does the child have preexisting medical, psychological, or developmental problems?
- Does the child have a current health care provider? When was the last time the child saw a health care provider? Has this child been seen by EMS for a previous concern?

Communicating with the child and caregivers

Method and style of communication are very important when dealing with situations surrounding possible child maltreatment. Judgmental and accusatory questioning may only serve to threaten the caregiver and incite defensiveness or aggression. Maintaining objectivity is very important in managing interactions with the child and caregiver. The provider should avoid challenging the child or caregiver on the proposed history and mechanisms for observed injuries.

Documentation

Accurate, detailed, and concise documentation of the scene, a complete physical examination of the child, and history from the caregiver and child are vitally important. Responses and statements made by the child and the caregiver should be placed in quotes. Conflicting histories should be noted. The objective findings documented by the prehospital provider frequently become very important in the investigation of suspected child maltreatment. Concerns should be carefully communicated to the hospital personnel taking over care of the patient from the EMS providers.

Medical conditions that may be confused with child abuse

Numerous medical conditions may present with signs and symptoms that may be confused with child maltreatment. Some of these conditions may have already been identified in the child's history. For example, a child with a blood clotting disorder such as hemophilia is more prone to bruising; however, this should not be interpreted to mean that these children have not been abused.

Young children may have skin markings that have the appearance of purplish bruising but are congenital melanosis ("Mongolian spots"). These markings are usually found on the lower back and buttocks but can also be on other parts of the body. The caregivers are usually able to give a history of these markings as being present since birth.

Sexual abuse

Sexual abuse represents the third most common form of child maltreatment. Research and statistics describing EMS response to child sexual abuse calls are minimal; therefore, it is unknown how frequently these types of calls are encountered in the prehospital environment and under what conditions. Because it is rare for an acute case of child sexual abuse to present to medical care, it is reasonable to expect that EMS response will also be relatively rare. EMS providers may respond to a call only to find that there is no medical emergency. A caregiver may call EMS not knowing what other action to take or may simply have no transportation options to access medical care for the child. It is important to understand the dynamics of how child sexual abuse is often disclosed in order to respond appropriately.

Children frequently do not disclose abuse when it happens. It may be weeks, months, or even years before a child is able to disclose being sexually abused. Smith et al. found that almost half of all women they interviewed who had sustained rape as a child did not disclose the rape within 5 years of the assault and 28% had never disclosed to anyone until surveyed in their study [10]. Children who are verbal often do not disclose sexual abuse due to threats or other manipulation by the abuser, who is often a trusted relative or friend.

One of the more common concerns a caregiver may mention is that the child's genital area appears red or irritated. Other concerns may involve a caregiver or other family member observing suspicious contact or inappropriate touching of the child.

Once there is an EMS response to a child sexual abuse call, it becomes vital that the medical, psychosocial, and safety needs of the child and family are addressed. This is a very complex process and requires a multidisciplinary and specialized approach. It is impossible for the EMS responder to address the many issues surrounding this type of event. Some communities have established protocols to address this type of response. When there is no local medical protocol, the best course of action is to transport these children to medical care.

Acute medical and forensic interventions are seldom indicated due to the rarity of immediate disclosure or discovery of child sexual abuse. Locales and communities may also have differing time-frames for defining "acute" for the purposes of immediately evaluating child sexual abuse (72–96 hours is more common but some may consider acute up to120 hours). However, the presence of any of the following within the established acute time-frame warrants having the child medically evaluated:

- discovery or disclosure of suspected sexual abuse occurring within the specified acute time-frame
- anogenital pain, bleeding, discharge
- contact with the suspected perpetrator within the specified acute time-frame
- other extragenital findings concerning for trauma such as bruises, abrasions, etc.
- a distressed child and/or caregiver.

The greatest responsibilities for the EMS provider are identification of concerns, crisis intervention, and careful documentation. If at all possible, the history from the caregiver should not be taken in front of the child if the child is verbal and capable of understanding. If possible, it is preferable to talk with the child alone. Many issues concerning the credibility of the child's history and disclosure of sexual abuse will arise as the child moves through the medical, social, and legal systems. A limited interview of the child should be conducted to ascertain areas of discomfort or pain. Probing questioning of the disclosure and details surrounding the abuse are better left to professionals who are skilled in the area of child interviewing for the purposes of documenting and diagnosing sexual abuse.

If a child spontaneously begins to give the history, allow him or her to do so, and document the history as carefully as possible. Use quotes to differentiate the child's verbatim words from other documentation because the response and the record may become a vital document in legal proceedings.

With acute events, preservation of any evidence on the child's body should be attempted by carefully handling the child and any clothing the child is wearing. Articles such as diapers, clothing, and the child's bedding and blankets may yield the best source of recoverable evidence and should be protected and preserved. If law enforcement is at the scene, officers should take possession of these items. If law enforcement is not present then the EMS provider should place each item in a separate brown paper bag, labeling each bag with the patient's name, date, time of recovery, and provider's signature. The items may then be turned over to the appropriate medical or hospital staff on arrival to medical care. The EMS provider should document the evidence recovered and to whom it was turned over.

Responding to intimate partner violence calls

It is not unusual for EMS to respond to calls involving intimate partner violence (IPV) (see Chapter 60). Concerns for child maltreatment should always be considered when responding to calls where IPV is occurring and children are part of the family unit. Children who reside in homes in which IPV is present are at increased risk of being maltreated and neglected, as well as suffering significant emotional and psychological harm from witnessing the abuse [11]. Appropriate measures should be undertaken to address safety concerns for these children and should involve collaboration with law enforcement, child welfare services, and medical oversight.

Medicolegal duties

All states and territories in the United States require reporting suspicions of child abuse. Prehospital providers should have a good understanding of how legal requirements guide reporting in their respective states or jurisdictions. Accurate and detailed written documentation is vital in conveying important information to which the prehospital provider may be privileged based on his or her unique position in the continuum of care. A thorough summary of the assessment and suspicions should be relayed to receiving physicians, nurses, and social workers.

Conclusion

Emergency medical services providers are in an excellent position to provide valuable information in the recognition, documentation, and ultimate intervention in cases of child maltreatment, but it is likely that prehospital personnel need more training in recognizing and managing child maltreatment than is typically provided [12]. Field personnel frequently have the opportunity to observe the home and/or the scene and note consistencies or inconsistencies that accompany the history provided by caregivers. EMS providers often see or hear things at the scene or en route that are suspicious and need follow-up or further investigation. Accurate documentation of the history and observations made is vital in the comprehensive assessment of child maltreatment.

References

1 US Department of Health and Human Services, Administration for Children and Families, Administration on Children, Youth and Families, Children's Bureau. Child Maltreatment 2011. Available at: www.acf.hhs.gov/programs/cb/research-data-technology/statistics-research/child-maltreatment

2 Deans KJ, Thackeray J, Askegard-Giesmann JR, et al. Mortality increases with recurrent episodes of nonaccidental trauma in children. *J Trauma Acute Care Surg* 2013;75:161–5.

3 Child Maltreatment Prevention Scientific Information. Definitions. Available at: www.cdc.gov/violenceprevention/childmaltreatment/definitions.html

4 Kos L, Shwayder T. Cutaneous manifestations of child abuse. *Pediatr Dermatol* 2006;23:311–20.

5 Peters ML, Starling SP, Barnes-Eley ML, et al. The presence of bruising associated with fractures. *Arch Pediatr Adolesc Med* 2008;162:877-81.

6 Maguire S, Mann MK, Sibert J, et al. Can you age bruises accurately in children? A systematic review. *Arch Dis Child* 2005; 90:187–9.

7 American Humane Association, Brittain C. *Understanding the Medical Diagnosis of Child Maltreatment: A Guide for Nonmedical Professionals.* Oxford: Oxford University Press, 2005.

8 Alexander RC, Surrell JA, Hohle SD. Oven burns to children: an unusual manifestation of child abuse. *Pediatrics* 1987;79: 255–60.

9 Cooperman D, Merten D. Skeletal manifestations of child abuse. In: Reece RM, Ludwig S (eds) *Child Abuse: Medical Diagnosis and Management,* 2nd edn. Philadelphia: Lippincott Williams & Wilkins, 2001, pp.123–56.

10 Smith DW, Letourneau EJ, Saunders BE, et al. Delay in disclosure of childhood rape: results from a national survey. *Child Abuse Neglect* 2000;24:273–87.

11 Kelleher K, Gardner W, Coben J, et al. Co-occurring Intimate Partner Violence and Child Maltreatment: Local Policies/Practices and Relationships to Child Placement, Family Services and Residence. US Department of Justice. 2006. Available at: www.ncjrs.gov/pdffiles1/nij/grants/213503.pdf

12 Markenson D, Tunik M, Cooper A, et al. A national assessment of knowledge, attitudes, and confidence of prehospital providers in the assessment and management of child maltreatment. *Pediatrics* 2007;119:e103–e108.

CHAPTER 63

Ethical challenges

Dave W. Lu and James G. Adams

Introduction

Emergency medical services providers make ethical decisions on a daily basis [1]. They frequently deal with issues of patient refusal, confidentiality, the treatment of minors, and other challenging ethical dilemmas. The fast-paced prehospital work environment compounds the complexity because difficult decisions often need to be made without having all the necessary information and without sufficient time for extended consideration and debate. An understanding of the principles of medical ethics, however, can help guide EMS providers on the front lines when faced with ethical questions.

Emergency medical services medical directors, physicians, and personnel should be familiar with the prevailing statutes of their respective state and local governments because ethical debate may be moot if the law renders a ready decision. However, because individual cases vary widely, the law leaves many ethical questions unanswered. There are important differences between ethics and the law. The law attempts to ensure order by establishing rules that are derived from social values. The law, however, does not attempt to enforce every moral value. Following legal rules alone, therefore, may be ethically insufficient. For example, EMS providers not infrequently encounter patients who refuse care. Although the minimal legal standard requires a signature of release by the informed patient, the signature alone may be ethically insufficient. From an ethical and professional standpoint, it is important to explore the patient's understanding, concerns, and perhaps alternative options for treatment in order to ensure that the patient is appropriately cared for. It is important to remember that the law establishes rules and regulations based on societal values but it does not mandate the full display of the highest ethical behaviors.

This chapter will introduce core medical ethics principles and demonstrate how they can be applied to common ethical dilemmas encountered in the prehospital setting.

Refusal of treatment and transport

Case #1: EMS responds to a 45-year-old unhelmeted man who was struck by a car while riding his bicycle with his two young sons. The patient is found thrashing about on the ground, with signs of head trauma. When EMS providers attempt to transport the patient to the ambulance, the patient repeatedly refuses care, instead only asking about the whereabouts of his children, who are unharmed and remain at his side. The patient is clearly disoriented and unable to engage the paramedics in any sustained manner. One of the EMS providers asks if the patient can be treated and transferred against his will.

Case#2: EMS is dispatched to the home of a 90-year-old woman with known end-stage lung cancer who is complaining of shortness of breath. Upon their arrival, EMS intervention is refused by a cachectic but lucid patient who is very aware of her medical condition. She explains that she has been recently discharged from the hospital after extensive discussions with her oncologist regarding her preference to spend her remaining days at home. She understands that her progressive shortness of breath is a result of her end-stage lung cancer and that she will likely die from the disease in the near future. The patient's sons and daughters admit that they had initiated the 9-1-1 call because they felt their mother appeared extremely uncomfortable. The patient adamantly refuses any transfer to the hospital, while her family demands that EMS providers "do something" to help her.

Autonomy is a core principle of medical ethics [2]. Individuals are assumed to have the right to self-determination, even if their decisions result in harm to themselves. Patient refusal of care may apply to a specific course of treatment (e.g. insertion of a peripheral IV) or plan for further care (e.g. patient refusing transportation to the closest hospital in favor of a different facility). For EMS providers, patients have capacity to make their own medical decisions when the following criteria are fulfilled [3,4].

1 The patient must have sufficient information about his or her medical condition.
2 The patient must understand the risks and benefits of available options, including the option not to act.
3 The patient must have the ability to use the above information to make a decision in keeping with his or her personal values.

Emergency Medical Services: Clinical Practice and Systems Oversight, Second Edition. Volume 1: Clinical Aspects of EMS.
Edited by David C. Cone, Jane H. Brice, Theodore R. Delbridge, and J. Brent Myers.
© 2015 NAEMSP. Published 2015 by John Wiley & Sons, Inc. Companion Website: www.wiley.com\go\cone\naemsp

4 The patient must be able to communicate his or her choices.

5 The patient must have the freedom to act without undue influence from other parties, including family and friends.

If any of the above criteria are not met, EMS providers should balance their respect for the patient's limited decision-making capacity with their obligation to act in the patient's best interest. A great challenge for EMS providers is to expertly assess decision-making capacity in order to understand when a refusal is informed and when it is an impulsive gesture of a person who lacks capacity due to severe psychiatric disease, intoxication, or overwhelming medical illness [5]. For example, medical conditions such as hypoglycemia, head trauma, and sepsis can make patients impulsive, restless, angry, and antagonistic such that there may be confusion regarding their ability to reason. If EMS providers believe a patient lacks decision-making capacity (as opposed to competence, which is a legal determination), actions should be taken to ensure the patient's safety and best interest. In this regard, EMS personnel must operate under the rubric of beneficence, another core principle of medical ethics [2].

In situations of refusal of care, providing unwanted treatment over the objection of a patient with sufficient decision-making capacity may render the EMS provider guilty of battery [6]. Conversely, an impulsive or incompletely informed refusal leading to lack of treatment and transport leaves the provider liable for negligence. It is therefore strongly recommended that whenever EMS providers defer transport or treatment due to a patient's refusal of care, the patient's decision-making capacity should be explicitly documented in the medical record, with special attention to the information that was specifically communicated and understood by the patient. Similarly, when EMS providers act in the patient's best interest and treat or transport a patient who refuses care but who is deemed to have insufficient decision-making capacity, the conditions leading to this determination should be carefully documented. EMS providers must remember that it is not the responsibility of patients to prove they have decisional capacity; it is the responsibility of the provider to identify any impairment of such capacity.

The patient in case #1 clearly did not exhibit signs of decision-making capacity, likely secondary to the head trauma he sustained. EMS providers would be acting ethically to deny his refusal of care and instead act in his best interest by treating and transporting him to a hospital for definitive care.

The patient in case #2, though critically ill, still possessed full decision-making capacity when questioned by EMS personnel. She demonstrated that she sufficiently understood her medical condition, the risks and benefits of refusing further medical care, and how these decisions were in keeping with her personal values of wishing to die at home surrounded by her family and friends. For this patient, her decision to refuse further care is compatible with the EMS provider's ethical obligation to respect a patient's autonomy. Although the patient's family may disagree with the patient's decision, EMS responders would be acting ethically by respecting her wishes not to be transported to a hospital.

Triage decisions

Case #3: EMS providers are en route to a patient who called 9-1-1 after falling down on the wet floor of a supermarket when they witness a motor vehicle collision at an intersection they had just crossed. It is clear to the paramedics that the occupants of the vehicles suffered injuries, although the severity of the injuries was still undetermined. Calls are just coming in regarding the current accident. One of the EMS providers in the ambulance asks if they should stop to assist at the accident because the 9-1-1 call they are responding to did not appear too serious.

Emergency medical services systems are designed to encourage the best use of scarce and valuable resources in a given environment. They are operated by individuals with an organized and overarching view of the entire needs of a community at any given time. Paramedics dispatched to calls do not have the luxury of this knowledge and as such should not make triage and rationing decisions on an *ad hoc* basis. EMS providers should, however, report any unexpected events that they encounter and ask for appropriate instruction.

In case #3, the individual at the supermarket may have been much more seriously injured than the paramedics were led to believe. The ethically appropriate action would be for EMS personnel to ask if they should be reassigned to the motor vehicle accident, given their proximity to the incident, and await further instruction from dispatchers and supervisors, who likely have better information regarding other available resources. Of course, if EMS providers encounter a clear and immediate life threat outside their original assignment, it would be reasonable to render assistance. But other than in these extreme and rare circumstances, individual EMS personnel should refrain from varying from designated triage and response assignments.

Emergency medical services providers should also refrain from dissuading patients from seeking transport to a hospital for definitive care. Paramedics may encounter patients who they feel are not ill enough to warrant care in an emergency department. EMS personnel, however, should be strongly cautioned against such action, because they are not trained to render formal medical diagnoses and decide if someone needs a formal medical evaluation [7,8]. Comments to patients such as "he probably will be fine and can avoid waiting for hours in the emergency room" are unwise and outside the EMS scope of practice. EMS physicians, on the other hand, are in a better position to determine if no further care is needed than what is being provided at the scene. Depending on the nature of the EMS physician's role in the system, it may be reasonable for the physician to encourage non-transport in certain circumstances. This may be an expected role for the EMS physician in the case of a mass casualty event that involves fairly large numbers of uninjured or minimally injured patients. The physician may be able to assess and "clear" these patients at the scene, avoiding unnecessary transports that will burden both the EMS system and the receiving facilities.

Confidentiality

Case #4: Paramedics respond to a call from the home of a prominent local politician after he was found passed out in the bathroom by his wife. At the scene it becomes clear to the EMS providers that the individual is severely intoxicated. After transfer to a local hospital, EMS providers are asked to comment on the circumstances of the politician's hospital visit by reporters from the local media.

Health care providers, through the nature of their work, have unique access to the private lives of patients. In order to maintain an honest working patient–caregiver relationship, patient trust in his or her health care providers must not be breached. Although there may be exceptions to this rule (e.g. criminal investigations, patients who admit to suicidal or homicidal ideation, suspected child or elder abuse, and patients who pose a public health threat), health care providers should exercise caution in revealing information to those who do not share a therapeutic relationship with the patient.

When EMS providers are asked to comment on the medical care delivered to any patient, they should exercise caution in what they reveal to media sources. EMS providers may do well to defer all questions to a specially designated media spokesperson, such as the agency's public information officer, who is well versed in sophisticated media relations. Had the EMS providers in case #4 stated that the patient "will be fine in a few hours," speculation would arise as to the nature of the hospital visit. Even seemingly benign comments about a patient's medical condition can be misconstrued. Likewise, health care providers should exercise restraint when asked by curious family members, friends, or colleagues about a prominent figure's medical condition. Not only would revealing such information represent a breach of patient confidentiality and trust, but strict and enforceable rules exist to discourage curious onlookers without a direct therapeutic relationship from accessing private patient information.

Truth telling and error disclosure

Case #5: EMS providers are called to a restaurant where a 55-year-old man with multiple food allergies complains of hives and itching. Intending to administer diphenhydramine, the EMS provider mistakenly administers 1 mg of 1:1,000 epinephrine IV, resulting in the patient's hospital admission for monitoring of multiple non-sustained runs of ventricular tachycardia. The patient is ultimately discharged without incident. The EMS provider asks the medical director if the error should be disclosed to the patient.

Truth telling is important under all circumstances, but more so when upsetting news and information regarding medical errors are disclosed. Many professional societies, patient safety experts, and standard practice guidelines recommend disclosure [9]. There are many reasons favoring the disclosure of harmful errors to patients. Disclosure supports truth telling, patient autonomy, and informed decision making, and is consistent with patients' preferences [10]. Patients want to know about errors even when the harm is minor, and expect a full explanation and an apology

[10]. Patients also seek acknowledgment of the pain and suffering that was caused by the error, along with reassurance that recurrences will be prevented. In addition, disclosing errors promotes patient safety, as it enables the critical appraisal of the conditions leading to errors and the development of interventions to prevent recurrences.

When errors are disclosed, the patient and family must sense honesty in the communication. Patients can often tolerate mistakes, but they will not tolerate providers who do not care. Information regarding errors must be explained to the patient in the proper context, even though the provider's natural instinct may be to cover up mistakes. This is a precarious maneuver both professionally and legally, especially if the patient or family later discovers the error. Many patients who file medical malpractice claims do so because they believe that disclosure was absent or inadequate and see legal action as their only option for finding out what happened [11].

Historically, providers were advised not to disclose errors to patients out of fear that offering an apology or an admission of fault would precipitate malpractice suits. Recent research suggests this assumption may be unfounded [12]. Health care organizations that have adopted robust disclosure programs are reporting favorable outcomes in the number of claims filed, litigation costs, and time to resolution [12]. In addition, 35 states and the District of Columbia have adopted laws making medical apology inadmissible as a statement of fault, with some states even requiring the disclosure of serious unanticipated outcomes to patients [13]. These developments have led many risk managers and malpractice insurers to strongly advocate for disclosure.

When disclosing a harmful medical error to a patient and his or her family, the provider should focus the conversation around the needs of the patient [9,10]. The provider needs to present information in a fashion that the patient and family can comprehend. Patients should be told the facts surrounding the event, what steps have been taken to address any medical repercussions, and plans to prevent recurrences. Finally, the provider should apologize and express regret for the error. It takes expertise to know how to disclose errors and communicate them properly, and in case #5, EMS providers should work closely with their EMS system leadership in handling these sensitive issues.

Personal risk

Case #6: EMS responds to a call from a local bar where a man was reportedly assaulted during a brawl. On arrival, paramedics observe multiple intoxicated bystanders shouting angrily at each other, some of whom are wielding empty glass bottles. One such bystander calls to EMS providers to help the injured patient inside the bar. Police have not yet arrived on scene.

Emergency medical services providers frequently encounter situations where the risk of physical harm is present. Although it is impossible to eliminate all potential dangers in the daily work of EMS personnel, reasonable caution can and should be exercised such that risks are minimized. Although the paramedics in case #6 may feel the need to attend to the injured individual, there is no moral requirement for health care providers to submit themselves to significant self-endangerment. The EMS responder should exercise proper judgment in determining what is reasonable and what is foolhardy. When possible, law enforcement officers should become involved to ensure a safe and secure scene. EMS providers have an ethical obligation to not place either themselves or others at undue additional harm.

Training and research

Case #7: EMS providers respond to a call from a nursing home and find a 75-year-old man who has been asystolic for an unknown period of time. EMS providers pronounce death at the scene after the patient begins showing early signs of rigor mortis and dependent lividity. En route to the hospital morgue, one of the paramedics asks if he can intubate the deceased patient using new equipment as part of a study on prehospital intubations conducted by a local academic medical center.

Continued education for health care providers is essential for quality patient care. Standards of training should be followed to ensure proper use of time and resources. In the case of practicing procedures on the recently deceased, out of respect for patient autonomy and dignity even when the individual is no longer living, consent from appropriate family members or a designated proxy should be obtained [14,15]. EMS providers operate with a significant level of trust from the public and all efforts should be undertaken to not compromise that confidence.

Similarly, caution should be exercised when performing research on patients who cannot give informed consent. In the prehospital and emergency setting, it is difficult, if not impossible, to obtain prospective informed consent from patients in order to enroll them in research trials [16,17]. In recognition of the need for this type of research to take place while concurrently preserving patient autonomy, the Food and Drug Administration (FDA) in conjunction with the Department of Health and Human Services (DHHS) have established clear rules for how such research should be conducted [18]. Among the many requirements for an exception from informed consent for research, the most prominent stipulation mandates that study investigators consult with the community in which the research will be conducted and that there will be close oversight of the clinical investigation by a data monitoring committee as well as an institutional review board [19]. Moreover, study investigators should obtain informed consent from the patient or his or her next of kin whenever and as early as possible. These FDA/DHHS regulations are particularly stringent because when research can only be conducted without the informed consent of subjects, every effort must be made to ensure patient autonomy is protected (see Volume 2, Chapter 45 for additional details).

In case #7, without having obtained prior consent from the patient's next of kin, it would be ethically inappropriate for the paramedic to practice intubating the deceased patient using the experimental equipment. In addition, had the patient even qualified for the research study, EMS personnel should ensure all procedures and protocols are closely followed in order to protect the patient's best interests.

Treatment of minors

Case #8: EMS providers are asked to respond to a call from a 15-year-old girl complaining of painful vaginal bleeding. Upon arrival to the house, the patient reports that her parents are both still at work and that they do not know about her approximately 3-month pregnancy. The paramedics discover a large amount of what appears to be active bleeding and the tearful patient is notably pale and diaphoretic. One of the EMS providers asks if they can treat and transport the patient to a hospital without first informing her parents.

Minors, defined as persons under the age of 18, are legally incapable of giving consent. Instead, they rely on a parent or guardian for informed consent. The few exceptions to this rule apply to a special population of emancipated minors, which is a state-specific definition that usually includes those who are married or by legal decree separated from their parents; those who are pregnant or have had a child; and those who have served in the armed forces [20]. Depending on state laws, EMS personnel can also treat non-emancipated minors without parental consent in special circumstances, such as when a minor seeks care for mental illness, substance abuse, pregnancy, or sexually transmitted diseases [21]. In these potentially stigma-laden situations, the risks in overriding parental consent are outweighed by concerns of individual privacy and benefits to public health. Each state operates under different policies and EMS personnel should be familiar with their local jurisdiction's conditions in which non-emancipated minors can seek care without parental consent.

In contrast to the emancipated minor, a special category of minor who may be able to offer limited consent for his or her own care is the mature minor. The mature minor (usually 14 years and older) is emotionally and intellectually sophisticated enough to be able to appreciate the nature of the illness along with the risks and benefits of the proposed treatment [20]. A mature minor's preferences should be taken into account when making treatment decisions [21]. In some cases, a minor originally and incorrectly determined to be emancipated may meet standards for mature minor status. Because the mature minor may not be able to provide complete consent, including both the parents and mature minor in medical decisions is optimal.

Many times EMS providers may be asked to care for minors who injure themselves either without the physical presence of a parent or when the guardian for one reason or another is incapable of consenting for the child. In these cases, an "emergency exception" is invoked such that health care providers are able to treat minors in a timely manner to prevent morbidity and mortality under the rubric of implied consent [21]. Because definitions of conditions that deserve an emergency exception vary from case to case, when in doubt, it is usually preferable for EMS providers to treat and transfer the minor to a hospital when no parent is present. When possible, it is preferable to postpone major medical interventions until the minor's parents can be involved.

In case #8, EMS providers can ethically treat and transport the patient without prior parental consent. Not only is the patient critically ill and therefore appropriate for treatment under the emergency exception, but by virtue of her pregnancy the patient can be evaluated as an emancipated minor and seek care without parental consent.

When the parent is present and disagrees with the medical decisions of EMS providers, the providers should remember to act first under the principle of the patient's best interest. If paramedics believe the minor is placed in significant and immediate risk by the parent's medical decisions, they can treat and transport the patient under a temporary protective custody. Protective custody of a minor should be taken only as a last resort and always in close consultation with the direct medical oversight physician and law enforcement personnel. If temporary protective custody of the patient is truly necessary, EMS personnel should remember that the parents do not subsequently lose all decision-making rights on behalf of their child. Paramedics should still involve and seek the consent of the parents in the remainder of the care of the patient as much as possible.

When EMS providers and parents are in agreement over the medical care of the minor, providers should still inform the patient of the medical decision process as much as possible. Even young children can understand the basics of medical care and all efforts should be made to involve them on an age-appropriate level.

Conclusion

The cases provided in this chapter illustrate the wide variety of ethical issues that EMS providers encounter on a regular basis. EMS providers should become proficient with the basic principles of medical ethics. In addition, the exercise of ethical judgment should always be performed in conjunction with knowledge of local laws and professional guidelines. Finally, EMS providers must remember to practice excellent communication skills when dealing with potentially complicated issues of patient care.

References

1 Becker TK, Gausche-Hill M, Aswegan AL, et al. Ethical Challenges in emergency medical services: controversies and recommendations. *Prehosp Disaster Med* 2013;28:488–97.

2 Beauchamp TL, Childress JF (eds). *Principles of Biomedical Ethics*, 7th edn. New York: Oxford University Press, 2012.

3 Magauran BG Jr. Risk management for the emergency physician: competency and decision-making capacity, informed consent, and refusal of care against medical advice. *Emerg Med Clin North Am* 2009;27:605–14.

4 Buchanan A. Mental capacity, legal competence and consent to treatment. *J R Soc Med* 2004;97:415–20.

5 Chow GV, Czarny MJ, Hughes MT, Carrese JA. CURVES: a mnemonic for determining medical decision-making capacity and providing emergency treatment in the acute setting. *Chest* 2010;137: 421–7.

6 Woolley S. Jehovah's Witnesses in the emergency department: what are their rights? *Emerg Med J* 2005;22:869–71.

7 Hauswald M. Can paramedics safely decide which patients do not need ambulance transport or emergency department care? *Prehosp Emerg Care* 2002;6:383–6.

8 Silvestri S, Rothrock SG, Kennedy D, et al. Can paramedics accurately identify patients who do not require emergency department care? *Prehosp Emerg Care* 2002;6:387–90.

9 Lu DW, Guenther E, Wesley AK, et al. Disclosure of harmful medical errors in out-of-hospital care. *Ann Emerg Med* 2013;61:215–21.

10 Gallagher TH, Waterman AD, Ebers AG, et al. Patients' and physicians' attitudes regarding the disclosure of medical errors. *JAMA* 2003;289:1001–7.

11 Mazor KM, Reed GW, Yood RA, et al. Disclosure of medical errors: what factors influence how patients respond? *J Gen Intern Med* 2006;21:704–10.

12 Mello MM, Gallagher TH. Malpractice reform – opportunities for leadership by health care institutions and liability insurers. *N Engl J Med* 2010;362:1353–6.

13 Mastroianni AC, Mello MM, Sommer S, et al. The flaws in state 'apology' and 'disclosure' laws dilute their intended impact on malpractice suits. *Health Aff (Millwood)* 2010;29:1611–19.

14 Schmidt TA, Abbott JT, Geiderman JM, et al. Ethics seminars: the ethical debate on practicing procedures on the newly dead. *Acad Emerg Med* 2004;11:962–6.

15 Sperling D. Breaking through the silence: illegality of performing resuscitation procedures on the "newly-dead". *Ann Health Law* 2004;13:393–426.

16 Jansen TC, Kompanje EJ, Bakker J. Deferred proxy consent in emergency critical care research: ethically valid and practically feasible. *Crit Care Med* 2009;37:S65–8.

17 Schmidt TA, Nelson M, Daya M, et al. Emergency medical service providers' attitudes and experiences regarding enrolling patients in clinical research trials. *Prehosp Emerg Care* 2009;13:160–8.

18 Nichol G, Powell J, van Ottingham L, et al. Consent in resuscitation trials: benefit or harm for patients and society? *Resuscitation* 2006; 70:360–8.

19 Mosesso VN Jr, Brown LH, Greene HL, et al. Conducting research using the emergency exception from informed consent: the Public Access Defibrillation (PAD) Trial experience. *Resuscitation* 2004; 61:29–36.

20 Baren JM. Ethical dilemmas in the care of minors in the emergency department. *Emerg Med Clin North Am* 2006;24:619–31.

21 Committee on Pediatric Emergency Medicine and Committee on Bioethics. Consent for emergency medical services for children and adolescents. *Pediatrics* 2011;128:427–33.

CHAPTER 64
End-of-life issues

Aaron Case, Dana Zive, Jennifer Cook, and Terri A. Schmidt

Memento Mori – Remember Death!*[1]

Introduction

The EMS system was designed to respond to emergencies to prevent disability and untimely death. With the aging of the population, EMS resources are now frequently called for patients with serious, life-threatening illness and for patients at or near the end of life. Many patients may not want the potentially life-extending interventions that are directed by standard EMS protocols [2]. A Canadian study found that nearly 10% of cardiac arrest calls were for patients with a terminal illness. In 63% of these cases, there was either a verbal (by family) or written request for no resuscitation [3]. Similarly, a Washington state study found that families of dying, terminally ill patients often called EMS because "they didn't know what else to do." Fewer than 10% of those patients had state-recognized formal written requests to withhold resuscitation, but a protocol allowing verbal and informally written requests to withhold resuscitation resulted in a significant decrease in unwanted interventions [4]. In addition, the American Heart Association reports that roughly 360,000 out-of-hospital cardiac arrests (OHCA) occur annually, with 60% treated by EMS professionals.

The chance of survival from OHCA is generally poor [5]. Survival rates vary based on the presenting rhythm, with survival from ventricular fibrillation ranging from 11% to 25%,[6,7] and overall survival to hospital discharge for all presenting rhythms being much smaller, and in some systems approaching zero [8]. There is also evidence that patients who do not have return of spontaneous circulation in the field have a very low likelihood (0.4%) of survival to hospital discharge [9]. Thus, EMS professionals need to determine whether the OHCA patient desires resuscitation, and to compassionately interact with family in the aftermath of a death in the field.

The EMS physician must design protocols to determine which patients should have attempts at cardiopulmonary resuscitation (CPR), or other life-sustaining interventions, and those who should not. (See Figure 64.1 for an example of one such protocol.) Considering the goals and ethical principles of medicine while remaining consistent with applicable local laws and regulations, these protocols should take into consideration patient preferences as well as the likelihood that the interventions will benefit the patient. It is not reasonable to assume that every patient found in cardiac arrest should undergo attempts at resuscitation, nor that everyone for whom resuscitation was attempted should be transported to the hospital.

The basic ethical principles on which modern medicine is founded include respect for patient autonomy, beneficence, non-maleficence, and justice [10]. Decisions about resuscitation are generally based either on the principle of respect for autonomy or on beneficence. Respect for patient autonomy requires honoring patient preferences for or against treatments, including advanced airway support, CPR, and transport to the hospital when those preferences are known. Based on both beneficence and non-maleficence, an intervention should not be performed if there is no chance that it will benefit the patient.

The American College of Emergency Physicians' position statement stipulates, "All emergency medical services (EMS) systems should have a policy addressing their response to 'Do Not Attempt Resuscitation' (DNAR) orders and other advance directives ..." and "If the patient's preferences regarding resuscitation are clear, they should be respected. Patient preferences to refuse resuscitative efforts can be communicated directly by the patient, or by an advance directive, a valid DNAR order, or by the patient's legal representative. Unofficial documentation may be considered when determining patient preferences" [11].

The number of states authorizing out-of-hospital DNAR orders increased from 11 in 1992 [12] to 42 in 1999 [13]. As of 2002, most United States EMS systems did not have palliative care protocols [14]. In the last few years states have been implementing Physician Orders for Life-Sustaining Treatment (POLST) programs to document and honor patient preferences

---

* In the 4th century AD, a group of monks lived as hermits in the deserts of Egypt, Palestine, Arabia, and Persia. These monks used *memento mori* as a common greeting.

Emergency Medical Services: Clinical Practice and Systems Oversight, Second Edition. Volume 1: Clinical Aspects of EMS.
Edited by David C. Cone, Jane H. Brice, Theodore R. Delbridge, and J. Brent Myers.
© 2015 NAEMSP. Published 2015 by John Wiley & Sons, Inc. Companion Website: www.wiley.com\go\cone\naemsp

Clackamas and Washington County, Oregon Death & Dying Protocol

A. DEATH IN THE FIELD

Purpose: To define under what conditions treatment can be withheld or stopped.

Resuscitation efforts may be withheld if:

1. The patient has a "DNR" order.
2. The patient is pulseless and apneic in a mass casualty incident or multiple patient scene where the resources of the system are required for the stabilization of living patients.
3. The patient is decapitated.
4. The patient has rigor mortis in a warm environment.
5. The patient is in the stages of decomposition.
6. The patient has skin discoloration in dependent body parts (dependent lividity).

Traumatic Cardiac Arrest:

1. A victim of trauma (blunt or penetrating) who has no vital signs in the field may be declared dead on scene. If opening the airway does nor restore vital signs/signs of life, the patient should NOT be transported unless there are extenuating circumstances.

2. A cardiac monitor may be beneficial in determining death in the field when you suspect a medical cause or hypovolemia: A narrow complex rhythm (QRS < .12) may suggest profound hypovolemia, and may respond to fluid resuscitation.

3. At a trauma scene, the paramedic should consider the circumstances surrounding the incident, including the possibility that a medical event (cardiac arrhythmia, seizure, and hypoglycemia) preceded the accident. When a medical event is suspected, treat as a medical cardiac event. VF should raise your index of suspicion for a medical event.

4. In instances prior to transport where the patient deteriorates to the point that no vital signs (i.e. pulse/respiration) are present, a cardiac monitor should be applied to determine if the patient has a viable cardiac rhythm. A viable rhythm especially in patients with penetrating trauma may reflect hypovolemia or obstructive shock (tamponade, tension pneumothorax) and aggressive care should be continued.

Medical Cardiac Arrest:

1. If the patient's EKG shows asystole or agonal rhythm upon initial monitoring, and after at least two lead changes, the patient, in the paramedic's best judgment, would not benefit from resuscitation:

   a. The PIC should determine DIF and notify the Medical Examiner or Law Enforcement;

   OR

   b. Begin BLS procedures, and contact OLMC with available patient history, current condition, and with a request to discontinue resuscitation.

2. If after the airway is established and the asystole protocol has been exhausted the patient persists in asystole, (confirm in 3 leads) consider termination of efforts. The PIC may declare the patient to be dead in the field.

3. The patient who has PEA and has not responded to the initial cycle of ACLS may be determined to be dead at the scene after appropriate consultation with OLMC.

4. All patients in VF should be treated and transported.

Notes & Precautions:

1. ORS allows a layperson, EMT or Paramedic to determine "Death in the Field"
2. The EMS provider is encouraged to consult OLMC if any doubt exists about the resuscitation potential of the patient.
3. A person who was pulseless or apneic and has received CPR and has been resuscitated, is not precluded from later being a candidate for solid organ donation.
4. $ETCO_2$ may be a useful adjunct in the decision to terminate resuscitation with PEA. An $ETCO_2$ of 10 or less in patients in PEA after 20 minutes of ACLS resuscitation does not correlate with survival.
5. Survival from trauma arrest is low, but not completely zero.

B. POLST ORDERS AND DECISION MAKING

1. In the pulseless and apneic patient who <u>does not meet</u> DEATH IN THE FIELD criteria, but is suspected to be a candidate for withholding resuscitation, begin CPR and contact OLMC.
2. A patient with decision-making capacity or the legally authorized representative has the right to direct his or her own medical care and can change or rescind previous directives.

Figure 64.1 Example EMS palliative and end-of-life protocol. Source: Selected portions of Metro Regional EMS Consortium Patient Treatmen Protocols 2014. Reproduced with permission of Clackamas County Emergency Medical Services.

3. EMS providers may honor a Do Not Resuscitate (DNR) order signed by a physician, nurse practitioner or physician assistant. DNR orders apply only to the patient in cardiopulmonary arrest and do not indicate the types of treatment that a person not in arrest should receive. POLST was developed to convey orders in other circumstances.

4. Physician Orders for Life-Sustaining Treatment (POLST):

    The POLST was developed to document and communicate patient treatment preferences across treatment settings. While these forms are most often used to limit care, they may also indicate that the patient wants everything medically appropriate done. **Read the form carefully!** When signed by a physician (MD or DO), nurse practitioner, or physician assistant, POLST is a medical order and EMS providersare directed to honor it in their Scope of Practice unless they have reason to doubt the validity of the orders or the patient with decision making capacity requests change. If there are questions regarding the validity or enforceability of the health care instruction, begin BLS treatment and contact OLMC [OAR 847-035-030 (7)] If the POLST is not immediately available, a POLST form as documented in the Electronic POLST registry hosted at MRH (503-494-7333) may also be honored.

    - Section A: Applies only when patient is in cardiopulmonary arrest
    - Section B: Applies in all other circumstances
    - For a POLST form to be valid it must include:

        i. Patient's name
        ii. Date signed (forms do not expire)
        iii. Health care professional's signature (patient signature is optional)

5. The legally authorized representative may make decisions for the patient who is unable to make medical decisions. However, when in doubt or for unresolved conflict on the scene contact OLMC. The order is:
    a. A legal guardian
    b. A power of attorney for health care as designated by the patient on the Oregon advance directive
    c. Spouse or legal domestic partner
    d. Adult children
    e. Parent

6. Death with Dignity Act:

    If a person who is terminally ill and appears to have ingested medication under the provisions of the Oregon Death with Dignity Act, the EMS provider should:

    a. Provide comfort care as indicated.
    b. Determine who called 9-1-1 and why (i.e. to control symptoms or because the person no longer wishes to end their life with medications).
    c. Establish the presence of DNAR orders and/or documentation that this was an action under the provisions of the Death with Dignity Act.
    d. Contact OLMC.
    e. Withhold resuscitation if:DNAR orders are present, and there is evidence that this is within the provisions of the Death with Dignity Act and OLMC agrees.

C. PATIENTS ENROLLED IN HOSPICE AND DYING PATIENTS

1. Look for POLST forms (contact Registry if needed) and attempt to honor patient preferences. Always provide comfort measures.

2. If patient is enrolled in hospice and the patient has not already done so, contact hospice if possible.

3. EMS providers cannot take medical orders from a hospice nurse but their advice is often invaluable and may be followed with direction from OLMC.

4. Treat dying persons with warmthand understanding. Do not avoid them. Allow them to discuss their situation, but do not push them to talk.

5. Many dying people are not upset by discussions of death as long as you do not take away all of their hope.

6. Touching a dying person is important. Use words like "death". Do not use meaningless synonyms.

7. Ask the person how you might help.

8. Give factual information.

9. Be aware of your own fears regarding death and admit when a dying person reminds you of a loved one. If a particular person is too disturbing, have your partner or other members of the responding team take over.

Figure 64.1 *Continued*

D. CARE OF GRIEVING PERSONS

Resuscitation phase:
1. As time allows give accurate and truthful updates about the patient's prognosis. If available, assign one person to interact with and support family members.
2. Consider gently remove children from the resuscitation area.
3. Depending upon the emotional state of family members, consider allowing them to watch and/or participate in a limited and appropriate way.
4. If family or friends were doing CPR prior to your arrival, commend their efforts.
5. If family or friends are disruptive consider removing them or try assigning simple tasks, such as helping bring in the stretcher, holding doors open, telling other family about the event and calling the doctor or minister.
6. Be respectful. Make requests. Don't give orders.

Once death is determined:
1. Treat the recently dead with respect.
2. Tell family and friends of the death honestly. Use the words "death" or "dead". Avoid using euphemisms such as "passed away" or "gone".
3. Avoid using past tense terms when speaking to survivors of the recently dead.
4. Allow family and friends to express their emotions. Listen to them if they want to talk but don't push them.
5. Give factual information.
6. Genuine warmth and compassion will be more helpful than almost anything else for survivors. Don't feel it necessary to say the "right" things. Listening often provides grieving people with the most comfort.

Focusing on survivors:
1. See to it that survivors have a support system present before you leave. Consider calling TIP through EMS Dispatch, if available in your jurisdiction. Call friends, family, clergy, or neighbors to be with them. Respect the survivor's wishes to be alone.
2. Explain the next steps to them after you have pronounced death. This will include the police coming to make reports, possibly the medical examiner, and the possible need for an autopsy in certain instance.
3. Contact the Medical Examiner's office before moving or altering the body (as soon as possible).
4. Allow family and friends to say their good-byes if possible.
5. A chaplain may be helpful in assisting with survivors. It is advisable to call early, as the chaplains do not have code-3 capabilities.
6. Help survivors make decisions such as which people should be called. If they ask you to make calls, try to comply, mention the need to find a funeral home, if one has not already been chosen. Clergy may also be helpful with this decision.

E. DEATH OF A CHILD:

1. Do not accuse the parents of abuse or neglect, but take careful note of the patient's surroundings and the general physical condition of the child.
2. Do not be overly silent, which may imply guilt to the parents.
3. Ask the parents only necessary questions and do not judge or evaluate them. Do not tell them what they "should have" been doing before your arrival.
4. Remind parents to arrange for child care of other children.
5. Listen carefully to their statements and answer only with accurate information.
6. If there is a police investigation, tell the parents that this is routine.
7. Successful management of child deaths requires supportive, compassionate and tactful measures.

Figure 64.1 *Continued*

regarding both resuscitation and other life-sustaining treatments [15]. EMS agencies in King County, Washington, have developed protocols that allow EMS professionals to withhold resuscitation if the patient has a preexisting terminal condition and the patient, family, or caregivers indicates, in writing or verbally, that the patient did not want resuscitation [4]. This protocol allows EMS professionals to withhold resuscitation based on verbal information without physician consult. The authors interviewed involved EMS professionals and found that most report the decision to withhold to be easy, and that they do not receive objections or complaints about that decision.

Advance directives

An advance directive is a written document, completed by the patient when he or she has decision-making capacity, expressing future wishes and/or appointing a surrogate decision maker. (See Figure 64.2 to compare documents indicating patient preferences). Advance directives have not been as effective as people had hoped [16]. The two main types of advance directives are living wills and durable powers of attorney for health care. Since 1991, the Patient Self-Determination Act has required all hospitals that accept Medicare and Medicaid funds to provide

Document	Advance Directive	Do Not Attempt Resuscitation (DNR/DNAR) orders	POLST (Physician Order for Life Sustaining Treatment)
Who completes	Patient	Health professional*	Health professional*
Who needs one	All adults	Person with advanced illness	Person with advanced illness
When they apply	Future time	Pulseless and apneic person	Current time
Guide EMS	Usually not	Yes	Yes
Guide hospital	Yes	Yes	Yes

*After discussion with patient and/or surrogate decision maker and based on the patient's goals and values

Figure 64.2 Comparison of advance directives, DNR/DNAR orders, and POLST. *After discussion with patient and/or surrogate decision maker and based on the patient's goals and values.

information about and develop policies for implementation of advance directives. Although there has been an increase in advance care planning since then, in many cases advance directives are still lacking when patients are transferred to emergency departments (EDs) [17–20]. One study found that many ED patients have never thought about advance directives or prefer that families make the decisions at the time of an event [21].

An expert panel has recommended that, "in the absence of signs of irreversible death, patient preferences regarding resuscitation should be the most important consideration of EMS personnel" [22]. EMS personnel need to make rapid decisions about attempting resuscitation for patients who are *in extremis*. Often the patients are unable to verbalize preferences about treatment and EMS professionals must make these time-critical decisions based on written instructions, when available. Unfortunately, written instructions are not always completed, or are unclear, which may be why systems such as King County now allow verbal statements.

One type of advance directive, the living will, expresses the wishes of patients regarding life-sustaining procedures in the event of conditions such as permanent coma or terminal illness. Living wills are theoretical documents that may state, for example, that the person would not want resuscitation if he or she is terminally ill, death is imminent, and resuscitation would only prolong the dying process. Because of these restrictive phrases, living wills are often difficult for EMS professionals to apply to decisions about specific life support measures [23,24] and in many cases health care providers do not follow them [25]. In at least one state, these documents explicitly do not apply except in a hospital or clinic setting [26], and one author has suggested that they may be misinterpreted as applying when they do not [27]. Living wills are not precise enough to predict all scenarios and consequently cannot outline appropriate guidance for all potential care situations [28,29].

Another form of patient-completed advance directive is the durable power of attorney for health care, which gives another person the authority to make decisions if the patient is unable to make decisions either temporarily or permanently. The person designated in the power of attorney becomes a legally recognized proxy decision maker. When a durable power of attorney exists, EMS protocols may allow the designated person to make decisions regarding the patient's medical care. Immunity is generally granted to providers who carry out the proxy's decision in good faith, but it is always wise to know local laws. Some states allow surrogates without a specific health care power of attorney to make decisions about resuscitation and end-of-life care for incapacitated patients, and others do not. Appointing surrogates who are aware of the patient's preferences can be effective, as long as the surrogate and the documentation confirming their status can be found at the time of an emergency.

Do Not Resuscitate orders

Unlike living wills and health care powers of attorney, DNAR orders are written by health care professionals to indicate that resuscitation should not be attempted in the patient who is pulseless and apneic. A national survey of EMTs found that 89% of respondents were willing to honor a state-approved DNAR order and that 77% of those surveyed had local protocols for termination of resuscitation in the out-of-hospital setting [30]. Although DNAR orders only apply when the patient is pulseless and apneic, many primary care providers, who complete the orders for their patients, believe that they apply in other circumstances and that intubation and cardioversion are not appropriate in a patient with DNAR orders [31].

There is variability in honoring DNAR orders. One EMS study found that even with DNAR orders present, resuscitation was attempted 21% of the time [32]. Some states have had success with their DNAR programs [33] but problems remain. For example, some states use a DNAR bracelet program requiring EMS professionals to honor these DNAR orders and providing immunity from liability for honoring the order [34]. However, one study suggests that bracelet DNAR programs are used infrequently [24].

In addition, advance directives and DNAR orders may not be available when EMS arrive and often do not accompany patients to the ED [18,35,36]. On the other hand, there are EMS systems that allow responders to accept verbal requests from family to withhold resuscitation.

Out-of-hospital DNAR programs typically provide only orders about resuscitation with no guidance for patients who are breathing and have a pulse. It is often hard for out-of-hospital providers to know what interventions are appropriate for the seriously ill patient who is not in cardiopulmonary arrest but cannot speak for himself or herself and does not have a surrogate present. A recent study found that half of patients with DNAR orders wanted comfort measures only, but half wanted higher levels of care [37].

The Physician Orders for Life-Sustaining Treatment program

In 1991, a group of Oregon health care professionals and organizations, including EMS and long-term care providers, began development of the Physician Orders for Life-Sustaining Treatment (POLST) program (states use various names including POLST, POST, MOLST, LaPOLST). The goal of this program is to honor patient end-of-life care preferences by turning those preferences into medical orders that can be implemented as patients transition between multiple care settings, such as from home or long-term care to the ED [27,36,38–42]. POLST is intended for patients with serious illness or frailty. The POLST form (see Figure 64.3 for an example) is a brightly colored set of medical orders designed to be placed in a prominent location. It provides clear guidance for resuscitation as well as a range of medical interventions, in contrast to advance directives and DNAR orders. The form is divided into several sections, the first two of which are especially helpful in the emergency setting. The national POLST Taskforce oversees POLST initiatives and endorses programs. There are 43 states that have or are developing POLST programs and as of August 2013, 15 programs were endorsed by the National POLST Taskforce [15]. The National Quality Forum noted that, "Compared with other advance directive programs, POLST more accurately conveys end-of-life preferences and yields higher adherence by medical professionals" [43]. Communities have found that POLST is an effective means of conveying patient preferences [44].

States have begun to develop electronic registries to facilitate access to POLST forms. The first statewide POLST-only registry was initiated in Oregon in December 2009. Legislatively enacted, the registry accepts POLST forms signed throughout the state and provides access to verbal orders for EMS, emergency departments, and acute care units through a non-public 24/7 call center. The legislation enacting the registry also mandated submission of completed forms by signers unless patients opt out. By July 2013, the Oregon registry had received over 150,000 forms for nearly 90,000 Oregonians, and over 2,500 emergency calls [45]. The Oregon registry's operations and patient matching algorithm have been found to limit release of "false-positive" matches [46] and also helped understand the EMS implications of the registry [47].

Several other states have developed registries or electronic mechanisms for accessing POLST forms or other documents like advance directives. In a 2011 report on behalf of the National POLST Paradigm Task Force, POLST registry efforts are outlined in seven states: California, Idaho, New York, Oregon, Utah, Washington, and West Virginia [48].

Studies indicate that POLST is effective in communicating patient preferences [38,49–51]. Studies in long-term care settings found that having a POLST form prevents unwanted life-sustaining treatments and hospitalization, and orders regarding resuscitation are typically followed, though medical intervention orders were followed less consistently [48,52–54]. One study surveyed a random sample of EMS professionals in Oregon to evaluate their experiences and attitudes regarding the use of the POLST form. Nearly three-quarters of respondents in this study had treated at least one patient with a POLST form, and in nearly half of the cases in which a POLST form was present, the EMS professionals used it to change the treatment plan, often avoiding interventions that the patient did not want [35]. Thus, the POLST paradigm is one model program for expressing patient preferences and helping EMS professionals to determine the best level of intervention for the patient.

Hospice and EMS

Hospice care focuses on the treatment of pain and other uncomfortable symptoms, as well as the patient's emotional and spiritual needs. Hospice is a benefit of Medicare when a physician determines that the person likely has less than 6 months to live and the patient is no longer seeking curative treatment. In the United States, most hospice care is provided at home. A patient enrolled in hospice generally has a nurse who is on call 24/7, and is encouraged to call that nurse for any problem that arises. Nonetheless, patients or their families often call EMS in times of crisis. When they do, the hospice nurse can be a great resource. Contacting the hospice nurse can help to alleviate the patient's and family's distress and provide solutions other than transport to an ED.

Care of the grieving survivors

The responsibility of EMS professionals does not end with the death of a patient. Once a person is determined to be dead at the scene, the survivors who are present become our patients. The survivors may have both physical and psychological needs. When a person dies, the remaining spouse has an increased risk of death [55,56]. EMS professionals have a responsibility to inform family members of a death in a compassionate manner and to provide care and comfort to the survivors. Most survivors find EMS professionals to be supportive and are accepting of a death in the field without the need for transport [57] and families accept the non-transport of loved ones found in asystole [58]. A study of survivors found that the most frequently reported complaints concerned a lack of information and questions left unanswered [59].

West Virginia Physician Orders
for Scope of Treatment (POST)

This is a Physician Order Sheet based on the person's medical condition and wishes. Any section not completed indicates full treatment for that section. When need occurs, <u>first</u> follow these orders, <u>then</u> contact physician.

Last Name/First/Middle Initial
Address
City/State/Zip
Date of Birth (mm/dd/yyyy) ___/___/___	Last 4 SSN	Gender ☐M ☐F

A
Check One Box Only

CARDIOPULMONARY RESUSCITATION (CPR): Person has no pulse <u>and</u> is not breathing.
☐ <u>R</u>esuscitate (CPR)   ☐ <u>D</u>o <u>N</u>ot Attempt <u>R</u>esuscitation (DNR/no CPR)

When not in cardiopulmonary arrest, follow orders in **B**, **C**, and **D**.

B
Check One Box Only

MEDICAL INTERVENTIONS: Person has pulse and/<u>or</u> is breathing.

☐ **Comfort Measures** Treat with dignity and respect. Keep clean, warm, and dry. Use medication by any route, positioning, wound care and other measures to relieve pain and suffering. Use oxygen, suction and manual treatment of airway obstruction as needed for comfort. **Do not transfer to hospital for life-sustaining treatment. Transfer <u>only</u> if comfort needs cannot be met in current location.**

☐ **Limited Additional Interventions** Includes care described above. Use medical treatment, antibiotics, IV fluids and cardiac monitoring as indicated. Do not use intubation or mechanical ventilation. **Transfer to hospital if indicated. Avoid intensive care unit.**

☐ **Full Interventions** Includes care above. Use intubation, advanced airway interventions, mechanical ventilation, and cardioversion as indicated. **Transfer to hospital if indicated. Include intensive care unit.**
Other Orders: _____

C
Check One Box Only in Each Column

MEDICALLY ADMINISTERED FLUIDS AND NUTRITION: Oral fluids and nutrition must be offered as tolerated.

☐ **No IV fluids** (provide other measures to assure comfort)   ☐ **No feeding tube**
☐ **IV fluids for a trial period of no longer than** _____   ☐ **Feeding tube for a trial period of no longer than** _____
☐ **IV fluids long-term if indicated**   ☐ **Feeding tube long-term**
Other Orders: _____

D

Discussed with:
☐ Patient/Resident   ☐ Health care surrogate   ☐ MPOA representative   ☐ Spouse
☐ Court-appointed guardian   ☐ Parent of Minor   ☐ Other: _____ (Specify)

Authorization
☐

INITIAL BOX if you agree with the following statement: If I lose decision making capacity and my condition significantly deteriorates, I give permission to my MPOA representative/surrogate to make decisions and to complete a new form with my physician in accordance with my expressed wishes for such a condition or, if these wishes are unknown or not reasonably ascertainable, my best interests.

Registry Opt-In
☐

INITIAL BOX if you agree to have your POST form, do not resuscitate card, living will and medical power of attorney form (if completed) submitted to the WV e-Directive Registry and released to treating health care providers. REGISTRY FAX - 304-293-7442

Signature of Patient/Resident, Parent of Minor, or Guardian/MPOA Representative/Surrogate (Mandatory)	Date

Signature of Physician	
Physician Name (Print Full Name)	**Physician Phone Number**
Physician Signature (Mandatory)	**Date and Time**

FORM SHALL ACCOMPANY PATIENT/RESIDENT WHEN TRANSFERRED OR DISCHARGED

©Center for End-of-Life Care, Robert C. Byrd Health Sciences Center of West Virginia University, P.O. Box 9022, Morgantown, WV 26506, 1-877-209-8086
2012 rev

Di ti R i   FAX 304 293 7442

Figure 64.3 Example POST (POLST) form. Source: West Virginia Physicians Orders for Scope of Treatment form. Reproduced with permission of West Virginia Center for End-of-Life Care.

Death notification can be stressful for EMS professionals [60]. A recent Canadian study found that paramedics find death notification stressful and think that they need more education in this area [61]. Deaths from violent crime, drunk driving crashes, or suicides, or the death of a child, increase the provider's distress regarding notification [62]. A 2009 survey of EMS professionals found that only 48% felt prepared to communicate death to family [63]. A 16-hour workshop based on the Emergency Death Education and Crisis Training (EDECT) program, with a 2-hour session on death notification, divided EMS professionals into three groups: long intervention, short intervention, and control. The authors found that after the training, 92% of those in the long intervention group felt that their training was adequate, compared with 43% in the short intervention group and 21% in the control group [64]. Although this study did not test whether or not death notification skills can be improved, it did show that education can improve EMS professionals' comfort with death notification. A final study by these authors also suggested that behaviors can be changed [65]. One recent study of a 90-minute education model found that educating paramedics to use a structured communication model improved confidence and competence in delivering death notification [66].

Other studies have analyzed emergency physicians, the group most likely to become EMS physicians and medical directors. Most emergency physicians report that they have insufficient education on how to perform death notification [67]. A study of emergency medicine residents showed that role-playing increases their comfort with death notification [68]. Another study found that most respondents recommend that education on death notification be part of Advanced Cardiac Life Support courses [69].

Conclusion

Just as EMS medical directors have an obligation to ensure high-quality medical care by the EMS professionals that they supervise, they also have an obligation to ensure high-quality, compassionate, and medically appropriate end-of-life care. This includes protocols and education to determine when and when not to provide resuscitation and other life-sustaining treatments, often based on patient preferences, which are documented by various means. The POLST paradigm is a proven and growing method for communicating end-of-life wishes. Additionally, EMS professionals must provide support to the grieving survivors left behind.

References

1 Merton, T. *The Wisdom of the Desert*. New York: New Dimensions, 1960.
2 Innes G, Wanger K. Dignified death or legislated resuscitation? *Can Med Assoc J* 1999;161:1264–5.
3 Guru V, Verbeek PR, Morrison LJ. Response of paramedics to terminally ill patients with cardiac arrest: an ethical dilemma. *Can Med Assoc J* 1999;161:1251–4.
4 Feder S, Matheny RL, Loveless RS Jr, et al. Withholding resuscitation: a new approach to prehospital end-of-life decisions. *Ann Intern Med* 2006;144:634–40.
5 Go SA, Mozaffarian D, Roger VL, et al. Heart disease and stroke statistics – 2013 update: a report from the American Heart Association. *Circulation* 2013;127:e6–e245.
6 Warner LL, Hoffman JR, Baraff LJ. Prognostic significance of field response in out-of-hospital ventricular fibrillation. *Chest* 1985;87:22–8.
7 Bonnin MJ, Pepe PE, Kimball KT, et al. Distinct criteria for termination of resuscitation in the out-of-hospital setting. *JAMA* 1993;270:1457–62.
8 Dunne RB, Compton S, Zalenski RJ, et al. Outcomes from out-of-hospital cardiac arrest in Detroit. *Resuscitation* 2007;72:59–65.
9 Kellerman AL, Hackman BB, Somes G. Predicting the outcome of unsuccessful prehospital advanced cardiac life support. *JAMA* 1993;270:1433–6.
10 Beauchamp TL, Childress JF. *Principles of Biomedical Ethics*, 5th edn. Oxford: Oxford University Press, 2001.
11 American College of Emergency Physicians. Ethical issues of resuscitation. *Ann Emerg Med* 2008;52:593.
12 Adams J. Prehospital do-not-resuscitate orders: a survey of polices in the United States. *Prehosp Disaster Med* 1993;8:317–22.
13 Sabatino CP. Survey of state EMS-DNR laws and protocols. *J Law Med Ethics* 1999;27:297–315.
14 Ausband SC, March JA, Brown LH. National prevalence of palliative care protocols in emergency medical services. *Prehosp Emerg Care* 2002;6:36–41.
15 Available at: www.polst.org/
16 Castillo LS, Williams BA, Hooper SM, et al. Lost in translation: the unintended consequences of advance directive law on clinical care. *Ann Intern Med* 2011;154:121–8.
17 Lahn M, Friedman B, Bijur P, et al. Advance directives in skilled nursing facility residents transferred to emergency departments. *Acad Emerg Med* 2001;8:1158–62.
18 Jackson EA, Yarzebski JL, Goldberg RJ, et al. Do-not-resuscitate orders in patients hospitalized with acute myocardial infarction: the Worcester Heart Attack Study. *Arch Intern Med* 2004;164:776–83.
19 Llovera I, Mandel FS, Ryan JG, et al. Are emergency department patients thinking about advance directives? *Acad Emerg Med* 1997;4:976–80.
20 Llovera I, Ward MF, Ryan JG, et al. Why don't emergency department patients have advance directives? *Acad Emerg Med* 1999;6:1054–60.
21 Grudzen CR, Liddicoat R, Hoffman JR, et al. Developing quality indicators for the appropriateness of resuscitation in prehospital atraumatic cardiac arrest. *Prehosp Emerg Care* 2007;11:434–42.
22 Abramson N, de Vos R, Fallat ME, et al. Ethics in emergency cardiac care. *Ann Emerg Med* 2001;37:s195–s200.
23 Partridge RA, Virk A, Sayah A. Field experience with pre-hospital advance directives. *Ann Emerg Med* 1998;32:589–93.
24 Danis M, Southerland LI, Garrett JM, et al. A prospective study of advance directives for life-sustaining care. *N Engl J Med* 1991; 324:882–8.
25 Silveira MJ, Buell RA, Deyo RA. Prehospital DNR orders: what do physicians in Washington know? *J Am Geriatr Soc* 2003;51:1435–8.
26 Mirarchi FL. Does a living will equal a DNR? Are living wills compromising patient safety? *J Emerg Med* 2007;33:299–305.
27 Bomba PA, Vermilyea D. Integrating POLST into palliative care guidelines: a paradigm shift in advance care planning in oncology. *J Natl Compr Canc Netw* 2006;4:819–29.
28 Marco CA, Schears RM. Prehospital resuscitation practices: a survey of prehospital providers. *J Emerg Med* 2003;24:101–6.

29 Perkins HS Controlling death: the false promise of advance directives. *Ann Intern Med* 2007;147:51–7.

30 Lerner EB, Billittier AJ, Hallinan K. Out-of-hospital do-not-resuscitate orders by primary care physicians. *J Emerg Med* 2002;23:425–8.

31 Iserson KV. A simplified prehospital advance directive law: Arizona's approach. *Ann Emerg Med* 1993;22:1703–10.

32 Becker LJ, Yeargin K, Rea TD, et al. Resuscitation of residents with do not resuscitate orders in long-term care facilities. *Prehosp Emerg Care* 2003;7:303–6

33 Leon MD, Wilson EM. Development of a statewide protocol for the prehospital identification of DNR patients in Connecticut including new DNR regulations. *Ann Emerg Med* 1999;34:263–74.

34 Morrison RS, Olson E, Mertz KR, et al. The inaccessibility of advance directives on transfer from ambulatory to acute care settings. *JAMA* 1995;274:478–82.

35 Schmidt TA, Hickman S, Tolle SW, et al. The Physician Orders for Life-Sustaining Treatment (POLST) Program: Oregon emergency medical technicians' practical experiences and attitudes. *J Amer Geriatr Soc* 2004;52:1430–4.

36 Dunn PM, Nelson CA, Tolle SW, et al. Communicating preferences for life-sustaining treatment using a physician order form. *J Gen Intern Med* 1997;12:102.

37 Fromme EK, Zive D, Schmidt TA, et al. POLST registry do-not resuscitate orders and other treatment preferences. *JAMA* 2012;307:34–5.

38 Dunn PM, Schmidt TA, Carley MM, et al. A method to communicate patient preferences about medically indicated life-sustaining treatment in the out-of-hospital setting. *J Am Geriatr Soc* 1996;44:785–91.

39 Citko J, Moss AH, Carley M, et al. The National POLST Paradigm Initiative. *J Pall Med* 2011;14:241–2.

40 Abrahm JL. Advances in palliative medicine and end-of life care *Annu Rev Med* 2011;62:187–99.

41 Meier DE, Beresford L. POLST offers next stage in honoring patient preferences *J Pall Med* 2009;12:291–5.

42 Bomba PA, Kemp M, Black JS. POLST: an improvement over traditional advance directives. *Cleve Clin J Med* 2012;79:457–64.

43 Hammes BJ, Rooney BL, Gundrum JD, et al. The POLST Program: a retrospective review of the demographics of use and outcomes in one community where advance directives are prevalent. *J Pall Med* 2012;15:77–85.

44 Anonymous. *A Framework and Preferred Practices for Palliative and Hospice Care Quality: A Consensus Report.* Washington, DC: National Quality Forum, 2006.

45 Oregon POLST Registry. Available at: www.or.polst.org/registry#registry-information-for-healthcare-professionals

46 Olszewski EA, Newgard CD, Zive D, et al. Validation of physician orders for life-sustaining treatment: electronic registry to guide emergency care. *J Am Geriatr Soc* 2012;60:1384–6.

47 Schmidt TA, Olszewski EA, Zive D, et al. The Oregon physician orders for life-sustaining treatment registry: a preliminary study of emergency medical services utilization. *J Emerg Med* 2013;44:796–805.

48 Zive D, Schmidt TA. Oregon POLST Registry. Pathways to POLST Registry Development: Lessons Learned 2011. Available at: www.polst.org/wp-content/uploads/2012/12/POLST-Registry.pdf

49 Hickman SE, Nelson CA, Perrin NA, et al. A comparison of methods to communicate treatment preferences in nursing facilities: traditional practices versus the Physician Orders for Life-Sustaining Treatment Program. *J Am Geriatr Soc* 2010;58:1241–8.

50 Hickman SE, Nelson CA, Koss AH, et al. Use of the Physician Orders for Life-Sustaining Treatment (POLST) Paradigm Program in the hospice setting. *J Pall Med* 2009;12:133–41.

51 Hickman SE, Nelson CA, Moss, AH, et al. The consistency between treatments provided to nursing facility residents and orders on the physician orders for life-sustaining treatment form. *J Am Geriatr Soc* 2011;59:2091–9.

52 Tolle SW, Tilden VP, Nelson CA, et al. A prospective study of the efficacy of the physician order form for life-sustaining treatment. *J Am Geriatr Soc* 1998;46:1097–102.

53 Caprio AJ, Rollins VP, Roberts E. Health care professionals' perceptions and use of the medical orders for scope of treatment (MOST) form in North Carolina nursing homes. *J Am Med Dir Assoc* 2012;13:162–8.

54 Lee MA, Brummel-Smith K, Meyer J, et al. Physician orders for life-sustaining treatment (POLST): outcomes in a PACE program. Program of All-Inclusive Care for the Elderly. *J Am Geriatr Soc* 2000;48:1343–4.

55 Helsing KJ, Szklo M. Mortality after bereavement. *Am J Epidemiol* 1981;114:41–52.

56 Helsing KJ, Szklo M, Comstock GW. Factors associated with mortality after widowhood. *Am J Public Health* 1981;71:802–9.

57 Schmidt TA, Harrahill MA. Family response to out-of- hospital death. *Acad Emerg Med* 1995;2:513–18.

58 Edwardsen EA, Chiumento S, Davis E. Family perspective of medical care and grief support after field termination by emergency medical services personnel: a preliminary report. *Prehosp Emerg Care* 2002;6:440–4.

59 Merlevede E, Spooren D, Henderick H, et al. Perceptions, needs and mourning reactions of bereaved relatives confronted with a sudden unexpected death. *Resuscitation* 2004;61:341–8.

60 Norton RL, Bartkus E, Schmidt TA, et al. Survey of emergency medical technicians' management of death in the field. *Prehosp Disaster Med* 1992;3:235–41.

61 Douglas L, Cheskes S, Fledman M, Ratnapalan S. Paramedics' experiences with death notification: a qualitative study. *J Param Prac* 2012;4:533–9.

62 Stewart AE, Harris Lord J, Mercer DL. A survey of professionals' training and experiences in delivering death notifications. *Death Stud* 2000;24:611–31

63 Stone SC, Abbott J, McClung CD, et al. Paramedic knowledge, attitudes, and training in end-of-life care. *Prehosp Disaster Med* 2009;24:529–34.

64 Smith-Cumberland TL, Feldman RH. EMTs' attitudes toward death before and after a death education program. *Prehosp Emerg Care* 2006;10:89–95.

65 Smith-Cumberland T. The evaluation of two death education programs for EMTs using the theory of planned behavior. *Death Stud* 2006;30:637–47.

66 Hobgood C, Mathew D, Woodyard DJ, et al. Death in the field: teaching paramedics to deliver effective death notifications using the educational intervention "GRIEV_ING". *Prehosp Emerg Care* 2013;17:501–10.

67 Schmidt TA, Tolle SW. Emergency physicians' responses to families following patient death. *Ann Emerg Med* 1990;19:125–8.

68 Schmidt TA, Norton RL, Tolle SW. Sudden death in the ED: educating residents to compassionately inform families. *J Emerg Med* 1992;10:643–7.

69 Jones K, Garg M, Bali D, et al. The knowledge and perceptions of medical personnel relating to outcome after cardiac arrest. *Resuscitation* 2006;69:235–9.

CHAPTER 65

Termination of resuscitation in the out-of-hospital setting

Laurie J. Morrison, Ian R. Drennan, and P. Richard Verbeek

Introduction

The irreversible cessation of life may be difficult to determine with complete confidence, particularly in the austere environment of out-of-hospital emergency care. As a result, clear protocols should be implemented in each EMS agency outlining when to attempt resuscitation and when to terminate resuscitation efforts.

When distinctive protocols do not exist, decision making is left to the discretion of the paramedic and the direct medical oversight physician at the point of care. The literature suggests that this leads to bias and inconsistency in care across similar patients [1].

There is limited evidence to guide when to start resuscitation. Yet a large body of work, including external validation across different geographical regions, exists to guide the development of local protocols to provide a consistent approach to termination of resuscitation in adult out-of-hospital non-traumatic cardiac arrest.

Adult out-of-hospital cardiac arrest

When to start resuscitation

There are three criteria that must be met to start resuscitation in the prehospital setting.

1 Provider safety is assured.
2 The patient is not obviously dead.
3 The patient does not have a "Do Not Attempt Resuscitation" directive (DNAR) that meets local policy.

The issues related to provider safety and policy and directives governing provider safety are dealt with in other chapters. The Uniform Determination of Death Act, which has been adopted by many states, and endorsed by both the American Bar Association and the American Medical Association, states that "an individual who has sustained either: 1) irreversible cessation of circulatory and respiratory functions; or 2) irreversible cessation of all functions of the entire brain, including brain stem, is

dead. A determination of death must be made in accordance with accepted medical standards" [2]. Although this statement attempts to define death, it still leaves the determination of the condition to the vague criterion of "accepted medical standards" as well as the provider's definition of "irreversibility."

When to withhold resuscitation

In most jurisdictions, obvious death with no need to attempt resuscitation is defined by legislation or by medical directives. An unpublished survey of the Resuscitation Outcomes Consortium (ROC) services was completed prior to establishing the ROC Epistry data set [3]. Definitions of obvious death were similar across the >280 services (Box 65.1).

As demographics continue to shift toward an aging population, end-of life decisions may be made in advance more commonly in patients calling EMS. A study in 2008 of cancer patients suggested that 37% had had these discussions in advance, which resulted in decreased ventilation, rates of resuscitation, and ICU admission, and increased hospice enrollment for end-of-life care [4]. Most importantly, these conversations resulted in better quality of life for patients and their caregivers. The various platforms facilitating patient decision making need to be considered when establishing medical directives concerning attempting resuscitation. These include living wills, health care advance directives, or (when combined) comprehensive health care advance directives [5,6] (see Chapter 64).

Seattle medical directives have been altered to include verbal DNAR as well as written DNAR. Employing a before-and-after design, Feder demonstrated 50% reduction in resuscitation rates when the directive enabled paramedics to not attempt cardiac arrest resuscitation in patients with a history of terminal illness, under the care of a physician at the time, and with a written DNAR or family requesting a DNAR [7,8]. This would have a positive effect on the survival rates from out-of-hospital cardiac arrest as these patients would be removed from the denominator.

In a system with explicit medical directives pertaining to obvious death and prescribed end-of-life autonomy in decision

Emergency Medical Services: Clinical Practice and Systems Oversight, Second Edition. Volume 1: Clinical Aspects of EMS.
Edited by David C. Cone, Jane H. Brice, Theodore R. Delbridge, and J. Brent Myers.
© 2015 NAEMSP. Published 2015 by John Wiley & Sons, Inc. Companion Website: www.wiley.com\go\cone\naemsp

Box 65.1 Example of obvious death medical directive

Resuscitation is not warranted where there is evidence of obvious death as defined as:
Rigor mortis
Lividity
Transection
Decapitation
Decomposition

Box 65.2 Termination of resuscitation of non-traumatic adult OHCA at scene is recommended when:

The patient has received the full (BLS or ALS) resuscitation protocol and the patient has not been transported from the scene and:
1 Did not receive a shock at any time during the resuscitation, **AND**
2 Did not achieve a prehospital return of spontaneous circulation, **AND**
3 Did not suffer an EMS-witnessed OHCA.

making, all other victims of out-of-hospital cardiac arrest (OHCA) should receive full resuscitation.

When to terminate resuscitation in adult non-traumatic OHCA

To understand the evidence for termination of resuscitation (TOR) rules, one must understand the definition of medical futility. Objective criteria for establishing medical futility were defined in 1990 as interventions that impart a <1% chance of survival [9].

In adult non-traumatic OHCA, there is a validated decision rule to guide TOR for BLS [10] (Box 65.2). This rule has been externally validated in the United States, Canada, Europe, and Japan [11–16].

The BLS rule has also been proposed and externally validated as the "Universal Rule" for all levels of providers [12,15,16], for all non-traumatic OHCA (Box 65.2). This reduces confusion in a service with a tiered response and enables simpler implementation strategies. The rules have been validated under the 2005 and 2010 resuscitation guidelines without any change in their performance accuracy [12]. It makes sense that any intervention in the prehospital setting (new drug, new device, or new step-by-step process of care) that potentially increases survival would first and foremost increase the rates of return of spontaneous circulation (ROSC) or enable ventricular fibrillation (VF) more often and increase the potential to receive a shock. Either of these outcomes would make the patient ineligible for TOR, and the rate of transport to hospital would rise. Thus, as scientific advances improve resuscitation outcomes, more patients will meet the criteria for transport instead of termination.

Adult patients with cardiac arrest attributed to an obvious cause such as lightning strike, mechanical suffocation, poisoning, near drowning, etc. should be treated via the prehospital resuscitation protocol and transported to ensure they are given the full benefit of interventions unique to the etiology of their arrests. These arrests were routinely excluded from all the studies pertaining to TOR rules.

Implementation issues related to termination of resuscitation

The 2010 Guidelines from the American Heart Association and the 2011 position paper from the National Association of EMS Physicians advocate for the implementation of the TOR rule to reduce the transport of futile resuscitations and provide a more consistent approach to all non-traumatic OHCA patients [17,18]. EMS medical directives relating to TOR need to be tailored in how they are implemented locally, taking system nuances into consideration; however, the medical directive must include the rule as validated with all three components after full prehospital resuscitation by a resuscitation protocol which is guideline compliant [19,20]. For example, if medics did not remain on scene to complete their resuscitation protocol and instead took a scoop-and-run approach, there would be insufficient time to complete the resuscitation protocol. Thus, there is insufficient time to adequately assess if the patient achieves ROSC or received a shock at any time. Termination of resuscitation would be premature and not compliant with the rule. Another example pertains to a medical directive that removed the first and third criteria, instructing the providers to terminate if no ROSC was achieved in the prehospital setting. This was explored in an analysis of the Toronto ROC data and it was found that resuscitation should not be terminated for patients who did not achieve ROSC but did receive shocks or had their arrests witnessed by EMS [21,22]. The survival rate in this group was 3.5%, which exceeds futility. It would be cavalier to reduce the TOR rule to no ROSC as it denies potential survivors the opportunity for transport and continued resuscitation.

Sasson et al. published a number of barriers to TOR protocol implementation, including changing legislation and local EMS remuneration practices to enable EMS services and their medical directors to implement the TOR decision rule [21]. It is essential that both of these barriers are addressed and corrected locally pior to implementation using the body of science and current position statements. Education should include a consistent approach to the use of TOR rules, and include sensitivity and grief counseling for providers who will be providing death notification to the families. Helping medical directors and colleagues understand the current body of knowledge should address the fear of litigation for medical directors and myths relating to the ability of EMS personnel to provide death notification and the effects on family members. Numerous studies have demonstrated that providers are comfortable with terminating resuscitation in the field, comfortable with conveying the news to family, and effective at doing it [7,23,24]. Furthermore, it has been established that family members are receptive to this approach to care and do not suffer any long-term emotional or psychological effects [25–27].

Pediatric out-of-hospital cardiac arrest

When to start resuscitation

In the case of children (aged 17 years or younger), decisions regarding when to resuscitate, how long to continue, and when to terminate resuscitation are based on fewer available data than we have for adults. Nevertheless, the available data indicate that, with the exception of posttraumatic arrest, EMS providers should attempt to resuscitate any pediatric patient who does not have obvious signs of irreversible death (e.g. lividity, rigor mortis or decomposition) or in the special circumstance of a valid DNAR order [25,28,29].

Due to the low occurrence and increased stress involved in pediatric resuscitation, it may occasionally be difficult for paramedics to reliably discern clinical signs of futility. In fact, in many cases that were later found at the emergency department (ED) to have already developed signs of lividity or rigor mortis, paramedics had found it difficult to truly discern these conditions in the field and therefore attempted resuscitation [29].

Recent literature has shown that survival to hospital discharge in pediatric patients greater than 1 year old is higher (9.1% for children aged 1–11 years and 8.9% for those aged 12–19 years) than survival in both infants (<1 year, 3.3%) and adults (4.6%) [30], suggesting that pediatric OHCA survival is improving [30–32].

When to terminate resuscitation

With regard to the decisions to terminate efforts in pediatric patients, no reliable clinical predictors have been sufficiently evaluated in the out-of-hospital setting to accurately predict pediatric resuscitation success or failure, and no decision rules derived for adult prehospital TOR have been evaluated in the pediatric population [17]. Furthermore, compared to adults, pediatric patients have been shown to have increased rates of survival from non-shockable rhythms [30,32,33], a cornerstone of many TOR decision rules used in the adult population. Published studies of pediatric OHCA have demonstrated that unwitnessed cardiac arrests, arrests without bystander cardiopulmonary resuscitation (CPR), and arrests with initial non-shockable rhythms are associated with decreased survival [28–31]. However, none of these variables alone or in combination has been shown to accurately predict futility. A lack of prehospital ROSC is also strongly associated with mortality [29,30,34], suggesting that, as with adult cardiac arrests, prehospital providers should focus on the delivery of high-quality CPR during initial resuscitation efforts instead of resorting to a scoop-and-run approach. In a prospective study of about 300 consecutive pediatric OHCAs, on-scene ROSC was never achieved in 267 children despite aggressive attempts at ACLS for more than a half hour, and none of these children survived [29].

The exact duration of CPR prior to recommending TOR is unknown. The absence of spontaneous circulation within 20–30 minutes of ACLS initiation has been associated with poor survival (unless there is hypothermia or persistent VF) [28,29,31,35–37]. However, current data are inconsistent and further research is needed to determine any specific cut-off values. A recent study of 138 pediatric OHCAs showed a median duration of CPR of 18.5 minutes in survivors compared to 41 minutes in non-survivors; however, survivors were reported with up to 64 minutes of resuscitation [34]. Cut-off values and predictive factors must be interpreted cautiously as emerging in-hospital treatments such as postarrest therapeutic hypothermia [38] and the use of extracorporeal membrane oxygenation (ECMO) [39,40] may result in good neurological outcome in patients who were once considered futile.

The concept of on-scene termination of resuscitative efforts for children is further complicated by the psychosocial effect on the family and the psychological discomfort of the EMS providers [24,25,41].

Health care professionals often find it more psychologically challenging to withdraw CPR attempts rather than not starting resuscitation in the first place [42]. A blinded survey of EMS personnel regarding comfort levels with on-scene pronouncement was reported using a rating scale of 1 (not comfortable) to 10 (very comfortable) [24]. The study found that veteran paramedics (n = 201) are very comfortable (average score 10) with the pronouncement of an adult on scene, but not with pronouncement of a child (average score 2). Accordingly, with the greater availability of in-hospital support services for the families of pediatric patients and the EMS providers' potential concerns with on-scene pronouncement, termination of resuscitative efforts for children may be best performed in the hospital. Nevertheless, it has also been emphasized that once medical futility is determined, EMS personnel should take care during transport not to create additional risks in traffic, and in-hospital personnel might adopt modified procedures that limit further resuscitation and resource use [24,25]. In addition, in some cases of suspected sudden infant death syndrome, unwarranted resuscitative efforts and hospital transport may compromise a potential crime scene investigation.

With limited and inconsistent evidence to terminate resuscitation, current guidelines do not recommend the use of TOR rules or specific criteria for pediatric OHCA [17,43,44]. In the absence of clear criteria, EMS providers should employ explicit definitions of obvious death to dictate when to start resuscitation and to continue resuscitation while transporting to the hospital, seeking consultation with direct medical oversight as required.

Adult traumatic cardiopulmonary arrest

Among the greatest challenges in EMS is decision making around the patient who is found to be experiencing a traumatic cardiopulmonary arrest. Whether traumatic arrest is the result of blunt or penetrating trauma, the prognosis for survival (approximately 2%) is dismal, but not futile as defined by an overall survival rate <1% [9,45].

The decision whether to withhold or terminate resuscitation of the traumatic arrest patient is fraught with emotion since patients are typically young and the circumstances surrounding the event often occur unexpectedly in public and unsecure settings, and can be subject to intense immediate and prolonged public and media scrutiny. In addition, there is a need for EMS providers to act quickly and decisively in an environment where it can be difficult to determine whether the patient has a detectable pulse [46].

Contrary to non-traumatic cardiopulmonary arrest, there are no prospectively derived and validated clinical decision rules to guide EMS providers on whether to withhold resuscitation of the traumatic arrest patient, or circumstances where it might be reasonable to terminate resuscitation after failed attempts to achieve ROSC in the field or during transport. Nevertheless, some observational studies have identified factors that are associated with futility such as the absence of organized electrocardiographic activity often described as asystole [45,47–53] and EMS provider CPR for greater than 10-15 min without ROSC [48,51,53–57]. Whereas, other observational studies suggested an increased survival was associated with the presence of normal sinus rhythm, pupillary responses, or visible respiratory effort, especially in penetrating trauma patients [46,52,58]. The challenge in making recommendations is that the literature reports >1% survival rates for victims of blunt and penetrating trauma even in the presence of dire clinical findings such as asystole [51,52,57,59]. It appears as if no single criterion unequivocally distinguishes between survivors and non-survivors of traumatic arrest.

Despite these challenges, NAEMSP and the American College of Surgeons Committee on Trauma (ACSCOT) have published joint position statements and supporting resource documents (initially in 2003[60] and updated in 2012 [45,61,62]) to provide guidance on withholding resuscitation and termination of resuscitation of adult traumatic arrest patients. The 2012 position statements provide separate recommendations for withholding resuscitation and TOR (see Boxes 65.3 and 65.4 below). The components of the position statements are a combination of operational design recommendations that are largely common sense, as well as a number of patient care assessment and intervention recommendations that resulted from a structured literature review focusing on clinical factors that are associated with outcomes of traumatic arrest.

Experience with the 2003 position statements has shown that there is a wide variation in their application, with several large EMS systems transporting traumatic arrest patients contrary to the recommendations [63]. Specific factors leading to this variation were not reported; however, this observation has resulted in a call to identify and address barriers to implementation as a way to increase compliance with these recommendations. This is important since the consequences of non-compliance have resulted in high rates of transport of futile patients, as evidenced by one study from a single center that reported only a single

---

Box 65.3 NAEMSP-ACSCOT 2012 position on withholding resuscitation in traumatic cardiopulmonary arrest

- It is appropriate to withhold resuscitative efforts for certain trauma patients for whom death is the predictable outcome.
- Resuscitative efforts should be withheld for trauma patients with injuries that are obviously incompatible with life, such as decapitation or hemicorporectomy.
- Resuscitative efforts should be withheld for patients of either blunt or penetrating trauma when there is evidence of prolonged cardiac arrest, including rigor mortis or dependent lividity.
- Resuscitative efforts may be withheld for a blunt trauma patient who, on the arrival of EMS personnel, is found to be apneic, pulseless, and without organized electrocardiographic activity.
- Resuscitative efforts may be withheld for a penetrating trauma patient who, on arrival of EMS personnel, is found to be pulseless and apneic and there are no other signs of life, including spontaneous movement, electrocardiographic activity, and pupillary response.
- When the mechanism of injury does not correlate with the clinical condition, suggesting a non-traumatic cause of cardiac arrest, standard resuscitative measures should be followed.

Source: Millin 2011 [43]. Reproduced with permission of NAEMSP.

---

survivor amongst 294 transported patients who met criteria for withholding or termination of resuscitation. This patient survived with a neurologically compromised state [57].

When to withhold resuscitation (Box 65.3)

The withholding resuscitation recommendations are unchanged from the 2003 position statement and are meant to identify blunt and penetrating trauma patients who by consensus have no meaningful chance (with the previous caveats) of survival and therefore do not warrant implementation of resuscitation procedures or transport. Ultimately, these patients can be left at the scene in the custody of authorities, thereby preserving forensic evidence to support investigations into the cause and circumstances related to the death.

Clinical application of the recommendations on withholding resuscitation requires sufficient assessment to determine the presence or absence of vital signs, pupillary response, respiratory effort, and spontaneous movement. It also requires the application of a cardiac monitor to determine the presence or absence of organized electrocardiographic activity. The lack of a precise definition in the recommendations as to what constitutes organized electrocardiographic activity reflects a similar lack of precision in the literature. Conservatively, one would interpret this to mean asystole, although it has been proposed that any heart rhythm at a rate less than 40 is uniformly associated with non-survival [50].

Importantly, these recommendations fall within the scope of practice of BLS and ALS providers. From an operational perspective, it is important to establish that this assessment does not constitute initiation of resuscitation; otherwise, there will be the potential for disagreement as to what constitutes withholding resuscitation. Of note in these recommendations is the added requirement for penetrating trauma patients to have no other signs of life. This relates to reports of survival in penetrating trauma patients with asystole who exhibited other signs of life [51,52,58].

When to terminate resuscitation (Box 65.4)

The clinical aspects of the position statement regarding TOR are meant to identify traumatic arrest patients who meet the criteria for resuscitation but do not achieve ROSC after adequate trials of CPR and other resuscitative procedures as dictated by the EMS providers' scope of practice and medical protocols. This is because both blunt and penetrating traumatic arrest patients who do not achieve ROSC have close to zero probability of survival despite further attempts at resuscitation in the hospital, including resuscitative thoracotomy. The duration of an "adequate trial" of CPR is not precisely defined. Traditionally 15 minutes has been supported as a cut-off; however, as reported in the 2012 position statement, the collective literature suggests that only 0.75% of traumatic arrest patients with more than 10 minutes of CPR survive to hospital discharge with good neurological status [45]. This low rate of survival suggests 10 minutes is a reasonable trial of CPR. It is somewhat difficult to conclude whether penetrating trauma patients (especially those with thoracic injuries) should have a longer trial of CPR before considering TOR since many studies do not differentiate between penetrating and blunt trauma in their patient populations. Yet,

reports of survival in patients with CPR for greater than 10 minutes tend to favor penetrating trauma patients [53,57].

It should be noted that contrary to 2003, the 2012 position statement does not specifically mention whether TOR should be considered in patients with EMS-witnessed traumatic arrest who fail to achieve ROSC after 10–15 minutes of prehospital resuscitation. The reason for this is not mentioned; however, it is important to acknowledge since about 37% of traumatic arrest patients fall within this category [57]. Unfortunately, most literature regarding prehospital traumatic arrest simply describes the presence or absence of arrest in the field but not its timing. Given only one neurologically compromised survivor out of 110 patients with EMS-witnessed TCPA [57], it seems reasonable to apply the TOR recommendations to this group as well.

Prehospital TOR of traumatic arrest patients is operationally challenging because CPR (and most other procedures) should typically be performed during transport (scoop and run). Therefore, application of TOR protocols under these circumstances would likely lead to many patients qualifying for TOR during transport. Moreover, many patients in urban settings would likely arrive at trauma facilities prior to "adequate" trials of CPR being completed. Development of TOR protocols during transport predictably will require consultation and support from a wide variety of stakeholders including the EMS agencies, medical oversight physicians, trauma centers, regulatory agencies, law agencies, and the medical examiners. Local protocols would also have to include the specific destination (e.g. morgue, coroner's office, emergency department) once TOR has been implemented. In urban settings, it may be that the best local solution once transport has been initiated is to continue resuscitation and leave the decision for TOR to the receiving trauma center.

While the 2012 position statement advocates for active physician oversight in developing and locally implementing TOR, there is no specific statement indicating the need for direct (online) medical oversight. While identifying patients who qualify for withholding resuscitation seems reasonably straightforward and ostensibly could be implemented without direct medical oversight, TOR appears more complex, especially since other resuscitative measures beyond CPR are typically performed. To ensure compliance with the recommendations and EMS provider comfort with implementing TOR, it may be that direct medical oversight would provide additional value to making the final decision.

A number of patient groups experiencing extenuating circumstances are noted in the guidelines which are not specifically addressed. This may be largely because the available literature has excluded them from study or the available information is scant and incomplete. Examples of these patient groups include pediatric patients, patients with environmental injuries, pregnant patients, and patients where the mechanism of injury does not correlate with the clinical condition. Many services will implement resuscitation and transport of these patients without regard for TOR recommendations, which is appropriate given the lack of literature.

Trauma TOR

Box 65.4 NAEMSP-ACSCOT 2012 position on TOR of traumatic cardiopulmonary arrest

- A principal focus of EMS treatment of trauma patients is efficient evacuation to definitive care, where major blood loss can be corrected. Resuscitative efforts should not prolong on-scene time.
- EMS systems should have protocols that allow EMS providers to terminate resuscitative efforts for certain adult patients in traumatic cardiopulmonary arrest.
- TOR may be considered when there are no signs of life and there is no ROSC despite appropriate field EMS treatment that includes minimally interrupted CPR.
- Protocols should require a specific interval of CPR that accompanies other resuscitative interventions. Past guidance has indicated that up to 15 minutes of CPR should be provided before resuscitative efforts are terminated, but the science in this regard remains unclear.
- TOR protocols should be accompanied by standard procedures to ensure appropriate management of the deceased patient in the field and adequate support services for the patient's family.
- Implementation of TOR protocols mandates active physician oversight.
- TOR protocols should include any locally specific clinical, environmental, or population-based situations for which the protocol is not applicable. TOR may be impractical after transport has been initiated.
- Further research is appropriate to determine the optimal duration of CPR before terminating resuscitative efforts.

Source: Millin 2011 [43]. Reproduced with permission of NAEMSP.

For patients who are transported to trauma centers in accordance with the position statement, it is important for EMS providers to appreciate that arrival at a trauma center does not dictate that a resuscitative thoracotomy will be performed. Rather, the recommendations identify patients who *may* qualify for resuscitative thoracotomy, and transport to a trauma center gives the option to the trauma team.

It should be noted that the literature on resuscitative thoracotomy is largely based on reports from Level I trauma centers that have experience and expertise in performing this procedure. It is logical to conclude, despite the absence of supporting literature, that the survival of traumatic arrest patients would be <1% in those who must be transported to non-Level I trauma centers. This would suggest that prehospital traumatic arrest TOR protocols may be more appropriately applied in rural EMS settings.

Conclusion

The decision of when to start or terminate resuscitation is fraught with inconsistency if left to the discretion of the individual provider or direct medical oversight. There is a body of knowledge that guides medical directors on an approach to TOR in adult OHCA of non-traumatic origin. The TOR rule is sanctioned by NAEMSP and AHA. Implementation includes addressing legislation and remuneration barriers, employing targeted education techniques, local planning with

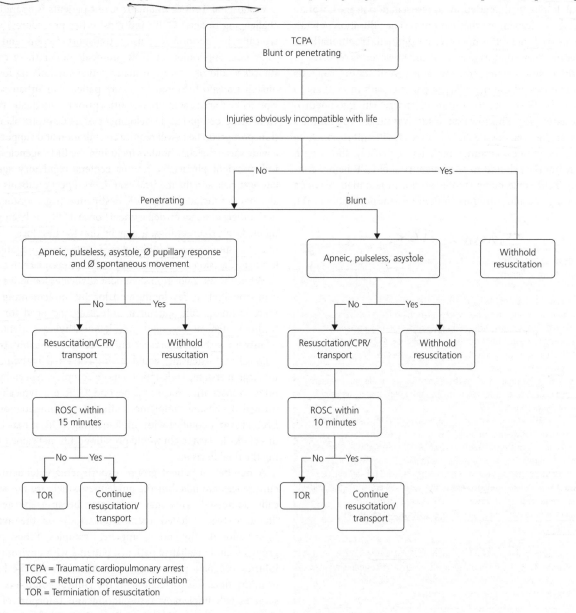

Figure 65.1 Clinical flow chart outlining the key components of the 2012 NAEMSP-ASCOT position statement on withholding or termination of resuscitation in traumatic cardiopulmonary arrest.

local authorities who share responsibility for death notification in the community (police, ambulance, fire, emergency departments, primary care physicians, and coroner's office) and engaging the physicians involved in direct medical oversight to assure common understanding, agreement, adoption, and adherence. All other cardiac arrests of a unique and obvious non-traumatic etiology such as near-drowning or overdose who fit the criteria to start resuscitation should be transported with ongoing resuscitation to benefit from etiology-specific interventions.

In the case of pediatric OHCA, there is a paucity of literature informing when to start and when to stop. Without signs of obvious death as defined by a medical directive, EMS personnel should attempt resuscitation in all cases of pediatric cardiac arrest. Factors such as unwitnessed arrests, non-shockable rhythms, and longer resuscitative efforts are all associated with poor outcomes; however, there are currently no accurate determinants of futility in pediatric cardiac arrests. Adult TOR guidelines have not been validated in the pediatric population and current cardiac arrest guidelines do not support the use of specific criteria to terminate resuscitation. Due to a lack of research examining pediatric TOR, each case should be examined on an individual basis in consultation with medical oversight, or transported to the hospital with continued resuscitation.

The science on when to withhold or terminate resuscitation of traumatic patients is less defined than for non-traumatic OHCA. All evidence is observational and has not been subjected to a clinical decision rule analysis. There appears to be no single clinical finding that universally distinguishes between survivors and non-survivors from either blunt or penetrating traumatic arrest. Recently updated guidelines have been published that provide a working tool for EMS medical directors to develop protocols to address these issues. A clinical flow chart outlining the key components of the 2012 NAEMSP-ASCOT position statement on withholding or termination of resuscitation in traumatic cardiopulmonary arrest is illustrated in Figure 65.1.

References

1 Eckstein M, Stratton SJ, Chan LS. Termination of resuscitative efforts for out-of-hospital cardiac arrests. *Acad Emerg Med* 2005;12:65–70.
2 Uniform Determination of Death Act. Available at: www.uniformlaws.org
3 Morrison LJ, Nichol G, Rea TD, et al. Rationale, development and implementation of the Resuscitation Outcomes Consortium Epistry-Cardiac Arrest. *Resuscitation* 2008;78:161–9.
4 Wright AA, Zhang B, Ray A, et al. Associations between end-of-life discussions, patient mental health, medical care near death, and caregiver bereavement adjustment. *JAMA* 2008;300:1665–73.
5 Cerminara KL, Bogin SM. A paper about a piece of paper. Regulatory action as the most effective way to promote use of physician orders for life-sustaining treatment. *J Legal Med* 2008;29:479–503.
6 Payne JK, Thornlow DK. Clinical perspectives on portable do-not-resuscitate orders. *J Gerontol Nurs* 2008;34:11–16.
7 Feder S, Matheny RL, Loveless RS Jr, Rea TD. Withholding resuscitation: a new approach to prehospital end-of-life decisions. *Ann Intern Med* 2006;144:634–40.
8 Kellermann A, Lynn J. Withholding resuscitation in prehospital care. *Ann Intern Med* 2006;144:692–3.
9 Schneiderman LJ, Jecker NS, Jonsen AR. Medical futility: its meaning and ethical implications. *Ann Intern Med* 1990;112:949–54.
10 Morrison LJ, Visentin LM, Kiss A, et al. Validation of a rule for termination of resuscitation in out-of-hospital cardiac arrest. *N Engl J Med* 2006;355:478–87.
11 Richman PB, Vadeboncoeur TF, Chikani V, et al. Independent evaluation of an out-of-hospital termination of resuscitation (TOR) clinical decision rule. *Acad Emerg Med* 2008;15:517–21.
12 Morrison LJ, Verbeek PR, Zhan C, et al. Validation of a universal prehospital termination of resuscitation clinical prediction rule for advanced and basic life support providers. *Resuscitation*. 2009;80:324–8.
13 Sasson C, Hegg AJ, Macy M, et al. Prehospital termination of resuscitation in cases of refractory out-of-hospital cardiac arrest. *JAMA* 2008;300:1432–8.
14 Ong ME, Jaffey J, Stiell I, Nesbitt L. Comparison of termination-of-resuscitation guidelines for basic life support: defibrillator providers in out-of-hospital cardiac arrest. *Ann Emerg Med* 2006;47:337–43.
15 Ruygrok ML, Byyny RL, Haukoos JS. Validation of 3 termination of resuscitation criteria for good neurologic survival after out-of-hospital cardiac arrest. *Ann Emerg Med* 2009;54:239–47.
16 Skrifvars MB, Vayrynen T, Kuisma M, et al. Comparison of Helsinki and European Resuscitation Council "do not attempt to resuscitate" guidelines, and a termination of resuscitation clinical prediction rule for out-of-hospital cardiac arrest patients found in asystole or pulseless electrical activity. *Resuscitation* 2010;81:679–84.
17 Morrison LJ, Kierzek G, Diekema DS, et al. Part 3: ethics: 2010 American Heart Association Guidelines for Cardiopulmonary Resuscitation and Emergency Cardiovascular Care. *Circulation* 2010;122:S665–75.
18 Millin MG, Khandker SR, Malki A. Termination of resuscitation in nontraumatic cardiopulmonary arrest. *Prehosp Emerg Care* 2011;15:542.
19 Berg RA, Hemphill R, Abella BS, et al. Part 5: adult basic life support: 2010 American Heart Association Guidelines for Cardiopulmonary Resuscitation and Emergency Cardiovascular Care. *Circulation* 2010;122:S685–705.
20 Neumar RW, Otto CW, Link MS, et al. Part 8: adult advanced cardiovascular life support: 2010 American Heart Association Guidelines for Cardiopulmonary Resuscitation and Emergency Cardiovascular Care. *Circulation* 2010;122:S729–67.
21 Sasson C, Forman J, Krass D, et al. A qualitative study to identify barriers to local implementation of prehospital termination of resuscitation protocols. *Circ Cardiovasc Qual Outcomes* 2009;2:361–8.
22 Drennan I, Lin S, Sidalak D, Morrison LJ. Survival in out-of-hospital cardiac arrest patients without a prehospital return of spontaneous circulation. *Circulation* 2012;126:A195.
23 Morrison LJ, Verbeek PR, Vermeulen MJ, et al. Derivation and evaluation of a termination of resuscitation clinical prediction rule for advanced life support providers. *Resuscitation* 2007;74:266–75.

24 Hall WL 2nd, Myers JH, Pepe PE, et al. The perspective of paramedics about on-scene termination of resuscitation efforts for pediatric patients. *Resuscitation* 2004;60:175–87.

25 Delbridge TR, Fosnocht DE, Garrison HG, Auble TE. Field termination of unsuccessful out-of-hospital cardiac arrest resuscitation: acceptance by family members. *Ann Emerg Med* 1996;27:649–54.

26 Edwardsen EA, Chiumento S, Davis E. Family perspective of medical care and grief support after field termination by emergency medical services personnel: a preliminary report. *Prehosp Emerg Care* 2002;6:440–4.

27 Schmidt TA, Harrahill MA. Family response to out-of-hospital death. *Acad Emerg Med* 1995;2:513–18.

28 Donoghue AJ, Nadkarni V, Berg RA, et al. Out-of-hospital pediatric cardiac arrest: an epidemiologic review and assessment of current knowledge. *Ann Emerg Med* 2005;46:512–22.

29 Sirbaugh PE, Pepe PE, Shook JE, et al. A prospective, population-based study of the demographics, epidemiology, management, and outcome of out-of-hospital pediatric cardiopulmonary arrest. *Ann Emerg Med* 1999;33:174–84.

30 Atkins DL, Everson-Stewart S, Sears GK, et al. Epidemiology and outcomes from out-of-hospital cardiac arrest in children: the Resuscitation Outcomes Consortium Epistry – Cardiac Arrest. *Circulation* 2009;119:1484–91.

31 Young KD, Gausche-Hill M, McClung CD, Lewis RJ. A prospective, population-based study of the epidemiology and outcome of out-of-hospital pediatric cardiopulmonary arrest. *Pediatrics* 2004; 114:157–64.

32 Kaneko H, Hatanaka T, Nagase A, et al. Children perform better than adults after out-of-hospital cardiac arrest. *Resuscitation* 2012;83:e31.

33 Nadkarni VM, Larkin GL, Peberdy MA, et al. First documented rhythm and clinical outcome from in-hospital cardiac arrest among children and adults. *JAMA* 2006;295:50–7.

34 Moler FW, Donaldson AE, Meert K, et al. Multicenter cohort study of out-of-hospital pediatric cardiac arrest. *Crit Care Med* 2011; 39:141–9.

35 Schindler MB, Bohn D, Cox PN, et al. Outcome of out-of-hospital cardiac or respiratory arrest in children. *N Engl J Med* 1996;335:1473–9.

36 Li CJ, Kung CT, Liu BM, et al. Factors associated with sustained return of spontaneous circulation in children after out-of-hospital cardiac arrest of noncardiac origin. *Am J Emerg Med* 2010;28:310–17.

37 Lopez-Herce J, Garcia C, Dominguez P, et al. Outcome of out-of-hospital cardiorespiratory arrest in children. *Pediatr Emerg Care* 2005;21:807–15.

38 Bernard SA, Gray TW, Buist MD, et al. Treatment of comatose survivors of out-of-hospital cardiac arrest with induced hypothermia. *N Engl J Med* 2002;346:557–63.

39 Morris MC, Ittenbach RF, Godinez RI, et al. Risk factors for mortality in 137 pediatric cardiac intensive care unit patients managed with extracorporeal membrane oxygenation. *Crit Care Med* 2004;32:1061–9.

40 Thalmann M, Trampitsch E, Haberfellner N, et al. Resuscitation in near drowning with extracorporeal membrane oxygenation. *Ann Thorac Surg* 2001;72:607–8.

41 Medical, moral, legal, and ethical aspects of resuscitation for the patient who will have minimal ability to function or ultimately survive. American College of Emergency Physicians, Dallas, Texas. *Ann Emerg Med* 1985;14:919–26.

42 Melltorp G, Nilstun T. The difference between withholding and withdrawing life-sustaining treatment. *Intensive Care Med* 1997; 23:1264–7.

43 Millin MG, Khandker SR, Malki A. Termination of resuscitation of nontraumatic cardiopulmonary arrest: resource document for the National Association of EMS Physicians position statement. *Prehosp Emerg Care* 2011;15:547–54.

44 Lippert FK, Raffay V, Georgiou M, et al. European Resuscitation Council Guidelines for Resuscitation 2010 Section 10. The ethics of resuscitation and end-of-life decisions. *Resuscitation* 2010;81:1445–51.

45 Millin MG, Galvagno SM, Khandker SR, et al. Withholding and termination of resuscitation of adult cardiopulmonary arrest secondary to trauma: Resource document to the joint NAEMSP-ACSCOT position statements. *J Trauma Acute Care Surg* 2013;75:459–67.

46 Pickens JJ, Copass MK, Bulger EM. Trauma patients receiving CPR: predictors of survival. *J Trauma* 2005;58:951–8.

47 Aprahamian C, Darin JC, Thompson BM, et al. Traumatic cardiac arrest: scope of paramedic services. *Ann Emerg Med* 1985;14:583–6.

48 Esposito TJ, Jurkovich GJ, Rice CL, et al. Reappraisal of emergency room thoracotomy in a changing environment. *J Trauma* 1991; 31:881–5; discussion 885–7.

49 Stratton SJ, Brickett K, Crammer T. Prehospital pulseless, unconscious penetrating trauma victims: field assessments associated with survival. *J Trauma* 1998;45:96–100.

50 Battistella FD, Nugent W, Owings JT, Anderson JT. Field triage of the pulseless trauma patient. *Arch Surg* 1999;134:742–5; discussion 745–6.

51 Powell DW, Moore EE, Cothren CC, et al. Is emergency department resuscitative thoracotomy futile care for the critically injured patient requiring prehospital cardiopulmonary resuscitation? *J Am Coll Surg* 2004;199:211–15.

52 Seamon MJ, Fisher CA, Gaughan JP, et al. Emergency department thoracotomy: survival of the least expected. *World J Surg* 2008; 32:604–12.

53 Moore EE, Knudson MM, Burlew CC, et al. Defining the limits of resuscitative emergency department thoracotomy: a contemporary Western Trauma Association perspective. *J Trauma* 2011; 70:334–9.

54 Fulton RL, Voigt WJ, Hilakos AS. Confusion surrounding the treatment of traumatic cardiac arrest. *J Am Coll Surg* 1995;181:209–14.

55 Pasquale MD, Rhodes M, Cipolle MD, et al. Defining "dead on arrival": impact on a level I trauma center. *J Trauma* 1996;41:726–30.

56 Moriwaki Y, Sugiyama M, Toyoda H, et al. Cardiopulmonary arrest on arrival due to penetrating trauma. *Ann R Coll Surg Engl* 2010; 92:142–6.

57 Mollberg NM, Glenn C, John J, et al. Appropriate use of emergency department thoracotomy: implications for the thoracic surgeon. *Ann Thorac Surg* 2011;92:455–61.

58 Rhee PM, Acosta J, Bridgeman A, et al. Survival after emergency department thoracotomy: review of published data from the past 25 years. *J Am Coll Surg* 2000;190:288–98.

59 Deasy C, Bray J, Smith K, et al. Traumatic out-of-hospital cardiac arrests in Melbourne, Australia. *Resuscitation* 2012;83:465–70.

60 Hopson LR, Hirsh E, Delgado J, et al. Guidelines for withholding or termination of resuscitation in prehospital traumatic cardiopulmonary arrest: joint position statement of the National Association of EMS Physicians and the American College of Surgeons Committee on Trauma. *J Am Coll Surg* 2003;196:106–12.

61 National Association of EMS Physicians and American College of Surgeons Committee on Trauma. Termination of resuscitation for adult traumatic cardiopulmonary arrest. *Prehosp Emerg Care* 2012;16:571.

62 National Association of EMS Physicians and American College of Surgeons Committee on Trauma. Withholding of resuscitation

for adult traumatic cardiopulmonary arrest. *Prehosp Emerg Care* 2013;17:291.

63 Brywczynski J, McKinney J, Pepe PE, et al. Emergency medical services transport decisions in posttraumatic circulatory arrest: are national practices congruent? *J Trauma* 2010;69:1154–9; discussion 60.

CHAPTER 66

Family and bystanders

Lynne Dees

Introduction

By its nature, EMS has been a reactive profession in that emergency responders have been prepared to respond quickly and work efficiently to attend to ill and injured individuals. A focus upon good health practices, including patient and family education and injury and illness prevention, has not yet become a vital mission in the profession. In addition, the lack of attention to social consequences of chronic illness in initial physician education [1] and the psychosocial aspects of health and illness has produced a similar void in paramedic education. Although most EMS providers acquire familiarity with patient psychology through street experience, social issues such as those involving family, social isolation, bystanders, and cultural sensitivity have been given short shrift in the education of EMS professionals.

Family support in patient care

Communication with and inclusion of family members is a topic in medical education that has not previously been a significant focus. Hartmann et al. [2] noted that training medical students and physicians in communicating with families is an essential task for the future. Families are increasingly involved in patient decision making. Similarly, family dynamics is usually not addressed in EMS education, particularly the differences in ethnic groups. Overall, EMS trainees rarely receive in-depth information regarding various cultural beliefs about health and illness, the sick role, and attitudes about health care providers.

Emergency medical services students have been taught almost exclusively what to do *to* patients, suggesting that all are *in extremis*. However, patient care involves more than medical knowledge and technical expertise. Talking to patients has served the sole purpose of accessing the history and chief complaint and then for advising the patient of procedures that would be performed. Establishing rapport and reaching common ground were absent in the repertoire of yesterday's paramedics and EMTs. EMS courses similarly lacked information regarding

communication with families. Providers were taught how to assertively inform family members that a loved one had died, but otherwise, interacting with and incorporating the family into patient care decisions has been limited to enlisting their help in convincing an unwilling patient who needed to go to the hospital or querying about history and medications in the unresponsive patient. EMS should now adopt trends seen in other medical settings. "The core features of family-centered health care are the acknowledgment of the unique strengths, resources and needs of all family members, and the emphasis placed on partnership between the patient, the family, the doctor and other service providers" [1]. No longer is the emphasis upon what is done *to* the patient, but what medical personnel can do *for* the patient, family, and other caregivers, all working as a team.

The threshold for accessing EMS is lower than for other medical professionals, excepting perhaps family physicians and/or the emergency department. EMS may be the first and only contact with a medical professional for a variety of chronic and/or acute patient misfortunes and therefore is considered one component in the health care safety net [3,4]. Even so, EMS providers tend to "scoop and run" and historically have not established short- or long-term relationships with their patients, families, and/or caregivers. However, as primary care providers have discovered, engaging the patient's family may be of assistance in several ways. First, it may engage those who can provide support to the patient, whether by monitoring diet and adherence to a medicine regime, serving as watchdogs for specific signs and symptoms of a worsening condition, or by creating a safer, more pleasant, and healthier environment for the patient. Second, acknowledging the family establishes trust and exhibits good will in caring for the patient. One of the normative cultural values in the Latino culture is *personalismo*, which refers to warm, personal relationships, including those expected with the physician or medical provider [5]. Finally, family-centered involvement solidifies the continuum of care and creates a cohesive unit whereby strength is achieved through larger numbers of individuals focused upon the patient's best interest.

Emergency Medical Services: Clinical Practice and Systems Oversight, Second Edition. Volume 1: Clinical Aspects of EMS.
Edited by David C. Cone, Jane H. Brice, Theodore R. Delbridge, and J. Brent Myers.
© 2015 NAEMSP. Published 2015 by John Wiley & Sons, Inc. Companion Website: www.wiley.com\go\cone\naemsp

In 2010, 56.7 million people or 18.7% of the US population were living with disabilities [6]. In addition to coordination of care between medical providers, coordination of care should also include the families and other caretakers of these patients [7]. EMS providers are frequently dependent upon families and caretakers of patients for information and history and occasionally must deal with multiple family members, not all of whom necessarily agree on their family member's care or who may not be equally informed. Coordination of patient care often requires medical personnel to interact with more than one family member, particularly for pediatric or impaired patients. Often, the EMS providers' management of the patient includes the decisions of the medical power of attorney. As a member of the health care team, EMS providers must work to improve communication in their arena of care. Even in an emergency setting, use of appropriate principles of interviewing and conversation with patients and their families can guide the EMT and paramedic toward relevant clinical decisions.

For those patients who are technology dependent or have special needs, and for those with chronic or terminal illnesses being cared for at home, family members provide a rich resource of information regarding that which is normal for their loved one, including level of consciousness, color, respiratory status, or vital signs. Increasing numbers of patients are being cared for at home rather than in institutions, and their caretakers are taught how to perform skills and troubleshoot devices such as tracheostomies, IV pumps, urinary catheters, and ventilators. In addition, implanted devices such as defibrillators, pacemakers, and left ventricular assist devices and procedures such as peritoneal dialysis are increasingly encountered by EMS providers responding to 9-1-1 calls. Although in-depth knowledge of the technology that supports these patients may be out of the scope of training for the EMT and paramedic, he or she should rely upon family members or other caretakers for assistance in managing these devices and/or patients. As an integral member of the health care team, the EMS provider should not view requesting assistance or information from the patient or patient's care provider regarding unfamiliar technology as a point of incompetence, but rather as an overlap in the team approach to patient care.

The inclusion of family members in patient decisions and care is paramount to improving a patient's health. However, the EMS professional should proceed cautiously while gathering patient information from the family or caregiver. Family members may insist that they are familiar with the patient's recent activities or medical history, and may possess inaccurate or irrelevant information for the current emergency problem, thus incorrectly shaping the paramedic's diagnosis and treatment [8]. Therefore, the EMS provider must filter incoming information and temper the influence of family members in order to avoid tunnel vision. Finally, a dispute between the patient and some or all family members may create friction and disagreement at the scene. In this setting of conflict, the EMT or paramedic must make sense out of the dynamics, avoid taking sides, identify each person's agenda, and orchestrate the scene in order to reach common ground [9].

Even with family present, a patient has rights of autonomy, confidentiality, and privacy. A frustrating situation for EMS providers includes the scenario where the family adamantly directs the EMS crew to treat and/or transport their loved one while the cognizant and competent patient refuses assistance. Furthermore, a patient may not want his health information or condition revealed to other family members. Adolescent patients may not wish to discuss their sexual or substance use histories in the presence of parents. Even pediatric patients may not admit the truth surrounding an incident for fear of punishment. A family member, just because of his or her relationship with the patient, is not automatically entitled to medical information regarding an ill or injured spouse and may not understand the legal ramifications involved.

Conversely, the family may not want the patient's condition revealed to the patient him- or herself, such as in the case of late-stage cancer, as seen in some Asian, Jewish, Italian, Navajo, Pakistani, and Hispanic communities [10] where cancer is seen as a curse and a social stigma [11]. Many cultures value family-based decisions over autonomy for management of the patient, although patient autonomy is currently the prevailing norm in the United States. *Familismo* in the Latino culture is loyalty to the family and priority over the individual [5], a viewpoint seen also in Middle Eastern and Japanese cultures [12], among others. EMS providers should consider this cultural viewpoint when family members are present during patient contact.

Despite the maturing of the EMS profession from its modern beginnings in the 1960s, this cohort remains mostly Anglo and male. Recent demographics for EMS providers in the United States include 75% Caucasians and 72% males [13]. In contrast, by mid-century, Caucasian European descendants will begin to constitute a population minority [14]. The current population majority in the United States is shifting toward a diverse mix of individuals from various cultures, ethnicities, races, and faiths.

Understanding family relationships forms the foundation for integration of family into patient care. Family dynamics vary depending upon culture, ethnicity, socioeconomic and educational level, and even geographical location. In some families, love is synonymous with dependence and closeness while in other families, love is expressed by allowing members to be independent [15]. The presence of family at the emergency scene simultaneously presents a unique opportunity and a challenge. Many EMS providers have felt frustration when attempting to interview and assess a patient while a roomful of chattering relatives looms at elbow's length and answers questions for the patient. Such behavior may result from the patient's culture and/or upbringing. Most patient-to-EMT contact occurs within a personal and intimate distance of 4 feet, which is the norm for the middle-class Anglo culture. However, other cultures and ethnic groups favor a much closer personal space, which may unnerve the EMT. Large, extended families such as the Roma (Gypsies) may cluster around the patient at arm's length to provide support [16].

Family dynamics as well as health beliefs are affected by culture. Paternalism exists in many Middle Eastern and Latino cultures, and Asian and Romani cultures revere their elders [10,16]. Therefore, the EMT may need to address the male figurehead or elder, while in certain matriarchal African cultures the oldest female may serve as the patient's spokesperson. In situations relating to women's problems, a female family member may be included in the history taking. The EMS provider should be aware that the cultural mores of a traditional Muslim female patient prohibit examination by a male medical provider.

Cultural competency refers to possessing knowledge and awareness of and respect for other cultures and ethnic groups [17]. An individual's culture has a direct effect upon health beliefs, values, and practices. Culture also shapes patients' and families' confidence in and viewpoint of modern medicine and health care professionals. The EMS medical director can promote cultural sensitivity and competency by encouraging EMS providers of different races and ethnicities to disseminate information about their culture/race to the other providers along with appropriate continuing education, exposure to, and discussion of different ethnicities and cultural beliefs.

Social isolation

Human beings are social creatures, even in individualistic societies such as the United States, which may be a survival mechanism lingering from the early days of mankind. Survival improved when individuals lived with and depended upon each other during times of duress and lack of food. Propagation of the species depended upon survival at least to reproductive age. In modern society, social ties continue to support survival in hard times [18] and may also forestall morbidity and mortality. Compared to time spent on other daily activities, individuals report being happiest when socializing and relaxing with friends and intimate partners [19]. The human desire for social interaction is so prevalent that people regularly devise perceived and non-reciprocal relationships with characters in books, movies, video games, and even deities [20].

Interest in the effect of social ties upon health has experienced a dramatic surge since the mid-1970s [21,22] although recognition of the social environment as a factor affecting health stems from Hippocrates [23]. Clinical risk factors have long been associated with mortality, including modifiable factors such as tobacco use, hypertension, sedentary lifestyle, obesity, and hypercholesterolemia. However, social isolation has emerged as a contributory risk factor as overwhelming as unhealthy lifestyle choices and disease. Berkman and Syme [24] found that the mortality risks for men and women who lacked social and community ties reached 2.3 and 2.8 respectively. A recent study with 16,849 non-institutionalized adult participants identified social isolation, determined by being unmarried, not affiliated with clubs or organizations, having infrequent social contact and infrequent participation in religious activities, as predicting early demise [25]. Low levels of social support have been found to be associated with an increase of unhealthy lifestyles [26] and a greater incidence of suicide ideation [27]. Why do social ties mitigate morbidity and mortality? Social ties may simply help to buffer life's stresses, and social interaction may encourage individuals to follow socially accepted health principles such as regular doctor visits, preventive health practices, exercise, abstinence from tobacco use, and reduced ingestion of alcohol.

What exactly is social isolation? Seeman [22] defined it as disengagement from social ties, institutional connections, or community participation. The terms *socially isolated* and *lonely* are not necessarily synonymous; rather, loneliness may be more accurately synonymous with *perceived* social isolation. Loneliness has been described as the social equivalent of physical pain, hunger, and thirst [20]. Several studies have identified *perceived* social isolation or loneliness as more contributory to poor health and increased mortality than physical social isolation [18,20,28,29]. Whereas a socially isolated individual may not feel at all lonely, a lonely person may actually be surrounded by attentive family and friends. A patient's perception may predict negative health issues more closely than actual circumstances.

Social isolation and poor physical health influence each other. Individuals may become socially isolated due to another cause such as increased age, frailty, immobilization, illness, mental deficiencies, disfigurement, social marginality, remote location, poverty, language barrier, or lack of education. Chronic conditions and worsening health may lead to social isolation as the patient becomes less mobile and less likely to participate in activities with others. Isolated patients may experience time distortion which affects their sleep-wake cycle, appetite and eating habits, or taking of prescribed medications, all of which ultimately worsen both physical and mental health. Physical barriers may also exacerbate social isolation. Factors such as stairs, heavy doors, inability to ambulate, lack of transportation, absence of nearby supermarkets and pharmacies, or residence in a high crime area or a remote location may further isolate an individual.

Conversely, a patient's inherent social isolation or perception of loneliness may contribute to physical or mental illness which worsens and ultimately perpetuates into increased social isolation. The individual may ultimately feel social demise as he or she moves farther from fulfilling a valued role in the community and/or family [30].

The population in the United States is aging; in 2011, 73.5% were under the age of 55 while 26.5% were 55 and over [31]. Additionally, the number of persons 80 years old and over is projected to double by 2050 [32]. Hence, senior citizens are poised to represent the largest sector of socially isolated individuals due to their increased risk of health issues, potential lack of mobility, and loss of their social support system, whether it includes friends, family members, or work colleagues who reduce or curtail contact, move away, or die.

In addition, the increasing number of special needs patients may represent a unique category of isolated individuals. In 2010, 56.7 million individuals in the US possessed a disability [6]. Both patients with disabilities along with the families caring for them may become victims of social isolation, because of difficulty motivating, marginalization due to the disability, or lack of time to socialize due to continual or complex patient care.

In 2009 in the US, there were an estimated 36,698,670 EMS responses [33]. Emergency providers often represent the first point of contact in an individual's access of the health care system. In the EMS setting, exploration of a patient's social history has not been included in initial paramedic education curricula. However, the identification of sociological factors has now become one of the essential assessment steps of the responding EMT and/or paramedic. The National EMS Education Standards [34] include psychosocial assessment for patients , specifically in the geriatric and other special patient populations. Assessment and management of sociological factors are becoming more important for improving and maintaining health.

In 2011, the US continued to lead the world in health care costs per capita, at $8508 [32]. Costly hospital admissions and readmissions in addition to frequent non-essential summoning of the 9-1-1 EMS system are at last being addressed. The patient who appropriately manages his or her health and complies with prescribed diet, medications, and physical activity often does so with social support. Attentiveness and adherence to a prescribed medical regime represent the primary step in not only cost-cutting but also the patient's immediate and long-term well-being.

Emergency medical services providers are in an opportune position to recognize social isolation while on scene of an emergency or during a home visit. Community paramedics can either access assistance for the patient or relate significant findings of the social history assessment to the receiving facility, which may ultimately lead to definitive management. EMS personnel have informally promoted health while operating on emergency runs, such as illustrating to parents how to secure their children in child safety seats, identifying household hazards to patients and their families, or correcting erroneous health myths. Health promotion may be achieved in a variety of ways. While O'Donnell [35] identified health promotion as the science and art of assisting individuals in changing their lifestyles to promote optimum health, the Ottawa Charter for Health Promotion [36] cites health promotion as creating environments conducive to healthy behaviors. Paramedics, in the mobile health care setting, are positioned to recognize both lifestyle and environmental obstacles to good health.

The medical director sets the standard, culture, and environment for EMS providers in his or her system. Proactive steps taken by the medical director can prepare the providers for success in identifying socially isolated individuals in their community. The National EMS Education Standards [34] include health screening and referrals as components of patient assessment along with knowledge of public health principles including epidemiology, health promotion, and illness and injury prevention. With the advent of expanded scope of care by providers such as community paramedics, interventions may be initiated at the level of street medicine.

In non-critical emergency responses where life and death interventions are not required, EMS providers could assess the patient's social history with instruments such as the Berkman-Syme Social Network Index (SNI), or modified SNI scale that focuses upon marriage/partnership, frequency of contact with friends and family, group membership, and frequency of religious participation [24]. The UCLA Loneliness Assessment [37] is a brief 20-question research instrument that paramedics may also utilize during home visits in non-critical situations.

Therapy for social isolation is beyond the current scope of training for EMS providers. The emergency setting in which EMS currently functions is not conducive to in-depth sociological or psychological interventions. However, EMS providers can communicate findings to appropriate contact persons who can then mobilize support services for those individuals who appear at high risk for undesired social isolation, with its physical and psychological ramifications. Referral should be made to community health workers, such as promotores who serve as community health workers in the Hispanic populations, or support groups such as Sisters in Support Together against Substances, Alcoholics Anonymous, Narcotics Anonymous, and Big Brothers Big Sisters. Most public health departments and hospitals maintain a list of social services available to community members in need. Finally, "2-1-1 US" is a system designed to assist individuals with access to health and human services in their communities [38]. Services provided include basic human necessities, support for older and disabled persons, and physical and mental health resources.

The EMS medical director should encourage development of assessment skills that encompass both the psyche as well as the physical self. In addition, observable clues to social isolation in the patient's affect and surroundings should be discussed. Finally, EMS providers should have opportunities to attend educational events and classes for exposure to specialists in the field of psychosocial health.

Bystanders

Nowhere in a medical delivery setting is the issue of bystanders more of a compelling consideration than in EMS. Unfortunately, bystander management is a topic that may not have been covered in initial EMS education. The unsecure setting of many EMS calls, including highways, businesses, schools, and street corners, lends itself to public involvement and potential interference in patient care. Providers may encounter difficulty in keeping bystanders out of the treatment area or scene. Safety concerns in EMS primarily focus upon the responders themselves and the patient. However, on-scene duties include the consideration of bystanders' safety and well-being. When a life hazard such as traffic, violence, or hazardous materials threatens the safety of onlookers, EMS personnel should summon law enforcement for assistance so that they may focus upon patient care.

One of the most perplexing situations for EMS personnel is the offer of assistance for or direction of patient care by a physician bystander. Self-identified medical personnel often offer assistance at the scene of an accident or sick person which places the EMT and paramedic in a difficult situation as they are likely unfamiliar with the individual and his or her credentials. EMS providers, although functioning under the guidance of a medical director who is likely an emergency medicine specialist, are often poorly prepared to manage the conflict of their responsibilities with an individual who possesses a higher level of medical training. Many feel intimidated by an on-scene physician, whether it is in person or via telephone. In fact, many paramedics view sending an on-scene physician away while managing a critical patient to be an extremely risky act. To complicate matters further, despite position statements by the American Medical Association (AMA), American College of Emergency Physicians (ACEP), and National Association of EMS Physicians (NAEMSP) regarding unsolicited medical personnel at emergency scenes, a vast majority of physicians are unfamiliar with these guidelines [39] and/or with the capabilities and responsibilities of EMS providers in general. Physicians who are not familiar with the EMS setting may not appreciate the Spartan nature of the prehospital environment. At times, the EMT and/or paramedic may be asked to follow orders by the patient's physician by telephone, which further complicates decision making.

Consider an especially difficult scenario for the EMS provider who is called to a patient in cardiac arrest but lacking in any definitive signs of death. Both the family present and the individual on the phone stating that she is the patient's primary care provider state that the patient has a Do Not Resuscitate order but the document is not present. Both the family and the patient's physician on the telephone are requesting that you do not begin resuscitative efforts. The situation has both ethical and legal ramifications for the EMS provider.

Physician presence on an EMS scene may also occur in clinic or office where the paramedics are summoned to transfer the patient to another facility such as the ED, nursing facility, or the patient's home. The physician may direct the EMS crew to perform patient procedures that are not in their standard of care or to transport the patient to a hospital which, in the EMTs' opinion, is not capable of managing the patient's condition or is not the closest appropriate facility. In some cases, the physician may advise the EMS crew to perform no patient care and to just transport the patient. A more disconcerting scenario is represented by a physician who is at a patient's side in a nonprofessional setting such as in a residence or on the golf course. Guidance for these types of scenarios should originate from the medical director and become part of the protocol or policies (Figure 66.1). Additionally, the medical director should guide

EMS providers as to how to manage bystander medical providers with respect and tact.

In some cases, consideration of the bystanders may affect the timing and/or location of detailed patient assessment and care. For example, injuries in settings such as restaurants, concerts, or public events may require quickly moving the patient to a more private area such as the ambulance before administering definitive care. Dramatic injuries occurring in front of sporting event crowds require EMTs to modify procedures in consideration of that which is not only best for the patient, but also for the coaches, team mates, family, and spectators [40]. In settings such as rodeos and contact sports, the injured participant may insist upon walking out of the arena rather than being carried on a stretcher. In part, this action is for the benefit of the spectators and team mates.

While it may be advantageous to dismiss bystanders, they may actually provide crucially needed assistance at an emergency scene. Much has been written about the bystander effect, a phenomenon where the presence of other bystanders decreases the probability that an individual will assist in a critical situation [41,42]. However, Fischer et al. [43] found that a bystander was more likely to assist if (a) there were larger numbers of bystanders, (b) the bystanders were all males, (c) the bystanders were strangers to each other, and (d) if the bystander perceived a high cost for intervening to him- or herself. However, a paucity of research exists regarding bystander involvement in conjunction with the presence of emergency responders. Anecdotally, most EMS providers could more likely recount situations where they had been inundated with helpful bystanders than not. If bystander assistance is enlisted, EMS providers must maintain patient confidentiality and privacy. Emergency personnel should remember that spectators often photograph or videotape scene activities. EMS should strive to protect patients' privacy, especially in the case where it may be impossible to move the patient to a more secure area.

Bystanders may also be helpful in recounting the history of an event or in locating involved individuals who may have left the scene prior to the arrival of EMS. Neighbors may offer additional information about when a shut-in patient was last seen. If adequate rescue personnel are present, one of them should take charge of talking to bystanders to elicit information while other rescuers provide patient care. Using this approach will assist in bystander management and keep them out of the way of the rescuers.

Bystanders, even though well-meaning, may be injured while wandering into a dangerous scene or into traffic. In any situation, an onlooker may become a patient him- or herself, due to injury or to fainting or suffering a medical emergency. Additionally, while potentially interfering with patient care, they may become hostile toward the rescuers, especially on a volatile or grisly scene or one involving extreme levels of grief (Figure 66.2). Bystander responses may be driven by their knowledge level and/or culture. Unfortunately, little written guidance exists regarding management of and communication with bystanders,

On-scene physician form

This EMS service would like to thank you for your effort and assistance. Please be advised that the EMS Professionals are operating under strict protocols and guidelines established by their medical director and the State of North Carolina. As a licensed physician, you may assume medical care of the patient. In order to do so, you will need to:

1. Receive approval to assume the patient's medical care from the EMS agencies online medical control physician.
2. Show proper identification including current North Carolina Medical Board Registration/ Licensure.
3. Accompany the patient to the hospital.
4. Carry out any interventions that do not conform to the EMS agencies protocols. EMS personnel cannot perform any interventions or administer medications that are not included in their protocols.
5. Sign all orders on the EMS Patient Care Report.
6. Assume all medico-legal responsibility for all patient care activities until the patient's care is transferred to another physician at the destination hospital.
7. Complete the "Assumption of Medical Care" section of this form below

Assumption of medical care

I, _____ ,MD; License #: _____ ,
    (Please print your name Here)

have assumed authority and responsibility for the medical care and patient management for

_____ .
                    (Insert patient's name here)

I understand that I must accompany the patient to the emergency department. I further understand that all EMS personnel must follow north carolina EMS rules and regulations as well as local EMS system protocols.

_____ , MD Date: _____ / _____ / _____ Time: _____ AM/PM
    (Physician signature here)

_____ , EMS   _____ Witness
    (EMS lead crew member signature here)   **(Witness signature here)**

Figure 66.1 Form for on-scene physicians. Source: North Carolina Chapter, American College of Emergency Physicians. Reproduced with permission of North Carolina Chapter, American College of Emergency Physicians.

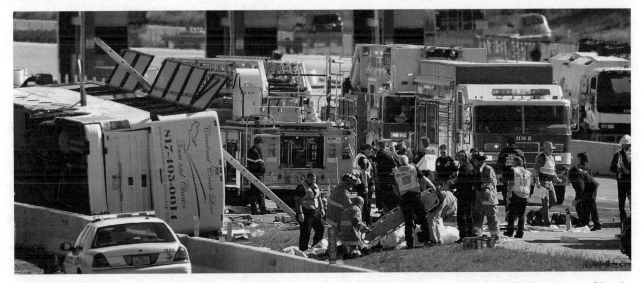

Figure 66.2 Mass casualty scenes attract large numbers of bystanders. Source: Tom Fox, The Dallas Morning News. Reproduced with permission of Tom Fox.

including mobilizing and enlisting their cooperation. When appropriate, EMS providers should use the same principles of mutual respect, tolerance, and clear, concise communication that are used with patients and their families.

Finally, bystander physicians and onlookers at emergency scenes present specific challenges for rescue personnel above and beyond their primary concern of patient care. Although bystanders may require management, organization, and, at times, removal from the scene, they may prove invaluable in settings with large numbers of sick or injured such as a natural or man-made disaster scene. EMS systems and medical directors should proactively prepare for integration of physicians and other medically trained bystanders to assist in these cases, and also to provide education regarding bystander management for the more routine EMS calls.

References

1 Gorter JW, Visser-Meily A, Ketelaar M. The relevance of family-centered medicine and the implications for doctor education. *Med Educ* 2010;44:332–4.

2 Hartmann M, Bäzner E, Wild B, et al. Effects of interventions involving the family in the treatment of adult patients with chronic physical diseases: a meta-analysis. *Psychother Psychosom* 2010;79:136–48.

3 Cooney DR, Millin MG, Carter A, et al. Ambulance diversion and emergency department offload delay: resource document for the National Association of EMS Physicians position statement. *Prehosp Emerg Care* 2011;15:555–61.

4 Taylor TB. Threats to the health care safety net. *Acad Emerg Med* 2001;8(11):1080–7.

5 Flores G. Culture and the patient–physician relationship: achieving cultural competency in health care. *J Pediatr* 2000;136(1):14–23.

6 US Census Bureau. Americans with disabilities: 2010. Available at: www.census.gov/prod/2012pubs/p70-131.pdf

7 Bodenheimer T. Coordinating care, a perilous journey through the health care system. *N Engl J Med* 2008;358:1064–71.

8 Henderson AC. Patient assessment in emergency medical services: complexity and uncertainty in street-level patient processing. *J Health Hum Serv Adm* 2013;35:505–42.

9 Lang F, Marvel K, Sanders D, et al. Interviewing when family members are present. *Am Fam Physician* 2002;65:1351–4.

10 Searight HR, Gafford J. Cultural diversity at the end of life: issues and guidelines for family physicians. *Am Fam Physician* 2005;71:515–22.

11 Thomas VN, Saleem T, Abraham R. Barriers to effective uptake of cancer screening among Black and minority ethnic groups. *Int J Palliat Nurs* 2005;11:562–71.

12 Mobeireek AF, Al-Kassimi F, Al-Zahrani K, et al. Information disclosure and decision-making: the Middle East versus the Far East and the West. *J Med Ethics* 2008;34:225–9.

13 National Highway Traffic Safety Administration. EMS workforce for the 21st century: A final report. Available at: www.ems.gov/workforce.htm

14 Ikeda J, Wright J. Pediatrics in a culturally diverse society. *Pediatr Basics* 1998;85:12–25.

15 Biordi DL, Nicholson NR. Social isolation. In: Larsen PD, Lubkin IM (eds)*Chronic Illness: Impact and Intervention*, 7th edn. Sudbury, MA: Jones and Bartlett, 2009.

16 Vivian C, Dundes L. The crossroads of culture and health among the Roma (Gypsies). *J Nurs Scholarsh* 2004;36:86–91.

17 Juckett G. Cross-cultural medicine. *Am Fam Physician* 2005;72:2267–74.

18 Kelly BJ, Lewin TJ, Stain HJ, et al. Determinants of mental health and well-being within rural and remote communities. *Soc Psychiatry Psychiatr Epidemiol* 2011;46:1331–42.

19 Kahneman D, Krueger AB, Schkade DA, et al. A survey method for characterizing daily life experience: the day reconstruction method. *Science* 2004;306:1776–80.

20 Hawkley LC, Cacioppo JT. Loneliness matters: a theoretical and empirical review of consequences and mechanisms. *Ann Behav Med* 2010;40:218–27.

21 Seeman TE. Health promoting effects of friends and family on health outcomes in older adults. *Am J Health Promot* 2000;14:362–70.

22 Seeman TE. Social ties and health: the benefits of social integration. *Ann Epidemiol* 1996;6:442–51.

23 Dubos R. *Mirage of Health: Utopias, Progress, and Biological Change.* New York: Harper, 1959.

24 Berkman LF, Syme SL. Social networks, host resistance, and mortality: a nine-year follow-up study of Alameda County residents. *Am J Epidemiol* 1979;109:186–204.

25 Pantell M, Rehkopf D, Jutte D, et al. Social isolation: a predictor of mortality comparable to traditional clinical risk factors. *Am J Public Health* 2013;103:2056–62.

26 Piwoński J, Piwoński A, Sygnowska E. Is level of social support associated with health behaviors modifying cardiovascular risk? Results of the WOBASZ study. *Kardiol Pol* 2012;70:803–9.

27 Handley TE, Inder KJ, Kelly BJ, et al. You've got to have friends: the predictive value of social integration and support in suicidal ideation among rural communities. *Soc Psychiatry Psychiatr Epidemiol* 2012;47:1281–90.

28 Cacioppo JT, Hawkley LC, Norman G J, Berntson GG. Social isolation. *Ann NY Acad Sci* 2011;1231:17–22.

29 Wilson C, Moulton B. *Loneliness among Older Adults: A National Survey of Adults 45+*. Knowledge Networks and Insight Policy Research. Washington, DC: AARP, 2010.

30 Watson E. Dead to the world. *Nurs Times* 1988;84:52–4.

31 US Census Bureau. Selected social characteristics in the United States: American community survey 1 year estimates. Available at: http://factfinder2.census.gov/faces/nav/jsf/pages/index.xhtml

32 Organization for Economic Cooperation and Development. *Public Health Expenditure Per Capita.* Available at: www.oecd.org/els/health-systems/oecdhealthdata2013-frequentlyrequesteddata.htm

33 National Highway Traffic Safety Administration. *National EMS Assessment. EMS Update.* Available at: www.ems.gov/pdf/2012/Newsletter_Fall_2012.pdf

34 National Highway Traffic Safety Administration. *National Emergency Medical Services Education Standards.* US Department of Transportation. Available at: www.ems.gov/EducationStandards.htm

35 O'Donnell MP. Definition of health promotion: Part III: Expanding the definition. *Am J Health Promot* 1989;3:5.

36 Epp L. *Achieving Health for All: A Framework for Health Promotion in Canada.* Toronto: Health and Welfare, 1986.

37 Russell D. UCLA Loneliness Scale (Version 3): Reliability, validity, and factor structure. *J Pers Assess* 1996;66:20–40.

38 2-1-1-US. Available at: www.211us.org/about.htm

39 Barishansky RM, O'Connor K, Perkins TJ. Is there a doctor in the house? Addressing bystander physician involvement on scene. *EMS World*. Available at: www.emsworld.com/article/10324273/

40 Augustine JJ. Out at home. *EMS World*. Available at: www.emsworld.com/article/10320417/out-at-home

41 Darly JM, Latańe B. Bystander intervention in emergencies: diffusion of responsibility. *J Pers Soc Psychol* 1968;8:377–83.

42 Latańe B, Nida S. Ten years of research on group size and helping. *Psychol Bull* 1981;89:308–24.

43 Fischer P, Krueger JI, Greitemeyer T, et al. The bystander effect: a meta-analytic review on bystander intervention in dangerous and non-dangerous emergencies. *Psychol Bull* 2011;137:517–37.

CHAPTER 67

Analgesia

Michael T. Hilton and Paul M. Paris

Introduction

Pain and suffering are not confined within hospital boundaries. Pain is a common complaint of patients cared for by EMS providers. It is estimated that 20% of the approximately 15 million patients transported by EMS annually in the United States experience moderate-to-severe pain [1]. Although prehospital personnel are usually focused on the ABCs, the treatment of pain should be considered an important priority in the care of ill and injured patients [2,3].

Most studies of EMS analgesia practices show that many patients with moderate-to-severe pain do not receive analgesia in the prehospital phase of their care. NAEMSP currently recommends that EMS systems have a policy to address prehospital pain management [3]. The initial statement in NAEMSP position paper is, "NAEMSP believes that the relief of pain and suffering of our patients must be a priority for every EMS system. Adequate analgesia is an important step for achieving this goal. NAEMSP believes that every EMS system should have a clinical care protocol to address prehospital pain management. Adequate training and education of prehospital personnel and EMS physicians should support the pain management protocol." Prehospital pain protocols should address the following issues.

1 Mandate for pain assessment
2 Tools for pain measurement
3 Indications and contraindications for prehospital pain management
4 Non-pharmacological interventions for pain management
5 Pharmacological interventions for pain management
6 Patient monitoring and documentation before and after analgesia
7 Transferring information to the receiving medical facility [4]

The challenge of treating pain in the prehospital setting is to use agents and techniques that are not only effective but safe and do not lead to physiological compromise or a delay in diagnosis upon arrival in the ED [5,6]. Because of inordinate fears of "masking the diagnosis" and the desire to prevent side-effects, many EMS systems have opted for little or no use of pharmacological analgesics. Providing analgesia has been largely ignored in prehospital care education [1].

Few EMS texts devote significant attention to this topic. Many systems do not have protocols to treat pain and suffering, other than that from ischemic chest pain [7]. Many prehospital providers are frustrated by being unable to offer patients more than the "bite the bullet" approach to providing relief from acute pain. For those systems with reasonable analgesia protocols, the majority of patients are still untreated or undertreated. Many paramedic attitudes have been suggested as reasons for this inadequate treatment of pain [8].

Prehospital pain management is a fertile area for study. Current research topics include barriers to prehospital analgesia, interventions to address barriers, non-opioid alternative analgesics (e.g. ketamine, IV acetaminophen), and alternative routes for pain relief, such as intranasal and transmucosal routes that can be used by basic providers as well as field-based ultrasound-guided nerve blocks that can be useful in wilderness settings or in prolonged extrications [9].

Literature review

Several studies have shown that oligoanalgesia is more the rule than the exception in prehospital care. One of the most dramatic studies was performed by White et al. in the city of Akron in the late 1990s [10]. At that time, the EMS system had standing orders for either the administration of morphine sulfate, 2–5 mg IV push, or nitrous oxide, 50% self-administered. During the study period, 1,073 patients with suspected extremity fractures were identified. Of this large number of patients, only 18 received analgesia: 16 patients received nitrous oxide and two received morphine. McEachin reported on several different EMS agencies transporting patients to a single hospital in Michigan [11]. Of 124 patients suspected of having lower extremity fractures, only 22 (18.3%) received parenteral analgesia. Many of these patients (38.4%) were triaged from an ALS response to a BLS transport.

Emergency Medical Services: Clinical Practice and Systems Oversight, Second Edition. Volume 1: Clinical Aspects of EMS.
Edited by David C. Cone, Jane H. Brice, Theodore R. Delbridge, and J. Brent Myers.
© 2015 NAEMSP. Published 2015 by John Wiley & Sons, Inc. Companion Website: www.wiley.com\go\cone\naemsp

Hennes et al. reported results from prehospital analgesia practice in Milwaukee where a review of 5,383 patients with acute pain showed that morphine was administered in only 258 patients (4.8%) [12]. Of those patients with extremity fractures, 37 of 351 (10.5%) received morphine, and morphine was given to only seven of 258 children (3.0%). In patients with burn injury, 16 of 130 (12.3%) received morphine; only one of 12 children received it. Similar findings showing lack of analgesic administration or oligoanalgesia have been replicated in other studies [13,14].

The benefits of prehospital analgesia are not only physiological. It improves the perception of quality of care provided by EMS. One study showed that 80% of patients reported the overall quality of EMS care to be excellent when they rated their pain management as excellent. Prehospital analgesia also dramatically decreases the time-to-analgesic administration, ranging from 60 to 120 minutes earlier, when compared to analgesic administration being deferred to the emergency department [15–17].

Evans made the poignant statement, "To allow a patient to suffer unnecessary pain does harm to the patient – a violation of the first ethical principle of medicine" [18]. In a 1999 editorial, the late Peter Baskett states, "The blame for 'oligoanalgesia' must be laid at the door of physicians in authority who have, through ignorance, underplayed the physiologic and psychological benefits of analgesia and overplayed the potential of deleterious side effects of agents that are commonly available" [19].

Opioids

Opioids are the best class of pharmacological agents to treat acute pain in all areas of medicine, including the prehospital environment. (See Box 67.1 for a list of desirable characteristics, most but not all of which are found in the opioids.) Osler referred to opioids as "God's own medicine" [20]. The properties that make opioids desirable in the field include rapid onset, high potency, titrateability, relative safety, and reversibility. Morphine sulfate has been used for ischemic chest pain in the field for the past three decades. Over the past several years, fentanyl has gained increased usage. In many EMS systems, it is now the most commonly used opioid for non-cardiac pain. In emergency departments and in the field, it is increasingly replacing morphine for myocardial ischemia and chest pain. For many types of pain, opioids can be titrated by the IV route to produce safe and effective analgesia and can be administered by the intramuscular and intranasal routes as well [21,22]. One of the major benefits of opioids is that most side-effects can be rapidly reversed with an opioid antagonist, such as naloxone, which is carried by most EMS systems for use in opioid overdoses. With all opioids, EMS systems must adhere to Food and Drug Administration guidelines for monitoring and documenting possession and use. Specialized critical care transport teams seem to provide analgesia and achieve significant pain relief more frequently than described in routine ground-based EMS systems [23].

Fentanyl

Fentanyl has several properties that make it well suited for prehospital use. It is one of the only opioids that does not cause a release of histamine, thereby preventing potential exacerbation of reactive airway disease, and reducing the chance of inducing significant hemodynamic changes. Fentanyl is very lipid soluble, and it crosses the blood–brain barrier quickly, reaching its peak effect within a few minutes. Its half-life is shorter than most other opioids with a duration of action less than 1 hour. Fentanyl does not cause any decrease in cardiac contractility. Like all opioids, however, it can decrease sympathetic tone and if a patient's blood pressure is dependent on the sympathetic nervous system, fentanyl can cause some hypotension, but this is relatively uncommon.

Kanowitz reported on the use of fentanyl in 2,129 prehospital patients with an average titrated dose of 118 μg, with a range of 5 to 400 μg [24]. Only 12 patients had any vital sign abnormalities during the drug's duration of action, and most of these were relatively minor, with only one patient receiving naloxone reversal. This one patient was an 83-year-old woman with a hip fracture who received two doses of 100 μg fentanyl and had some respiratory depression while in the ED that was immediately reversed with 0.4 mg of naloxone without any adverse effects. There were no significant complications or deaths as a result of prehospital use of fentanyl. The authors concluded that fentanyl effectively decreased pain scores without causing significant vital sign changes, thereby allowing it to be used safely and effectively for prehospital pain management. Several studies have also been reported showing the safe and effective use of fentanyl in ground and air transport of adult and pediatric patients [25,26].

Fentanyl has a short half-life and duration of action of 60 minutes or less. Opioid-induced hypotension is rare with fentanyl, but in patients who are only able to maintain normal systemic pressure due to extreme sympathetic drive, fentanyl can blunt the sympathetic response and theoretically lower blood pressure. Should this occur, fluid administration is typically all that is needed, but alpha-adrenergic agents can be used to help to restore blood pressure. The safe and effective use of oral transmucosal use of fentanyl has been described in the battlefield setting [27].

Box 67.1 Desired characteristics of analgesics

In choosing an analgesic for the field, desirable properties include:
- Safety
- Efficacy
- Ease of administration
- Rapid onset
- Short duration
- Low abuse potential for patient and staff
- Reversible

Fentanyl also has been used via the intranasal route through an atomizer device [28]. In some systems, fentanyl is replacing morphine as the opioid of choice for ischemic cardiac chest pain.

Morphine

Morphine has been widely used in EMS systems for the past three decades. Initially it was largely restricted to the treatment of ischemic cardiac pain, but its indications have expanded to a wide variety of pain states. Despite the potential for a multitude of side-effects related to the prehospital use of morphine, the literature does not suggest that these have been a major clinical issue. Morphine has the advantage of having a wide margin of safety when it is used in careful IV titrated fashion [29]. It is safe in patients with liver disease and for acute pain and can be used safely in renal disease. Morphine does not decrease cardiac contractility but does decrease preload and afterload and therefore should be used with caution in any patient who has borderline or frank hemodynamic instability. It is important to titrate the dose to the analgesia accomplished.

Opioid agonist-antagonists

Some characteristics of the opioid agonist-antagonist class of analgesics make them ideally suited for prehospital use. Drugs in this group include nalbuphine and butorphanol. The primary benefits of this class are the ceiling on respiratory depression, minimal euphoria and limited abuse potential, lack of biliary spasm, and minimal hemodynamic effects. Stene et al. described the prehospital use of nalbuphine in 46 patients with moderate-to-severe pain due to multiple trauma, burns, fractures, and intraabdominal conditions [30]. The agent was partially to completely effective in 89% of patients and was without any major untoward effects. Nalbuphine also causes very minimal, if any, hemodynamic changes. Since that early study, others have confirmed the value of IV nalbuphine in the field [31,32]. Another advantage of this drug is that it is not a controlled substance, easing some of the paperwork required when using morphine. Butorphanol is now available as a nasal spray [33,34]. This agent and route of administration have many theoretical benefits in the prehospital environment, but studies have yet to be reported on the field use of nasal butorphanol.

The use of the agonist-antagonist class of analgesics in the field may result in patients in the ED requiring somewhat higher doses of pure opiate agonists to achieve adequate analgesia [35].

Nitrous oxide

Nitrous oxide-oxygen mixtures fulfill many of the properties desired for a prehospital analgesic [36–38]. Several field studies have demonstrated the safety and efficacy of self-administered 50% nitrous oxide in prehospital care [39–41]. All studies have confirmed that the majority of patients with moderate-to-severe pain from a variety of sources will achieve significant pain relief. In unpublished data from use in the city of Pittsburgh in

the past two decades, over 4,000 patients have been treated without any significant major adverse effects. Significant analgesia is achieved in approximately 80% of patients. In a rural EMS system, a nitrous oxide-oxygen mixture led to pain relief in 85% of patients for which it was used [42].

One of the major advantages of the use of nitrous oxide is that it is relatively devoid of serious side-effects. Its major side-effect has been nausea, noted in four patients in a study by Ducasse et al., which also found that numerical rating scores decreased significantly with use of a nitrous oxide-oxygen mixture [43]. In 1994, an alert entitled "Controlling exposure of nitrous oxide during anesthetic administration" provided guidelines to prevent environmental levels from exceeding their recommended standards. In a moving vehicle, or one with a fan, short-term administration should be safe for the providers, although well-designed protocols must be written and followed when using this gas mixture. A prototype of a nitrous oxide protocol is shown in Box 67.2; it includes the absolute and relative contraindications to nitrous oxide administration [44].

Recently, Australian authors conducted a systematic review of the safety literature related to the use of 50% nitrous oxide [45]. They identified 12 randomized clinical trials investigating the use of 50% nitrous oxide compared with placebo. They conclude, "Nitrous oxide at a concentration of 50% is an effective and safe form of analgesia. The side effect profile of this agent suggests that it could be used by adequately trained laypersons in the prehospital setting. The question of nitrous oxide use by basic EMTs or by even lesser trained individuals such as rescue teams or ski patrol is a legitimate question, particularly in parts of the world where there is a dearth of prehospital advanced life support personnel."

Ketamine

Ketamine is a dissociative anesthetic that is structurally related to phencyclidine, and it has some unique properties. The dissociative state produced by ketamine is characterized by analgesia and amnesia, while preserving airway protective reflexes [46–48]. Because ketamine is a bronchodilator, it can be used to treat severe asthma [49,50]. It can be used as a field anesthetic for unusual situations, such as field amputations [51], dislocation reductions, or prolonged or complicated extrications. It has also been described as a useful agent for field surgical procedures during disasters, especially among children [52].

Although this agent has had little indication for routine prehospital use, recently, at subdissociative dosages, it has been studied as a primary analgesic agent. The intranasal administration of S-ketamine has been described in Scandinavia [53,54]. It has also been studied as an adjunct agent to decrease the dose of opioid needed to achieve pain relief in the emergency department [55]. Polomano and others describe the use of low-dose IV ketamine in patients with pain from complex combat injuries, showing it to be safe and effective.

Box 67.2 Nitrous oxide/non-cardiac pain protocol[44]

The following protocol for the non-cardiac analgesia use of nitrous oxide stresses the psychological support that can be provided by prehospital caregivers.
- Develop a rapport with the patient with appropriate reassurance and encouragement.
- Properly prepare the equipment necessary to administer the gas.
- Offer nitrous oxide to the patient if there are no contraindications to its use. The patient should self-administer the gas via a mask or mouthpiece. NOTE: When using nitrous oxide-oxygen mixtures, remember that it induces a trance-like state in patients, thereby making them particularly sensitive to suggestion. This can be used to increase the therapeutic effect of the gas, but caution must be exercised because idle conversation may be misinterpreted by the patient and have detrimental effects. Sample instructions would be: "We're going to give you some oxygen with pain-relieving medicine in it to help relieve your discomfort. To get the medicine, you have to hold the mask (or mouthpiece) firmly to your face and breathe normally. In a minute or two, you will feel calm and relaxed and you may feel a little drowsy. Your arms and legs may feel a little heavy as you begin to feel more comfortable. Just relax and let the medicine work for you."
- Immobilization and splinting if necessary.
- Gentle handling and movement.
- Monitor the patient's vital signs every 5–10 minutes.

Contraindications
- Obvious intoxication
- Altered level of consciousness
- Pregnancy (except during labor)*
- Suspected pneumothorax
- Decompression sickness
- Suspected bowel obstruction
- Patients with blood pressure less than 90 mmHg or respirations less than 8/min
- Chronic obstructive pulmonary disease (COPD)*
*This is a relative contraindication

Notes
All inflow ventilating fans must be operating in the patient compartment during administration of this agent.
Studies have shown that female dental assistants have a higher rate of spontaneous abortions than a control group if they work around nitrous oxide. The exact risk is not clear but it would seem to be a reasonable policy for female prehospital providers who are considering pregnancy or may possibly be pregnant to limit their total time in the patient care compartment of the ambulance when nitrous oxide is being used.
It is also desirable for EMS systems to monitor the use of the agent with a log and consider using a locking system to limit the temptation of providers abusing the agent.

Non-steroidal antiinflammatory agents

Currently, few EMS systems routinely use aspirin or other non-steroidal antiinflammatory (NSAID) drugs. Aspirin is now the standard of care as an antiplatelet drug in the treatment of acute coronary syndrome by field personnel, but rarely is aspirin used for pain management. NSAIDs are particularly well suited for

treatment of ureteral and biliary colic [56]. These drugs may also potentiate the analgesic action of opiates [57].

Although these agents do not work as quickly as opiates, if given at the scene they will frequently have beneficial effects before the patient arrives at the hospital and definitely before the time that analgesic agents will be administered in the hospital. These agents should not be considered as a substitute for opiates and nitrous oxide but as another helpful adjunct with selected indications. The major side-effects to consider with a single-dose use in the field would be allergic reactions and platelet inhibition. They should therefore be withheld in the field if the patient has known allergies to NSAIDs or if the anti-platelet effect may exacerbate an underlying problem.

Acetaminophen

Acetaminophen is rarely carried on ambulances or used in the prehospital setting. Acetaminophen, like the NSAIDs, is an effective analgesic, especially in combination with opioids. One potential side-effect, although not likely after a single dose in the field, is the exacerbation of asthma. It is also well known to precipitate acute hepatic failure in patients with underlying liver disease or as a cumulative dose. A single dose in the field is unlikely to lead to acute hepatic failure, but caution would still be advised in these patients. Intravenous acetaminophen is increasingly being used in the hospital and has been studied in the postoperative setting [58].

Communication techniques

The most ignored aspect of providing prehospital relief to those with pain and suffering is the powerful effects that can result from therapeutic communication techniques [59]. These techniques can be mastered by all providers and can bring a significant degree of comfort to patients without use of pharmacological agents. Jacobs points out that many patient responses to an injury or illness are occurring at an unconscious level and that "every word, phrase, sentence, pause, voice inflection, and gesture can initiate automatic psychophysiologic effect" [60]. An example of a suggested dialogue for a patient with burns is as follows.

"I'll bet you can imagine some place you'd rather be than here. As a matter of fact, go ahead and do that now while we get you bandaged up. Think of your favorite place. When you are there in your mind's eye, look around and notice all the things there are to notice. Listen to the sounds. Feel the good feelings. There might even be a special aroma you can smell. When you are really experiencing that place, let me know by raising your index finger. Good."

Although many prehospital providers may feel uncomfortable with guided imagery techniques such as this, they all should recognize the powerful implications of their verbal and nonverbal communication. Providers should be capable of engaging patients in a way that distracts them from their injury or illness.

Distraction can also be very helpful while prehospital providers are performing potentially painful interventions, such as starting an IV line or splinting a fracture. Music has been shown to be effective in decreasing the pain of laceration repair in EDs and could be adapted for use on an ambulance.

Words should be chosen carefully when communicating; *mild discomfort* is more useful than terms such as *bee sting*, *prick*, or *shot*.

Assesment of pain

Objective assessment of pain can be difficult because it is a subjective symptom. The degree of pain cannot be gauged simply by observing vital signs or facial expressions. The pain literature repeatedly documents the unreliability of both vital signs and facial expression in assessing the severity of pain. For pediatric patients, EMS providers often underestimate pain [61]. However, easy-to-use tools are available for adult and pediatric patients that are based upon patient self-report. According to NAEMSP position statement "Prehospital pain management," self-report scales are "the most reliable indicator of pain " [62]. These scales allow not just the quantification of pain at one point in time, but also for monitoring the change in the level of pain over time and after analgesic administration. A helpful technique is to use a 1–10 ("no pain" to "unbearable pain") numerical rating scale (NRS), which is a completely verbal scale. This scale is very easy to use for patients who can speak and are fluent in the same language as the prehospital provider. Alternative scales include the verbal rating scale (VRS) and visual analog scale (VAS). These scales require printed diagrams so are more cumbersome. However, they can be useful for patients who are unable to speak or who are fluent in languages other than that of the prehospital provider. The instructions and diagrams for these two scales can be preprinted in any language.

The VRS has five listed pain levels and the patient is asked to pick the one that describes his or her pain. The VAS has a line that is 100 mm long, with "no pain" listed on the left and "maximal pain" written on the right. The patient is asked to indicate where along the line his or her own pain level lies. According to "Prehospital pain management," one-dimensional pain scales that can be used for pediatric patients include the Color Analogue Scale (in which colors indicate the intensity of pain) and the Faces Pain Scale (in which cartoon facial expressions indicate the intensity of pain). The Faces Pain Scale also may be useful for non-English-speaking patients or those with limited English comprehension skills.

Pitfalls

The major pitfall regarding analgesia is the attitude that it should not be provided in the field but should wait for hospital evaluation. Safe and effective prehospital pharmacological and non-pharmacological techniques are appropriate for the majority of patients with pain. These techniques will not "mask" the diagnosis or worsen the patient's condition. Pain is subjective and should be measured by the patient's words and not expectations of how much a patient should be suffering for a given condition.

Another pitfall is to believe that there is a "uniform" dose of analgesic that will bring elimination of pain when using pharmacological therapy. Particularly with the use of opioids, there is tremendous interpatient variability. The best way to approach pain control is to titrate the medication, monitoring for side-effects and efficacy, until the desired result is reached.

A particularly common pitfall is the belief that the degree of pain can be gauged by vital signs or facial expressions. The pain literature repeatedly documents the unreliability of either vital signs or facial expression in assessing the severity of pain. The only scale that should be used is verbal expression. A helpful technique to use is a 1–10 verbal analog scale, with 10 representing the worst pain the patient has ever experienced. For pediatric patients, using other methods, EMS providers underestimate pain [61].

Another pitfall is to fail to distract the patient while performing painful procedures. Just the opposite usually occurs, with the provider calling attention to every step of the procedure, using terms that are intended to soften the insult but usually actually magnify it.

Studies have identified many barriers to prehospital analgesia. These include lack of "significant objective signs," concern for malingering, aiming simply to "take the edge off," and concern about administering dosages of morphine greater than 5 mg [63]. Specifically in pediatric patients, unfamiliarity with pediatric patients and protocols, insufficient education in pediatrics, difficulty in medication administration in uncooperative pediatric patients and inability to assess pain in children have been reported as barriers to analgesia [64–66].

Protocol changes have been attempted as a means to improve prehospital analgesia rates by removing protocolized barriers, such as the need for a medical oversight order or restrictive assessment categories (e.g. only allowing analgesics for extremity injury or cardiac chest pain). Removing the need for medical oversight order has been found to increase time to analgesic administration. Neither of these protocol changes has been shown to increase the number of patients receiving analgesia to any clinically important amount [67,68]. The lack of efficacy of these changes is not surprising considering that they do not address the identified barriers to prehospital analgesia. However, educating prehospital providers about pain management may be a more efficacious route to improving prehospital analgesia because such interventions can address the barriers to analgesia. This has been proven to be the case in multiple studies, showing improved understanding of pain management principles and a significant improvement in prehospital pain treatment after educational interventions [69,70].

Conclusion

Treating acute pain and relieving suffering should be a primary mission of all health care providers. Unfortunately, EMS personnel have not been given the tools or training to satisfactorily accomplish this worthy goal. Although patient "safety" and "doing no harm" must always be considered, these should not be used as excuses for "doing no good" for patients with acute pain treated in the field.

References

1 Mclean SA, Maio RF, Domeier RM. The epidemiology of pain in the prehospital setting. *Prehosp Emerg Care* 2002:6:402–5.

2 Paris PM, Stewart RD (eds) *Pain Management in Emergency Medicine.* Norwalk, CT: Appleton & Lange, 1987, p.313–21

3 Clinical Practice Guideline. *Acute Pain Management: Operative or Medical Procedures and Trauma.* AHCPR Pub. No. 92-0032. Rockville, MD: Agency for Health Care Policy and Research, US Department of Health and Human Services, 1992.

4 Alonso-Serra HM, Wesley K. National Association of EMS Physicians Standards and Clinical Practices Committee. Prehospital pain management. *Prehosp Emerg Care* 2003;7:482–8.

5 Verdile VP, Stewart RD. The prehospital management of pain. In: May HL (ed) *Emergency Medicine,* 2nd edn. Boston: Little, Brown, 1992, pp.626–30.

6 Stewart RD. Analgesia in the field. *Prehosp Disaster Med* 1989;4:31–5.

7 Dailey M, French D. Sedation and analgesia for the prehospital emergency medical services patient. In: Burton JH, Miner J (eds) *Emergency Sedation and Pain Management.* New York: Cambridge University Press, 2008, pp.255–9.

8 Walsh B, Cone DC, Meyer EM, et al. Paramedic attitudes regarding prehospital analgesia. *Prehosp Emerg Care* 2013;17:78–87.

9 Lippert SC, Nagdev A, Stone MB, et al. Pain control in disaster settings: a role for ultrasound-guided nerve blocks. *Ann Emerg Med* 2013;61:690–6.

10 White LF, Cooper JD, Chambers RM, Gradisek RD. Prehospital use of analgesia for suspected extremity fractures. *Prehosp Emerg Care* 2000;4:205–8.

11 McEachin CC, McDermott JT, Swor R. Few emergency medical services patients with lower-extremity fractures received prehospital analgesia. *Prehosp Emerg Care* 2002;6:406–10.

12 Hennes H, Kim MK, Pirrallo RG. Prehospital pain management: the comparison of providers' perceptions and practices. *Prehosp Emerg Care* 2005;9:32–9.

13 Albrecht E, Taffe P, Yersin B, et al. Undertreatment of acute pain (oligoanalgesia) and medical practice variation in prehospital analgesia of adult trauma patients: a 10yr retrospective study. *Br J Anaesth* 2013;110:96–106.

14 Galinski M, Picco N, Hennequin B, et al. Out-of-hospital emergency medicine in pediatric patients: prevalence and management of pain. *Am J Emerg Med* 2011;29:1062–6.

15 Abbuhl FB, Reed DB. Time to analgesia for patients with painful extremity injuries transported to the emergency department by ambulance. *Prehosp Emerg Care* 2003;7:445–7.

16 McEachin CC, McDermott JT, Swor R. Few emergency medical services patients with lower-extremity fractures receive prehospital analgesia. *Prehosp Emerg Care* 2002;6:406–10.

17 Swor R, McEachin CM, Seguin D, Grall KH. Prehospital pain management in children suffering traumatic injury. *Prehosp Emerg Care* 2005;9:40–3.

18 Evans WO. The undertreatment of pain. *Indiana Med* 1988;81: 848–50.

19 Baskett PJ. Acute pain management in the field. *Ann Emerg Med* 1999;34:784–5.

20 Karnad AB. Treating cancer pain. *N Engl J Med* 1994;331: 199–201.

21 Gray A, Johnson G, Goodacre S. Paramedic use of nalbuphine in major injury. *Eur J Emerg Med* 1997;4:136–9.

22 Paris PM, Weiss LD. Narcotic analgesics: the pure agonists. In: Paris PM, Stewart RD (eds) *Pain Management in Emergency Medicine.* Norwalk, CT: Appleton & Lange, 1988, pp.125–56.

23 Frakes MA, Lord WR, Kociszewski C, et al. Factors associated with unoffered trauma analgesia in critical care transport. *Am J Emerg Med* 2009;27:49–54.

24 Kanowitz A, Dunn TM, Kanowitz EM, et al. Safety and effectiveness of fentanyl administration for prehospital pain management. *Prehosp Emerg Care* 2006;10:1–7.

25 DeVellis P, Thomas SH, Wedel SK, et al. Prehospital fentanyl analgesia in air-transported pediatric trauma patients. *Ped Emerg Care* 1998;14:321–3.

26 Garrick JF, Kidane S, Pointer JE, et al. Analysis of the paramedic administration of fentanyl. *J Opioid Manag* 2011;7:229–34.

27 Wedmore IS, Kotwal RS, McManus JG, et al. Safety and efficacy of oral transmucosal fentanyl citrate for prehospital pain control on the battlefield. *J Trauma Acute Care Surg* 2012;73:S490–5.

28 O'Donnell DP, Schafer LC, Stevens AC, et al. Effect of introducing the mucosal atomization device for Fentanyl use in out-of-hospital pediatric trauma patients. *Prehosp Disaster Med* 2013: 28:520–2.

29 Bruns BM, Dieckmann R, Shagoury C, et al. Safety of prehospital therapy with morphine sulfate. *Am J Emerg Med* 1992;10:53–7.

30 Stene JK, Stofberg L, MacDonald G, et al. Nalbuphine analgesic in the prehospital setting. *Am J Emerg Med* 1988;6:634–9.

31 Hyland-McGuire P, Guly HR. Effects on patient care of introducing prehospital intravenous nalbuphine hydrochloride. *J Accid Emerg Med* 1998;15:99–101.

32 Chambers JA, Guly HR. Prehospital intravenous nalbuphine administered by paramedics. *Resuscitation* 1994;27:153–8.

33 Joyce TH, Kubicek MF, Skjonsby BS, Jones MM. Efficacy of transnasal butorphanol titrate in postepisiotomy pain: a model to assess analgesia. *Clin Ther* 1993;15:160–7.

34 Diamond S, Freitag FG, Diamond ML, et al. Transnasal butorphanol in the treatment of migraine headache pain. *Headache Quarterly, Cut Ther and Res* 1992;3:164–70.

35 Houlihan KP, Mitchell RG, Flapan AD, Steedman DJ. Excessive morphine requirements after prehospital nalbuphine analgesia. *J Accid Emerg Med* 1999;16:29–31.

36 Stewart RD. Nitrous oxide. In: Paris PM, Stewart RD (eds) *Pain Management in Emergency Medicine.* Norwalk, CT: Appleton & Lange, 1988, pp.221–39.

37 Burton JH, Stewart RD. Nitrous oxide. In: Paris PM, Grass JA (eds). *Textbook of Acute Pain Management.* Philadelphia: W.B. Saunders. (in preparation)

38 Paris PM, Yealy DM. Pain management. In: Marx J, Hockberger R, Walls R et al (eds) *Rosen's Emergency Medicine,* 5th edn. St Louis, MO: Mosby Year Book, 2002.

39 Johnson JC, Atherton GL. Effectiveness of nitrous oxide in rural EMS system. *J Emerg Med* 1991;9:45–53.

40 Yealy DM, Paris PM, Kaplan RM, et al. The safety of prehospital naloxone administration by paramedics. *Ann Emerg Med* 1990;19: 902–5.

41 Donen N, Tweed WA, White D, et al. Prehospital analgesia with Entonox. *Can Anaesth Soc J* 1982;29:275–9.

42 Johnson JC, Atherton GL. Effectiveness of nitrous oxide in a rural EMS system. *J Emerg Med* 1991;9:45–53.

43 Ducasse JL, Siksik G, Durand-Bechu M, et al. Nitrous oxide for early analgesia in the emergency setting: a randomized, double-blind multicenter prehospital trial. *Acad Emerg Med* 2013;20:178–84.

44 Mosesso V, Stewart RD, Paris PM, et al. City of Pittsburgh ALS Protocols (adaptation), 1994.

45 Faddy SC, Garlick SR. A systematic review of the safety of analgesia with 50% nitrous oxide: can lay responders use analgesic gases in the prehospital setting? *Emerg Med J* 2005;22(12):901–8.

46 Bennett CR, Stewart RD. Ketamine. In: Paris PM, Stewart RD (eds) *Pain Management in Emergency Medicine*. Norwalk, CT: Appleton & Lange, 1988, pp.295–310.

47 Green SM, Rothrock SG, Lynch EL, et al. Intramuscular ketamine for pediatric sedation in the emergency department: safety profile in 1,022 cases. *Ann Emerg Med* 1998;31:688–97.

48 Green SM, Clem KJ, Rothrock SG. Ketamine safety profile in the developing world – survey of practitioners. *Acad Emerg Med* 1996;3:598–604.

49 Sarma VJ. Use of ketamine in acute severe asthma. *Acta Anaesthesiol Scand* 1992;36:106–7.

50 Jahangir WM, Islam L. Ketamine infusion for post-operative analgesia in asthmatics: a comparison with intermittent meperidine. *Anesth Analg* 1993;76:45–9.

51 Bioin JF. Infusion analgesia for acute war injuries: a comparison of pentazocine and ketamine. *Anaesthesia* 1984;39:560–4.

52 Dick W, Hirlinger WK, Mehrkens HH. Intramuscular ketamine: an alternative treatment for use in disaster? In: Manni C, Magnalini, SI (eds) *Emergency and Disaster Medicine: Proceedings of the Third World Congress in Medicine, 1983*. Berlin: Springer-Verlag, 1985, pp.167–72.

53 Graudins A, Meek R, Egerton-Warburton D, et al. The PICHFORK (Pain InCHildren Fentanyl OR Ketamine) trial comparing the efficacy of intranasal ketamine and fentanyl in the relief of moderate to severe pain in children with limb injuries: study protocol for a randomized controlled trial. *Trials* 2013;14:208.

54 Johansson J, Sjoberg J, Nordgren M, et al: Prehospital analgesia using nasal administration of S-ketamine – a case series. *Scand J Trauma Resusc Emerg Med* 2013;21:38.

55 Ahern TL, Herring AA, Stone MB, Frazee BW. Effective analgesia with low-dose ketamine and reduced dose hydromorphone in ED patients with severe pain. *Am J Emerg Med* 2013;31: 847–51.

56 Goldman G. Biliary colic treatment and acute cholecystitis prevention by prostaglandin inhibitor. *Dig Dis Sci* 1989;34:809–11.

57 Paris PM, Yealy DM. Pain management. In: Marx J, Hockberger R, Walls R (eds) *Rosen's Emergency Medicine: Concepts and Clinical Practice*, 6th edn. Philadelphia: Elsevier Mosby, 2006, pp.2913–37.

58 Khalili G, Janghorbani M, Saryazdi H, Emaminejad A. Effect of preemptive and preventive acetaminophen on postoperative pain score: a randomized, double-blind trial of patients undergoing lower extremity surgery. *J Clin Anesth* 2013;25:188–92.

59 Goldfarb B. Prehospital pain management: providing physical and psychological care. *Prehosp Care Reports* 1992;2:73–80.

60 Jacobs TJ. *Patient Communications*. Englewood Cliffs, NJ: Brady, 1991.

61 Luger TJ, Lederer W, Gassner M, et al. Acute pain is underassessed in out-of-hospital emergencies. *Acad Emerg Med* 2003;10:627–32.

62 Alonso-Serra HM, Wesley K, National Association of EMS Physicians Standards and Clinical Practices Committee. Prehospital pain management. *Prehosp Emerg Care* 2003;7:482–8.

63 Walsh B, Cone DC, Meyer EM, Larkin GL. Paramedic attitudes regarding prehospital analgesia. *Prehosp Emerg Care* 2013;17: 78–87.

64 Hennes H, Kim MK, Pirrallo RG. Prehospital pain management: a comparison of providers' perceptions and practices. *Prehosp Emerg Care* 2005;9:32–9.

65 Murphy A, Barrett M, Cronin J, et al. A qualitative study of the barriers to prehospital management of acute pain in children. *Emerg Med J* 2014;31(6):493–8.

66 Williams DM, Rindal KE, Cushman JT, Shah MN. Barriers to and enablers for prehospital analgesia for pediatric patients. *Prehosp Emerg Care* 2012;16:519–26.

67 Fullerton-Gleason L, Crandall C, Sklar DP. Prehospital administration of morphine for isolated extremity injuries: a change in protocol reduces time to medication. *Prehosp Emerg Care* 2002;6:411–16.

68 Pointer JE, Harlan K. Impact of liberalization of protocols for the use of morphine sulfate in an urban emergency medical services system. *Prehosp Emerg Care* 2005;9:377–81.

69 Bowman WJ, Nesbitt ME, Therien SP. The effects of standardized trauma training on prehospital pain control: have pain medication administration rates increased on the battlefield? *J Trauma Acute Care Surg* 2012;73:S43–8.

70 French SC, Chan SB, Ramaker J. Education on prehospital pain management: a follow-up study. *West J Emerg Med* 2013;14: 96–102.

CHAPTER 68

Point-of-care testing in EMS

Alix J.E. Carter

Introduction

Technology has evolved such that many laboratory-based analyses can now be performed on portable (sometimes hand-held) devices, allowing testing at the point of care. Point-of-care testing (POC) is emerging across many settings in health care. Broadly addressing the setting of emergency care, the advantages may include reduction in time to treatment for emergency conditions, and improved flow through increasingly congested emergency departments. There is discussion of the potential benefits offered by introducing POC testing to the prehospital setting. Advantages may include earlier initiation of life-saving treatment, as well as enabling more informed destination choices. The wide variety of POC testing options may save money and make the practice of EMS more efficient and effective. However, it is a balance of costs and benefits. The discussion contains three subissues: what is the reliability of the emerging technology of POC, can that reliability translate to rugged prehospital conditions, and, most importantly, will it make a difference to patients? There may be a fourth issue in the subtext: what this means to the scope and education of EMS professionals.

Is POC right for EMS?

There are a number of advantages, at both patient and system level. POC may allow more targeted and earlier intervention. This may enable more appropriate regionalized destination strategies. It may even stretch to evidence-based non-transport, and the application of new therapies in the field. POC may have a particular role in community paramedicine (Box 68.1).

There are some disadvantages as well. POC may carry medicolegal risk, with a need for development of a robust quality assurance/improvement plan. There is concern for scope creep, and that POC represents just another fancy toy. There is skepticism that POC testing will contribute to EMS being used as doctor or nurse replacement in the reform of health care.

Furthermore, the incentive to "stay and play" must be considered, and whether the possibility of longer scene time would be mitigated by more efficient overall system utilization is unknown. The implications for a change in the training of EMS providers, to include a foundation of pathophysiology sufficient to troubleshoot and understand the implications of positive and negative tests, must be a factor in the decision to introduce POC testing.

Is this particular test right for my service?

Is the POC test valid and reliable?

A good diagnostic test moves the clinician from diagnostic uncertainty to greater certainty. If the pretest probability of disease is low or high enough, there is no point in doing a test that costs money and may carry risk – at a minimum, the risk of false positive (or negative), at worst, a risk of harm by adverse reaction. For each test, there is a need to ascertain the sensitivity and specificity, and/or positive and negative predictive value. The issue of whether the result will change clinician actions is also important. The presence (or absence) of action may be on the basis of evidence-based criteria, local practice, and/or system design. For example, if field trauma triage protocols are not structured to incorporate the results of a lactate or cranial scanning for hemorrhage, there is no sense in putting these tools in the field. They are expensive, they need maintaining, and it will be frustrating for the field provider to produce data on which he or she cannot act.

How practical is this POC test?

The system must consider an estimate of the upfront and ongoing costs, and weigh these against other system priorities. Consider whether the test will work in an ambulance. On a system level, assess the potential effect on performance or process measures, and the capacity of the system to handle required changes to infrastructure, for example training, follow-up, CQI infrastructure. Multiple factors go into the decision as to whether introducing a given POC is right for your EMS system (Box 68.2).

Emergency Medical Services: Clinical Practice and Systems Oversight, Second Edition. Volume 1: Clinical Aspects of EMS.
Edited by David C. Cone, Jane H. Brice, Theodore R. Delbridge, and J. Brent Myers.

Specific POC tests for consideration in the EMS setting

Medical devices in the United States are regulated by Food and Drug Administration (FDA). POC tests, as with other laboratory testing devices, fall under the FDA Clinical Laboratory Improvement Amendments (CLIA). CLIA sets standards for

quality assurance and categorizes testing based on how complex it is for the analyst to run the test (e.g. training, knowledge, interpretation). The categorization (waived, moderate, or high complexity) has implications for who can use the tests, and the quality oversight infrastructure required. Box 68.3 provides more detail on the implications, and a note is made in the individual discussion as to the CLIA complexity category of a POC test (www.fda.gov/Medical Devices/DeviceRegulation andGuidance/IVDRegulatory Assistance/ucm124105.htm). EMS systems in other settings need to investigate local regulations as they apply to medical devices. In all settings, the general discussion in this chapter with regard to important questions and infrastructure still applies.

Prehospital ultrasound

Please see Volume 1, Chapter 69 for further detail. All of the general discussions regarding POC in this chapter can be applied.

Box 68.1 Considerations for POC in community paramedicine

Rule in	Initiation of treatment depending on system design and goals of care, alternatively would activate the emergency response system
Rule out	Greater potential with longer contact times, return visits, old records
Exclusive to community paramedicine	Role for urinalysis, peak flow test, occult blood testing of emesis or stool, blood chemistry? Could brain natriuretic peptide have a role as in the emergency department?

Box 68.2 POC key questions

Validity	How well the POC performs compared to the laboratory version of the test
Test characteristics	Sensitivity/specificity or positive/negative predictive value of the POC version of the test
Effect on patient outcome	What is known about the clinical implications or effects of this POC?
System responsiveness	The capacity within the system design/protocols to change the course of action in response to the POC result
Logistics	Whether the test or reagents require refrigeration Shelf-life of these products in or out of the fridge Battery or corded power supply, battery life, and charging times Weight of the device For flight EMS, special issues of air pressure and electromagnetic interference
Ongoing costs	Software updates/licensing Per-use costs for strips or cartridges Generally a new cost, not mitigated by replacement of an older process
Reimbursement	Likely no billing code for POC yet – significant issue for leadership of some systems
Quality assurance	Risk of false negatives/positives, of treating test but not whole patient Performance measures should be defined a priori, be clearly articulated and measurable, and have clinical meaning Examples: (1) percentage of patients with condition X got test Y, e.g. percentage of head injury patients get the cranial infrascanner, or (2) benchmarking of mortality for condition X Caution: Measuring one thing in isolation may give false impressions; for example, the scene time may be slightly longer but the time to definitive care shorter, and both measures are required to understand the effects
Initial and continuing education	Both initial and ongoing training will be important. Determination of minimum skill level to use a POC test appropriately may have implications for initial provider education as well
Restocking/outdating	Shelf-life before expiry Deployment strategy that will increase the stock in areas of greater usage, and/or cycle stock nearing expiry to high-usage areas Does method of storage have an effect on shelf-life and can you optimize this?
Calibration	To be incorporated in the training, restocking, and quality improvement plans, as well as budget implications for calibration materials if applicable
Scene/transport time	Considerations such as: Whether test will need to be calibrated on scene, and how long that might take Any mandatory transmission of the results and/or online consultation Do longer scene times generate one or more of: better patient outcomes, shorter time to definitive care, avoidance of unnecessary lights and sirens transports, or prolonged transports to specialty centers? If the test rules a condition in or out, a change in action should result: a field triage protocol should permit bypass directly to a specialty center, or conversely transport to the closest facility instead of a specialty center

Box 68.3 FDA-CLIA implications for EMS POC testing

CLIA-waived	Home use tests such as pregnancy and blood glucose; also urinalysis, fecal occult blood
	These can be used by EMS without any regulatory concerns (all the discussion in this chapter still applies, however)
CLIA moderate-complexity	About 70% of POC tests are "CLIA-moderate complexity"
	Moderate complexity testing must be overseen by:
	• a lab director, who must be a physician with lab training (not all physicians would qualify)
	• a technical and clinical consultant; this can be a physician or a PhD-level scientist with significant experience in laboratory testing – a suitable physician could fill all roles. The technical consultant must be available on an as-needed basis and is responsible for selecting test methods and establishing their performance characteristics, implementing quality assurance, evaluating the competency and performance of testing personnel, and providing training
	EMS providers should qualify to perform moderate-complexity POC; regulations state such personnel must have, at minimum, high school diplomas and documentation of satisfactory completion of training appropriate to the testing performed, which may have been obtained either formally or informally on the job
CLIA high-complexity	High-complexity tests, fortunately, are unlikely to be utilized in the POC setting. The regulatory requirements would be a significant barrier to use in EMS
Not regulated by FDA-CLIA	Non-invasive (e.g. laser hematocrit), breath tests (e.g. *H. pylori*, alcohol), drugs of abuse – workplace, monitoring devices (e.g. blood pressure)
	These tests can be used by the lay public or EMS

Detection of coagulopathy
Is it valid?
In terms of accuracy as compared to laboratory testing, and ease of use at the point of care, the best POC test appears to be INR/PT, better than aPTT, hemoglobin, or fibrinogen [1]. One important exception is coagulopathy from platelet inhibition; POC remains limited, as does the ability to reverse anticoagulation [2].

Is it logical/feasible for EMS?
Point-of-care testing for INR/PT performs with comparable sensitivity to the standard tests, returning a result in a matter of seconds. The machines are expensive, and per-use cost is in the range of $9 USD (www.cliawaived.com/web/Basic_Metabolic_Status.htm). This POC test is CLIA-moderate complexity.

Will it matter clinically?
In trauma
There are two types of coagulopathy to consider in trauma: that from anticoagulant/antiplatelet medications and that induced by trauma itself. EMS should already be addressing the root causes of mortality in trauma-induced coagulopathy, through prevention of hypothermia and targeted /low-pressure resuscitation (goal systolic blood pressure 85 mmHg). In-hospital strategies such as blood transfusion, cryoprecipitate, fresh frozen plasma, and recombinant factor VIIA are not easily translated to the field, with the need for refrigeration being a major limitation [3]. Treatment of hypoperfusion may be the most important factor [4]. In terms of medication-induced coagulopathy, head-injured patients are at particular risk from oral anticoagulation [5]. A potential action would be notification of the trauma center to call for fresh frozen plasma or initiate a massive transfusion protocol. Supratherapeutic INR could factor into field

trauma triage. Vitamin K may have a role in the specific case of oral anticoagulation with warfarin, and could potentially be administered in the field.

In stroke
German researchers have used INR POC testing in the field in an on-scene stroke diagnosis and treatment protocol, with a reduction in time to needle [6,7]. However, these studies also had portable computed tomography (CT), and the EMS team included a paramedic, a physician, and access to a neuroradiologist. That being said, it suggests that the use of POC INR testing is feasible. If it affected regional stroke triage and/or the activation of a stroke protocol at the receiving facility, it would have clinical importance in our EMS systems.

Troponin
Is it valid and reliable?
The manufacturer's instructions state the device should be on a flat, stable surface during measurement. Fortunately, Venturini et al. found no significant difference between measurement of the same sample in the ED or the moving ambulance [8].

Is it practical?
Manipulating the tiny cartridge could be challenging, but several studies suggest it can be done. As the results take 10–15 minutes, it is suggested that the test be initiated on scene but to transport while awaiting results. Issues of cost are not negligible. One of the assays, the iSTAT, is in the range of US$11,000, and US$15 per use. The iSTAT cartridges only have a shelf-life of 2 weeks without refrigeration (www. abbottpointofcare.com/). This POC test is CLIA-moderate complexity.

Will it make a difference clinically?

In chest pain

A paramedic-based EMS system in Denmark has demonstrated increased diagnostic clarity for chest pain patients, with nine of 78 patients triaged directly for primary percutaneous coronary intervention (PCI) based primarily on the positive POC troponin T in the setting of an equivocal ECG or bundle branch block of uncertain origin [9]. This study also suggests good prehospital feasibility of troponin T POC testing with a 97% success rate in 958 attempts. The sensitivity was only 31%; this likely is related to the fact that 65% of patients had symptoms for less than 2 hours, making it very early in the troponin rise. A low sensitivity, or greater utility as a rule-in for ambiguous patients, is supported by other work [10,11].

Troponin along with creatine kinase-MB, myoglobin, negative ECG, and low-risk assessment was used to rule out acute myocardial infarction with at least 6 hours of chest pain [12]. In this Israeli EMS system there are both a physician and a paramedic on scene.

Evidence for use as a rule-out in the prehospital setting is lacking; there is perhaps a greater role in a community paramedicine setting where contact times can be longer and follow-up options may exist. As a rule-in, studies have shown increased detection and improved access to definitive care, particularly for those with non-diagnostic ECGs.

In stroke

Prehospital POC troponin T and N-terminal pro brain natriuretic peptide (NT-proBNP) have been suggested as predictors for stroke mortality in a Slovenian physician-based EMS system [13]. The authors of this study argue that this predicts patients who need more intensive monitoring. However, it is unclear whether this would affect our current EMS standard stroke care.

Lactate

Is it reliable?

A POC lactate test is available and valid/reliable in both adults and children [14,15]. High prehospital lactate was significantly associated with the need for critical care during admission, and a high lactate (>2.0 mmol/L) occurred in the presence of normal vital signs in 13% of children [14]. POC lactate as a triage tool has been supported in other studies, posited as more accurate than traditional field triage measures like SBP <90 mmHg [16–18].

Is it practical?

The hand-held meters use a drop of blood, from fingerstick, with results in 15 seconds for newer models (60 seconds for older), and have been shown to function at a range of altitudes and temperatures. The estimated per-use cost is approximately US$1.80 to $2.80 for Lactate Pro or Lactate Plus, plus the cost of the machine which was $280 for Lactate Plus and $600 for Lactate Pro 2 (LP2).

The test strips for the LP2 also calibrate (www.fact-canada.com/LactatePro/lactate-pro-portable-analyzer.html) [16]. The LP devices claim to be the only CLIA-waived lactate POC.

Will it make a difference clinically?

In trauma

Addition to the triage algorithm would help identify patients in need of more aggressive intervention, particularly those with "occult hypoperfusion" which might otherwise result in failure to resuscitate adequately and triage to a trauma center.

Conversely, could a normal prehospital lactate (1.0 mmol/L or less) be used to avoid overtriage? Shah et al. showed that no patient with normal vital signs, a normal Glasgow Coma Scale score, and a lactate less than 1 mmol/L needed critical care [14].

In sepsis

Prehospital POC lactate testing as part of a sepsis alert protocol was found to reduce mortality [19]. In this study lactate and systemic inflammatory response criteria formed a prehospital protocol to detect and aggressively manage sepsis; this produced a "sepsis alert" with dedicated staff in the emergency department prepared for the patient's arrival, and an aggressive prehospital and in-hospital management of the patient.

Brain natriuretic peptide (BNP)

Studies are heterogeneous in care provided and in definition of "prehospital." No conclusion can be drawn.

Carbon monoxide (CO)

Most common in the EMS/fireground environment, two options for POC CO detection exist: an end-exhalation breath analysis and a pulse cooximeter. Both have been tested in this environment and found to be feasible to deploy [20–22]. Notable limitations to validity include baseline CO in smokers, and the inability to detect peak or cumulative exposure. Actions that would result in meaningful clinical and system effects could include recognition of clinically significant acute exposure, rule-in or rule-out need for transport and oxygen, and consideration of hyperbarics.

Capnography

Is it valid and reliable?

With good correlation to blood gas and multiple uses in the EMS environment, capnography is viewed by many as "standard of care" [23].

Is it practical/feasible?

Qualitative capnography detectors can be placed on the endotracheal tube to detect expired carbon dioxide as evidence of proper tube placement. Quantitative capnography is an integrated feature in many monitor-defibrillator packages. Sensors can be in-line with the endotracheal tube-ventilation tubing when positive pressure ventilation is being used, and intranasal sensors are also available to monitor for hypoventilation in patients who are breathing spontaneously but sedated.

Will it make a difference clinically?

Uses of capnography include titration of ventilation, particularly in brain-injured or lung disease patients [24,25]. Safety indications include recognition of misplaced or dislodged endotracheal tubes [26,27]. Novel applications include recognition of return of spontaneous circulation [28,29].

Near-infrared cranial scanner

This scanner uses near-infrared transcranial spectroscopy, in adults and children, to enable detection of intracranial hemorrhage. One advantage is that it does not require the technical expertise needed for ultrasound, although a disadvantage is the limitation to one disease.

Is it valid and reliable? Is it feasible?

Sensitivities are quoted as 100% in a pediatric intensive care unit and 88.9% in an EMS setting [30,31,33]. Specificities are in the range of 80%. It has been demonstrated to be feasible for use in the prehospital setting (Figure 68.1).

Will it make a difference?

None of the studies has suggested it can replace CT for diagnosis, but it may have some utility in triage to or away from trauma centers, or assignment of triage acuity scales.

Integration

A number of "tests" done routinely in EMS such as temperature, blood glucose, and oxygen saturation would qualify as POC. Considerations of training, quality improvement, cost, validity,

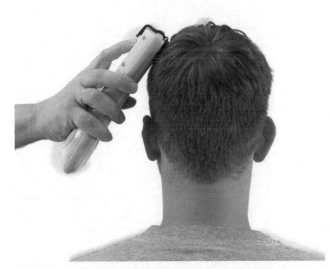

Figure 68.1 Cranial infrascanner application. Source: InfraScan Inc. Reproduced with permission of InfraScan Inc.

practicality, and clinical significance should apply to them all. There are also a number of devices which are not strictly speaking POC but figure into implementation:
- audio communication (beyond VHF/UHF radio, cell phone)
- real-time vital signs/electrocardiogram
- picture transmission
- video streaming
- interface of POC tests with tablets and cell phones
- integrated monitor-defibrillator
- real-time telemedicine link, including potential to interact [34].

A network of optimized information technology capabilities could greatly enhance EMS capacity to get the right care to the right patient at the right time [35]. The capabilities of the information technology world have moved light years, and EMS can learn a lot from enterprises like banking, couriers, and taxis [35].

The potential for POC to improve quality and efficiency of EMS care is real. Careful consideration will be important to ensure valid, reliable POC tests are implemented with positive effects on outcomes.

References

1 Hagemo JS. Prehospital detection of traumatic coagulopathy. *Transfusion* 2013;53:48S–51S.

2 Bansal V, Fortlage D, Lee J, et al. A new clopidogrel (Plavix) point-of-care assay: rapid determination of antiplatelet activity in trauma patients. *J Trauma* 2011;70:65–9.

3 Stein DM, Dutton RP. Uses of recombinant factor VIIa in trauma. *Curr Opin Crit Care* 2004;10:520–8.

4 Brohi K, Cohen MJ, Ganter MT, et al. Acute coagulopathy of trauma: hypoperfusion induces systemic anticoagulation and hyperfibrinolysis. *J Trauma* 2008;64:1211–17.

5 Ott MM, Eriksson E, Vanderkolk W, et al. Antiplatelet and anticoagulation therapies do not increase mortality in the absence of traumatic brain injury. *J Trauma* 2010;68:560–3.

6 Weber JE, Ebinger M, Rozanski M, et al. Prehospital thrombolysis in acute stroke: results of the PHANTOM-S pilot study. *Neurology* 2013;80:163–8.

7 Walter S, Kostopoulos P, Haass A, et al. Diagnosis and treatment of patients with stroke in a mobile stroke unit versus in hospital: a randomised controlled trial. *Lancet Neurol* 2012;11:397–404.

8 Venturini JM, Stake CE, Cichon ME. Prehospital point-of-care testing for troponin: are the results reliable? *Prehosp Emerg Care* 2013;17:88–91.

9 Sorensen JT, Terkelsen CJ, Steengaard C, et al. Prehospital troponin T testing in the diagnosis and triage of patients with suspected acute myocardial infarction. *Am J Cardiol* 2011;107:1436–40.

10 Di Serio F, Lovero R, Leone M, et al. Integration between the telecardiology unit and the central laboratory: methodological and clinical evaluation of point-of-care testing cardiac marker in the ambulance. *Clin Chem Lab Med* 2006;44:768–73.

11 Leshem-Rubinow E, Abramowitz Y, Malov N, et al. Prehospital cardiac markers in defining ambiguous chest pain. *Arch Intern Med* 2011;171:2056–7.

12 Roth A, Malov N, Golovner M, et al. The "SHAHAL" experience in Israel for improving diagnosis of acute coronary syndromes in the prehospital setting. *Am J Cardiol* 2001;88:608–10.

13 Hajdinjak E, Klemen P, Grmec S. Prognostic value of a single prehospital measurement of N-terminal pro-brain natriuretic peptide and troponin T after acute ischaemic stroke. *J Int Med Res* 2012;40:768–76.

14 Shah A, Guyette F, Suffoletto B, et al. Diagnostic accuracy of a single point-of-care prehospital serum lactate for predicting outcomes in pediatric trauma patients. *Pediatr Emerg Care* 2013;29:715–19.

15 Guyette FX, Gomez H, Suffoletto B, et al. Prehospital dynamic tissue oxygen saturation response predicts in-hospital lifesaving interventions in trauma patients. *J Trauma Acute Care Surg* 2012;72:930–5.

16 Vandromme MJ, Griffin RL, Weinberg JA, et al. Lactate is a better predictor than systolic blood pressure for determining blood requirement and mortality: could prehospital measures improve trauma triage? *J Am Coll Surg* 2010;210:861–7, 867–9.

17 Jansen TC, van Bommel J, Mulder PG, et al. The prognostic value of blood lactate levels relative to that of vital signs in the pre-hospital setting: a pilot study. *Crit Care* 2008;12:R160.

18 Karon BS, Scott R, Burritt MF, Santrach PJ. Comparison of lactate values between point-of-care and central laboratory analyzers. *Am J Clin Pathol* 2007;128:168–71.

19 Guerra WF, Mayfield TR, Meyers MS, et al. Early detection and treatment of patients with severe sepsis by prehospital personnel. *J Emerg Med* 2013;44:1116–25.

20 Cone DC, MacMillan DS, Van Gelder C, et al. Noninvasive fireground assessment of carboxyhemoglobin levels in firefighters. *Prehosp Emerg Care* 2005;9:8–13.

21 Piatkowski A, Ulrich D, Grieb G, Pallua N. A new tool for the early diagnosis of carbon monoxide intoxication. *Inhal Toxicol* 2009; 21:1144–7.

22 Dunn KH, Devaux I, Stock A, Naeher LP. Application of end-exhaled breath monitoring to assess carbon monoxide exposures of wildland firefighters at prescribed burns. *Inhal Toxicol* 2009;21:55–61.

23 Phelan MP, Ornato JP, Peberdy MA, et al. Appropriate documentation of confirmation of endotracheal tube position and relationship to patient outcome from in-hospital cardiac arrest. *Resuscitation* 2013;84:31–6.

24 Krauss B. Capnography in EMS. A powerful way to objectively monitor ventilatory status. *JEMS* 2003;28:28–30, 32–8, 41.

25 Wampler D. Capnography as a clinical tool. The capnography waveform is a key vital sign when determining treatment for patient in the field. *EMS World* 2011;40:37–43.

26 Katz SH, Falk JL. Misplaced endotracheal tubes by paramedics in an urban emergency medical services system. *Ann Emerg Med* 2001;37:32–7.

27 Silvestri S, Ralls GA, Krauss B, et al. The effectiveness of out-of-hospital use of continuous end-tidal carbon dioxide monitoring on the rate of unrecognized misplaced intubation within a regional emergency medical services system. *Ann Emerg Med* 2005;45: 497–503.

28 Hatlestad D. Capnography as a predictor of the return of spontaneous circulation. *Emerg Med Serv* 2004;33:75–80.

29 Pokorna M, Necas E, Kratochvil J, et al. A sudden increase in partial pressure end-tidal carbon dioxide (P(ET)CO(2)) at the moment of return of spontaneous circulation. *J Emerg Med* 2010; 38:614–21.

30 Ghalenoui H, Saidi H, Azar M, et al. Near-infrared laser spectroscopy as a screening tool for detecting hematoma in patients with head trauma. *Prehosp Disaster Med* 2008;23:558–61.

31 Kahraman S, Kayali H, Atabey C, et al. The accuracy of near-infrared spectroscopy in detection of subdural and epidural hematomas. *J Trauma* 2006;61:1480–3.

32 Kessel B, Jeroukhimov I, Ashkenazi I, et al. Early detection of life-threatening intracranial haemorrhage using a portable near-infrared spectroscopy device. *Injury* 2007;38:1065–8.

33 Salonia R, Bell MJ, Kochanek PM, Berger RP. The utility of near infrared spectroscopy in detecting intracranial hemorrhage in children. *J Neurotrauma* 2012;29:1047–53.

34 Bergrath S, Rossaint R, Lenssen N, et al. Prehospital digital photography and automated image transmission in an emergency medical service – an ancillary retrospective analysis of a prospective controlled trial. *Scand J Trauma Resusc Emerg Med* 2013;21:3.

35 Landman AB, Rokos IC, Burns K, et al. An open, interoperable, and scalable prehospital information technology network architecture. *Prehosp Emerg Care* 2011;15:149–57.

CHAPTER 69

Ultrasound applications in EMS

Rachel Liu

Introduction

Clinician-performed ultrasound has proven crucial for the evaluation of critical disease. Improvements in size, weight, cost, user-friendliness, and communications have allowed the enthusiasm for hospital ultrasound to migrate into the out-of-hospital arena. With increasing evidence that ultrasound can play a role in out-of-hospital emergency care, this diagnostic modality has been used in international explorations on all continents, in challenging high-altitude expeditions, on cruise ships, in hyperbaric chambers, and even in outer space on the International Space Station [1].

Ultrasound-guided diagnosis of critical conditions in the field has the potential for improving triage decisions, hastening therapy prior to hospital arrival, avoiding unnecessary or harmful treatments, and expediting transport to correct facilities. Prehospital ultrasound has been described in advanced ground and flight EMS systems, in military medicine for both service personnel and civilians, in austere or underdeveloped environments, and in mass casualty situations. Non-physicians with limited medical backgrounds have demonstrated the ability to perform and interpret ultrasounds with adequate training. Despite the recognition of a need for field use of point-of-care ultrasound, its routine incorporation into prehospital algorithms has not yet been established.

Why prehospital ultrasound?

Bedside ultrasound performed by non-radiologists has been well described to accelerate diagnosis and patient management, ultimately decreasing hospital lengths of stay and reducing costs [2]. Out-of-hospital ultrasound has facilitated improvements in diagnostic accuracy [3] but outcomes research has not been performed within this setting. The potential for extrapolation of similar outcomes using prehospital ultrasound is intriguing. Prehospital diagnosis of a grave illness may lead to immediate procedural care, direct admission to relevant specialty centers,

and prevention of secondary transfers. Ultrasound-assisted triage may allow more stable patients to be redistributed away from overwhelmed centers and visibly guide immediate resuscitative interventions in the field [4,5].

Settings of field use

In the United States, EMS crews are primarily staffed with non-physicians using a "scoop and run" transport philosophy, providing basic resuscitation while delivering patients to the nearest appropriate facilities. Some European countries, however, use physician personnel on board their EMS vehicles or mobilize specific physician units to direct medical management and allocate resources. EMS physicians are increasingly common in the US as well. These units may spend longer in the field providing treatment prior to transport [3]. Therefore, the utility and feasibility of prehospital ultrasound may differ depending upon practice environment. The concept of ultrasound assistance enabling rapid, accurate care before hospital arrival remains the same regardless of which system is employed.

Indications

The 2008 American College of Emergency Physicians policy statement regarding emergency ultrasound lists the following examinations as core emergency ultrasound applications: trauma, intrauterine pregnancy, abdominal aortic aneurysm (AAA), cardiac and volume status, biliary, urinary tract, deep venous thrombosis (DVT), soft tissue and musculoskeletal, thoracic, ocular, and procedural guidance [1]. Prehospital use in many of these areas is described in the following sections.

Trauma

The area of most extensive study regarding prehospital ultrasound is the Focused Assessment with Sonography in Trauma (FAST) examination to detect traumatic cardiac tamponade and

Emergency Medical Services: Clinical Practice and Systems Oversight, Second Edition. Volume 1: Clinical Aspects of EMS.
Edited by David C. Cone, Jane H. Brice, Theodore R. Delbridge, and J. Brent Myers.
© 2015 NAEMSP. Published 2015 by John Wiley & Sons, Inc. Companion Website: www.wiley.com/go\cone\naemsp

intraperitoneal bleeding [6,9 13]. The current standard is for the FAST exam to be performed immediately upon arrival to the trauma center during advanced trauma life support physical examination surveys. However, Walcher et al. demonstrated that performing prehospital FAST (PFAST) ultrasounds at the trauma scene changed management in 30% of patients with a 93% sensitivity and 99% specificity for detecting intraperitoneal free fluid [6]. Identification of free fluid enabled providers to reduce patient blood loss by providing permissive hypotension, and non-essential therapies were avoided to shorten time to surgery. Advance notification of PFAST results was provided to receiving hospitals, which then activated surgical teams when needed. In 22% of patients, the choice of receiving hospital was changed based on the ultrasound findings. Due to the results of this study, one major German air rescue provider incorporated PFAST into its algorithm for trauma management [6]. Other studies have demonstrated successful paramedic performance of the PFAST exam while en route, on ground or in air, without prolonging time to transport [4,10,14].

Of note, ultrasound cannot distinguish blood from ascitic fluid or pinpoint exact areas of bleeding. It is not sensitive in the detection of retroperitoneal fluid, organ injury, or hollow viscus injury. These limitations of ultrasound may cause delayed or missed fluid detection on out-of-hospital or triage FAST exam [15–17]. It remains to be seen whether positive findings on a PFAST exam in the United States would alter management as illustrated in the Walcher study [6], since many trauma centers in the US have immediate response by trauma teams and protocols in place to mobilize operating theaters quickly.

The FAST detection of pericardial fluid may have more potential for prehospital intervention. A dramatic case report details the course of a 17-year-old 26-week pregnant female suffering from a stab injury. Despite field chest tube placement with evacuation of air and blood, the patient's vital signs declined. Ultrasound revealed a significant amount of pericardial fluid, which was immediately drained in the field and again in the emergency department. The patient ultimately survived, largely due to prehospital intervention [18]. Similarly, another report describes how in-ambulance paramedic detection of traumatic pericardial effusion and subsequent alerting of the receiving team facilitated direct operative intervention [11]. These cases highlight the potential for the PFAST exam to change prehospital practice and guide on-scene resuscitative therapies.

Pulmonary

While the Extended FAST exam (eFAST), including evaluation of pleural sliding, has been imprinted into emergency department and trauma protocols, it has not become standard in the prehospital environment. Adoption of sonographic pneumothorax evaluation may be invaluable in the trauma setting, as physical exam findings and ancillary monitoring have proven insensitive or difficult to discern in a noisy ambulance or helicopter [5,7,8,19]. Detection may facilitate prehospital needle thoracostomy and prevent development of tension pneumothorax. Additionally,

ruling out pneumothorax avoids unnecessary procedures and their sequelae, allowing focus on other resuscitative efforts [5].

Equally, assessments of lung sliding and pleural effusion have become useful adjuncts in the management of acute dyspnea. Zechner et al. report a common scenario encountered by prehospital personnel: a patient with a history of both chronic obstructive pulmonary disease (COPD) and congestive heart failure (CHF) presenting in severe respiratory distress with wheezing. When pulmonary edema was discovered via on-ambulance sonographic B-lines, treatment was immediately altered to discontinue terbutaline and proceed with urapidil (an alpha$_1$-antagonist), enabling rapid improvement in the patient's clinical status [20]. Subsequently, a German group developed a prehospital chest protocol to evaluate undifferentiated dyspnea. Using the subxiphoid cardiac view, bilateral coronal views, and bilateral anterior intercostal views, this protocol investigates pericardial or pleural effusion, pneumothorax, and right heart distension for pulmonary embolus. Providing supportive information in 68% of their patients and most useful for finding pleural effusion in decompensated CHF, prehospital ultrasound guided emergency physician management at the hospital [8].

Another area of rising interest is sonographic confirmation of endotracheal tube placement as an adjunct to capnometry. Brun et al. describe verification of tube position during cardiopulmonary resuscitation (CPR) by viewing bilateral pleural sliding when there was sudden absence of end-tidal CO_2 detection and limited ability to perform auscultation due to noise in the vehicle [21].

Prehospital lung ultrasound appears useful in revealing the presence or absence of pneumothorax, detecting pulmonary edema, narrowing diagnosis among differing respiratory disease processes, identifying pleural effusion, and as a supplement to current respiratory monitoring techniques.

Cardiac

Dedicated prehospital cardiac examination is very amenable to ultrasound. Brun et al. illustrate prehospital use of transthoracic echo for evaluation of shock in a patient with prior cardiac surgery presenting with dyspnea, tachypnea, crackles on exam, and hypotension. Ultrasound revealed pericardial effusion with thrombus in contact with the right ventricular free wall causing diastolic collapse of the right heart from a vitamin K antagonist overdose. The prehospital team notified the receiving hospital to prepare prothrombin complex concentrates in advance of arrival, and shortened time to drainage by the cardiac surgeons [22].

Out-of-hospital groups have also diagnosed pulmonary embolus from acute right heart strain [8] and examined cardiac output using non-physicians with tele-ultrasonography [23]. The same challenges that affect interpretation of in-hospital echocardiography exist, such as differentiating between acute versus chronic right heart strain, epicardial fatty tissue versus small pericardial effusion, and stable versus unstable pericardial effusion. These physiological processes may require a more in-depth level of training [7,8].

The main area of prehospital cardiac research stems from literature suggesting that absence of cardiac activity on bedside echocardiography predicts unsuccessful resuscitation in cardiac arrest [24,25]. Thus there has been some focus on prehospital echocardiography performed by non-physicians for field pronouncement of death and avoidance of costly resuscitative efforts or misdirected allocation of resources [12,24]. This has been further supported by a prospective study showing only a 3.1% (one patient out of 32) survival to hospital admission of cardiac arrest patients who displayed cardiac standstill on prehospital echo. In situations where uncertainties in decision to stop resuscitation are influenced by downtime, presence of bystander CPR, duration of resuscitation, ECG rhythm, age, or persistence of pulseless electrical activity (PEA), having a visible and reproducible prognostic parameter is useful. Although this study supports the idea that prolonged resuscitative efforts in the field may be futile when cardiac standstill is seen, there appears to be a small subgroup of people who survive to hospital admission, and the authors recommend not basing prehospital resuscitation on one single initial scan [25].

Abdominal

Within the emergency department setting, bedside ultrasound has been a rapid and accurate adjunct for diagnosis of AAA, renal colic, and cholecystitis. There are few reports of ultrasound for these disease processes in out-of-hospital settings. Prehospital ultrasound as a tool for investigation of abdominal or flank pain in the suspected abdominal aortic aneurysm may enhance admission decisions and reduce the potential for secondary transfer [26]. An Australian helicopter retrieval team describe use of in-flight ultrasound in a man with suspected inferior myocardial infarction (MI). He had already received aspirin and enoxaparin prior to ultrasound-guided discovery of AAA. His management was changed to administration of fresh frozen plasma (FFP) for reversal of these agents and arrangements were made for direct transfer to the vascular team through advance notification to the receiving hospital [27]. Other groups have successfully trained medic crews to evaluate the abdomen for AAA [10,27] but the incidence of prehospital discovery and subsequent changes in patient outcomes have not been demonstrated. Out-of-hospital physicians utilizing ultrasound have changed management plans in hurricane disaster relief and in expeditions to the Amazon jungle when evaluating causes of abdominal disease [28].

Obstetrics

Evaluation of obstetric emergency is an area that may significantly benefit from prehospital ultrasound. A case series demonstrated the utility of ultrasound during air medical transfer where ambient noise creates difficulties in auscultating fetal heart rate. One case in particular highlighted the appropriate prevention of air medical transport in a patient displaying fetal distress due to premature rupture of membranes with prolapsed cord. When the flight team discovered intermittent fetal bradycardia on ultrasound, the

transport was aborted and the patient went straight to the operating theater, averting fetal demise in this initially unrecognized condition [29]. Diagnosis of ruptured ectopic pregnancy was confirmed by sonographic right upper quadrant free fluid in a patient with a reportedly normal pregnancy. Presence of free fluid heightened the suspicion of the prehospital team, who arranged immediate laparotomy during which a uterine rupture from myometrial implantation was discovered [30].

Musculoskeletal

Emergency medical technicians have successfully detected the presence of simulated fractures [31], and ultrasound detection of fractures has been useful in combat environments [12]. These suggest diagnostic and therapeutic ultrasound implications particularly in remote environments where traditional diagnostic imaging is not available. Unstudied prehospital ultrasound applications include detection and reduction of shoulder dislocations, hip dislocations, pediatric fractures, and muscle and tendon injuries, and in nerve block analgesia.

Prehospital ultrasound protocols

Prehospital ultrasound protocols have been developed for the evaluation of life-threatening conditions. The Prehospital Assessment with Ultrasound for Emergencies (PAUSE) protocol includes a heart and thorax examination for pericardial effusion, pneumothorax, and cardiac motion with systematic guidance of resuscitative efforts [7]. An integrative sonographic trauma survey has been proposed to identify multi-injury pathologies in the setting of mass casualty or combat. The CAVEAT examination assesses the chest for pneumothorax, hemothorax, and pericardial tamponade, the abdomen for FAST detection of hemoperitoneum, the inferior vena cava for qualitative volume assessment, and targeted extremity evaluation for detection of fracture. As each of the components within this protocol has been demonstrated using non-physicians, it is presumed that this protocol may be incorporated into the medic skill set [13]. Supplementation of EMS training programs with easy-to-follow algorithms using pictorial aids may enable the implementation of prehospital ultrasound evaluation for resuscitation.

Other

In addition to detection of fluid in pleural, pericardial, and peritoneal cavities, Lapostolle et al. evaluated DVT and vascular flow disruptions in an out-of-hospital setting. This study found that ultrasound examination improved diagnostic accuracy in 67% of cases [3]. Ultrasound has been used to diagnose high-altitude pulmonary edema and high-altitude cerebral edema in the Himalayas using thoracic and ocular ultrasound respectively, although with experienced physicians and not with mountain medics [32]. Groups have explored prehospital transcranial Doppler use for assessment of brain injury and neurological disease [33]. Procedural applications like peripheral intravenous access and abscess evaluations may also be useful in out-of-hospital scenarios [12]. Ultrasound-guided thoracentesis and paracentesis are anecdotally common in settings without other radiographic capabilities.

Disaster and mass casualty triage

Mass casualty incidents require fast, reliable triage of large numbers of patients using limited resources. The chaotic environment, relative lack of medical personnel, and destruction of existing infrastructure can prevent early treatment of injured patients. The ability of ultrasound to identify patients who would benefit most from intervention could lessen uncertainties of physical exam findings in these situations. Placing diagnostic capability into the hands of first responders may be useful in future disaster strategies to augment triage accuracy, enhance mobilization of resources, improve allocation of scarce resources, and facilitate destination decisions.

The few studies that have examined the above are understandably retrospective. Chart analysis of trauma patients at a Level I trauma center found that 20 of 286 patients triaged as "yellow" in the simple triage and rapid treatment (START) method had positive FAST findings, with possible delayed hemoperitoneum identified in 7% of total patients. However, only six patients received operative management within 24 hours, with both over- and undertriage as significant problems. Because it is unclear if positive FAST findings would alter management in this setting, the study did not support the use of routine FAST as a secondary triage tool [34].

Others have illustrated the usefulness of the FAST exam as a diagnostic and triage adjunct. Ultrasound was used as a screening modality for free fluid in the 1998 Armenian earthquake [16]. Renal Doppler ultrasound performed at triage guided management of severe acute crush injuries in the aftermath of a 1999 Turkish earthquake [15,35], and ultrasound proved crucial in the identification of hemoperitoneum, hemothorax, intimal tear of the femoral artery, DVT, and deep tissue hematoma in both triage and middle-late stage assessment of patients admitted during the 2010 Wenchuan earthquake [17].

The most recent case illustration highlights the usefulness of emergency department triage by ultrasound during the 2013 Boston Marathon bombing. An emergency medicine resident went bed-to-bed performing ultrasound and tagging results to the patient. The authors note that both triage and acute care for these patients were "crucially informed" by the results of bedside ultrasound and recommended its implementation in disaster planning [36].

Military

The potential for out-of-hospital ultrasound use by military medics in the field is considerable, especially in the recognition of occult blood loss occurring in conditioned soldiers to prevent late-stage shock [13] and in possible sonographically guided coagulation of internal bleeding [37]. Army National Guard medics (EMT-B level) have successfully performed limited echocardiography for detection of cardiac activity [24]. Military non-physician medics have performed fracture evaluation, FAST with pneumothorax examination, ocular, renal, vascular, and obstetric examinations. In addition, ultrasound training has been incorporated into the curriculum for special operator medics [37].

Role of non-physicians/EMS training

Multiple studies have established that non-physician personnel are capable of quickly learning and demonstrating proficiency with ultrasound in a wide variety of applications, in diverse environmental settings, and in differing modes of EMS transport [7–10,23–26].

Training has encompassed a number of different methods including lectures, proctored hands-on sessions, before and after examinations, refresher sessions, OSCE assessments, web-based modules, flashcards, and tele-ultrasound guidance. Course times vary from as little as 2 minutes for fracture evaluation instruction to 1 day for FAST teaching, with cardiac and lung training reported from 10 minutes to 2 hours [4–7,10,14, 23,24]. Instruction for paramedics or ultrasound-naïve physicians outside the United States appears longer, from 8-hour to 100-hour programs for the FAST exam [4,6,9] and 2-day courses for the thoracic exam [38]. Currently, there is no consensus on the optimal training time or method required to adequately train non-physician personnel, and no study to date has compared different training methods for EMS personnel.

Tele-ultrasound

Tele-ultrasound may become a valuable data transmission tool which takes advantage of a centralized expert's sonographic skills and disperses acquisition and interpretation of images to multiple unskilled providers. Tele-ultrasound has been described in remote locations and aboard the International Space Station [23]. In an American study examining feasibility, 51 paramedics with no prior ultrasound experience received a 20-minute didactic session covering orientation and the FAST examination. With tele-ultrasound guidance, they performed complete FAST exams in a median time of 262 seconds [39]. Although real-time clinical translation during EMS transport is required, this technology shows promise.

Feasibility of ultrasound in the field

Apart from operator skill and already known limitations of ultrasound as a diagnostic modality, several recurring limitations appear in field use which may prevent adequate completion of an ultrasound examination. Flight medics reported insufficient time to complete scanning. Screen visibility was hindered by bright ambient light, and physical restrictions arose from lack of space. Patient parameters such as obesity and combativeness prevented imaging, and battery or machine failure contributed to unsuccessful acquisition [14,19]. Similar factors affect on-ground transport: difficult spatial arrangements, sunlight, battery problems, and a requirement for probe handling to be ambidextrous [8]. In addition, harsh environmental conditions deprioritized ultrasound performance and optimal views were limited by presence of pacer pads, cervical collars, or splints [19,40].

With ground transport, multiple examination completion times are longer and measurements may be less precise when completed in a moving vehicle, but these may not be statistically or clinically significant when compared with stationary performance [26]. Other studies have shown that ultrasound can be completed without prolonging transport time [6,8]. Despite these limitations, authors who have examined prehospital ultrasound feasibility have shown positive overall results and demonstrated the modality's utility in the field.

Technological advances have allowed machinery to decrease in cost, weight, and bulk. Recent development of pocket-sized devices, wearable transducers, and in-clothing tele-ultrasound devices illustrates this, but perpetual improvements need to be made. Portable ultrasound devices need to be robust enough to operate in extremes of temperature while maintaining reasonable battery life, and inbuilt alternative power sources (e.g. solar energy) need to be considered. Displays that provide good visibility in bright light conditions with rapid boot-up time and simplified controls need to be incorporated. In addition, expanded image storage space and intrinsic capabilities for image transmission such as wireless internet or Bluetooth need to be included [28].

Future directions

European expert consensus groups have recognized prehospital ultrasound as one of their top research priorities [41]. Recent literature has shown achievable diagnostic accuracy in non-physician hands and presented examples of patient care facilitation in treatment and transport decisions, thus supporting the use of prehospital ultrasound in varying EMS systems, in austere or impoverished settings, in combat and disaster environments, and in large recreational settings. Many of these studies involve small numbers of providers or small numbers of patients. The documented benefits of ultrasound in a hospital setting need to be reproduced in high-powered, larger-scale scenarios in the EMS literature. More permanent integration of ultrasound use within EMS systems, and development of longitudinal standardized curricula within EMS training, need to be established. Within this realm, questions surrounding the most efficacious way to teach first responders the most applicable ultrasound examination types to learn, and the optimal way to approach quality assurance of

prehospital users, need to be answered. Ultimately, large-scale demonstration of the clinical improvement that prehospital ultrasound can produce in patient care needs to be established, and patient-centered outcomes both within and outside the hospital need to be documented.

References

1 American College of Emergency Physicians. Policy Statement: emergency ultrasound guidelines. *Ann Emerg Med* 2009;53:550–70.

2 Melniker LA, Leibner E, McKenney MG, et al. Randomized controlled clinical trial of point-of-care, limited ultrasonography for trauma in the emergency department: the first sonography outcomes assessment program trial. *Ann Emerg Med* 2006;48:227–35.

3 Lapostolle F, Petrovic T, Lenoir G, et al. Usefulness of hand-held ultrasound devices in out-of-hospital diagnosis performed by emergency physicians. *Am J Emerg Med* 2006;24:237–42.

4 Press GM, Miller SK, Hassan IA, et al. Evaluation of a training curriculum for prehospital trauma ultrasound. *J Emerg Med* 2013;45:856–64.

5 Noble VE, Lamhaut L, Capp R, et al. Evaluation of a thoracic ultrasound training module for the detection of pneumothorax and pulmonary edema by prehospital physician care providers. *BMC Med Ed* 2009;9:3.

6 Walcher F, Weinlich M, Conrad G, et al. Prehospital ultrasound imaging improves management of abdominal trauma. *Br J Surg* 2006;93:238–42.

7 Chin EJ, Chan CH, Mortazavi R, et al. A pilot study examining the viability of a prehospital assessment with ultrasound for emergencies (PAUSE) protocol. *J Emerg Med* 2013;44:142–9.

8 Neesse A, Jerrentrup A, Hoffmann S, et al. Prehospital chest emergency sonography trial in Germany: a prospective study. *Eur J Emerg Med* 2012;19:161–6.

9 Nelson BP, Chason K. Use of ultrasound by emergency medical services: a review. *Int J Emerg Med* 2008;1:253–9.

10 Heegaard W, Hildebrandt D, Spear D, et al. Prehospital ultrasound by paramedics: results of field trial. *Acad Emerg Med* 2010;17:624–30.

11 Heegaard W, Hildebrandt D, Reardon R, et al. Prehospital ultrasound diagnosis of a traumatic pericardial effusion. *Acad Emerg Med* 2009;16(4):364.

12 Nelson BP, Melnick ER, Li J. Portable ultrasound for remote environments, Part II: current indications. *J Emerg Med* 2011;40:313–21.

13 Stawicki SP, Howard JM, Pryor JP, et al. Portable ultrasonography in mass casualty incidents: The CAVEAT examination. *World J Orthop* 2010;1:10–19.

14 Melanson SW, McCarthy J, Stromski CJ, et al. Aeromedical trauma sonography by flight crews with a miniature ultrasound unit. *Prehosp Emerg Care* 2001;5:399–402.

15 Ma OJ, Norvell JG, Subramanian S. Ultrasound applications in mass casualties and extreme environments. *Crit Care Med* 2007;35:S275–9.

16 Sarkisian AE, Khondrkarian RA, Amirbekian NM, et al. Sonographic screening of mass casualties for abdominal and renal injuries following the 1988 Armenian earthquake. *J Trauma* 1991;31:247–50.

17 Dan D, Mingson L, Jie T, et al. Ultrasonographic applications after mass casualty incident caused by Wenchuan earthquake. *J Trauma* 2010;68:1417–20.

18 Byhahn C, Bingold TM, Zwissler B, et al. Prehospital ultrasound detects pericardial tamponade in a pregnant victim of stabbing assault. *Resuscitation* 2008;76:146–8.

19 Roline CE, Heegaard WG, Moore JC, et al. Feasibility of bedside thoracic ultrasound in the helicopter emergency medical services setting. *Air Med J* 2013;32(3):153–7.

20 Zechner P, Aichinger G, Rigaud M, et al. Prehospital lung ultrasound in the distinction between pulmonary edema and exacerbation of chronic obstructive pulmonary disease. *Am J Emerg Med* 2010;28:389.e1–2.

21 Brun P, Bessereau J, Cazes N, et al. Lung ultrasound associated to capnography to verify correct endotracheal tube positioning. *Am J Emerg Med* 2012;30:2080.e5–6.

22 Brun P, Chenaitia H, Gonzva J, et al. The value of prehospital echocardiography in shock management. *Am J Emerg Med* 2013;31:442.e5–e7.

23 Hamilton DR, Sargsyan AE, Martin DS, et al. On-orbit prospective echocadiography on international space station crew. *Echocardiography* 2001;28:491–501.

24 Backlund BH, Bonnett CJ, Faragher JP, et al. Pilot study to determine the feasibility of training army national guard medics to perform focused cardiac ultrasonography. *Prehosp Emerg Care* 2010;14:118–23.

25 Aichinger G, Zechner PM, Prause G, et al. Cardiac movement identified on prehospital echocardiography predicts outcome in cardiac arrest patients. *Prehosp Emerg Care* 2012;16:251–5.

26 Snaith B, Hardy M, Walker A. Emergency ultrasound in the prehospital setting: the impact of environment on examination outcomes. *Emerg Med J* 2011;28:1063–5.

27 Mazur SM and Sharley P. The use of point-of-care ultrasound by a critical care retrieval team to diagnose acute abdominal aortic aneurysm in the field. *Emerg Med Australas* 2007;19:71–5.

28 Nelson BP, Melnick ER, Li J. Portable ultrasound for remote environments, Part I: feasibility of field deployment. *J Emerg Med* 2011;40:190–7.

29 Polk JD, Merlino JI, Kovach BL, Mancuso C, Fallon WF. Fetal evaluation for transport performed by air medical teams: a case series. *Air Med J* 2004;23(4):32–4.

30 Galinski M, Petrovic T, Rodrigues A, et al. Out-of-hospital diagnosis of a ruptured ectopic pregnancy: myometrial embryo implantation, an exceptional diagnosis. *Prehosp Emerg Care* 2010;14:496–8.

31 Heiner J, McArthur TJ. The ultrasound identification of simulated long bone fractures by prehospital providers. *Wilderness Environ Med* 2010;21:137–40.

32 Fagenholz PJ, Murray AF, Noble VE, et al. Ultrasound for high altitude research. *Ultrasound Med Biol* 2012;38:1–12.

33 Chenaitia H, Squarcioni C, Marie BP, et al. Transcranial sonography in prehospital setting. *Am J Emerg Med* 2011;29:1231–3.

34 Sztajnkrycer MD, Baez AA, Luke A. FAST Ultrasound as an adjunct to triage using the START mass casualty triage system: a preliminary descriptive study. *Prehosp Emerg Care* 2006;10:96–102.

35 Keven K, Ates K, Yagmurlu B, et al. Renal doppler ultrasonographic findings in earthquake victims with crush injury. *J Ultrasound Med* 2001;20:675–9.

36 Kimberly HH, Stone MB. Clinician-performed ultrasonography during the Boston marathon bombing mass casualty incident. *Ann Emerg Med* 2013;62:199–200.

37 Hile DC, Morgan AR, Laselle BT, et al. Is point-of-care ultrasound accurate and useful in the hands of military medical technicians? A review of the literature. *Mil Med* 2012;177:983–7.

38 Brooke M, Walton J, Scutt D, et al. Acquisition and interpretation of focused diagnostic ultrasound images by ultrasound-naïve advanced paramedics: trialing a PHUS education programme. *Emerg Med J* 2012;29:322–6.

39 Boniface KS, Shokoohi H, Smith ER, et al. Tele-ultrasound and paramedics: real-time remote physician guidance of the focused assessment with sonography for trauma examination. *Am J Emerg Med* 2011;29:477–81.

40 Hoyer HX, Vogl S, Schiemann U, et al. Prehospital ultrasound in emergency medicine: incidence, feasibility, indications and diagnosis. *Eur J Emerg Med* 2010;17:254–9.

41 Rudolph SS, Sorensen K, Svane C, et al. Effect of prehospital ultrasound on clinical outcomes of non-trauma patients – a systematic review. *Resuscitation* 2014;85:21–30.

Safety and Quality

CHAPTER 70

Culture of patient safety

Blair L. Bigham and P. Daniel Patterson

"First, do no harm" (origin unclear)

Introduction

Thousands of patients are treated by EMS providers each day. For most of these patients, their exposure to the health care system will improve their well-being. However, some will experience unintentional harm or be put at risk of being harmed. The sentinel Institute of Medicine paper *To Err is Human: Building a Safer Health System* brought to light the effects these risks and harms can have on patients and systems throughout the health care industry [1]. Since the release of this paper, health care systems and practitioners from a broad spectrum of fields have worked towards understanding the threats to patient safety, researching factors that contribute to unintentional harm and developing methods to reduce, eliminate or mitigate accidental harm.

The term *adverse event* describes an occurrence that resulted in unintended and detrimental morbidity or mortality (patient harm). Adverse events are thought to stem from systemic weaknesses, individual behaviors, or a combination of the two. It has been estimated that one-third of patients admitted to acute care hospitals experienced at least one adverse event [2]. The uncontrolled and time-sensitive prehospital setting offers unique challenges that make adverse events all the more likely to occur.

The concept of EMS as high-reliability organizations (operating relatively error-free operations over a long period of time) is new. Long ago embraced by the nuclear power, aviation, and military industries, high-reliability organizations avoid catastrophes, consistently make safe decisions, and have high-quality, reliable operations. This chapter summarizes the challenges and risks of emergency medical care delivered in the field, presents mechanisms that can address these challenges and reduce these risks, and provides a framework for becoming highly reliable.

There is considerable research and theory focused on the predictors of error and adverse events in high-risk settings. Health care has borrowed from this work and adopted many of the concepts and practices that improve safety. Programs widely used in health care, such as the Agency for Healthcare Research and Quality's TeamSTEPPS, are based on this prior research and theory [3]. Many of these programs or interventions may be active in the hospitals where medical directors practice. Below is an overview of the most common and widely accepted concepts in safety, which may aid medical directors in their efforts to adopt, adapt, or develop programs specifically for their EMS organizations and systems.

How accidents happen

The Swiss cheese model

Several factors can affect patient safety in EMS, and rarely does any one factor act alone to create an adverse event. These factors may be human, relying on people to either commit or omit certain functions, or systemic, depending on procedures, administrative controls, or engineering and design. When people and systems function properly, these aspects work to protect patients from hazards. However, weaknesses can occur. The Swiss cheese model [4] likens these weaknesses to holes in slices of Swiss cheese; many layers of Swiss cheese slices rarely line up to have a hole that one could peer through, but when the slices align in just the right way, a trajectory through the cheese opens up, and an adverse event can occur (Figure 70.1). The model attributes these holes to two conditions: active failures, where unsafe acts are committed by people, and latent conditions referred to as systemic flaws in design or processes that allow hazards to be present. When active failures and latent conditions align in the right manner, an adverse event can occur.

System factors

While human error often contributes to adverse events, humans are considered the last piece of cheese in the Swiss cheese model. As humans are, by nature, not highly reliable, additional slices of cheese are installed in organizations to make processes safer. These system factors can include the workplace culture itself, written

Emergency Medical Services: Clinical Practice and Systems Oversight, Second Edition. Volume 1: Clinical Aspects of EMS.
Edited by David C. Cone, Jane H. Brice, Theodore R. Delbridge, and J. Brent Myers.
© 2015 NAEMSP. Published 2015 by John Wiley & Sons, Inc. Companion Website: www.wiley.com\go\cone\naemsp

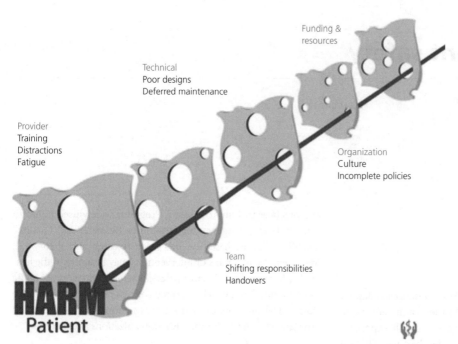

Funding &
resources

Technical
Poor designs
Deferred maintenance

Provider
Training
Distractions
Fatigue

Organization
Culture
Incomplete policies

Team
Shifting responsibilities
Handovers

HARM
Patient

Figure 70.1 The Swiss cheese model of accidents. Multiple approaches are taken to avoid patient harm. If each layer of defense fails, an adverse event can occur. Careful analysis of the "slices" can lead to increased slices or reduced holes. Source: Reason 2000 [4]. Reproduced with permission of the BMJ.

policy and procedure, training in process and best practice, and technological solutions or engineering modifications that account for human fallibility. Examples of system factors that may lead to ambulance collisions include policies that require lights and sirens use, poor training in emergency vehicle operation, a culture that glorifies speedy driving, and vehicles with poor reflective markings [5]. Examples of system-level safety improvements to these problems include evidence-based algorithms that recommend judicious lights and sirens use, provision of special vehicle operator training, a culture that emphasizes safety over speed, and ambulances with science-guided reflective markings [5].

Many different organizations work together to ensure EMS services are provided to the community. This includes all the partner organizations that contribute to a tiered response, including municipal fire and police agencies, ambulance dispatch centers, base hospitals providing medical oversight, and receiving hospitals. With these multiple groups come inherent opportunities for miscommunication and adverse events to occur. Fragmented oversight of the system could lead to a situation where the same adverse event goes unrealized and occurs repeatedly. Interagency collaboration and training can improve team performance [6].

Human factors and ergonomics

Human traits that contribute to adverse events are known as *human factors* [7]. Examples of human factors that can have negative effects on patient safety include complacency, fatigue, eyesight, and inattention [8]. However, it is important to remember that human factors also contribute to safety, as human action or inaction is often the last "slice of cheese" protecting patients. Examples include seeking clarification from a partner or developing strong habit patterns for checking medication concentrations.

Task fixation is a common human factor that can contribute to error in EMS. Commonly termed "tunnel vision," it can occur during endotracheal intubation or 12-lead ECG acquisition. Here, providers are so focused on a task perceived to be important that changes in the patient condition, such as desaturation, or competing priorities, such as chest compressions, can be excluded from thought. Many EMS procedures involve many actions and decisions. When the *critical step* is completed, it is common for downstream sequential actions to be forgotten. An example would be failure to release a tourniquet after placing an intravenous cannula.

Another term used alongside human factors is *ergonomics*. This refers to physical human limitations, and is most commonly employed in developing work environments that complement the human body. Applying ergonomic science has brought about color- and font-coded medications, advanced "track system" stairchairs, and cardiopulmonary resuscitation (CPR) metronomes. A classic example of a common adverse event that was addressed using human factors and ergonomic science is that of the tourniquet; previously made of latex that was a similar tone to Caucasian skin, phlebotomists and other health care workers were known to leave tourniquets applied after collecting blood. By changing the color of tourniquets to bright blue, the incidence of forgetting to remove tourniquets dropped dramatically. The visual cue of the bright blue was all that was required to help providers remember the step of tourniquet release.

Communication is also a key component to safety [9]. Not being heard, or being heard incorrectly, can lead to a task not being performed, the wrong task being performed, or a task being performed in the wrong way. Examples include medication errors and procedures being performed on the wrong limb. Callouts are used to ensure clear communication among all members of a team. Yelling "Clear!" prior to discharging a defibrillator is an example of a callout. A *readback* occurs when the receiver repeats the message from the sender. For example:

> Paramedic A: "Please give 5 milligrams of morphine"
> Paramedic B: "Ok, giving 5 milligrams of morphine"
> Paramedic A: "Yep, thank you"

When a readback does not happen, the sender should challenge the receiver to make sure he or she interpreted the message correctly. For example:

> Paramedic A: "Did you hear me ask you to give 5 milligrams of morphine?"

Judgment and clinical thinking

There is limited research describing the actions, inactions, and clinical decision making of EMS personnel in relation to safety. Prehospital care providers exercise clinical decision-making skills on each and every call. Two key outcomes of these decisions are working diagnoses and treatment plans. Often protocols and guidelines are used to help field clinicians arrive at an accurate working diagnosis, which increases the likelihood that a correct treatment plan will be initiated.

However, error exists in this area. Physicians are estimated to make a misdiagnosis in 10–15% of cases, and this is likely higher in emergency medicine [10]. Over 100 biases contribute to error in emergency medicine and can be related to cognitive pathways used by emergency workers to arrive at decisions [11]. The first is the intuitive pathway, developed through repeated experience. In this pathway, patterns are recognized quickly, and interventions are applied without much thought. While this serves paramedics well, there will be times when intuition is wrong. Following an analytical pathway can improve reliability in decision making by applying conscious, deliberate thought processes to a clinical situation. While this may take longer, the process of careful examination and testing can improve upon the intuitive pathway. Analytical reasoning is resource intensive, and requires a certain state of mind that can be clouded by stress, workload, and human factors such as personal stress, sleep patterns, and diet [12].

By understanding how emergency physicians and prehospital care providers think in the clinical setting, we can start to appreciate how patient safety is safeguarded by making sound clinical decisions, and how poor decisions can lead to disaster. Remembering that nearly all clinical staff want to perform well and improve patients' lives, it is important to examine poor clinical decisions from a system perspective and not place blame on individuals. Addressing clinical decision making is best done with educational strategies that train clinicians how to think critically. Described as the "ability to engage in purposeful, self-regulatory judgment" [13], this construct permits clinicians to make treatment decisions based on the analytical pathway when needed, specifically to "double check"

and override the intuitive pathway. An example of this metacognition would be when a paramedic walks into a residence and sees a patient who is diaphoretic, clutching his chest. Intuitively the paramedic may think "Oh, this guy is having a STEMI!" but the analytical process of obtaining a 12-lead ECG and inquiring about risk factors and incident history may elucidate a scenario more suggestive of aortic dissection, pulmonary embolism, or cocaine toxicity.

Croskerry describes the development of critical thinking which, while not innate, can be "taught and cultivated, but even accomplished critical thinkers remain vulnerable to occasional undisciplined and irrational thought" [12].

In contrast to hospital settings, there is a stunning lack of epidemiological data pertaining to adverse events in the prehospital setting, despite a recognized need to better understand patient safety in EMS systems [14,15]. While there is some evidence documenting medical error by prehospital care providers [16], research from time-sensitive areas in the hospital, such as the critical care unit or emergency department, can also shine a light on adverse events that likely occur in the field as well. In one retrospective chart review of 15,000 cases, the emergency department was the most prevalent location in the hospital for negligent adverse events to occur [17] and others have made efforts to establish definitions and measurements for error in emergency medicine [18].

Patient safety in EMS

The unique environment

Emergency medical services personnel often work in small, poorly lit spaces in an environment that is chaotic, unfriendly, and challenging for time-sensitive health care interventions; indeed, it is often the dangerous nature of the environment that has led to the call for help. Unlike a hospital, emergency scenes can be filled with distracters that can increase the odds that an adverse event will occur. Physical characteristics of these scenes include loud noises, poor lighting, uncontrolled movement of people and vehicles, and small spaces. Language barriers, noise, stress, and medical conditions may limit effective communication between providers and their patients. Providers often work from compact bags rather than large, well-labeled cabinets and drawers. This limitation reduces the opportunity to place visual cues or organize equipment for optimal performance.

In addition to these challenging environmental factors, emotional stressors are often heightened by the presence of panicked family members and curious bystanders, and a lack of human and medical resources. The time-sensitive nature of EMS care further compounds these physical and emotional stressors. Further, EMS work can be complicated by multiple handoffs from BLS providers to ALS providers to air ambulance crews and finally to hospital staff. Lastly, EMS work is round the clock, and often EMS workers endure 12-, 14-, or 24-hour shifts with few opportunities for meals or rest [19]. This can lead to fatigue, which is known to play a role in adverse event incident rates [8,20]. The arena in which EMS providers work is rich with opportunities for adverse events attributed to provider or system errors.

Importantly, unintentional error can have profoundly negative effects on EMS providers [21,22]. Increased stress, time away from work, family disruptions, job burnout, divorce, depression, and suicide in health care workers have all been correlated to adverse events [22].

Defining patient safety in EMS

There is no common language used to define adverse events in the EMS setting, making general discussion and comparisons challenging. The World Health Organization defines patient safety as the "reduction of risk of unnecessary harm associated with health care to an acceptable minimum" [7]. The term "acceptable minimum" refers to the collective notions given current knowledge, resources available, and the context within which care was delivered weighed against the risk of non-treatment or other treatment [7]. In other words, the acceptable minimum risk fluctuates based on the context of the health care delivery system. What may be considered an unacceptable risk in an operating theatre may be an acceptable risk in the prehospital setting, and vice versa.

Harm need not occur for patient safety principles to apply; potential risks of unintended harm, termed *near misses*, are of core interest as they represent opportunities to implement safer practices before harm has been inflicted. Examples of near misses include drawing up, but not administering, the wrong medication, or charging a defibrillator when a patient has a palpable pulse.

Sometimes, the distinction between patient safety and clinical efficacy can be difficult. The efficacy of specific treatments for specific diseases, such as albuterol for asthma or needle thoracostomy for tension pneumothorax, is excluded from the realm of patient safety, while drug dosing errors and diagnostic errors surrounding these treatments are included.

Adverse events are commonly categorized as *active failures*, involving humans at the point of care, or *latent conditions*, where contributing factors facilitated the human-driven error to occur. An example of an active failure would be a paramedic calculating a drug dose incorrectly. Examples of latent conditions could be the lack of preloaded medications, long work hours, and poor training [4].

Measuring adverse events in EMS

The very nature of EMS creates complex challenges to measuring adverse event rates [23,24]. Currently, recognition of adverse events is achieved in one of three ways. First, an EMS provider recognizes that an error has occurred. Second, another health care provider, such as a receiving hospital physician, recognizes an adverse event. Lastly, retrospective quality assurance measures rely on documentation review (chart review) to identify adverse events.

Often, adverse events go unrecognized. Once providers transport a patient to an emergency department or an inpatient bed, they return to service in their community. Often, providers will transport patients to several different hospitals during a shift. These aspects of EMS work make patient follow-up difficult, and adverse events that do not present immediately are difficult if not impossible to realize. In addition, privacy legislation often prohibits EMS services from accessing outcomes on patients transported to hospital as some interpret the legislation in such a way that it excludes the paramedic and the EMS service from the "circle of care."

Emergency department staff caring for individuals may not realize the role EMS played in a patient safety incident and may not be familiar with a process to report such events even if they suspected it was attributed to EMS care. Efforts to calculate adverse event rates in EMS may require extension into the emergency department and include hospital outcomes to truly understand the scope of adverse events associated with prehospital care.

If recognized, adverse events must then be reported. Until recently, formal adverse event reporting processes were lacking in most EMS systems. Today, reporting systems remain heterogeneous and underutilized. Providers often admit they do not report adverse events for fear of punitive action by employers or medical directors [22]. Others report feeling ashamed, and fear humiliation in the face of their colleagues. To combat this human tendency, many EMS systems use anonymous adverse event reporting systems [25]. EMS providers also express a willingness to report but often complain about the complexity or inconvenience involved in certain electronic or paper-based reporting tools [6]. To benefit from recognized adverse events, organizations must foster a culture where adverse event and near-miss reporting is encouraged and develop convenient platforms that facilitate reporting. The term *just culture* is applied to describe an environment where unintentional human error is supported rather than penalized.

Currently there is no uniform method for measurement or a national dataset to quantify the rate of adverse event rates in EMS systems [23,24]. The lack of a common language to define adverse events in EMS makes comparing literature difficult. Few EMS systems have attempted to measure the incidence of adverse events, and those that have done so have relied on self-reported adverse event rates provided in retrospective surveys [16,26–28]. Without a framework for defining, classifying, and reporting adverse events, there is no way of knowing the true incidence of adverse events in the prehospital setting. Recent research focused on measurement validity provides a foundation from which to fill this gap in structure and standardization [23]. This problem is not unique to EMS, and has been described in the hospital and mental health settings as well [1,7,29].

The major problems

Scientific literature

A systematic review published in 2012 compiled 88 peer-reviewed articles that investigated patient safety in EMS [30]. The articles identified seven key themes related to patient harm

Table 70.1 Patient safety themes in the literature (2011)

Theme	# articles
Clinical judgment	13
Adverse events and error reporting	22
Ground vehicle safety	6
Aircraft safety	9
Interfacility transport	16
Field intubation	16

in the EMS setting and mostly studied low-hanging fruit – topics that are easy to define and retrospectively measure (Table 70.1). The methods and quality of the articles were highly variable, and only one was a randomized controlled trial. Populations studied included patients of all ages, from neonatal to geriatric, as well as the providers themselves. Conditions studied ranged from "all-callers" to specific patient subgroups. Both 9-1-1 and interfacility encounters were studied, and providers ranged from EMTs to physicians [30].

In the only randomized controlled trial [31], safety outcomes for patients >59 years of age who received treatment from standard paramedics versus extended scope paramedics who had received additional training in the management of low acuity conditions were studied.

Patient safety outcomes studied in the literature ranged from physiological variables (heart rate, blood pressure, oxygen saturation, etc.) and equipment malfunction (defibrillators, stretchers, aircraft, etc.), to perceived barriers in self-reporting adverse events (culture, fatigue, policies, etc.) [30]. Other outcomes examined patient discourse (readmission, death, etc.), information exchange (in dispatch, at transfer of care, etc.), and technical skill accuracy (medication dose calculation, endotracheal intubation success rates, etc.) [30].

The literature and the experts: a disconnect

As part of a large, multiphase study into patient safety in EMS, the Canadian Patient Safety Institute and EMS Chiefs of Canada conducted qualitative research with EMS experts following completion of the 2012 systematic review [6,30,32]. The objective was to triangulate the findings of the systematic review with knowledge users working in clinical and administrative positions in the EMS industry. However, the experts interviewed were surprised by the systematic review findings [32]. Generally, they considered that the literature studied matters that were not priority issues in safety. For examples, ground vehicle collisions and endotracheal intubation featured prominently in the literature, but experts felt these were studied because of the dichotomous nature and "sexiness" of the topics. Core problems were felt to be more complex and difficult to measure.

Clinical judgment was felt to be the greatest threat to patient safety. Citing "scope creep," where additional skills and responsibilities are added to EMS provider practice without the requisite foundational education, experts felt that good clinical judgment was the best attribute of a provider. Strong foundational training

and years of experience were thought to contribute to strong clinical decision making. The second topic felt to be affecting safety is an "identity crisis" in EMS where it is torn between the health care industry and the public safety industry. Fundamental cultural differences between these two industries were thought to be exploitable to improve safety. For example, the emphasis on speed in public safety may not benefit patients clinically and may in fact cause harm. Similarly, the hierarchy that can be present in public safety chains of command may lead to a lack of communication between providers that can allow recognized harms to happen [32].

The emphasis placed on judgment and culture by the experts has been poorly studied, yet some evidence supports their convictions [5]. Providers with more experience or education tend to make fewer errors than their inexperienced or lesser trained counterparts, and organizational culture has been found to be closely associated to adverse event rates, reporting rates, and the ability of systems to improve safety metrics.

Just culture and adverse event reporting

In recognition of human factors and previously discussed systemic deficits that contribute to adverse events, safety experts advocate for a "just culture" in health care organizations [33]. The most important step in creating a safe culture is the establishment of justice. In a "just" culture, a term coined by David Marx, a system of shared accountability exists where an organization is responsible for safe *system and process design*, and employees are responsible for *safe choices and behaviors*. Rather than operating in a *"blame and shame"* environment, where employees feel frightened of reporting safety concerns and human error, in a just culture employees trust the leaders to respond fairly to employee concerns and behaviors. In turn, leaders act when human error is anticipated by establishing system-level solutions to support employee operations and prevent adverse events. Employees are expected to make safe choices and utilize the tools and processes implemented by leaders. In this collaborative environment, maximum safety can be achieved.

Employee reporting is critical to achieving maximum safety [34]. Using an iceberg to illustrate this importance, EMS leaders are aware of only the tip of the iceberg when it comes to safety challenges in EMS systems, while field providers are aware of the ice beneath the surface. To encourage adverse event and near-miss reporting, several steps can be taken as an EMS agency develops a safety culture [25].

- The use of anonymous adverse event report systems has been successful in demonstrating the commitment of leaders to developing trust with employees. By not identifying those who report, the perceived threat of punitive action is removed.
- Reporting must be made easy to do. The use of complex, password-protected reporting tools using mandatory data fields often results in non-compliance due to perceived hassle or time required to report.

- Each report of an adverse event or near miss should feature a "closed loop" where the person who reported the concern receives a synopsis of investigations and actions taken to establish system-level improvements. This will reinforce reporting behavior and lead to grassroots support of the reporting system.
- Praise those who come forward. It takes remarkable courage to admit error, especially in the EMS environment. Highlight staff who come forward as being exceptional, professional, brave, and caring.

Fostering a just culture will encourage reporting, but processes must be in place to make sure that reports do not get ignored. A safety management system, described later in this chapter, features processes that facilitate reporting, trigger key actions that mitigate harm, mandate the systems-level search for root causes that could be addressed, assign responsibility to follow up with stakeholders and implement safety solutions and feedback pathways to reinforce reporting and analyze the actions of individuals and the organization itself. Several successful adverse event tools have been implemented by various groups. For example, an online publically accessible form is run by the State of Pennsylvania [35]and the Center for Leadership, Innovation and Research in EMS operates the EMS Voluntary Event Notification Tool (EVENT) used by several agencies in both the US and Canada [36].

A just system does not necessitate a blame-free system. Three levels of behavior can be considered in hierarchical fashion [25].

1 **Human error**: an inadvertent action; inadvertently doing other that what should have been done; slip, lapse, mistake.
2 **At-risk behavior**: a behavioral choice that increases risk where risk is not recognized, or is mistakenly believed to be justified.
3 **Reckless behavior**: a behavioral choice to consciously disregard a substantial and unjustifiable risk.

By carefully analyzing an adverse event, leadership can then select appropriate responses to the unsafe behavior. Such responses may be only to console, to provide additional training or reminders, or, in the case of reckless behavior, to respond punitively. In a just culture, employee and leader responsibilities can reach a balance and striving for safety excellence becomes a shared vision of everyone in the organization.

Evaluating organizational safety culture

Given the difficulty with detecting and quantifying adverse events, there is great interest and wide-scale acceptance for the measurement of workplace safety culture as a barometer of safety conditions in the health care workplace. Organizational (workplace) safety culture refers to the shared meaning, language and metaphors, rituals and convictions, beliefs, attitudes, behaviors, and norms adopted and displayed by workers regarding safety [37]. Attention to and research of workplace safety culture originated in high-risk industries such as nuclear power, manufacturing, and aviation [38]. Since 1980, more than 140 studies have been completed on workplace safety culture in health care settings [39].

The most commonly used tool for measuring safety culture is a survey of front-line workers [40]. Multiple survey tools are available, including the Safety Attitudes Questionnaire (SAQ), the Agency for Healthcare Research and Quality safety culture survey, and others [40]. Most tools assess multiple components of safety culture and provide a score to indicate positive or non-positive perceptions of safety. These scores are commonly used for benchmarking purposes and to evaluate the effect of a safety focused intervention. The SAQ is a frequently used tool that has been adapted for diverse settings, including the prehospital setting [41].

Few studies have examined the safety culture of EMS organizations. The first known study showed that an adaptation to the SAQ, in the form of the EMS-SAQ, would provide reliable and valid data [41]. A follow-up study deployed the EMS-SAQ to 61 diverse EMS agencies, exposed wide variation in safety culture scores across EMS agencies, and provided base-rate data for comparison/benchmarking purposes [42]. A third study demonstrated a linkage between EMS-SAQ scores and safety outcomes, including injury, errors, adverse events, and safety-compromising behaviors [43]. Related efforts demonstrate the utility of adapting other safety culture tools for application in the EMS setting [44].

Higher, more positive safety culture scores have been linked to air medical EMS agencies, private free-standing EMS systems, smaller organizations with fewer employees (e.g. ≤50), and EMS organizations with fewer total patient contacts [42]. Lower, or non-positive scores, have been linked to urban ground-based models, hospital-based systems, larger organizations with >101 employees, and agencies that amass >10,000 annual patient contacts [42]. Administrators of EMS agencies may examine their safety culture and gather base-rate data for benchmarking by deploying the EMS-SAQ survey tool, available free to all [42].

Changing organizational culture

Change in workplace safety culture begins with and is sustained by upper management. The renowned father of patient safety, Dr Lucian Leape, emphasized the importance of the role of leadership in the following statement: "Over and over again, we have observed process and quality improvement efforts implemented but ultimately fail because the CEO did not lend support to the initiatives" [45].

Whether recognized or not, our leaders set the example for employees to follow [46]. Their visibility or lack thereof, tone of message, communication or lack thereof, and commitment to safety infiltrate the workforce and affect behavior. Some key attributes of a positive safety culture and supportive leadership structure include:

- safety as a core value and philosophy of the organization and leadership
- safety principles/assumptions known and adhered to by the workforce and proclaimed by leadership
- presence, operation, and support for an internal safety management system
- integrity to safety reporting and management and commitment from the leadership for safety improvement
- amnesty for reporting and a blame-free culture
- empowerment of safety leaders within the front-line workforce
- constant monitoring and improvement in safety [46].

Change does not and cannot begin with front-line employees [46]. Unfortunately, disconnects can exist between what leadership perceives as the workplace safety culture and what the front-line workers perceive [47]. Often times, leaders perceive a much higher (more positive) safety culture while workers perceive the culture to be much lower [47]. This disconnect must be addressed and not ignored. High-level management must also decide that safety is a priority and that the time, resources, and commitment required to improve safety will be provided, or change will not occur [46].

Safety management systems in EMS

Safety management systems are formal, organized programs within or across high-reliability organizations. They must have written policies and procedures in place, prescribe responsibility, authority, accountability and expectations, ensure strong record keeping, encourage deliberate and early recognition of potential problems, and support quick intervention to address hazards and manage risk. The collection and analysis of data are used to support and advance safety goals and assure progress is being made. Audit/investigations are a component of assurance. While medical directors may not have control over all aspects of the safety of EMS operations, they can play a role in continual improvement and change management. Lastly, safety must be promoted throughout the organization through training, communication, and cultural integration. This starts by seeking out safety-focused qualities in job candidates, training staff in just culture, and socializing them into an organization that supports and in fact demands safe behavior.

In some systems, medical directors will have a great deal of control over the design and day-to-day operations of a safety management system. Others will have only a small role. Regardless of the degree of control, medical directors can ensure that there is a data collection process so that all members of an organization can and do report adverse events and near misses. Further, medical directors can play a role in using these data to seek continuous improvements.

The International Helicopter Safety Team's safety management system (SMS) toolkit lists the following methods of promoting safety [25].

- Publish a statement of the commitment of the leadership to the SMS.
- Leaders should demonstrate their commitment to SMS by example.
- Communicate the output of the SMS to all employees.
- Provide training for personnel commensurate with their level of responsibility.
- Define competency requirements for individuals in key positions.
- Document, review, and update training requirements.
- Share "lessons learned" that promote improvement of the SMS.
- Have a safety feedback system with appropriate levels of confidentiality that promotes participation by all personnel in the identification of hazards.
- Implement a "just culture" process that ensures fairness and open reporting in dealing with human error.

The future of patient safety in EMS

The past decade has seen patient safety become a focus of the EMS industry. Numerous national initiatives to improve patient safety in the EMS industry are under way. Several researchers from both paramedic and physician backgrounds have begun to build a solid body of knowledge and meaningful frameworks from which to drive further academic study. The EVENT anonymous reporting system has spread to include several jurisdictions in both Canada and the US [36]. In addition to a plethora of literature about patient safety in other health care settings, a white paper entitled *Patient Safety in EMS: Advancing and Aligning the Culture of Patient Safety in EMS* was a large initiative published by the Canadian Patient Safety Institute in 2009 [6]. Following this, the National Highway Traffic Safety Administration launched a "Culture of Safety" initiative that describes the issue of patient safety in EMS as "an urgent problem of unknown scope" and expands the issue of patient safety into that of public safety and provider safety. Indeed, the triad of patient, provider and the public are all at risk when ambulances crash en route to hospital.

Commonly, both the Canadian and American strategy documents identify a lack of data-driven decision making as a major obstacle to improving safety in EMS, and addressing this will be a focus of the next decade. In addition to sound safety data systems, just culture, adverse event reporting, provider and leader education, safety standards and resources, and collaboration between organizations and regulators are priorities as EMS agencies seek to become highly reliable [48].

Conclusion

The EMS industry is fraught with challenges by the very nature of responding to emergencies in the field. Physical and emotional stressors can challenge providers in their technical skills, cognitive thinking, and communication tasks. Several latent environmental and system factors exist that make EMS scenes ripe with opportunity for adverse events to occur, and the system of care involves several organizations that do not share common leadership or culture. This fragmented characteristic of EMS delivery requires extensive collaboration amongst many agencies to identify potential system attributes that can lead to adverse events, recognize adverse events through front-line staff engagement, create a just culture, and employ safety management systems to engineer and implement solutions that can prevent adverse events from occurring. Through collaboration and the fostering of a just culture, data-driven decisions will allow EMS agencies to achieve higher reliability and offer the safest care to the patients they serve.

References

1 Kohn L, Corrigan J, Donaldson M. *To Err is Human: Building a Safer Health System: Committee on Quality of Health Care in America.* Washington, DC: Institute of Medicine, 1999.

2 Classen DC, Resar R, Griffin F, et al. Global trigger tool shows that adverse events in hospitals may be ten times greater than previously measured. *Health Aff (Millwood)* 2011;30:581–9.

3 US Department of Health and Human Services. TEAMSTEPPS. Available at: http://teamstepps.ahrq.gov

4 Reason J. Human error: models and management. *BMJ* 2000; 320:768–70.

5 Brice J, Studnek JR, Bigham BL, et al. EMS provider and patient safety during response and transport: proceedings of an Ambulance Safety Conference. *Prehosp Emerg Care* 2012;16:3–19.

6 Bigham BL, Maher J, Brooks SC, et al. *Patient Safety in Emergency Medical Services: Advancing and Aligning the Culture of Patient Safety in EMS.* Edmonton, Canada: Canadian Patient Safety Institute, 2010.

7 Runciman W, Hibbert P, Thomson R, et al. Towards an international classification for patient safety: key concepts and terms. *Int J Qual Health Care* 2009;21:18–26.

8 Patterson PD, Weaver MD, Frank RC, et al. Association between poor sleep, fatigue, and safety outcomes in emergency medical services providers. *Prehosp Emerg Care* 2012;16:86–97.

9 Thomas EJ. Improving teamwork in healthcare: current approaches and the path forward. *BMJ Qual Saf* 2011;20:647–50.

10 Berner ES, Graber ML. Overconfidence as a cause of diagnostic error in medicine. *Am J Med* 2008;121:S2–23.

11 Croskerry, P. A universal model of diagnostic reasoning. *Acad Med* 2009;84:1022–08.

12 Croskerry P. From mindless to mindful practice – cognitive bias and clinical decision making. *N Engl J Med* 2013;368:2445–8.

13 Abrami PC, Bernard RM, Borokhovski E, et al. Instructional interventions affecting critical thinking skills and dispositions: a stage 1 meta-analysis. *Rev Educ Res* 2008;78:1102–34.

14 O'Connor RE, Slovis CM, Hunt RC, et al. Eliminating errors in emergency medical services: realitites and recommendations. *Prehosp Emerg Care* 2002;6:107–13.

15 Patient safety in emergency medical services: roundtable report and recommendations. Available at: http://saem.org/newsltr/2002/mar-apr/nhtsa.pdf

16 Hobgood C, Bowen JB, Brice JH, Overby B, Tamayo-Sarver JH. Do EMS personnel identify, report, and disclose medical errors? *Prehosp Emerg Care* 2006;10:21–7.

17 Thomas EJ, Studdert DM, Burstin HR, et al. Incidence and types of adverse events and negligent care in Utah and Colorado. *Med Care* 2000;38:261–71.

18 Handler JA, Gillam M, Sanders AB, Klasco R. Defining, identifying and measuring error in emergency medicine. *Acad Emerg Med* 2000;7:1183–8.

19 Patterson PD, Weaver MD, Hostler D, et al. The shift length, fatigue, and safety conundrum in EMS. *Prehosp Emerg Care* 2012;16:572–6.

20 Australian Commission on Safety and Quality in Health Care. *Safe Staffing and Patient Safety Literature Review.* Report for the Australian Council for Quality and Safety in Health Care. Available at: www.safetyandquality.gov.au

21 Cushman JT, Fairbanks RJ, O'Gara KG, et al. Ambulance personnel perceptions of near misses and adverse events in pediatric patients. *Prehosp Emerg Care* 2010;14:477–84.

22 Fairbanks RJ, Crittenden CN, O'Gara KG, et al. Emergency medical services provider perceptions of the nature of adverse events and near-misses in out-of-hospital care: an ethnographic view. *Acad Emerg Med* 2008;15:633–40.

23 Patterson PD, Lave JR, Martin-Gill C, et al. Measuring adverse events in helicopter emergency medical services: establishing content validity. *Prehosp Emerg Care* 2014;18(1):35–45.

24 Patterson PD, Weaver MD, Abebe K, et al. Identification of adverse events in ground transport emergency medical services. *Am J Med Qual* 2012;27:139–46.

25 Greene M, Bigham B, Patterson D. *Best Practices in EMS: Safety Management Systems in EMS: An Implementation Guide*, 2012. Available at: www.fitchassoc.com/download/Safety_Mgmt_Systems_EMS.pdf

26 Hobgood C, Weiner B, Tamayo-Sarver JH. Medical error identification, disclosure, and reporting: do emergency medicine provider groups differ? *Acad Emerg Med* 2006;13:443–51.

27 Hobgood C, Xie J, Weiner B, Hooker J. Error identification, disclosure, and reporting: practice patterns of three emergency medicine provider types. *Acad Emerg Med* 2004;11:196–9.

28 Vilke GM, Tornabene SV, Stepanski B, et al. Paramedic self-reported medication errors. *Prehosp Emerg Care* 2007;11:80–4.

29 Bowers L. The expression and comparison of ward incident rates. *Issues Ment Health Nurs* 2000;21:365–74.

30 Bigham BL, Buick JE, Morrison M, et al. Patient safety in emergency medical services: a systematic review of the literature. *Prehosp Emerg Care* 2012;16:20–35.

31 Mason S, Knowles E, Freeman J, Snooks H. Safety of paramedics with extended skills. *Acad Emerg Med* 2008;15:607–12.

32 Atack L, Maher J. Emergency medical and health providers' perceptions of key issues in prehospital patient safety. *Prehosp Emerg Care* 2010;14:95–102.

33 Patterson PD, Huang DT, Fairbanks RJ, et al. Variation in emergency medical services workplace safety culture. *Prehosp Emerg Care* 2010;14:448–60.

34 Gallagher JM, Kupas DF. Experience with an anonymous web-based state EMS safety incident reporting system. *Prehosp Emerg Care* 2011;16:36–42

35 Pennsylvania State. EMS safety event reporting system. Availabe at: http://ems.health.state.pa.us/EMSEventSystem/EMSEventDataEntry.aspx?

36 Center for Leadership, Innovation and Research in EMS. EMS voluntary event notification tool. Available at: http://event.clirems.org/

37 Guldenmund FW. The nature of safety culture: a review of theory and research. *Saf Sci* 2000;34:215–57.

38 Helmreich RL, Merritt AC. *Culture at Work in Aviation and Medicine: National, Organizational, and Professional Influences.* Burlington, VT: Ashgate Publishing Company, 1998.

39 Halligan M, Zecevic A. Safety culture in healthcare: a review of concepts, dimensions, measures and progress. *BMJ Qual Saf* 2011;20:338–43.

40 Colla JB, Bracken AC, Kinney LM, Weeks WB. Measuring patient safety climate: a review of surveys. *Qual Saf Health Care* 2005;14:364–6.

41 Patterson PD, Huang DT, Fairbanks RJ, Wang HE. The emergency medical services safety attitudes questionnaire. *Am J Med Qual* 2010;25:109–15.

42 Patterson PD, Huang DT, Fairbanks RJ, et al. Variation in emergency medical services workplace safety culture. *Prehosp Emerg Care* 2010;14:448–60.

43 Weaver MD, Wang HE, Fairbanks RJ, Patterson PD. The association between EMS workplace safety culture and safety outcomes. *Prehosp Emerg Care* 2012;16:43–52.

44 Eliseo LJ, Murray KA, White LF, et al. EMS providers' perceptions of safety climate and adherence to safe work practices. *Prehosp Emerg Care* 2012;16:53–8.

45 Grazier KL. Interview with Lucian Leape, adjunct professor of health policy, Department of Health Policy and Management, Harvard School of Public Health. *J Healthcare Manag* 2008; 53:73–7.

46 McKinnon RC. *Changing the Workplace Safety Culture.* Boca Raton, FL: CRC Press, 2014.

47 Huang DT, Clermont G, Sexton JB, et al. Perceptions of safety culture vary across the intensive care units of a single institution. *Crit Care Med* 2007;35:165–76.

48 American College of Emergency Physicians. National EMS culture of safety. Available at: www.emscultureofsafety.org/

CHAPTER 71

A historical view of quality concepts and methods

Dia Gainor and Robert Swor

Introduction

Anyone on a journey of learning about quality will find the roadside littered with acronyms and mysterious terms; ISO, SPC, and Six Sigma are just a few. This chapter will provide the reader with an understanding of the evolution and types of quality initiatives that have appeared during the 20th century. In addition to literacy about common quality improvement (QI) systems in contemporary use, EMS system leaders and others involved in quality should have a fundamental understanding about the setting, concepts, and progression of quality initiatives in recent history. This chapter will highlight the origins and approach of quality systems found in the United States through the hospital, manufacturing, and government influences that shaped them into what they are today.

Key differences between the approaches undertaken in the industrial and manufacturing settings and their resulting systems illustrate the opportunities from which EMS and other components in the health care system may benefit. This chapter will describe the genesis and "systems" of quality assessment and improvement that have been or can be adopted by organizations interested in enhancing their performance. To the extent that a person, agency, or tool was instrumental in the discovery or development of the system, they will be addressed in context.

The evolution of quality concepts and methods

Prior to the 20th century, activities most closely related to quality assurance emerged in medicine and manufacturing in very similar ways: societies or "guilds" of like practitioners or craftsmen formed on a community or jurisdictional basis [1,2]. These societies set standards and reviewed the performance of individual members, acting against or expelling members for unacceptable performance or behavior. Early in their legislative

formation (some as early as the late 1700s), many states yielded the authority to credential physicians to medical societies [2]. Although this was largely an effort to protect the profession, it likely assured some level of quality through the development of community standards of care.

The landscape of medicine and manufacturing began to change in different ways in the early 20th century. By 1900, in the United States it was common for states to establish boards and effect physician licensure as a function of the state. This migration marked the beginning of one approach to assuring quality in health care: regulation. The regulatory approach was marked by the states' decisions to mandate licensure of hospitals by their state health departments, beginning early in the 1900s [2]. Licensure activities typically include some form of application, inspection to assure conformity with minimum standards, correction of conditions that fail to meet the minimum standard, issuance of a credential for a time-limited duration, and a cyclical repetition of these steps in order to perpetuate the license.

During the same time frame, medicine in the United States was revolutionized by the work of Sir William Osler, attributed with the "learning science" approach to assuring quality in health care [3]. While Osler's work did not label him as a quality pioneer *per se*, the nature of his work at the University of Pennsylvania and then as the first professor of medicine at Johns Hopkins University led to his recognition as an expert diagnostician who viewed consideration of the patient's state of mind and the underlying disease as equally important. His lasting effect was through changes in learning and curricula for physicians: increased patient contact while in medical school, use of laboratory findings, and authorship of his novel principles in a text that was considered a cornerstone in physician education through the 1920s [4]. Dr Osler's work channeled the focus of medical institutions and physicians towards education as a means of improving quality evidenced by morbidity and mortality reviews, grand rounds, and clinicopathological conferences that abounded in the health care industry as a result [3].

Emergency Medical Services: Clinical Practice and Systems Oversight, Second Edition. Volume 1: Clinical Aspects of EMS.
Edited by David C. Cone, Jane H. Brice, Theodore R. Delbridge, and J. Brent Myers.

The field of medicine witnessed other advances in the early 1900s indicative of a learning science predilection. In 1910 the Carnegie Foundation published the Flexner Report, which accused the industry of educational malpractice through "enormous over-production of uneducated and ill trained medical practictioners" [5]. Although this report has been questioned in more modern times in terms of both methods and comprehensiveness, the report is acknowledged as creating a significant focus on improving medical education quality and causing fundamental changes in medical education and practice structure [6].

Another health care quality history landmark was a 1910 proposal by a physician named Ernest Codman. Dr Codman's concept, called the "End Result System of Hospital Standardization" [7], involved tracking every patient outcome by the attending physician and investigation into the causes of poor outcomes. This was viewed as an antagonistic evaluation of surgeons' competencies and Harvard University withdrew Codman's medical staff privileges at Massachusetts General, with the leadership refusing to implement the system. Although other publications describe Codman resigning in disgust and establishing a private hospital where the end-result system was aggressively implemented and published [8], assessments of the effect of Codman's concepts agree on one fact: they became a founding objective of the American College of Surgeons (ACS) [7–9].

The founder of the ACS, Dr Franklin Martin, was a colleague of Codman's who embraced his proposal; the concept of minimum standards for hospitals became part of the ACS' objectives at the outset. Within 5 years, the "Minimum Standard for Hospitals" was published and the ACS began inspecting hospitals; only 13% of the nearly 700 initially inspected met the five-point criteria [7,9]. Presumably, hospitals were willing to undergo this form of peer review, and with a shift in focus from the individual physician to the facility as a whole, the ACS process met less resistance than Codman's system. Since hospitals were expected to modify their practices based on experiences exploring the minimum standards, this process is characterized as another example of a "learning science" tradition within the health care environment [3].

In the meantime, a completely different approach to assurance of quality was evolving in the early 1900s in the manufacturing sector of the United States: treating management as a "science." As the Industrial Revolution entered its second wave of impact in the United States, formally trained engineers and other scientists were common in the workplace. Attention shifted from exclusive focus on mechanical issues such as conveyor belt function and scrap management to more elusive issues such as worker productivity and human motivation. Frederick Taylor, an American industrial engineer, made a compelling statement in his 1911 treatise: "We can see and feel the waste of material things. Awkward, inefficient, or ill-directed movements of men, however, leave nothing visible or tangible behind them" [10]. Frederick Taylor's work was considered a foundation for the field that is now referred to as scientific management [11].

Manufacturing and other industries found value in the work of Taylor and his contemporaries, laying the cornerstone of scientific management deep within businesses. Their approach placed greater value on the scientific assessment of operations using quantitative approaches, including the use of mathematical models, rules of motion, and standardization of tools and implements. While there was recognition that cooperation had to exist between employees and supervisors, scientific management introduced change by observing work processes and redesigning the steps, tools, and human actions associated with the task [12].

By 1920, the Flexner Report had been credited for medical schools having more tailored entrance requirements, more diverse medical student bodies, and refined curricula; more striking was the fact that 60 out of 155 medical schools in the nation closed during this period [6]. Fundamentally, the contemporaneous efforts of both Mr Flexner and Dr Osler brought dramatic changes to the thinking and process associated with learning, and both yielded perceptions and beliefs that the quality of medical care was improved strictly as a result of the change in education that took place.

Another milestone in the history of US health care that ultimately became a mechanism for assuring quality was the licensure of hospitals, evolving during this timeframe as a Department of Health function in individual states. The 1920s was the only decade of exclusive regulation (primarily in the form of police powers to protect the health and safety of patients) by the states before the federal government began preempting states' laws related to governance of hospitals [2].

Meanwhile, scientific management rapidly grew as the favored approach in the post-World War I industrial environment that was experiencing increasing demand for goods and services and growing organizations [12]. Fortunately, this predominantly engineering focus was complemented by the birth of the behavioral school of management thought when what is now known as the Hawthorne Studies took place at Western Electric's Hawthorne plant in suburban Chicago [13]. The industrial sector of the United States was laying the groundwork for quantitative workload management and performance considerations tempered by an understanding of human relations and workplace psychology.

In the 1920s, Western Electric was also incubating several other processes and pioneers that ultimately made significant contributions to quality science evolution. Primarily a manufacturer of electrical and telephone system components, Western Electric was one of the largest corporations in the United States and one of the few with international presence [14]. Walter Shewhart, an engineer, carefully developed and tested methods that forced leadership to rethink inspection of finished products as the sole means of assuring quality. He devised a statistical method of monitoring and analyzing processes, allowing for the correction of conditions before a defective product was made. His original, elegantly simple concept proposal of a control chart was presented to Western Electric management on a single page of paper in 1924 [15].

Within 2 years, Western Electric had established a "quality" department, and appointed Joseph Juran, a young engineer, to lead the unit. Other Shewhart contemporaries were perfecting sampling techniques and by 1931, Shewhart published *Economic Control of Quality of Manufactured Product* [16]. Regarded today as a foundational text for the study of quality engineering through statistical process control, the work had relatively little impact outside Western Electric and its research branch, known as Bell Telephone, in its first 10 years. Another scientist exposed to these principles during work at Western Electric ultimately carried the first banner on the value of quality management to the outside world: W. Edwards Deming [14].

After his experience at Western Electric, Deming invited Shewhart to lecture with him in the late 1930s at the US Department of Agriculture Graduate School [17]. Shewhart had continued his statistically centered focus on quality (which also led to his definition of the Plan-Do-Check-Act cycle) and published *Statistical Method from the Viewpoint of Quality Control* [15]. Deming transferred to the US Census Bureau to assist with sampling techniques and in 1940, he implemented the first statistical process control use in an environment outside manufacturing as he managed clerical operations in the US Census Bureau during the 1940 census [17].

Meanwhile, Juran continued his work in quality management in the Bell system, training and publishing handbooks for employees [14]. In the 1940s Juran published his conceptualization of the "Pareto Principle," hypothesizing that management challenges could be classified and prioritized following an 80%/20% pattern [1]. This principle had actually been published more than 40 years earlier in a series of texts on economics by the politically riddled economist Vilfredo Pareto, who postulated that a universal logarithmic formula governed the distribution of wealth [18]. Professor Pareto's formula asserts that 20% of the people in a jurisdiction (any jurisdiction, anywhere in the world) hold 80% of the wealth. While empirical studies conducted since have reinforced this, the concept was adopted by Juran to distinguish between the issues (80%) over which supervisors had control, versus the reminder (20%) over which the workforce had control. Juran's and others' adoption of Pareto's assertion for other management beliefs drew criticism [19] but Juran maintained that studies performed in the 1950s and 1960s also supported his application, which further evolved into the reference during root cause analysis to the "vital few" and "trivial many" [1].

These three already productive parents of quality management – Shewhart, Deming, and Juran – may have fathered a very different beginning for total quality management than they eventually did had their lives and the work of the US government not been detoured by the onset of World War II. The federal "War Department" supporting the deployed armed services had two needs requiring them to reach out into the private sector: materiel and expertise. Subject matter experts were solicited from large businesses to assist with federal administrative functions, including Joseph Juran [20]. Deming's transfer from census work to the War Department resulted in the concepts of sampling and control charting as requirements for materiel suppliers [17]. These standards, essential for quality assurance and conformity of goods and services provided throughout the country, evolved into formal specifications that became commonly referred to as "MIL STD" (military standards) or MIL specs. These MIL procedures dictated sampling, machine calibration, schematic, and quality control practices [21] in the interest of avoiding defects, or errors, in products or processes. The counterpart sentiment of employee value and involvement was evidenced by the introduction of the practice of "quality circles" on factory floors by the late 1940s [22].

Medicine learned and benefited "on the job" at war: physics and genetics (courtesy of the atom bomb), antibiotics, and unprecedented organized care behind the lines were key improvements but nonetheless individual discoveries or accomplishments, not the result of an overall strategy to improve quality *per se*. Military publications emphasize that the overall specialization of providers in subsets of skills, acceleration of training, and provider preparation for disease and trauma care not routine in typical practice settings became the focus as the military became the single largest producer or preparer of medical providers. In 1939 alone, the prewar mobilization of the "Medical Department," a subordinate entity within the War Department, required an explosive increase of enlisted medical personnel and officers from less than 11,000 to 140,000 [23].

After the war, the American public's definition of quality health care was abundant health care [24]. The ACS continued to assess hospitals' conformity to basic minimum standards, having assessed over 3,000 hospitals by the early 1950s [25]. In a transition not unlike that of the shift for physician credentialing from societies to state regulatory bodies, ACS joined forces with the American Hospital Association, the American Medical Association, and others to form the Joint Commission on the Accreditation of Hospitals (JCAH) in 1952 [7]. The perspective was retrospective and geared towards confirming a standard of care through conformity of practices [26], not error prevention. It would be nearly 20 years before the JCAH retuned its standards to achieve "optimal achievable" versus "minimum essential" levels of quality [7].

A more commonly known aspect of quality management history in the late 1940s was the impact of Deming on the Japanese manufacturing sector. Less commonly known is that Deming went there as part of an entourage sent by the War Department to help rebuild Japan's postwar infrastructure – by studying agricultural challenges [17]! Another source cites the reason as assisting with Japanese population estimation for the US government [27] but it is nonetheless often overlooked that Deming did not go to Japan as a quality guru initially. It was during his visits that he convinced a rising Japanese statistician of the value of using statistics in the industrial sector. Deming returned to Japan five times to teach and consult with the blessing of the Supreme Commander of the Allied Forces; Shewhart was the preferred instructor, but he was unavailable.

Deming's presentations, ultimately referred to as the "Deming Method," urged a statistical approach to managing quality. Juran followed, doing numerous presentations for Japanese executives as well [1]. His training centered on his professional conclusions at that point: systems of quality management were an absolute necessity for a successful organization. "Made in Japan" had historically meant low-cost, shabby products. By the 1960s, the influence of Juran and Deming was clear as the Japanese achieved market leadership in the automobile and electronic sectors [28]. Engineering schools in the US were incorporating statistical quality control classes into their curricula, but the US was behind the quality curve.

While other new thinking evolved in the regulatory and industrial sector of the United States, such as "good manufacturing practices" and "management by objectives," an international organization that would have a lasting effect on quality in the US was being birthed: "ISO." The International Organization for Standardization published its first technical standards (numbering in the hundreds) in the 1950s. The value and purpose of the ISO, presently composed of representatives of 148 countries' national standards institutes, are best stated in its own "What if Standards Didn't Exist?" literature:

> "If there were no standards, we would soon notice. Standards make an enormous contribution to most aspects of our lives – although very often, that contribution is invisible. It is when there is an absence of standards that their importance is brought home. For example, as purchasers or users of products, we soon notice when they turn out to be of poor quality, do not fit, are incompatible with equipment we already have, are unreliable or dangerous. When products meet our expectations, we tend to take this for granted. We are usually unaware of the role played by standards in raising levels of quality, safety, reliability, efficiency and interchangeability – as well as in providing such benefits at an economical cost."

During the 1960s ISO issued thousands of standards using an elaborate but well-orchestrated system of subject matter experts and technical committees [29].

Standards and requirements for hospitals took a dramatic turn in the 1960s as well. Congress enacted a requirement of JCAH accreditation for hospitals participating in Medicare and Medicaid [7]. Soon afterwards, utilization review committees (staffed by hospitals' own clinicians) were mandated by Medicare. Intended to prevent fraud in reimbursement practices, this was the first vestige of performance assessment on a system-wide basis. These committees had no criteria to use in their evaluation processes, no incentive to thrive, and no mechanism for interfering with reimbursement. By 1970, despite resistance by the AMA, the federal government had introduced professional standards review organizations (PSROs) [9].

There is greater evidence of quality-related efforts in health care than manufacturing in the 1970s. Stagnation or poorly channeled energies in US manufacturing quality control efforts were apparent as focus on productivity and quotas was greater than customer preferences and satisfaction. Foreign producers (especially Japan) had eclipsed the US with design-based and systems approaches to quality. Manufacturing productivity in the US was increasing only half as fast as in Japan. American executives traveled to Japan in an effort to capture and replicate the Japanese success, but they returned with individual tools such as quality circles and missed the overall system underlying the industry advantage [30].

The 1970s saw a quality thinking breakthrough in the health care industry as a physician named Avedis Donabedian introduced the paradigm of structure, process, and outcomes as a means of organizing and assessing quality. Beginning with an article in 1966 and with a pinnacle of three volumes in the early 1980s, Donabedian effectively refocused the questions on health care quality and provided a framework that would bring some order to an otherwise complex set of issues faced in hospital settings. Despite his death in 2000, his body of knowledge lives on in eight books, over 50 journal articles [31], and countless references to structure, process, and outcomes.

The 1970s were also the formative years of EMS systems in the US. Congress acknowledged the value of EMS systems in 1973 in the EMS Systems Act (Public Law 93-154), which stipulated that one of the 15 essential components of an EMS system was review and evaluation "of the extent and quality of the emergency health care services provided" [32]. In what may be the only administratively oriented EMS text published in the 1970s, Jelenko and Frey refer to process and outcomes in EMS as "a little explored area" [33]. During this decade the first peer-reviewed articles specific to quality of out-of-hospital care were published in US journals, totaling 26 articles by 1979 [34].

In 1980 a documentary catapulted quality into the spotlight in the US as only television can do. *If Japan Can…Why Can't We?* featured Deming and the quality methods he had taught the Japanese. His telephone ringing off the hook the next day indicated that Americans in the manufacturing sector finally understood that it took a systematic approach [27]. The US Navy was awakened by two Navy Personnel Research and Development Center psychologists, one of whom saw the documentary and the other who went to a Deming lecture in 1981. Four years of planning ensued, and by 1985 a program was launched that was very successful, ultimately gaining considerable momentum. Even the name "total quality management" was born in the Navy; the label was recommended by a behavioral scientist as a more palatable alternative to the common reference in Japan, "total quality control" [30].

Total quality management (TQM) enjoyed over a decade of heralding, book publishing, seminar offerings, and consultant opportunities. However, concrete definitions and applications were elusive, and while many organizations could embrace the concept and value of improved quality, training was likely to result in increased knowledge but no tangible skills. In addition to Deming's 14 points, akin to "rules of the road " [30], other constructs emerged. A journal article describing TQM use in the public sector listed the principles as management commitment, employee empowerment (teams, training), fact-based decision making (the seven statistical tools, statistical process control, etc.), continuous improvement, and customer focus [35].

The Joint Commission on Accreditation of Hospitals, about to change its name to the Joint Commission on Accreditation of Healthcare Organizations (JCAHO), influenced health care institutions in the 1980s as a quality "assurance" plan became part of the JCAHO inspection. Additionally, the PSROs evolved into regional professional review organizations with more binding standards and a contractual scope of work required to be updated periodically under contracts with the US Health Care Financing Administration [9]. These efforts were largely retrospective inspection techniques, although in 1986 the JCAHO formed a not-for-profit consulting subsidiary, Quality Healthcare Resources [7]. Both the JCAHO and the AMA published models for quality assurance processes and systems, although the AMA guidelines focused almost exclusively on peer review activities [36]. The JCAHO has continued with additional performance improvement initiatives to present as a primary influence on hospital-based quality assessment.

Little awakening to quality in EMS was evident in the 1980s. Only 36 articles related to quality in EMS were published between 1980 and 1989, up marginally from the previous decade [34]. The comprehensive *Systems Approach to Emergency Medical Care*, published in 1983, devoted an entire chapter to the subject of operational and clinical evaluation. While the chapter thoroughly addressed program evaluation models, structure, process, and outcomes, and offered an exhaustive list of references [32], it probably was not ferreted out by EMS administrators interested in quality since it was buried in a voluminous textbook. The "pop" EMS administration text of the decade, *Managing Emergency Medical Services* by Newkirk and Linden, had a chapter entitled "Quality Control" but its focus was on employee appraisals and retrospective reviews of emergency responses. Most notable about the era was that both the National Association of EMS Physicians and the American College of Emergency Physicians conducted EMS-specific quality improvement conferences and published textbooks on the subject.

The very foundation of quality efforts in the US was re-poured in 1987 as the result of two separate projects of national and international origin: ISO 9000 and the Malcolm Baldrige National Quality Award Program. As described earlier in this chapter, the ISO focused almost exclusively on manufacturing and product standards initially; it would have a profound effect on organizations interested in quality management when "generic management system standards" were issued [29]. Some of the early reaction in the US was negative. Despite the influence and contribution of US work in quality to the ISO 9000 family of standards, misconceptions hampered its acceptance. Some of these myths included that these were "foreign" standards not appropriate to US businesses, a source of voluminous paperwork, and weak in their specificity about statistical methods [37].

ISO 9000 can be thought of as a header or book title, with the underlying chapters (ISO 9001, ISO 9002, etc.) containing the details of quality systems, management, and elements characteristics. The standards were written generically in an attempt to make them applicable to any business setting. Following the 1994 revision of the standards, nearly 400,000 organizations worldwide met or exceeded the standards and proved themselves with external validation and registration. Given the complexity of quality management issues, the content of the "chapters" of the standard had expanded to over 20 different standards and documents. When it was revised beginning in 2000, the standards' names and content changed accordingly.

ISO 9000:2000 "Quality management systems – Fundamentals and vocabulary"
ISO 9001:2000 "Quality management systems – Requirements"
ISO 9004:2000 "Quality management systems – Guidance for performance improvement" [29]

For some organizations pursuing ISO 9000 and the associated registration was a necessity in order to do business in or with a European country; for others it was a programmed way to implement or formalize quality improvement initiatives. Several European governments chose to embrace quality as a national initiative, often endorsing or elevating that country's ISO 9000 equivalent as a national standard [37]. In the United States, however, a completely different initiative evolved: the legislation that ultimately became the Malcolm Baldrige National Quality Improvement Act of 1987 (Public Law 100-107) comprised only four pages of text [38].

The original Act called for awards to be issued to small business and "companies." In the late 1990s, the National Board for Quality Promotion (NBQP) responded to the education and health care communities by publishing criteria unique to those sectors. The core content is largely the same, however, with adjustments made to terminology to reflect what is typical in that sector. For example, the criterion labeled "Customer and Market Focus" in the business criteria is named "Focus on Patients, Other Customers, and Markets" in the Health Care Criteria for Performance Excellence. The remaining categories in the health care criteria are:

- leadership
- strategic planning
- measurement, analysis, and knowledge management
- staff focus
- process management
- organizational performance results [35].

In his cover letter accompanying the 2004 criteria, the director of the BNQP addresses the value and utility of the criteria in efforts to "align resources and approaches, such as ISO 9000, Lean Enterprise, Balanced Scorecard, and Six Sigma; improve communication, productivity, and effectiveness; and achieve strategic goals" [39]. This emphasizes that the Baldrige criteria are a framework or architecture, not a quality system in and of themselves. While that may have been the bone of contention for Deming, it speaks to the utility that the criteria may have for

EMS agencies as a starting point when coupled with a body of knowledge about quality management.

Motorola, one of the winners of the Baldrige Award the first year, had an important quality armament that led to its success in the BNQP application process: Six Sigma.* An outgrowth of their TQM processes in the mid-1980s, Six Sigma was launched in January 1987 after a senior engineer made a proposal to the CEO [40] in a manner reminiscent of Shewhart's one-page proposal about the concept of control charts. Motorola was committed to unprecedented levels of improvement, and a new system of achieving and measuring that degree of change was needed.

Sigma is the name of the Greek symbol used in statistics to represent the standard deviation of the true population mean. Under a normal curve, about 65% of values will fall within one standard deviation on either side of the center, or average value, 95.5% will fall within two standard deviations, and so forth. Typically we don't refer to or calculate beyond three standard deviations, since 99.7% of values are captured at that point. The Six Sigma philosophy, however, is very concerned about the 0.27% beyond that boundary when it is an important process. While one-quarter of 1% may seem like an infinitesimally small number to worry about, it actually calculates as 1 out of 370. In high-stakes manufacturing and other public and private sector industries, ways of measuring and expressing 1 out of 1,000, 1 out of 10,000, and 1 out of a million would be a necessity.

Leaving the specifics to more detailed texts on the topic [41], "sigma quality level" or "sigma level" are ranges that account for some common variation occurring in a process, but allow measurement at that greater level of specificity. So, at four sigma, our process is defective in 6,210 out of 1 million events or opportunities; at five sigma, only 233 out of a million fail to meet our expectations; and at the Six Sigma level, 3.4/1,000,000 events result in a misadventure or defect [42]. The US airline industry is often used as an example of attaining Six Sigma level quality when evaluating fatality rates of passengers: the death of 19 passengers after one or more of the 9.8 million scheduled departures in 2003 equates to just over two deaths per million flights [43].

Six Sigma is much more than its measurement system, however. It is a framework of pursuing quality solutions based on both process analysis and statistical analysis under the lens of the customer's expectations. This balance allows for true diagnosis of the problem an organization is trying to solve, and is applied on a project-by-project basis [44]. Motorola discovered that its utility was not limited to the manufacturing floors. Its early utilization proved that Six Sigma could be leveraged for business, administrative, and service functions. Through an alliance with IBM, Texas Instruments, and Xerox, a system of executing Six Sigma projects was defined, allowing other organizations to adopt and deploy this powerful business strategy [41]. This has created a common platform on which Six Sigma

learning and comparison can take place across not only different organizations but even disparate disciplines.

Somewhat evocative of Shewhart's Plan-Do-Check-Act cycle, Six Sigma projects follow a prescribed sequence of steps, entitled Define, Measure, Analyze, Improve, and Control. Each of the steps has important subprocesses that assure identification of characteristics critical to customers, thorough investigation of root causes, a complete understanding of the nature and frequency of the problem, mathematical modeling that allows for hypothesis testing, acceleration of detection and feedback loops, diagnosis of the condition, selection and trials of solutions, and control systems to assure the problem does not recur. The approach can be applied to any situation where an organization wants to accelerate a process, reduce the cost of a process, or reduce the number of events that do not meet a specification [41,42,44].

General Electric brought Six Sigma into the national spotlight in the late 1990s with annual reports and speeches to shareholders revealing the extraordinary savings and successes the organization was enjoying as a result of its Six Sigma deployment [42]. Two-thirds of Fortune 500 firms initiated Six Sigma programs during the same time frame [44]. Six Sigma is gaining popularity among health care and other industries, including Johnson & Johnson, Cigna, Blue Cross and Blue Shield licensees, hospitals such as the Mayo Clinic, and many more since its disciplined approach translates well into virtually any setting. Its methodology is ultimately powerful in facilitating a transition for organizations to an evidence-driven way of doing business with technical advantages that distinguish it from TQM and other quality predecessors [41].

Institute of Medicine

Perhaps no other organization has had such a profound effect on health care quality in the 21st century as the Institute of Medicine (IOM). The IOM is the medical arm of the National Academy of Sciences (NAS) and is an independent, non-profit organization, whose mission is to give authoritative, unbiased information to decision makers and the public [45]. The IOM convenes expert committees to critically evaluate and summarize information on issues central to health care, publishing their summaries.

Primum non nocere

To Err is Human – Building a Safer Health System was published in 1999 and documented the magnitude and effect of medical errors in health care [45]. Identifying medical errors as the sixth most common cause of death in the US garnered tremendous media attention and, predictably, governmental scrutiny. Congress began hearings on this issue and other authors and countries embarked on further study to assess the scope of medical errors. A subsequent report by the World Health Organization identified that one in ten patients receiving medical care will suffer preventable injury [46]. The IOM report called for the establishment of a Center for Patient Safety and

---

*Six Sigma is a registered trademark and service mark of Motorola, Inc.

other efforts to focus the attention of the health care system. This initial report fundamentally changed the dialogue of how medical care was assessed and provided in this country.

Crossing the Quality Chasm: Creating a New Health System for the 21st Century, published in 2001, called for a fundamental redesign of the American health care system to improve quality [47]. It focused on the need for a systems approach to optimize health care, and identified that "the nation's health care delivery system has fallen far short in its ability to translate knowledge into practice and to apply new technology safely and appropriately." It identified specific aims for a revitalized health care system, creating a system that is:

- **safe**: avoiding injuries to patients from the care that is intended to help them
- **effective**: providing services based on scientific knowledge to all who could benefit, and refraining from providing services to those not likely to benefit. patient centered: providing care that is respectful of and responsive to individual patient preferences, needs, and values, and ensuring that patient values guide all clinical decisions
- **timely**: reducing waits and sometimes harmful delays for both those who receive and those who give care
- **efficient**: avoiding waste, including waste of equipment, supplies, ideas, and energy
- **equitable**: providing care that does not vary in quality because of personal characteristics such as gender, ethnicity, geographic location, and socioeconomic status.

The report identified ten rules for redesign based on the above care principles. It called for the Agency of Healthcare Quality and Research to develop care processes for 15 common health care conditions, to develop a listing of those conditions, and to work with stakeholders to develop action plans to implement this process. Other key principles espoused included the application of evidence to health care, expanding the use of information technology, and aligning payment policies with quality improvement. These topics have become the foundation of the philosophical, technological, and financial changes in the modern health care system. Much of health care has now coalesced around the core principle of evidence-based practice. The need for information technology has revolutionized medicine through the dramatic implementation of electronic health care records. Finally, the call for payment to be aligned with health care quality has been foundational in the evolution of payment for health care services to hospitals and other providers.

Pay for performance and public reporting

Public reporting of quality of care was a concept developed through a collaboration of hospitals, the Association of American Medical Colleges, and CMS [48]. This "voluntary" program's purpose was to invigorate quality efforts by allowing competitors and the public to compare selected quality measures of hospitals. It was linked to the annual Medicare update (payment adjustment) by CMS, and as a result 98% of all hospitals agreed to participate in the program. It allowed the public to access hospital process and outcome data through a public website. Initial data were reported in 2003 and compared hospital performance regarding the care of patients with congestive heart failure, myocardial infarction, and pneumonia. This program has continued to grow dramatically, and now includes measures of emergency care, patient satisfaction, and many other measures of health care performance.

Pay for performance, also known as value-based purchasing, evolved through the first decade of the 21st century to improve the value for health care dollar spent. While it addresses the laudable goal of improving health care system efficiency, the driving force for this initiative was both economic (decrease waste and improve expenditures on necessary care) and political (legislators can demonstrate fiscal responsibility). Two subsequent IOM reports led the way for this rather fundamental change in health care quality initiatives. The first, a 2006 report on "preventing medication errors," recommended incentives to align patient safety goals with provider, industry and insurer profitability [49]. The second, *Rewarding Provider Performance: Aligning Incentives in Medicare* (2006), identified that the health care system doesn't recognize or reward the coordination of care [50]. Nor did it reflect the value of health care in patient care quality. The report recommended pay for performance programs as an "immediate opportunity" to align incentives for performance improvement. A key driver for this economic initiative was Congress which, in enacting the Deficit Reduction Act of 2005, called for CMS to develop a plan for "value-based purchasing" by 2009 [51]. One example of this approach to reimbursement was to pay hospitals an incremental incentive for care of a specific type of disease. If patients sustaining myocardial infarctions received timely reperfusion (door to balloon angioplasty within 90 minutes) in a reliable manner (>90% of the time), hospitals would receive an incremental increase in CMS payment. In at least one analysis, Lindenauer et al. demonstrated a modest (2.6–4.1%) improvement in quality measures for hospitals participating in a pay for performance program, compared to those that did not [52].

Though conceptually sound, clinicians, academicians, and administrators identified a host of concerns regarding relative value of interventions, appropriate measures of quality, additional administrative burden of data collection, and data accuracy. An additional concern was raised regarding case mixes and the relative effect that higher acuity, such as seen in tertiary care hospitals, might have on efficiency of care and on outcomes. Finally, a universal concern was raised regarding the ethical concern that programs focused on outcomes may misalign incentives for care between physicians and patients. A noncompliant diabetic with an elevated hemoglobin A1C, for example, may result in a decreased payment to their physician, who in turn may decide to refuse to care for that patient.

Such concerns did not dissuade payers (primarily CMS) from implementing such programs and they have, in fact, continued to expand programs that require payment for meeting certain thresholds (e.g. 100% rate of aspirin administration for patients with acute myocardial infarction). To address concerns of providers, the US Department of Health and Human Services (DHHS) awarded a contract to the National Quality Forum (NQF) to establish a portfolio of quality and efficiency measures (core measures) that will allow the federal government to more clearly see how and whether health care spending is achieving the best results for patients and taxpayers. The contract is part of a provision in the Medicare Improvements for Patients and Providers Act of 2008. The NQF is a private-sector, consensus-based standard-setting organization composed of a variety of stakeholders whose mission is to define goals for performance improvement, standard setting, and public reporting of performance [53].

The Affordable Care Act

The Affordable Care Act (ACA) [54] was enacted in March 2010 and promises to fundamentally change the American health care system more than any other legislation since the enactment of Medicare. The ACA will also result in a dramatic expansion in the use of electronic medical records in health care, which should facilitate data retrieval for quality efforts and improve access to outcome data for evaluation of care. As of this writing, the ACA has not become fully implemented, and the authors are speculating as to its future effect on health care quality, other than to opine that it will be profound.

Conclusion

Emergency medical services in the US are still in their adolescence of incorporating quality improvement as a mainstream activity. This historical review illustrates the strengths and effects of different approaches, including learning science, regulation, management science, and systems of quality assessment and performance improvement. Hospitals and manufacturing firms followed very different paths over the last century, allowing the reader to recognize origins and cycles in various systems and put them to use appropriately. Health care quality initiatives have now moved dramatically into the public view, and quality and reimbursement, through pay for performance initiatives, have become inextricably linked. EMS organizations will need to integrate quality principles developed in industry and medicine to improve system operations, financial viability, and patient outcomes.

References

1 Juran JM. *Juran on Leadership for Quality: An Executive Handbook.* New York: Free Press, 1989.

2 Burde H. The implementation of quality and safety measures: from rhetoric to reality. *J Health Law* 2002;35:263–81.

3 Merry MD, Crago MG. The past, present and future of health care quality. *Physician Exec* 2001:27(5):30–5.

4 McCall N (ed). *The Portrait Collection of Johns Hopkins Medicine: Celebrating the Contributions of William Osler,* 1993. Available at: www.medicalarchives.jhmi.edu/osler/biography.htm

5 Flexner A. *Medical Education in the United States and Canada: A Report to the Carnegie Foundation for the Advancement of Teaching,* Bulletin No. 4. New York: Carnegie Foundation for the Advancement of Teaching, 1910.

6 Hiatt MD. The amazing logistics of Flexner's fieldwork. *Medic Sent* 2000;5:167–8.

7 Joint Commission on Accreditation of Healthcare Organizations. *Our History.* Available at: www.jointcommission.org/about_us/history.aspx

8 Neuhauser, DV. Heroes and martyrs of quality and safety. Qual Saf Health Care 2002;11:104–5.

9 McIntyre D, Rogers L, Heier EJ. Overview, history, and objectives of performance measurement. *Health Care Fin Rev* 2001;22:7–21.

10 Taylor FW. *The Principles of Scientific Management 1911.* New York: Cosimo Classics, 2006.

11 Schermerhorn JR. *Management for Productivity,* 3rd edn. New York: John Wiley and Sons, 1989.

12 Szilagyi AD Jr. *Management and Performance,* 2nd edn. Glenview, IL: Scott, Foresman, 1981.

13 Adams SB, Butler OR. *Manufacturing the Future: A History of Western Electric,* 2nd edn. Cambridge, UK: Cambridge University Press, 2008.

14 BellSystemMemorial.com. USA: David Massey, c.1997–2013. Available at: www.beatriceco.com/bti/porticus/bell/bellsystem_history.html

15 Shewhart WA. *Father of Statistical Control.* Milwaukee, WI: American Society for Quality, 2004. Available at: www.asq.org/join/about/history/shewhart.html

16 NIST/SEMATECH. *NIST/SEMATECH e-Handbook of Statistical Methods,* 2012. Available at: www.itl.nist.gov/div898/handbook/

17 Deming WE. *A Mission Pursued on Two Continents.* Milwaukee, WI: American Society for Quality, 2004. Available at: http://asq.org/about-asq/who-we-are/bio_deming.html

18 Hafner AW. Pareto's principle: the 80-20 Rule, 2001. Available at: www.bsu.edu/libraries/ahafner/awh-th-math-pareto.html

19 Fonseca GL, Ussher L. Profile: Vilfredo Pareto. Available from: http://cepa.newschool.edu/het/profiles/pareto.htm

20 Joseph M. *Juran: A Search for Universal Principles.* Milwaukee, WI: American Society for Quality, 2004. Available at: http://asq.org/about-asq/who-we-are/bio_juran.html

21 Juran JM. The history of managing for quality in the United States. In: Juran JM (ed) *A History of Managing for Quality.* Burr Ridge, IL: Irwin Professional Publishing, 1995.

22 Schmidt WH. *The Race Without a Finish Line: America's Quest for Total Quality.* Ann Arbor, MI: Proquest, 1992.

23 Mullins WS (ed in chief). *Medical Training in World War II.* Washington, DC: Surgeon General, US Army, 1976. Available at: http://history.amedd.army.mil/booksdocs/wwii/medtrain/

24 Bennett L, Slavin, L. *Continuous Quality Improvement: What Every Health Care Manager Needs To Know.* Cleveland, OH: Case Western Reserve University, 2002. Available at: www.cwru.edu/med/epidbio/mphp439/CQI.htm

25 Wellborn J. The JCAHO Timeline. *Med Leg Rev* 2000;2:2.

26 Tabladillo M. *Quality Management Climate Assessment in Healthcare* [dissertation]. Atlanta, GA: Georgia Institute of Technology, 2002.

27 Dobyns L, Crawford-Mason C. *Quality or Else.* Boston, MA: Houghton Mifflin, 1991.

28 Kinlaw DC. *Continuous Improvement and Measurement of Total Quality.* San Diego, CA: Pfeiffer and Co, 1992.

29 International Organization for Standardization. Available at: www.iso.org/

30 Dobyns L, Crawford-Mason C. *Thinking About Quality: Progress, Wisdom, and The Deming Philosophy.* New York: Random House, 1994.

31 Frenk J. Avedis Donabedian. *Bull World Health Organ* 2000;78:1475.

32 Boyd DR, Edlich RF, Micik S (eds). *Systems Approach to Emergency Medical Care.* Norwalk, CT: Appleton-Century-Crofts, 1983.

33 Jelenko C, Frey CF. *Emergency Medical Services: An Overview.* Bowie, MD: Robert J. Brady Company, 1976.

34 Gunderson M. External accountability. *EMSMJ.* Available at: www.emsvillage.com/articles/article.cfm?id=1617

35 Martin L. Total quality management in the public sector. *Nat Product Rev* 1993;10:195–213.

36 McDowell RM. Concepts in EMS quality management. In: Swor RA (ed) *Quality Management in Prehospital Care.* St Louis, MO: Mosby Lifeline, 1993, pp.14–28.

37 Johnson PL. *ISO 9000: Meeting the New International Standards.* New York: McGraw-Hill, 1993.

38 Public Law 100-107: The Malcolm Baldrige National Quality Improvement Act of 1987. Available at: www.quality.nist.gov/PDF_files/Improvement_Act.pdf

39 US Department of Commerce. *Baldrige National Quality Program.* Gaithersburg, MD: US Department of Commerce. Available at: www.baldrige.nist.gov

40 Barney M. Motorola's second generation. *Six Sigma Forum Mag* 2002:1:13–16. Available at: www.kellogg.northwestern.edu/course/opns430/modules/quality_management/Mot_Six_Sigma.pdf

41 Bertels T (ed). *Rath & Strong's Six Sigma Leadership Handbook.* Hoboken, NJ: John Wiley, 2003.

42 Breyfogle FW, Cupleo JM, Meadows B. *Managing Six Sigma.* New York: John Wiley, 2001.

43 National Transportation Safety Board. *Aviation Accident Statistics.* Washington, DC: National Transportation Safety Board, 2012. Available at: www.ntsb.gov/data/aviation_stats.html

44 DeFeo JA, Barnard WW. *Six Sigma Breakthrough and Beyond.* New York: McGraw-Hill, 2004.

45 Kohn LT, Corrigan JM, Donaldson MS. *To Err is Human: Building a Safer Health System.* Washington, DC: National Academies Press, 2000, p.312.

46 World Health Organization. *10 Facts on Patient Safety.* Available at: www.who.int/features/factfiles/patient_safety/en/index.html

47 Institute of Medicine. *Crossing the Quality Chasm: A New Health System for the 21st Century.* Washington, DC: National Academies Press, 2001. Available at: http://www.nap.edu/openbook.php?record_id=10027&page=R1

48 Hospital Compare. Washington, DC: Department of Health and Human Services, 2013. Available at: www.medicare.gov/hospital compare/search.html

49 Institute of Medicine. *Preventing Medication Errors.* Washington, DC: National Academies Press, 2006. Available at: www.nap.edu/catalog.php?record_id=11623

50 Institute of Medicine. *Rewarding Provider Performance: Aligning Incentives in Medicare.* Washington, DC: National Academies Press, 2006. Available at: www.nap.edu/catalog.php?record_id=11723#toc

51 Deficit Reduction Act of 2005. S. 1932 Section 5001 Public Law No. 109-171. Available at: http://origin.www.gpo.gov/fdsys/pkg/PLAW-109publ171/html/PLAW-109publ171.htm

52 Lindenauer PK, Remus D, Roman S, et al. Public reporting and pay for performance in hospital quality improvement. *N Engl J Med* 2007;356:486–96.

53 National Quality Forum. *Who We Are.* Available at: www.quality forum.org

54 Patient Protection and the Affordable Care Act. Public Law No. 111–148, 124 STAT 119, 111th Congress. Available at: http://itcaon line.com/wp-content/uploads/2011/06/PubLaw-111-148.pdf

CHAPTER 72

Defining, measuring, and improving quality

Kevin E. Mackey and Scott S. Bourn

"Quality is not an act; it is a habit" (Aristotle)

Introduction

Quality in EMS can be analogous to UFOs. Some are sure they have seen them and can describe them in detail. Others believe in their existence but have never seen them. Still others doubt their existence entirely or refuse to believe they are possible. But everyone agrees that, although often difficult to define, quality is an essential component of a vibrant EMS community. This chapter will describe current knowledge about quality and improvement, and then apply those principles to EMS. Throughout the chapter, examples will be provided to make the theory tangible, and specific suggestions will be offered to help medical directors and clinical leaders apply the principles to their own practices.

Quality in EMS

Traditional descriptions of EMS quality have frequently had a narrow focus on specific objectives rather than overall system performance. For example:

- **patient-centric**: administration of aspirin to chest pain patients
- **paramedic-centric**: number of successful versus failed intubations monthly
- **community-centric**: recognition of coronary ischemic discomfort for STEMI patients
- **organization-centric**: percentage of patients cared for by an organization who received oxygen.

In 2001, the Institute of Medicine published *Crossing the Quality Chasm* and described health care quality as safe, effective, patient-centered, timely, efficient, and equitable [1]. Five years later, this same organization, in the seminal report *Emergency Medical Services at the Crossroads*, described EMS as fragmented and stated that EMS quality is "highly inconsistent from one town, city, or region to the next" [2]. The report went on to assert that there is no agreed-upon national measure for quality and no consensus for who oversees or is accountable for quality.

The challenge for EMS leaders is to move quality in EMS, be it a state, region or a local EMS community, urban, rural, volunteer, wilderness, military, or interfacility operation, from a myth to a reality that continuously drives excellent, patient-centered care. In responding to that challenge, it will be important to remember that quality is a journey, not a destination; a process of assessment and reassessment, change, and adaption to continuously improve the delivery of the product (in this case, comprehensive and coordinated expert care) to the consumer. It is all about improvement, never being satisfied that the product is perfect.

The science of quality and performance improvement

The science of improvement had its origins in manufacturing, where quality is based on reliable execution of optimal processes. W. Edwards Demings was a statistician, professor, and consultant who spent a large part of his life teaching corporate leaders how to improve design and product quality. In the early 1980s, Deming was recruited to jump-start a quality movement in the failing Ford Motor Company. Within 3 years, Ford had undergone a massive internal transformation and surpassed General Motors in sales and profits. In 1987, President Ronald Reagan awarded Deming the national Medal of Technology for his contribution in improving quality workmanship within the technology sector of the United States.

Deming believed that the ability to create improvement requires knowledge about the subject at hand (making cars or practicing medicine) combined with what he referred to as the System of Profound Knowledge. The System of Profound Knowledge asserts that improvement requires an understanding

Emergency Medical Services: Clinical Practice and Systems Oversight, Second Edition. Volume 1: Clinical Aspects of EMS.
Edited by David C. Cone, Jane H. Brice, Theodore R. Delbridge, and J. Brent Myers.
© 2015 NAEMSP. Published 2015 by John Wiley & Sons, Inc. Companion Website: www.wiley.com\go\cone\naemsp

of the interaction of four factors that affect processes and outcomes. The descriptions below offer EMS examples for each.

- **Appreciation of a system**: having an understanding of the interactions of a system and how they affect the outcome or quality measures. The EMS system is rather large, and includes dispatch, first responders, fire (including hazmat and special operations), hospitals, public health, mental health, and the EMS authority, as well as the health care provider and the patient. Any successful improvement effort must recognize the role each of these system elements plays in creating the outcome.

- **Knowledge of variation**: understanding what is a "normal variation" within a system compared to what is unexpected or unpredictable. Blood glucose levels offer a good example for describing the knowledge of variation. A patient whose daily glucose levels have fluctuated between 84 and 106 over the past 2 weeks does demonstrate variation, but the narrowness of the range suggests that it is the result of normal variations in diet and metabolic functions. This is referred to "common cause" variation because it affects all people and does not reflect a metabolic system that is "out of control." In contrast, a patient whose daily glucose levels have fluctuated wildly between 84 and 320 during the same timeframe likely has what Deming referred to as "special cause" variation – not common to all people, and likely reflective of a system that is "out of control." *Successful quality efforts identify and focus on reducing special cause variation and DON'T waste time and resources trying to "fix" common cause variation.* Like all other systems, EMS has a lot of common cause variation: cardiac arrest survival, skills success rates by paramedics, or on-scene intervals – performance varies week to week or month to month. Statistical tools such as process control charts are used to identify variation that is *not* common cause (such as consistent differences in cardiac arrest survival between communities). Understanding and reducing special cause variation is what process improvement, and this chapter, is all about.

- **Building knowledge**: understanding the system under consideration and using that understanding to predict what improvement efforts will successfully reduce special cause variation. The knowledge-building process not only refers to making informed predictions *before* beginning improvement efforts, but also the continued gathering of information on how interventions actually affected the system. For this reason, efforts to create system improvement need to be structured in a way that enables the effect of change to be carefully measured. The Plan-Do-Study-Act (PDSA) cycle is the strategy for systematically testing changes within the system and building additional knowledge, and will be discussed below.

- **Human behavior**: how humans behave and react to given circumstances. What are the "human" factors contributing to the special cause variation? And how will they respond to the proposed changes? Will there be resistance? Human behavior is often underappreciated when change efforts are undertaken, especially in a large and diverse system like EMS.

Careful consideration of all four aspects of the System of Profound Knowledge will guide quality leaders in developing a change or improvement within the system.

The Model for Improvement

Application of Deming's principles to actually solve quality problems requires a structural framework that can guide the process and set parameters. Fortunately, there is a powerful tool available that can be used to guide and drive the process of quality improvement. The Associates in Process Improvement (Austin, Texas) developed this tool several years ago and it is currently used in education, health care, and public and private business to drive change and improvement. Although there are other guides and tools available, the Model for Improvement was adopted by the Institute of Healthcare Improvement as its "weapon of choice" to promote a balanced and healthy approach to improving quality within health care systems, including EMS. Use of this model within your system to define, measure, and ultimately improve quality is a major focus of this chapter.

The Model for Improvement (Figure 72.1) begins with three basic questions, each of which is foundational to understanding and defining the target of the improvement effort.

1. **Aim**: *What are we trying to accomplish?* Aim statements are very specific and address the topics of "What?," "By when?," and "For whom?" The aim should ideally possess qualities that will keep the intent of the aim on those things that matter. First, the aim should be *patient-centered*. The delivery of quality patient care is the driver of EMS and our quality initiatives should reflect that belief. Second, the aim should be focused on a practice with *wide special cause variation*, meaning that some providers (or communities) perform well while others do not. There is no benefit to patients in focusing

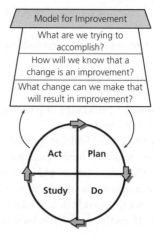

Figure 72.1 Model for Improvement. Source: Langley G, Moen R, Nolan K et al. *The Improvement Guide: A Practical Approach to Enhancing Organization Performance*, 2nd edn. San Francisco: Jossey-Bass, 2009, p.24. Reproduced with permission of John Wiley & Sons, Inc.

improvement on practices that all providers do well (only common cause variation). While ultimately it is beneficial to address issues that virtually no one does well, it is a very difficult place to *begin* performance improvement efforts because there are no "best practices" available to learn from. Instead, it is wise to begin with issues that have broad variability. Finally, the aim should be *evidence based and backed by solid, foundational literature and best practices*. Selecting aims that have an adequate evidence base reduces the controversy around the interventions that will be tested to improve performance. Consider the following EMS improvement aim that meets these criteria.

- To improve the percentage of patients in respiratory distress who are normally oxygenated to 95% by March 31st.

2 **Measure:** *How will we know that a change is an improvement?* The measure becomes the lens through which all potential change strategies are viewed to determine whether they will actually create the desired result. Like aim statements, measurement statements must be very specific and describe *how* the change will be measured. There are several characteristics of good measures. First, as with the aim, metrics should be *patient-centered* whenever possible. EMS metrics have traditionally been provider centered, but often there is a corresponding (better) patient-centered metric. For example, many EMS systems have long used the intubation success rate as an important measure; the patient-centered metric would be adequate ventilation and oxygenation as measured by $EtCO_2$ and SpO_2. Shifting to these measures takes the focus off the caregiver and shifts it appropriately to the patient, and also reduces the risk of unintended consequences associated with caregiver-centered metrics such as choosing to not attempt intubation in a challenging case in order to maintain a high success rate. Health care metrics have evolved to a focus on patient outcomes and patient harm related to the care provided by health care professionals. EMS metrics for quality must do the same. In addition, measures should be *specific and numerical*. Consider the following measures for the aims described in the previous section.

- To improve the percentage of patients in respiratory distress whose SpO_2 is >90% at the final assessment of the EMS encounter to a target SpO_2 of 95% at the final assessment of the EMS encounter by March 31st.

3 **Change:** *What changes can be made that will result in an improvement?* At its core, change is driven by a *prediction* about what change could be made within the system that would achieve the aim as evaluated by the measures. There are several attributes of effective changes. First, they require development, meaning that they have as their foundation the framework offered by Deming's System of Profound Knowledge: built upon an understanding of the system and knowledge of variation, influenced by knowledge, and informed by sensitivity to the human factors involved. They also must be amenable to evaluation, meaning that the change itself can be measured in addition to the outcome. For example, to improve the percentage of patients in respiratory

distress whose SpO_2 is >90%, a change that might be predicted to achieve the aim might be administration of oxygen in a higher percentage of patients. In addition to the outcome (SpO_2), it would be possible to measure what percentage of patients actually received supplemental oxygen. Finally, successful changes require an *effective strategy for implementation*. To continue with the supplemental oxygen administration example, *how* will the goal of increasing the number of patients who receive oxygen be achieved? This may involve assuring that oxygen is available in all ambulances, training crews on how to administer oxygen and why it is important, and monitoring oxygen administration during the implementation phase to track progress. Unfortunately, many systems begin their attempts at quality improvement by going straight to implementation; they look for changes within the system or organization without having a clear understanding first of what they are trying to accomplish and if what they are trying to accomplish is measureable. If, however, the approach is first evaluated from a proper aim with measureable objectives, then the real fun can begin with brainstorming and a free flow of ideas that fills a whiteboard.

For a system, provider group, or organization to be successful at implementing a robust, patient-centered, well-defined, and measurable quality project, there must be a *champion*, or leader, who has the focus and vision to accomplish what lies ahead. Often, but not always, that person is the medical director or another EMS physician. This individual needs to have oversight of patient care and have the knowledge, skills, and ability to drive change. But the champion is just the start. Once an aim is identified, it is important to identify additional individuals and groups who need to participate in order to effectively execute a change and measure the effect on the aim. These individuals will likely vary and might include representatives of the provider group, emergency responders, hospitals, public health, mental health, law enforcement, the local EMS authority, state officials, and others. Each aim will differ in participants, but each will require a leader, or champion, of the quality system.

Tools for success

The System of Profound Knowledge and Model for Improvement provide an excellent framework for guiding improvement, but their success is enhanced through the use of several tools that improve understanding of the *causes* of quality challenges, the *drivers* of successful improvement, and the *process* for testing and adopting change. These tools will be illustrated using the following sample aim: *By August 1st, achieve a 10% reduction in the delay of transport of STEMI patients to STEMI centers.*

Diagramming cause and effect

One of the elements of the System of Profound Knowledge is *appreciation of the system*: understanding the elements of the care delivery system and how they affect the quality of care provided. Before embarking on a quality improvement measure, it is helpful to take a moment and look at how inputs either directly or indirectly affect, or cause, an outcome. This is a good time to assemble all team members, go to the whiteboard, and brainstorm everything that contributes to the outcome. Kaoru Ishikawa, a Japanese industrialist who worked closely with W. Edwards Demings to redesign the Kawasaki shipyards and catapult Japan into becoming a world leader, developed the *fishbone diagram* [3]. The fishbone diagram, also known as a *cause and effect diagram,* is an excellent tool for identifying factors that contribute to special cause variation.

The fishbone starts by identifying the problem. This is listed as the "head" of the fish. As major causal categories are brainstormed, they are added as larger "fishbones" that make up the skeleton. As the discussion continues, factors that have influence over these causal categories are listed as smaller "bones" of the overall skeleton. If brainstorming begins to stall, consider some "generic" causal categories recommended by the American Society for Quality [4].

- Methods
- Equipment
- People
- Materials
- Measurement
- Environment

Figure 72.2 illustrates a sample fishbone chart for delays in transport of STEMI patients to designated centers.

Identifying opportunities for change

Once cause and effect are better understood, it is time to identify how to drive improved performance. While fishbone diagrams are tools to clarify "problems," *driver diagrams* are used to organize "solutions" and are informed in many ways by the elements of the fishbone diagram. A driver diagram lists broad ideas that influence the aim. These are referred to as the "primary drivers." Under each primary driver are "secondary drivers" or those things that influence the primary drivers. Most driver diagrams list at least three primary drivers and can have a multitude of secondary and even tertiary drivers. Figure 72.3 is a sample driver diagram for STEMI.

Driver diagrams are important tools for answering the question *what changes can be made that result in improvement?* Opportunities for change that are relevant within a specific system can be quickly identified in the list of secondary drivers. For example, for communities that are early in their STEMI system development it might be important to focus on secondary drivers associated with the primary driver "Develop infrastructure to support STEMI care," such as increasing community awareness or designating STEMI centers. Other systems that have already developed the infrastructure may want to focus their improvement efforts on improving rapid STEMI care and transport or reliable hospital care. A well thought-out driver diagram can literally serve as a roadmap for improvement over several years as changes are instituted one secondary driver at a time.

Systematically testing change: the PDSA model

The driver diagram offers a strategy for selecting opportunities for improvement by identifying secondary drivers that theoretically affect outcomes and are relevant to the system under consideration. The next step is to systematically test these changes to see if they bring about the desired improvement. The key to conducting these tests is that they be performed on a smaller scale, with a limited number of participants or sites. This enables the change to be tested, measured, and modified as

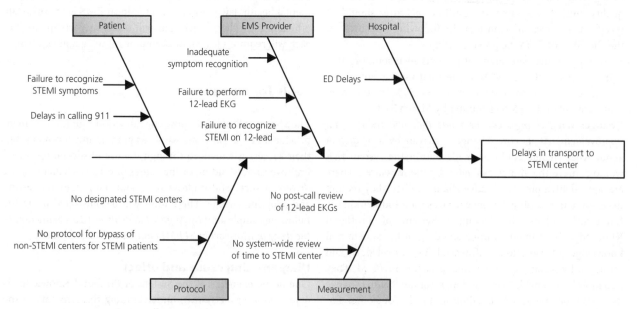

Figure 72.2 Fishbone diagram: delays to STEMI center.

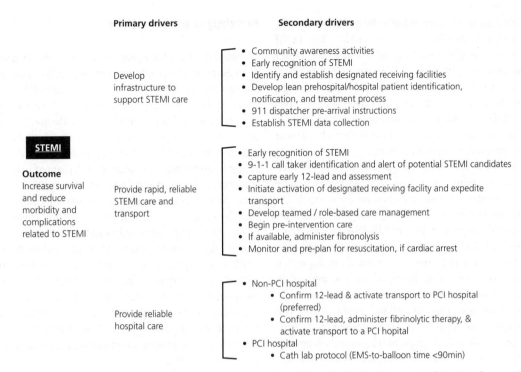

Figure 72.3 Driver diagram: delays to STEMI center. Reproduced with permission of American Medical Response and TrueSimple.

needed before rolling out any changes across a company, community, region, or state. The goal of this small-scale testing process is to identify if change to "X" produced improvement in result "Y."

Western Electric employed Walter Shewhart, a physicist and statistician, and a mentor of W. Edwards Deming, in the 1920s. Shewhart used the scientific method of inductive and deductive reasoning to develop a very simple method to evaluate change. The process he developed is called the *Plan-Do-Study-Act (PDSA) cycle* (see Figure 72.1).

- **Plan**: identify the objective (aim and measure) and predict the outcomes or improvements of the change. Selection of which change to test is informed by the driver diagram. One of the keys to successful PDSA is to begin with small tests of change. For example, returning to the goal of shortened time to STEMI center, a small test of change might be to use a visual prompt placed on the cardiac monitor screen ("ACTIVATE STEMI CENTER") to see whether it affects time to activation. Of course, part of the planning is to identify what measures will be used to gauge success; in many cases during small tests of change the measures will be more focused around process (the crew remembered to activate the STEMI system) than outcomes (shortened time to STEMI center).
- **Do**: execute the planned change. As noted before, execute on a small scale first. For example, it would be useful to try the prompt on the cardiac monitor screen with one crew for 1 week.
- **Study**: gather information to determine the effect of the test. In the early stages this could be as simple as asking the crew if they saw the prompt on the cardiac monitor. Was it visible?

Did it have the desired effect? Did they actually have any cases in which they activated the STEMI center and, if they did, did the prompt help? As the test progresses (see the section below), the size and length of the test increase and usually the data collected become more outcome oriented. Ultimately, as the PDSA cycles evolve, the data will be the actual measure identified in the aim: reduction of time to STEMI center. During these later stages it will also be important to visually assess the data using tools like run and control charts. But in the early stages of testing, the data collected are more related to processes and crew effects.

- **Act**: quality improvement requires *action*. At this point, decisions are made whether to make adjustments and send the process through another PDSA cycle, or to adapt/abandon the changes made. In the early stages of the PDSA process there will be tests that fail and need to be abandoned. Other tests may be somewhat successful but need to be adapted (for example, the font size in the on-screen prompt may need to be made larger). Successful tests are adopted. Adoption in early testing means that the test is broadened to more crews, while in the later stages adoption may result in creation of new policies and procedures for the system. Most process changes require multiple PDSA cycles. With each "spin of the cycle" fine-tuning and tweaking of the processes can be accomplished to maximize the desired outcome.

Visual display of data to identify real change

As noted previously, the world is filled with variation. One of the real challenges of process improvement and using PDSA cycles is mistaking common cause variation for real improvement; it can be tempting to ascribe a decrease in time to STEMI activation rates in a single week to a successful PDSA rather than common cause variation. Graphical display of data offers two tools to assist with longitudinal measurement of change, both short and long term. These graphic representations also help to reestablish or refocus a particular aim, and provide concrete input that can be used to show others and garner support for the particular direction a change is headed.

One method of diagramming change is a *run chart*, which graphs a numerical change over time. On the x-axis is time (days, months, minutes, seconds, etc.) and on the y-axis is the measure of interest (temperature, ETCO$_2$, Glasgow Coma Scale scores, etc.), with the high and low cut-offs of the y-axis being 20% above and 20% below the highest and lowest measures, respectively. Once each data point is inserted in sequential order, common cause variation becomes evident, and when actual sustained improvement occurs it is visually apparent. Depending upon the aim, the slope of the graphical data will determine if change has occurred and if that change is desired. A neutral or random slope will represent that no real change has transpired. More information about run charts, as well as examples, can be found at the American Society for Quality website (http://asq.org/training/run-chart_RCASQ.html) and in the "Putting it all together" section below.

Once adequate data are available to demonstrate the mean and common cause variation, a *control chart* can be created (http://asq.org/learn-about-quality/data-collection-analysis-tools/overview/control-chart.html). The control chart looks like a run chart (time along the x-axis, variable of interest on the y-axis), but also has "control lines" that typically represent two standard deviations above and below the mean. These control lines create visual delineations between common cause and special cause variation; sustained change outside the control lines represents special cause variation, and may signal significant results from a process change.

Putting it all together

To better illustrate the material covered in this chapter, let's look at an example of a quality problem that exists in a fictitious EMS community. Dr Smith is the medical director of the sole transport provider for a large urban community. There are three trauma centers serving this community. Over the past several months the trauma quality council, chaired by Dr Smith, has noted multiple instances of field-activated patients arriving at the trauma center hypothermic. Dr Smith uses 2 years of historical data to construct a run chart and finds that, as suspected, a distinct negative slope has developed over the past 5 months, representing what he believes is a special cause variation (Figure 72.4). The quality council has convened to address this trend.

In a brainstorming session, Dr Smith and his team construct a fishbone diagram to list as many causal factors affecting the patient's temperature as possible (Figure 72.5). Once this is completed, Dr Smith's team builds a driver diagram to begin to assimilate solutions to the hypothermia problem fleshed out in the fishbone diagram (Figure 72.6). Recall that the fishbone diagram evaluates the problem and the driver diagram organizes potential solutions.

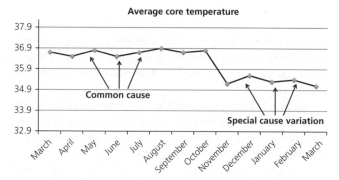

Figure 72.4 Dr Smith's run chart showing common cause variation and special cause variation.

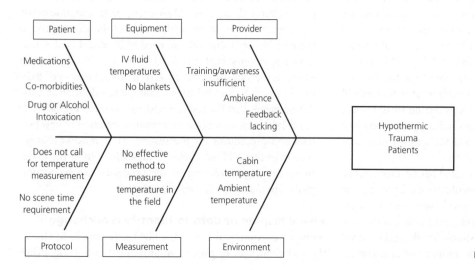

Figure 72.5 Dr Smith's fishbone diagram.

Secondary drivers   Primary drivers

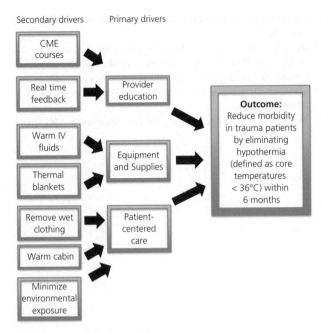

Figure 72.6 Dr Smith's driver diagram.

Average core temperature

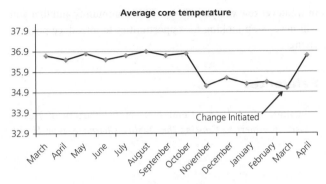

Figure 72.7 Dr Smith's run chart after implementing changes.

upper and lower limits of normal. This completes the changes and provides Dr Smith with a method to track progress.

Strategies for Success

DO:
- focus on the system, not individual caregivers
- clearly identify things that matter (patient-centered objectives)
- use run charts (or similar tools) to detect "disturbances in the force"
- develop aims with clearly defined goals and timelines
- thoughtfully select measures that match the aim
- get lots of input from front-line caregivers during the planning stage of the PDSA cycle
- be patient. Change is sometimes slow
- remember that most quality successes don't come from identifying *what* to do. The goal is *reliability*. The challenge is *how* to follow the evidence with every patient encounter, every caregiver, every day.

DON'T:
- change too many variables at once (you won't know what changes had positive effects and what changes had negative effects)
- build an improvement project around irrelevant aims
- get discouraged.

Next, the quality council, with the guidance and input of the provider educator, selects two simple and small changes to be introduced in 25% of the transport units (trialing the change in a small subset is key to flushing out hiccups or complications with the new change). Using the PDSA model, Dr Smith and the educator develop the following aim and measure: first measured core temperature on trauma patients delivered by EMS of 36 °C within 4 weeks time. From the driver diagram, the team decides to add thermal blankets and use the heaters in the passenger compartments of the ambulance. The team then identifies a small group to test these changes, and develops provider training in the use of blankets and passenger compartment heaters on all trauma patients. Dr Smith decides to test this change in the northeastern section of the community, which transports 20% of the trauma calls

At the end of each week, Dr Smith gathers and plots the prior week's data. He also spends time discussing the effect of the changes with his providers involved in the evaluation. He might ask if the use of the heater is simple and if there is any effect on the care they deliver. He might also ask if the blankets are easy to access and if they interfere with patient care in any way. Dr Smith would most certainly provide feedback about the data he is observing, reinforcing the change and/or looking for new directions to head. At the conclusion of the study period, Dr Smith repeats the run chart to evaluate if any change has occurred (Figure 72.7). He discovers that in fact a positive slope has appeared on the run chart, suggesting the changes he implemented did in fact begin correcting the issue of hypothermic trauma patients and he could potentially accomplish his aim.

Moving forward, Dr Smith institutes company-wide training on the new changes, and continues plotting his data on a run chart to assess progress. When enough data are available, Dr Smith constructs a control chart defining an average as well as

Conclusion

In this chapter, we looked at a comprehensive, patient-centered, balanced, and highly effective approach to defining, measuring, and improving quality in an EMS system. The details outlined in this chapter are widely applicable to all types of EMS communities and systems. The journey of improvement has a beginning but has no end. The opportunities to improve are boundless but each positive change brings a multitude of rewards not only for the system but most importantly for the patient. We hope that the tips, tools, and techniques discussed herein will guide you in whatever role you play in your EMS community and that you will never stop looking for opportunities to introduce positive change.

References

1 Institute of Medicine, Committee on the Quality of Health Care in America. *Crossing the Quality Chasm: A New Health System for the 21st Century.* Washington, DC: National Academy Press, 2001.

2 Institute of Medicine, Committee on the Future of Emergency Care in the US Health System. *Emergency Medical Services at the Crossroads.* Washington, DC: National Academy Press, 2006.

3 Ishikawa Diagram. Available from http://en.wikipedia.org/wiki/Ishikawa_diagram

4 Tague NR. *The Quality Toolbox*, 2nd edn. Milwaukee: ASQ Quality Press, 2005, pp.247–9.

CHAPTER 73

Data management and information systems

Greg Mears

Introduction

Emergency medical services, along with health care in general, has progressed in the last decade from a paper-based documentation system to an electronic health record. The short-term goals for this evolution were to improve operational efficiencies, with a strong focus on billing and risk management. The long-term goal should be integrated health information systems that support the "Iron Triangle" of health policy: improving access, improving quality, and controlling cost [1].

In the next 10 years, health information systems will continue to evolve. Current medical devices and software that function as tools in service delivery and patient care of an EMS system will become true members of the health care team. Devices and software will become real-time assistants assuring patient safety, providing recommendations based on evidence-based guidelines, and ultimately improving operational effectiveness and efficiency.

By embracing this new health care doctrine and infrastructure, EMS will no longer be isolated as an expensive source of transportation. It will be held accountable for response times, service quality, medical care, and cost or value to the customer (citizen). EMS will be held to standards based on an overall "system of care" approach, integrated with other health care specialties. EMS must prove its effect on patient outcome as a justification for its existence. Finally, EMS will be truly integrated with the rest of the health care system at the local, regional, state, and federal levels through the exchange of health information [2].

Historical foundations

The US Department of Health, Education, and Welfare defined 15 components of an EMS system within the 1973 EMS Act [3]. Although an information system was not listed as one of the 15 components, each component was shaped or defined as a piece in a puzzle. The puzzle, when completed, requires a significant amount of data to interact and monitor each of the pieces or components through a coordinated patient record. It was not until 20 years later that the National Highway Traffic Safety Administration (NHTSA) developed a consensus document defining 81 data elements important to an EMS information system [4]. The purpose of the Uniform Prehospital Dataset (version 1.0) was to allow EMS systems to benchmark their service, patient care, personnel performance, patient outcome, and data linkage with other organizations or larger datasets. Perhaps even more important than the data elements themselves was the creation of a standard definition for each element, critical for any information system.

In 1996, NHTSA published the EMS Agenda for the Future, which addressed EMS as a community-based health management system, fully integrated with the overall health care system [5]. The goal of the agenda was to improve the quality of community health, resulting in more appropriate use of acute health care resources. To meet this goal, the agenda recommended development of 14 distinct attributes of EMS, one of which was information systems. Formal recommendations within the information systems attribute were as follows.

- EMS must adopt a uniform set of data elements and definitions to facilitate multisystem evaluations and collaborative research.
- EMS must develop mechanisms to generate and transmit data that are valid, reliable, and accurate.
- EMS must develop and refine information systems that describe the entire EMS event so that patient outcomes and cost-effective issues can be determined.
- EMS should collaborate with other health care providers and community resources to develop integrated information systems.
- Information system users must provide feedback to those who generate data in the form of research results, quality improvement programs, and evaluations.

The EMS Agenda for the Future Implementation Guide [6] was published by NHTSA in 1998 and reinforced the concept that an EMS information system is the backbone connecting every component of the EMS system.

Emergency Medical Services: Clinical Practice and Systems Oversight, Second Edition. Volume 1: Clinical Aspects of EMS.
Edited by David C. Cone, Jane H. Brice, Theodore R. Delbridge, and J. Brent Myers.
© 2015 NAEMSP. Published 2015 by John Wiley & Sons, Inc. Companion Website: www.wiley.com\go\cone\naemsp

In 1991, an international consensus group published the "Recommended guidelines for uniform reporting of data from out-of-hospital cardiac arrest: the Utstein style" [7]. As the first major document to specifically address EMS systems and their performance with respect to patient outcome, the Utstein criteria were a standard dataset with standard definitions for measuring and reporting cardiac arrest survival across systems. The Utstein criteria required the exchange of information between the dispatch center, the EMS system, and the hospital. A revised version was published in 2004 unifying the hospital, prehospital, and pediatric templates, providing a more usable standard for outcomes measurement [8]. A second revision of the Utstein dataset is under way.

The first formal funding for an EMS information system came in 2001. Based on a 1999 Health Resources Services Administration Emergency Medical Services for Children program feasibility study demonstrating it was possible to create an organized EMS data system, NHTSA formally funded the National EMS Information System Project (NEMSIS). The NEMSIS project has four primary goals and objectives.

- Establish a standardized national EMS dataset that is used to document the EMS service delivery, personnel performance, and care for every EMS event in the nation.
- Establish an electronic EMS documentation system in every local EMS system to support service delivery and clinical care operations.
- Establish a state EMS database in every state where a portion of the data collected by each local EMS system can be aggregated to support state EMS regulatory and disaster management functions.
- Establish a national EMS database where a portion of the data maintained by each state's EMS database can be aggregated to support federal EMS program, educational, fiscal, and advocacy needs.

NHTSA Uniform Prehospital Dataset (Version 2.2.1) is currently in use with more than 400 data elements defined [9]. This national standard has been adopted in principle by all 56 US states and territories. At the time this chapter was written (fall, 2013), a total of 43 states have operational state data systems that are NEMSIS compliant and submit data to the national EMS database. In 2012, 19,831,189 records were added to the national EMS database, submitted to state repositories by 8,448 local EMS agencies [10]. This represents 54% of the 36,698,670 EMS responses and 42% of the 19,971 EMS agencies identified by the National EMS Assessment in 2011 [11]. Every state and US territory has a goal, pending resources and funding, to establish a NEMSIS-compliant state EMS data system.

Data are used differently at each level of EMS (local, state, and national). A national dataset was identified consisting of data elements especially relevant to describing EMS at the national industry level which can be used to better target EMS needs, national policy, advocacy, educational curricula, and reimbursement. Each state EMS office works with its local EMS agencies to define a state EMS dataset that can be implemented locally. At the state level, EMS data determine how state and federal resources are applied, target legislative initiatives and funding, assure EMS coverage and service delivery, develop and maintain educational programs, and promote performance improvement initiatives that ultimately assure quality patient care. Locally, EMS data are used to determine resource allocation, service delivery, personnel performance, and patient care.

Beginning in 2005, NHTSA funded the NEMSIS Technical Assistance Center (TAC), which houses the national EMS database and provides technical assistance to states implementing NHTSA dataset. The TAC ensures that software programs used to document EMS care at the local level are compliant with the current NEMSIS standard. In 2006, four states (North Carolina, Minnesota, Mississippi, and New Hampshire) began providing data into the national EMS database. Today, more records are received each month than were received in that complete initial year of data collection. Information on NEMSIS and access to the web-based reports associated with the National EMS Database can be found online at www.nemsis.org. In addition, an aggregate NEMSIS research dataset is released each year and can be accessed at www.nemsis.org/reportingTools/request NEMSISData.html.

In 2012, NHTSA Uniform Prehospital Dataset was revised to Version 3.0. As the dataset was revised through EMS industry consensus, it was also processed through the Standards Developing Organization (SDO), HL7, and included the federally required migration to ICD-10. The NEMSIS HL7 CDA is now ready to be approved by the American National Standards Institute (ANSI) as a US health care standard. ANSI approval is a requirement to be included in the National Healthcare Information Infrastructure (NHII) initiative that has a presidential mandate for all health care entities to be using integrated electronic health records by 2014. The implementation of integrated electronic health records empowers health information exchange, a key component of the Affordable Care Act and US health care reform.

In 2006, the Institute of Medicine released *Emergency Medical Services at the Crossroads* [12] reflecting a very detailed evaluation of EMS, including the current organizational structure, EMS service delivery, and financing of EMS services and systems from a national perspective. Recommendations from the report specifically addressed the need for standardized EMS data and information systems, including:

- the development of evidence-based categorization systems for EMS, emergency departments, and trauma centers based on adult and pediatric service capabilities
- the development of evidence-based model prehospital care protocols for the treatment, triage, and transport of patients
- the development of evidence-based indicators for emergency and trauma system performance
- the development of demonstration programs to promote regionalization, coordination, and accountability of EMS and trauma care systems

- the development of integrated and interoperable hospital, EMS, public safety, emergency management, and public health communications and data systems
- the National Coordinator for Health Information Technology should fully involve prehospital EMS leadership in the discussions about design, deployment, and financing of the NHII
- federal agencies that fund emergency and trauma care research should target an increased share of research funding for prehospital EMS research, with an emphasis on systems and outcomes research.

Existing registries and health care databases

Health care databases

Trauma registries serve as valuable descriptive and quality management tools for trauma centers and trauma systems. Containing detailed information regarding the course and management of patients within the trauma system, trauma registries capture some EMS data. A link with EMS data is extremely important to complete the description of trauma care from event through hospital discharge or rehabilitation. The American College of Surgeons Committee on Trauma maintains the National Trauma Data Bank (NTDB), a standardized dataset based on the National Trauma Data Standard. Developed in cooperation with NEMSIS and incorporating the same data element definitions as NHTSA Uniform Prehospital Dataset, the NTDB currently contains more than 5 million records from trauma centers in the United States and Puerto Rico [13]. Access to the NTDB can be obtained through the American College of Surgeons website at www.facs.org.

Currently the Centers for Disease Control and Prevention's Paul Coverdale National Acute Stroke Registry is active in 11 states documenting the incidence, treatment, and outcome of stroke [14]. Data associated with EMS care are critical to stroke registries to understand and optimize stroke systems of care. Outcome data from stroke registries are also critical for EMS to evaluate their service delivery and care.

ST-elevation myocardial infarction (STEMI) registries are being implemented to document incidence, treatment, and outcome including clinical performance parameters such as time from onset of symptoms until definitive care or reperfusion. Integration with EMS data provides a complete picture of STEMI care from first medical contact to patient outcome.

The Cardiac Arrest Registry to Enhance Survival (CARES) focuses on improving the survival associated with out-of-hospital cardiac arrest (OHCA). CARES is housed at Emory University and while it was initially funded through the Centers for Disease Control and Prevention (CDC), it is currently funded through combination of for-profit and non-profit organizations. Data collection through CARES began in 2005 and is currently implemented within 40 communities within 26 states, including eight state-wide implementations. More than 40 EMS agencies and 900 hospitals currently participate in CARES [15].

The Cardiac Arrest Registry to Enhance Survival helps local EMS administrators and community leaders establish and improve a cardiac arrest system of care. One unique attribute of CARES is its interface with hospitals to obtain OHCA outcomes. Hospitals are given access to the web-based application. When an OHCA victim is brought to a specific hospital, email notification prompts the hospital to log in to the system and securely enter the patient's outcome. This method has allowed EMS agencies using CARES to obtain outcome information on well over 95% of their OHCA events.

Several other health care-related databases and information systems exist at local, state, and national levels. Most states have some form of hospital insurance or admission/discharge database. These databases may or may not capture information on patients who are not admitted to the hospital, such as those seen in the emergency department and released. Each state maintains vital statistics and medical examiner's databases that record information on all births and deaths. Most states also have some form of public health and/or injury surveillance database. The amount of information and usefulness of these databases vary greatly from state to state.

Law enforcement database

At the state and national level, motor vehicle crash data are collected and maintained through either the US Department of Transportation or law enforcement. The various state motor vehicle departments also maintain databases of information with respect to drivers and vehicles. Both of these data sources have potential interaction with EMS information systems.

NHTSA has a program, known as the Crash Outcomes Data Evaluation System (CODES), which uses probabilistic linkage to match state data from law enforcement, EMS, and the emergency department or hospital. CODES uses a collaborative approach to generate medical and financial outcome information relating to motor vehicle crashes, and uses this outcome-based data as the basis for decisions related to highway traffic safety. CODES has been in existence since 1992, and it is currently working with 16 states [16].

Disaster and preparedness data systems

The National Hospital Available Beds for Emergencies and Disasters (HAvBED) Project consists of a standardized dataset to monitor hospital bed availability. The system provides a national hospital bed tracking system that can be used to address any surge of patients during a mass casualty event. The system is maintained by the Office of the Assistant Secretary for Preparedness and Response within the Department of Health and Human Services. Information on the HAvBED project can be found online at https://havbed.hhs.gov/v3/.

Several events, beginning with the terrorist attacks of 11 September 2001, increased the national attention given to public health emergency preparedness. These events underscored the need for an emergency "surge" or supplemental health care workforce that can be mobilized to respond immediately to a mass casualty event that overwhelms existing health care resources. The Emergency System for Advance Registration of Volunteer Health Professionals (ESAR-VHP), administered on the state level, verifies health professionals' identification and credentials so that they can respond more quickly when disaster strikes. Information on ESAR-VHP can be found online at www.phe.gov/esarvhp/Pages/default.aspx.

Public health surveillance data systems

Events over the past decade, including the potential for terrorist acts using chemical or biological weapons, and concerns of an influenza pandemic, have increased the national attention given to public health surveillance systems. The CDC provided initial funding for these systems and still serves a role in their coordination. Most states maintain some type of public health surveillance data system which monitors public health and other health care-related data in an effort to provide early event detection and a timelier public health response. Data being used for surveillance vary from state to state but include data sources such as poison center call data, EMS event data, emergency department data, pharmacy sales data, and school attendance data. Additional information on public health surveillance data systems can be found at www.cdc.gov/surveillancepractice/.

EMS information system design

The raw material for information is data. Information systems collect and arrange data to serve particular purposes. Following the recommendations of the EMS Agenda for the Future, uniform data elements with uniform definitions which can describe an entire EMS event are the goal of an EMS information system. An EMS event begins with layperson or patient recognition of a problem, which leads to activation of the system through the 9-1-1 or communications center. The end of an EMS event is the transfer of care of a patient to another health care provider outside the EMS system, EMS release of the patient from care, patient refusal of EMS care, or death. To measure and draw conclusions through research, patient outcomes, quality management, or evaluation, the end of an EMS event must include information regarding emergency department care, hospital care, and final disposition.

Information systems must also provide a mechanism for storage and retrieval of EMS events in the form of historic medical records. The knowledge of previous medical care or EMS usage can be crucial in true acute care situations when little patient information can otherwise be obtained. A movement within health care reform is the development of regional health care information organizations and accountable care organizations which unite health care providers through policy and information technology to allow individual health care information to flow and be visible across organizations. Information should be available to each health care provider in a format that can be accessed prior to or during patient care.

An EMS information system must be able to include data from several sources. The communication center can provide time-related data, such as dispatch and arrival times, dispatch complaint information, vehicle response information, and other emergency medical dispatch (EMD) data. EMD protocols identify general demographics of the patient, the chief complaint, the protocol used for the response, and prearrival instructions. A patient or event identifier should be established to link these data with the EMS patient care record.

The Utstein criteria and NHTSA Uniform Prehospital Dataset, when combined, give an important definition standard to prehospital data points. It is important to work within these recommendations to create an environment where information can be linked with other databases, systems, and registries. Through this uniform data, standardized evaluation, research, and outcome measures can be obtained. These two datasets fundamentally recommend only a subset of their data, known as a "minimum dataset." For complete documentation of an EMS event, other data elements must be created to include standards of medical care documentation, such as current medications taken by the patient, drug allergies, medical and injury-related risk factors, examination results, narrative interactions or treatment exceptions, and disposition details or instructions. As EMS moves outside its traditional treatment and transport modalities, the need to create a medical document with the consideration of treatment and referral or treatment and non-transport must be addressed. This requires increased documentation of disposition instructions and patient education.

Information collected during an EMS event can be improved through the use of medical devices. Information collected by a medical device, stored, and later downloaded into the information system is essential to the future of EMS information systems. Direct data collection from medical devices removes many of the inherent data entry errors, improves the completeness of the medical record, and frees personnel to provide patient care. Currently, prehospital medical devices do not have a universal capability to transfer all their numeric and waveform data to information systems outside their proprietary software, but a standardized solution is incorporated into NEMSIS Version 3. Often a single EMS system will have multiple devices from multiple manufacturers performing the same function. This duplication forces a system to have the proprietary software from each manufacturer to download and archive data, limiting the ability to combine and functionally use the data, especially if waveforms from monitors/defibrillators are included. This same problem makes it impossible to create an electronic medical record in a timely manner for use immediately after patient care, and makes the retrieval of previous EMS events for comparison extremely difficult. Manufacturers must work to implement NEMSIS Version 3 as an open architecture where device data, both alphanumeric and waveform, can be moved from database to database within an information system in a time frame to allow electronic record retrieval or generation.

Information systems must be designed to interface with the other health care providers participating in a patient's care. Communication with emergency departments and hospitals is critical to the linkage between the EMS and other health care databases, while assuring patient confidentiality and health information security. It is only through these linkages that systems of care and patient outcomes can be measured and improved. States should work toward improving EMS law and regulations so that information can flow in both directions. The future of EMS is dependent on the ability to obtain outcome information in a timely manner.

Emergency medical services systems are now, more than ever, in a position of financial accountability; they are held accountable for their service quality, patient care, and finances. All EMS information systems should incorporate information required for billing and reimbursement in a format that will allow interaction with billing software and fulfill government regulations for Medicare reimbursement.

Finally, EMS data collection and use must be based on system design and workflow. It is impossible to separate EMS operations from patient care. Failure to consider these two issues together will result in incomplete data, useless information, and failure of the information system. Many EMS data collection systems have failed for the lack of understanding and consideration of the end user and workflow.

EMS system types

Stout was the first to describe models of EMS delivery and management through the analysis of several urban-based EMS systems [17]. Using methods at the time known as system status management, he postulated that the ideal size for EMS efficiency was a population base of just more than 1 million people. High-performance EMS implementations now commonly use both predictive and real-time data analysis within their dispatch and administrative software to manage resources on a case-by-case basis.

To be successful, EMS information systems must be based on standards and yet mirror the diversity of the EMS systems they serve. When implementing an EMS information system, it is critical to consider each and every attribute of the EMS system. The amount, method, and mechanism for data collection and data analysis are very different for each system. Information system design is critical to measurement and analysis when patient outcomes and system design are compared between urban and rural EMS implementations.

Emergency medical services data must also be considered from a time perspective. Documentation of an EMS event should include information regarding the entire EMS event, from dispatch through disposition (with or without transport). This involves preevent information, the actual patient encounter, and the postevent disposition and documentation. Data should be defined and analyzed based on sound business principles

including documentation with the ability to analyze performance at three levels: the EMS agency, the EMS health care professional, and the patient. EMS data must take into account the system workflow. Definitions of data must be clear and understandable, collection must be as automated as possible, and should have a positive effect on the system's performance by improving the provider's time with each patient, improving the treatment and care for individuals, and providing real-time (or near real-time) feedback to the system and personnel.

EMS operations from a data perspective

An EMS event begins with the recognition, by a victim or bystander, of a medical or traumatic event that requires medical care. There is an established workflow from 9-1-1 call activation through hospital discharge, each of which has a unique time-stamp. These time-stamps, describing the "action" times of an EMS response, document when the call arrived in the dispatch center; when the responders were alerted to the call, and when the responding unit(s) rolled out of the station, arrived at the scene, arrived at the patient, departed the scene, arrived at the receiving facility, and was or were again ready for service.

Computer-aided dispatch (CAD) entry is critical to the documentation and analysis of EMS system response. Dispatch centers still using radio-acknowledged time-stamps are less accurate than those with automated GIS-based systems. EMS agencies should be electronically importing data from the dispatch center into their EMS patient care reports (PCRs) so these data are available for EMS service delivery and patient care documentation, peer review, and performance improvement initiatives.

Public safety answering point

Early in the chain of events, a public call into the public safety answering point (PSAP) is processed through a series of computerized data management systems. Dispatch priority can be assigned to the EMS call based on the response to a few key questions asked by the dispatcher. A high-priority call can involve a multiple agency and multiple vehicle response. Data sharing among responders may involve voice, alpha-pagers, mobile data printers, and mobile data terminals. Voice communication to responders provides a traditional medium for communicating information (scene safety, patient condition, and other hazards). Although communications interoperability has improved with the lessons learned from 11 September 2001, most communities are still working to fully integrate emergency communication systems across all public safety agencies.

An important measure of system effectiveness is a reasonable and consistent response time. To achieve the optimum response time for any EMS event, the EMS agency must navigate the shortest distance and/or most efficient route to the event, and if necessary, to the destination health care facility. Technology in the dispatch center and the response unit should assist in call assignment to the closest unit, suggest the best route from the EMS unit's current location, and record key time-stamps for event documentation. A modern CAD system with supplemental automated vehicle locators and in-vehicle navigation can determine the closest unit and direct the responders via an electronic map with the shortest distance of travel.

In some emergency situations, such as motor vehicle crashes, commercial services implemented within motor vehicles can automatically notify the closest PSAP when a vehicle crash occurs. Systems such as On-Star provide automated collision notification services as well as the GPS location of the vehicle and a voice operator interaction to its subscribers. Data collected through these vehicle telemetry systems can also predict the possibility of serious injury based on the force of impact associated with the motor vehicle crash. This information can be used by the dispatch center to determine the level of EMS response that is appropriate for the event [18].

One other important data component of an EMS dispatch center is EMD, a structured question-and-answer approach by the dispatcher to obtain key information and assure the appropriate EMS service level and response urgency to the event. EMD also provides guidance to dispatch centers on how to prioritize events when requests are made at the same time or are stacked awaiting EMS responses. Finally, using EMD prearrival instructions, medical care such as CPR can be relayed over the phone to the scene while EMS is en route. There are key EMD data elements associated with each EMS event that should be collected and incorporated into the EMS data system and its performance improvement process.

EMS systems for 2020: a look at the future

Personnel 2020

In the year 2020, EMS personnel are now equipped with hand-held multifunctional devices capable of assessing and monitoring vital signs (non-invasive blood pressure, pulse oximetry, pulse, respiratory rate, cardiac rhythm, 12-lead ECG, carbon dioxide and/or carbon monoxide levels, tissue perfusion, hemoglobin, and blood glucose) to evaluate patients. The device is quickly attached to the patient and automatically performs these functions while EMS personnel spend time interviewing the patient and performing the needed physical exam and treatment. As they perform their assessment and provide treatment, personnel enter data into a second portable device that allows data to be entered in a combination of ways. Verbal information is entered by voice recognition. Treatment and procedures are entered by a combination of touch screen and radiofrequency-identified medications and supplies. Scanning the barcode of the patient's driver license or personal ID enters the patient's demographic data and assigns the patient a tracking identifier for follow-up and tracing activity. While the patient assessment and care are under way, the data collected are continuously monitored to guide the EMS professional based on the patient's medical problem and the treatment protocols in use. Patient errors are minimized with the assistance of software decision support, avoiding the administration of contraindicated medications, medications to which the patient is allergic, etc.

During the response and transport associated with the EMS event, software within the vehicle is also monitoring the vehicle and occupants for safety. Using "black box" type technology, similar to what has been used on aircraft for decades, the EMS vehicle is monitored based on the driving behavior of the EMS professional. As acceleration, speed, stopping force, and other parameters are monitored during the event, the driver is provided with signals and alerts to assure the safety of the occupants within the EMS vehicle and the other vehicles in its path.

The hand-held device then communicates back to a central database through a wireless interface to determine if this patient has received EMS services in the past and, if so, provides the most recent past medical history, medication, and allergy list. It imports all other pertinent information in the system into the PCR to minimize data entry by personnel. The advanced monitoring device communicates with the hand-held data unit through a wireless or Bluetooth connection to complete the PCR. Dispatch, 9-1-1, and EMD data are electronically retrieved and imported in to the PCR over the wireless network. EMS personnel choose from a list of destinations, and the event and patient care information are automatically relayed to the receiving hospital where it is visible during the transport to the receiving facility prior to the arrival of the EMS unit. If a life-threatening, time-dependent illness or injury is associated with the event, the appropriate trauma, STEMI, or stroke team is activated.

On arrival to the emergency department, the EMS PCR is electronically reviewed based on the type of event, the patient's primary medical condition, and the treatment protocols used to assure that all of the required documentation is complete, prompting or querying for any missing data. The completed PCR is then finalized using a combination of electronic and touch screen signatures. Once the report is finalized, it is electronically transmitted into the hospital electronic medical records system (using the NEMSIS HL7 CDA). The PCR is also relayed to any other EMS administrative areas, assuring the EMS unit is restocked, performance improvement processes are reviewed, and the EMS event is electronically billed within the same workday. The PCR data are stored centrally on a database with a web browser/internet interface.

Concerned about another call that has just been paged out, the EMS personnel quickly restock the ambulance based on the list of used supplies provided on the hand-held data unit's tabulations, and a crew member activates the button on the hand-held unit, signifying they are back in service. At the end of the day, the EMS provider generates a quality management report from this specific call, which indicates all care was provided appropriately based on the complaint and protocol and the patient was admitted for definitive care.

EMS information system components

Dataset

An EMS information system must begin with a well-structured and defined dataset. Patient care data can be divided into four broad categories.

- Patient information: demographics, billing information, medical history
- Surveillance data: injury risk/mechanism, cardiac arrest, review of systems
- Current diagnostic/physiological monitoring: vital signs, physical exam
- Interventional: procedures and treatment (pharmacology), disposition

Hardware

Modern computer technology has done much to remove barriers to collecting and using data across devices and various types of hardware. Most databases can either exist in, or move data back and forth through, desktop computers, cloud-based servers, hand-held personal digital assistants, and other medical devices. The design of any information system should include specifications that provide for this data exchange.

Software

Software associated with EMS information systems often is grouped into three components. There is the "front-end" user interface where users interact with the information system to view or enter information. There is a database that serves as the nerve center for the storage and retrieval of information. Finally, there is a "back-end" which provides a user interface for report generations and data analysis.

The front-end user interface for an EMS information system can vary in its implementation. It may consist of a simple form that will allow the user to view or enter information, but quality EMS software will do much more. Good user interfaces will assist the users in their task of data entry or retrieval. Based on the patient's medical problem, the EMS service provided, and the treatment protocol, the user interface should guide the user through the documentation workflow. Using business logic and decision support, the software can improve documentation quality, completeness, and speed.

The database component of the software often does much more than store and retrieve data based on the user interface. It is often at the database level that external data from dispatch, medical devices, external medical records, and other data sources are imported or exchanged, and that linkage of records is accomplished. Examples of linkage could be the linkage between an EMS PCR and an emergency department database so that the outcome of the EMS patient can be connected with the EMS care and event. Finally, some of the analysis and calculations of the EMS data are done at the database level so that notifications and messaging can occur to EMS units, professionals, and administrators.

The back-end user interface is typically associated with the generation of reports or data analysis. Report generators can be very open, allowing the user to move information and explore the data very loosely, or very specific, allowing minimal interaction other than the generation of a preconfigured report. Some EMS PCR solutions allow access to their data from third-party reporting and analysis tools such as Crystal Reports or Microsoft Excel. Complex statistical analysis, business modeling, GIS mapping, and other detailed trending often require specialized software.

Almost all information systems (in or out of EMS and health care) are moving toward internet-based solutions via hosted or cloud-based software. The advantage of a cloud-based solution is that the hardware, software, security, and availability of the application are combined into a single solution. Since the system is centrally hosted, it is maintained by experts in the specific software and information technology. This frees the EMS agency from having to maintain complex and costly information technology staff in house. Cloud-based solutions are often more economical initially as there is no hardware to purchase and can be more easily budgeted as the maintenance cost is often based on an ongoing monthly fee.

As each EMS information system is implemented locally and matures, there is a shift in focus from data entry to data use. As EMS systems begin using data, performance improvement programs are implemented. These programs evaluate the service delivery, personnel performance, and patient care provided. Although a formal discussion of performance improvement is provided elsewhere in this textbook (see Chapters 71, 72, and 74 of this volume), EMS data systems are key to the success of these programs.

Maintenance

All computers and computer software require ongoing maintenance and support. EMS information systems are no exception. The nature of EMS, being unpredictable with disparate locations and conditions, provides many opportunities for equipment and software failure, malfunction, or system overload. Cloud-based EMS implementations have extensive back-up and security components and are recommended if the information technology resources for the EMS agency are limited.

With any EMS information system, a formal educational program, support, and maintenance structure must be planned, developed, and maintained. The quality and service provided in this one area will determine the success and failure of an EMS information system.

Security

The security of an EMS information system is critical and can be split into two areas: security and confidentiality of the patient's information, and that of the EMS system's information. EMS system security is important for many reasons. EMS is a political entity and is subject to public and private scrutiny. EMS is also a component of the health care system that comes with a significant amount of medicolegal risk. EMS is also often in a competitive market where details of operational and system issues, if made available outside the agency, could be detrimental. Finally, EMS, as part of the health care system, is responsible for peer review, performance improvement, and benchmarking. This process provides a continuing analysis of patient care and system operations to optimize service delivery and care.

An EMS information system should be designed from the ground up to provide top-level security to the EMS system and its personnel. Policies and procedures should be developed that define access and use of the system, complete with appropriate disciplinary actions to assure their compliance.

Any information system that aggregates data from multiple EMS systems should have adequate policies and procedures in place to prevent the identity of EMS systems from being disclosed to any outside agencies, or the public, without the consent of that EMS agency.

Patient security is also critically important to an EMS information system. Policies and procedures should be developed and implemented to provide appropriate access by EMS personnel in need of patient data but also to protect the patient from undue or unnecessary exposure.

In 2000, the US Department of Health and Human Services released regulations protecting patients and health care data that are transmitted electronically. This regulation (the Health Insurance Portability and Accountability Act, or HIPAA) has significant implications for all of health care, including EMS. This Act provides detailed requirements relating to health care information that is collected by any health care entity. Much of the document addresses electronic transactions with respect to reimbursement, but there are significant sections on patient confidentiality and security. From an EMS information system perspective, HIPAA basically divides security and confidentiality into four major components.

- Patient privacy and confidentiality
- User policy and procedure
- Physical security
- Software security

Clear definitions are provided stating when a patient's record can be released from the health care provider. Within the HIPAA regulation, the data elements that can be used to identify a patient are defined, as well as the process and procedures heath information systems must follow to protect patient-identifiable information.

Any health care data or information system must have a detailed policy and procedure describing who, when, where, how, and why any personnel can access the system. Any such must meet the physical security requirements of HIPAA, including issues such as locked files, controlled access, and entry logs. Finally, any health care information that is transmitted electronically must meet the HIPAA requirements, including issues such as user authentication and data encryption.

Elements of successful information systems

There are several qualities that can be identified in successful information systems. The design must start by defining what information is needed and can actually be collected. Each of these data points must be identified and defined through a consensus of the front-end data entry personnel as well as the back-end data maintenance and processing personnel. The methods of data entry must be considered based on the equipment, training, experience, and education of the EMS provider.

As data points are defined, classifications or schemes must be derived to allow information to be sorted into useful groups. This is a difficult process, in that no standard diagnostic or reimbursement coding system was designed with EMS as a primary user. EMS documents are based on chief complaint, rather than diagnosis; providers at all levels have difficulty in translating EMS records into usable ICD-9 or ICD-10 code parameters. The depth of these coding systems is much too complex for day-to-day operations. It is critical for the success of an EMS information system to have a standardized problem-based classification scheme, which can objectively and reliably cross over to other EMS and data systems. This will also be the foundation for true EMS billing and reimbursement based on services provided, rather than transportation of a patient from one location to another.

The introduction of any new data system requires planning and patience. There is no "off the shelf" solution for EMS that does not require significant configuration and testing to assure it is functional and meets the needs of the EMS agency. Once the software is configured and tested, every staff member must be trained both initially and in an ongoing fashion as updates and changes to the software occur.

A successful implementation requires designated technical and operational staff who represent both the front-end and back-end users. Whether the system is installed locally or via a cloud-based solution, 24/7/365 support from the software provider is mandatory. Locally created systems will need similar support mechanisms.

If ambulance-based hardware is part of the project, care for safety (airbag clearance and locked mounts), security, lighting (visible in night and day), and power must be addressed. New wireless technologies are expanding connected devices in areas where traditional "wire-based" connections were costly or impossible.

References

1 The Patient Protection and Affordable Care Act (PPACA), Pub. L. No. 111-148, 124 Stat. 119. 2010.

2 Mears G. Emergency medical services information systems. *NC Med J* 2007;68;266–7.

3 Emergency Medical Services Systems Act 1973. Public Law 93-154, Title XII of the Public Health Services Act. Washington, DC, 1973.

4 National Highway Traffic Safety Administration. *Uniform Pre-Hospital Emergency Medical Services (EMS) Data Conference: Final Report.* Washington, DC: National Highway Traffic Safety Administration, 1994.

5 National Highway Traffic Safety Administration. *Agenda for the Future (DOT HS 808 441)*. Washington, DC: US Department of Transportation, 1996.

6 National Highway Traffic Safety Administration. *Agenda for the Future. Implementation Guide. (DOT HS 808 711)*. Washington, DC: US Department of Transportation, 1998.

7 Cummins RO, Chamberlain DA, Abramson NS, et al. Recommended guidelines for uniform reporting of data from out-of-hospital cardiac arrest: the Utstein Style. *Ann Emerg Med* 1991;20:861–74.

8 Jacobs I, Nadkarni V, Bahr J, et al. Cardiac arrest and cardiopulmonary resuscitation outcome reports: update and simplification of the Utstein templates for resuscitation registries. *Resuscitation* 2004;63: 233–49.

9 National Highway Traffic Safety Administration Uniform Prehospital Dataset, Version 2.2.1 Data Dictionary, 2006. Available at: www.NEMSIS.org

10 National EMS Information System (NEMSIS). Available at: www. NEMSIS.org

11 Federal Interagency Committee on Emergency Medical Services. *2011 National EMS Assessment*. Washington, DC: US Department of Transportation, National Highway Traffic Safety Administration, 2012. Available at: www.ems.gov

12 Institute of Medicine. *Emergency Medical Services at the Crossroads*. Washington, DC: Institute of Medicine, 2006.

13 American College of Surgeons. National Trauma Data Bank Annual Report, 2013. Available at www.facs.org

14 Schwamm LH, Pancioli A, Acker JE, et al. Recommendations for the establishment of stroke systems of care: recommendations from the American Stroke Association's Task Force on the Development of Stroke Systems. *Stroke* 2005;36:690–703.

15 McNally B, Robb R, Mehta M, et al. Out-of-hospital cardiac arrest surveillance – Cardiac Arrest Registry to Enhance Survival (CARES), United States, October 1, 2005–December 31, 2010. *MMWR Surveill Summ* 2011;60:1–19.

16 Johnson SW, Walker J. *NHTSA Technical Report: The Crash Outcomes Data Evaluation System (CODES). DOT HS 808 338*. Washington, DC: Department of Transportation, National Highway Traffic Safety Administration, 1996.

17 Stout JL. System status management: the strategy of ambulance placement. *JEMS* 1983;8:22–32.

18 Bachman LR, Preziotti GR. *Automated Collision Notification (ACN) Field Operational Test (FOT) Evaluation Report*. Washington, DC: Department of Transportation, National Highway Traffic Safety Administration, 2001.

CHAPTER 74

EMS quality improvement and the law

Maria B. Abrahamsen

Introduction

Two principal legal issues are raised by performing quality improvement (QI) activities in any health care setting, including EMS. The first issue is the extent to which information generated by or for the body and individuals that perform QI may be kept confidential. The second question is whether participants in QI activities face liability as a result of their participation. These issues are addressed by statute in some (but by no means all) states, and the scope and nature of statutory protection differ significantly from state to state. By analogizing to the more fully developed law relating to QI in the *hospital* setting, however, it is possible to provide some practical suggestions aimed at protecting the prehospital QI process and those who participate in it.

Confidentiality of quality improvement materials

Reasons for confidentiality

Those who perform QI reviews, and those who are the subject of such reviews, generally wish to protect QI data from public disclosure, including release for use in legal proceedings or to the media. Those legislatures and courts that have elected to protect the confidentiality of QI information typically are motivated by a desire to encourage candid review by assuring QI participants that the results will not be made public and may not be used in litigation against the subject of review. In other words, the purpose of confidentiality is to promote candid evaluation and protect the effectiveness of the *QI process,* thereby improving the quality of health care available to the public. The individual providers who are the subjects of QI activities are the ancillary beneficiaries of such confidentiality. The National Association of EMS Physicians has adopted a position statement endorsing statutory protection for the confidentiality of EMS patient safety and quality information because such protections promote learning and foster a culture of safety [1].

However, courts and legislatures are also influenced by countervailing considerations. There are strong public policies in favor of giving consumers access to health care quality data, and making all relevant information available to the parties to litigation in order to enhance the likelihood of a just result. Each state attempts to reconcile these conflicting public policies in its statutes and court decisions relating to the confidentiality of QI records [2].

State confidentiality statutes

Participants in EMS QI should familiarize themselves with the statute, if any, in their state that governs the confidentiality of QI materials. Unless QI materials are made confidential by state statute, they are likely to be (a) subject to subpoena and other forms of pretrial discovery, (b) admissible as evidence at trial (assuming the materials are relevant and otherwise satisfy generally applicable requirements for the admission of evidence), and (c) subject to public disclosure under the state's freedom of information statute if they come into the possession of a state governmental agency.

Who conducts protected QI?

Emergency medical services QI may be conducted by hospitals individually, by EMS agencies individually, or by a centralized body responsible for the quality of care throughout an emergency medical system or on a regional or state-wide basis. The availability of confidentiality may depend on who conducts EMS QI.

A majority of states have enacted statutes that grant *hospital* peer review records at least limited confidentiality. When EMS QI is conducted by a hospital, participants should confirm that the emergency medical care they review is within the scope of the statutory definition of "hospital" QI.

A number of states have adopted statutes that expressly protect the confidentiality of records of *centralized* review of EMS that is conducted by a private or governmental body that is responsible for monitoring the care provided by *multiple* prehospital providers. Such statutes typically also protect the records of QI activities that are conducted by providers themselves [3]. For example, the Florida legislature has expressly provided that, "The investigations, proceedings and records of a committee

Emergency Medical Services: Clinical Practice and Systems Oversight, Second Edition. Volume 1: Clinical Aspects of EMS.
Edited by David C. Cone, Jane H. Brice, Theodore R. Delbridge, and J. Brent Myers.
© 2015 NAEMSP. Published 2015 by John Wiley & Sons, Inc. Companion Website: www.wiley.com\go\cone\naemsp

providing quality assurance" regarding EMS "shall not be subject to discovery or introduction into evidence in any civil action or disciplinary proceeding" conducted by the state or by an agency that employs emergency medical personnel [4]. The same Florida statute provides that persons who attend a meeting of an emergency medical review committee are not permitted or required to testify in any such civil or disciplinary proceeding regarding information relating to the committee, except for information from external sources that was presented to the committee. A number of states have established state-wide or state-appointed EMS QI bodies, and have enacted statutes that grant confidentiality to the records of these statutorily mandated QI bodies [5].

A significant number of states protect the confidentiality of QI conducted by a *single* EMS provider with respect to its own services [6]. Often it is not clear whether these confidentiality statutes, which expressly apply to an individual provider's activity, also cover QI that is conducted on a centralized basis, such as where a committee of representatives of the state or local EMS authority performs QI. In states that protect only the records of individual providers, QI providers might attempt to bring themselves within the protection of the statute by having each participating provider sign a simple form that delegates the provider's QI functions to the centralized EMS QI committee. While this approach is largely untested, there is strong appeal to the theory that if QI is confidential when conducted independently by individual providers, it should also be equally protected when performed (perhaps more effectively and efficiently) on a centralized basis by a group of such providers.

Research revealed only one reported court decision that addresses the confidentiality of EMS peer review materials. In McCoy v. Hatmaker, 135 Md App 693, 763 A2d 1233 (2000), the Maryland Court of Special Appeals upheld a lower court decision protecting the confidentiality of a fire department's records. The fire department employed an EMT who allegedly had violated state-wide EMS protocols when providing emergency care to a motorist who died. The motorist's estate sued the EMT and his municipal employer for wrongful death. In the course of that litigation, the plaintiff subpoenaed the report of an investigation of the incident/death that was conducted by the EMT's supervisor. The fire department refused to release the record to the plaintiff on the grounds it was confidential "medical review" and protected against discovery by Maryland's medical review committee statute. The Maryland statute protects the confidentiality of the proceedings and records of committees that review the quality or necessity of health care or the competence or performance of providers; the statute is generic and does not apply expressly to EMS. The Court of Special Appeals agreed with the fire department and observed (135 Md App at 726, 763 A2d at 1251):

> Although medical review committees are most often associated with hospitals or other traditional health care facilities, a review by the Fire Department would constitute a protected action, when as here, the fundamental purpose of the review was the improvement of health care services provided by the Fire Department paramedics.

Extent of confidentiality created

State peer review confidentiality statutes also vary with respect to the scope of confidentiality each creates. The principal variables include the following.

- **Type of information protected**: data submitted *to* QI body, body's deliberations, and/or its conclusions; written records only, or also prohibit oral disclosure of QI information (including testimony).
- **Type of QI protected**: prospective (such as development of protocols and policies), concurrent, and/or retrospective review.
- **Whose records are protected**: specified bodies only, or any individual and/or body that performs a QI function.
- **Type of disclosure prohibited**: pretrial discovery, admission as evidence at trial, Freedom of Information Act (FOIA) requests, and/or voluntary disclosure by QI body. For example, the Rhode Island emergency medical transportation services peer review statute (General Laws 1956, §23-4.1-18) prohibits discovery and admissibility of EMS peer review records in any lawsuit *except* "litigation arising out of the imposition of sanctions upon a [sic] emergency medical technician," and peer review records may be used as evidence *against* an EMT to show the EMT furnished care contrary to a restriction or supervision that had been imposed with respect to the EMT.
- An absolute prohibition against disclosure, or a "privilege" that may be waived by the provider who is the subject of review and/or by the QI body. If disclosure is prohibited by law, the statute may prevent use of QI information in any and all proceedings or only in specific types of cases, such as professional liability actions and/or other types of personal injury lawsuits against providers.

Participants in EMS QI can be effective advocates for confidentiality legislation that incorporates broad protection with respect to each of the variables outlined above.

Federal confidentiality statute

Confidentiality protection for EMS QI materials may also be available under federal law. Patient safety organizations (PSOs) were created under the 2005 Patient Safety and Quality Improvement Act (PSQIA) which amended the federal Public Health Service Act to improve patient safety and reduce the incidence of adverse events [7]. The PSQIA creates comprehensive confidentiality for "patient safety work product," which is defined broadly to include virtually all information that is collected or generated by providers for submission to a PSO, or by a PSO. To qualify as a PSO, an organization must be an independent entity whose primary activity is to improve patient safety and the quality of health care delivery. A PSO must satisfy a number of requirements, including collecting and analyzing patient safety work product from multiple providers in a standardized manner for comparison purposes, and utilizing these data to provide direct feedback to providers and assist providers to minimize patient risk. An organization qualifies as a PSO only if it applies to and is certified as such by the federal government. Patient safety work product is made confidential by the PSQIA and is protected from discovery or admissibility in federal, state, and local litigation and protected against disclosure under the FOIA.

Emergency medical transportation agencies and emergency medical personnel are not in the statutory list of examples of "providers" under the PSQIA. However, "providers" is defined broadly as all individuals and entities "licensed or otherwise authorized under state law to provide health care services." This definition is sufficiently expansive to include emergency medical personnel and agencies.

The PSQIA has been interpreted by the courts to provide significant protection to the confidentiality of patient safety work product. For example, reports of pharmacy dispensing errors submitted by a chain drug store to a certified PSO were determined to be privileged documents under the PSQIA and not discoverable even in a lawsuit filed by a state health professional licensing agency to enforce its subpoena for the drug store's "incident reports" relating to a specific pharmacist [8].

Practical steps to enhance confidentiality

The measures that will enhance the confidentiality of QI records will vary from state to state and will depend on the state's specific statute and case law. Nevertheless, the following general considerations are relevant in all jurisdictions.

What are the defined elements of QI?

The bylaws and written policies of individual prehospital providers and of centralized EMS agencies should include an expansive list of the committees and individuals who are responsible for QI (such as the centralized agency's chief medical officer, QI committee, and governing body). Bylaws and policies should also describe each QI function (such as retrospective reviews and provider credentialing) as constituting "peer review" or whatever alternative terminology the applicable state statute uses to define confidential records. A court is more apt to respect the confidentiality of QI materials if there is evidence that a clearly organized QI system exists and that the records in question were generated by that system.

By whom are QI data collected and analyzed?

Quality improvement data should be collected and analyzed *only* by individuals or committees that have been formally assigned a QI function, as described above. If, for example, providers are asked to prepare summaries or incident reports that will be utilized in QI, the QI policies should expressly state that these documents constitute QI materials. Access to QI documents should then be limited to formally designated QI participants.

Neither state statutes nor reported court decisions address the effect on peer review or on confidentiality when the same patient is treated in multiple settings. For example, a patient might be transported to Hospital A by Ambulance 1, and then transferred to Hospital B for tertiary care by Ambulance 2. The individual hospitals and prehospital providers that treated the patient might be asked to share their QI records with one another, or a state-wide or regional EMS QI body might undertake review of the quality of care provided in all settings. Any transfer of QI records and any centralized QI activities should be supported by a written policy or other documentation that emphasizes the confidential and privileged nature of the records that are generated and shared.

How are QI records maintained and distributed?

As a general rule, courts are willing to protect QI records from public disclosure only if the health care provider who holds the record has also respected the confidentiality of the records. A court will not look with sympathy on a request, for example, that QI committee minutes be protected from subpoena if the minutes were freely distributed by the provider to those without a "need to know" before receiving the subpoena. All QI documents that the participants hope to protect (such as QI committee minutes and reports) should be appropriately marked (for example, with the notation "Confidential/Peer Review Materials"). The terminology chosen for the notation should track the language of the state's confidentiality statute. Some providers print each page of QI materials on special paper that contains such a notation.

If the QI committee is required to report its activities or findings to other bodies that are not clearly covered by a peer review confidentiality statute, the committee's reports should be concise and should not contain information that the committee wishes to protect against subpoena or other public disclosure. Particular care should be taken when releasing QI information to *public* bodies, such as county and state agencies, because records in the possession of public bodies are frequently subject to public disclosure under a state freedom of information act, unless protected by a specific exemption.

To reduce the chance that QI records will be inappropriately distributed and the privileged nature of such records waived, it is good practice to collect copies of all QI materials at the end of meetings of QI bodies unless it is essential that committee members take such materials with them. Responsibility for maintaining QI records should be centralized, and access to such records should be limited to individuals who need them in order to perform assigned QI functions. It is preferable if access to confidential records is governed by a written policy.

Example

The importance of clearly defining what constitutes QI data, and for whom the data are collected, is illustrated by two court decisions that arose under the same statute that makes confidential the "data and records collected by or for an individual or committee" granted a hospital peer review duty. A court held that this statute did *not* protect the confidentiality of data regarding the outcome of a form of hyperalimentation because the data had been collected independently by a physician and *later* turned over to a hospital QI committee [9]. The court rested its decision on the fact that the data were not *initially* gathered at the request of a person or committee assigned a QI function. The court held that data (which were not created *by* or *for* a peer review body) could not be converted into confidential material by subsequently turning them over to a peer review body. However, in another case interpreting the same statute, the court held that hospital incident reports constituted confidential QI materials which could not be subpoenaed. The court based its decision in this second case on evidence that the reports were generated for the purpose of reducing morbidity and mortality and, pursuant to hospital policy, were submitted to the hospital's safety and/or QI committees [10].

In short, the likelihood that data can be kept confidential is significantly enhanced if the QI body identifies in advance in written policies the types of data that are considered confidential and if access to such data is limited to those who have been formally granted QI duties.

Liability

Types of potential liability

Individuals who submit information to an EMS QI body and those who serve as its members frequently express concern regarding the potential for liability as a result of their participation in QI. The following types of claims are the most likely to arise as a result of QI.

- A defamation (libel or slander) claim by the provider who is the subject of review, particularly if QI information regarding the provider is disclosed in a manner contrary to a confidentiality statute. A successful defamation claim requires evidence that the defendant, knowing that the information was false or at least negligently failing to ascertain the facts, transmitted to a third party false information regarding the plaintiff which harmed the plaintiff's reputation. In other words, distribution of *truthful* information is not defamation.
- An antitrust claim and/or claim of wrongful interference with business relationships by a provider who experienced licensure discipline and/or adverse publicity as a result of QI; for example, a claim that competing providers misused the QI process to eliminate the plaintiff from the market or to secure plaintiff's customers for themselves.
- A claim by a patient who is injured while receiving emergency medical services that QI was performed negligently, as a result of which proper protocols were not in place or an incompetent provider was permitted to continue to practice.

Immunity statutes

In order to encourage candid participation in the QI process, a number of states have enacted statutes that provide immunity from liability arising from the performance of EMS QI [11]. The principal variables among such immunity statutes include the following.

- **Persons covered**: members of a QI body, those who furnish information to a QI body, those who investigate on behalf of or otherwise counsel or assist a QI body, and/or the body itself.
- **Prerequisites to immunity**: no malice, good faith, and/or reasonable belief that action was warranted by facts known.
- **Types of claims protected against**: claims for monetary damages only, all civil claims, or all civil and criminal claims.

Immunity statutes do not preclude a plaintiff from *filing a lawsuit* against QI participants. The existence of an immunity statute does not even necessarily ensure that a lawsuit will be *dismissed* at an early stage (e.g. on motion for summary judgment) because there may be factual disputes as to whether the defendants satisfy the statutory requirements for immunity. However, immunity statutes increase the number of facts the plaintiff must prove in order to succeed in his or her lawsuit; for example, the existence of an immunity statute might require the plaintiff to prove that the defendants acted in bad faith while participating in QI. Most importantly, immunity statutes decrease the risk that a QI participant can be held liable for damages to a provider or patient as a consequence of the QI activity.

Common law protection

In addition to specific immunity statutes, the courts have developed certain principles that protect against liability in cases alleging defamation or interference with business relationships. There is common law protection (or, in legal parlance, a "privilege") against defamation liability for communications that are made in good faith and in the reasonable belief that the communication was necessary in order to fulfill a moral or legal duty, provided the disclosure is limited to appropriate individuals and proper subject matter. Similarly, where a person acts to protect a public interest or for other laudable purposes, he or she may be protected by the courts from a claim of interference with business relationships, especially if the defendant's actions were reasonable in light of the threatened harm. Common law privileges of this sort generally are not well defined and are highly dependent upon the facts of each case. Nevertheless, where QI participants act reasonably for the purpose of improving health care available to public, and are not motivated by self-interest, they may be protected from liability by common law privileges.

Practical steps to reduce risk of liability

The risk that those who conduct EMS QI or those who furnish information to a QI body will incur liability as a result of such participation may be reduced by the following measures.

- Define broadly in the QI body's bylaws and procedures who is charged with QI duties, and comply strictly with these documents when conducting QI activities. This will enhance the likelihood that review activities will be deemed part of official quality improvement and therefore qualify for any available immunity and/or privilege. For example, the Rhode Island EMS peer review statute (General Laws 1956, §23-4.1-18) limits statutory immunity to members of a "duly appointed peer review board operated pursuant to written bylaws" and to those who communicate information to such a board.

- Do not permit the QI process to be misused. QI participants should diligently avoid use of the QI process for any purpose other than improvement of patient care. In order to avoid even the appearance that QI is being used for anticompetitive purposes, try to avoid having providers participate in decisions from which they might benefit financially.
- Preserve the confidentiality of QI records. By doing so, the QI body will reduce the risk that the reputation of a provider who is the subject of review will be harmed and thereby also reduce the risk of a successful claim of defamation or interference with business relationships.

Conclusion

Participants in EMS QI should familiarize themselves with the laws of their state regarding the confidentiality of QI materials and immunity from liability for QI participants. If the QI confidentiality and/or immunity statutes have been interpreted by state courts (whether in the context of QI conducted by an EMS organization or any other type of provider), QI participants should also be familiar with these rulings. The policies, minutes, reports, and other documents of the bodies that conduct QI should be drafted in a manner that maximizes the likelihood that confidentiality and immunity will apply to the QI bodies' activities and QI should be conducted with consideration for the consequences to confidentiality and immunity. QI participants in states that do not presently have confidentiality or immunity statutes covering EMS quality improvement should consider seeking enactment of such statutes.

Acknowledgment

The author acknowledges with gratitude the research assistance provided by law student Jacquelyn Godin.

References

1 NEAMT Position Statement: Protecting Patient Safety and Quality Information, adopted February 8, 2013.
2 *State* courts are obliged to follow the QI confidentiality statutes of their state when ruling on the discoverability or admissibility of QI records. However, when *federal* courts hear lawsuits that are based on federal statutes (such as the federal civil rights or antitrust laws or the Constitution) the federal courts must consider, but are not obliged to follow, state evidentiary laws, including state QI confidentiality statutes. Therefore, a *federal* court may order the disclosure of QI records despite the existence of a strong peer review confidentiality statute.
3 See, for example, Louisiana, LSA-R.S. 40:2845.1, covering the trauma registry, licensing board and its committees, any regional commission, any emergency medical services council, all providers, and "any other group or committee whose purpose is to monitor and improve quality care pursuant to" the Louisiana emergency response network statute; Montana, MCA 50-6-415; and New York, NY CLS Pub Health §3006.
4 Fla. Stat. §401.425(5).
5 For example, the following statutes create confidentiality for state-wide or state-approved EMS QI bodies: Colorado, C.R.S. 25-3.5-704(2)(h) covering the state's continuing quality improvement system and regional emergency medical and trauma advisory councils, Delaware, 16 Del. C. §9707 covering the state's Trauma System Committee, Emergency Medical Services Oversight Committee, and their subcommittees; Iowa, Iowa Code §147A.25 regarding a state-appointed system evaluation and quality improvement committee; Maine, 32 M.R.S. §92-A covers EMS quality assurance committees that are approved by a state EMS board; Michigan, MCLA §333.20919 requires each state-appointed medical control authority to have in place a quality improvement program that qualifies for statutory confidentiality; New Hampshire, RSA 153-A:9 applies to a state-wide trauma medical review committee and its subcommittees; and Washington, Rev. Code Wash. §70.168.090 covers state-mandated regional EMS QI committees.
6 Illinois, 210 ILCS 50/3.110; Louisiana, La. R.S. 13:3715.3; Michigan, MCLA §331.531 et. seq. and §333.20175(6); Montana, MCA 50-6-415; and Wis. Stat. §146.38.
7 Patient Safety and Quality Improvement Act of 2005, PL 109-41, July 29, 2005, 119 Stat 424. Some states have included patient safety organizations under their own peer review statutes. See VA Code Ann. §8.01-581.17 (2011).
8 *Dep't of Fin. & Prof'l Regulation v. Walgreen Co.*, 2012 IL App (2d) 110452, 970 N.E.2d 552.
9 Marchand v. Henry Ford Hospital, 398 Mich. 163, 247 NW2d 280 (1976).
10 Gallagher v. Detroit-Macomb Hospital Association, 171 Mich. App. 761 (1988).
11 See, for example, Delaware, 16 Del. C. §9707(c); Illinois, 201 ILCS 50/3.110(b); Louisiana, La. R.S. 13.3715.3; Maine, M.R.S. §92-A; Michigan, MCLA §331.533 et. seq; and New Hampshire, RSA 153-A:9.III. The federal Health Care Quality Improvement Act of 1986 (42 U.S.C. §§11101-11152) creates qualified immunity for the participants in certain forms of peer review. This federal statute is unlikely to provide immunity for EMS QI activities, however, because (1) it protects only against claims brought by *physicians* (defined as MD and DO), (2) covers only professional review actions of a "health care entity," which is defined as an entity that both provides health care (or a professional society) and follows a formal peer review process; and (3) covers only actions that adversely affect a physician's clinical privileges or membership in a health care entity.

Appendix
The Core Content of Emergency Medical Services Medicine

The EMS Examination Task Force, American Board of
Emergency Medicine

Debra G. Perina MD, Chair, Editor, EMS Subspecialty
Examinations

Peter T. Pons MD, Editor, EMS Subspecialty Examinations

Thomas H. Blackwell MD

Sandy Bogucki MD PhD

Jane H. Brice MD

Carol A. Cunningham MD

Theodore R. Delbridge MD

Marianne Gausche-Hill MD

William C. Gerard MD

Matthew C. Gratton MD

Vincent N. Mosesso Jr MD

Ronald G. Pirrallo MD

Kathy J. Rinnert MD

Ritu Sahni MD

American Board of Emergency Medicine

Anne L. Harvey PhD

Terry Kowalenko MD

Alpine Testing Solutions

Chad W. Buckendahl PhD

Lisa S. O'Leary PhD

Myisha Stokes

December 15, 2011

The *Core Content of EMS Medicine* is used with the permission of the American Board of Emergency Medicine, copyright 2011.

Please address correspondence regarding this manuscript to:

Anne L. Harvey PhD
American Board of Emergency Medicine 3000 Coolidge Road
East Lansing, MI 48823
571.332.4800, ext. 304
aharveyabem.org

The Core Content of Emergency Medical Services Medicine

Preamble

On September 23, 2010, the American Board of Medical Specialties (ABMS) approved Emergency Medical Services (EMS) as a subspecialty of Emergency Medicine. As a result, the American Board of Emergency Medicine (ABEM) is planning to award the first certificates in EMS Medicine in the fall of 2013. The purpose of subspecialty certification in EMS, as defined by ABEM, is to standardize physician training and qualifications for EMS practice, to improve patient safety and enhance the quality of emergency medical care provided to patients in the prehospital environment, and to facilitate integration of prehospital patient treatment into the continuum of patient care.

In February 2011, ABEM established the EMS Examination Task Force to develop the Core Content of EMS Medicine (Core Content) that would be used to define the subspecialty and from which questions would be written for the examinations, to develop a blueprint for the examinations[1], and to develop a bank of test questions for use on the examinations. The Core Content defines the training parameters, resources, and knowledge of the treatment of prehospital patients necessary to practice EMS Medicine. Additionally, it is intended to inform fellowship directors and candidates for certification of the full range of content that might appear on the examinations.

Development of the Core Content

To develop the Core Content, the Task Force began with previous versions of content outlines developed by the National Association of EMS Physicians (NAEMSP) and ABEM as part of the application to the ABMS for a subspecialty in EMS Medicine. The Task Force began the process of development by generating an inclusive list of potential content and coming to

---

[1]The examination blueprint defines the percent of questions in each content category. The examination blueprint for the EMS Subspecialty can be found at www.abem.org.

Emergency Medical Services: Clinical Practice and Systems Oversight, Second Edition. Volume 1: Clinical Aspects of EMS.
Edited by David C. Cone, Jane H. Brice, Theodore R. Delbridge, and J. Brent Myers.
© 2015 NAEMSP. Published 2015 by John Wiley & Sons, Inc. Companion Website: www.wiley.com/go/cone/naemsp

consensus on both the list and its organization. The outline was then crossed with the Accreditation Council on Graduate Medical Education (ACGME) and American Board of Medical Specialties (ABMS) six core competencies of medicine[2] to assure that all of the competencies were addressed.

The rationale for the organization was to cover the full breadth of EMS Medicine with as little overlap in content categories as possible. Nonetheless, the Task Force found that many aspects of the daily practice of EMS Medicine could easily fall into more than one category. As a result of the discussion, the Core Content is divided into four broad categories: 1.0 Clinical Aspects of EMS Medicine, 2.0 Medical Oversight of EMS, 3.0 Quality Management and Research, and 4.0 Special Operations. Each of these categories is further divided into broad topics, with examples and subtopics listed below each of the topics.

To validate the work of the Task Force, and to further refine the list of content, the Task Force conducted a survey of clinically active EMS Physicians to determine the frequency and importance of each of the content listings. (Manuscript in preparation.) The Task Force retained sections that are not a large part of every EMS medical system, such as wilderness medicine, as it was felt that they constitute an important aspect of EMS Medicine that all candidates for certification should know.

Future Development of the Core Content

The Core Content is intended to be a living document, in keeping with the ever-evolving practice of EMS Medicine. ABEM anticipates regular updates to the Core Content, with publication every two to five years. Suggested changes to the Core Content can be addressed to examcontentabem.org.

The Core Content of EMS Medicine[3]

	ACGME[4] and ABMS[5] Core Competencies					
	Patient Care	Medical Knowledge	Practice-based learning	Professionalism	Interpersonal Skills	System-based Practice
1.0 CLINICAL ASPECTS OF EMS MEDICINE						
1.1 TIME/LIFE-CRITICAL CONDITIONS	X	X	X			X
1.1.1 Cardiac Arrest	X	X			X	
1.1.1.1 General management	X	X			X	
1.1.1.2 Resuscitate in the field vs. transport	X	X	X			X
1.1.1.3 Post-resuscitation care	X	X	X			X
1.1.2 Airway Compromise/ Respiratory Failure	X	X				
1.1.2.1 Devices for securing airway	X	X				
1.1.2.2 Portable ventilator management	X	X				
1.1.2.3 Pros and cons of drug-assisted intubation	X	X				
1.1.2.4 Tracheotomy complications	X	X	X			
1.1.3 Hypotension and Shock	X	X				
1.1.3.1 Diagnosis with limited ancillary testing	X	X				
1.1.4 Altered Mental Status	X	X				
1.2 INJURY	X	X				
1.2.1 Trauma	X	X				X
1.2.1.1 Care of the trapped patient	X	X				
1.2.1.2 Protocols delineating shortened scene time	X	X				X
1.2.1.3 Resuscitation in the field vs. rapid transport to trauma center	X	X				X
1.2.1.4 Field trauma triage	X	X				X
1.2.1.5 Management of spine trauma (application of spinal immobilization, selective immobilization)	X	X				
1.2.1.6 Management of burns	X	X				
1.2.1.7 Management of crush injuries	X	X		X	X	
1.2.2 Orthopedics	X	X				
1.2.2.1 Fractures and dislocations	X	X				
1.2.2.1.1 Splinting using non-traditional materials	X	X				
1.2.2.1.2 Reductions without anesthetics	X	X			X	

[2]Found at http://www.acqme.orq/acWebsite/dutyHours/dhdutyhoursCommon PRO7012007dutyhoursCommonPRO7012007.pdf and http://www.abms.orq/ Maintenance of Certification/MOC competencies.aspx
[3]Used with permission of the American Board of Emergency Medicine, copyright 2011.

[4]Accreditation Council for Graduate Medical Education (ACGME)
[5]American Board of Medical Specialties (ABMS)

Continued

	ACGME[4] and ABMS[5] Core Competencies					
	Patient Care	Medical Knowledge	Practice-based learning	Professionalism	Interpersonal Skills	System-based Practice
1.2.3 Traumatic Brain Injuries	X	X				
1.2.3.1 Management of severe head injuries	X	X	X			X
1.2.3.2 Management of concussions	X	X				
1.2.3.3 Sideline management for team medics/physicians	X	X			x	X
1.2.4 Assault — Domestic/Sexual/Elder Abuse/Child Abuse	X	X		X	X	X
1.2.4.1 Safety					x	X
1.2.4.2 Evidence preservation and reporting		X				X
1.2.5 Environmental	X	X				
1.2.5.1 Cold-related illnesses	X	X				
1.2.5.1.1 Hypothermia	X	X				
1.2.5.1.1.1 Clinical diagnosis without the use of a thermometer	X	X				
1.2.5.1.2 Frostbite	X	X				
1.2.5.1.2.1 Protection of injury vs. re-warming	X	X				
1.2.5.2 Heat-related illnesses	X	X				
1.2.5.2.1 Methods to cool a patient in the field	X	X				X
1.2.5.3 High altitude injury (e.g., high altitude pulmonary edema, high altitude cerebral edema)	X	X				
1.2.5.3.1 Protection of the rescuer from high altitude injury	X	X				
1.2.5.3.2 Portable hyperbaric chamber	X	X				
1.2.5.3.3 Field prophylaxis and treatment	X	X				
1.2.5.4 Near-drowning, submersion, and diving injuries	X	X	X			
1.2.5.4.1 Initial management in water	X	X				X
1.2.5.5 Lightning and electrical injuries	X	X				X
1.2.5.5.1 Reverse triage	X	X				
1.3 MEDICAL EMERGENCIES	X	X				
1.3.1 Respiratory	X	X				
1.3.1.1 Shortness of breath	X	X				
1.3.1.1.1 Use of portable non-invasive ventilation devices	X	X				
1.3.1.1.2 Field identification of chronic obstructive pulmonary disease (COPD)	X	X				
1.3.1.1.3 Assisted ventilation	X	X				
1.3.1.1.4 Use of capnometry and capnometry waveforms in diagnosis	X	X				
1.3.1.2 Pneumothorax	X	X				
1.3.1.2.1 Identifying without ancillary testing	X	X				
1.3.1.2.2 Management with occlusive dressings and alternative drain devices	X	X				
1.3.2 Cardiovascular	X	X				
1.3.2.1 ST elevation myocardial infarction (STEMI)	X	X				
1.3.2.1.1 Utilization of electrocardiogram (ECG) in the field	X	X				X
1.3.2.1.2 Use of oxygen (e.g., how much to use; demand vs. supply)	X	X				X
1.3.2.1.3 Methods of revascularization in the field	X	X				
1.3.2.2 Acute exacerbation of congestive heart failure (CHF)	X	X				
1.3.2.2.1 Use of portable non-invasive ventilation devices	X	X				
1.3.2.2.2 Field identification of CHF	X	X				
1.3.2.2.3 Field use of vasopressors and inotropes without confirmed diagnosis	X	X				
1.3.2.2.4 Assisted ventilation	X	X				
1.3.2.3 Implantable cardiac devices	X	X				
1.3.2.3.1 Use of magnets for management of devices	X	X				
1.3.3 Neurological	X	X				
1.3.3.1 Stroke	X	X				
1.3.3.1.1 Prehospital stroke scales	X	X				
1.3.3.2 Management of seizures	X	X				

Continued

Continued

	ACGME[4] and ABMS[5] Core Competencies					
	Patient Care	Medical Knowledge	Practice-based learning	Professionalism	Interpersonal Skills	System-based Practice
1.3.4 Diabetic Emergencies	X	X				
1.3.4.1 Glucagon, oral/intravenous glucose	X	X				
1.3.4.2 Protocols for treat & release	X	X				X
1.3.5 Renal	X	X				
1.3.5.1 Hemodialysis	X	X				
1.3.5.1.1 Use of dialysis access for resuscitation	X	X				
1.3.5.1.2 Uncontrolled hemorrhage from shunt site	X	X				
1.3.5.1.3 Special considerations for hyperkalemia	X	X				
1.3.6 Obstetric and Gynecologic Emergencies	X	X				
1.3.6.1 Perinatal issues	X	X				
1.3.6.1.1 Control of seizures in eclampsia	X	X				
1.3.6.1.2 Placental abruption	X	X				
1.3.6.1.3 Placenta previa	X	X				
1.3.6.2 Childbirth	X	X				
1.3.6.2.1 High risk vs. normal delivery	X	X				
1.3.6.2.2 Managing home birth catastrophes	X	X				
1.3.6.2.3 Post-partum hemorrhage	X	X				
1.3.6.2.4 Breech/shoulder dystocia in the field	X	X				
1.3.6.2.5 Umbilical cord prolapse	X	X				
1.3.6.3 Vaginal hemorrhage	X	X				
1.3.6.3.1 Packing in the field	X	X				
1.3.6.4 Ectopic pregnancy	X	X				
1.3.6.4.1 Effect of clinical diagnosis on transport decisions	X	X				X
1.3.7 Poisoning/Toxicologic Emergencies	X	X				
1.3.7.1 Clinical management of toxins	X	X				
1.3.7.1.1 Carbon monoxide	X	X				
1.3.7.1.2 Cyanide	X	X				
1.3.7.1.3 Chlorine	X	X				
1.3.7.1.4 Hydrofluoric acid	X	X				
1.3.7.1.5 Organophosphates	X	X				
1.3.7.1.6 Mustards and other blister agents	X	X				
1.3.7.1.7 Phosgene	X	X				
1.3.7.1.8 Hydrocarbons	X	X				
1.3.7.2 Knowledge of poisons, antidotes, chemical properties of hazardous materials, effects of radiation exposure, and approach to initial decontamination	X	X				
1.3.7.3 Caustic substance ingestion	X	X				
1.3.7.3.1 Prehospital airway management options	X	X				
1.3.7.4 Decontamination	X	X				
1.3.8 Dermatology	X	X				
1.3.8.1 Use of bum dressings for desquamating disease	X	X				
1.3.9 Communicable Diseases	X	X				
1.3.9.1 General	X	X				
1.3.9.1.1 Knowledge of prehospital personal protective equipment (PPE)	X	X				
1.3.9.1.2 Isolation of persons with suspected infectious agents (e.g., severe acute respiratory syndrome [SARS])	X	X				X
1.3.9.1.3 Use of prehospital providers for mass vaccination programs	X	X				X
1.3.9.2 Multi-drug resistant organisms (MDR05)	X	X				
1.3.9.2.1 Protection in the field (e.g., PPE, decontamination of ambulances)	X	X				
1.3.9.3 Category A bioterrorism agents	X	X				
1.3.9.3.1 Hemorrhagic fevers	X	X				
1.3.9.3.2 Smallpox	X	X				
1.3.9.3.3 Plague	X	X				
1.3.9.3.4 Ricin	X	X				

Continued

		ACGME[4] and ABMS[5] Core Competencies					
		Patient Care	Medical Knowledge	Practice-based learning	Professionalism	Interpersonal Skills	System-based Practice
1.3.9.4	Emerging infections	X	X				
1.3.9.4.1	Pandemic viral illnesses	X	X				
1.3.9.4.2	SARS	X	X				
1.3.9.5	Quarantine	X	X				
1.3.10	**Behavioral Emergencies**	X	X				
1.3.10.1	Managing combative patients	X	X				
1.3.10.1.1	Use of restraints (chemical vs. mechanical)	X	X				
1.4	**SPECIAL CLINICAL CONSIDERATIONS**	X	X	X			X
1.4.1	**Airway Management in Adverse Conditions**	X	X	X			X
1.4.1.1	Low light	X	X	X			X
1.4.1.2	Atypical patient position	X	X	X			X
1.4.1.3	Minimal backup	X	X	X			X
1.4.1.4	Sub-optimal suction in the absence of standard equipment	X	X	X			X
1.4.2	**Procedures**	X	X				
1.4.2.1	Airway	X	X				
1.4.2.1.1	Opening airway with head-tilt/chin-lift method	X	X				
1.4.2.1.2	Opening airway with jaw thrust method	X	X				
1.4.2.1.3	Insertion of oropharyngeal & nasopharyngeal airways	X	X				
1.4.2.1.4	Bag-valve-mask	X	X				
1.4.2.1.5	Glottic airways	X	X				
1.4.2.1.6	Supraglottic airways	X	X				
1.4.2.1.7	Continuous positive airway pressure (CPAP)	X	X				
1.4.2.1.7.1	Use of prehospital CPAP devices	X	X				
1.4.2.1.8	Airway intubation adjuncts	X	X				
1.4.2.1.9	Direct laryngoscopy with endotracheal intubation	X	X				
1.4.2.1.10	Nasal intubation	X	X				
1.4.2.1.11	Facilitated intubation without paralytics	X	X				
1.4.2.1.12	Rapid sequence intubation (RSI) and use of paralytics	X	X				
1.4.2.1.13	Cricothyroidotomy	X	X				
1.4.2.1.14	Control of post-tonsillectomy hemorrhage	X	X				
1.4.2.2	Cardiovascular	X	X				
1.4.2.2.1	Placement of peripheral intravenous lines	X	X				
1.4.2.2.2	Access or placement of central venous lines in the field	X	X				
1.4.2.2.3	Placement of intraosseous lines	X	X				
1.4.2.2.3.1	Adult	X	X				
1.4.2.2.3.2	Pediatric		X				
1.4.2.2.4	Prehospital administration of thrombolytics for STEMI	X	X				
1.4.2.2.5	Transport directly to percutaneous coronary intervention (PCI)-capable hospital	X	X				
1.4.2.2.5.1	Helicopter EMS (HEMS) activation	X	X				
1.4.2.2.6	Pericardiocentesis without ultrasound guidance or other guidance device	X	X				
1.4.2.2.7	Balloon pump management	X	X				
1.4.2.3	Trauma	X	X				
1.4.2.3.1	Needle thoracostomy	X	X				
1.4.2.3.2	Tube thoracostomy	X	X				

Continued

Continued

	ACGME[4] and ABMS[5] Core Competencies					
	Patient Care	Medical Knowledge	Practice-based learning	Professionalism	Interpersonal Skills	System-based Practice
1.4.2.3.3 Pericardiocentesis without ultrasound guidance or other guidance device	X	X				
1.4.2.3.4 Control of life threatening hemorrhage	X	X				
1.4.2.3.5 Application of traction devices	X	X				
1.4.2.3.6 Wound care management	X	X				
1.4.2.3.7 Field trauma triage	X	X				
1.4.2.3.8 Application of cervical collar and backboard	X	X				
1.4.2.3.9 Selective spine immobilization	X	X				
1.4.2.3.10 Controlled hyperventilation for management of impending brain herniation in head trauma	X	X				
1.4.2.4 Obstetrics	X	X				
1.4.2.4.1 Normal delivery of a fetus	X	X				
1.4.2.4.1.1 Challenges of prehospital deliveries	X	X				
1.4.2.4.1.2 Resource allocation with increasing number of multiple births	X	X				X
1.4.2.4.2 Management of abnormal presentations of fetus	X	X				
1.4.2.4.3 Management of post-partum hemorrhage	X	X				
1.4.2.4.4 Pre/post-mortem cesarean section	X	X				
1.4.2.5 Point of care testing	X					
1.4.2.6 Ultrasound use in EMS	X	X				
1.4.2.6.1 Focused assessment with Sonography for Trauma (FAST) examination	X	X				
1.4.2.6.2 Line placement	X	X				
1.4.2.6.3 Cardiac activity for field termination of resuscitation	X	X				
1.4.3 Pain Assessment and Management in the Field	X	X				
1.4.4 Flight Physiology	X	X				
1.4.4.1 Effect of altitude on patient management	X	X	X			X
1.4.4.2 Effect of altitude on the healthcare provider		X	X			X
1.4.5 Pediatrics	X	X				
1.4.5.1 Controversies over airway management	x	X				
1.4.5.2 Pediatric trauma	x	X				X
1.4.5.3 Specialized equipment	x	X				
1.4.5.4 Unique issues related to consent	x	X		X	X	X
1.4.5.5 Maltreatment	x	X		X	X	
1.4.5.6 Apparent life-threatening event (ALTE)	x	X				
1.4.5.7 Seizure mimics	X	X				
1.4.5.8 Special needs children	X	X				
1.4.5.8.1 Technology dependent	X	X				
1.4.6 Geriatrics	X	X				
1.4.6.1 Geriatric trauma	X	X				
1.4.6.2 Polypharmacy	X	X	X			X
1.4.6.3 Maltreatment	X				x	X
1.4.7 Bariatric Issues	X	X			X	
1.4.7.1 Equipment					x	X
1.4.7.2 Procedure challenges	X	X				
1.4.8 End-of-Life Issues	X	X		X	X	X
1.4.8.1 Hospice	X			X	X	X
1.4.8.2 DNR/DNI/Advanced Directives/Physician Orders for Life Sustaining Treatment (POLST)	x			X	X	X
1.4.9 Social Issues				X	X	X
1.4.9.1 Isolation syndrome				X	X	X
1.4.9.2 Family centered care				X	X	X
1.4.9.3 Management of bystanders while caring for patient				X	X	X
1.4.10 Termination of Resuscitation	X	X		X	X	X

Continued

	ACGME[4] and ABMS[5] Core Competencies					
	Patient Care	Medical Knowledge	Practice-based learning	Professionalism	Interpersonal Skills	System-based Practice
1.5 SPECIAL CONSIDERATIONS FOR EVALUATION, TREATMENT, TRANSPORT, AND DESTINATIONS	X	X	X			X
1.5.1 Time-Life Critical Conditions	X	X	X			X
1.5.2 Special Patient Populations		X	X		x	X
2.0 MEDICAL OVERSIGHT OF EMS						
2.1 MEDICAL OVERSIGHT	XX		X	X	X	X
2.1.1 Medical Oversight of EMS Systems	XX		X	X	X	X
2.1.1.1 Direct medical oversight	X	X		X	X	X
2.1.1.1.1 Provision of direct patient care	X	X				
2.1.1.1.2 Physician directed care via radio or phone	X	X		X	X	X
2.1.1.1.3 Physician directed care in person	X	X		X	X	X
2.1.1.1.4 Telemedicine	X				x	X
2.1.1.2 Indirect medical oversight	XX		X	X	X	X
2.1.1.2.1 Evidence guided development of medical care protocols	X	X	X		x	X
2.1.1.2.2 Quality improvement programs	X	X	X		x	X
2.1.1.2.3 Determination of medical necessity in the field	X	X	X		x	X
2.1.1.3 Assessment of provider competence and fitness for duty	X			X	X	X
2.1.2 Legal Issues	X			X	X	X
2.1.2.1 Definition of a patient	X			X	X	X
2.1.2.2 Mandatory reporting issues	X	X		X	X	X
2.1.2.3 Determination and/or pronouncement of death	X	X		X	X	X
2.1.2.4 Capacity to refuse care	X	X		X	X	X
2.1.2.4.1 Understand the elements of informed consent and informed refusal	X	X	X	X	X	
2.1.2.4.2 Understand the difference between capacity and competence	X	X	X	X	X	
2.1.2.5 Federal regulations impacting EMS						X
2.2 EMS SYSTEMS	X	X			x	X
2.2.1 Public Safety Answering Points			X	X	X	X
2.2.1.1 Pre-arrival instructions	X	X		X	X	
2.2.1.2 Dispatch	X	X	X	X	X	X
2.2.1.2.1 Use of lights and sirens	X		X	X	X	X
2.2.1.2.2 Prioritization of response (e.g., determining local needs based on local resources)	X	X	X	X	X	X
2.2.1.2.3 Tiered-response			X			X
2.2.2 Design of System Components						X
2.2.2.1 Response and transport vehicles						X
2.2.2.2 EMS provider levels						X
2.2.2.3 Service delivery models						X
2.2.2.4 Equipment design and supply issuesx`						X
2.2.3 Delivery Systems with Special Considerations						X
2.2.3.1 Urban EMS						X
2.2.3.2 Rural EMS						X
2.2.3.3 Wilderness EMS						X
2.2.3.4 Volunteer EMS						X
2.2.3.5 Inter-facility transport						X
2.2.3.6 Military EMS						X
2.2.3.7 Air medical						X
2.2.3.8 International EMS						X
2.3 EMS PERSONNEL						X
2.3.1 Scope of Practice Models						X
2.3.1.1 Military/federal government medical personnel						X
2.3.1.2 State vs. national						X
2.3.1.2.1 Levels of providers						X
2.3.1.3 Field capabilities						X
2.3.2 Education			X			X
2.3.2.1 Theories of adult learning			X			X
2.3.2.2 Education delivery models			X			X

Continued

	ACGME[4] and ABMS[5] Core Competencies					
	Patient Care	Medical Knowledge	Practice-based learning	Professionalism	Interpersonal Skills	System-based Practice
2.3.2.3 Provider training programs			X			X
2.3.2.3.1 Initial education			X			X
2.3.2.3.2 Continuing education			X			X
2.3.2.4 Accreditation of training programs			X			X
2.3.2.5 Remediation and work force re-entry			X			X
2.3.3 EMS Provider Health and Wellness	X	X		X	X	X
2.3.3.1 Occupational culture of safety	X	X		X	X	X
2.3.3.1.1 Occupational health	X	X		X	X	X
2.3.3.1.2 Knowledge of regulations and standards (e.g., National Fire Protection Association [NFPA] 1582, Ryan White Act, Occupational Safety and Health Administration [OSHA] requirements)			X			X
2.3.3.1.3 Emergency incident rehabilitation	X		X	X	X	X
2.3.3.1.4 Awareness of ergonomic factors			X			X
2.3.3.1.5 Disordered sleep and work schedule				X	X	X
2.3.3.1.6 Prevention and intervention for psychologically stressful events				X	X	X
2.3.3.1.7 Emergency vehicle operations	X		X	X		X
2.3.3.2 Exposure to communicable disease	X	X	X	X	X	X
2.3.3.2.1 Standard PPE precautions	X	X				
2.3.3.2.2 Appropriate use of PPE for various infectious agents (contact vs. droplet vs. airborne precautions)	X	X				
2.3.3.2.3 Body substance exposure	X	X				
2.3.3.2.3.1 Knowledge of Centers for Disease Control and Prevention (CDC) guidelines for human immunodeficiency virus (HIV) and other blood-borne pathogens	X	X	X			
2.3.3.2.3.2 Medical director liaison role between hospital and EMS agency	X	X				
2.3.3.2.4 Post-exposure prophylaxis and testing	X	X				
2.3.3.2.5 Occupational health screening (e.g., tuberculosis, hepatitis)	X	X				
2.4 SYSTEM MANAGEMENT				X	X	X
2.4.1 System Finance						x
2.4.1.1 Allocation of resources						x
2.4.2 Legislation and Government						x
2.4.2.1 Working with government and public health agencies					x	X
2.4.2.2 Knowledge of state EMS laws						X
2.4.2.3 Understanding of healthcare law			X			X
2.4.3 Public Health		X	X			X
2.4.3.1 Specialty hospital designations and transport of patient		X	X			X
2.4.3.2 Field triage issues		X	X			X
2.4.3.3 Public access to defibrillation (PAD)		X	X			X
2.4.3.4 Issues of hospital diversion and bypass		X	X			X
2.4.3.5 Integration of EMS with community public resources and social services	X		X			X
2.4.4 System Status Management		X				X
2.4.4.1 Response times	X		X			X
2.4.5 Service Delivery Models						X
2.4.6 Patient Safety	X	X				X
2.4.7 Ethics in EMS	X			X	X	
3.0 QUALITY MANAGEMENT AND RESEARCH						
3.1 QUALITY IMPROVEMENT PRINCIPLES AND PROGRAMS			X			X
3.1.1 Data Collection, Management, and Analysis			X			X

Continued

	ACGME[4] and ABMS[5] Core Competencies					
	Patient Care	Medical Knowledge	Practice-based learning	Professionalism	Interpersonal Skills	System-based Practice
3.1.2 **Quality Improvement Programs**			X			X
3.1.3 **Evidence-based Practice**			X			X
3.2 **RESEARCH**			X			X
3.2.1 **Informed Consent (e.g., Use of FDA "Final Rule" or Exception to Informed Consent)**			X			X
3.2.2 **Fundamental Knowledge of Biostatistics and Epidemiology**			X			X
4.0 **SPECIAL OPERATIONS**						
4.1 **MASS CASUALTY MANAGEMENT**	X		X			X
4.1.1 **Incident Command System (ICS)**	X				x	X
4.1.1.1 Integration with fire ICS/medical operations					x	X
4.1.2 **Triage**	X	X				X
4.1.3 **Mass Casualty Management**	X	X		X	X	X
4.1.3.1 Local, state, federal assets	X	X		X	X	X
4.1.3.2 Regional resource allocation and management	X					
4.1.3.3 Role of emergency management agencies			X			X
4.2 **CHEMICAL/BIOLOGICAL/RADIOLOGICAL/NUCLEAR/ EXPLOSIVE (CBRNE)**	x	X	X			X
4.2.1 **Toxic Exposure/Poisoning/Hazardous Materials (HAZMAT)**	X	X	X	X	X	X
4.2.1.1 Need for HAZMAT team/antidotes	X	X				X
4.2.1.2 Field identification of toxins/hazardous materials	X	X				X
4.2.1.3 Field/provider/patient decontamination	X	X				X
4.2.1.4 Protecting the public (containment)/public health concerns				X	X	X
4.2.1.5 Resuscitation during contamination while wearing PPE	X	X				X
4.2.1.6 Knowledge of various levels of PPE			X			X
4.2.1.7 Knowledge of federal law enforcement reporting requirements		X				
4.2.1.8 Knowledge of poisons, antidotes, chemical properties of hazardous materials, radiation and effects of exposure	X	X				
4.2.2 **Immediate Danger to Life and Health (IDLH) Environments**	X	X				
4.2.2.1 Knowledge of asphyxiation and other gas and fire hazards	X	X				
4.2.3 **Explosive Incidents**						X
4.2.3.1 Improvised Explosive Devices (IEDs) and terrorist activity		X				
4.2.3.2 Community risk assessment						X
4.2.3.3 Integration with search and rescue						X
4.2.4 **Weapons of Mass Destruction and Related Injury**	X					
4.2.4.1 Secondary devices and scene safety						X
4.3 **MASS GATHERING**	X	X				X
4.3.1 **Disaster Planning and Operations**			X			X
4.3.2 **Human Resource Needs in Disaster Response**	X	X				X
4.3.2.1 Care teams	X	X				X
4.3.2.2 Physician placement	X	X				X
4.3.3 **Training and Drills**			X			X
4.3.4 **Design of Temporary Treatment Facilities**						X
4.3.4.1 Level of care						X
4.3.4.2 Ingress/egress						X
4.3.5 **Equipment Needs**						X
4.3.5.1 **Communications**				X	X	
4.3.5.2 **Integration of telecom systems with existing EMS system**	X					
4.4 **DISASTER MANAGEMENT**	X	X				X
4.4.1 **National Incident Management System (NIMS) & National Response Framework**						X
4.4.1.1 NIMS 100,200, 700, 800						X

Continued

Continued

	ACGME[4] and ABMS[5] Core Competencies					
	Patient Care	Medical Knowledge	Practice-based learning	Professionalism	Interpersonal Skills	System-based Practice
4.4.2 Catastrophic Events						X
4.4.2.1 State and federal criteria for disaster declaration						X
4.4.2.2 State emergency mutual aid compacts						X
4.4.3 Health and Medical Resources						X
4.4.3.1 National Disaster Medical System (NDMS)						X
4.4.3.2 Specialized teams						X
4.4.3.3 Non-governmental agencies						X
4.4.3.4 Regional medical response corps						X
4.4.3.5 State and federal assets						X
4.4.4 Special Response Considerations						X
4.4.4.1 Allocation of scene resources			X			X
4.4.4.2 Provider credentialing issues				X		X
4.4.4.3 Altered standards of care			X		x	X
4.5 EMS SPECIAL OPERATIONS	X	X				X
4.5.1 Tactical	X	X				X
4.5.1.1 Low or no light environment of care	X	X				X
4.5.1.2 Care in a hostile environment	X	X				X
4.5.1.3 Care with limited supplies	X	X				X
4.5.1.3.1 Hemostatic agent use	X	X				
4.5.1.3.2 Airway management in low or no light	X	X				
4.5.1.4 Remote assessment	X	X				X
4.5.1.5 Knowledge of tactical combat casualty care	X	X				X
4.5.1.6 Operational considerations for provider & casualty	X	X				X
4.5.2 Casualty Evacuation	X	X				X
4.5.2.1 Evacuation triage	X	X				X
4.5.2.2 Conventional EMS vs. unconventional transport modalities	X	X				X
4.5.2.3 Knowledge of ground, sea, and air transport	X	X				X
4.5.2.4 Potential for delayed/prolonged evacuation	X	X				X
4.5.3 Limited Patient Access Situations	X	X				
4.5.3.1 Confined space care (OSHA definition)	X	X				
4.5.3.2 Extrication	X	X				
4.5.4 Wilderness EMS Systems	X					X
4.5.4.1 Management of traumatic and medical disorders in a wilderness environment	X	X				
4.5.4.2 Evacuation/non-traditional transport	X	X				
4.5.4.3 Multi-agency response					X	
4.5.4.4 Survival skills and ability to operate independently in remote/wilderness environments					X	

Index

Page numbers in *italic* denote figures, those in **bold** denote tables.

Emergency Medical Services: Clinical Practice and Systems Oversight, Second Edition. Volume 1: Clinical Aspects of EMS.
Edited by David C. Cone, Jane H. Brice, Theodore R. Delbridge, and J. Brent Myers.
© 2015 NAEMSP. Published 2015 by John Wiley & Sons, Inc. Companion Website: www.wiley.com\go\cone\naemsp